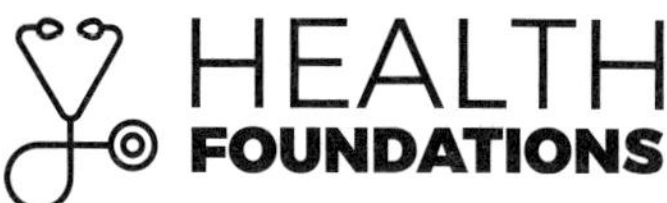

personal HEALTH

A POPULATION PERSPECTIVE

Michele Kiely, DrPH
Associate Dean for Research
City University of New York Graduate School of Public Health and Health Policy
New York, New York

Meredith G. Manze, MPH, PhD
Assistant Professor
Department of Community Health and Social Sciences
City University of New York Graduate School of Public Health and Health Policy
New York, New York

P. Christopher Palmedo, PhD, MBA
Associate Professor
City University of New York Graduate School
Department of Community Health and Social Sciences
City University of New York Graduate School of Public Health and Health Policy
New York, New York

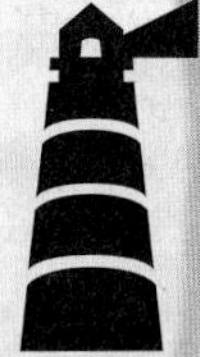

JONES & BARTLETT
LEARNING

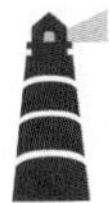

World Headquarters
Jones & Bartlett Learning
5 Wall Street
Burlington, MA 01803
978-443-5000
info@jblearning.com
www.jblearning.com

Jones & Bartlett Learning books and products are available through most bookstores and online booksellers. To contact Jones & Bartlett Learning directly, call 800-832-0034, fax 978-443-8000, or visit our website, www.jblearning.com.

Substantial discounts on bulk quantities of Jones & Bartlett Learning publications are available to corporations, professional associations, and other qualified organizations. For details and specific discount information, contact the special sales department at Jones & Bartlett Learning via the above contact information or send an email to specialsales@jblearning.com.

09966-9

Production Credits
VP, Product Management: David D. Cella
Director of Product Management: Michael Brown
Product Manager: Sophie Fleck Teague
Product Specialist: Danielle Bessette
Associate Production Editor: Alex Schab
Senior Marketing Manager: Susanne Walker
Production Services Manager: Colleen Lamy
Manufacturing and Inventory Control Supervisor: Amy Bacus
Composition: codeMantra U.S. LLC
Cover Design: Kristin E. Parker
Text Design: Kristin E. Parker
Director of Rights & Media: Joanna Gallant
Rights & Media Specialist: Merideth Tumasz
Media Development Editor: Shannon Sheehan
Cover Image (Title Page, Chapter Opener):
© Hero Images/Getty Images
Printing and Binding: LSC Communications
Cover Printing: LSC Communications

Library of Congress Cataloging-in-Publication Data
Names: Kiely, Michele, author. | Manze, Meredith, author. | Palmedo, Chris, author.
Title: Personal health: a population perspective / Michele Kiely, Meredith Manze, and Chris Palmedo.
Description: First edition. | Burlington, Massachusetts: Jones & Bartlett Learning, [2019]
Identifiers: LCCN 2018023089 | ISBN 9781284099652 (paperback)
Subjects: LCSH: Health. | BISAC: MEDICAL / Public Health.
Classification: LCC RA776 .K4856 2019 | DDC 613—dc23
LC record available at https://lccn.loc.gov/2018023089

6048

Printed in the United States of America
23 22 21 20 19 10 9 8 7 6 5 4 3 2

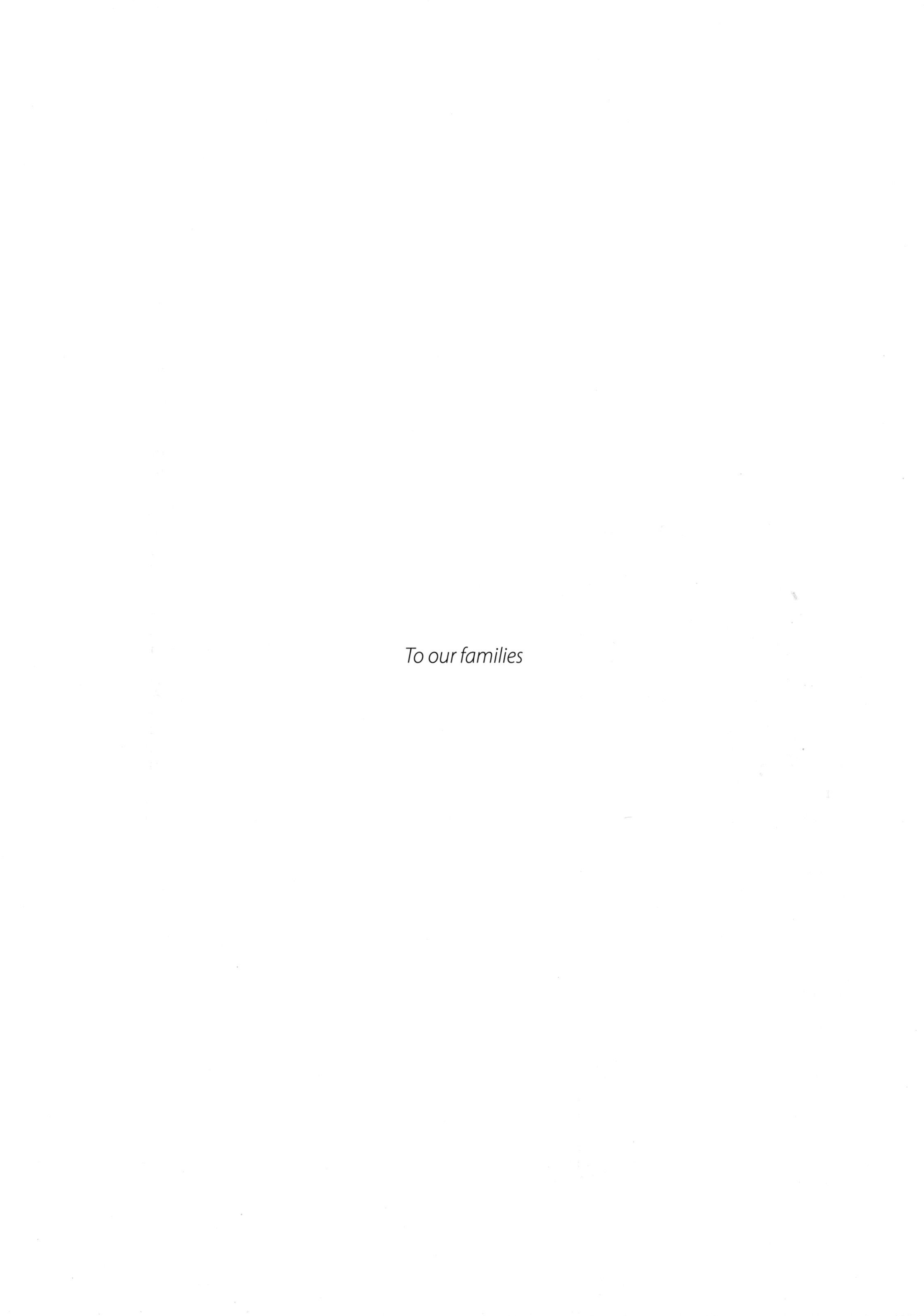

To our families

© Hero Images/Getty Images

Brief Contents

© Hero Images/Getty Images

Contents

Acknowledgments

The authors would like to express their gratitude to the many people who contributed to this book. The following individuals provided support, discussed fine points, and willingly gave of their expertise by providing feedback, suggestions, and administrative support: Beth Ansel, Renaisa Anthony, Deana Brooksher, Matthew Caron, Ayman El-Mohandes, Elizabeth Geltman, Maureen Giese, Sally Guadagno, Jamie Handlovits, Amelia Joy, Eric Joy, Woodie Kessel, John L. Kiely, Danielle Krushnic, Eleni Murphy, Tamar Pacht, Kelly Palmedo, Sage Palmedo, Deepika Rao, Lindsey Sousa, Barry Zitin, and Melinda Zitin. We beg forgiveness if there is anyone whose name we failed to mention.

Foreword

Reading this book and using it as a study guide will be a unique experience for you. The authors of this book have used both the microscope and the telescope to help you understand the risks and opportunities that surround us. These risks and opportunities exist within us, tempered by the world in which we live, and can influence our health in ways that we feel and know—and in other ways that are hidden but are just as important.

Regardless of the area you choose to study or your career direction, broadening your understanding of how to remain healthy and enhance the health of those around you is a skill and an asset that will stay with you indefinitely. This enhanced awareness of health and its implications for an individual's development, the resourcefulness of a community, the well-being of a city, and the resilience of a nation is confirmed both theoretically and empirically. The authors cover many topics, some social, some biological, some cultural. It may surprise you to discover just how many factors affect our health as individuals and populations.

Some of the factors the authors address manifest directly in how you feel about yourself today—how active, how happy, or restful you may be, or how anxious or how tired you may feel. These same characteristics may also apply to your family, your neighborhood, your community, as well as your village or your city.

The authors wrote this book with the intention of building a knowledge base as well as creating a broader understanding of health and well-being. Their focus is on the entire life span, but particularly on college-aged individuals. They explain what is healthful or what may be dangerous for you, as an individual or for the population as a whole. Avoiding health risks and preventing the health challenges is only possible when you know what they are. Making the best choices today for you, your friends, and your family may turn into a habit that you will embrace and practice for many years to come.

You may be taking a health course to fill a distribution requirement or because you intend to choose it as a career. Regardless, this book will help you understand more about the variety of professional domains that serve the health of individuals and populations. This book could be your entry point. It may lead you in the right direction if you want to be a doctor, a nurse, a physical therapist, or another career that supports health needs either in a clinical setting or community. However, careers in the health professions span beyond those in a clinical setting. Examples include health educators, social workers, environmental health specialists, public health officials, and health managers. Many of these professionals treat people who are sick or protect individuals who are healthy. Regardless of their career, they should always have an eye on what health means for larger groups of people and populations. These factors could have an impact not just on health, but also on productivity, well-being, social cohesiveness, and economic productivity. Health is not just about your temperature today or how many calories you have consumed; it is also about how dynamic you may be and how fulfilling your life is. I hope that you will develop new perspectives on many aspects of your life and the society in which we live and how this affects your health. I also hope you develop a deeper understanding of how health behavior and the environment impact your life and future.

This book will increase your curiosity about health and its implications. It will be a stepping stone toward making better choices, remaining aware, and understanding the risks that surround you. Enjoy reading it, and maybe you will keep it as your bedside table companion.

Ayman A. E. El-Mohandes, MD, MPH
Dean
City University of New York Graduate School of Public Health and Health Policy
New York, New York

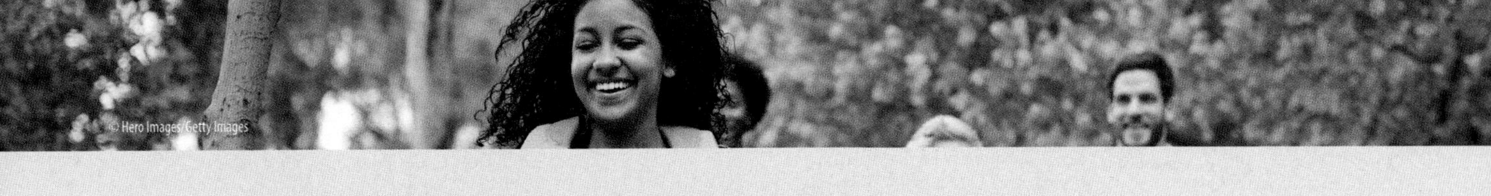

Reviewers

Ari Fisher, MA
Senior Instructor
Louisiana State University, Baton Rouge
Baton Rouge, Louisiana

Julie Gast, PhD
Professor
Utah State University
Logan, Utah

Eliza MacDonald, MPA, AT, ATC
Affiliate Faculty Member
Grand Valley State University
Allendale, Michigan

Pardess Mitchell, EdD
Assistant Professor, Department Chair
Harper College
Palentine, Illinois

Julianne Murphy, PhD
Department Chair
Triton College
River Grove, Illinois

Yuliya Shneyderman, PhD
Assistant Professor
Borough of Manhattan Community College
New York, New York

How to Use This Book

In addition to including the most current information concerning general health, each chapter includes helpful learning aids for both students and instructors. Utilizing these features for classroom and/or blog discussions and debates, or as individual reflective writing assignments, can help to drive stronger comprehension and retention of core concepts while reinforcing critical thinking skills.

Each chapter begins with a list of **Chapter Objectives** to help you focus on the most important concepts in that chapter.

CHAPTER OBJECTIVES

- Review key concepts to help understand terminology used in this text.
- Define health in the broader context.
- Explain how our environment influences the health choices we make.
- Describe the meaning of health across the life span.
- Review the theories of health behavior.
- Explore the meaning of race and racism and why they are important health issues.

In Summary sections can be found at the end of each chapter to reinforce concepts introduced in the chapter.

In Summary

Every day you make choices that impact your health. Those choices are not made in a vacuum; they are influenced by the environment around you. Researchers have proposed theories of health behavior that attempt to explain how people make decisions about their health behaviors. These theories are helpful because public health practitioners want to understand how to help people make healthier choices.

This chapter introduces key concepts and terms fundamental to understanding health. The concept of health across the life span helps you understand that the choices you make, as well as the external environment around you, affect your health. The concept of race is a social, not biological, construct. The consequences of racism on health are devastating.

We also consider health determinants that are not always obvious. Where you live is important. It influences your sense of well-being, your health, your happiness, and other choices about your life. Furthermore, understanding what will make you happy is critical to living a healthy life.

Key terms are bolded in the text and listed at the end of each chapter. Terms are defined in the margins and in the glossary at the end of the book.

Key Terms

built environment
cancer
congenital anomalies
cutoff value
discrimination
epidemiologists
focus groups
heart disease
incidence
population health
prevalence
race
racism
screening tests
randomized controlled trials
social determinants of health
sudden infant death syndrome (SIDS)

Try It! applies topics from the text to your daily life.

TRY IT!

Create a Budget

Give yourself a "healthy diet" budget. What food choices would you make if you had $3.00 per day to spend? What about $6.00 per day? Or $10.00 per day? Try to come up with a grocery list for a week's worth of groceries based on those numbers. [Hint: Look on the Internet to come up with suggestions if you need to. This is an exercise many have tried!]

Fact vs. Fiction debunks popular health myths and explores controversies.

FACT VS. FICTION

Camera Enforcement of Speed Limits

Myth: Speed cameras are just a way for cities to make money and don't make people slow down.

Fact: Speeding is a factor in most collisions, especially ones where there are injuries and fatalities. Encouraging people to slow down helps to reduce or eliminate injuries and fatalities. Like many cities resorting to cameras to monitor speeding, in 2007, police in Rockville, Maryland, installed two cameras to detect speeders in front of a local high school. It was one of the city's worst speeding locations. About 2,800 vehicles pass the cameras every day. When the cameras were first installed, there were approximately 75 citations issued per day; 2 years later, it is only 16 per day. The cameras in front of the high school were placed there after someone speeding through the school zone killed a student who was crossing the street.

By the Numbers displays relevant—and often surprising—statistics to further your understanding of topics discussed in the text.

BY THE NUMBERS

Heart Attacks in the United States

Every 43 seconds, someone in the United States has a heart attack.[29]

Up for Debate describes current controversies in public health to engage students in discussions.

UP FOR DEBATE

Should the United States Allow Direct-to-Consumer Advertising?

In the United States, there are several categories of pharmaceutical drugs that require a prescription, and are unavailable for you to purchase off the shelf from the store. And yet, drug companies can still market those products directly to you by advertising on TV, in magazines, and through social media. What do you think about that?

Nearly every other country in the world bans prescription drug companies from marketing directly to consumers. The United States and New Zealand are the only two countries that allow **direct-to-consumer advertising** (DTC) of prescription drugs. In other nations, if a drug requires a prescription, it cannot be advertised to the public. The reasoning is that because regulations restrict people from buying drugs directly from a store or pharmacy without a prescription, drug companies should not be permitted to "sell" directly to consumers.

Pharmaceutical companies argue that DTC advertising increases knowledge, encourages patient–physician communication, reduces the stigma of certain disorders by placing them widely open in the public, and represents freedom of speech.[18]

Physicians have indicated that direct-to-consumer advertising has both positive and negative effects on patients and on public health.[19] In recent years, the physician community has begun to organize in greater opposition to the practice.

In 2015, the American Medical Association (AMA) voted to ban DTC advertising, citing concerns about the negative impact of commercially driven promotions, and the role marketing costs play in rising drug prices. The AMA also argued that DTC marketing increased demand for new and more expensive drugs, even when these drugs may not be appropriate.[20] Meanwhile, a spokesperson for the pharmaceutical manufacturers trade association (PhRMA) said that DTC advertisers design their advertising to "provide scientifically accurate information to help patients better understand their health care and treatment options."[19]

In many cases, drug companies market their products, not to get patients to seek the medication, but to get them to request their particular brand when generic (non–brand name) versions of the drug are available. The generic drugs are less expensive than the brand name ones being advertised.

Along with issues of treatment, DTC advertising has cost implications, both for individuals and the nation's health system. One drug, Neulasta, for example, can cost $5,000 per injection in the United States, generating $4.6 billion in sales in 1 year for its manufacturer, Amgen.[21] This level of profit makes the total DTC advertising spending in 2015 of approximately $5 billion for the entire industry[21] seem cost-effective!

What do you think? Should prescription drug ads be banned from the eyes of consumers, or do consumers have the right to receive the most professionally produced and effective communications possible from the manufacturers? After all, the call to action is not to "buy," but to "ask your doctor."

Going Upstream provides insights to help students think about predisposing factors to health, particularly social determinants of health.

GOING UPSTREAM

Why Are People of Color at Higher Risk for Cardiovascular Diseases?[36]

Several theories exist as to why people of color, particularly Black men and women, are at higher risk of developing cardiovascular diseases and dying from them. One theory is that this population has higher rates of obesity and diabetes, which can lead to CVD. Another theory is that a gene common among African Americans may make this group more sensitive to salt. However, it is clear that a large part of this disparity exists due to barriers to diagnosis and treatment. Social determinants of health, including inequalities in income, education, and access to care, discussed throughout this book, disproportionately affect people of color and contribute to these barriers to cardiovascular care.

Tales of Public Health are real-life public health stories, to bring a human face to the concepts described.

TALES OF PUBLIC HEALTH

The White Potato: In or Out?

Mashed? Baked? Fried? Boiled? The white potato, or *Solanum tuberosum*, is a member of the perennial nightshade family, which includes tomatoes, eggplant, and chili peppers. Originally from the Andes mountains, it is now cultivated throughout the world, and its place on the American table has been unanimously accepted for centuries.

That changed in 2015, when the simple white potato found itself at the center of a fierce argument in Washington, DC. The debate called into question whether the potato is nutritious enough to be included in the federal nutrition assistance program for pregnant women and their newborn babies.

The **Women, Infants, and Children (WIC)** program provides nutrition at the crucial time in human development when human growth and cellular resilience are taking shape—in the womb and during the first few years of childhood. The program provides vouchers for mothers, which can be spent only on foods deemed "exceptionally nutritious" by the USDA, such as milk, cereal, eggs, fruits, vegetables, beans, and peanut butter. The USDA takes its guidance from the National Academy of Medicine (NAM), a nongovernmental nonprofit organization that provides unbiased guidance for policy decisions related to health and health care.

In 2006, the medical and nutritional scientists at the NAM determined that potatoes were not healthy enough to be considered a "crucial" food for women and postpartum babies and thus ineligible for WIC reimbursement. For the potato industry, the financial implications were enormous. WIC had distributed around $7 billion in vouchers in 2006,[42] and removing an item from WIC funding has a major effect on jobs and profits for large industrial food producers, as well as small farmers, whether they're raising potatoes or peanuts.

After a long campaign of communications, lobbying, and financial contributions, the potato industry got what it wanted. In February 2015, the NAM announced that white potato would be returned to the list of approved WIC foods. It was a victory for the potato farmers, but what about the health impact? In the United States, most potatoes are whipped, deep-fried, or processed into chips and other products that are not "crucial" nutrition for pregnant women and new mothers. This was the concern expressed by the American Public Health Association, which protested that this was not a "health" decision but one based on political and financial influence. The American Academy of Pediatrics (AAP) said they were "tremendously concerned" about industry intervening in WIC regulations. The AAP argued that including potatoes would "override the sound scientific judgment of our nation's leading nutrition science experts."[43] New York University nutrition professor Marion Nestle wrote, "I have a hard time believing that WIC recipients are suffering from lack of potatoes in their diets. Potatoes are fine foods, but highly caloric when prepared in the usual ways. Encouraging WIC recipients to choose leafy greens and other vegetables seems like a good idea."[44]

The food industry has influenced USDA dietary guidelines since the first recommendations in 1894. This influence has been in lobbying Congress, funding nutrition research, and forming partnerships with professional nutrition organizations.

Each sector of American life (governments, companies, nonprofit organizations) has a different perspective on health, and in America, the public and private sectors both have influence on our diets. Reaching a better understanding of these areas through critical discussion and open reporting may help all of us to become healthier eaters, and consequently, healthier people.

Discussion Questions and Activities at the end of each chapter encourage students to discuss, ponder, and critically analyze their own feelings and opinions about the information presented in the book.

Student Discussion Questions and Activities

1. Placing limits on the sale of tobacco and establishing smoke-free workplace laws are two examples of laws and policies intended to reduce cancer rates in the United States. What are some other policies you can think of that may help more people avoid cancer?
2. What would you do or say if a parent or grandparent told you they had cancer? How would you talk to them? Would you feel comfortable making recommendations or offering to help? If so, what might be some ways you might offer to help?
3. Why do you think that CVDs are so highly prevalent in the United States if there are ways to change behavior and lifestyle to effectively reduce one's risk?
4. Think about what you normally eat. Does it include foods high in sugar, fat, and salt? How hard do you think it would be to change to a healthier diet?
5. Consider changes people need to make to lower their risk of type 2 diabetes. Do you need to make those changes? Design a program for yourself or friends to lower the risk of type 2 diabetes.
6. Imagine you have asthma. How do you control the symptoms?
7. Imagine what a day would be like if you had COPD and had to take an oxygen tank with you everywhere you went. How would that effect what you do every day?

Because of these features, we believe that *Personal Health: A Population Perspective* is particularly user-friendly and will encourage student motivation and learning.

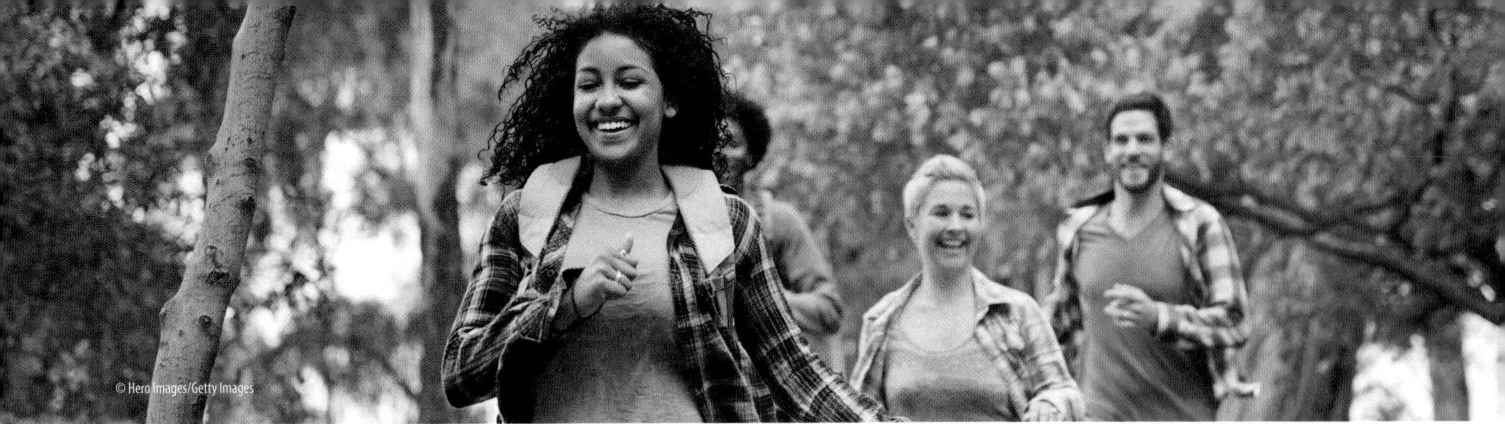
© Hero Images/Getty Images

CHAPTER 1
Health: An Introduction

CHAPTER OBJECTIVES

- Review key concepts to help understand terminology used in this text.
- Define health in the broader context.
- Explain how our environment influences the health choices we make.
- Describe the meaning of health across the life span.
- Review the theories of health behavior.
- Explore the meaning of race and racism and why they are important health issues.

Health isn't merely the absence of disease—it is much broader than that! You may know what it feels like to be healthy, but can you explain what health is to someone else? In 1948, the World Health Organization (WHO) defined health as "a state of complete physical, mental, and social well-being and not merely the absence of disease or infirmity."[1] This definition hasn't changed over time, although we now know to add environmental factors into the definition.[1] Health is a balance between the individual and his or her environment.[2]

Together, we will learn about many aspects of health—both personal health and population health—from the choices you can make on a personal level to the state of health of the world around you. We will take a look at your personal health, and we will also help you understand health from a family, community, and global perspective. You will learn about how to make healthy choices and, hopefully, will choose those over less healthy ones. Perhaps you will be inspired to help others make healthy choices and to help the world become a healthier place in which to live.

Most health issues affect all of us, whether we are directly affected (having a disease or health disorder) or indirectly affected (smoking by others in public places or laws requiring helmet use for motorcycle riders). Because we are not alone in our struggle for good health, scientists and researchers look at our health issues collectively, using the term **population health**. Throughout this book, we will show you how your health and your choices impact, and are impacted by, the health and choices of those around you—both physically nearby and through the interconnectivity of the global population.

population health The health outcomes of a group of individuals, including the distribution of such outcomes within the group. This field of study includes health outcomes, patterns of health determinants, and policies and the interventions that link them. It is an approach that aims to improve the health of an entire human population.

POPULATION HEALTH VERSUS PUBLIC HEALTH

Population health—the health of a population over the life course.
Public health—the health of a whole society; a discipline focused on the development and application of preventive strategies and interventions to achieve a state of population health.

The distinction between population health and public health is that population health describes the situation, whereas public health includes the plans, strategies, and actions required to achieve the population's health.

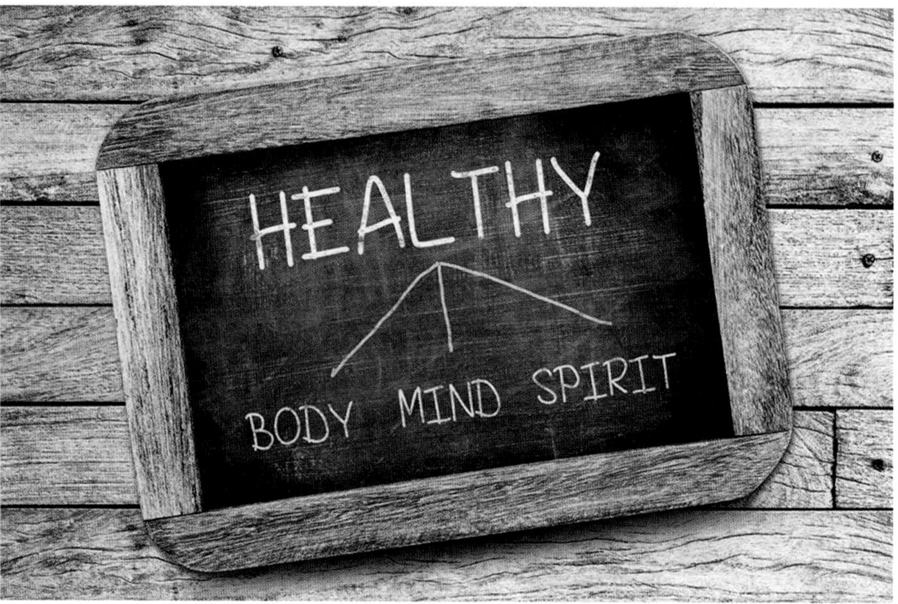

Body, mind, and spirit.

Personal Health Choices in a Societal Context

Most of us think about the health choices we make every day: what to eat, whether and how much to exercise, how much sleep to get, whether to smoke. We all know that making health choices is not always easy! Look at the data in the By the Numbers box.

When viewing health statistics, the questions often raised are: Why do people make unhealthy choices, and whose fault is it when they do? For the answer, we usually point to personal responsibility; after all, we each choose how much

BY THE NUMBERS

Healthy or Unhealthy Choices?

The most recent National Health Report from the Centers for Disease Control and Prevention (CDC) found that approximately 25% of adults smoke, although among youth, it declined between 2005 and 2013 to a record low of 15.7%. Approximately 35% of adults and 17% of youth suffer from obesity. Only 21% of adults met the recommended levels of physical activity. On the flip side, during the 2012–2013 influenza season, vaccination rates reached highs among children and adults, including among pregnant women.[3]

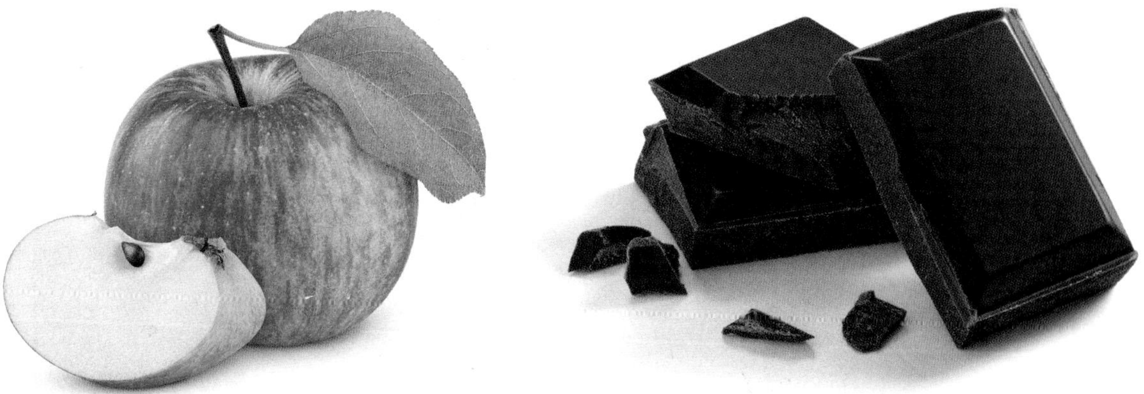

FIGURE 1-1 Fruit versus chocolate: Which would you choose?

we eat or exercise. Yet, research shows that the environment in which we live strongly affects how easy or hard it is to make healthy decisions. *Environment*, in this context, can refer to your city, neighborhood, school, or home—any place where you spend your time.[4] Think about your own environment. How easy or difficult is it for you to find healthy, fresh food? Are you close to a gym or park where you can exercise? How is the air quality where you live? An important population health goal is to design environments that encourage people to make healthy choices.

Research shows that while people understand the importance of eating healthy foods, they often opt for less healthy choices. One study found that participants were "dynamically inconsistent" in their choice between healthy and unhealthy snacks. When asked what they would choose 1 week in the future, 74% picked a healthy choice (fruit). When the following week arrived, 70% chose chocolate over fruit (**FIGURE 1-1**). Current hunger level contributed to participants' future choices. That is, participants who were hungry, even when choosing for the future, were more likely to choose chocolate over fruit.[5]

Another study explored how bite size influences overall food consumption. Researchers collected data in a restaurant and manipulated bite size by providing diners with small or large forks. They found that people consumed more when using smaller rather than larger forks. They hypothesized that in a restaurant setting, factors that relate to the experience of eating impact diners' choices. In a controlled lab study, when those factors are absent, the pattern of results is reversed.[6] Another series of studies showed how plate size affects the amount of food we consume.[7] Researchers found that people with larger bowls served themselves approximately 30% more cereal than did people given smaller bowls. They also found that people tend to eat the same percentage of food regardless of plate size. How much a person ate depended on the plate size—the bigger the plate, the more food eaten. In American culture, plate size has increased over time. As illustrated in **FIGURE 1-2**, plate size, and thus how many calories a diner will consume, varies with plate size, which depends where the person is eating. These studies demonstrate the importance of the structure of our options in affecting the choices we make.

If we want everyone (all adults) to eat healthy diets, we need to begin early and we need to make healthy choices affordable to those with less money. Two issues affecting healthy diets are cost and quality. A 2013 study reviewed data from 10 countries and found that eating healthy was more expensive.

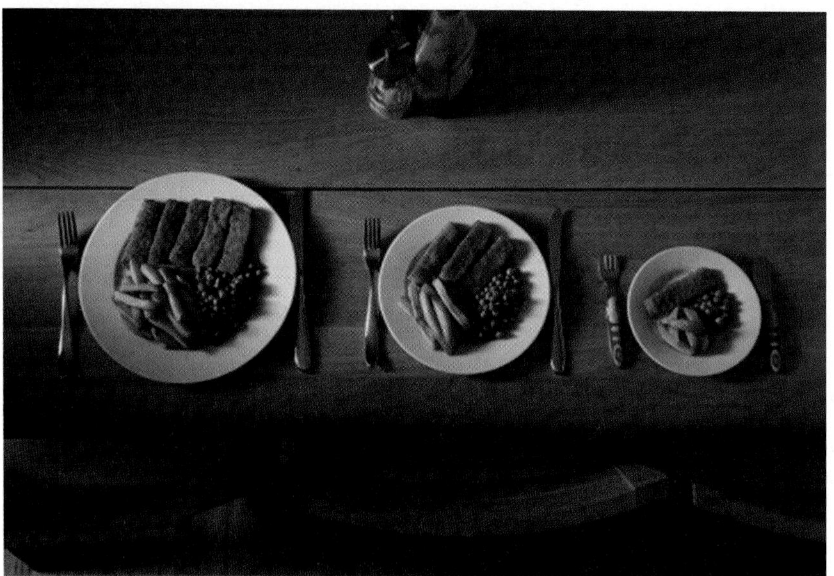

FIGURE 1-2 Plate size varies depending on where you are eating.

BY THE NUMBERS

Organ Donation

Are you an organ donor? In the United States, an average of 22 people die each day waiting for an organ transplant. People of every age, from infants to seniors, give and receive organ donations. In 2014 alone, 29,532 people received an organ transplant. Yet the gap between the number of people donating organs and those who need them is widening.[8] Although a 2012 national survey showed that 94.9% of U.S. adults support or strongly support donation, only 60.1% had granted permission on a driver's license.[9] In countries where the default is opt out (actively choose to not donate organs) rather than opt in (actively choose to donate organs), the rate of organ donation is much higher because people tend to go with the default option.[10] **FIGURE 1-3** shows how much a difference this opt-out factor can make.

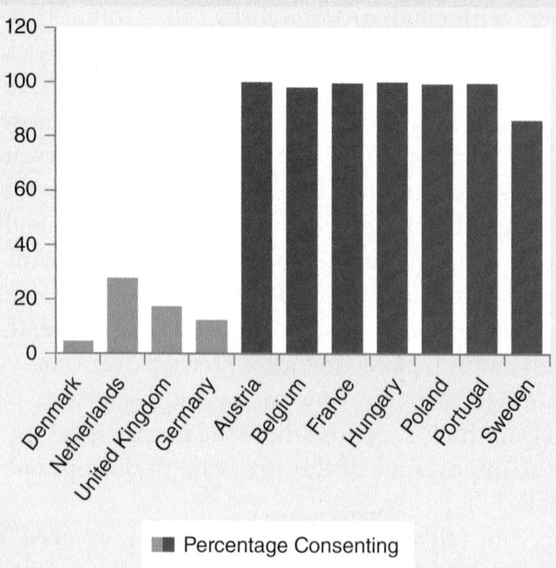

FIGURE 1-3 Opting in versus opting out of organ donation.

The healthiest diets cost $1.50 more per person, per day. The largest difference in price was found for healthy versus less healthy meat/protein. The researchers also found smaller but statistically significant differences in prices for snacks/sweets, grains, fats/oils, and dairy.[11] With the idea of helping kids eat healthier, in 2012 school lunches in the United States were redesigned to make healthy choices more accessible. A study that evaluated students' responses to the healthier lunch options found that most students liked the choices.[12] Another study that reviewed how food options changed between 2006–2007 and 2013–2014 found that the percentage of schools that regularly offered healthful items, such as vegetables (other than potatoes), fresh fruit, salad bars, whole grains, and more healthful pizzas, increased significantly. In addition, the number of schools offering less-healthy foods, such as fried potatoes, regular pizza, and high-fat milks, decreased significantly. While these changes are good news, they are not uniform. Schools in the West were significantly more likely to offer salad bars than were schools elsewhere. Majority-Black or majority-Latino schools were significantly less likely to offer fresh fruit than were predominantly White schools. Schools with low socioeconomic status were significantly less likely to offer salads regularly than were schools with middle or high socioeconomic status.[13] This disparity is one of the population health inequities that must be addressed.

TRY IT!

Create a Budget

Give yourself a "healthy diet" budget. What food choices would you make if you had $3.00 per day to spend? What about $6.00 per day? Or $10.00 per day? Try to come up with a grocery list for a week's worth of groceries based on those numbers. [Hint: Look on the Internet to come up with suggestions if you need to. This is an exercise many have tried!]

The importance of environment to our health also applies to physical activity. As schools became more accountable for student success, recess was frequently viewed as expendable. Yet, the American Academy of Pediatrics views recess as a necessary break from the rigors of concentrated, academic challenges in the classroom. Additionally, it offers cognitive, social, emotional, and physical benefits.[14] The physical, health, and emotional benefits of exercise continue into adulthood, but communities, workplaces, and governments need to support citizens to make healthy choices. Examples of programs that have worked are community programs that encourage citizens to walk more, point-of-decision signs that are designed to help people choose stairs over the elevator, worksite wellness programs that support physical activity, and cities that build bicycle lanes and walking paths. Having access to places and opportunities for physical activity and the knowledge that these opportunities exist are crucial.[15]

TRY IT!

How to Encourage Physical Activity?

What programs are in place in your environment to encourage physical activity? If you had the resources to do so, what changes would you make in your community to increase participation in physical activity?

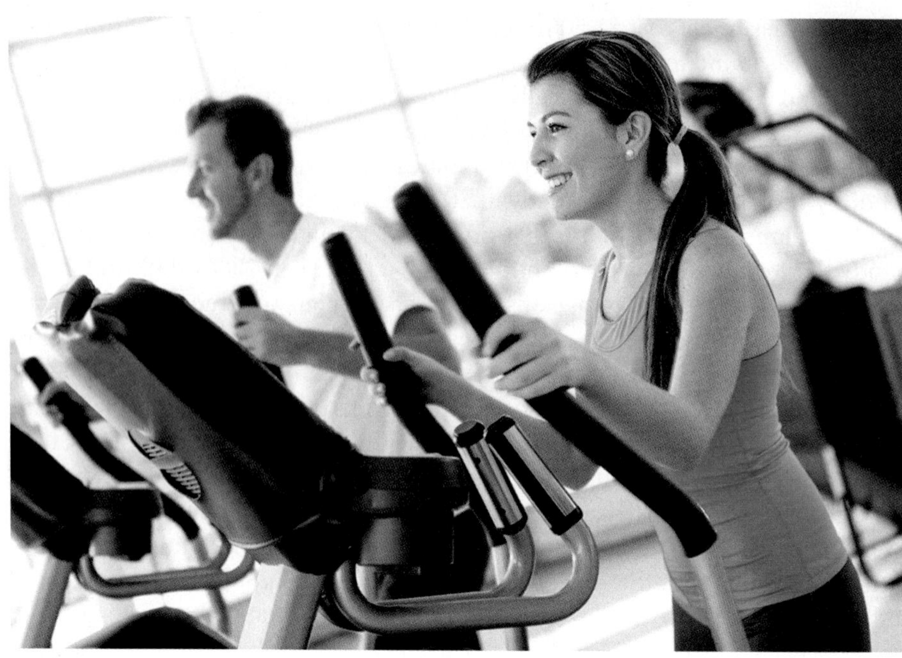

Theories of Health

So far, we have examined how the environment can influence the choices we make. Did you ever think about how you make the choices you do? Researchers want to understand health behavior as well as how to develop interventions to improve the health of individuals and communities. There are many theories that address changing a specific behavior, such as promoting safe sex or discouraging excess alcohol consumption. Let's look at the most important theories of health behavior and health behavior change. For each theory, we will examine a study from the medical literature to illustrate how researchers have used that theory to study health behavior change.

Social-Ecological Model

The social-ecological model (or socioecological model) is a theory-based framework (an idea that explains what is observed) for understanding how multiple levels of personal and environmental factors influence behaviors. In 1988, Dr. Kenneth McLeroy proposed this model for health promotion. It focuses on both individual and social environmental factors as targets for health promotion interventions. The model assumes that a change in the social environment will cause a change at the personal level.[16]

The social-ecological model describes the interaction between the individual, the group/community, and the physical, social, and political environments,[17–19] and it explains how each of those factors impacts health (**FIGURE 1-4**). Because of its broad applicability, the social-ecological model has been used to address areas of public health, including nutrition and physical activity,[20] **cancer**,[21] violence prevention,[22] diabetes,[23] and cardiovascular disease.[24]

cancer A malignant growth or tumor resulting from the abnormal division of cells.

The social-ecological model has five levels: individual, interpersonal, community, organizational, and policy/enabling environment. **TABLE 1-1** provides a brief description of each level. Individual behaviors both shape and are shaped by the social environment. The most effective approach to population health prevention and control uses a combination of interventions at all levels of the model.

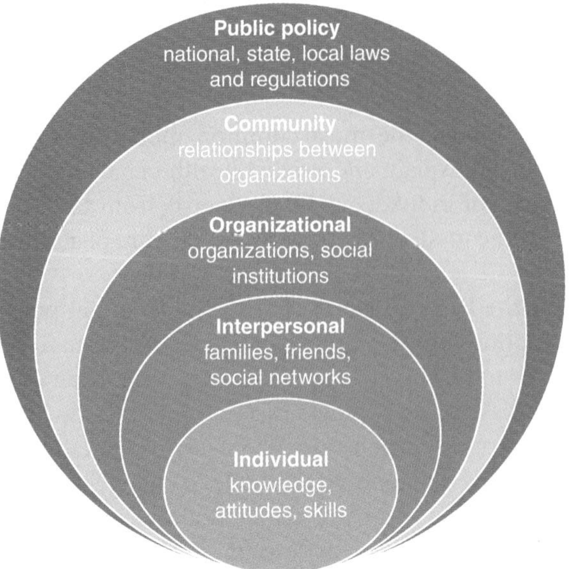

FIGURE 1-4 Social-Ecological Model.

Reproduced from Violence Prevention : The Social-Ecological Model: A Framework for Prevention, Centers for Disease Control and Prevention (CDC). Retrieved from http://www.cdc.gov/ViolencePrevention/overview/social-ecologicalmodel.html

TABLE 1-1 A Description of the Social-Ecological Model

Social-Ecological Model Level	Description
Individual	Characteristics of an individual that influence behavior change, including knowledge, attitudes, behavior, self-efficacy, developmental history, gender, age, religious identity, racial/ethnic identity, sexual orientation, economic status, financial resources, values, goals, expectations, literacy, stigma, and others
Interpersonal	Both formal and informal social networks and social support systems that can influence individual behaviors, including family, friends, peers, coworkers, religious networks, customs, or traditions
Organizational	Organizations or social institutions with rules and regulations for operations that affect how, or how well, services are provided to an individual or group
Community	Relationships among organizations, institutions, and informational networks within defined boundaries, including the built environment (e.g., parks), local associations, community leaders, businesses, and transportation
Policy/Enabling Environment	Local, state, national, and global laws and policies, including policies regarding the allocation of resources for health and access to healthcare services, restrictive policies (e.g., high fees or taxes for health services), or lack of policies, that affect an individual

A research team utilized the social-ecological model to examine urban social stress and exposure to violence as predictors of poor quality of life for adolescent and young mothers during pregnancy and postpartum. The team found that higher social stress predicted lower mental and physical quality of life during pregnancy. The associations were significantly stronger for mothers exposed to violence. Population health interventions within each of the social-ecological model levels need to work to improve the young women's lives, including stress reduction and teaching pregnancy and parenting programs to tailor their work to address violence.[25]

The Health Belief Model

The Health Belief Model, the most common model used to explain health behavior,[26] attempts to explain and predict health behaviors by focusing on the attitudes and beliefs of individuals. Psychologists from the U.S. Public Health Service developed the model to understand the failure of a tuberculosis screening program.[27]

The basis for the Health Belief Model is the idea that people's behavior is due to four perceptions: how serious they believe a disease to be, whether they believe themselves to be susceptible to a disease, the value of a new behavior in decreasing the risk of developing a disease, and an individual's belief in his or her ability to adopt a new behavior. There are also cues to action, which are events, people, or things that motivate people to change their behavior, such as an advertisement warning pregnant women not to drink alcohol.

The last part of the Health Belief Model is self-efficacy, a person's belief in his or her ability to do something. A picture of the Health Belief Model is presented in **FIGURE 1-5**, and an example of the Health Belief Model is presented in **TABLE 1-2**.

A 2015 study used the Health Belief Model to study minority adolescents' use of testing for HIV (human immunodeficiency virus; the virus that causes AIDS). The researchers used a survey followed by focus groups to assess perceptions about HIV testing. Only 15% of participants thought that it was *somewhat likely* or *very likely* they would get HIV (perceived susceptibility), although 73% of participants thought HIV was a very serious problem for someone their age. Rather than being a motivating factor to get tested, the seriousness of HIV made many adolescents afraid to get tested and find out if they were HIV positive (perceived severity). Participants in both the survey and the focus groups acknowledged the importance of getting tested to avoid spreading the disease to others (perceived benefit). Adolescents reported barriers to getting tested, including privacy concerns, waiting for results, and stigma associated with getting an HIV test (perceived barriers). The students acknowledged few cues to action for getting tested. The researchers concluded

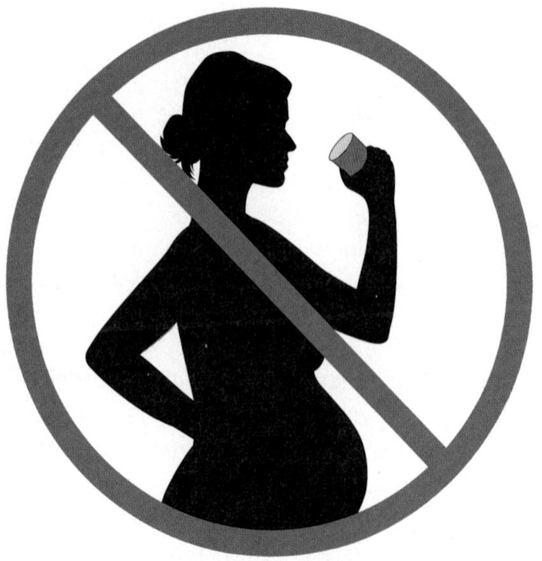

Don't drink alcohol when you are pregnant.

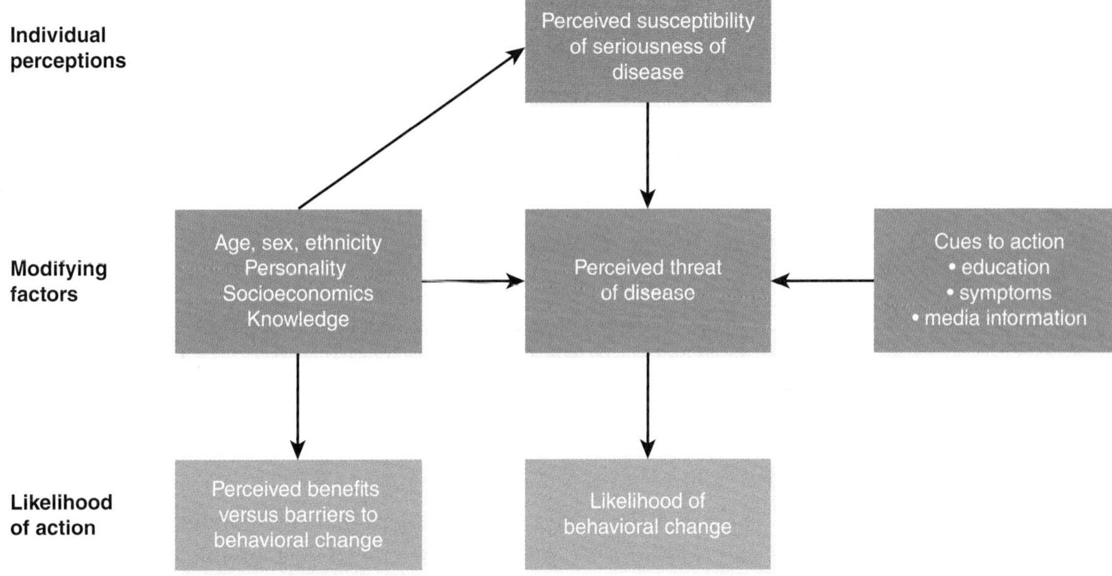

FIGURE 1-5 Health Belief Model.

Data from Glanz, K., Rimer, B.K. & Lewis, F.M. (2002). Health Behavior and Health Education. Theory, Research and Practice. 52. San Fransisco: Wiley & Sons.

TABLE 1-2 An Example of the Health Belief Model

Concept	Behavior: Using a Designated Driver
1. Perceived susceptibility	Individual believes she will get caught if she drinks and drives.
2. Perceived severity	Individual believes that the consequences of drinking and driving, such as getting caught or having a crash, are serious enough to try to avoid.
3. Perceived benefits	Individual believes that when it is not her turn to be the designated driver, she can enjoy herself without worry.
4. Perceived barriers	Individual's personal barriers to using a designated driver may include lack of independence or privacy.
5. Cues to action	Signs posted for DUI (driving under the influence) enforcement areas.
6. Self-efficacy	Individual is confident that someone will be willing to be the designated driver.

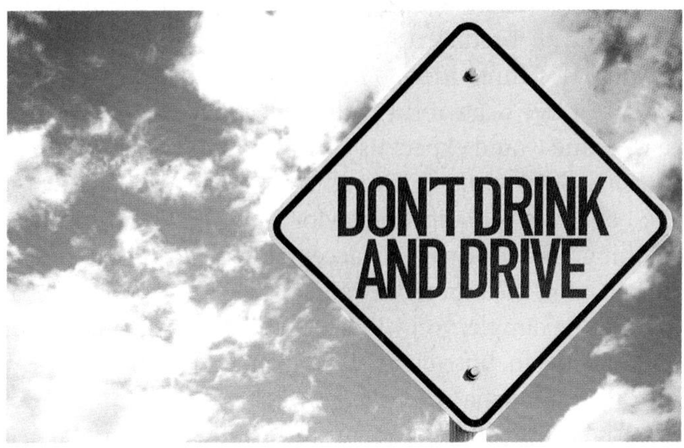

Don't drink and drive.

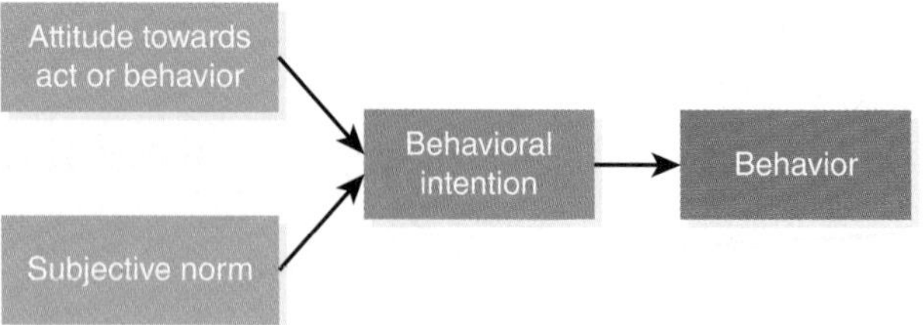

FIGURE 1-6 Theory of Reasoned Action.

that there was a need to design interventions to address adolescents' perceived barriers to HIV testing and to increase access to and knowledge about HIV testing.[28]

Theory of Reasoned Action

The Theory of Reasoned Action describes how people decide to act in a certain way (**FIGURE 1-6**). According to the theory, people consider their actions before they decide on their behavior. This theory assumes that individuals will usually act upon their intentions. The two major attributes are an individual's attitude toward a behavior (i.e., whether it is right or wrong) and an individual's beliefs concerning social pressures to either engage or not engage in the behavior.[29,30]

A study tested the applicability of the Theory of Reasoned Action in predicting whether college students would act as whistle-blowers within the setting of fraternity or sorority hazing. Researchers gave the participants a survey with three scenarios, varying in level of severity (*not severe, moderately severe, most severe*), describing a hypothetical hazing situation. Results showed that the Theory of Reasoned Action provided a sound basis for predicting whistle-blowing intentions. The level of severity moderated students' intentions. For both the *moderately severe* and the *most severe* scenarios, the perceived severity of hazing really did affect a participant's intention to report hazing. Student participants were less likely to report *not severe* hazing. Although this model is not usually used in ethical decision-making contexts, the results indicated the Theory of Reasoned Action could be used to explain the students' intentions.[31]

Theory of Planned Behavior

Professor Icek Azjen extended the Theory of Reasoned Action to the Theory of Planned Behavior,[32] which links beliefs with behavior. The intention to perform in a certain way can be predicted by a person's attitudes toward the behavior. This theory comprises three ideas: (1) A person's attitude toward a behavior will influence his or her behavior; (2) the *normative component*—that is, what other people we value would expect us to do—will influence the individual; and (3) *perceived behavior control*, which is the degree to which a person feels able to control the behavior, will affect behavior (**FIGURE 1-7**). Essentially, the more you like something, the more socially acceptable it is, and the more control you have over the behavior, the more likely you are to do it. If you are at a football or basketball game, for example, you will likely cheer for your team even if you are not really a big sports fan, but you are less likely to do so in a library.

A study from California examined the Theory of Planned Behavior and texting while driving in college students. The students who participated were of all races and ethnicities, were age 18 years or older, owned a cell phone, and drove a car. Over 70% of the sample reported that within the past week they

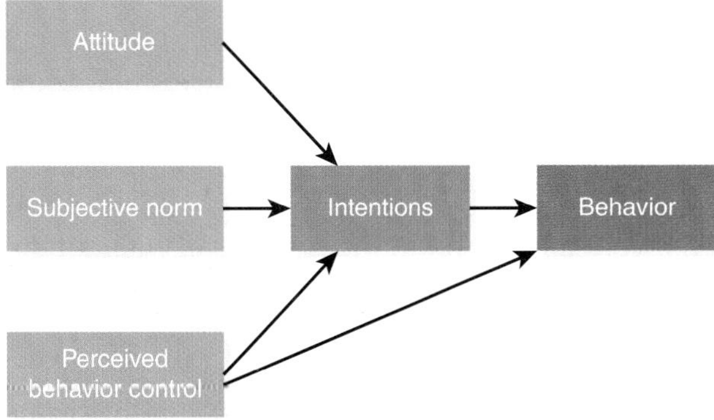

FIGURE 1-7 Theory of Planned Behavior.

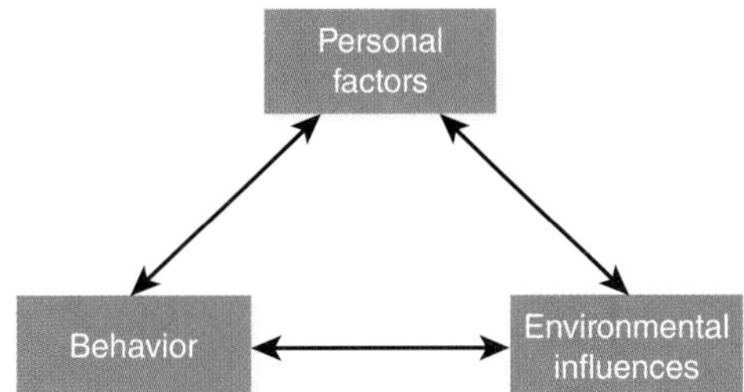

FIGURE 1-8 Social Cognitive Theory.

had talked on their cell phone and had sent and received text messages "at least a few times" while driving. Only 27% reported being stopped by police. Twenty-six percent reported reading or sending texts and having to slam the brakes to avoid hitting another car or a pedestrian(s) as a result within the past month. Attitude was the strongest factor that predicted intention. Intention changed the relationship of willingness to text while driving on students' perceived belief that they could control their behavior. That is, the more the student intended not to text while driving, the greater their belief that they could change their behavior increased. These findings highlight the usefulness of the Theory of Behavior Change to understand where to focus change interventions to stop texting while driving.[33]

Social Cognitive Theory

Social cognitive theory is a model of behavior from the work of Albert Bandura.[34,35] Basically, learning occurs in a social context, and much of what people learn comes from watching others. Social cognitive theory has been used for organizational behavior, athletics, and mental and physical health (**FIGURE 1-8**).

A study from North Carolina wanted to develop short educational videos to motivate teens with asthma to be more involved during their doctor visits. The researchers used social cognitive theory to develop the videos. To do this, they conducted **focus groups**. Four groups consisted of teens with asthma, four groups of parents of teens, and seven groups of physicians. The subject matter for the videos came from themes proposed in the focus groups. Based on the results, teen newscasters narrated six short videos with different themes: (1) how to get mom off your back, (2) asthma triggers, (3) staying active with asthma, (4) tracking asthma symptoms, (5) how to talk to your doctor, and (6) having confidence with asthma.[36] The researchers concluded that the teens, parents, and providers gave them insight into developing the videos to increase the teens' involvement during their medical visits.

focus groups Small number of people brought together with a moderator to discuss a specific topic. They aim at generating discussion instead of on individual responses to formal questions, and produce preferences and beliefs that may be expected from a larger population. The group may be deliberately selected.

The Transtheoretical Model

The Transtheoretical Model conceptualizes the process of intentional behavior change.[37,38] It includes ideas from other theories.

The stages of change are the core principles of the Transtheoretical Model. When people modify their behavior, they go through a series of steps. Each step is required before moving on to the next stage. Often, individuals repeat the stages or regress to an earlier stage from later ones. The stages are precontemplation (person is not yet ready for change), contemplation (person is getting ready for change), preparation (person is ready for change), action (person makes the change), and maintenance (person maintains the change) (**FIGURE 1-9** and **TABLE 1-3**).

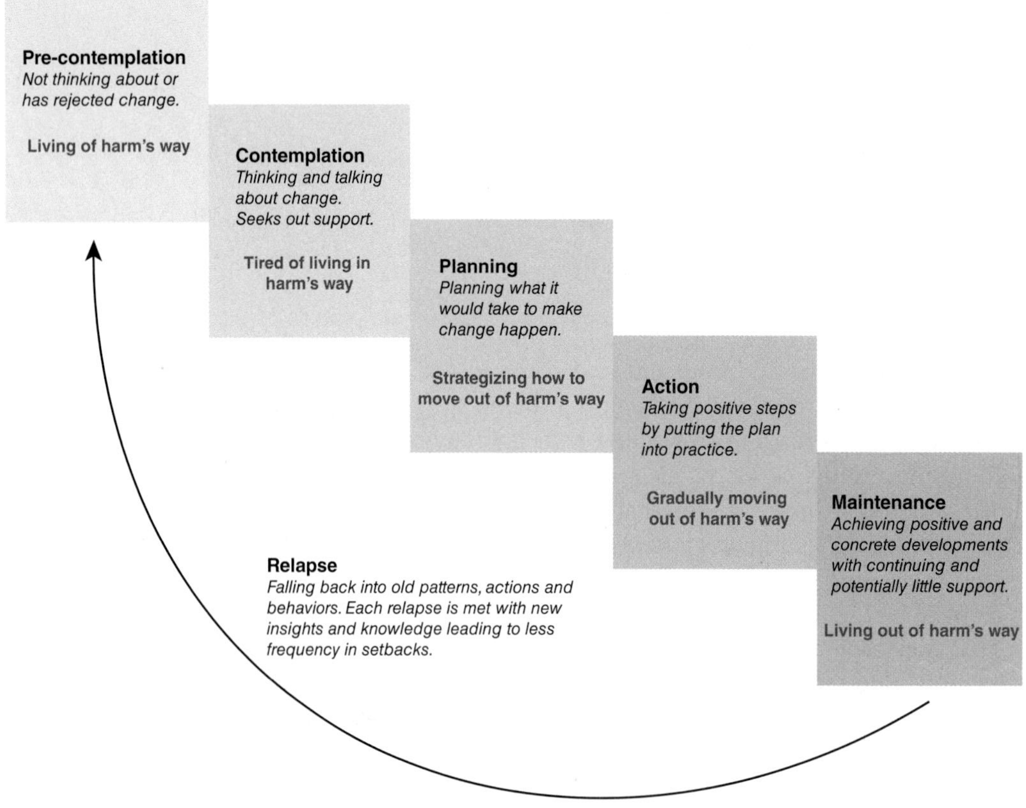

FIGURE 1-9 The Transtheoretical Model.

TABLE 1-3 A Description of the Transtheoretical Model

Transtheoretical Stage of Change	Description	Example
Precontemplation (not ready)	People in the precontemplation stage do not intend to take action in the near future. Being uninformed or less than adequately informed about the consequences of one's behavior may result in a person being in the precontemplation stage.	If someone is trying to change a behavior, such as stopping cigarette smoking, multiple attempts to quit can demoralize a person about his ability to change.

Contemplation (getting ready)	Contemplation is the second stage, where a person intends to change his or her behavior within the next 6 months. The person is more aware of the pros and cons of changing.	Our person who wants to quit smoking knows the benefits but understands how hard it is and many of the downsides. This weighing between the costs and benefits of changing can cause ambivalence so that the person remains at this stage for a long period.
Preparation (ready)	Preparation is the stage in which people plan to take action in the immediate future, usually within the next month. These people may have a plan.	Our person trying to quit smoking may take a health education class, talk to his physician about a prescription for medicine to help quit, or encourage friends to support him in his efforts.
Action	Action is the stage in which people have modified their behavior, usually within the past 6 months.	In our example, reduction in the number of cigarettes or switching to e-cigarettes, low-tar, and low-nicotine cigarettes do *not* count as *actions*. Only totally not smoking counts as the desired action.
Maintenance	Maintenance is the stage where people have modified their behavior and are working actively to prevent relapse.	Our now ex-smoker is not tempted to have a cigarette and increasingly feels confident that he will not return to smoking.

Two other parts of the Transtheoretical Model are decision making and self-efficacy.[39] Irving Janis and Leon Mann conceptualized decision making as a balance of potential gains and losses. Self-efficacy is also addressed in social cognitive theory.[34,35] It reflects people's belief that they can maintain their behavior change.

Weiss and colleagues[40] applied the Transtheoretical Model to bicycle helmet use among middle school, high school, and college students in Phoenix, Arizona. Forty-three percent of the students were in precontemplation, 17% were in either contemplation or preparation, 16% were in either action or maintenance, and 24% had used a bicycle helmet in the past but had relapsed to an earlier stage. Compared with students in precontemplation, students in the contemplation stage were disproportionately younger. The researchers concluded that the Transtheoretical Model was a useful framework for designing interventions aimed at increasing bicycle helmet use in children and adolescents.

Health Across the Life Span

Health begins at conception and continues through birth, childhood, adulthood, and old age. In utero, health depends on genetic makeup, a mother's health before she gets pregnant, and her behavior and choices while she is pregnant. In childhood, our health depends on love and support from parents; good nutrition, including access to clean water; enough physical activity; and quality health care and immunizations. As we grow into the teen and early adult years, beyond the basic physical health considerations of these groups, choices regarding tobacco, sexual activity, drinking, and illegal substance use will affect our health. When we move into parenthood (or not), we have to make choices about contraceptive practices, prenatal care, breastfeeding, and preventive services. Finally, as we get older, our health needs change further. Nutrition and exercise remain important; we also have concerns about chronic diseases. Screening and knowledge about chronic diseases like cardiovascular disease, diabetes, and cancer as well as other conditions are important. For some people, mental health care is an issue that needs to be addressed. Depending on the particular diagnosis, mental health services may or may not be needed. Access to high-quality health care for both preventive care and treatment is important.

When we think about health across the life span, there is an almost unlimited number of topics to cover. Because many of these issues are covered in the following chapters, we will describe only a few here, touching on issues across the life span.

Children

BY THE NUMBERS

Under Age 5 Mortality

Globally in 2016, there were 5.6 million deaths among children under 5 years of age.[41] As many as that may seem, we have come a long way. In 1955, just over 60 years earlier, there were 20.6 million deaths among children under age 5 years.[42]

In the United States, many people take for granted the factors that influence child survival, such as access to clean water, food that is clean and nutritious, and access to good primary health care. Think about your own childhood and whether you had access to clean water, healthy food, and primary health care. Were these readily available or were they a struggle for your family? As the WHO says, biology and environment determine a child's fate. A child's risk of dying "is influenced biologically by its gender, its natural defenses and its nutrition; and by its physical, microbial, social and cultural environments. The living conditions of families, the **prevalence** and modes of transmission of infectious disease agents and the nutritional status of the child are among the strongest immediate determinants that set the different levels of under-five mortality rates around the world."[42]

prevalence The total number of cases of a health condition, exposure, or other variable related to health, known to have existed over a period of time.

The leading causes of death among children under 5 years of age in the United States are **congenital anomalies**, prematurity, unintentional injuries, **sudden infant death syndrome (SIDS)**, and pregnancy complications.[43] In low- and middle-income countries, children under 5 years of age die from preterm birth complications, pneumonia, birth asphyxia, diarrhea, and malaria. About 45% of the deaths in developing countries are linked to malnutrition.[44]

congenital anomalies A structural or functional anomaly (e.g., metabolic disorders) that occurs during intrauterine life and can be identified prenatally, at birth, or later in life. Also known as a birth defect, congenital disorder, or congenital malformation.

sudden infant death syndrome (SIDS) The sudden unexplained death of an infant younger than 1 year old. The cause remains unexplained after a complete investigation.

Teen Pregnancy

The most recent report from the CDC shows that teen pregnancy rates are declining.

There is a strong association between age of having a baby and the mother's socioeconomic well-being. Simply put, the younger a woman is when she delivers her first child, the worse her economic future is. Pregnancy and delivery increase the likelihood of female students dropping out of high school. Only half of teen mothers graduate high school by age 22 years, compared to 90% of girls who do not become adolescent mothers. Adolescent mothers are less likely to marry, and when they do work, they earn less money.[46] There are costs to the children of teenagers as well. Children of teenage mothers are at higher risk of dropping out of high school, having more health problems, becoming a teenage parent, and being unemployed as a young adult.

BY THE NUMBERS

Teen Births

In the United States in 2015, there were 229,715 babies born to teenagers 15 to 19 years of age. This means that there were 22.3 births for every 1,000 women age 15 to 19 years. Three-quarters of teen pregnancies are unplanned. The U.S. teen pregnancy rate is higher than that in other Western industrialized countries.

The overall rate of decline was 8% from 2014 to 2015. Declines were seen for all races and for Hispanics.[45] Among 15- to 19-year-olds, teen birth rates decreased as follows:

- 10% for Asian/Pacific Islanders
- 9% for non-Hispanic Blacks
- 8% for Hispanics
- 8% for non-Hispanic Whites
- 6% for American Indian/Alaska Natives

Adults

In the United States, for those 45 years old or older, the two leading causes of death are **heart disease** and cancer.[43] (See the chapter "A Growing Challenge: Chronic Diseases" for a more comprehensive discussion of each of these.)

heart disease A broad category of conditions relating to disease of the cardiovascular system, including vessels and heart structures. Coronary artery disease is the most common type, and it is the leading cause of death for both men and women in the United States—and across the world.

Heart Disease

Coronary artery disease, the most common type of heart disease, is the *number one* killer of both men and women in the United States—and across the world.[43,47]

Coronary artery disease develops when the major blood vessels that carry oxygen-rich blood to the heart become damaged. This happens because plaque builds up in the arteries, decreasing blood flow to the arteries. Eventually, the decreased blood flow may cause chest pain (angina), shortness of breath, or other symptoms. If the artery becomes blocked, a heart attack results (**FIGURE 1-10**).

Coronary artery disease usually develops over decades. People may be unaware that they have a problem until there are symptoms or a heart attack occurs. However there are actions that people can take to minimize their risk of heart disease. As we will discuss here, it is amazing how important our lifestyle choices are for remaining healthy. Important lifestyle choices include[48]:

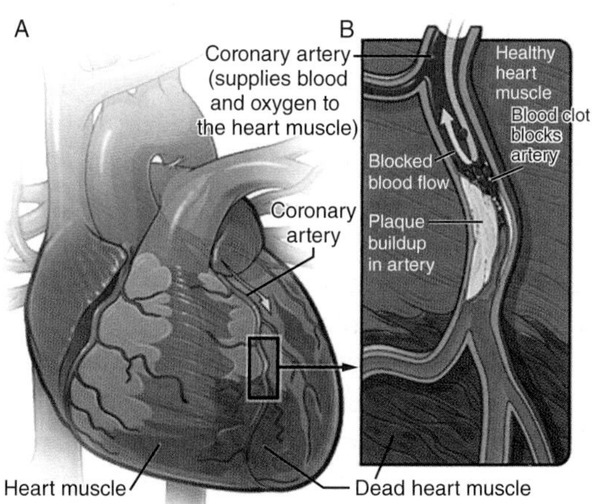

FIGURE 1-10 Heart showing muscle damage and a blocked artery.

Reproduced from Heart Disease: Symptoms, Diagnosis, Treatment, NIH MedLine Plus. Retrieved from https://medlineplus.gov/magazine/issues/winter09/articles/winter09pg25-27.html.

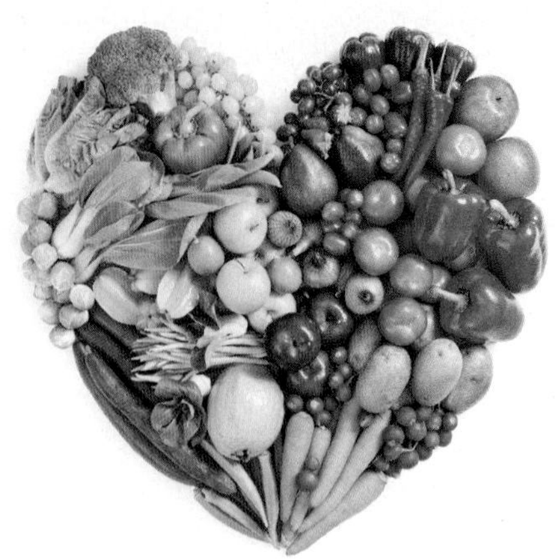

© ifong/Shutterstock.

1. Quit smoking! Smoking can raise your risk for coronary artery disease and heart attack and worsen other coronary artery disease risk factors.
2. Eat a heart-healthy diet. Eat five servings a day of fruits and vegetables. Eat fish high in omega-3 fatty acids (i.e., salmon, tuna, and trout) twice a week. Choose fat-free or low-fat dairy products, legumes (e.g., kidney beans, lentils, chickpeas), and whole grains. Minimize saturated fat, trans-fat, and sugary foods and beverages.
3. Maintain a healthy weight. The ideal body mass index is between 18.5 and 24.9.
4. Manage stress. A common trigger for a heart attack is an emotionally upsetting event. Cope with stress in a healthy way, such as meditation or a physical activity. Try a stress management program or relaxation therapy. Talking about things with friends and family is often helpful.
5. Exercise regularly. Any exercise is better than no exercise, but everyone should aim for 2.5 hours of moderate-intensity aerobic exercise or 1.25 hours of vigorous aerobic exercise per week. The more active you are, the more you'll benefit![48]

Cancer

Cancer is a collection of related diseases that can occur anywhere in the body. In cancer, the orderly process by which cells grow and die goes awry. Either the cells grow and divide when they should not or they do not die when they should.[49] Many cancers form solid tumors. Cancers of the blood, such as leukemias, usually do not form solid tumors. Cancerous tumors are malignant, meaning they spread into nearby tissues. Additionally, as the tumors grow, cancerous cells sometimes break off and move to other parts the body.[49]

incidence The number of new cases of a disease over a specified period of time.

There are more than 100 types of cancer. Cancer types are typically designated according to the organ or system affected.[49] The **incidence** of cancer is 454.8 cases per 100,000 men and women per year, and the mortality rate is 171.2 per 100,000 men and women per year. Mortality is highest among African American men (261.5/100,000) and lowest among Asian/Pacific Islander women (91.2/100,000). (Rates cited here are based on 2008–2012 cases and deaths.)[50]

The overall death rate for cancer has declined since the early 1990s, as physicians and scientists now understand more about how to lower risks for cancer as well as treat cancers when they occur. From 2004 to 2013, cancer death rates have decreased by 1.8% per year among men and 1.4% per year among women.[50]

When you see your healthcare professional, he or she will likely tell you all of the following ways to lower your risk for cancer. You will also read more

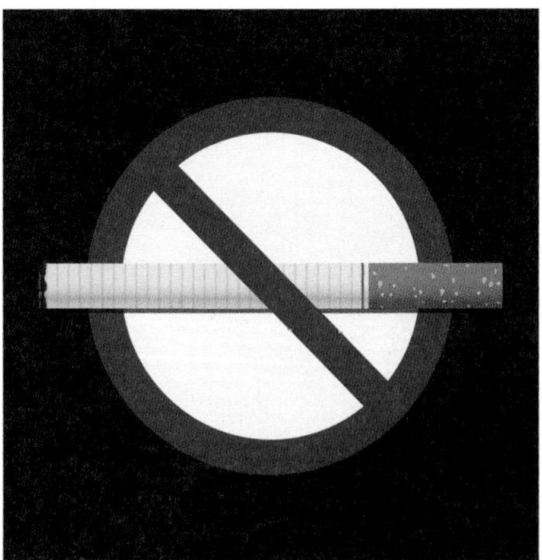

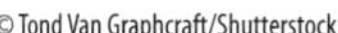

© Tond Van Graphcraft/Shutterstock.

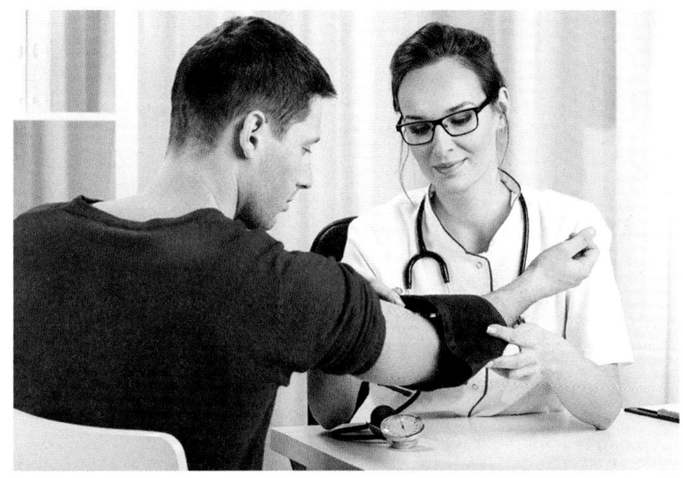

© ESB Professional/Shutterstock.

about these recommendations later. Your chances of developing cancer are affected by the lifestyle choices you make. Following these tips will help you to be healthy beyond helping you to lower your cancer risk[51]:

1. Don't use tobacco of *any* kind. Smoking raises your risk for cancer of the lung, mouth, throat, larynx, pancreas, bladder, cervix, and kidney. Chewing tobacco raises your risk for oral cancers and pancreatic cancer. Exposure to secondhand smoke increases your risk of lung cancer.
2. Eat a healthy diet, including lots of fruits and vegetables as well as whole grains and beans. Drink alcohol in moderation, if you drink at all. According to the National Institute on Alcohol Abuse and Alcoholism, *moderate* means drinking no more than two drinks per day for men and one drink per day for women.[52] One drink is defined as 12 ounces of beer, 5 ounces of wine, or 1½ ounces of distilled liquor.[53] Limit the amount of processed meat you eat.
3. Maintain a healthy weight and exercise regularly.
4. Protect yourself from the sun. Avoid the midday sun, seek shade, and use sunscreen. Avoid tanning beds and sun lamps.
5. Get immunized against hepatitis B and human papillomavirus (HPV).
6. Avoid risky behaviors. Practice safe sex and don't share needles.
7. Get regular medical care. Take your healthcare provider's recommendations for screening tests seriously.[51]

Social Determinants of Health and Health Inequities

Although it is important to follow the recommendations in the preceding lists, our health begins with our families. It continues with our homes, neighborhoods, schools, and communities. As you will read here, taking care of ourselves by eating a nutritious diet, being physically active, not smoking, wearing seat belts, getting immunizations and recommended **screening tests**, and seeing a healthcare professional when we are sick all influence our health. But less obvious factors, such as our access to high-quality schools and to social and economic opportunities, also determine our health. The cleanliness of the water we drink, the food we eat, and the air we breathe are all important, as are our neighborhood and the **built environment** in which we live. Our social

screening tests A simple test usually performed to identify those in a population who have or are likely to develop a specified disease.

built environment The physical environments where communities live and interact, including parks, sidewalks, green space, and housing.

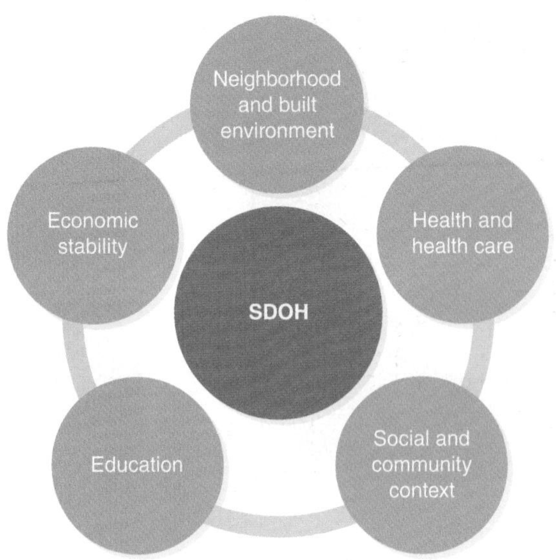

FIGURE 1-11 Social determinants of health.

Reproduced from Social Determinants of Health , HealthyPeople.gov. Retrieved from https://www.healthypeople.gov/2020/topics-objectives/topic/social-determinants-of-health.

interactions when we are out in the world and our relationships with other people all play an important part in our mental and physical health. All of these factors help explain why some people are healthier than others (**FIGURE 1-11**).

There is a wider set of forces and systems that shape daily life for people in this country and around the world. Part of the **social determinants of health** is the economic policies and government structure in the country in which we live, as well as the social norms of our society.[54] Although there are individual choices we make about our own health, there are also important material, social, political, and cultural conditions that determine our lifestyles and behaviors. As a society, we must reduce socioeconomic and racial inequities for everyone to enjoy good health.[55]

social determinants of health The circumstances in which people are born, grow, live, work, and age. They are shaped by the distribution of money, power, and resources at global, national, and local levels.

Health and Wealth

The poorer health experienced by those with lower incomes is not merely a problem of access. If that were true, the passage of the Affordable Care Act would eliminate disparities moving forward. But evidence from many other countries that have universal health care, including Canada, the United Kingdom, and virtually all of Europe and many other nations around the world, tells us that offering health insurance to all members of a society does not guarantee equalities in health. When comparing the well-off to the very rich, there are disparities between these two groups as well, with the very rich being healthier.[56]

The situation is not simply the poor versus everyone else. Data from the Gallup-Sharecare Well-Being Index demonstrates that while those with low income have worse health outcomes than the wealthier, those with high incomes are consistently healthier than middle-class families (**TABLE 1-4**).[57] In addition to specific diagnoses, the overall well-being increases as income rises.[57]

Race

People make many assumptions, good or bad, attributed to race. But, contrary to what people may think, **race** is a sociocultural concept, not a biological one. A person's racial group cannot be identified by blood type,[58,59] skin color,[60,61] ancestry,[62] or genes.[63,64]

race A sociocultural concept, not a biological one, that has emerged as a way to categorize and rank groups.

Because skin is one of our most visible features, we use it to divide people into racial categories.[61] As noted, skin color is not just *a* trait by which people define population differences; it is *the* trait.[60] The idea of race was invented as a

TABLE 1-4 Physical Health Indicators by Income Group

Health Condition	Low Income	Middle Class	High Income
Obesity	32.0%	27.9%	21.7%
Diabetes	16.1%	10.1%	6.7%
High blood pressure	36.4%	29.0%	23.6%
High cholesterol	29.3%	26.4%	25.3%
Heart attack	7.2%	3.5%	2.2%
Asthma	15.9%	10.5%	9.2%
Cancer	7.7%	6.9%	6.0%
Diagnosis of depression	29.0%	15.2%	10.2%

Data from Mendes, E. (2010, October 18). In U.S., health disparities across incomes are wide-ranging. Gallup-Healthways Well-Being Index. Well-Being. Retrieved from http://www.gallup.com/poll/143696/Health-Disparities-Across-Incomes-Wide-Ranging.aspx

way to categorize and rank groups.[65] It is a concept that has molded our economy, laws, and social institutions.[65]

It is difficult to talk about race. We have, through our history and culture, made race the determinant of devastating consequences. As you will discover, in this book, we mention race frequently. We do so because of the devastating consequences that categorizing people based on race has inflicted on our population and on the population's health. The idea of race is only a few hundred years old.[65] In 1619, Jamestown colonist John Rolfe traveled to the Court of London with his new wife Pocahontas. Because Pocahontas was a princess, this marriage caused a scandal. Seventeenth-century England was a very feudal society and people's status was fixed at birth. Maintaining social order was so important that they had laws regulating the clothing people could wear, defining their class. No one was upset that Rolfe had married an Indian. His marriage to Pocahontas was unthinkable because people of that time could not accept that a person of royalty would marry a commoner.[66]

Just because someone is *Black*, does not automatically make the person African American. He or she could be African, Afro-Caribbean, or Afro-European, for example. Likewise, someone who was born in the United States but whose parents were born and raised in Africa would correctly be called African American, even if that person is White.

TRY IT!

Where Is Your Family From?

Do you know your ancestry? Companies like Ancestry DNA, Family Tree DNA, and 23andMe will provide you with DNA results to help track your ancestry (for a fee). To view recent videos that show how some people get some surprising results from DNA analysis, search for the following on YouTube:

"Momondo: The DNA Journey"

"An open world begins with an open mind"

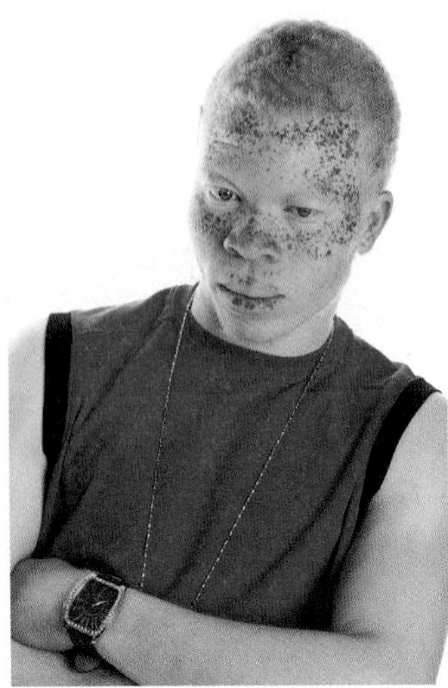

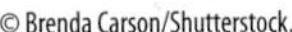

© Brenda Carson/Shutterstock.

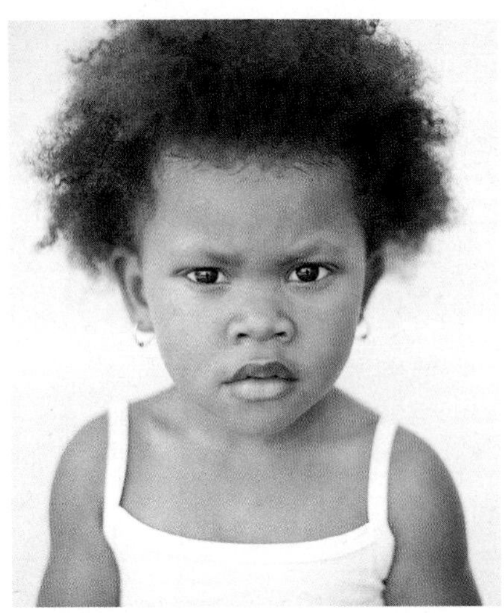

© pamelaoliveras/RooM/Getty.

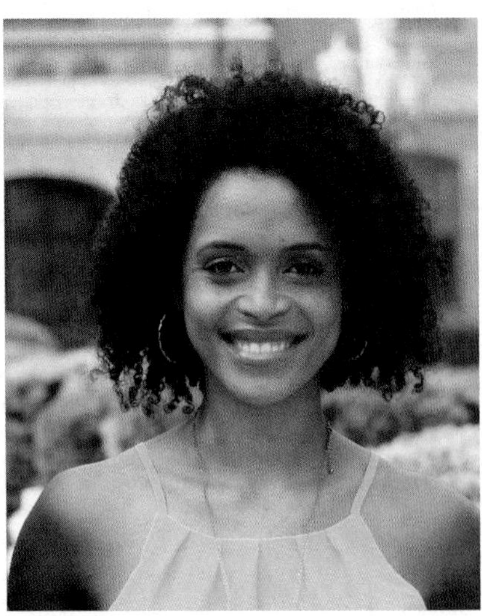

Courtesy of Anna Nzuzki Kiely; Photographer: Jean Pierre Vertil.

Skin color is an adaptation to geography. The closer people's ancestors were to the equator, the darker their skin. Variation in human skin color is an adaptive trait that correlates closely with geography and the sun's ultraviolet radiation. The amount of melanin in a person's skin determines how brown he or she is. Melanin is a natural sunscreen. It protects people from the harmful effects of ultraviolet radiation. As people migrated away from the tropics to colder areas with less sunlight, they developed lighter-colored skin. Lighter skin allowed ultraviolet rays to penetrate and produce vitamin D.[67] Based on our current understanding of genetics, inheritance of skin color is controlled by multiple genes working in combination. As a result, skin tones range from very pale to rich dark browns.

Another factor that has historically influenced skin color is diet. The native people of Alaska and Canada retain their darker skin even though they live in areas with low ultraviolet rays. Their diet, rich in vitamin D from seafood, provides an alternate source of vitamin D.[67]

As we talk about the consequences of how racial designations affect health, in general, we use the term African American to denote people whose skin is brown and whose ancestors came from Africa, although we understand that this designation is imprecise. Indeed, other designations will also be used. When we reference data with more precise designations, we use those terms, and when we refer to comparisons from published works, we use the terms the authors used.

Race and Income

There is massive financial and economic disparity across the races at every income level (**FIGURE 1-12**). According to a Pew Research Center report, from 2010 to 2013, White households' median wealth rose 2.4%, to $141,900. (*Median* refers to the midpoint; in this instance half the families are above this point and half are below. It indicates how the "typical" family is doing.) Over that same period, the median wealth in Black households declined to $11,000 and in Hispanic households declined to $13,700. That is a 13-fold wealth gap, the widest it has been since 1989.[68]

The other factor that helps explain the widening gap is where people invest their money. Real estate makes up a large portion of the wealth of Blacks and Hispanics. After the last recession, financial markets rebounded more than housing did. Because Whites are more likely to own stocks than are people of color, this added to the wealth gap. Additionally, the median income of minority households fell 9% between 2010 and 2013. During that same period, the median income of Whites fell by 1%.[68]

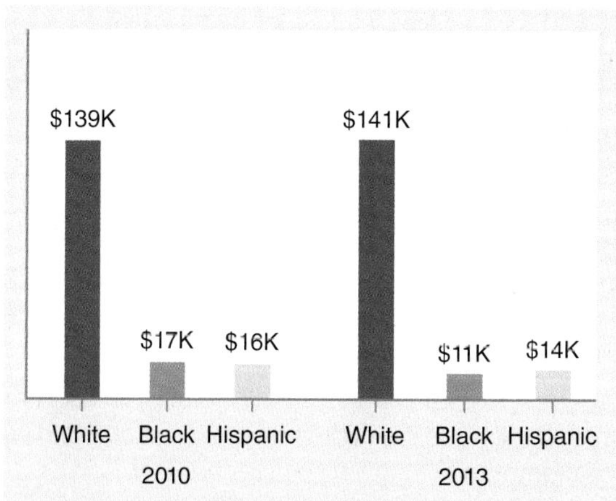

FIGURE 1-12 Race and ethnicity strongly predict wealth.

Data from https://www.washingtonpost.com/news/get-there/wp/2014/12/12/white-people-have-13-dollars-for-every-dollar-held-by-black-americans/?tid=a_inl

GOING UPSTREAM

We Are the 99 Percent

The disparity between the richest and poorest Americans has been increasing over time. "We Are the 99 Percent" is a website about income inequality, wealth concentration, and the economic system. As a measure of the inequality that exists in this country, think about the following:

- *Inequality impact.* Due in part to economic factors, students from low-income families with high test scores are no more likely to complete college than students from high-income families with low test scores.[69]
- *Inequality impact.* Extreme inequality causes many other social problems, like decreases in life expectancy, math proficiency, literacy, social mobility, and education and increases in infant mortality, homicides, imprisonment, teenage births, social distrust, obesity, mental illness, drug addiction, and debt.[70]
- *Wealth concentration.* Over one-third of Americans who are born to parents at the bottom of the income ladder remain very poor for their entire lives.[71]
- *Wealth concentration.* In America today, the number one factor predicting how wealthy you will be is not whether or not you went to college, but whether or not your parents are wealthy.[71]
- *Income inequality.* In 2009, the richest 74 Americans earned as much as the 19 million lowest paid Americans combined.[72]
- *Income inequality.* In 2010, the wealthiest 1 percent of Americans took home 24 percent of all U.S. income.[73]
- When politicians say that helping the rich will help everyone below them, they are not telling the truth.

BY THE NUMBERS

Wealth

Wealth is the value of all a person's assets of worth, which can be determined by taking the total market value of all physical and intangible assets owned, then subtracting all debts. The wealth gap is determined by dividing the median wealth of the wealthier group by the median wealth of the poorer group. In our example, the gap between the median White household wealth compared to that of the median Black household is $141,900/$11,000 = 12.9.

racism Prejudice, discrimination, or antagonism directed against someone of a different race based on the belief that one's own race is superior.

discrimination Unfair treatment of a person based on the person's race, ethnicity, gender, religious beliefs, sexual orientation, or other personal characteristics.

Black Lives Matter: A Public Health Issue?

Racism has not disappeared from the United States. The fact that the country elected an African American president not once but twice does not mean racism has gone away. People of color face **discrimination** every day in many different ways, from profiling by stores to unarmed individuals being killed by police despite presenting no real threat. The news is filled with stories of

BY THE NUMBERS

Fatal Encounters With Police

The Root used data reported by the *Washington Post*, Fatal Encounters, *The Guardian's* The Counted project, and the Cato Institute's National Police Misconduct Reporting Project from 2007 to 2017.[74]

If you think the playing field is level for all people in the United States, think again. Even when police officers are charged with a crime, they are rarely convicted by judges and juries.

- They found only three cases of a White police officer serving time for killing an African American (in one case, three officers were charged with killing a 92-year-old grandmother).
- Between 2005 and 2017, there were 49 people killed by police who were indicted for their crimes, of whom 33 were Black. Only five of the police officers were convicted, giving a 12% homicide conviction rate for Black victims.
- Since June 2007, there have been approximately 10,000 police shootings, yet only five White police officers have been imprisoned for killing a Black person.
- In 2015, police killed 1,146 victims. Of those, 307, or 7.69/1,000,000 people, were Black. Not a single police officer was convicted for an on-duty killing.

violence against communities of color; yet all too often, charges brought against the perpetrators of these violent acts are dismissed if the perpetrator is White.

In 1998, the American Public Health Association released a policy statement on the impact of police violence on public health. They noted then, and it is still true today, that "police brutality and excessive use of force are widely reported and have a disproportionate impact on people of color [and that there is] significant morbidity and mortality associated with these events."[75]

As discussed in the previous section, there is a strong relationship between race and income. We also know that people who are poor and less privileged have worse health and die much younger than people who are rich and more privileged. As noted, the socioeconomic inequalities in health and mortality are very large. These inequalities have existed for a long time, even though we

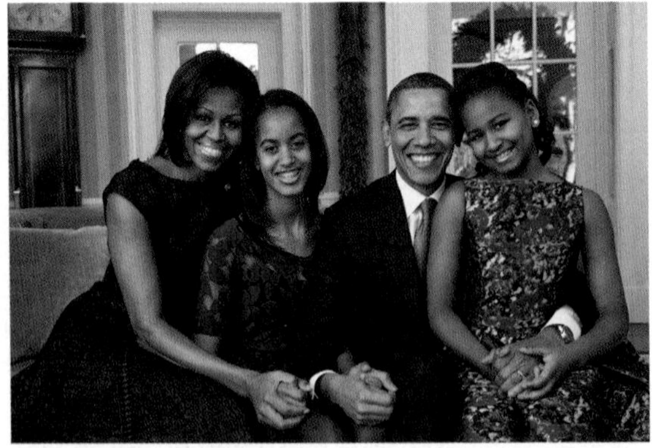

Former President Barack Obama and family.

Official White House Photo by Pete Souza.

The American Public Health Association is an organization for public health professionals. The organization speaks out for public health issues and policies backed by science. Their mission is to "improve the health of the public and achieve equity in health status."

have addressed many of the causes, such as overcrowding and poor sanitation.[76] Rates of poor pregnancy outcome, cancer, and cardiovascular disease are significantly different by socioeconomic status and by race.

As discussed, race is a social construct that holds devastating repercussions for communities of color, and this makes racism a social determinant of health. If we understand that racism is a system that unfairly disadvantages some individuals and communities, and advantages others,[77] then the consequences of living in a racially stratified society are evident when health outcomes demonstrate disparities along racial lines. There are many examples of these disparate outcomes, including higher rates of infant mortality among Blacks, higher rates of deaths caused by heart disease and stroke, and a shorter life expectancy for Blacks in comparison with Whites.[78] These disparities are a consequence of racism.

GOING UPSTREAM

Experiences of Racism

Consider a study from California, where researchers conducted focus groups to study women's experiences of racism. Researchers found that women experienced racism throughout their lives. The racism they experienced as children was particularly salient and enduring. They continued to experience the effects as adults, directly and vicariously, in seeing their children suffer. The women experienced interpersonal, institutional, and internalized forms of racism. They had behavioral, emotional, cognitive, and bodily responses to the racism. Finally, the women acknowledged being vigilant in anticipation of future racism toward themselves and toward their children. The stress these women and other women of color experience contributes to poor birth outcomes.[79]

Racism is institutionalized, racism is interpersonal, and racism is internalized. Institutional racism comes in the form of structural barriers that make society unequal. Institutions include governments, organizations, schools, banks, and courts of law, any of which may treat certain groups of people negatively because of their race. When schools in poor communities, filled predominantly with students of color, are not as good as schools in affluent neighborhoods, that is institutionalized racism. When the societal norm is that people who are White can get better jobs than people of color, that is institutionalized racism. When people are privileged simply because their skin is a lighter color, that is institutionalized racism.

Interpersonal racism is what happens between people. When an individual is not welcome into a home because of his or her color, that is interpersonal racism. When someone makes an assumption about another based on his or her race, that is interpersonal racism. Interpersonal racism can be intentional or unintentional, but even if it is unintentional, it is still racism. When individuals internalize the messages that they are less than equal or somehow unworthy simply because of the color of their skin, that is internalized racism.[80]

There is a large body of medical literature verifying that discrimination impacts people's health.[81–91] Exposure to discrimination is a risk factor for poor health, even among children.[81] Skin color is a dominant factor that impacts self-reported health,[85] and the darker a person's skin, the more discrimination he or she experiences.[84]

"The most certain test by which we judge whether a country is really free is the amount of security enjoyed by minorities."
—**John E. E. Dalberg**, Lord Acton, *The History of Freedom in Antiquity*, 1899.[92]

Social Justice

The definition of social justice is "promoting a just society by challenging injustice and valuing diversity."[93] A just society will exist when all people have a right to equitable treatment, support for their human rights, and a fair allocation of community resources. Applied to health, this means that everyone deserves equal rights and opportunities, including the right to good health.[93]

We live in a society where many of the diseases that threaten our health and well-being are preventable. Unfortunately, there is an unequal distribution of money, power, and resources that helps maintain a divided society. Some inequities affect health, for better or for worse, depending on what side of the divide a person lives on. The division includes access to safe housing, jobs with living wages, quality education, nutritious and affordable food, a safe place to be physically active, and access to high-quality, respectful, and affordable health care.

GOING UPSTREAM

Is It a Level Playing Field?

If schools were a level playing field, discipline would be administered evenly across all students and discipline rates would show no difference based on race or ethnicity. However, discipline rates do show differences and it matters because this starts early and continues through life. Unfortunately, as school administrators and teachers have reported, most discipline policies do not lead to improvements in behavior.

What is striking is not that there is a racial divide in discipline, but how early it starts, how pervasive it is, and how it continues.

An article from the *Seattle Times* found that short-term suspension rates for Black elementary students were four times that for White students.[94] Or, consider a story from Georgia where two 12-year-old girls, one Black, and one White, got into trouble for writing graffiti on the walls of the gym bathroom. Both girls were suspended for a few days and requested to pay a $100 fine. The White girl's family paid the fine, but the Black girl's family could not. A few weeks after the disciplinary hearing, the Black girl was charged in juvenile court with a trespassing misdemeanor and potentially a felony. In a plea bargain, she admitted to criminal trespassing, spent her summer on probation, with a 7:00 p.m. curfew, and completed 16 hours of community service.[95]

The Center for the Study of Race and Equity in Education at the University of Pennsylvania found that in 13 Southern states, Blacks made up only 24% of students enrolled in public school, but 48% of the students who were suspended and 49% of the students' expelled.[96] In 84 of the school districts across the Southern states, 100% of the suspended students were Black. As you can see from **TABLE 1-5**, the proportion of Black students suspended greatly exceeded the

TABLE 1-5 Percentage of Black Students Enrolled and Suspended in Southern States[96]

State	Blacks as a % of Students Enrolled	Blacks as a % of Students Suspended	Differential (% Suspended/% Enrolled)
Alabama	34%	64%	1.9
Arkansas	21%	50%	2.4
Florida	23%	39%	1.7
Georgia	37%	67%	1.8
Kentucky	11%	26%	2.4

Louisiana	45%	67%	1.5
Mississippi	50%	74%	1.5
North Carolina	26%	51%	2.0
South Carolina	36%	60%	1.7
Tennessee	23%	58%	2.5
Texas	13%	31%	2.4
Virginia	24%	51%	2.1
West Virginia	5%	11%	2.2

Data from Penn Graduate School of Education. Center for the Study of Race & Equity in Education. Disproportionately Disciplined: Black Student Suspension Rates in the American South. 2018. Retrieved from: https://equity.gse.upenn.edu/sites/default/files/GSE_HarprSspnsnInfo_R5.pdf

proportion such students represent in a school. The consistency of the findings across all these states suggests that for Black students the playing field is definitely not level.[96]

Students who are disciplined unfairly are more likely to fall behind in their schoolwork, more likely to drop out of school, and more likely to end up in jail or prison. A study from the Bureau of Justice found that Black males received harsher sentences than White males after accounting for the facts of the case. The study also found that disparities increased between 2005 and 2012 (the years of the study).[97]

Think about how such disparities make individuals feel. Has this ever happened to you? Have you seen it happen to a peer? The stress of being made to feel less than worthy contributes to poor health outcomes.

In his book, *A Theory of Justice*, author John Rawls describes how it is unlikely that society will achieve equal outcomes for all members. Rawls maintains that this reality is acceptable if every person has a reasonable opportunity to achieve optimal outcomes. As this argument applies to health, if all members of society have safe housing, jobs that pay a living wage, equal access to education, nutritious food, physical activity, and high-quality health care, it is still unlikely that everyone will be equally healthy; however, that scenario is acceptable because everyone has an equal opportunity for health.[98]

If we consider the past and much of the present, we realize that the differences we see in health are due to racism and discrimination that make the opportunity for equity currently impossible.

Why Is Change Important?

Imagine a world where we don't judge others—a place where all races, genders, and people who look different than ourselves are judged by who they are as people rather than how they look. We need to remove the perception of "normal" and "acceptable." Imagine a world where there is no hate or discrimination. Imagine a world where instead of spending time and energy on fearing or ridiculing others, people simply accept others and move on to far more important things. There will always be people different than you, but it is important to embrace diversity. To witness one man's journey from racism to understanding, search for "James Rainey Reformed Racist on Oprah" on YouTube.

Although we have focused mainly on race, discrimination can be based on many factors. Many people face discrimination on a regular basis, including women, LGBTQ (lesbian, gay, bisexual, transgender, queer and/or questioning) individuals, religious minorities, and individuals with disabilities.

Being LGBTQ often means facing discrimination, which may manifest as verbal abuse, being ignored while waiting for service at a restaurant or store, or an outright refusal of service from a public entity. For example, a local bakery that refuses to make a wedding cake for a same-sex couple. Although partially repealed a year later, the North Carolina legislature on March 23, 2016, passed a law (HB2) that prevented transgender people from using bathrooms that correspond with their gender identity.[99]

GOING UPSTREAM

Experiencing Discrimination

"We have an insanely long way to go [for equality]. I am happy enough to be a white, cisgender, gay male; as such, I face much less prejudice than many members of the LGBTQIA+ community. That said, I experience it on almost a daily basis and I look like a somewhat affluent member of the white middle class. Can you imagine how much worse it would be if I were a person of color?"

—**Derrick De Lise**, author, activist, chef, and Culinary Institute of America alumnus[100]

Individuals with a disability face discrimination every day. Some examples include the assumption that if you have a physical disability, you are not intelligent; lack of physical access to buildings; wheelchair quotas for concert venues, airplanes, city buses, and amusement park rides; nondisabled people

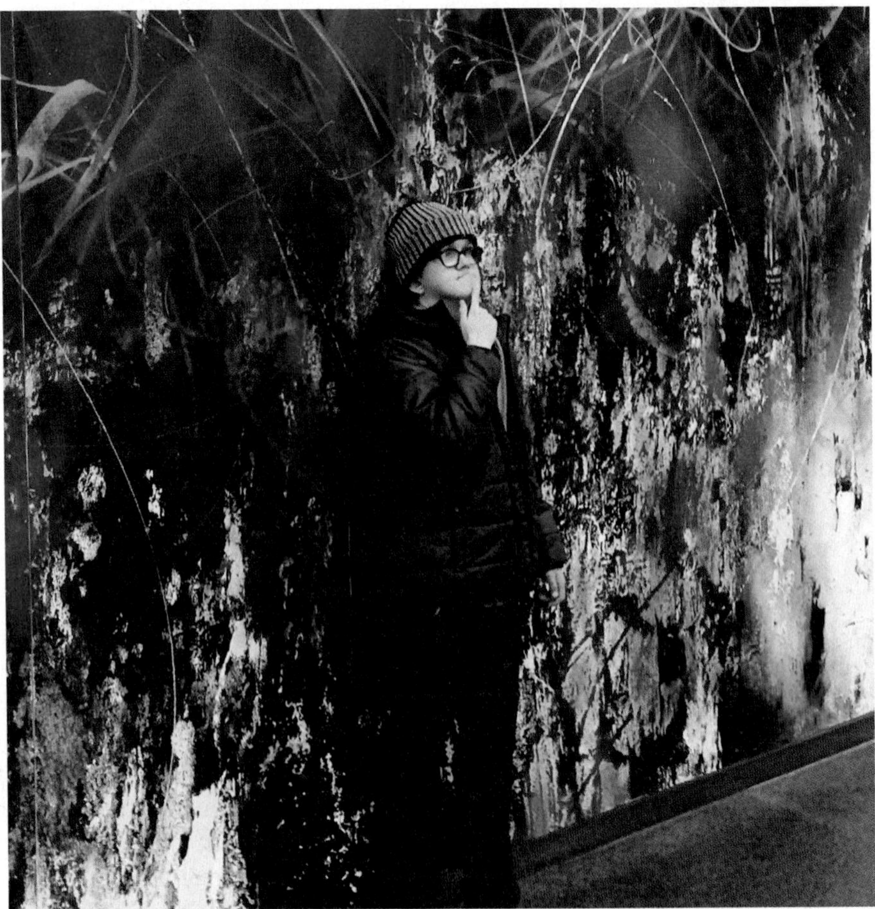

Dylan Foyster

Courtesy of Traci and Dylan Foyster.

parking in handicapped parking spots; and people acting like the disabled person is invisible.[101] People shout at the blind as if they were deaf. Many people assume that someone with intellectual impairments will not understand negative comments about them or stares from curious people. It is important to remember that everyone has feelings and wants acceptance.

Discrimination has a significant negative effect on health. Many groups in society are the targets of frequent discrimination, both overt and subtle. Mental health outcomes include stress, depression, and anxiety. Physical health outcomes of discrimination include hypertension, obesity, high blood pressure, substance use, and self-reported poor health. Repeated exposure to discrimination is a chronic stressor that erodes a person's protective mechanisms and increases the likelihood of physical illness. The more severe and the more frequent the discrimination, the more negative the mental and physical health outcomes.[102]

Location, Location, Location: The Importance of Where We Live

How many times have you moved? We are a mobile society. The average American moves every 7 years. This means that 40 to 50 million people move each year. Of these people, 15 to 20 million individuals are making *big* moves—to a new city, county, or state. This is important, because where you live increasingly shapes your life and your opportunities.[103] Think about how many moves you have made in your life. Are you above or below the average?

Where you live matters, especially if you are poor. As the *New York Times* puts it, the rich live longer everywhere; for the poor, geography matters. In some areas, the poor live as long as their middle-class neighbors. In other areas, those with the lowest incomes die young.[104] (See the interactive map available at this reference.) Between 2001 and 2014, the gap between the life spans of the rich and the poor grew wider. Life expectancy increased continuously with income. American men earning in the top 1% of income lived 15 years longer than men in the bottom 1%. Among women, the gap was 10 years. Additionally, the inequality in life expectancy has increased over time. While individuals in the top 5% of income gained approximately 3 years of life expectancy, those in the bottom 5% experienced no gains.[105] The authors identified five factors associated with substantial upward mobility, many related to policies at the local level. These factors include (1) less segregation by income and race, (2) lower levels of income inequality, (3) better schools, (4) lower violent crime rates, and (5) a higher proportion of two-parent households. The location in which a person lives was more important for boys than for girls and for lower-income children than for rich children.[106]

Noise Pollution

How loud is it where you live? We regard noise as unwanted or disturbing sound. It can interfere with sleeping or conversation and can impact a person's health. Housing close to sources of noise (e.g., highways, trains, airports, sirens, factories) is obviously less desirable, and therefore, less costly. Thus, if you can afford to live where it is quiet, it is likely that is what you will choose.

Approximately 22 million workers in the United States are exposed to hazardous work-related noise.[107] Research has shown noise exposure to be related to type 2 diabetes mellitus,[108] hearing loss,[107] decreased sleep, and decreased performance of manual activities.[109]

When looking for a place to live, of all the factors you might consider, the noise level of an apartment can be difficult to anticipate. However, a website called howloud.com provides a "soundscore" based on traffic activity, airport activity, and local noise sources (e.g., restaurants, schools, stores) to inform you about whether the neighborhood is calm, active, or busy.[110] Note that some variables cannot be included in this assessment, including how noisy or quiet other tenants are or whether the apartment faces the street or the back of a building. The score rates an address from 0 to 100, with a higher score reflecting less noise.

TRY IT!

Noise

How noisy is where you live? Search for how loud and compare your perceptions with your addresses' score.

Move to Opportunity Experiment

What about where you grew up? A study by the Equality of Opportunity Project found that there is a wide variation in the ability of an individual to improve his or her economic status across different places in the United States. The researchers in this study mapped the ability to change economic status by county all across the United States. Children from lower-income families who live in the southeastern United States, on average, stayed in that income bracket. Across much of the Great Plains, with the exception of some large Native American reservations, children had a better than average chance of moving to higher income brackets.[111]

The researchers also studied how the neighborhood where one lives affects a person's ability to improve his or her income. The project found that every year of exposure to a better environment improved a child's chance of success. The researchers also reanalyzed data from a study called the Moving to Opportunity experiment, designed by the U.S. Department of Housing and Urban Development. Between 1994 and 1998, approximately 4,600 families living in high-poverty public housing projects in five large U.S. cities were randomly assigned to one of three groups. One group received a subsidized housing voucher that required moving to an area with less than 10% poverty. The second group received standard housing vouchers with no requirements. The third group retained their access to public housing but did not receive a voucher.[112] Adults in the first group had greatly improved mental and physical health.[113] As shown in **FIGURE 1-13**, the children who were younger than

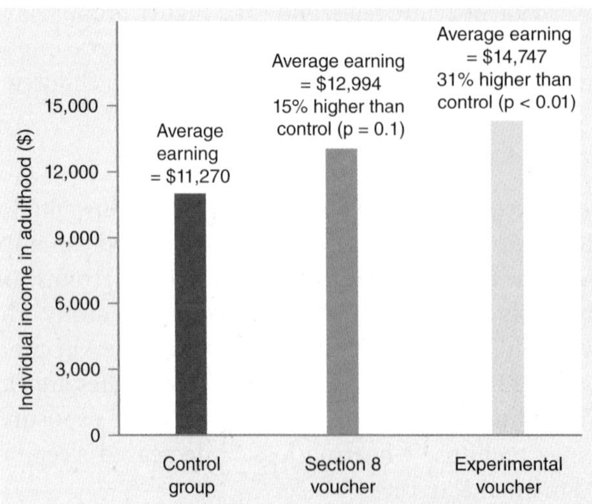

FIGURE 1-13 Cost-effective policy: The Move to Opportunity study increased the earnings of children.

13 years when they moved had higher incomes in adulthood. Children who were age 13 to 18 years when they moved to a lower-poverty neighborhood had an insignificant or slightly worse outcome in terms of income. The economic gains from moving declined steadily as children got older at the time of the move.[112] The gains from moving at a young age were robust regardless of gender or city of residence or race/ethnicity. The researchers estimated that moving a family to a low-poverty area when a child is young translates into a total lifetime increase in earnings of $302,000. Importantly, the findings suggest that integrating disadvantaged families into mixed-income communities may reduce poverty for the children and grandchildren of those disadvantaged families.[112]

What Is Happiness?

You probably know when you're happy and when you're not. But look around your classroom and ask your classmates what makes them happy. You will likely get many different answers because defining happiness is not easy. There are thousands of articles in the medical literature about being happy. The Declaration of Independence (1776) describes it as a fundamental and inalienable right. Yet the pursuit of happiness is elusive.

So what makes us happy? What have researchers discovered?

It's Partly Your Genes

Although not entirely, to some extent genes do control your happiness.[114–116] Researchers estimate that genes might be responsible for between one-third and one-half of a person's happiness.[114,117] Bartels and colleagues estimate that the amount of happiness inherited genetically is almost twice as high for females (41%) as for males (22%).[115] Gatt, Burton, Schofield, Bryant, and Williams suggest there are common genetic factors that contribute to a sense of well-being and satisfaction with life.[118]

While some people are born with sunnier personalities, even sunny people are not happy all of the time. Additionally, people who are not genetically predisposed to happiness can learn to be happier.

Do you believe you know what does or will make you happy?

Being Rich

There is no doubt that having money makes life easier, but does money actually make you happy? Surprisingly, not so much! A study from Princeton University found that the income required to improve one's chances of happiness is about $75,000 a year. The lower a person's annual income is below that number, the unhappier the person is. But no matter how much more a person makes than the $75,000, it does not make him or her happier.[119] Being rich is not like what you see on TV. In real life, most people who are rich work for their money, and many work all the time. And while money can buy quality health care, it cannot buy health.[120]

Spending Time With Good Friends

Spending quality time with good friends is an important part of a happy life.[121] Taking time off to relax will also keep your stress levels low. It is important to prioritize the time you spend with friends and not wait for special occasions to get together—call up your friends today and make a plan!

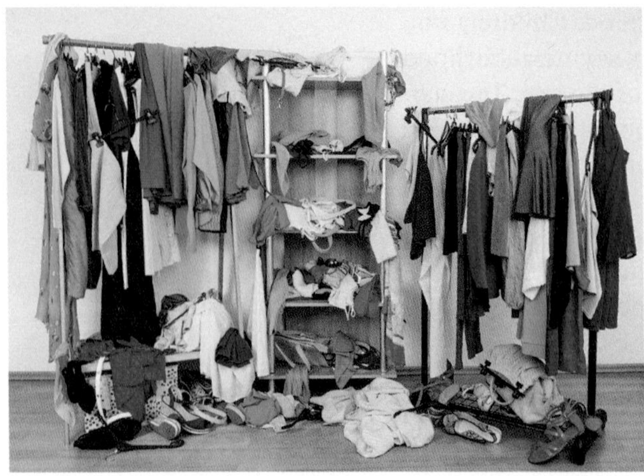
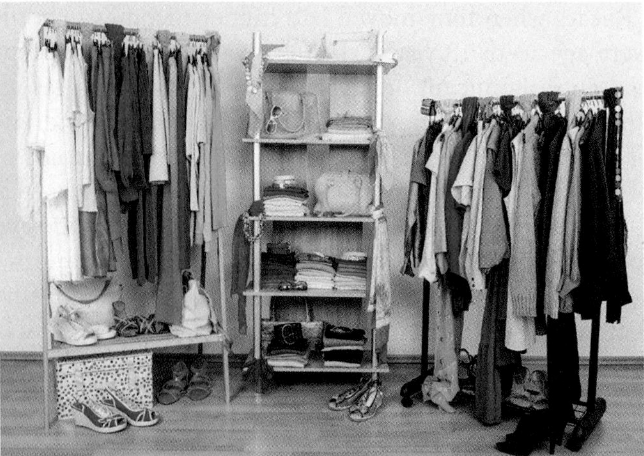

FIGURE 1-14 Before and after decluttering.

Getting Your Room/Apartment Organized

It may not be your favorite way to spend the day, but organizing certainly is gratifying. Cleaning out the clutter and creating a usable space will give you a sense of achievement that is guaranteed to boost your well-being (**FIGURE 1-14**). Perhaps the junk we live with clutters our minds as well.[122]

Losing Weight

There is no doubt that if you are overweight, weight loss is good for you. But it does not seem to make people happy; nor should it. If weight loss is not making people happy, that could explain, at least in part, why many people struggle to keep weight off. As Roberto and colleagues suggest, when you are trying to lose weight, changes in brain chemistry, metabolism, and hunger make it difficult to definitively lose weight.[123]

Being healthy and exercising, even without losing weight, will make you healthier than the person who does not exercise.[124] The goal is for your blood pressure, cholesterol, blood sugar, and other indicators to fall within a healthy range. A person who feels healthy is more likely to be happy.[125]

Smile!

As simple as this suggestion seems, smiling has been scientifically proven to make you feel happy. It is something like the saying, when you smile, the world smiles with you.[126]

Happiness and a Meaningful Life

Martin Seligman is the founder of Positive Psychology and promotes the idea that a happy life is one that is pleasurable, engaging, and meaningful. Seligman found that the most satisfied, upbeat people are those who had discovered and exploited their unique combination of strengths. People who use their energies to lead engaging and meaningful lives are more likely to be happy than individuals who focus on immediate pleasure.[127]

What does this mean for you? Do what you love. An activity that makes you happy and helps you ignore outside stressors is good. Activities that provide something of a challenge, such as playing a musical instrument, bring reward. Participation in social activities can both bring happiness and increase your well-being.

Being satisfied with your life is important as you get older. In a 9-year study, older individuals rated questions about their life satisfaction over time. The participants responded annually over the course of the study, also answering questions about age, gender, education, health conditions, smoking status, physical activity, and depressive symptoms. As participants' life satisfaction increased, the risk of mortality decreased. Some people's satisfaction with their life varied over the course of the study. People whose satisfaction was low had increased mortality risk, while people who were satisfied with their life had lower mortality risk. Individuals in the group with both low satisfaction and high variability in satisfaction were at greatest risk of mortality over the course of the study.[128]

Key Health Concepts

It is a good idea to understand how researchers and other experts in the field define and discuss health. Once you understand the concepts that underlie the subject of health, reading and digesting the facts and figures presented here will be much easier. Each of these concepts is introduced briefly.

Rates Versus Numbers

The concept of rates is important when discussing health. Rates are different than numbers because rates consider the size of the population, which allows us to make comparisons. We can use rates to measure time as well as numbers. Rates are statements of frequency (e.g., disease frequency) that allow comparisons between groups of people. For example, let's consider the number of cases of a fictional illness called "madpox disease." In City A there are 100 cases, and in City B there are only 40 cases (**TABLE 1-6**). This suggests to us that madpox disease is a greater problem in City A than in City B, right?

To make a meaningful comparison, however, we must determine the prevalence of the disease in each city, which means that we need to know each city's population. We discover that City A has a population of 40,000 residents, while City B has 8,000 residents. That changes the picture a bit. To arrive at the disease prevalence, we must divide the number of cases in each city by the population (**TABLE 1-7**).

When we compare the prevalence in the two cities, it is clear that madpox disease is actually a much greater problem in City B, due to its smaller population, than in City A, even though the total number of cases is greater in City A.

TABLE 1-6 Existing Cases of Madpox Disease in Cities A and B

	Existing Cases
City A	100
City B	40

TABLE 1-7 Prevalence of Madpox Disease in Cities A and B

	Existing Cases	Population	Prevalence
City A	100	40,000	.0025
City B	40	8,000	.0050

TABLE 1-8 Existing Cases of Madpox Disease and Population in Cities A and B With Prevalence as a Rate

	Existing Cases	Population	Prevalence (as a decimal fraction)	Prevalence (per 1,000 population)
City A	100	40,000	.0025	2.5/1,000
City B	40	8,000	.0050	5.0/1,000

Because we are talking about people, a number as small as 0.005 is not particularly useful on its own. Such small numbers are common when interpreting the prevalence of rare diseases. To raise numbers to a more useful value, **epidemiologists** multiply the prevalence rate by 1,000, which for most diseases yields a number larger than 1 (**TABLE 1-8**). The prevalence can now be described as being "per 1,000." There are diseases that are so rare that the multiplier used is 1,000,000 and prevalence is discussed as "per 1,000,000."

epidemiologists Individuals who study the causes and distributions of disease among local and global populations. They not only focus on preventing and controlling the spread of communicable diseases, but also on understanding how to prevent chronic diseases.

Neither city has exactly 1,000 residents, but by using the "per 1,000" convention, we now have a clearer picture of the prevalence of madpox among residents in each city. You can see how presenting the information as a rate is much more informative than simply stating a total,[129] and how it changes our original view that madpox was a greater problem in City A than in City B. It also allows you to determine whether the comparison you are making is truly comparable.

Incidence Versus Prevalence

Researchers often refer to disease frequency in population health. They talk about disease frequency in terms of incidence and prevalence. Incidence is the number of *new* cases of a disease over a specified period (e.g., 100 cases over 2 years). However, it is difficult to measure incidence because the exact time of the beginning of an illness is hard to pinpoint. As we have already noted, prevalence is the total number of cases, per population size, known to have existed over a period.[129] For example, a 2008 study found that among college students, 306/1,000 had smoked a water pipe in the past year.[130] We will primarily discuss prevalence as we look at population health.

FIGURE 1-15 illustrates the relationship between incidence and prevalence. As incidence (new cases) increases, so does prevalence. If we are discussing an infectious disease, such as malaria or the flu, when people get the condition again, prevalence increases. If people die of the condition, the prevalence decreases.

Randomized Controlled Trials

randomized controlled trials A study design that randomly assigns participants to either an intervention group or a control group. The control may be a standard practice, a placebo ("sugar pill"), or no intervention at all. As the study is conducted, the only expected difference between the control and experimental groups is the outcome variable being studied.

When researchers want to know if a treatment (or intervention) will improve disease outcomes in individuals or communities, they employ an intervention study. Investigators make comparisons between a group receiving a new, innovative intervention (the intervention group) and a group receiving an older intervention (the control group) or no intervention (also called a control group).

Many people regard **randomized controlled trials** as the absolute best, or "gold standard," for judging the benefits of interventions (treatment).[131] A randomized controlled trial is a kind of study that randomly assigns participants into one of two groups, either an intervention group or a control group.

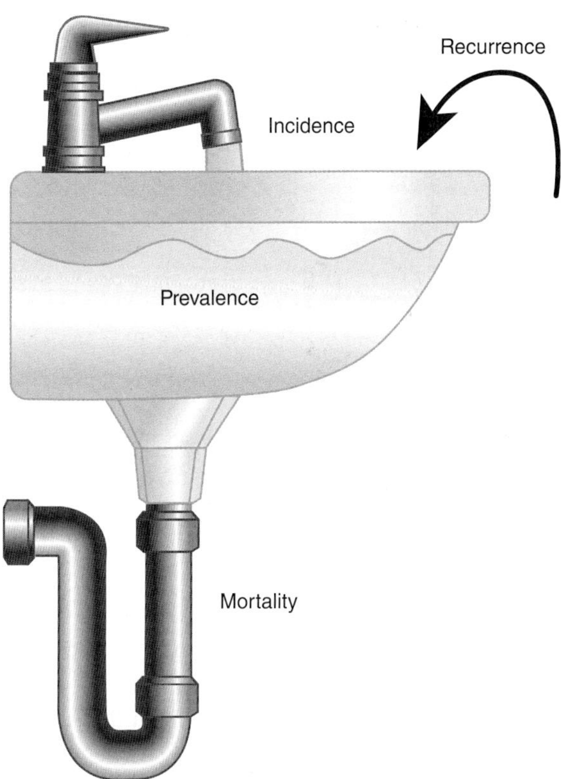

FIGURE 1-15 The relationship between incidence and prevalence.

The control group may receive the standard practice, such as the usual medical care; a placebo, which is a treatment that is deliberately ineffective, such as giving someone a "sugar pill"; or no intervention at all. When correctly done, after randomization (i.e., the process of dividing the participants so that each person has an equal chance of being assigned to either group) but before the intervention, the characteristics of the two groups should be similar. Relevant characteristics depend on the purpose of the trial and may include, for example, age, gender, education, employment, usual exercise routine, diet, or prior medical history.

Statistical Significance

As you're reading this book, you will come across statements such as "This rate is significantly different than that rate." This refers to *statistical significance*, which means that differences found among groups are not likely to have occurred by chance. For example, consider a board game that uses two dice to determine how many spaces a player moves. Everyone rolls two sixes once in a while, but if on *every* turn one player rolls a double six, you will suspect the person's consistency is not just a matter of chance; you will look for a logical explanation—namely, that the person is cheating. So when we say that the difference between two things is statistically significant, we mean that we believe the difference cannot be attributed to chance—that there is a logical explanation for the difference.

Screening

Another concept important in population health is screening. Screening is a simple test usually performed to identify those in a population who have or are likely to develop a specified disease. For instance, newborn screening is

TABLE 1-9 Validity of Disease Screening

	Person Has Disease	Person Does Not Have Disease
Screening results are positive	True positive	False positive
Screening results are negative	False negative	True negative

the practice of testing every newborn for specific harmful or potentially fatal diseases that are not otherwise apparent at birth. When you are young and healthy, fewer screening tests are needed. As you age, however, screening tests are used more frequently. Common examples of screening tests are blood pressure measurements, cholesterol checks through blood analysis, diabetes screening, mammograms to screen for breast cancer, and Pap tests to screen for cervical cancer.

Sometimes, results of a screening can tell the healthcare professional if you are at low, medium, or high risk of developing a disease, but the results of other screening tests can be only positive or negative. An ideal screening test will identify everyone correctly. That is, people who have the disease will test positively on the screening test, and those who do not have the disease will test negatively on the screening test. In reality, though, the tests are not always 100% correct. Many factors affect whether a screening test is positive or negative, including the stage of the disease, the care with which the test was conducted, and medications a person is taking.

Screening is necessary for serious diseases like cervical cancer. Treatment often is both more effective and less invasive when disease identification occurs early. A good screening test is inexpensive, easy to administer, produces minimal discomfort for the patient, is reliable (provides consistent results), and is valid (distinguishes between people with a disease and those who are disease-free) (**TABLE 1-9**).

If you have a screening test that was positive, then your healthcare provider will perform a diagnostic test to determine if you have the disease. If it is a serious disease such as cancer, the **cutoff value** for a positive test is set low, because it is better to declare a test positive when the person does not have cancer than to declare a test negative when he or she does.

cutoff value The level at which the result of a diagnostic test is determined to be positive or negative.

Inequities

Inequity can generally be defined as a lack of fairness. The inequalities that we will discuss have much to do with existing sociocultural inequities, and you will see how they have an enormous impact on the population's health.

Everyone wants to be healthy. People who are poor may take good care of themselves but live in an environment that is bad for them. The environment in which people live can have an enormous impact on their health. Exposure to mold, pests such as rats and cockroaches, and poor air quality can raise the risk for diseases. Chronic stress and discrimination also affect a person's health. It is neither a coincidence nor surprising that people living in such environments and under such conditions have more health issues than do those who live in better conditions.

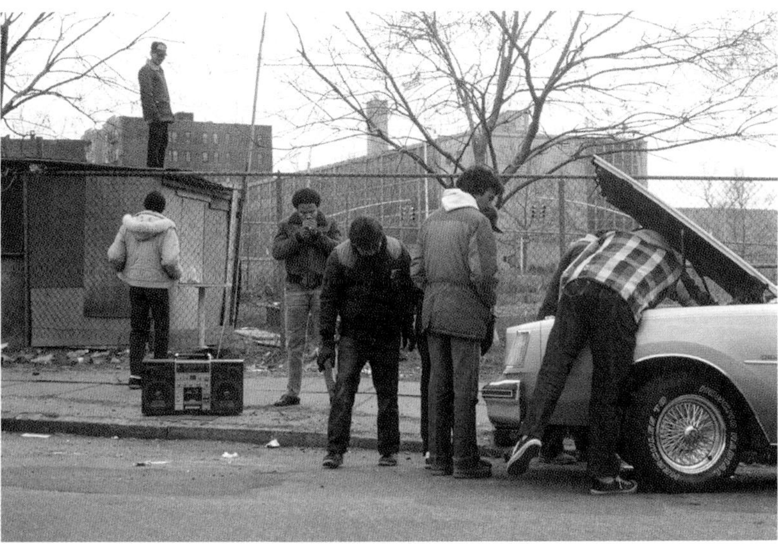

South Bronx, New York City.

According to the U.S. Census Bureau data, the 50 largest cities have significant income gaps between the rich and the poor. In 2015, the poorest cities in the United States were Louisville, Boston, Indianapolis, El Paso, Fresno, Baltimore, Tucson, Philadelphia, Memphis, Detroit, and Milwaukee. The causes for the poverty include high unemployment rate, lack of economic diversity, a relatively uneducated population, and poor-paying jobs (i.e., most available jobs pay minimum wages).[132] The poor neighborhoods in these and many other cities tend to be high in crime and air pollution and low in quality, affordable housing and services. They are the places in which people live when they cannot afford to live in healthier places. People end up in these neighborhoods when the resources and political power to make things better are absent. In disadvantaged neighborhoods, many residents have no choice but to be more concerned about everyday survival than what a nearby industry is doing. One of the results of these inequities is poor health. The disparities in health are due directly and indirectly to social, economic, cultural, and political inequities.[133]

In Summary

Every day you make choices that impact your health. Those choices are not made in a vacuum; they are influenced by the environment around you. Researchers have proposed theories of health behavior that attempt to explain how people make decisions about their health behaviors. These theories are helpful because public health practitioners want to understand how to help people make healthier choices.

This chapter introduces key concepts and terms fundamental to understanding health. The concept of health across the life span helps you understand that the choices you make, as well as the external environment around you, affect your health. The concept of race is a social, not biological, construct. The consequences of racism on health are devastating.

We also consider health determinants that are not always obvious. Where you live is important. It influences your sense of well-being, your health, your happiness, and other choices about your life. Furthermore, understanding what will make you happy is critical to living a healthy life.

Key Terms

built environment
cancer
congenital anomalies
cutoff value
discrimination
epidemiologists
focus groups
heart disease
incidence
population health
prevalence
race
racism
screening tests
randomized controlled trials
social determinants of health
sudden infant death syndrome (SIDS)

Student Discussion Questions and Activities

1. How would you define health? Why do you define it that way? How is your definition similar to, or different from, the definition given by the World Health Organization?
2. Consider the social-ecological model and how it explains the different factors that affect the choices a person makes. Give one example for each model level of an influence over your personal health decisions.
3. Compare the recommendations to protect yourself against heart disease and cancer. Many of these recommendations apply to your health in general. Which ones do you follow?
4. Think about where you grew up. It could be in a city, suburb, or town, or out in the country. (If you grew up out in the country, think about the nearest town.) Describe the neighborhoods—rich, poor, and in between—and how they differ.
5. Think about the Moving to Opportunity experiment. Do we as a society have an obligation to help others? Do you think the Moving to Opportunity plan should be implemented throughout the country?
6. Consider what makes you happy. Do you think being rich would make you happy?

References

1. World Health Organization. (n.d.). Preamble to the constitution of the World Health Organization as adopted by the International Health Conference, New York, 19–22 June, 1946; signed on 22 July 1946 by the representatives of 61 states (official records of the World Health Organization, no. 2, p. 100) and entered into force on 7 April 1948. Retrieved from http://www.who.int/about/definition/en/print.html
2. Sartorius, N. (2006). The meanings of health and its promotion. *Croatian Medical Journal, 47*(4), 662–664.
3. Johnson, N. B., Hayes, L. D., Brown, K., Hoo, E. C., Ethier, K. A., & Centers for Disease Control and Prevention. (2014). CDC national health report: Leading causes of morbidity and mortality and associated behavioral risk and protective factors—United States, 2005–2013. *Morbidity and Mortality Weekly Report, 63*(4), 3–27.
4. Stulberg, B. (2014). The key to changing individual behavior: Change the environment that gives rise to them. *Harvard Public Health Reviews, 2.*
5. Read, D., & van Leeuwen, B. (1998). Predicting hunger: The effects of appetite and delay on choice. *Organizational Behavior and Human Decision Processes, 76*(2), 189–205.
6. Mishra, A., Mishra, H., & Masters, T. M. (2012). The influence of bite size on quantity of food consumed: A field study. *Journal of Consumer Research, 38*(5), 791–795.
7. Van Ittersum, K., & Wansink, B. (2012). Plate size and color suggestibility: The Delboeuf illusion's bias on serving and eating behavior. *Journal of Consumer Research, 39*(2), 215–228.
8. Organdonor.gov. (2015). The need is real: Data. Retrieved from http://www.organdonor.gov/about/data.html
9. U.S. Department of Health and Human Services. (2013, September). 2012 National Survey of Organ Donation Attitudes and Behaviors. Retrieved from http://www.organdonor.gov/dtcp/nationalsurveyorgandonation.pdf
10. Johnson, E. J., & Goldstein, D. (2003). Medicine: Do defaults save lives? *Science, 302*(5649), 1338–1339.
11. Rao, M., Afshin, A., Singh, G., & Mozaffarian, D. (2013). Do healthier foods and diet patterns cost more than less healthy options? A systematic review and meta-analysis. *BMJ Open, 3*(12), e004277–004277.
12. Turner, L., & Chaloupka, F. J. (2014). Perceived reactions of elementary school students to changes in school lunches after implementation of the United States Department of

Agriculture's new meals standards: Minimal backlash, but rural and socioeconomic disparities exist. *Childhood Obesity, 10*(4), 349–356.

13. Turner, L., Ohri-Vachaspati, P., Powell, L., & Chaloupka, F. J. (2016). Improvements and disparities in types of foods and milk beverages offered in elementary school lunches, 2006–2007 to 2013–2014. *Preventing Chronic Disease, 13*, E39.
14. Murray, R., Ramstetter, C., & Council on School Health, American Academy of Pediatrics. (2013). The crucial role of recess in school. *Pediatrics, 131*(1), 183–188.
15. Centers for Disease Control and Prevention. (2011). Strategies to prevent obesity and other chronic diseases: The CDC guide to strategies to increase physical activity in the community. Retrieved from http://www.cdc.gov/obesity/downloads/PA_2011_WEB.pdf
16. McLeroy, K. R., Bibeau, D., Steckler, A., & Glanz, K. (1988). An ecological perspective on health promotion programs. *Health Education Quarterly, 15*(4), 351–377.
17. Israel, B. A., Schulz, A. J., Parker, E. A., Becker, A. B., Allen, A. J., & Guzman, J. R. (2003). Critical issues in developing and following community based participatory research principles. In M. Minkler & N. Wallerstein (Eds.), *Community-based participatory research for health* (pp. 53–76). San Francisco, CA: Jossey-Bass.
18. Sallis, J. F., Owen, N., & Fisher, E. B. (2008). Ecological models of health behavior. In M. Minkler, B. K. Rimer, & K. Viswanath K (Eds.), *Health behavior and health education* (4th ed., pp. 465–485). San Francisco, CA: John Wiley & Sons.
19. Wallerstein, N., & Duran, B. (2003). The conceptual, historical and practice roots of community-based participatory research and related participatory traditions. In M. Minkler & N. Wallerstein (Eds.), *Community-based participatory research for health* (pp. 27–52). San Francisco, CA: Jossey-Bass.
20. Lemacks, J., Wells, B. A., Ilich, J. Z., & Ralston, P. A. (2013). Interventions for improving nutrition and physical activity behaviors in adult African American populations: A systematic review, January 2000 through December 2011. *Preventing Chronic Disease, 10*, E99.
21. Centers for Disease Control and Prevention. (2015). Social ecological model—colorectal cancer control program. Retrieved from http://www.cdc.gov/cancer/crccp/sem.htm
22. Centers for Disease Control and Prevention. (2015). The social-ecological model: A framework for violence prevention. Retrieved from http://www.cdc.gov/ViolencePrevention/pdf/SEM_Framewrk-a.pdf
23. Chang, J., Guy, M. C., Rosales, C., Zapien, J. G., Staten, L. K., Fernandez, M. L., & Carvajal, S. C. (2013). Investigating social ecological contributors to diabetes within Hispanics in an underserved U.S.–Mexico border community. *International Journal of Environmental Research and Public Health, 10*(8), 3217–3232.
24. Balcazar, H., Wise, S., Rosenthal, E. L., Ochoa, C., Rodriguez, J., Hastings, D., . . . Flores, L. (2012). An ecological model using promotores de salud to prevent cardiovascular disease on the U.S.-Mexico border: The HEART project. *Preventing Chronic Disease, 9*, E35.
25. Willie, T. C., Powell, A., & Kershaw, T. (2016). Stress in the city: Influence of urban social stress and violence on pregnancy and postpartum quality of life among adolescent and young mothers. *Journal of Urban Health, 93*(1), 19–35.
26. Glanz, K., Rimer, B. K., & Lewis, F. M. (2002). *Health behavior and health education: Theory, research and practice.* San Francisco, CA: Wiley & Sons.
27. Hochbaum, G. M. (1958). *Public participation in medical screening programs: A socio-psychological study*. Public Health Service Publication No. 572. Washington, DC: Public Health Service.
28. Schnall, R., Rojas, M., & Travers, J. (2015). Understanding HIV testing behaviors of minority adolescents: A health behavior model analysis. *Journal of the Association of Nurses in AIDS Care, 26*(3):246–258.
29. Fishbein, M., & Azjen, I. (1975). *Belief, attitude, intention and behavior: An introduction to theory and research.* Reading, MA: Addison-Wesley.
30. Azjen, I., & Fishbein, M. (1980). *Understanding attitudes and predicting social behavior.* Englewood Cliffs, NJ: Prentice Hall.
31. Richardson, B. K., Wang, Z., & Hall, C. A. (2012). Blowing the whistle against Greek hazing: The theory of reasoned action as a framework for reporting intentions. *Communication Studies, 63*(2), 172–193.
32. Ajzen, I. (1985). From intentions to actions: A theory of planned behavior. In J. Kuhl & J. Beckmann (Eds.), *Action control: From cognition to behavior* (pp. 11–39). New York, NY: Springer-Verlag.
33. Bazargan-Hejazi, S., Teruya, S., Pan, D., Lin, J., Gordon, D., Krochalk, P. C., & Bazargan, M. (2016). The theory of planned behavior (TPB) and texting while driving behavior in college students. *Traffic Injury Prevention, 18*, 1–7.
34. Bandura, A. (1977). *Social learning theory*. Englewood Cliffs, NJ: Prentice Hall.
35. Bandura, A. (1986). *Social foundations of thought and action: A social-cognitive theory*. Englewood Cliffs, NJ: Prentice Hall.
36. Sleath, B., Carpenter, D. M., Lee, C., Loughlin, C. E., Etheridge, D., Rivera-Duchesne, L., . . . Tudor, G. (2016). The development of an educational video to motivate teens with asthma to be more involved during medical visits and to improve medication adherence. *Journal of Asthma*, 1–6.
37. Prochaska, J. O., & DiClemente, C. C. (1983). Stages and processes of self-change of smoking: Toward an integrative model of change. *Journal of Consulting and Clinical Psychology, 51*(3), 390–395.
38. Prochaska, J. O., DiClemente, C. C., & Norcross, J. C. (1992). In search of how people change: Applications to addictive behaviors. *American Psychologist, 47*(9), 1102–1114.
39. Janis, I. L., & Mann, L. (1977). Emergency decision making: A theoretical analysis of responses to disaster warnings. *Journal of Human Stress, 3*(2), 35–45.
40. Weiss, J., Okun, M., & Quay, N. (2004). Predicting bicycle helmet stage-of-change among middle school, high school, and college cyclists from demographic, cognitive, and motivational variables. *Journal of Pediatrics, 145*(3), 360–364.
41. World Health Organization. (2016). Under-five mortality. Retrieved from http://www.who.int/gho/child_health/mortality/mortality_under_five_text/en/
42. World Health Organization. (1998). World health report 1998—Life in the 21st century: A vision for all. Retrieved from http://www.who.int/whr/1998/en/
43. Centers for Disease Control and Prevention. (2016). Ten leading causes of death and injury. Retrieved from http://www.cdc.gov/injury/wisqars/leadingcauses.html
44. World Health Organization. (2016). Children: Reducing mortality. Retrieved from http://www.who.int/mediacentre/factsheets/fs178/en/
45. Centers for Disease Control and Prevention. (2018). About teen pregnancy. Retrieved from http://www.cdc.gov/teenpregnancy/about/

46. Hotz, V. J, McElroy, S. W., & Sanders, S. G. (1997). The impacts of teenage childbearing on the mothers and the consequences of those impacts for government. In R. Maynard (Ed.), *Kids having kids: The economic costs and social consequences of teen pregnancy* (pp. 55–94). Washington, DC: Urban Institute Press.
47. World Health Organization. (2014). The top 10 causes of death. Retrieved from http://www.who.int/mediacentre/factsheets/fs310/en/
48. National Heart, Lung, and Blood Institute. (2016). How can coronary heart disease be prevented or delayed? Retrieved from http://www.nhlbi.nih.gov/health/health-topics/topics/cad/prevention
49. National Cancer Institute. (2015). What is cancer? Retrieved from http://www.cancer.gov/about-cancer/understanding/what-is-cancer
50. National Cancer Institute. (2016). Cancer statistics. Retrieved from http://www.cancer.gov/about-cancer/understanding/statistics
51. Mayo Clinic. (2015). Cancer prevention: 7 tips to reduce your risk. Retrieved from http://www.mayoclinic.org/healthy-lifestyle/adult-health/in-depth/cancer-prevention/art-20044816
52. National Institute on Alcohol Abuse and Alcoholism. (2015). Drinking levels defined. Retrieved from https://www.niaaa.nih.gov/alcohol-health/overview-alcohol-consumption/moderate-binge-drinking
53. National Institute on Alcohol Abuse and Alcoholism. (n.d.). What is a standard drink? Retrieved from https://www.niaaa.nih.gov/alcohol-health/overview-alcohol-consumption/what-standard-drink
54. World Health Organization. (2016). Social determinants of health. Retrieved from http://www.who.int/social_determinants/en/
55. Marmot, M., & Allen, J. J. (2014). Social determinants of health equity. *American Journal of Public Health, 104*(suppl 4), S517–S519.
56. Clay, R. A. (2001). Wealth secures health. American Psychological Association. Retrieved from www.apa.org/monitor/oct01/wealthhealth.aspx
57. Mendes, E. (2010, October 18). In U.S., health disparities across incomes are wide-ranging. Gallup. Retrieved from http://www.gallup.com/poll/143696/Health-Disparities-Across-Incomes-Wide-Ranging.aspx
58. BloodBook.com. (n.d.). Racial and ethnic distribution of ABO blood types. Retrieved from http://www.bloodbook.com/world-abo.html
59. Zack, N. (2002). *Philosophy of science and race*. New York, NY: Routledge.
60. Khan, R. (2009, May 14). Skin color is not race: Gene expression. *Discover*. Retrieved from http://blogs.discovermagazine.com/gnxp/2009/05/skin-color-is-not-race/#.V_zvleArKVM
61. RACE. (2016). Only skin deep. Retrieved from http://www.understandingrace.org/humvar/skin_01.html
62. Ali-Khan, S. E., Krakowski, T., Tahir, R., & Daar, A. S. (2011). The use of race, ethnicity and ancestry in human genetic research. *HUGO Journal, 5*(1), 47–63.
63. Jorde, L. B., & Wooding, S. P. (2004). Genetic variation, classification and "race." *Nature Genetics, 36*(11 suppl), S28–S33.
64. Bamshad, M., & Guthery, S. L. (2007). Race, genetics and medicine: Does the color of a leopard's spots matter? *Current Opinion in Pediatrics, 19*(6):613–618.
65. Goodman, A. H., Moses, Y. T., & Jones, J. L. (2012). *Race: Are we so different?* Hoboken, NJ: Wiley-Blackwell.
66. Public Broadcast System. (2003). What is race? The race quiz. *RACE—The power of an illusion* [Documentary]. Retrieved from http://www.whatsrace.org/images/racequiz.pdf
67. Smithsonian Institution. (2016). Human skin color variation. The Smithsonian Institution's Human Origins Program. Retrieved from http://humanorigins.si.edu/evidence/genetics/human-skin-color-variation/modern-human-diversity-skin-color
68. Fletcher, M. A. (2014, December 12). White people have 13 dollars for every dollar held by Black Americans. *The Washington Post*. Retrieved from https://www.washingtonpost.com/news/get-there/wp/2014/12/12/white-people-have-13-dollars-for-every-dollar-held-by-black-americans/
69. Economic Policy Institute. (2011). The state of working America: mobility. Retrieved from http://www.stateofworkingamerica.org/fact-sheets/mobility/
70. Wilkinson, R. G., & Pickett, K. (2010). *The spirit level: Why greater equality makes societies stronger*. New York: Bloomsbury Press.
71. Mazumder, B. (May 2008). Upward Intergenerational Economic Mobility in the United States. Economic Mobility Project. Philadelphia, PA. Pew Charitable Trust Retrieved from http://www.pewtrusts.org/~/media/legacy/uploadedfiles/pcs_assets/2012/empreportsupward20intergen20mobility2008530pdf.pdf
72. Johnston, D. C. (2010). Scary new wage data. (p. 481-484) Retrieved from http://taxprof.typepad.com/files/129tn0481.pdf
73. Piketty, T. & Saez, E. 2007. Income and wage inequality in the United States, 1913–2002. In A. B. Atkinson & T. Piketty (Eds.), *Top Incomes over the 20th century* (pp. 141–225). Oxford: Oxford University Press.
74. Harriot, M. (2017). White men can't murder: Why white cops are immune to the law. *The Root*. Retrieved from http://www.theroot.com/white-men-cant-murder-why-white-cops-are-immune-to-the-1796309966
75. American Public Health Association. (1998). American public health association. Impact of police violence on public health. Retrieved from http://www.apha.org/policies-and-advocacy/public-health-policy-statements/policy-database/2014/07/11/14/16/impact-of-police-violence-on-public-health
76. Phelan, J. C., Link, B. G., & Tehranifar, P. (2010). Social conditions as fundamental causes of health inequalities: Theory, evidence, and policy implications. *Journal of Health and Social Behavior, 51*(Suppl), S28–S40.
77. Jee-Lyn Garcia, J., & Sharif, M. Z. (2015). Black lives matter: A commentary on racism and public health. *American Journal of Public Health, 105*(8), e27–e30.
78. Olshansky, S. J., Antonucci, T., Berkman, L., Binstock, R. H., Boersch-Supan, A., Cacioppo, J. T., . . . Rowe, J. (2012). Differences in life expectancy due to race and educational differences are widening, and many may not catch up. *Health Affairs (Millwood), 31*(8), 1803–1813.
79. Nuru-Jeter, A., Dominguez, T. P., Hammond, W. P., Leu, J., Skaff, M., Egerter, S., Jones, C. P., & Braveman, P. (2009). "It's the skin you're in": African-American women talk about their experiences of racism. An exploratory study to develop measures of racism for birth outcome studies. *Maternal and Child Health Journal, 13*(1), 29–39.

80. Jones, C. P. (2000). Levels of racism: A theoretic framework and a gardener's tale. *American Journal of Public Health, 90*(8), 1212–1215.
81. Sanders-Phillips, K., Settles-Reaves, B., Walker, D., & Brownlow, J. (2009). Social inequality and racial discrimination: Risk factors for health disparities in children of color. *Pediatrics, 124*(Suppl 3), S176–S186.
82. Hudson, D. L., Puterman, E., Bibbins-Domingo, K., Matthews, K. A., & Adler. N. E. (2013). Race, life course socioeconomic position, racial discrimination, depressive symptoms and self-rated health. *Social Science and Medicine, 97*, 7–14.
83. Meyer, J. D. (2014). Race-based job discrimination, disparities in job control, and their joint effects on health. *American Journal of Industrial Medicine, 57*(5), 587–595.
84. Perreira, K. M., & Telles, E. E. (2014). The color of health: Skin color, ethnoracial classification, and discrimination in the health of Latin Americans. *Social Science and Medicine, 116*, 241–250.
85. Garcia, J. A., Sanchez, G. R., Sanchez-Youngman, S., Vargas, E. D., & Ybarra, V. D. (2015). Race as lived experience: The impact of multi-dimensional measures of race/ethnicity on the self-reported health status of Latinos. *Du Bois Review, 12*(2), 349–373.
86. Monk, E. P., Jr. (2015). The cost of color: Skin color, discrimination, and health among African-Americans. *American Journal of Sociology, 121*(2), 396–444.
87. Bleser, W. K., Miranda, P. Y., & Jean-Jacques, M. (2016). Racial/ethnic disparities in influenza vaccination of chronically ill U.S. adults: The mediating role of perceived discrimination in health care. *Medical Care, 54*(6), 570–577.
88. Carliner, H., Delker, E., Fink, D. S., Keyes, K. M., & Hasin, D. S. (2016). Racial discrimination, socioeconomic position, and illicit drug use among U.S. Blacks. *Social Psychiatry and Psychiatric Epidemiology, 51*(4), 551–560.
89. Cuevas, A. G., O'Brien, K., & Saha, S. (2016). African American experiences in healthcare: "I always feel like I'm getting skipped over." *Health Psychology, 35*(9), 987–995.
90. Mukherjee, S., Trepka, M. J., Pierre-Victor, D., Bahelah, R., & Avent, T. (2016). Racial/ethnic disparities in antenatal depression in the United States: A systematic review. *Maternal and Child Health Journal, 20*(9), 1780–1797.
91. Walker, R. J., Strom Williams, J., & Egede, L. E. (2016). Influence of race, ethnicity and social determinants of health on diabetes outcomes. *American Journal of Medical Sciences, 351*(4), 366–373.
92. Dalberg, J. E. E. (1899). *The history of freedom in antiquity*. New York, NY: Wembly Press.
93. Robinson, M. (2016). What is social justice? Department of Government and Justice Studies, Appalachian State University. Retrieved from http://gjs.appstate.edu/social-justice-and-human-rights/what-social-justice
94. Rowe, C. (2015). Race dramatically skews discipline, even in elementary school. *The Seattle Times*. Updated March 18, 2016. Retrieved from http://www.seattletimes.com/education-lab/race-dramatically-skews-discipline-even-in-elementary-school/
95. Vega, T. (2014). Schools' discipline for girls differs by race and hue. *The New York Times*. Retrieved from https://www.nytimes.com/2014/12/11/us/school-discipline-to-girls-differs-between-and-within-races.html?mcubz=0
96. Smith E.J., Harper, S.R. (2015). Disproportionate impact of K-12 school suspension and expulsion on Black students in Southern states. University of Pennsylvania Center for the Study of Race and Equity in Education. Retrieved from https://equity.gse.upenn.edu/sites/default/files/publications/Smith_Harper_Report.pdf
97. Rhodes, W., Kling, R., Luallen, J., & Dyous, M. A. (2015). Federal Sentencing Disparity: 2005–2012. Bureau of Justice Statistics. Retrieved from https://www.bjs.gov/content/pub/pdf/fsd0512.pdf
98. Rawls, J. (2005). *A theory of justice*. New York, NY: Oxford Paperbacks.
99. Gordon, M., Price, M. S., & Peralta, K. (2016, March 26). Understanding HB2: North Carolina's newest law solidifies state's role in defining discrimination. *The Charlotte Observer*. Retrieved from http://www.charlotteobserver.com/news/politics-government/article68401147.html
100. De Lise, D. (2015, December 22). Dining out: Sometimes you have to wonder. *Huffington Post*. Retrieved from http://www.huffingtonpost.com/derrick-de-lise/dining-out-sometimes-you-_b_8845756.html
101. Carlson, T. (2013, December 27). 6 instances of discrimination people with disabilities face every day. *Huffington Post*. Retrieved from http://www.huffingtonpost.com/tiffiny-carlson/discrimination-people-disabilities-_b_4509393.html
102. Pascoe, E. A., & Richman, L. S. (2009). Perceived discrimination and health: A meta-analytic review. *Psychological Bulletin, 135*(4), 531–554.
103. Florida, R. L. (2008). *Who's your city? How the creative economy is making where to live the most important decision of your life*. New York, NY: Basic Books.
104. Irwin, N., & Bui, Q. (2016, April 11). The rich live longer everywhere. For the poor, geography matters. *New York Times*. Retrieved from http://www.nytimes.com/interactive/2016/04/11/upshot/for-the-poor-geography-is-life-and -death.html?_r=0
105. Chetty, R., Stepner, M., Abraham, S., Lin, S., Scuderi, B., Turner, N., . . . Cutler, D. (2016). The association between income and life expectancy in the United States, 2001–2014. *JAMA, 315*(16), 1750–1766.
106. Aisch, G., Buth, E., Bloch, M., Cox, A., & Quealy, K. (2015, May 4). The best and worst places to grow up: How your area compares. *The New York Times*. Retrieved from http://www.nytimes.com/interactive/2015/05/03/upshot/the-best-and-worst-places-to-grow-up-how-your-area-compares.html
107. Masterson, E. A., Bushnell, P. T., Themann, C. L., & Morata, T. C. (2016). Hearing impairment among noise-exposed workers—United States, 2003–2012. *Morbidity and Mortality Weekly Report, 65*(15), 389–394.
108. Dzhambov, A. M., & Dimitrova, D. D. (2016). Exposures to road traffic, noise, and air pollution as risk factors for type 2 diabetes: A feasibility study in Bulgaria. *Noise Health, 18*(82), 133–142.
109. Khajenasiri, F., Zamanian, A., & Zamanian, Z. (2016). The effect of exposure to high noise levels on the performance and rate of error in manual activities. *Electronic Physician, 8*(3), 2088–2093.
110. Soundscore. (2016). HowLoud. Retrieved from http://howloud.com/soundscore/
111. Kiersz, A. (2014, July 20). Equality of Opportunity Project map. *Business Insider*. Retrieved from http://www.businessinsider.com/equality-of-opportunity-project-map-2014-7
112. Chetty, R., Hendren, N., & Katz, L. (2015). The effects of exposure to better neighborhoods on children: New evidence from the Moving to Opportunity experiment. Retrieved from http://www.nber.org/papers/w21156

113. Ludwig, J., Duncan, G. J., Gennetian, L. A., Katz, L., Kessler, R. C., Kling, J. R., & Sanbonmatsu, L. (2013). Long-term neighborhood effects on low-income families: Evidence from moving to opportunity. *American Economic Review P&P, 103*(3), 226–231.
114. Dfarhud, D., Malmir, M., & Khanahmadi, M. (2014). Happiness & health: The biological factors—systematic review article. *Iranian Journal of Public Health, 43*(11), 1468–1477.
115. Bartels, M., Saviouk, V., de Moor, M. H., Willemsen, G., van Beijsterveldt, T. C., Hottenga, J. J., . . . Boomsma, D. I. (2010). Heritability and genome-wide linkage scan of subjective happiness. *Twin Research and Human Genetics, 13*(2), 135–142.
116. Bartels, M. (2015). Genetics of wellbeing and its components satisfaction with life, happiness, and quality of life: A review and meta-analysis of heritability studies. *Behavior Genetics, 45*(2), 137–156.
117. De Neve, J., Christakis, N. A., Fowler, J. H., & Frey, B. S. (2012). Genes, economics, and happiness. CESifo Working Paper Series No. 2946.
118. Gatt, J. M., Burton, K. L., Schofield, P. R., Bryant, R. A., & Williams, L. M. (2014). The heritability of mental health and wellbeing defined using COMPAS-W, a new composite measure of wellbeing. *Psychiatry Research, 219*(1), 204–213.
119. Luscombe, B. (2010, September 6). Study: Money buys happiness when income is $75,000. *TIME*. Retrieved from http://content.time.com/time/magazine/article/0,9171,2019628,00.html
120. Carlson, N. (2013). Does being rich make you happy? *Business Insider*. Retrieved from http://www.businessinsider.com/does-being-rich-make-you-happy-2013-12
121. Molcho, M., Gabhainn, S. N., & Kelleher, C. C. (2007). Interpersonal relationships as predictors of positive health among Irish youth: the more the merrier? *Irish Medical Journal, 100*(8), 33-36.
122. Buist, E. (2015). Why tidying up could change your life. *The Guardian*. Retrieved from https://www.theguardian.com/lifeandstyle/2015/may/01/do-something-decluttering
123. Roberto, C. A., Swinburn, B., Hawkes, C., Huang, T., Costa, S., Ashe, M., . . . Brownwell, K. D. (2015). Patchy progress on obesity prevention: Emerging examples, entrenched barriers, and new thinking. *Lancet, 385*(9985), 2400–2409.
124. Ortega, F. B., Lee, D. C., Katzmarzyk, P. T., Ruiz, J. R., Sui, X., Church, T. S., & Blair, S. N. (2013). The intriguing metabolically healthy but obese phenotype: Cardiovascular prognosis and role of fitness. *European Heart Journal, 34*(5), 389–397.
125. DeSalvo, K. B., Bloser, N., Reynolds, K., He, J., & Muntner, P. (2006). Mortality prediction with a single general self-rated health question. A meta-analysis. *Journal of General Internal Medicine, 21*(3), 267–275.
126. Chang, J., Zhang, M., Hitchman, G., Qiu, J., & Liu, Y. (2014). When you smile, you become happy: Evidence from resting state task-based fMRI. *Biological Psychology, 103*, 100–106.
127. Seligman, M. E., & Csikszentmihalyi, M. (2000). Positive psychology. An introduction. *American Psychologist, 55*(1), 5–14.
128. Boehm, J. K., Winning, A., Segerstrom, S., & Kubzansky, L. D. (2015). Variability modifies life satisfaction's association with mortality risk in older adults. *Psychological Science, 26*(7), 1063–1070.
129. MacMahon, B., & Pugh, T. F. (1970). *Epidemiology: Principles and methods* (pp. 57–72). Boston, MA: Little, Brown and Company.
130. Primack, B. A., Sidani, J., Agarwal, A. A., Shadel, W. G., Donny, E. C., & Eissenberg, T. E. (2008). Prevalence of and associations with waterpipe tobacco smoking among U.S. university students. *Annals of Behavioral Medicine, 36*(1), 81–86.
131. Barton, S. (2000). Which clinical studies provide the best evidence? The best RCT still trumps the best observational study. *BMJ, 321*(7256), 255–256.
132. Kennedy, B. (2015, February 18). America's 11 poorest cities. *CBS News*. Retrieved from http://www.cbsnews.com/media/americas-11-poorest-cities/
133. Adelson, N. (2005). The embodiment of inequity: Health disparities in Aboriginal Canada. *Canadian Journal of Public Health, 96*(suppl 2), S45–S61.

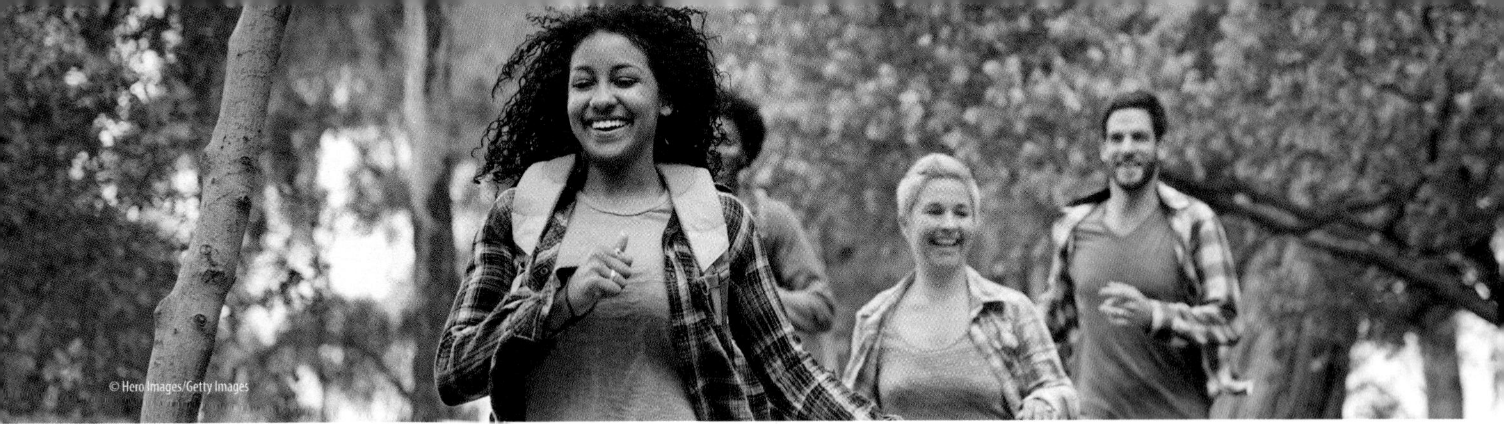
© Hero Images/Getty Images

CHAPTER 2

Starting With Food: Nutrition and Health

CHAPTER OBJECTIVES

- Convey the basic biological process of digestion and metabolism.
- Explain the roles and functions of macronutrients and micronutrients.
- Help develop skills for making healthier food decisions.
- Help develop a stronger understanding of the connection between social nutritional policies and population health outcomes.

You are what you eat. It is a centuries-old statement that remains true today for individuals, families, communities, and even nations.

What you put into your body affects your short-term and long-term energy levels, your mood, your physical performance, and even your long-term overall well-being. Your eating patterns can provide you with energy or sap energy from you. How your mind and body function is often a reaction to what you put into your body. This reaction also depends on your age, sex, weight, allergic disposition, past behaviors, and possibly even your mother's behavior before you were born.

The same is true for families and communities—collectively, we are what we eat. Research continues to discover differences in health outcomes among countries, regions, and even continents. The effects of **regional-level eating patterns** indicate that different cultures can have better overall health outcomes than others, due, in large part, to their diets. For example, the Mediterranean diet, high in vegetables and low in processed foods, seems to yield lower-than-average rates of chronic diseases and higher-than-average life expectancies.[1]

Different communities that are not far from each other can also see important differences in health outcomes. One neighborhood within a single city or town can have better outcomes compared to another only a quarter of a

regional-level eating patterns The diet typical to a given region. Studies of regional-level eating patterns indicate that some cultures can have better overall health outcomes than other cultures due, in large part, to their diets.

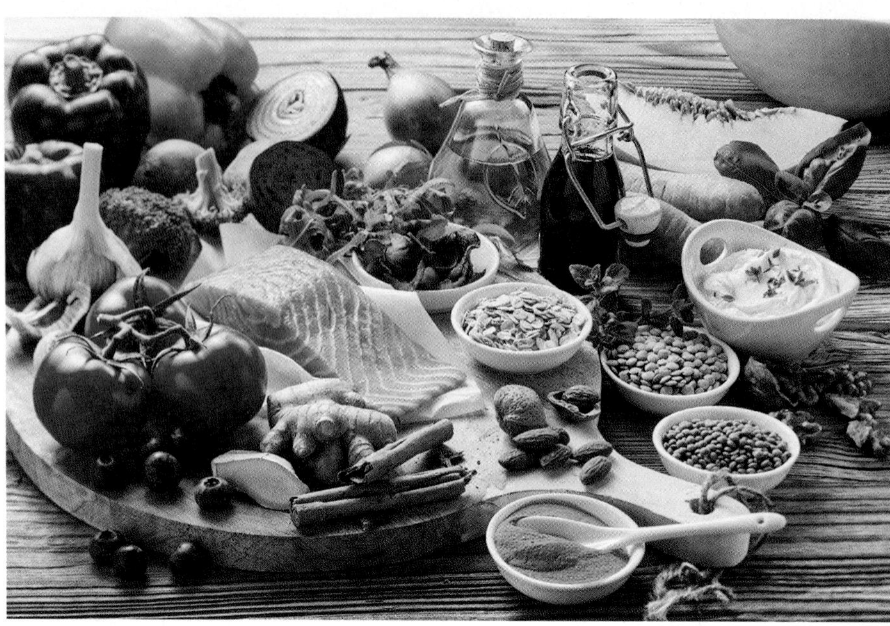

Diets high in vegetables, olive oils, and fish, and low in processed foods, are part of a "Mediterranean diet," shown to be associated with higher life expectancy.

mile away, or even just across a major street or train track. In many cases, these health differences arise from cultural, socioeconomic, and demographic factors, such as historical, institutional and racist policies, which may have led to the racial and ethnic health disparities that persist in that community. While each community has its own set of social and environmental factors that affect health disparities, these differences can be seen directly in **nutritional environments**. These environments—both healthy and unhealthy—in turn, affect diet-related population outcomes, including obesity, diabetes, heart disease, and cancer.

nutritional environments The environment where people purchase and eat food.

This chapter will discuss the basic science of nutrition and how we obtain energy, strength, and vitality through food. Because no person can achieve complete physical, mental, and social well-being in an otherwise unhealthy environment, the focus of the chapter will shift between the individual biological environment and the wider societal view. This will help us develop a more critical understanding of the important environmental and social factors that influence our personal nutritional choices and, consequently, our health.

TRY IT!

Pick two social settings—maybe two schools, two families, two neighborhoods, two different streets. Make five statements about which one of the two is healthier (i.e., smoking is more common in one, one population seems to be overweight, one seems to have higher levels of stress, etc.). Now, think about some factors that may be behind *why* the one seems to be healthier than the other. Does the healthier population have more or less average family income? Are there more fast-food places nearby? More parks? Does education play a role? Are there historical events (e.g., segregation) that may have shaped why these two places are different?

These kinds of observations can help us gain a better understanding about how the decisions we make as a society can help to ensure that everyone has access to the best nutritional environments possible.

Next, we will look at the social factors that influence our health over the course of our lives. There are important developmental periods for each of us, when nutritional choices are especially significant to our long-term health, and the health of our families and communities. The nutritional choices made by an average 58-year-old man are less impactful on long-term health than, for example, is the diet of a 2-year-old boy or an 11-year-old girl. What should that mean for the policies we establish?

Let's start with individual nutrition and consider how the food you eat turns to the energy that allows you to live and, hopefully, thrive.

Digestion and Absorption: What Happens When You Eat or Drink?

Early Stages of Digestion

Digestion begins the moment you put something in your mouth (**FIGURE 2-1**). The first stage, chewing, or mechanical digestion, is influenced by whether or not you have a healthy set of teeth. The health of your teeth will affect the kinds of foods you can eat and how well you break down solid foods. Oral health plays a role in nutritional status, just as sound nutrition is necessary to ensure healthy teeth. People deprived of adequate vitamin C and calcium early in life are, for example, more likely to develop unhealthy teeth as they grow older. Unhealthy teeth, in turn, will limit their ability to achieve nutritional balance over time, continuing the cycle throughout the life span.

For individuals and for populations, nutritional status affects teeth, and oral health affects nutritional status. Proper nutrition helps support healthy teeth, saliva, mucus, musculature, and enzymes that, in turn, help ensure healthy teeth, saliva, mucus, and digestive organs.

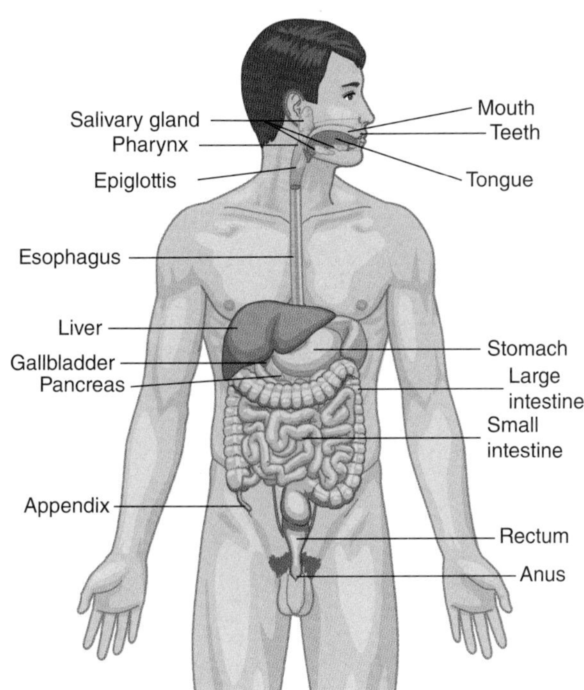

FIGURE 2-1 The digestive system.

JOIN THE ALLIANCE!

Tooth decay is the most common chronic childhood disease[1]

*More than **1 in 4 children** aged 2 to 5 years suffer from tooth decay[2]. When left untreated, tooth decay can significantly impact a child's current – and future – health, development and academic success.*

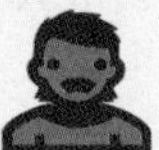

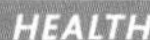

HEALTH

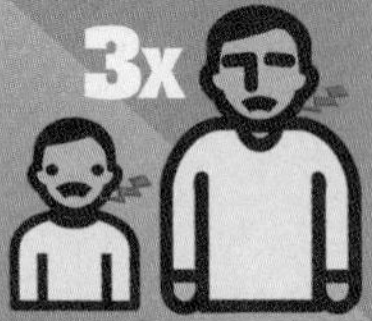

- *Children with early cavities in their primary teeth are nearly **3x more likely** to develop cavities in their adult teeth[3].*
- *In Canada, tooth decay accounts for one-third of all day surgeries performed on children between the ages of 1 and 5[4].*

DEVELOPMENT

- *Pain and infection caused by tooth decay can lead to problems with eating, speaking and learning[5].*
- *Rampant decay can adversely affect a child's quality of life, inhibit learning and social development and compromise self-esteem[6].*

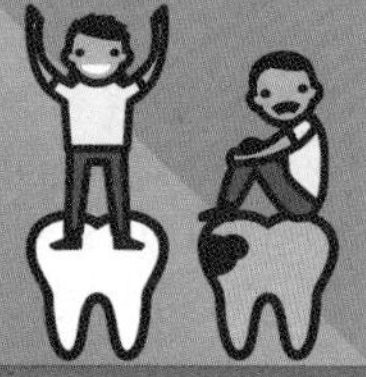

ACADEMIC SUCCESS

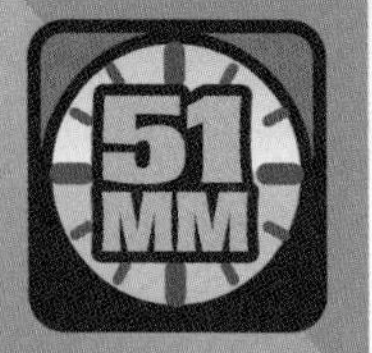

Oral health affects students' academic performance[7]. Tooth pain keeps many children home from school or distracted from learning:

- *More than **51 million hours** of school are lost each year in the U.S. due to dental problems[8].*
- *An estimated **2.26 million school days** are missed each year in Canada due to dental-related illness[9].*

PREVENTION

The best medicine is prevention

- ***First tooth, first dental visit**. Good oral health habits start early!*
- *Ensure children brush thoroughly twice a day with fluoride toothpaste.*

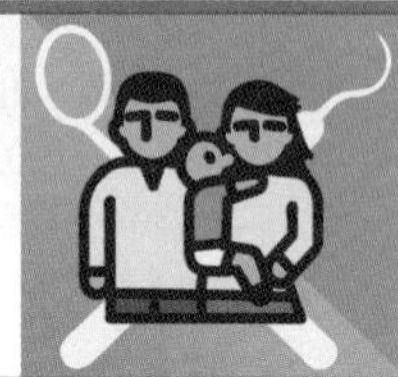

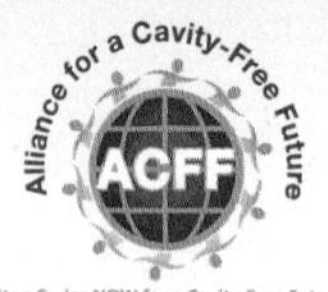

For more information visit us at www.AllianceForACavityFreeFuture.org or email us at admin@acffglobal.org

[1]American Academy of Pediatric Dentistry. Early Childhood Caries.
[2]National Children's Oral Health Foundation. Facts about decay.
[3]Research America! Children's Dental Health Research.
[4]Canadian Institute for Health Information. Treatment of Preventable Dental Cavities in Preschoolers: A Focus on Day Surgery Under General Anesthesia.
[5]National Children's Oral Health Foundation. Facts about decay.
[6]National Children's Oral Health Foundation. Facts about decay.
[7]Am J Public Health. The Impact of Oral Health on the Academic Performance of Disadvantaged Children.
[8]National Children's Oral Health Foundation. Facts about decay.
[9]National Children's Oral Health Foundation. Facts about decay.

The root of it all.

The body is an interconnected organism—every component affects everything else, and nothing is truly isolated. At a community and population level, the same is true. Our individual nutritional habits are inextricably connected to the places where we spend the most time and to the communities and cultures that influence us.[2]

During chewing, in addition to breaking food down mechanically, the mouth introduces salivary gland secretions and mucus, which break down foods for digestion and solubilize nutrients. Receptors transmit taste signals to your brain. Saliva also plays a role in oral hygiene, flushing away bacteria and releasing the enzymes that begin the process of digestion.

After foods are swallowed, they pass through a bundle of muscles within the esophagus called the upper esophageal sphincter, which secretes more mucus and keeps food from passing down your windpipe. The esophagus also warms the food to body temperature, which optimizes digestive efficiency.[3] The esophagus then channels food through the cardiac sphincter and into the stomach, which is where it is stored as food. The stomach's storage function allows you to eat a large meal and process the nutrients from that meal over the course of many hours.

The stomach is a powerful muscle that churns, grinds, and applies hydrochloric acid and enzymes to the food to prepare it for digestion. The digestion that takes place in the stomach is called the **predigestive process**. Acid destroys harmful bacteria and breaks down the food, while mucus protects the body's cells from the stomach acids. The chemical and enzymatic process converts foods into the fine liquid called chyme, which is released slowly into the intestine (also referred to as the gut), where the next phase of digestion occurs.

predigestive process The process by which the stomach churns, grinds, and applies hydrochloric acid and enzymes to ingested food to prepare it for digestion.

Through the Gut

The small intestine is a loosely coiled tube, approximately 20 feet long, held together by a fine membrane. It consists of three sections—the duodenum, the jejunum, and the ileum. Each has a different cellular and digestive function. The duodenum breaks down food, while the other two are responsible for absorbing nutrients into the bloodstream.

A wavelike motion of contractions moves food through the bowel and mixes it with digestive secretions. Along with the secretions from the pancreas, liver, and stomach, the intestinal wall also secretes important digestive enzymes. The enzymes accelerate, or catalyze, the breakdown of **macronutrients** and **micronutrients** during digestion (**FIGURE 2-2**).

Trillions of microscopic organisms live in our gut, and have an enormous influence on our health.[4] These bacteria, which form the body's **microbiome**, produce vitamins from our food, fight disease, and control our weight.[5] These microorganisms have been associated with improving our immune system and our mood and mental health.[6,7] Although research in this area is still relatively recent, scientists are beginning to discover that a diet rich in vegetables and fiber can encourage healthy function of our microbiome and consequently protect us from numerous diseases. A "probiotic" nutrition program encourages

macronutrients Carbohydrates, proteins, and fats that serve as the primary components of a healthy diet.

micronutrients Nutrients, mostly vitamins and minerals, that are essential for optimal health, although only in miniscule amounts. Micronutrients are important for the normal functioning of the body and enable many of the important chemical reactions that promote good health.

microbiome The environment created by the trillions of microscopic organisms living in our gut, which have an enormous influence on our health. They have been found to produce vitamins from our food, fight disease, and control our weight.

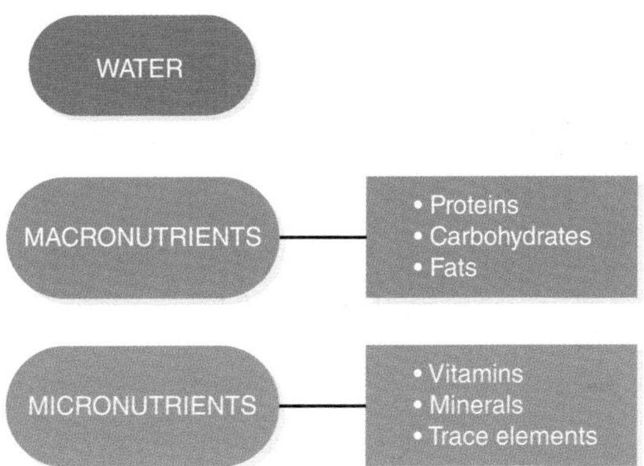

FIGURE 2-2 Macronutrients and micronutrients.

diets that promote a thriving microbiome. Early research indicates that foods such as kimchi, sauerkraut, kefir, and probiotic yogurts may encourage gut bacteria and lead to healthier immune systems, reduced weight gain, and possibly even reduced depression.[8–10]

Breaking Down and Building Up: The Metabolic Process

You have likely heard people referring to their metabolism and whether it is "fast" or "slow." Metabolism is the process the body uses to generate energy and maintain life. Metabolism consists of two fundamental stages. Catabolism is the phase that breaks down nutrients, creating energy through the process of cellular respiration. Anabolism is the constructive phase, where energy builds the proteins, nucleic acids, and cells that make up our body. Your body is metabolizing nutrients continuously. Your rate of metabolism depends on both the amount of exercise you get, and your age, sex, body size, and genetics.[11]

The amount of energy from food is measured in calories. Technically, the calorie we use for food energy is a "kilocalorie," based on 1,000 "small calories" from a measuring system rarely seen today. This is why you will sometimes see the food calorie symbolized as the "kcal." The more calories a meal has, the more energy you can spend—or store as fat.

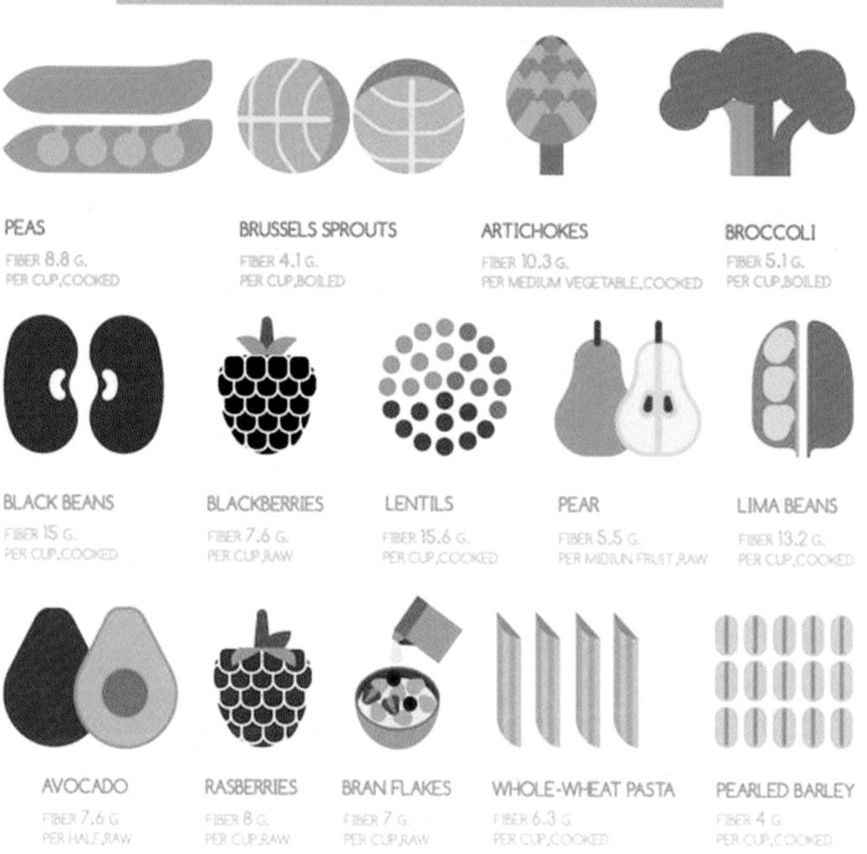

The current guidelines offered by the USDA Center for Nutrition Policy and Promotion offer a similar perspective on nutritional recommendations for Americans.

Courtesy of U.S. Department of Health and Human Services.

Into the Colon and Then Out

During the last part of the digestive process, the remaining components of the foods that were eaten but were not used for nutrition enter the large intestine, or colon. This is where water is absorbed from the remaining nondigestible waste to form feces, before being expelled via defecation.

Macronutrients and Other Key Components of Nutrition

Carbohydrates

Carbohydrates (also called "carbs") consist of carbon, hydrogen, and oxygen atoms (hence the term *carbo* + *hydrate*). Produced from the sun's energy, carbohydrates hold the energy found in fruits, grains, and plants, and serve as fuel for body and brain function. Carbohydrates are classified by the number of sugar units contained in each molecule. Most carbohydrates are either monosaccharides, containing 1 unit; disaccharides, containing 2 units; or polysaccharides, containing 10 or more units. Carbohydrates are sometimes classified as "simple" (monosaccharides and disaccharides) and "complex" (polysaccharides). **Complex carbohydrates** comprise a long chain of three or more sugars linked together, while carbohydrates in smaller pieces (one or two sugars) are referred to as "simple carbohydrates." Complex carbs, which generally contain more vitamins than simple carbs, include beans, peas, lentils, brown rice, and oatmeal. Simple carbs include sugar, white bread, and white rice. The body tends to digest and absorb **simple carbohydrates** more quickly than complex ones, which partially explains why simple carbs are more likely than complex carbs to end up stored in your body as fat.[12]

complex carbohydrates Sometimes referred to as "good" carbohydrates because they provide useful nutrients to the body, as compared to simple ("bad") carbohydrates, which are more easily converted to fat.

simple carbohydrates Sometimes referred to as "bad" carbohydrates because they are more easily converted to fat, as compared to complex ("good") carbohydrates, which provide useful nutrients to the body.

When you eat more carbohydrates than your body needs, the excess carbohydrates are converted into the compound glycogen, which the body stores in the liver and muscle tissues. Glycogen remains as a potential future source of energy and is stored as fat if not used during physical activity. While the time it takes for glycogen to be converted into fat varies from person to person, eating too much sugar or starch is an easy way to gain body fat.

Glycemic Index and Glycemic Load

While there is no simple way to evaluate the healthfulness of different types of carbohydrate, there are some useful ways to understand them. While "complexity" can be helpful, this classification can be deceiving, since some complex carbohydrates can cause greater blood sugar surges than less complex carbs. A measure called the **glycemic index** provides an indication of how powerfully foods affect blood sugar (glucose). Pure sugar has a glycemic index of 100 and raises a person's blood glucose level at the fastest rate possible. At the other end of the spectrum, carrots and peanuts are more slowly metabolized and cause a slower rise in blood glucose. Meat does not have a glycemic index because it contains no sugar and so does not increase blood glucose.

glycemic index A system that ranks food from 1 to 100 to indicate the food's effect on blood sugar (glucose) levels.

The glycemic index only provides information about the type of carbohydrate without providing information about how carbohydrate-heavy a food can be. Glycemic load, by contrast, classifies carbohydrates according to their impact on the body's blood sugar levels. For example, watermelons have a high

TABLE 2-1 Glycemic Index (GI)/Glycemic Load (GL) for Typical Serving Size (grams) for Common Foods

	Low GI	Medium GI	High GI
Low GL	Apple (120 g) (6/38) Carrot (80 g) (3/47) Peanuts (50 g) (0/7) Strawberries (30 g) (1/40) Hummus (30 g) (0/6)	Beets (60 g) (5/64) Cantaloupe (120 g) (4/65) Pineapple (120 g) (6/66)	Popcorn (20 g) (8/72) Watermelon (120 g) (4/72) Whole-wheat bread (30 g) (9/71)
Medium GL	Banana (12/52) Orange juice (8 oz) (12/50) Corn tortilla (12/52)	Boiled new potatoes (120 g) (12/57) Wild rice (120 g) (18/57)	Cheerios (30 g) (15/74) Shredded wheat (30 g) (15/75)
High GL	Macaroni (120 g) (23/47) Spaghetti (120 g) (20/42)	Couscous (120 g) (23/65) White rice (120 g) (23/64)	Baked potato (28/85) Cornflakes (120 g) (21/81)

Data from International tables of glycemic index (GI) and glycemic load (GL) values: 2008. (2008). *Diabetes Care, 32*(12), 2218–2283.

glycemic index because the type of carbohydrate is simple. However, the food itself is mostly water, so the glycemic load of watermelon is relatively low. In general, foods with a low glycemic index are healthy options, because they contain water, vitamins, and fiber in addition to the carbohydrate. Glycemic load, however, can provide more information about the readiness of carbs to be converted to blood sugar (and, if not counterbalanced with exercise, into fat). The lower the load, the better (**TABLE 2-1**).

While simple carbohydrates (monosaccharides) do not require further breakdown, enzymes (which usually end in "-ase") accelerate chemical reactions and break down foods for energy. Carbohydrates with fewer sugar units are sweeter tasting, while the more complex carbohydrates, consisting of more complex varieties of sugar units, have a starchier flavor. Simple carbohydrates include sugar, honey, fruits, syrups, and juices, while complex carbohydrates include peas, wheat, corn, lettuce, and grains.

Insulin

All digestible simple sugars and starches eventually get converted to glucose in our body. Most types of cells use glucose as their main fuel source. After we eat sugars or starches, our blood glucose level rises, which is where insulin becomes involved.

Insulin is a hormone—a chemical serving as a messenger—that regulates function from one part of the body to another. Insulin is produced and secreted by the pancreas, and its role is to regulate the body to either use glucose for energy or store it for future energy use. Insulin controls the blood glucose level from getting too high (hyperglycemia) or too low (hypoglycemia). Hyperglycemia is particularly dangerous and results if the body does not produce enough insulin or if the insulin is not as effective as it should be.

type 2 diabetes Previously called adult-onset diabetes, a condition that occurs when the cells become resistant to insulin. Blood sugar levels rise, and the pancreas responds. When the pancreas can no longer keep up with the demand and becomes exhausted, it loses control over blood sugar regulation, resulting in the diabetic condition.

Type 2 diabetes (previously called adult-onset diabetes) occurs when the cells become resistant to insulin. The pancreas responds to this by producing more and more insulin. When the pancreas can no longer keep up with the demand, and becomes exhausted, it loses control over blood sugar regulation, resulting in the diabetic condition.[13] Long-term complications of diabetes include chronic kidney failure, damage to the eyes, and foot ulcers, which can lead to amputation.

Diabetes is a powerful example of what can result from preventable poor nutritional environments, in households and in communities. Nutritional choices have consequences for community health, chronic disease, and financial stress. Both affected individuals and communities struggle to pay the long-term healthcare costs of nutrition-related conditions such as diabetes.

Fiber

Fiber is the nondigestible complex carbohydrates found in plant materials. There are two types: soluble (which will dissolve in water) and insoluble (which will not). Cellulose is insoluble fiber, and it is found in parts of plants such as wheat husks, apple peels, and leafy vegetables. Soluble fiber is found inside an apple or pear, for instance, and is often used to bind foods together.

Even though you do not digest fiber, it is highly beneficial for many reasons. It helps regulate sugar metabolism, removes toxins, encourages the growth of healthful bacteria in the lower gut, and provides bulk and moisture in the large intestine. The regulation of sugar metabolism is critical, because when fiber is not present, the absorption of sugar occurs more quickly than nature intended, and that can lead to excess weight gain or, if unchecked, to diseases such as type 2 diabetes and heart disease.[14]

During most of human history, people consumed as much as 100 to 300 grams of fiber per day. However, because the oils in fiber can cause spoiling and reduce shelf life, processing methods were developed to remove fiber from foods. Removing fiber made it easier for manufacturers to store and ship their products. Because of the increase in processed foods consumed in the Western diet over the past several decades, roughly half of Americans do not get the daily amount of fiber recommended by the National Academy of Medicine: 25 grams per day for women and 38 grams per day for men.[15] Because of the important role fiber plays in lowering cholesterol, maintaining healthy weight, controlling blood sugar, and maintaining bowel health, many nutrition scientists believe that consuming enough fiber is one of the most important dietary changes we can make to improve our health.[16–18]

In healthier populations, governments and communities discourage unnecessary food processing and encourage more affordable access to vegetables and other foods naturally rich in fiber. For individuals, this can mean incorporating more fresh fruits, vegetables, and grains into their daily diet. For communities and governments, it means establishing policies such as zoning laws ensuring that healthy foods are accessible to children and families—in schools, parks, and other public environments.

Lipids

Lipids, or fats, are macronutrients that are a necessary component of a healthy diet. Lipids are not soluble in water or blood, and must be transported through structures called lipoproteins.

Fatty acids are the basic building block of lipids and represent the densest form of our dietary energy, providing approximately 9 kilocalories (kcal) per gram—compared to carbohydrates and proteins, which both provide around 4 kcal per gram.[19] Because calories from carbohydrates are quickly burned, your fat stores are a crucial component of an efficient and well-functioning bodily system.[20]

Essential fatty acids are found primarily in meats, dairy, nuts, seeds, olives, and avocados. They are metabolized to give us energy when we need it and when we are not getting enough from our diet. Fats are important in transporting micronutrients, such as the fat-soluble vitamins A, D, E, and K. Fats are an essential component of the cell membrane and internal fatty tissues, which protect the vital organs from trauma and insulate them from temperature change.[21] Fatty tissue also helps regulate overall body temperature.

Each fat molecule is made of one glycerol molecule and three fatty acid chains. These chains can be either saturated, monounsaturated, or polyunsaturated. Fats consisting of a molecular structure where carbon is saturated with hydrogen are called "saturated" fats. **Unsaturated fats** are categorized as monounsaturated or polyunsaturated, depending on the number of carbon bonds in the molecule. **Saturated fats** are solid at room temperature and are often simply referred to as "fats" (e.g., butter, Crisco), while unsaturated fats remain liquid at room temperature and are called "oils" (e.g., olive oil, canola oil). Most food items contain a mixture of both saturated and unsaturated fatty acids, which explains why there can be both liquid and solid fats present in meats and even nuts.

unsaturated fats Fats that remain liquid at room temperature, referred to as "oils."

saturated fats Dietary fats that are solid at room temperature and often referred to simply as "fat."

fatty acids Saturated or unsaturated carboxylic acids with an even number of carbon atoms.

Only two **fatty acids** are known to be essential for humans (meaning they are necessary to sustain life): alpha-linolenic acid (an omega-3 fatty acid) and linoleic acid (an omega-6 fatty acid). Omega-3 fatty acids are polyunsaturated fatty acids that support numerous functions, such as blood function, brain development, and protection against heart disease and stroke. New studies indicate a protective function for other conditions such as cancer, bowel disease, and other autoimmune diseases, including lupus and rheumatoid arthritis.[22] Among the most abundant sources of omega-3 fatty acids are soybean oil, flaxseed oil, walnuts, brussels sprouts, kale, spinach, salad greens, and fatty fish, such as salmon and tuna.

Omega-6 fatty acids are also essential polyunsaturated fatty acids that our bodies cannot make themselves. They have been found to lower levels of low-density lipoprotein (LDL) cholesterol (so-called "bad cholesterol"), reduce inflammation, and otherwise protect against heart disease. Common sources of omega-6 fatty acids include safflower, corn, cottonseed, and soybean oils.

After digestion, most of the fats are carried in the blood and metabolized through different processes, referred to as lipolysis, beta-oxidation, and ketosis. Lipolysis and beta-oxidation occur in the mitochondria, producing energy, carbon dioxide, and water. Ketone bodies are molecules that result from producing energy from fat, and they can be toxic when produced in amounts too high for the body to process. **Ketosis** occurs when the rate of formation of ketones by the liver is greater than the ability of tissues to oxidize them. It occurs during prolonged starvation and when large amounts of fat are eaten in the absence of carbohydrates. This process is often exploited through low-carbohydrate diets, and it can be dangerous if it deprives the body of important nutrients that promote healthy body function and brain activity.

ketosis A metabolic process involving raised ketone body levels; it may occur in people with diabetes or those who follow a low-carb diet.

Proteins

Along with carbohydrates and lipids, protein is an essential macronutrient for the human body. Proteins are the critical building blocks of muscle and cellular tissue, and a source of fuel for energy. As a fuel source, proteins are as efficient as carbohydrates, containing 4 kcal per gram, although not as efficient as lipids (9 kcal per gram). Proteins are complex molecules (polymer chains) that consist of amino acids linked together. They are constantly being broken down and replaced through the amino acids we consume in our foods.

Proteins maintain cell structure and are critical for the function and regulation of all of the body's tissues, particularly muscle tissue, which is composed mostly of protein. Proteins help metabolize fat and produce the satiety that tells us when to stop eating. They also work with insulin to regulate the release of carbohydrates into the bloodstream, playing an important role in energy release, weight regulation, and the prevention of sugar-related diseases such as diabetes.

There are 20 different amino acids. Nine of these are called "essential," because we require them through our diet. The other 12 are made by our bodies using the energy produced from the essential ones.[14] Nearly all sources of meats, fish, dairy, and eggs contain sufficient quantities of the nine essential amino acids to sustain life. These foods are termed *complete proteins*. For vegans and vegetarians, it is more of a challenge to consume the complete requirements of protein. Although most vegans and vegetarians are in no danger of protein deficiency, it is more difficult for some to consume adequate levels of the amino acids lysine, methionine, and tryptophan their body needs. Vegans and vegetarians should seek a diversified combination of grains and proteins, such as beans and rice, millet and beans, brown rice and sunflower seeds, peanut butter with whole-grain bread, or grains with leafy green vegetables.

The body makes protein from the amino acids consumed through diet, or from storage in muscle. This is why the U.S. Department of Agriculture (USDA) recommends that adults consume at least 50 grams of balanced protein daily (the World Health Organization recommends 1/3 gram of protein per pound of body weight) to provide adequate energy and maintain lean muscle.

One way of classifying protein foods is according to the efficiency with which the body digests them and metabolizes them into energy. This measurement has been called the net protein utilization (NPU), or the ratio of

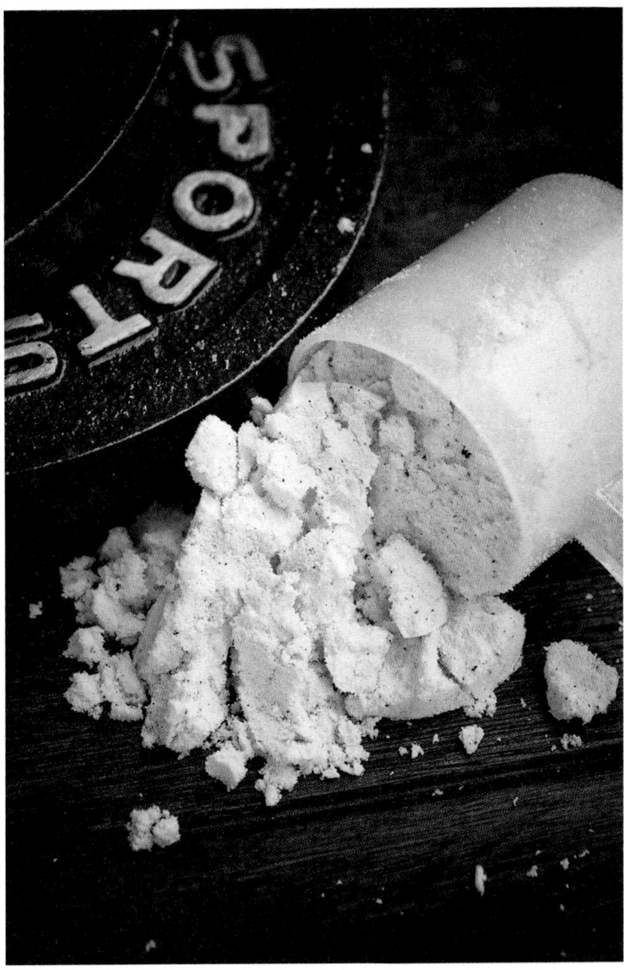

Protein powders.

UP FOR DEBATE

"Hope in a Can"—Are Protein Powders Worth It?

You see them in gyms, pharmacies, and grocery stores. They are particularly popular among young adults, teens, and moms. In fact, pregnant women are one of the fastest-growing consumer segments of this expanding industry. Often mixed with water or milk to form a shake, protein powders are now being used outside the realm of intense weightlifting workouts, as a meal replacement, in order to save time and money.[23]

The most common bases for protein powders are whey and soy. Whey is produced from milk and is a by-product of cheese making. Because whey contains all nine essential amino acids, it is a complete protein. However, despite the advantages of providing a dense source of protein in an easily consumable form, protein powders have a number of negative attributes.

For one thing, they're expensive. They also may be largely unnecessary. Medical professionals suggest that a diet with adequate meat, fish, dairy, nuts and/or beans is likely to contain enough protein for the body to fully recover and rebuild from nearly any vigorous workout. The body can break down only so much protein at a time—less than 1 gram per kilogram of body weight. The remaining energy is converted to fat or is excreted,[24] which may explain why many users of protein powders report stomach pain and discomfort. Another concern is the amount of sugar often contained in these products. Protein bars, such as Luna, Clif, and Balance, may contain as much as 30 grams of sugar per serving, so it is important to check the amount of sugars listed on the label.

A 2010 investigation by *Consumer Reports* confirmed that protein drinks can pose health risks due to the presence of harmful heavy metals.[23] In a test of 15 of the most popular powders, each drink contained high enough levels of lead, arsenic, cadmium, and/or mercury to concern the researchers. This poses a risk for pregnant women and people who consume more than one protein shake per day. Also of concern is the high level of soy, too much of which has been linked to endocrine disruption, hormone interference, and, in some cases, cancer, birth defects, and developmental disorders.[25]

Marketing campaigns for these powders—commonly seen in shopping malls—target teens and young adults, who are easily convinced by advertisers' inaccurate message that you need more than a balanced and healthy diet consisting of plenty of water to recover from a workout. Teens are particularly vulnerable to the promise of "hope in a can," as protein powders and shakes are most commonly used by boys 12 to 18 years of age.

Although protein supplementation has been found to be effective at promoting increases in mass and muscle endurance in high-intensity weight training programs, the money you spend on supplemental protein shakes can probably be more effectively spent elsewhere, with no adverse effect on your overall health.

What do you think? Do you take supplements? Do you think they are a marketing scam? Should they be more regulated? Or, is the "hope" they engender a good enough reason to allow them to be marketed as they are today, aggressively and boldly?

amino acid converted to proteins to the ratio of amino acids supplied. Eggs are considered to have protein with highest known NPU. Following eggs, in descending order, are fish, milk and cheese, brown rice, red meat, and poultry.[5]

Water—The Most Essential Nutrient of All

While water is sometimes misclassified as a macronutrient, rather than the chemical compound that it is, there is no dispute that water is essential to human life. While you can survive without food for weeks, you can survive without water for only a few days.

About three-fourths of all muscle tissue is composed of water, and water helps regulate body temperature, cushions bones and vital organs, and contributes critical functions to the digestive system, such as transporting nutrients and eliminating waste.

An analysis from the *Journal of the American Dietetic Association* estimated that the average sedentary adult should consume 4 to 8 pints (2 to 4 liters) of water by drinking pure water or consuming soups or water-rich fruits and vegetables such as citrus, cucumber, and peppers.[26] If your diet is healthy and well balanced, then drinking four 12-ounce glasses (about 1.4 liters) of water per day is probably enough to supplement what you are getting from fruits and vegetables.[27] Of course, that number increases the more physically active you are.

Research indicates that many Americans suffer from dehydration, or underconsumption of water, which can increase the risk of urinary diseases, obesity, cancers, asthma, and heart disease.[28] For public health professionals, the issue of dehydration can be particularly frustrating, given how plentiful and available water is throughout the United States. While many populations around the world struggle to gain access to clean and adequate water supplies, most people in the United States do not have that problem (Flint, Michigan, in the mid-2010s is an important exception). However, this country — and increasingly the world — does have a food and beverage industry dedicated to selling as much sugar-infused product as possible. The beverage industry is known to categorize highly sweetened sports and energy drinks as "healthy," even though the amounts of sugar contained in these drinks can prevent hydration! Furthermore, the health concerns of soft drinks may go beyond sugary drinks: Some scientists attribute the surprising connection between *diet* sodas and obesity as possibly related to the dehydrating effect of artificially sweetened drinks.[29]

In the United States, virtually every municipal water system produces water that is as safe and nutritious, and less expensive, as water sold in bottles. While water is not as heavily marketed as beverages tagged with terms such as "energy," "sports," and "vitamin," pure water is your best bet for a healthy beverage choice—before, during, and after exercise.

Micronutrients—Necessities in Small Bits

Micronutrients are the vitamins and minerals that are essential for optimal health, although only in miniscule amounts. While they do not provide energy the way carbohydrates, lipids, and proteins do, micronutrients are important for the normal functioning of the body, and they enable many of the important chemical reactions that promote good health.

Vitamins assist **metabolism**, growth, and development and help regulate and enhance cell function, working together with enzymes and other substances that are necessary for a healthy life. Vitamins are either fat-soluble or water-soluble. When consumed in excess, fat-soluble vitamins are stored in the body's fatty tissues and are therefore not excreted easily. You do not need to consume them as often as water-soluble vitamins, and because the body cannot flush them out as easily as water-soluble vitamins, fat-soluble vitamins can actually cause toxicity in large doses.

metabolism The process that occurs inside the body at the cellular and the physiological levels to generate energy and maintain life. Metabolism consists of two fundamental stages—catabolism and anabolism.

Water-soluble vitamins are excreted in urine when consumed in excess. For this reason, they need to be consumed regularly, ideally in food, and pose less of a threat from overconsumption. Although vitamins do not produce energy, some vitamins, such as some of the B vitamins, facilitate energy-producing chemical reactions initiated by micronutrients (**TABLE 2-2**).

Minerals are classified into macrominerals and microminerals (or trace minerals). Macrominerals are those that your body requires in relatively larger amounts and include calcium, potassium, iron, sodium, and magnesium. Iron, for example, is a constituent of hemoglobin, a protein molecule found in blood, which is why iron is an essential mineral for strong blood health. Microminerals include copper, zinc, and chromium—necessary in minute amounts for the function of enzymes in the body (**TABLE 2-3**).

TABLE 2-2 Important Vitamins, Recommended Daily Allowance (RDA),* Functions, and Sources

Vitamin	RDA, Men	RDA, Women	Best Sources	Functions
A (carotene)	900 µg	700 µg	Yellow or orange fruits and vegetables, liver, dairy products	Helps maintain skin, hair, and mucous membranes, eye function, bone and tooth growth
B_1 (thiamine)	1.2 mg	1.1 mg	Fortified cereals and oatmeal, meats, rice and pasta, whole grains, liver	Helps body release energy from carbohydrates during metabolism; aids in growth and muscle tone
B_2 (riboflavin)	1.3 mg	1.1 mg	Whole grains, green leafy vegetables, organ meats, milk, eggs	Helps body release energy from protein, fat, and carbohydrates during metabolism
B_6 (pyridoxine)	1.3 mg	1.3 mg	Fish, poultry, lean meats, bananas, prunes, dried beans, whole grains, avocado	Helps body build tissues; aids in metabolism of protein
B_{12} (cobalamin)	2.4 µg	2.4 µg	Meats, milk products, seafood	Aids cell development, functioning of nervous system, and metabolism of fat and protein
Folate (folic acid and folacin)	400 µg	400 µg	Green leafy vegetables, organ meats, dried peas, beans, lentils	Aids in genetic material development and in red cell production
Niacin	16 mg	14 mg	Meat, poultry, fish, enriched cereals, peanuts, potatoes, dairy products, eggs	Involved in carbohydrate, protein, and fat metabolism
C (ascorbic acid)	90 mg	75 mg	Citrus fruits, berries, vegetables (especially peppers)	Essential for bone and cartilage strength and for healthy muscles and blood vessels; helps maintain capillaries and gums; aids in absorption of iron
D	5 µg	5 µg	Fortified milk, sunlight, fish, eggs, butter	Aids in bone and tooth formation; helps maintain heart action and nervous system
E	15 mg	15 mg	Fortified and multigrain cereals, nuts, wheat germ, vegetable oils, green leafy vegetables	Protects blood cells, body tissue, and essential fatty acids from harmful destruction
K	120 µg	90 µg	Green leafy vegetables, fruit, dairy products, grains	Essential for blood clotting functions

µg, micrograms (one millionth of a gram, or one thousandth of a milligram); mg, milligrams.

*Average daily level of intake sufficient to meet the nutrient requirements of nearly most healthy people, also referred to as RDA.

Alan Freishtat-Certified Wellness Coach and Certified Personal Trainer www.alanfitness.com

TABLE 2-3 Important Minerals, Recommended Daily Allowance (RDA), Functions, and Sources

Mineral	RDA, Men	RDA, Women	Best Sources	Functions
Calcium	1,000 mg	1,000 mg	Milk and milk products	Aids in strong bones, teeth, muscle tissue; regulates heartbeat, muscle action, and nerve function; aids in blood clotting
Fluoride	4 mg	3 mg	Fluorinated water, teas, marine fish	Stimulates bone formation; inhibits or even reverses dental caries
Iodine	150 µg	150 µg	Seafood, iodized salt	Component of hormone thyroxine, which controls metabolism
Iron	8 mg	18 mg	Meats, especially organ meats, legumes	Aids in hemoglobin formation; improves blood quality; increases resistance to stress and disease
Magnesium	420 mg	320 mg	Nuts, green vegetables, whole grains	Helps maintain acid–alkaline balance; important in metabolism of carbohydrates, minerals, and sugar (glucose)
Potassium	4,700 mg	4,700 mg	Lean meat, vegetables, fruits	Helps maintain fluid balance; controls activity of heart muscle, nervous system, and kidneys
Selenium	55 µg	55 µg	Seafood, organ meats, lean meats, grains	Protects body tissue against oxidative damage from radiation, pollution, and normal metabolic processing
Zinc	11 mg	8 mg	Lean meats, liver, eggs, seafood, whole grains	Involved in digestion and metabolism; important in development of reproductive system; aids in healing

µg, micrograms; mg, milligrams.

Data from National Academy of Sciences, 2002.

TRY IT!

Making Sense of Nutrition Labels

The Nutrition Facts label is required on most packaged food sold in the United States and many other countries (**FIGURE 2-3**). In the United States, the label begins with standard serving measurement, followed by calories, and such components as fat, sodium, carbohydrates and protein. The U.S. Food and Drug Administration (FDA) updates the label periodically, in an effort to make it easier for people to understand what is on the label and in the package. The most recent changes include making the "servings per container" and "serving size" numbers in larger and/or bolder type. In addition, serving sizes were updated to be more realistic in reflecting the sizes people normally go with. You'll notice that 2,000 calories per day is used as a healthy number of calories that the average person of average size is meant to consume but, in reality, this number ranges dramatically, depending on age, sex, height, and your daily level of physical activity. The Ingredient List is ordered from the most to least, according to weight. Take a look at the U.S. FDA "Nutrition Facts" label below with its instructions from the U.S. Food and Drug Administration, and then find a label in your own kitchen and decide for yourself: Is it healthy or not? Why?

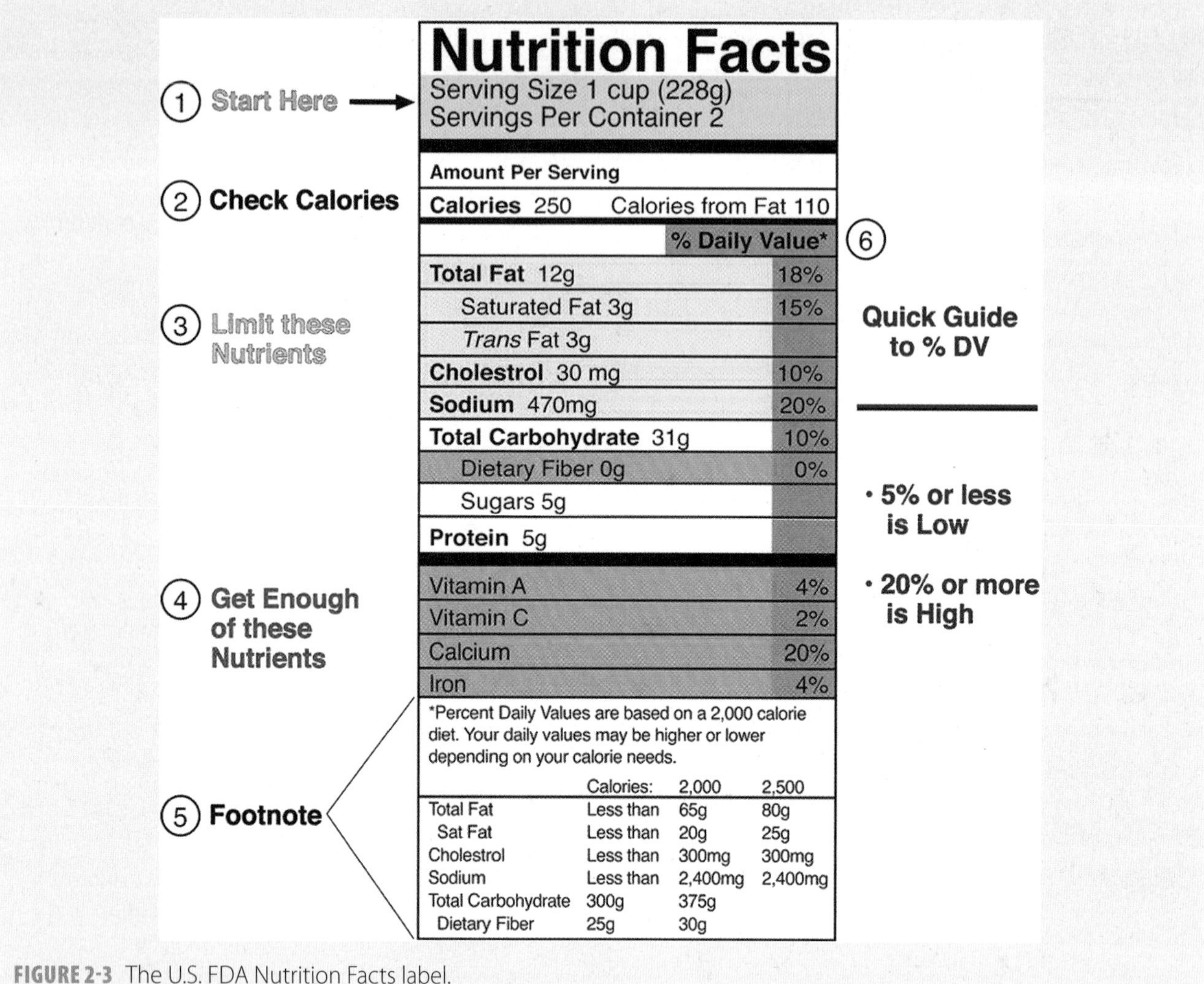

FIGURE 2-3 The U.S. FDA Nutrition Facts label.

Courtesy of U.S. Food and Drug Administration.

While not technically classified as micronutrients, phytochemicals are plant-based chemicals, many of which have been shown to benefit cell function and immunity. Foods that are naturally rich in phytochemicals are also rich in fiber and water and are naturally low in calories.

Eating Wisely—As Individuals and Communities

What should you do to eat well? With the thousands of nutrition-related studies completed each year, and at least as many nutrition experts, publications, and journals releasing new recommendations and advice for our benefit every single day, it can be challenging to know where to start. It seems like every day there is a new diet to try! The following are evidence-based, time-tested nutrition principles that are likely to stay relevant for many years to come.

Getting Your Nutrients From Food

According to the World Health Organization, the best way to prevent micronutrient malnutrition is to ensure that you eat a balanced diet that is adequate in every nutrient. However, maintaining such a diet tends to be easier with affluence: Wealthier families in the United States tend to consume a more complete intake of micronutrients, while families in lower-income communities consume a more nutrient-deprived diet.[30] This disparity may be related to differences in education levels, but it often relates to different nutritional opportunities between wealthier and less wealthy communities.

In developing nations around the world, and even many communities in the United States, the challenge of ensuring adequate nutrition is more difficult, making a process known as **food fortification** an important solution for this international issue. In fact, fortification has been used for nearly a century in industrialized countries as a means of restoring micronutrients lost by food processing. Do you know how your food is fortified? In the United States, examples of supplementation include adding vitamin D to milk, folic acid to bread, and iodine to salt.[31]

food fortification A method used for nearly a century in industrialized countries to restore micronutrients lost by food processing. In the United States, examples of supplementation include adding vitamin D to milk, folic acid to bread, and iodine to salt.

Yet year after year, researchers conclude that many forms of vitamin supplementation show no results—or worse—cause toxicity or bodily harm. A large clinical trial in 2015 showed no meaningful effect on cancer rates from a decade of vitamin C or E supplements. Another study found no benefit of vitamins C and E for heart disease. In 2014, a major trial studying whether selenium could lower a man's risk for prostate cancer was stopped when it was discovered that treatments may have been doing harm.[32] A Johns Hopkins School of Medicine review of 19 vitamin E clinical trials showed that high doses of vitamin E increased a person's risk of dying. Another study linked daily vitamin E to a higher risk of heart failure.[22] One systematic review concluded that there was no overall benefit of vitamin C for preventing colds. The review did, however, show a reduction in colds among extremely active people, such as marathon runners and soldiers exposed to significant cold or physical stress.[33]

Recent findings confirm a long-held understanding within the medical and public health community: It is safest, and best for your health, to get your micronutrients the way you get your macronutrients, through pure, unprocessed, healthy food. In fact, recent research has shown linkages between herbs and spices and important health benefits, such as cancer risk reduction and even modification of cancer tumor growth. A growing body of evidence points to herbs and spices as having multiple anticancer characteristics. Today, many ethnic cuisines are recognized for their reliance on herbs and spices for healing properties. For example, turmeric, cinnamon, basil, garlic, oregano, and ginger have all been found to have anticancer characteristics. Cherries, too, demonstrate anticancer benefits. Research continues to indicate that the phytochemical compounds in foods produce benefits that are unable to be replicated through nutritional supplements.[34] While taking vitamin supplements may help some people who are deficient in specific vitamins, the longstanding advice to "eat the rainbow" (i.e., a wide color variety of fruits, vegetables, and spices) has proven to be the best advice for getting the vitamins and minerals needed by the average person.

Some foods are so nutritionally dense that they are referred to as "superfoods." While there is no clear definition and no single list of foods that fall into this category, some examples of foods that have numerous health effects include spinach, kale, blueberries, almonds, and wild salmon.

Sugar: More Important to Avoid Than Ever

Over the past few decades, increasing evidence has linked the consumption of sugar, particularly soda and other sweetened drinks, to diabetes, heart disease, and cancers.[35] Research also indicates that sweet drinks play a significant role in driving current obesity trends. According to the USDA, the average American consumes more than 150 pounds of sugar per year. A century ago, it was only about 4 pounds.[36]

refined sugar A form of sugar made from sugar cane or sugar beets. Once the sugar is extracted, it is processed into white sugar. Also known as sucrose.

high-fructose corn syrup A popular sweetener used in sodas and other beverages. Inexpensive production of corn led to its development.

Refined sugar, found in foods and beverages in the form of sucrose or **high-fructose corn syrup**, leaches vitamins and minerals from the body through its digestion and elimination. Minerals such as sodium (from salt), potassium and magnesium (from vegetables), and calcium (from the bones) are all mobilized and expelled in combating the toxic effects of sugar, thus linking sugar consumption to general malnutrition.[37]

High-fructose corn syrup was first widely introduced to the U.S. market in 1975, and today, because of federal government subsidies, it is so cheap that it has found its way into breads, pretzels, cereals, and most condiments, sauces, and dressings found in the United States.[38]

Regularly eating or drinking refined sugar produces a continuously overactive condition where the body requires more and more minerals to rectify the imbalance resulting from the elimination of the sugar. To protect the blood, calcium is taken from the bones and teeth, which can cause decay and general weakening. Excess sugar is initially stored in the liver in the form of glucose (glycogen) but eventually affects every organ in the body. Because the liver's capacity is limited by sugar consumption, too much refined sugar makes the liver expand like a balloon. When this happens, the excess glycogen is returned to the blood in the form of fatty acids, leading to weight gain or, worse, obesity.[30] Sucrose and high-fructose corn syrup consumption are considered the primary causes of a public health issue referred to as the "metabolic syndrome," which is a combination of obesity, diabetes, hypertension, and cardiovascular disease. Metabolic syndrome affects approximately one-third of American adults and affects our economy through the reduced productivity among people affected by this combination of conditions.[35]

Researchers have also found that excess sugar consumption causes increases in triglycerides and decreases in high-density lipoprotein (HDL) cholesterol (often called "good cholesterol"), each of which can increase the risk of heart disease.[39,40]

Liquid Sugar: Soda, Sports Drinks, and Juice

Recent studies have suggested that an additional mechanism by which sugar-sweetened beverages may lead to weight gain is the low satiety of liquid carbohydrates and the resulting incomplete compensation of energy at subsequent meals. So, in more simple terms: People who consume sugar through liquid do not feel as full as if they had eaten the same number of calories through solid food. That is, you'd likely feel more full by eating one donut than by drinking three cans of Coca-Cola. This may be one of the reasons sweetened beverages are even more closely related to rising levels of obesity and weight gain in the United States than are food products such as candy and desserts.[30]

While there is no limit to the number of diet approaches (and diet books and videos) out there, many of the most popular fall into basic categories (**TABLE 2-4**). Overall, the healthiest diets encourage eating plenty of vegetables and avoiding refined sugar and bleached white flour. Getting enough exercise and drinking lots of water are as important to health as your diet, so be sure to combine them all for best results.

TABLE 2-4 Popular Diets

Basic Approach	Popular Names	Benefits	Concerns
Vegan/Vegetarian (vegan = no animal products [i.e., meat, cheese, eggs]; vegetarian = no meat)	Plant-based Alkaline	Practitioners say this diet leads to a greater sense of well-being. Associated with clear skin, colon health, heart health, reduced chronic diseases, and longevity. Positively associated with environmental health.	Getting adequate protein can be difficult for some people. Because sugars and processed foods can be consumed by some of these regimes, vegans/vegetarians can still have unhealthy diets.
Low carbohydrate	Atkins Paleo South Beach Dukan Low-carb	Can lead to rapid weight loss and high muscle-to-fat ratio.	Weight gain can return quickly if the diet cannot be sustained. The diet can be unhealthy if inadequate fiber is consumed.
Mediterranean (mostly natural foods such as vegetables, salads, fruits, pastas and rice, with meat eaten in moderation)	Mediterranean	Associated with heart health and longevity Avoids processed foods.	Weight loss can be difficult for some under this program – especially when flours and starches are not kept in check.
Gluten-free (no wheat of any kind)	Gluten-free Celiac disease diet	Avoids many unhealthy and fattening foods (donuts, pizza, cake, cookies, etc.). Provides relief for many people with allergies.	Many gluten-free substitutes contain more sugar and fat than the original wheat-based product. Many gluten-free products are highly processed.
Fasting (i.e., for one day or longer every few days)	Intermittent fasting 5:2 (5 days eating normally and 2 days completely or partially fasting)	Associated with weight loss, reduced chronic diseases, and increased mental acuity.	Can be dangerous and can cause malnutrition, and even death, if improperly done.

Selective Diets: The Common Good . . . and the Bad

You can see them in your local bookstore, in your grocery store, on Facebook, or in pop-up Internet ads: Diets are everywhere, and they promise everything. Consume a Mediterranean diet to achieve the longevity enjoyed by so many Greeks, Spaniards, and Italians. Eat a Paleolithic diet and become fit and strong like our hunter–gatherer ancestors. Different ways of eating are promoted by celebrities, athletes, and medical doctors and promise healthy weight, energy, and clean skin if you follow their strict—but delicious—path to dietary righteousness (**FIGURE 2-4**). But do they work? Why? How? Or, in many cases, why not?

Before considering these questions, it is important to note that, according to some estimates, at least 20% of people who start a specific dietary plan abandon it within 30 days, which can lead to a number of feelings relating to failure and despondency.[41]

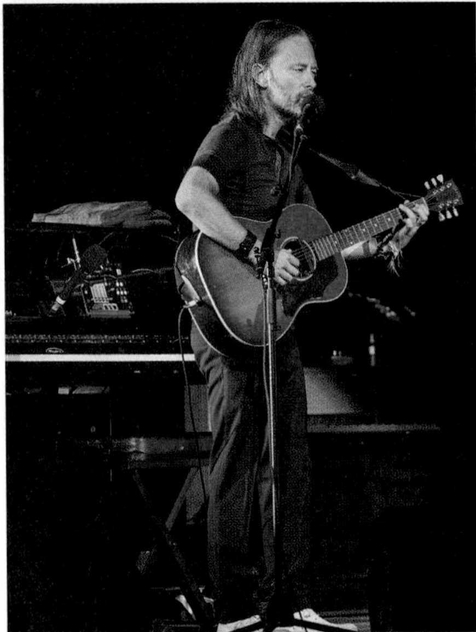
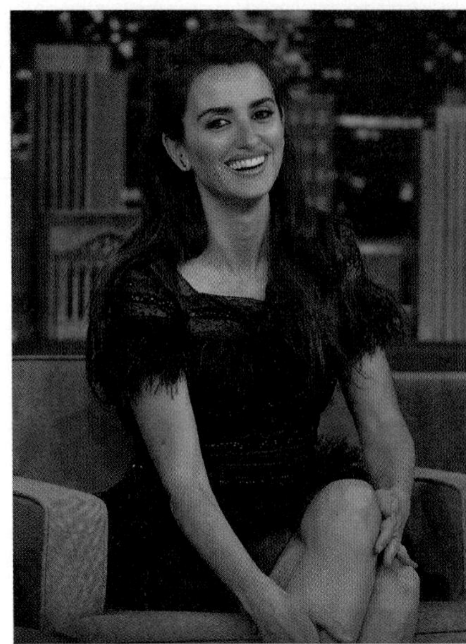
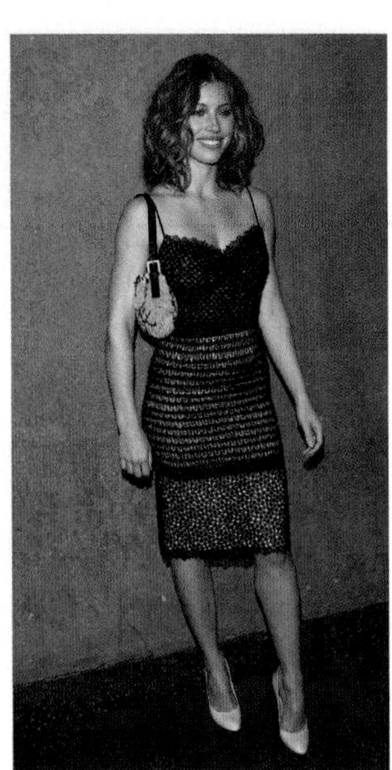

FIGURE 2-4 Examples of the many celebrities who have been associated with specific diets include Thom Yorke of Radiohead (vegan), Penelope Cruz (Mediterranean diet), and Jessica Biel (paleo).

Because diets can be associated with the idea of deprivation, they are likewise seen as something that has a beginning and an end, but the ideal "diet" is a pattern of eating that promotes health and can be sustained indefinitely. Many diets are difficult to adhere to but have been shown to be extremely satisfying for those who do so. These include vegan, vegetarian, and gluten-free diets, all of which can be adopted with success for better health, to avoid allergies, or for philosophical reasons. In the end, most health-promoting diets share some common elements.

TRY IT!

Common Elements of All Healthy Diets

1. Avoid processed foods, especially sugar and high-fructose corn syrup. These foods also include white flours, white breads, and pasta.
2. Eat a variety of raw green leafy vegetables, such as lettuce, spinach, and kale.
3. Seek out foods high in fiber (fruits, vegetables, beans, grains, and nuts).
4. Drink plenty of water.

These basic guidelines allow plenty of flexibility to build your diet around vegetarian preferences, or to include more meat protein. They are also consistent with the key principles of several popular regimens, such as the Atkins, South Beach, Paleolithic, gluten-free, vegan, and Full Plate diets, as well as guidelines from the U.S. government via the USDA (**FIGURE 2-5**).

University of California professor and nutrition author Michael Pollan provides a simple dietary mantra: "Eat food. Not too much. Mostly plants." This reminds us to avoid processed foods such as convenience store snacks and soda, which some would argue are so nutritionally compromised that they are not actually food.

Pollan's directive also encourages us to be aware of the amount of food we eat, indicating that diets high in nutrient-rich foods require fewer calories to achieve adequate cell growth and energy. Note, however, that for athletes and others who burn large amounts of energy, the "not too much" phrase is relative.

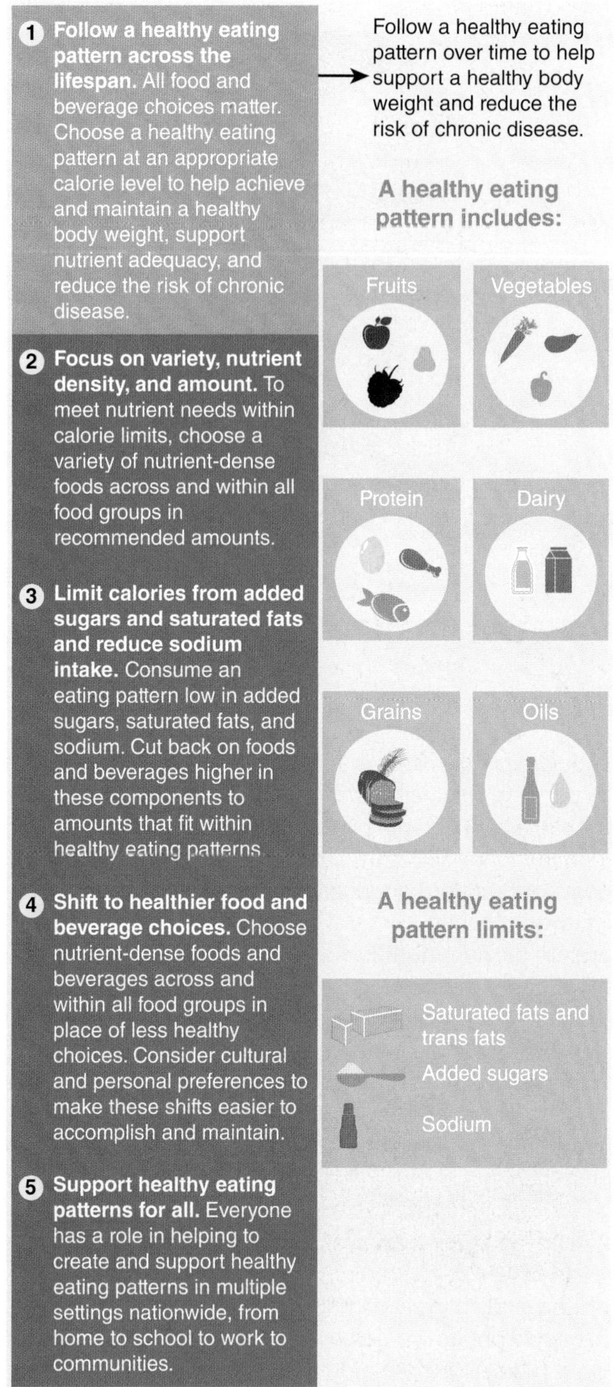

FIGURE 2-5 USDA dietary guidelines. The current guidelines offered by the USDA Center for Nutrition Policy and Promotion offer a similar perspective on nutritional recommendations for Americans.

Moving Ahead to Parenthood: The First Thousand Days

Research indicates that our health is determined by nutritional choices made for us early in life. We now know that our risk of chronic diseases such as type 2 diabetes, heart disease, stroke, and some cancers may be affected by the foods eaten right before and during a mother's pregnancy, and for the first years of a child's life.[45]

Women, Infants, and Children (WIC) A federal nutrition assistance program for pregnant women and their newborn babies. The program provides vouchers for mothers, which can be spent only on nutritious foods.

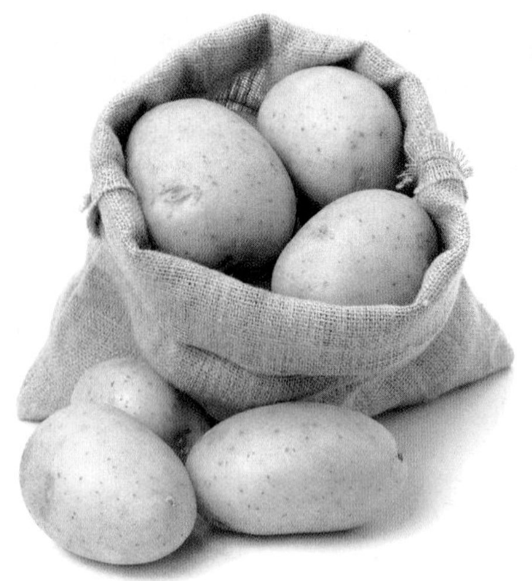

The seemingly innocuous white potato.

TALES OF PUBLIC HEALTH

The White Potato: In or Out?

Mashed? Baked? Fried? Boiled? The white potato, or *Solanum tuberosum*, is a member of the perennial nightshade family, which includes tomatoes, eggplant, and chili peppers. Originally from the Andes mountains, it is now cultivated throughout the world, and its place on the American table has been unanimously accepted for centuries.

That changed in 2015, when the simple white potato found itself at the center of a fierce argument in Washington, DC. The debate called into question whether the potato is nutritious enough to be included in the federal nutrition assistance program for pregnant women and their newborn babies.

The **Women, Infants, and Children (WIC)** program provides nutrition at the crucial time in human development when human growth and cellular resilience are taking shape—in the womb and during the first few years of childhood. The program provides vouchers for mothers, which can be spent only on foods deemed "exceptionally nutritious" by the USDA, such as milk, cereal, eggs, fruits, vegetables, beans, and peanut butter. The USDA takes its guidance from the National Academy of Medicine (NAM), a nongovernmental nonprofit organization that provides unbiased guidance for policy decisions related to health and health care.

In 2006, the medical and nutritional scientists at the NAM determined that potatoes were not healthy enough to be considered a "crucial" food for women and postpartum babies and thus ineligible for WIC reimbursement. For the potato industry, the financial implications were enormous. WIC had distributed around $7 billion in vouchers in 2006,[42] and removing an item from WIC funding has a major effect on jobs and profits for large industrial food producers, as well as small farmers, whether they're raising potatoes or peanuts.

After a long campaign of communications, lobbying, and financial contributions, the potato industry got what it wanted. In February 2015, the NAM announced that white potato would be returned to the list of approved WIC foods. It was a victory for the potato farmers, but what about the health impact? In the United States, most potatoes are whipped, deep-fried, or processed into chips and other products that are not "crucial" nutrition for pregnant women and new mothers. This was the concern expressed by the American Public Health Association, which protested that this was not a "health" decision but one based on political and financial influence. The American Academy of Pediatrics (AAP) said they were "tremendously concerned" about industry intervening in WIC regulations. The AAP argued that including potatoes would "override the sound scientific judgment of our nation's leading nutrition science experts."[43] New York University nutrition professor Marion Nestle wrote, "I have a hard time believing that WIC recipients are suffering from lack of potatoes in their diets. Potatoes are fine foods, but highly caloric when prepared in the usual ways. Encouraging WIC recipients to choose leafy greens and other vegetables seems like a good idea."[44]

The food industry has influenced USDA dietary guidelines since the first recommendations in 1894. This influence has been in lobbying Congress, funding nutrition research, and forming partnerships with professional nutrition organizations.

Each sector of American life (governments, companies, nonprofit organizations) has a different perspective on health, and in America, the public and private sectors both have influence on our diets. Reaching a better understanding of these areas through critical discussion and open reporting may help all of us to become healthier eaters, and consequently, healthier people.

Research first conducted in England in the 1980s[46] demonstrated how chronic diseases such as diabetes, high blood pressure, and heart disease can be "programmed" into people's bodies when they are deprived of important nutrients as fetuses and babies. Poor nutrition slows fetal growth and can cause stress during development that can affect long-term health. Low birth weight has been shown to increase the risk of heart disease and diabetes later in life by up to seven times.[47] The nutritional decisions we face as individuals are important to the health of our children. When we consider how these choices can be affected by disadvantaged living conditions, the challenge of making nutritious foods available and affordable to all people becomes a critical issue of public health.

The moment of conception through 2 years of age is when organs develop most quickly. Nutritional deprivation early on can lead to metabolism and hormonal feedback that makes the body gain weight or become more susceptible to heart attacks later in life. Research now indicates that our genes are affected by the conditions mothers experience before and during pregnancy.[46]

One illustration of this effect is "the Dutch Hunger Winter" of 1944–1945, when the people of Holland endured a devastatingly cold winter during World War II. A German blockade caused a major reduction in food to the region, and the entire population suffered severely. More than 20,000 people died, and those who survived experienced health problems for the rest of their lives. When the country recovered, the Dutch national health system tracked the outcomes of these people and their descendants for generations. They found that the children of malnourished mothers had higher obesity rates and a greater incidence of other health problems throughout their lives. Even the grandchildren of the malnourished pregnant mothers had more health problems than the rest of the population. This is termed an *epigenetic* effect—when changes in biology can be seen generations beyond a specific adverse experience.

epigenetics The process by which our genes respond to environmental cues; and while the genetic code does not change, the epigenetic biological responses, or "switches," can change as a result of nutritional scarcity or abundance in the womb.

Epigenetics is the process of our genes responding to environmental cues. While our genetic code does not change, the epigenetic ("epi" refers to "above" or "beyond" the gene) responses can change, based on stress or nutritional scarcity in the womb. These changes in genetic responses can be passed from mother to child, making children from disadvantaged nutritional environments more vulnerable to diseases.

This new research is important to help us reduce health disparities among people of different income levels and among different races and ethnicities.

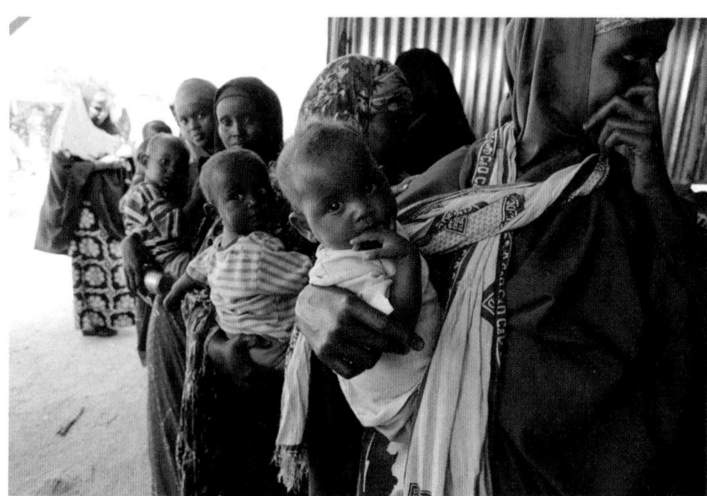

Health advocates all over the world are increasingly recognizing the importance of supporting nutrition for the first thousand days—from pregnancy through the second year of life.

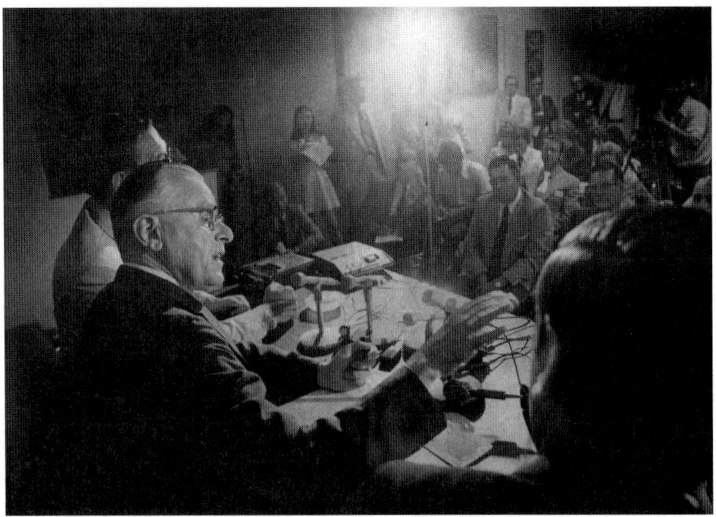

Secretary of Agriculture Earl Butz, foreground, takes questions from reporters in 1973.

GOING UPSTREAM

The Low Price of Soda and Fast Food

Why are spinach and blueberries more expensive than candy, chips, and soda? Finding the answer to this question can help us better understand how the United States can reduce its rates of obesity, diabetes, heart disease, and cancer.

The price differences between healthy and unhealthy foods did not happen by accident. They are the result of policy decisions made by the U.S. government over many years, some still in place today. The U.S. government passed the Agricultural Adjustment Act of 1933 to stabilize crop prices by controlling food overproduction. One way the government did this was by making subsidy payments to farmers. In 1974, the USDA introduced a new policy to encourage producers of corn, wheat, and soy to harvest as much as possible. Then Secretary of Agriculture, Earl Butz, orchestrated a complex system of payments that provided financial support for the overproduction of these commodities. It was the beginning of a long series of multibillion-dollar price supports for the food industry that coincided with a decrease in the number of small farms that produced diverse varieties of vegetables and other crops.

The subsidy system greatly influences our current food supply (**FIGURE 2-6**). One result is a consistent oversupply of cheap corn in the United States, which has led to massive production of high-fructose corn syrup as a sweetener of

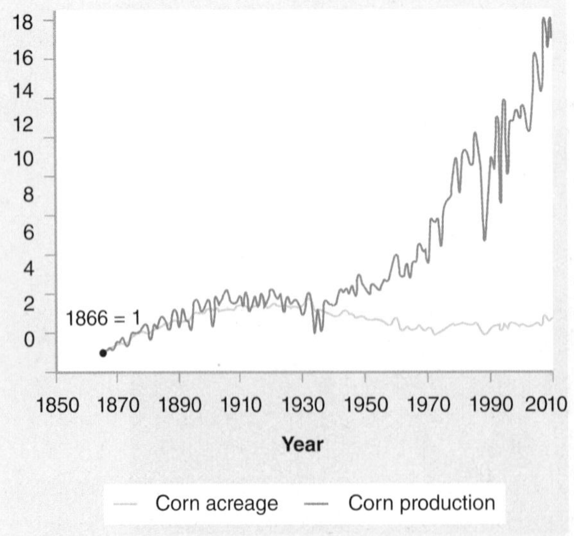

FIGURE 2-6 Corn acreage and production, 1870–2010. U.S. corn production and area farmed.

The Return of Nature: How Technology Liberates the Environment, U.S. Census Bureau (1975, 2012). http://thebreakthrough.org/index.php/journal/past-issues/issue-5/the-return-of-nature beverages and other foods. Corn also became a cheaper source of feed for cows, which used to be fed mostly on grass. While the stomach of the cow doesn't naturally digest corn, animal pharmaceuticals combined with cheap corn proved to be a more economical alternative for livestock farmers than the traditional grass feeding process. Cows raised on corn yield meat that is higher in calories and contains more harmful omega-6 fatty acids and fewer omega-3 fatty acids than cows raised on grass.[49]

In the 1980s, the United States became more restrictive over raw sugar imports, driving up the price of sugar and contributing to the widespread substitution of corn sweetener. This has resulted in lower prices for corn chips, corn-fed beef, and even fast-food items such as buns (sweetened with corn syrup) and shakes (often made with corn and soy). Cheap corn is now a key ingredient in numerous processed foods, from candy to breakfast cereals and soft drinks, all of which contribute to the type 2 diabetes plaguing the United States. Between 1985 and 2010 the price of beverages sweetened with high-fructose corn syrup dropped by 24%, while the price of fresh fruits and vegetables rose 39%.[50]

Americans now spend a smaller amount of their time preparing food than do people from any other nation in the world, and with each generation, they spend less and less time.[51] Food marketing practices, which invest approximately $2 billion per year on children alone, and disproportionally to minorities, also have a major influence over the consumption of unhealthy foods in the United States.[52]

The U.S. government works to improve health too, through policies such as food assistance and free lunch programs. But, as the editors of *Scientific American* noted, "Public money is working at cross-purposes: backing an overabundance of unhealthful calories that are flooding our supermarkets and restaurants, while also battling obesity and the myriad illnesses that go with it. It is time to align our farm policies with our health policies."[50]

Addressing the simple question of why your spinach is more expensive than your soda turns out to be more complex than it first seems. However it is a question that must be dealt with in order to create a sensible food policy system where the ultimate goal is the healthiest population possible.

Ensuring that every pregnant mother and every newborn baby receives adequate nutrition during the critical gestation and early developmental period may be one of the most effective ways we can use our public resources. Making sure our governments invest in this area may hold the greatest hope for achieving the best overall improved health for everyone, all over the world.[48]

Societal Choices: How Do We Improve Nutritional Options for Everyone?

Eating well is one of the best ways to prevent illness and disease later in life; it is an investment that pays off not only in terms of quality of life, but also financially, because illness and disease are expensive. The benefits of this investment apply to you as an individual, to your family, to your community, and to your country. The financial cost alone of nutrition-related conditions and illnesses such as obesity, diabetes, heart disease, and stroke run in the hundreds of billions of dollars in healthcare costs, increased depression, and reduced numbers of people who can be employed in such areas as public safety, law enforcement, and the military.[53,54]

Ensuring adequate nutrition for pregnant mothers and their children and making healthy choices available to everyone is not a simple process. Lower-income neighborhoods are particularly susceptible to being deprived of affordable healthy food choices. Areas high in fast-food outlets but low in grocery stores are often called **food deserts**, and they are more common in low-income areas of the nation, and the world, than in high-income areas.[55]

food deserts An area high in fast-food outlets but low in grocery stores.

So, what can we do to ensure that healthy food is easier to find and prepare than unhealthy food? What policy decisions can we make to improve nutritional environments for all children? These are the questions facing public health officials, politicians, corporations, public interest groups, and others who influence the nation's food system, and they are not easy.

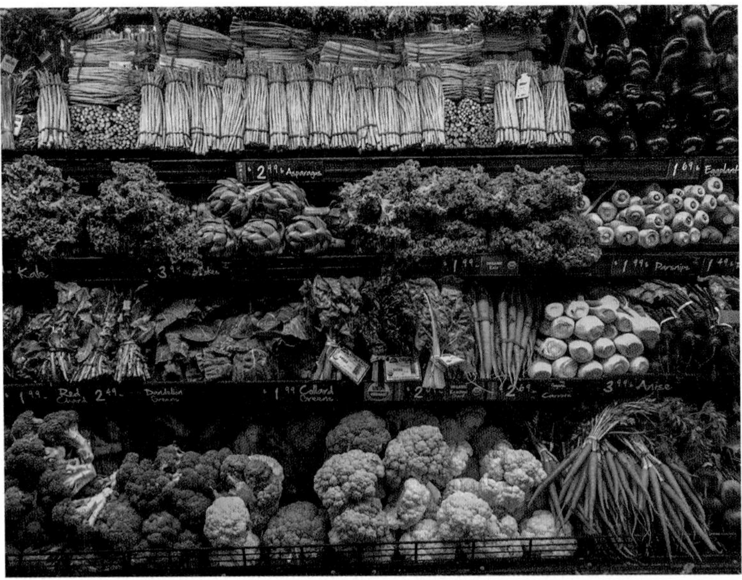

Wealthier neighborhoods are more likely to have stores like this.

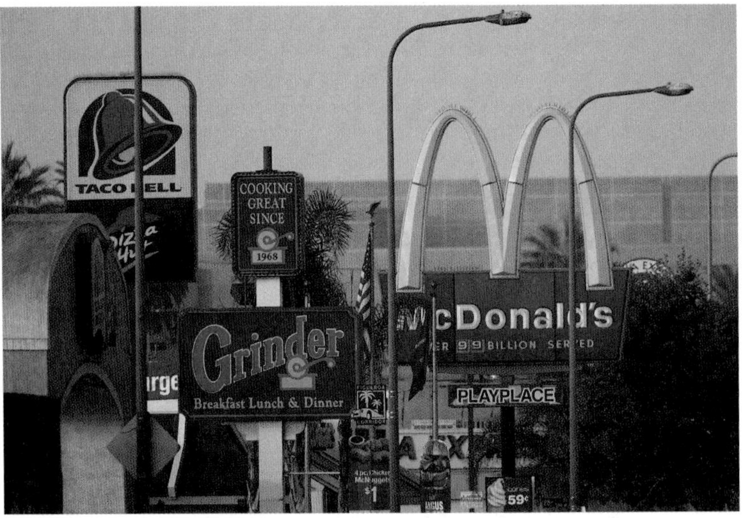

Lower-income neighborhoods tend to have a higher percentage of stores like this.

Addressing Food Subsidies

At the federal level, the policy area influencing the nutritional decisions faced by Americans is the national subsidy program, which determines the foods into which we invest our tax dollars. Currently, the United States channels billions of dollars into subsidizing the corn that makes high-fructose corn syrup cheap and plentiful (see the Going Upstream box). Addressing these subsidies could have a positive impact on the health of our nation. The U.S. government now prohibits farmers from using subsidies to grow fresh, healthy produce (which it labels "specialty crops"). Even now, our food system is encouraged to produce more soda, sweetened hamburger buns, and corn chips, and less organic produce.[56]

Confronting Food Marketing

The influence of major food producers is another important factor in the dietary habits of Americans. The largest food companies, such as Coca-Cola, Pepsi,

Mars, Kellogg, and Kraft, invest millions of dollars to study the brain's pleasure centers and calibrate products to "optimize" cravings in order to maximize revenues.[57] Marketing is another area that impacts food choices; as of 2015, food companies were estimated to have spent around $2 billion per year on advertising specifically to children.[58]

Menu Labeling

What if you had calorie information right on the menu when you were deciding what to order? As part of the Affordable Care Act, the FDA is implementing regulations that require all chain restaurants with more than 20 locations to provide point-of-sale information about the serving size and calories. Some cities and states have already implemented such policies. While research has yet to show major population-based behavior change, it is still too early to tell how much of an impact these regulations will have on consumer behavior—and health—over the long term.

Taxation

One of the efforts currently being debated to address this issue is excise taxation, or taxing harmful products to discourage their use. For example, in November 2014, Berkeley, California, residents passed the nation's first voter-approved soda tax, arguing that it would reduce diabetes and obesity among the population. States such as Vermont and Illinois have considered such taxes, following the lead of Berkeley, and of Mexico, which passed its own national tax on soda and sports drinks. Supporters feel that these taxes are important to improve the health of the population; however, opponents argue that such taxes are "regressive," meaning they unfairly punish low-income consumers. In 2016, the Philadelphia City Council passed a 1.5 cent-per-ounce tax on soda, energy drinks, and sports drinks. In one of his statements about the tax, Philadelphia Mayor Jim Kenney pointed out that "big soda companies have been marketing to poor neighborhoods for generations."[59]

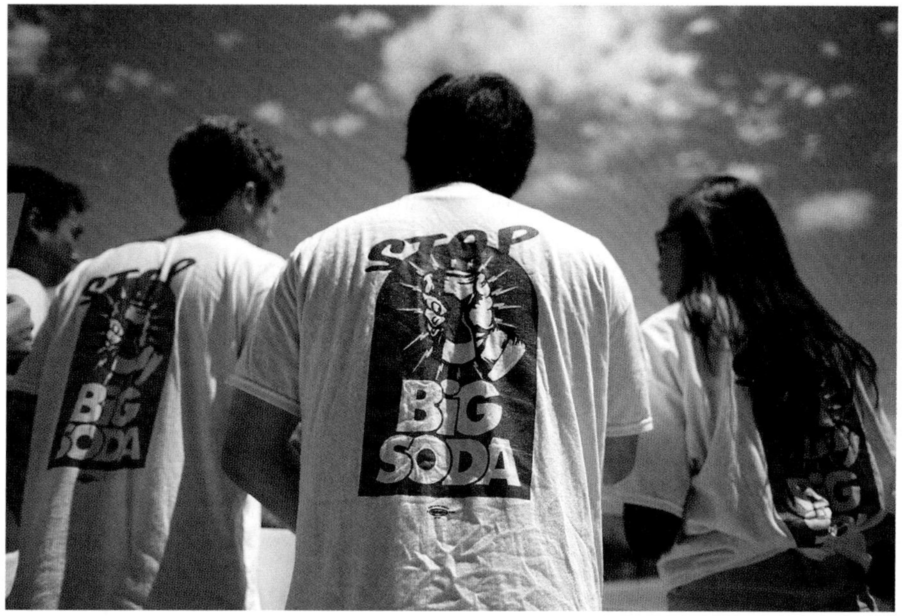

Health advocates rally in favor of a soda tax at San Francisco City Hall in 2014. That effort was unsuccessful, but Philadelphia passed a similar tax in 2016.

Warning labels on sugary drinks are another strategy that has been proposed by public health advocates, who clearly have taken some of their cues from the tobacco control efforts of the past few decades. Establishing schools, hospitals, and community centers as **sugar-sweetened beverage-free zones** is now being employed by more and more local communities. All of these efforts are intended to counterbalance the massive influence food companies have over the landscape of food choices available to Americans.

sugar-sweetened beverage-free zones An initiative to eliminate the sale of sugar-sweetened beverages from school campuses.

Procurement

Another policy area health advocates are looking at is procurement, or the purchasing rules established by public and private entities. Procurement policies address workplace food and beverage sources, including vending machines and cafeterias (for employees as well as students, prisoners, etc.), and can be vital to a policy strategy to improve public nutrition.[60] Private companies can adopt healthy food procurement policies, and so can city, state, and federal governments.

Seeking to improve a nation's nutrition through policy changes can result in major public impacts on health, but policy change can be controversial. Policy decisions, whether they seek to regulate human consumption, exert control over corporate marketing, or add costs through taxation, touch on fundamental tensions of individual freedom of choice, versus protecting the common good. As this chapter has discussed, food and nutrition decisions are not only personal but can also be highly political. Of course that does not mean we should avoid policy change; it simply means that these decisions are not easy. The way we as a society choose to navigate these choices will have effects on population health, now and into the future.

In Summary

Nutrition is one of the most important determinants of our own *personal* health. The nutritional choices available to our communities, towns, cities, and countries have a direct effect on the *public's* health. Just as our bodies require a complex and adequate balance of macronutrients and micronutrients, communities face decisions about how to best ensure that people have access to good nutrition. These decisions include how to ensure that mothers have strong nutrition options before, during, and after pregnancy. They also include figuring out how people, especially children, will not be inundated with highly processed and sweetened food options.

These decisions are not easy. Policies and marketing practices are in place today to encourage unhealthy eating. For example, government subsidies that make corn sweeteners a cheap option. Changing these policies can be difficult, but many people and government agencies are trying.

Developing a thorough understanding of population health nutrition requires learning about the biological functions of eating, drinking, and metabolism, as well as the governmental functions of how policies are established. Working to change nutritional environments requires education and action on both the individual and the societal fronts.

Key Terms

complex carbohydrates
epigenetics
fatty acids
food deserts
food fortification
glycemic index
high-fructose corn syrup
ketosis
macronutrients
metabolism
microbiome
micronutrients
nutritional environments
predigestive process
refined sugar
regional-level eating patterns
saturated fats
simple carbohydrates
sugar-sweetened beverage-free zone
type 2 diabetes mellitus
unsaturated fats
Women, Infants, and Children (WIC)

Student Discussion Questions and Activities

1. Look around at your community. In what contexts do you encounter foods that are processed or contain excess sugars, trans fats, and other unhealthy ingredients? How did they get there? What strategies do you recommend to shift the diets in your community from heavy on simple carbohydrates and processed foods to focused on more complex and nutrition-dense foods that are richer in fiber? What more "upstream" policies are there to improve the dietary patterns of Americans?
2. Who is in charge of the food decisions you make? Is it you alone? Your roommates? Your parents? How does government policy influence your choices? What about food companies' marketing and advertising? Do they give us what we want to buy, or do they determine what we want? Do the production and marketing practices of food companies influence what you eat? How?
3. How much control should be exercised over the marketing practices of food companies? Do individuals need to be responsible for their own choices, or is there a responsibility of food manufacturers to ensure that their products are not too unhealthy?
4. What role should for-profit corporations have over health and nutrition guidelines of the nation? What kinds of partnerships can there be between companies and governments to ensure the best health for Americans?
5. Are there decisions regarding the WIC program that can be made that are more impactful than the inclusion of the white potato? What foods should be included or excluded?

Food Journal

Make a food and nutrition journal for 1 week. Document both what you ate and its nutritional characteristics (as closely as you can estimate). For each meal or snack, document:

- Calories
- Carbohydrates
- Protein

- Fat
- Sugars (glucose, fructose, and sucrose) and what foods they come from
- Major micronutrients of note (vitamins and minerals)
- Pure water (completely pure or slightly flavored with fruit)

Also document the cost per week of your diet and assess your overall satisfaction with your nutrition choices. Consider the following:

- What does your diet tell you about yourself?
- What does your diet tell you about your community or where you live?
- Are there decisions you would have made differently now that you see what you ate over the course of a week?
- What areas did you feel were deficient or lacking? What areas were plentiful?
- How might you have had a more healthy or unhealthy diet if you could spend more money?
- Based on this experience, is there anything about your diet that you will change?

References

1. de Lorgeril, M., Salen, P., Martin, J. L., Monjaud, I., Delaye, J., & Mamelle, N. (1999). Mediterranean diet, traditional risk factors, and the rate of cardiovascular complications after myocardial infarction. *Heart Failure, 99*(6), 779–785.
2. Liska, D., & Bland, J. S. (2004). *Clinical nutrition: A functional approach* [Audiobook]. Princeton, NJ: Recordings for the Blind and Dyslexic.
3. Balch, P. (2006). *Prescription for nutritional healing*. New York, NY: Penguin.
4. Morgan, X. C., & Huttenhower, C. (2012). Human microbiome analysis. *PLoS Computational Biology, 8*(12), e1002808.
5. Bested, A. C., Logan, A. C., & Selhub, E. M. (2013). Intestinal microbiota, probiotics and mental health: From Metchnikoff to modern advances: Part II—contemporary contextual research. *Gut Pathogens, 5*(1), 1.
6. Smith, P. A. (2015, June 23). Can the bacteria in your gut explain your mood? *New York Times Magazine*. Retrieved from http://www.nytimes.com/2015/06/28/magazine/can-the-bacteria-in-your-gut-explain-your-mood.html?_r=0
7. Pollan, M. (2013, May 15). Some of my best friends are germs. *New York Times Magazine*. Retrieved from http://www.nytimes.com/2013/05/19/magazine/say-hello-to-the-100-trillion-bacteria-that-make-up-your-microbiome.html
8. Coman, M. M., Cecchini, C., Verdenelli, M. C., Silvi, S., Orpianesi, C., & Cresci, A. (2012). Functional foods as carriers for SYNBIO, a probiotic bacteria combination. *International Journal of Food Microbiology, 157*(3), 346–352.
9. Guzman, J. R., Conlin, V. S., & Jobin, C. (2013). Diet, microbiome, and the intestinal epithelium: An essential triumvirate? *BioMed Research International*. doi:10.1155/2013/425146
10. Dash, S., Clarke, G., Berk, M., & Jacka, F. N. (2015). The gut microbiome and diet in psychiatry: Focus on depression. *Current Opinion in Psychiatry, 28*(1), 1–6.
11. Haas, E. M. (2006). *Staying healthy with nutrition: The complete guide to diet and nutritional medicine*. New York, NY: Random House.
12. Garrison, R., Jr., & Somer, E. (1995). *The nutrition desk reference*. New Canaan, CT: Keats Publishing.
13. Livestrong.com. (2017, August 14). How does diabetes occur? Retrieved from https://www.livestrong.com/article/32042-diabetes-occur/
14. Michaud, D. S., Liu, S., Giovannucci, E., Willett, W. C., Colditz, G. A., & Fuchs, C. S. (2002). Dietary sugar, glycemic load, and pancreatic cancer risk in a prospective study. *Journal of the National Cancer Institute, 94*(17), 1293–1300.
15. Anderson, J. W., Baird, P., Davis, R. H., Jr., Ferreri, S., Knudtson, M., Koraym, A., . . . Williams, C. L. (2009). Health benefits of dietary fiber. *Nutrition Reviews, 67*(4), 188–205.
16. Slavin, J. L., & Beate, L. (2012). Health benefits of fruits and vegetables. *Advances in Nutrition, 3*(4), 506–516.
17. Kranz, S., Brauchla, M., Slavin, J. L., & Miller, K. B. (2012). What do we know about dietary fiber intake in children and health? The effects of fiber intake on constipation, obesity, and diabetes in children. *Advances in Nutrition, 3*(1), 47–53.
18. Turner, N. D., & Lupton, J. R. (2011). Dietary fiber. *Advances in Nutrition, 2*(2), 151–152.
19. Whitney, E. N., & Rolfes, S. R. (2007). *Understanding nutrition*. Belmont, CA: Wadsworth, Cengage Learning.
20. Dunford, M. (2006). *Sports nutrition: A practice manual for professionals*. Chicago, IL: American Dietetics Association.
21. Haas, E. M., & Levin, B., (2006). *Staying healthy with nutrition: The complete guide to diet and nutritional medicine* (p. 1168). Berkeley, CA: Celestial Arts.
22. Harvard T. H. Chan School of Public Health. (n.d.). Omega-3 fatty acids: An essential contribution. *The Nutrition Source*. Retrieved from https://www.hsph.harvard.edu/nutritionsource/omega-3-fats/
23. Grogan, S., 2016. *Body image: Understanding body dissatisfaction in men, women and children*. Abingdon, UK: Taylor & Francis.
24. Golden, M. H., Waterlow, J. C. & Picou, D., (1977). Protein turnover, synthesis and breakdown before and after recovery from protein-energy malnutrition. *Clin Sci Mol Med, 53*(5), 473-477.
25. Consumer Reports. (2010). *Health risks of protein drinks*. Retrieved from https://www.consumerreports.org/cro/2012/04/protein-drinks/index.htm Accessed: 4/18/2018

26. Kleiner, S. M. (1999). Water: An essential but overlooked nutrient. *Journal of the American Dietetic Association, 99*(2), 200–206.
27. Popkin, B., D'Anci, K. E., & Rosenberg, I. H. (2010). Water, hydration, and health. *Nutrition Reviews, 68*(8), 439–458.
28. Batmanghelidj, F., & Page, M. (2012). *Your body's many cries for water.* Old Saybrook, CT: Tantor.
29. Fowler, S. P., Williams, K., Resendez, R. G., Hunt, K. J., Hazuda, H. P., & Stern, M. P. Fueling the obesity epidemic? Artificially sweetened beverage use and long-term weight gain. *Obesity, 16*(8), 1894–1900.
30. Steinberger, J., Daniels, S. R., Eckel, R. H., Hayman, L., Lustig, R. H., McCrindle, B., . . . Council on Nutrition, Physical Activity, and Metabolism. (2009). Progress and challenges in metabolic syndrome in children and adolescents: A scientific statement from the American Heart Association Atherosclerosis, Hypertension, and Obesity in the Young Committee of the Council on Cardiovascular Disease in the Young; Council on Cardiovascular Nursing; and Council on Nutrition, Physical Activity, and Metabolism. *Circulation, 119*(4), 628–647.
31. Rosenberg, I. H. (2007). Further evidence that food fortification improves micronutrient status. *British Journal of Nutrition, 97*(6), 1051–1052.
32. Parker-Pope, T. (2008, November 20). News keeps getting worse for vitamins. *NYTimes.com.* Retrieved from http://well.blogs.nytimes.com/2008/11/20/news-keeps-getting-worse-for-vitamins/
33. Hemilä, H., & Chalker, E. (2013). Vitamin C for preventing and treating the common cold. *The Cochrane Library.* doi:10.1002/14651858.CD000980.pub4
34. Kaefer, C. M., & Milner, J. A. (2008). The role of herbs and spices in cancer prevention. *Journal of Nutritional Biochemistry, 19*(6), 347–361.
35. Simopoulos, A. P. (2013). Dietary omega-3 fatty acid deficiency and high fructose intake in the development of metabolic syndrome, brain metabolic abnormalities, and non-alcoholic fatty liver disease. *Nutrients, 5*(8), 2901–2923.
36. Centers for Disease Control and Prevention. (2015). *2014 national diabetes statistics report.* Retrieved from http://www.cdc.gov/diabetes/data/statistics/2014statisticsreport.html
37. Lustig, R. H. (2013). *Fat chance: The bitter truth about sugar.* London, UK: Fourth Estate.
38. Lustig, R. H. (2009). Sugar: The bitter truth. YouTube. Retrieved from https://www.youtube.com/watch?v=dBnniua6-oM
39. Boyles, S. (2010, April 10). High-sugar diet linked to cholesterol. WebMD. Retrieved from http://www.webmd.com/heart-disease/news/20100420/high-sugar-diet-linked-lower-good-cholesterol#1
40. Welsh, J., Sharma, A., Abramson, J. L., Vaccarino, V., Gillespie, C., & Vos, M. B. (2010). Caloric sweetener consumption and dyslipidemia among U.S. adults. *JAMA, 303*(15), 1490–1497.
41. Daily Mail Reporter. (2013, September 16). Diet starts today . . . and ends on Friday: How we quickly slip back into bad eating habits within a few days. Dailymail.uk. Retrieved from http://www.dailymail.co.uk/news/article-2421737/Diet-starts-today—ends-Friday-How-quickly-slip-bad-eating-habits-days.html
42. U.S. Department of Agriculture. (n.d.). WIC fact sheet. Retrieved from http://www.fns.usda.gov/sites/default/files/wic/WIC-Fact-Sheet.pdf
43. American Academy of Pediatrics. (n.d.). Statement opposing Congressional intervention in the WIC food packages. Retrieved from https://www.aap.org/en-us/advocacy-and-policy/federal-advocacy/Documents/AAPJointStatementOpposingCongressionalInterventioninWIC.pdf
44. Nestle, M. (2016, February 26). Potatoes. Food Politics Blog. Retrieved from http://www.foodpolitics.com/tag/potatoes/
45. Delisle, H. (2002). *Programming of chronic disease by impaired fetal nutrition: Evidence and implications for policy and intervention strategies.* World Health Organization. Retrieved from http://apps.who.int/iris/bitstream/10665/67126/1/WHO_NHD_02.3.pdf
46. Barker, D. J. (1990). The fetal and infant origins of adult disease. *BMJ, 301*(6761), 1111.
47. Negrato, C. A., & Gomes, M. B. (2013). Low birth weight: Causes and consequences. *Diabetology and Metabolic Syndrome, 5*(1), 1.
48. Braveman, P., & Barclay, C. Health disparities beginning in childhood: A life-course perspective. *Pediatrics, 124*(Suppl 3), S163–S175.
49. Hebeisen, D. F., Hoeflin, F., Reusch, H. P., Junker, E., & Lauterburg, B. H. (1992). Increased concentrations of omega-3 fatty acids in milk and platelet rich plasma of grass-fed cows. *International Journal for Vitamin and Nutrition Research, 63*(3), 229–233.
50. *Scientific American.* (2012, May 1). For a healthier country, overhaul farm subsidies. Retrieved from http://www.scientificamerican.com/article/fresh-fruit-hold-the-insulin/
51. Pollan, M. (2010, June 10). The food movement, rising. *The New York Review of Books.* Retrieved from http://www.nybooks.com/articles/archives/2010/jun/10/food-movement-rising/
52. Kovacic, W. E. (2008). *Marketing food to children and adolescents: A review of industry expenditures, activities, and self-regulation.* Federal Trade Commission. Retrieved from https://www.ftc.gov/sites/default/files/documents/reports/marketing-food-children-and-adolescents-review-industry-expenditures-activities-and-self-regulation/p064504foodmktingreport.pdf
53. Bauer, U. E., Briss, P. A., Goodman, R. A., & Bowman, B. A. (2014). Prevention of chronic disease in the 21st century: Elimination of the leading preventable causes of premature death and disability in the USA. *The Lancet, 384*(9937), 45–52.
54. Cawley, J., & Maclean, J. C. Unfit for service: The implications of rising obesity for U.S. military recruitment. *Health Economics, 21*(11), 1348–1366.
55. McGraw, T. (2013). Combating food deserts through incentivizing local businesses. *The Cornell Roosevelt Institute Policy Journal Center for Healthcare Policy, 15.*
56. Pollan, M. (2008, October 12). Farmer in chief. *New York Times Magazine.* Retrieved from http://michaelpollan.com/articles-archive/farmer-in-chief/
57. Freudenberg, N. (2014). *Lethal but legal.* New York, NY: Oxford Press.
58. Corbett, A. (2015). Blurred lines: The food marketing landscape and its effect on children's health. *2015 APHA Annual Meeting and Expo.* Chicago, IL. October 31–November 4, 2015.
59. Philadelphia first major city in U.S. to pass sugary drink tax. (2016, June 16). *NBC News.* Retrieved from http://www.nbcnews.com/nightly-news/video/philadelphia-first-major-city-in-u-s-to-pass-sugary-drink-tax-707171395512
60. Anderson, L. M., Quinn, T. A., Glanz, K., Ramirez, G., Kahwati, L. C., Johnson, D. B., . . . Task Force on Community Preventive Services. (2009). The effectiveness of worksite nutrition and physical activity interventions for controlling employee overweight and obesity: A systematic review. *American Journal of Preventive Medicine, 37*(4), 340–357.

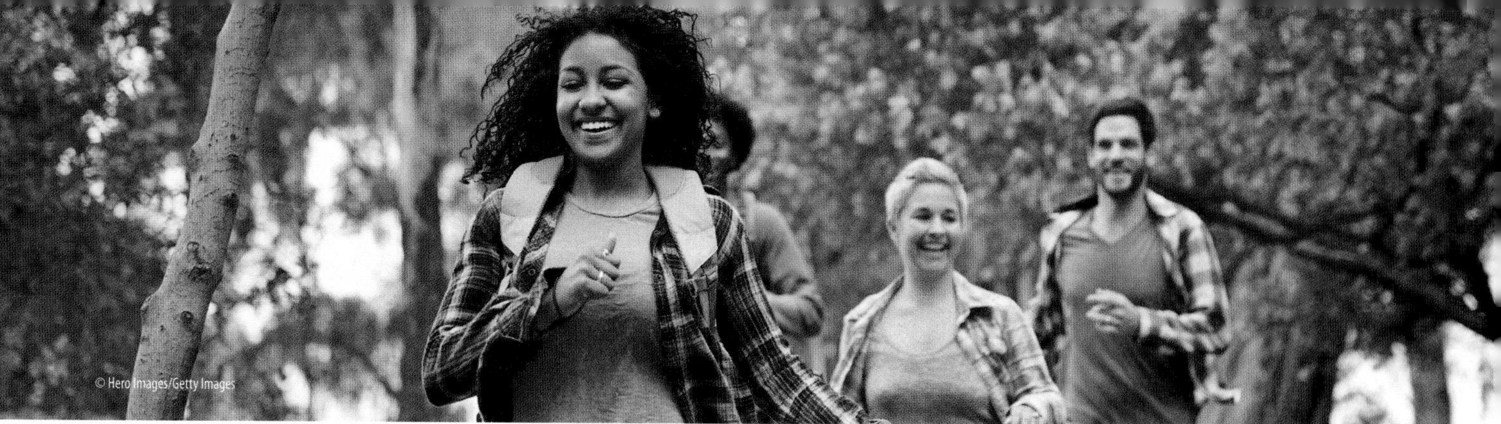
© Hero Images/Getty Images

CHAPTER 3

Let's Get Moving! Active Living for Better Health

CHAPTER OBJECTIVES

- Explain the benefits of exercise for physical, cognitive, and emotional health.
- Define key terms related to physical activity.
- Discuss and analyze the different forms of physical exercise.
- Discuss important behaviors to support exercise (stretching, breathing, rest, sleep).
- Explore key questions faced by communities to incorporate more societal opportunities for active living.

For most of us, the single best way to ensure good health, quality of life, and longevity is through **exercise**.[1,2] While eating well, making safe choices, and having good genes are all important, more and more evidence is showing us that exercise may be the most effective pathway to a lifetime of good health.[3] In fact, one recent study has shown that lack of exercise can be twice as deadly as obesity alone.[4]

exercise A form of physical activity that is usually planned, structured, and repetitive.

However exercise does much more than help you live longer. It improves your immune system, which can help you prevent colds, flu, and other communicable diseases. Activities like walking, running, biking, dancing, and weight training keep your muscles and bones strong, which helps you exercise more efficiently and allows you to reap more of the benefits that come from **physical activity**. Those benefits are numerous! Because exercise improves circulation, nutrient delivery, and toxin removal throughout your body, all of your organs benefit from exercise. Even your skin benefits, which explains the "glow" some people experience after working out, even after the perspiration has dried off.

physical activity The broad category of bodily movement that results in energy expenditure.

Exercise boosts blood flow to the brain and helps it receive and use oxygen and nutrients. This process enhances neurologic function, enabling you to think more clearly and perform better academically.[1,5–7] When the body exercises, the brain releases neurotransmitters such as serotonin and dopamine, which lead

endorphins Hormones that improve neurologic function and produce feelings of well-being and happiness.

to feelings of alertness and well-being. Exercise also activates the release of **endorphins** in the brain. Endorphins are hormones that improve neurologic function and produce feelings of well-being and happiness. People with depression have low levels of endorphins. Studies have found that there is a significant and positive relationship between physical activity and happiness, just as there is a correlation between lack of physical activity and feelings of anxiety and depression.[8,9]

People who exercise are less likely to develop cancer, particularly colon, breast, prostate, and lung cancers.[10] Some of the effects of exercise, such as body fat reduction and insulin regulation, seem to be what protects us against many forms of cancer. For example, when a person exercises, there is a reduction of blood estrogen level, and this appears to be one of the reasons that physical activity has been shown to help prevent breast cancer in women.[11] Likewise, exercise produces changes in digestive acids, which have been shown to specifically protect against colon cancer.[12]

metabolism The process that occurs inside the body at the cellular and the physiological levels to generate energy and maintain life. Metabolism consists of two fundamental stages—catabolism and anabolism.

Regular exercise also contributes to a consistent and healthy **metabolism**—the rate at which the body burns food for energy. Regulation of your metabolism is one of the key reasons exercise can help you prevent excessive weight gain.

If nothing else, exercise simply makes it easier to get around, and for many people, that can contribute to feelings of confidence and self-assurance.

Convinced yet? We hope so. But the benefits of exercise go beyond each person's individual health. The level at which we incorporate physical activity into our communities is an essential population health issue. Inactivity has been declared as one of the leading risk factors of death in the United States, and around the world.[13] Growing rates of sedentary lifestyles among the general population create a burden to society in doctor, hospital, and pharmaceutical expenses, government disability payments, and numerous other public costs. These can be people missing work from illness or disability, and family members needing to care for loved ones suffering from these health effects.

According to many experts, U.S. rates of obesity from inactivity and poor nutrition are now an issue of national security. In 2010, the retired chairs of the U.S. Joint Chiefs of Staff, John Shalikashvili and Hugh Shelton, testified that the nation is less able to defend itself than it once was. Currently, more than one-quarter of Americans ages 17 to 24 years are too overweight to serve in

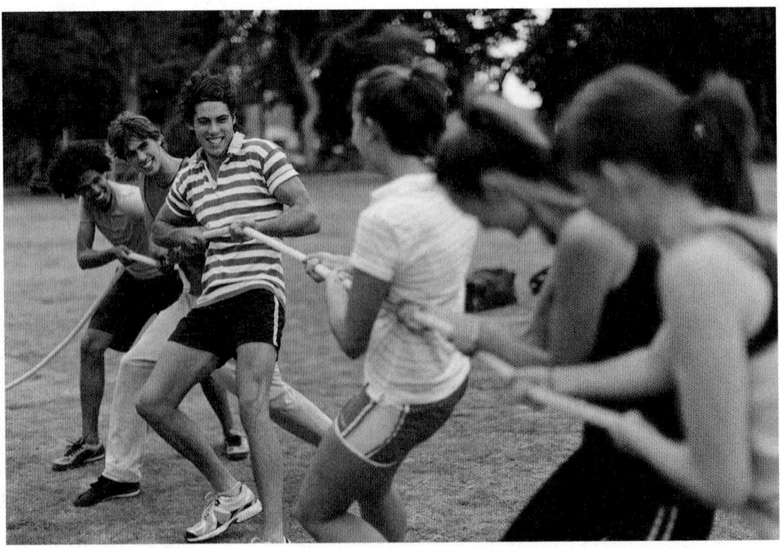

Exercise leads to self-confidence.

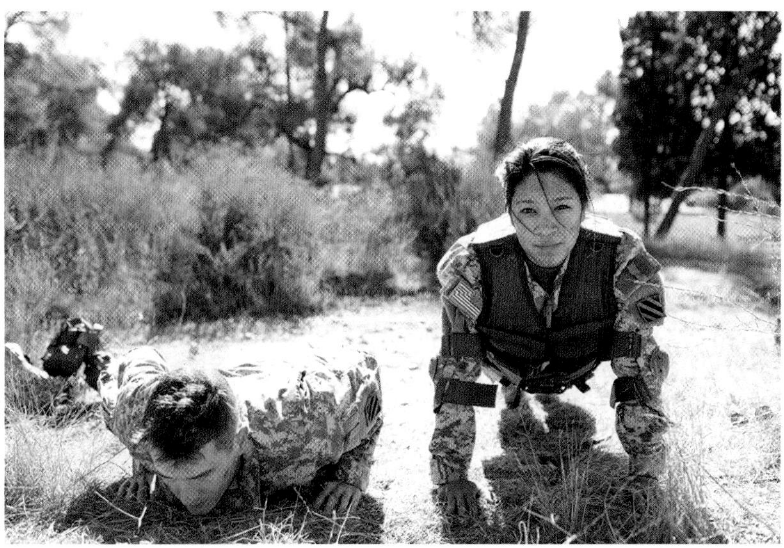

Public fitness is a military issue. Military disqualification and its effect on national security is an example of the indirect costs associated with the increase in sedentary lifestyles among Americans.

the military.[14] In 2015, Major General Allen Batschelet, in charge of U.S. Army Recruiting Command, revealed that 10% of Army recruits are disqualified from military service due to obesity and said that obesity is the most troubling issue in army disqualification because "the trend is going in the wrong direction."[15]

Society pays two types of costs associated with our obesity and obesity-related conditions: direct and indirect. Direct costs are health and healthcare services such as the surgeries and pharmaceutical drug therapies that result directly from sedentary lifestyles. These costs can stem from physical conditions, such as obesity, diabetes, heart disease, and cancer, but also from mental and emotional issues. There is a strong link between anxiety and depression and chronic inactivity.

Indirect costs include lost wages or other types of lost productivity that affect our overall economy when employees miss work from issues such as sickness and depression. Increased rates of health insurance from rising health expenses due to sedentary lifestyles are another indirect cost. Military disqualification and its effect on national security is also an example of the indirect costs associated with the increase in sedentary lifestyles among Americans.[16] In 2015, direct costs in the United States associated with inactivity were estimated to be over $100 billion.[17] The indirect costs, while difficult to quantify, bring the economic cost even higher.

Fitness or Exercise: What's the Difference?

While it is common to think of the terms **fitness**, *exercise*, and *physical activity* as interchangeable, there are subtle differences that affect how we promote active living on college campuses and throughout our communities.

fitness The ability to perform required activities to complete a task or a job.

In the 1980s, government policy and public health experts developed a health promotion plan to get more people to engage in exercise at least three times per week. The idea was to help people participate in running, aerobics, weight training, and other forms of intense exercise. Unfortunately, few people changed their behavior. People who already exercised regularly kept doing it, but those who did not were unlikely to start based on the marketing. Many people even reported feeling guilty or more depressed after being told they should be exercising more when they did not make the changes. So much for the well-being associated with exercise! Enter the **active living** perspective, which places more responsibility on those who have the power to create environments that are more likely to encourage people to move more vigorously and more frequently. By expanding the definition of physical activity to include using stairs, walking to work, gardening, or performing housework, efforts to promote active living began to increase among advocates for healthy living.

active living An expanded definition of physical activity that includes normal daily activities, such as using stairs, walking to work, gardening, or performing housework.

It is important to reach a basic understanding of the terminology to ensure that we are all talking about the same thing when it comes to fitness and exercise. *Physical activity* is the broad category of bodily movement that results in energy expenditure. This energy expenditure is usually measured in kilocalories, and can come through walking to work, household chores, or occupational activities such as waiting on tables or cleaning hotel rooms. Physical activity in daily life is often categorized into occupational, sports, conditioning, household, or other activities.

Exercise is a form of physical activity and is usually planned, structured, and repetitive. It involves objectives, such as maintaining fitness or performance goals. These goals may include running for distance, lifting specific amounts of weight, or losing weight. There is no precise point at which "physical activity" becomes "exercise." An activity becomes exercise when you plan to do it and think of it as exercise. Thus, household chores thought of as dull or tedious activities can become exercise when you think of them that way. Studies have shown that people who are conscious of the health benefits of activities like vacuuming are more likely to lose weight than those who did not think of the health benefits of the same activities. Attitude counts!

skill-related fitness A set of attributes that allows someone to respond to the physical demands of a particular skill or activity, such as construction or textile work. These attributes can be measured with specific tests, such as those measuring agility, speed, reaction time, and balance.

health-related fitness Fitness measures intended to ensure overall health.

Originally the term *fitness* meant the ability to perform required activities to complete a task or a job. This is now often called "skill-related" fitness, which means possessing a set of attributes that allow someone to respond to the physical demands of a particular skill or activity, such as construction or textile work. One can measure these attributes with specific tests, such as determining agility, speed, reaction time, and balance (the way the U.S. military uses such tests). "Health-related" fitness is more generally applied to maintaining physical health throughout the life span. Rather than occupational or **skill-related fitness**, this chapter is more focused on **health-related fitness**, and its components of cardiorespiratory fitness, musculoskeletal fitness, and **body composition**.

body composition The amount of body fat in proportion to overall weight. Body composition is improved through losing fat, increasing lean muscle, or a combination of both.

Being on the same page about our goals allows us to create the path to reach those goals. If our objective is to achieve fitness around specific tasks, it helps if we all agree what the tasks are, especially if someone else is evaluating our progress. We continue to learn more about the pathways to achieving success in different occupations and different sports. For example, new science tells us that **muscular strength** and weight training may be less beneficial for success in some sports, such as tennis or fencing, than we used to think. Likewise, as schools recognize that it may be less important that students graduate with the knowledge of how to throw a football than with an understanding of how to build **flexibility** through yoga poses, the approach to how we construct physical education classes must change.

muscular strength The ability of a muscle to exert force against resistance, which comes from the cells providing energy to the muscle fibers for different forms of contractions (concentric, eccentric, and isometric) that initiate power and strength.

flexibility The range of motion of a person's joints, the ability of the joints to move freely, and the mobility of the muscles, which allows for more movement throughout the person's body.

As you consider ways to begin or improve your individual activity habits, you may ask yourself what you want to achieve in the near term and the long term (however you choose to define those). This exploration will help you figure out the most effective and enjoyable ways to achieve your goals and objectives.[18–20]

Why Are We Less Active Now Than We Once Were?

Based on the Centers for Disease Control and Prevention's body mass index data, approximately one out of every eight preschool children in the United States is obese.[21] While there have been some signs of improvement in recent years, they are only small blips in an otherwise downward trend over the course of the 20th century and into the 21st. There seem to be several important rea sons we are less active than we used to be. For one thing, we are walking less due to the steady increase in the use of automobiles throughout the 20th century, and the parallel construction of car-centric neighborhoods that encourage driving to and from work, school, and grocery shopping.

Another critical factor seems to be the steady reduction in physically oriented jobs. During the 20th century, industrial machinery replaced much of the work previously done using human power. During this time, we started to see an increase in desk jobs involving computers and other technology designed to make work easier and more efficient. Between 1950 and 2012, the number of sedentary jobs increased more than 80%.[22] Screen time in front of computers and televisions among children has also increased since the 1970s, along with the amount of time spent in cars by their parents.[23]

Human inactivity is becoming a serious global concern. Lack of exercise alone has been linked to significant percentages of the world's cases of heart disease, diabetes, and cancers. According to the World Health Organization, sedentary lifestyles kill more than five million people each year. Latin America is particularly vulnerable, where the rate of physical inactivity is among the highest in the world.[24]

For all of these reasons, physical fitness has a direct and immediate connection to how we personally feel and how our society functions. Physical activity is now recognized as one of the most important issues in global health.[25]

Getting Started: What's Best for Me? What's Best for Us?

You have unique needs and interests, and physical activity can take many different forms. Your preferences, personal style, and physiological and athletic goals influence the type of exercise you want to do and how frequently you work out. Also, many people have different abilities and disabilities that influence the ways they exercise. While some people are devoted to rigorous exercise and feel comfortable doing it, others have different preferences. Many of us love the excitement and intense competition of a team sport like basketball, soccer, or football, while others prefer the solitude of running. Others seek inner peace and relaxation through the calm movements of tai chi or yoga.

These same issues apply to families, cultures, and nations. Governments grapple with decisions about which activities to promote and how to do it. Because school-based physical education is an effective way to increase physical activity among youth,[26] school districts must determine the amount of time that should be required for each child to spend on physical activity during an average day. Because not only is physical activity good for physical health; studies have shown that physical activity during school hours leads to better *academic* results, too.[27]

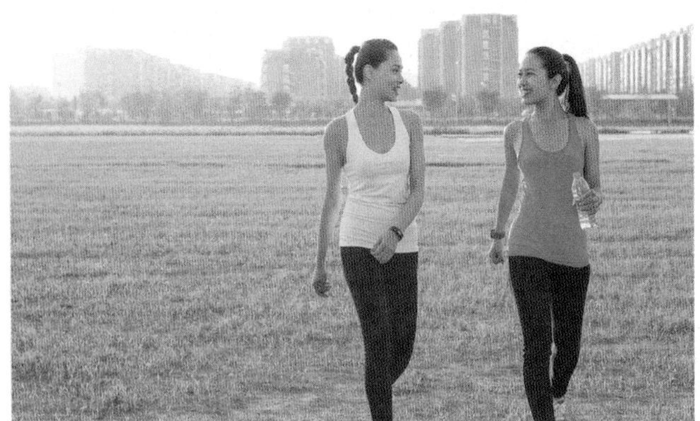

Parks have been shown to increase levels of physical activity among neighborhood residents and have also been shown to improve health beyond mere physical fitness.

One important public policy question is, "What should constitute physical activity?" This is becoming more relevant as trends change among students and as science teaches us more about the activities that are most effective at improving endurance, strength, flexibility, body composition, and well-being. High school and college physical education classes still tend to emphasize traditional sports such as soccer, basketball, and volleyball. But unfortunately, this can cause students who are less interested in these competitive activities to lose the motivation to participate, and even to lose interest in physical activity altogether.[28] Activities such as yoga, tai chi, qigong, and pilates are gradually being introduced in schools and colleges, providing students with more options and allowing people with different preferences and backgrounds to enjoy the benefits of physical fitness. These activities, in contrast to the emphasis on speed and coordination of traditional sports-oriented physical education courses, allow students to develop additional beneficial habits and skills, such as breathing and stretching (yoga), muscle-core stabilization and alignment (pilates), and balance and coordination (tai chi).

Public parks play an important role in facilitating physical activity.[26,29] They also contribute to human health in ways that go beyond activity. By promoting natural environments and serving as gathering places for family and friends, parks have been demonstrated to contribute to improving individual and public health.[30] For these reasons, communities must carefully consider questions about where parks should be located and the kinds of activities that should be encouraged in those parks. Such questions may seem obvious, but research continues to demonstrate that racial, ethnic, economic, and even gender disparities still exist in terms of who has access to parks and how those parks are used.[31] Too often, there is no process for community input regarding where parks or other recreation facilities should be located. It is a mistake not to ask the community about the facilities and activities they want and need. The good news is that cities and neighborhoods are increasingly looking at how our public spaces can encourage physical activities that community members will actually engage in. These efforts are sometimes called "community needs assessments."[32]

The Changing Nature of Physical Activity in the United States

Communities face other policy choices that can impact how physical activity is encouraged. When our roads are primarily built for cars with only minimal space for pedestrians or bicycles, it is no surprise that fewer people than we would like walk or ride bikes. But when a community converts a former railway line or crumbling aqueduct into a new walking and biking path, physical activity becomes more accessible to more people (**FIGURE 3-1**). Research tells us that people walk more when sidewalks are available and safe, and bicycle ridership increases when bike lanes are plentiful, wide, and separated from car traffic.[33,34]

When a new public building has a clear and accessible elevator but a stairway that is dark, hidden, and maybe a little scary, it's no wonder that people choose the elevator. When you consider that people may work in that building five days per week for several hours per day, this decision can translate to hundreds of thousands of steps during a single year and millions of calories that are not burned.

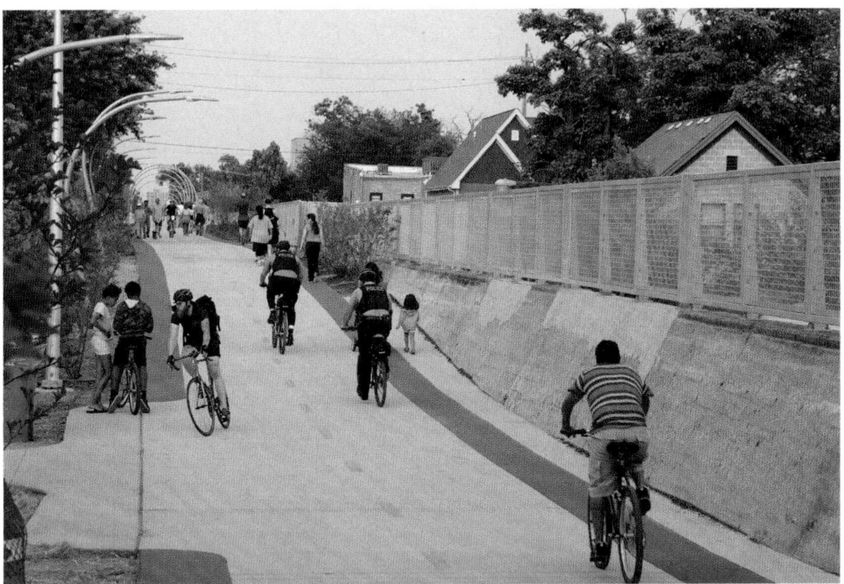

FIGURE 3-1 The Bloomingdale Trail. In 2015, when the city of Chicago converted 2.7 miles of elevated railroad track into the Bloomingdale Trail, it increased fitness opportunities for cyclists, runners, in-line skaters, and stroller-pushing parents.

GOING UPSTREAM

Racial Inequities in Physical Activity

Racial, ethnic, and income-based health inequities persist when it comes to environments that encourage or discourage physical activity. Studies show that African American, Hispanic, and other minority groups in the United States remain less likely to meet federal exercise guidelines than their White counterparts.[35,36] An important factor is racially segregated neighborhoods (**FIGURE 3-2**). Minority communities are still less likely than predominantly White neighborhoods to include social and physical environments that encourage activity.[36,37] These opportunities can include access to safe parks and playgrounds, quality recreational facilities, and well-constructed sidewalks and biking paths.

What are the causes of these inequities? In many cases, they come from explicitly racist 20th century policies, such as those practiced by the Federal Housing Administration (FHA), which was established by the U.S. Congress to insure private mortgages for homebuyers. In the middle of the 20th century, the FHA set policies that prohibited insuring mortgages in predominantly African American neighborhoods. This policy, called "redlining," occurred in most major cities across the United States, and it allowed racial segregation to grow even worse. The effects of these policies are still felt today, where people of color remain less likely to live near major parks and other areas where opportunities for recreation are safe and plentiful. While this situation is changing, the effects are still there well into the 21st century.

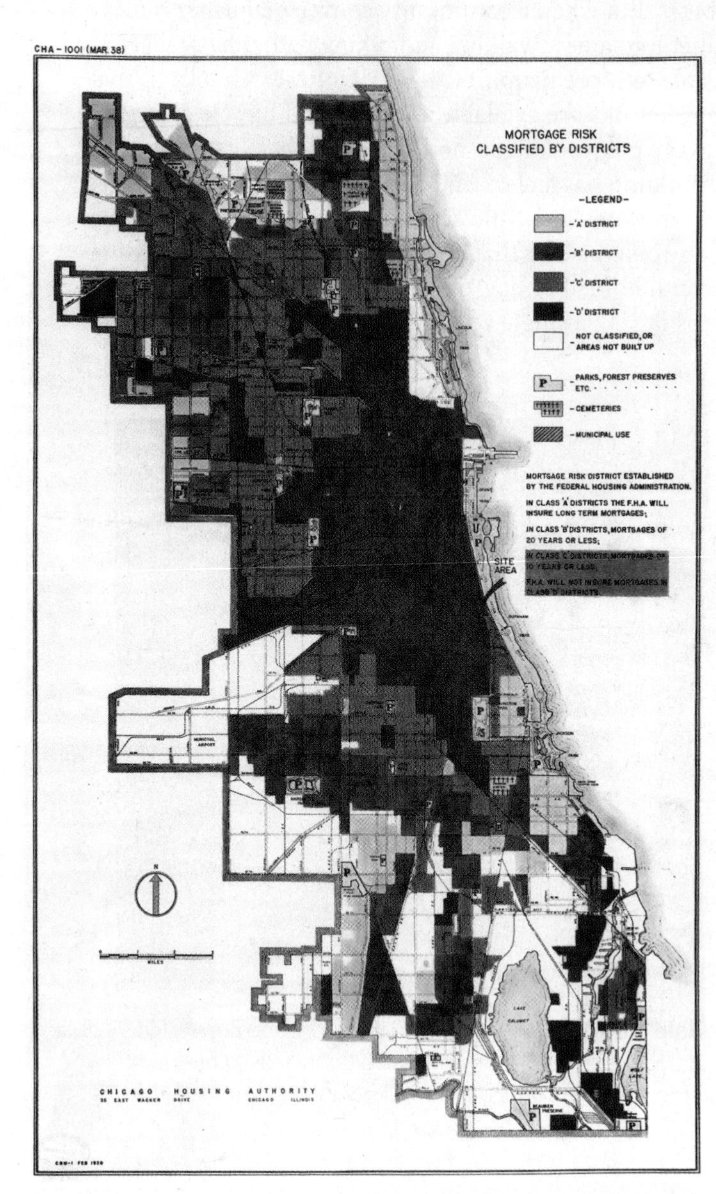

FIGURE 3-2 In the early 20th century, the Home Owners' Loan Corporation, an entity of the US Government, used maps to identify minority neighborhoods where home lending was to be discouraged. This policy, called "redlining," resulted in much lower home ownership within communities of color, and contributed to the racial and ethnic health disparities that persist across the US today.

Reproduced with permission from The University of Chicago Department of Art History

Finding Your Own Path to Fitness

This chapter presents some different ways that you can think about fitness, exercise, and physical activity. Our intent is to help you choose a path to fitness that you can enjoy, develop, and sustain over your entire life. As you think through the science, the general recommendations for physical activity, and the specific recommendations for different performance needs, you should be able to make some decisions about the best activities for you.

While moderate physical activity is good for your health, regular vigorous activity is even better. The U.S. Department of Health and Human Services (DHHS) guidelines recommend around 30 minutes of moderate activity per

TABLE 3-1 Examples of Moderate and Vigorous Physical Activity

Moderate Activity	Vigorous Activity
Walking: 30 minutes	Walking stairs: 15 minutes
Volleyball: 45 minutes	Shoveling dirt or snow: 15 minutes
Raking leaves: 30 minutes	Running or jogging: 15 minutes
Slow lap swimming: 20 minutes	Basketball: 20 minutes

U.S. Department of Health and Human Services, Centers for Disease Control and Prevention, National Center for Chronic Disease Prevention and Health Promotion. (1996). Physical activity and health: A report of the Surgeon General. Atlanta: USDHHS.

day for at least 5 days each week, or 75 minutes of vigorous activity per week, with at least 10 minutes spent per activity at a time. Of course, these activities can vary considerably. **TABLE 3-1** provides an approximate comparison between moderate and vigorous activity.

As you think about your path to fitness, you might ask the following: What policy choices would allow more people to experience the exhilaration that comes from vigorous activity? How can we get more communities to reap the benefits of sports and activity leagues? How do we ensure that a safe walk to work or school is available to everyone? What can we do to increase the use of stairs in our schools and public buildings?

In other words, what can we do to make fitness, exercise, and active living the easy and affordable choice, rather than the difficult or expensive one? After all, health should be accessible to everyone, and not a luxury, only available to some.

Starting From Within

Fitness and exercise are highly personal activities. What you choose to do depends on your motivations, your goals, your abilities, your interests, your personal style, and the environment you live in. These differences can be seen even among people who do the exact same exercise!

For example, Aisha, who is 21 years old, may choose to take a daily vigorous 5-mile run through her city because she likes the way she feels afterward for the rest of the day—physically and mentally. Jorge, 25 years old, may run the exact same distance on his college campus because he wants to maintain a healthy weight. Sheila, 23 years old, may run the same distance with the same frequency but for a completely different reason: to improve endurance in the off-season for her role on the varsity basketball team. In other words, there is no right or wrong reason to exercise. The functional and well-being benefits are limitless.

Physical Activity: Recommendations for Adults

In 1996, the U.S. Public Health Service released *Physical Activity and Health: A Report of the Surgeon General.*[38] This report incorporated research on fitness and exercise to determine the role of physical activity in preventing disease and make recommendations for the public. Along with showing that regular physical activity can reduce the risk of heart disease, diabetes, numerous cancers, anxiety, and depression, the report discussed the levels of exercise that yield the most benefits. It concluded that benefits begin to occur with the amount of activity required to walk briskly for 30 minutes per day— and increase with more vigorous activity or when the moderate activity is done for more time.

In 2008, the DHHS released a new report, *Physical Activity Guidelines for Americans*, which featured more comprehensive recommendations on physical activity for children, adults, and seniors.[39] Among the recommendations outlined in the guidelines were the following[39]:

- To begin to achieve health benefits from exercise, adults should engage in 2.5 hours of moderate-intensity activity or 1.25 hours (75 minutes) of vigorous-intensity activity (or a combination of the two) per week. Aerobic activities such as running, biking, or cross-country skiing should be done for at least 10 minutes at a time and should be spread throughout the week—not just one long session.
- To achieve even greater benefits, adults should increase activity to a total of 5 hours per week of moderate aerobic physical activity or 2.5 hours per week of vigorous activity.
- Even greater health benefits are seen when muscle strengthening activities involving all major muscle groups are done for at least 2 days per week in addition to the aerobic activities.

The Components of Health-Related Fitness

The concept of health-related physical fitness consists of the elements of fitness that most directly relate to good health. While skills-based components, such as a short sprint or a high jump, can give us good information about performance, they don't always give an indication of someone's overall health. Health-related fitness measures can do that, which is why we will be focusing on those components of fitness here.

UP FOR DEBATE

To Measure or Not?

Physical activity can be measured and evaluated in different ways. One way of quantifying exercise is to look at a measure called metabolic equivalents (METs), where 1 MET is the energy it takes to simply sit still. The average adult consumes about 1 calorie per every 2.2 pounds of body weight per hour when sitting quietly, so someone who weighs 160 pounds would burn approximately 70 calories an hour just sitting still. Moderate activities such as walking burn around five times as much energy as sitting, which would be 5 METs. Vigorous activities, such as running up an inclined treadmill can burn 6 to 10 METs. Of course, people have different levels of fitness, so the same activity can consume different MET levels for different people. Nevertheless, it remains an effective method for comparing types of activities.

Another way to measure fitness is through health-based and skill-based tests. Although they can be closely related, skill-based tests, such as a 40-yard sprint or a vertical jump, measure performance and are closely connected to athletic ability. Health-based tests tend to be more focused on measuring functional well-being, such as the range of motion of a shoulder or flexibility through the ability to touch one's toes when sitting on the floor with the legs straight out and parallel.

Many fitness tests include "norms," through which we can compare ourselves to others. While many people have no interest in completing such tests, others are curious about how they compare to their peers. For these reasons, such tests may be useful to some, while worthless to others. They are most appreciated by those who are interested in taking them, but they do allow us to develop an understanding of what the "baseline" measurements are from which we can improve. These tests should not be used to make people feel guilty, however. If you are in a "low" category, you simply have a lot of room to improve.

Sitting is now increasingly seen as a dangerous activity. As James Levine, MD, PhD, a researcher who has studied the effects of sedentary lifestyles for over 30 years, has said, "Sitting is more dangerous than smoking, kills more people than HIV, and is more treacherous than parachuting. We are sitting ourselves to death."[40] Research has concluded that long-term sitting can increase the risk of developing cancer, heart disease, and type 2 diabetes, to name just a few possible outcomes.[40] So, you can weigh into the debate for yourself and decide whether, and how intensely, to measure your exercise. But even if you do not take the time to measure every one of your movements, at least take time to move—as frequently and as much as possible.[41,42]

Health-related fitness includes the following components:

- Cardiorespiratory endurance
- Muscular strength
- Muscular endurance
- Flexibility
- Body composition

Cardiorespiratory Endurance

Cardiorespiratory endurance is the ability of your heart, blood vessels, and lungs to deliver oxygen and essential nutrients to your working muscles and remove toxins during vigorous physical activity. When you get that "huffing and puffing" feeling of exhaustion from running as fast as you can to get to class, you are experiencing the limits of your cardiorespiratory endurance.

In many ways, cardiorespiratory endurance is the most important health-related fitness component, as you can think of it as a measure of how efficiently your body functions. There is a close connection between cardiorespiratory endurance and the prevention of many poor health outcomes.

Regular aerobic activity improves your endurance. **Aerobic exercise** helps improve how the body uses oxygen. The word *aerobic* literally means "relating to or requiring oxygen," and can be defined as a continuous activity that elevates your heart rate to around 75% of your maximum rate. The longer you exercise and the higher your heart rate, the more aerobic capacity and endurance you build. **Anaerobic exercise** focuses on strengthening the muscles, while aerobic activity uses slow-twitch muscle fibers (more on that later). Anaerobic exercise burns more calories from fat than it does from **glycogen**; thus, this type of exercise leads to weight loss rather than muscle gain. Weight training is an anaerobic exercise, but so is short-distance sprinting or tennis. Anaerobic activities occur in short bursts and not one continuous stretch.

Cardiorespiratory endurance strengthens your heart and lungs and helps them to work more efficiently. Cardiorespiratory endurance improves your physical capacity to deal with stress and lowers your risk factors for numerous chronic diseases. Regular aerobic activity builds cardiorespiratory endurance and helps control obesity, high blood pressure, and high cholesterol. It can also cut your risk of developing heart disease in half.[43] Building cardiorespiratory endurance also helps reduce anxiety and depression and is your most effective method for keeping your body weight at a healthy level.

cardiorespiratory endurance The ability of the heart, blood vessels, and lungs to deliver oxygen and essential nutrients to the working muscles and remove waste products during vigorous physical activity.

aerobic exercise Exercise that helps improve how the body uses oxygen. The word *aerobic* literally means "relating to or requiring oxygen" and aerobic activity is commonly defined as continuous activity that elevates the heart rate to around 75% of its maximum rate.

anaerobic exercise Short-duration and high-intensity exercise that activates fast-twitch muscle fibers and strengthens muscles through activities such as sprinting, body building, and jumping.

glycogen A converted form of glucose that is stored in muscles and the liver.

Walking

Walking may be the easiest aerobic activity you can do, and several studies have proven that walking is good for your health. A consolidation of multiple studies has shown that regular walking reduces the risk of having a heart attack by 31%. To achieve the benefits of walking, all you have to do is walk 5 miles per week at a leisurely pace. If you walk even longer, and faster, you see even more health benefits, including weight loss and a decreased chance of suffering high blood pressure, diabetes, mental stress, dementia, cancer—even erectile dysfunction.[44]

How is walking technically different from running? "Racewalkers" must have at least one foot on the ground at all times. Runners are, at some point during their stride, suspended mid-air. Many serious walkers achieve significant health benefits, including improvements in hip mobility and upper body strength—often even above and beyond that of runners.

Walking outdoors seems to be especially beneficial for improving mood, with numerous studies looking at this issue from different perspectives.

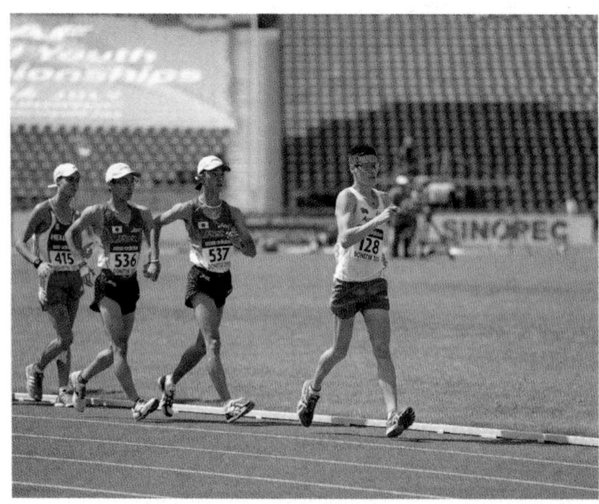

Racewalking—a serious sport. Walking is a great source of moderate exercise, and racewalking has been an Olympic event since 1904.

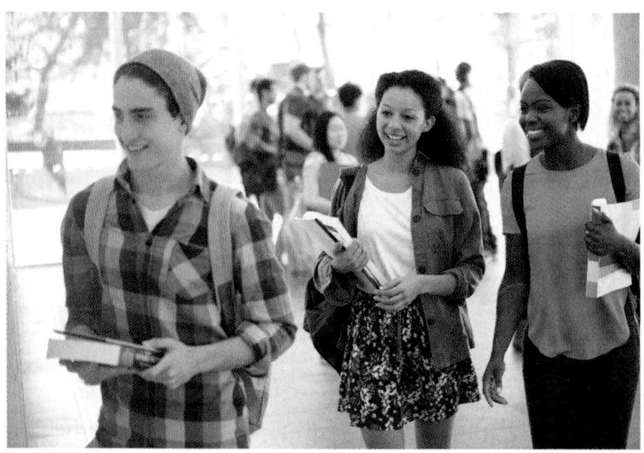

Walking on campus. Walking outdoors is especially beneficial for improving your mood. Walk your campus!

New research indicates that walking outside actually alters brain function in ways that improve emotional health. While walking on a treadmill is perfectly healthy, walking is even better when done outside.[45]

Running and Jogging

Although the American College of Sports Medicine (ACSM) has warned that running can put more strain on your back and knees than walking, there is evidence to indicate that the opposite is true. Regular jogging and running has been shown to reduce injuries and even heal the back and joints faster than if no running is done at all.[46] While weightlifting, soccer, and football have all been linked to early-onset knee arthritis and other injuries, the evidence shows that running does not lead to degeneration of the knees. In fact, a study at Stanford University found that regular running is more likely to lead to healthier knees than is remaining sedentary.[47] Of course, running can lead to falls, twisted ankles, and broken bones. Also, running too long and too often can lead to acute or overuse injury. One way of preventing such injury is to listen to your body; when it feels as though you may be overtaxing yourself, rest.

Along with the innumerable aerobic benefits that running provides, it is an extremely time-efficient way to get your exercise. In only 30 minutes, with no need to get yourself to a pool or a gym, you can have your daily workout over and done with. And it does not need to be 30 minutes. One study found that even 10 minutes per day of low-intensity running can extend life several years, when you compare it with not running at all.[48] The health and longevity benefits increase the more running you do, but after 2.5 hours of running per week (30 minutes per day, 5 days per week, for example), the benefits do not increase as quickly. This is why 2.5 hours has been called a "sweet spot" for weekly running levels.

One of the additional benefits of running is the so-called "runner's high"—a feeling of euphoria that runners can experience during their runs and long after the run is over. Scientists have found that during long jogs (at least 30 minutes) the prefrontal and limbic regions of the runner's brain produce the same endorphins felt with emotions like love. The body also produces endocannabinoids, similar to the chemical that produces the "high" of marijuana.[49] Some runners feel this sense of well-being most during their runs, while others insist the "high" stays with them throughout the day and is what gets some morning runners out of bed and onto the road at the dawn's earliest light.

UP FOR DEBATE

Wearables and Measurables: How Far Can You Go?

First invented in Japan in the 1960s, pedometers became popular in the early 2000s. Every night, people would read the numbers, write them down, and try to do better the next day. For many, the goal was 10,000 steps per day, a number agreed by many exercise researchers as a healthy target.[50]

Next came bracelets and apps that could track walking, running, biking, or skiing progress—how far and how fast you went, and where you traveled. Newer technologies are becoming smaller and more accurate and can be incorporated into patches that attach to a T-shirt or sports bra. Will your skin be next?

One of the questions facing society today is, how willing are we to allow this data to be used by others—employers, governments, or the company that makes each device? These technologies, formerly limited to individual data, can now provide information about millions of users. Companies such as Fitbit, Jawbone, Garmin, and Apple now have more aggregated information about exercise patterns than most public health departments. Researchers are now asking how we can harness all this information to encourage more and better activity. For example, if the data tells us too many bicyclists per day are trying to cross a bridge with inadequate bike lanes, this data could provide evidence of the need for wider lanes.

But when do we go too far? Would it be okay for a message to pop up while you are watching a video indicating that you have been sitting down for more than 3 hours without moving?

What do you think? Are you concerned about breaches of privacy? Are you okay with your data being part of a larger movement to encourage more healthy environments? What regulations and policies do you think should be in place today to encourage the best system of data collection and management in the future?

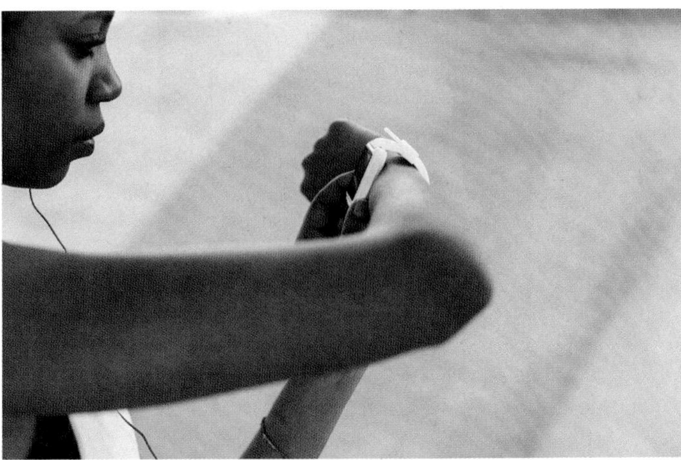

The quantified self. It is possible that even smart watches will seem clunky in the near future. What are the implications of these devices?

Swimming

From year to year, swimming has always been one of the top five most popular sports activities in the United States, and for good reason. There's none of the pavement-pounding that drives some people away from running, and it's relatively easy to do slowly. Many people report that they simply prefer water exercise to land activity.

It doesn't matter whether you prefer land or water, because the health benefits from swimming are similar to those that you get from walking, running, or cycling. Studies of swimmers have found the sport effectively reduces blood pressure and improves circulation, in the same way that other cardiorespiratory exercises do. And because of its steady temperature, water exercise hardly ever results in heat-based injuries, the way running in hot weather can.[51]

One side effect of swimming is that, for many people, it stimulates appetite more strongly than other exercises with the same level of exertion.[52]

Other Ways to Improve Cardiorespiratory Endurance

There's no limit to what you can do to improve your cardiorespiratory endurance: soccer, hockey, basketball, lacrosse, tennis, squash, cross-country skiing, rollerblading, hiking, dancing, and walking.

Muscular Strength

Muscular strength is the ability of a muscle to exert force against resistance, when your cells provide energy to your muscle fibers for contractions (concentric, eccentric, and isometric) that initiate power and strength. Muscular strength is an important health-related fitness component because it makes the day-to-day activities in life easier and more enjoyable. Muscle strength enhances basic activities, such as lifting and carrying things and helps you improve every higher-level activity you are involved in, from athletic performance to the performing arts.

There are numerous benefits to mild, moderate, or even intense strength training activities. Along with helping you maintain a fit and lean physique,[49,50]

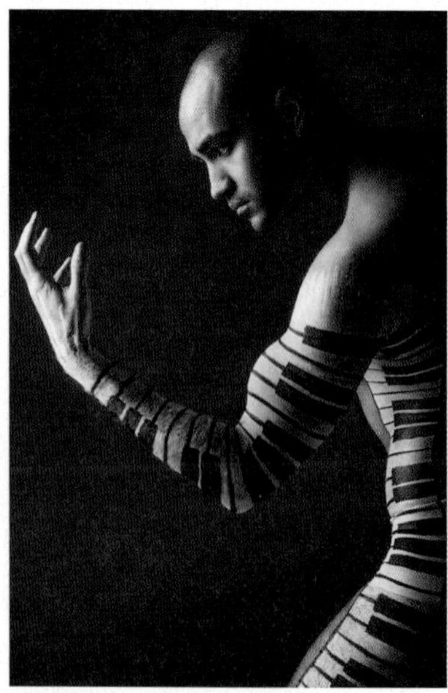

Weight training can enhance any physical activity. Emmanuel Vass is a classical pianist who "pumps iron" to stay in performance shape.

Photographer: Edward Taylor Model; Emmanuel Vass; Body art: Charlotte Mahdoodi.

it helps achieve healthier bone density, protect the skeletal system, and prevent chronic knee and back pain.[53] Weight training promotes a healthier metabolism and can play an effective role in maintaining a healthy weight, controlling blood sugar, and reducing diabetes. Unlike your fat tissue, muscle actually burns calories even when you are standing still. When you build more muscle, your resting metabolic rate becomes faster, which means you are burning more calories throughout the day, even when you are standing still.

When you work your major muscle groups, e.g., your back, chest, and shoulders, you are also training your smaller "stabilizer" muscles. Exercising these muscles, which is particularly effective when "free weights" are used, improves your balance and stability—both of which are important for day-to-day living and also for sports, public speaking, or playing music. Muscle training can also improve brain function.[53] Weight training can generate improvement for people of all ages from kids 6 years of age[52] to seniors 90 years of age and older.[53]

It may be difficult for a typical college student to understand this, but your body will not be as resilient in your later years as it is in your 20s and 30s. Building a healthy musculature now will reduce your risk of injury and improve your chances of a good quality of life long into the future.

How Muscle Growth Works

There are three types of muscles in the human body: smooth, cardiac, and skeletal. Smooth (also called involuntary) muscles are inside hollow organs such as the stomach, esophagus, and blood vessels. They are stimulated by involuntary neurogenic impulses. **Cardiac muscle** is the muscle that makes your heart function; it has both striated fibers, like the **skeletal muscle**, and smooth, involuntary muscles.

Skeletal muscle is what most people think about when they think of muscles. The muscles' myofibrils and sarcomeres form the fibers in the 650 skeletal muscles that lie beneath our skin. **FIGURE 3-3** shows some of the muscles most commonly involved in muscular strength training. Skeletal muscles receive signals from motor neurons, which direct the muscles to activate through contraction.

cardiac muscle A type of involuntary muscle tissue found only in the heart. This muscle constricts to remove blood from the heart and relaxes to fill the heart with blood.

skeletal muscle The muscle associated with muscle strength and endurance. These muscles contract when they receive signals from motor neurons, which direct the muscles to activate through contraction.

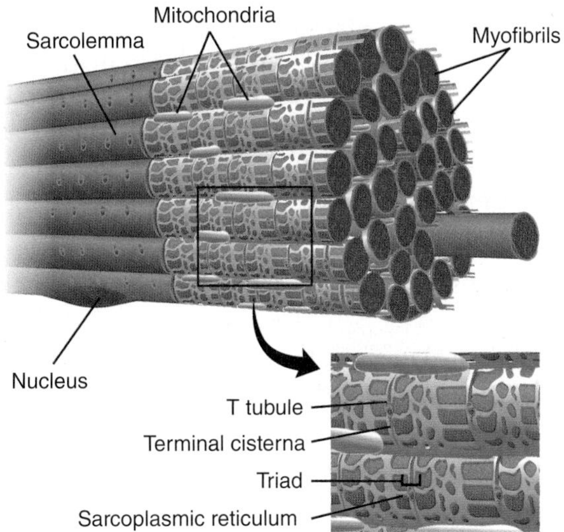

FIGURE 3-3 Skeletal muscle fiber.

One way a muscle gets stronger is by developing an ability to activate and contract more effectively. Motor unit recruitment, the process of activating the motor neurons in a muscle, determines a muscle's effectiveness. Motor unit recruitment improves through weight training.

Muscles strengthen by growing. When you work out with weights, you damage the muscles through natural stress and overload. After you stress the muscles during lifting, your body begins to repair the damaged fibers by forming new **muscle protein myofibrils**. The newly repaired myofibrils grow back with slightly increased thickness and in greater number, to create muscle growth (hypertrophy). Muscles continue to get stronger when you increase weight, repetitions, or sets. New forms of tension placed on the muscles can make the muscles even stronger.

muscle protein myofibrils A threadlike fiber that composes skeletal and cardiac muscle fibers.

Muscle growth occurs when the rate of muscle protein synthesis (growth) is greater than the rate of muscle protein breakdown. The soreness you experience after a workout, which can last for several days, comes from the localized muscle damage from stress and overload.

The process of strengthening the muscle occurs not during the weight training, but during recovery. That is why rest, diet, and rehabilitation, such as applying ice after hard workouts, is so important to the muscle-strengthening process.

Form Before Fitness: Technique Comes First!

Form and technique are absolutely critical elements to performing any physically demanding activity: from ballroom dancing to working with power tools. Before doing any exercise, it is important to learn the proper form and technique to ensure the most efficient, effective, and injury-preventive movements. Gym injury rates are higher among college students than the rest of the population.

Bad posture is one of the primary causes of workout-related injuries. It weakens the musculoskeletal structure over time and sets a bad precedent for your workout technique. This is why it is important to learn the basics of good posture, including the correct form for walking, running, sitting at a desk, or performing any activities you do for long periods (**FIGURE 3-4**). Ensuring good posture includes positioning your computer screen in a way that allows you to sit upright and comfortably.

Another cause of injury is lifting too much weight. Choosing the right weight is important to ensure proper posture. While guidelines depend on your own level of fitness and the specific exercise, the ACSM recommends performing a minimum of 8 repetitions for any weight training exercise. Except for very specific power-related goals, 8 to 12 repetitions of any exercise is ideal to accomplish your fitness, weight-maintenance, or performance-related goals.

Proper technique is critical to improving efficiency and reducing injury, and includes both posture and breathing. Here are some general guidelines to help you ensure proper posture for everything you do:

- Don't hunch your shoulders; keep them back and wide and relaxed, with your chest out.
- Pull your abdomen in slightly.
- For most lifting and pulling exercises, keep your feet about hip distance apart.
- Balance your weight evenly on both feet.
- Try not to tilt your head forward or backward or sideways. Keep it relatively straight.
- Don't forget to breathe and take some breaths before you start something difficult!

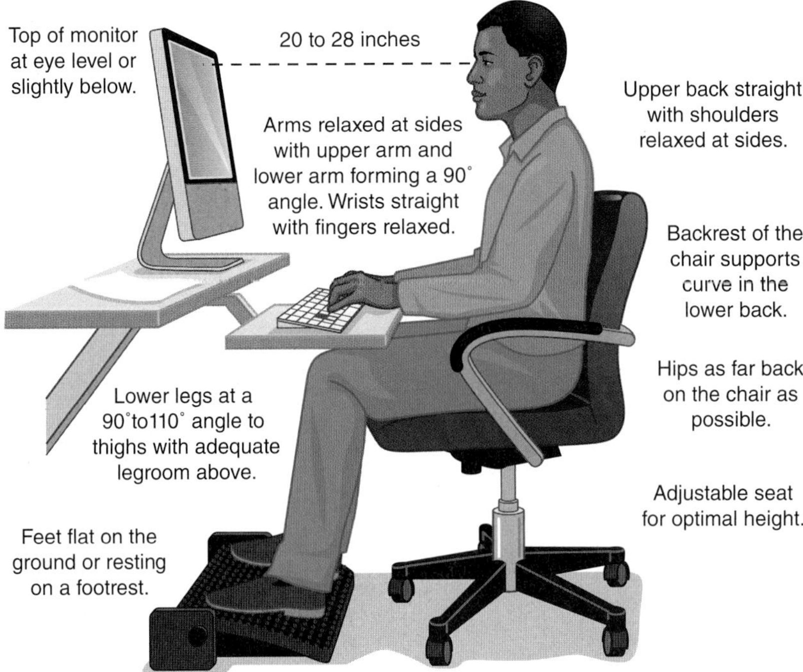

FIGURE 3-4 Proper sitting posture.

The following are a few exercises that can help you ensure proper posture and balance.

Advanced Reach. This exercise helps you align your hips with the rest of your body and trains the muscles in your pelvis and core to work together. To perform the exercise, start on all fours (your hands and knees). Raise your right leg straight back and point your toes. At the same time, bring your left arm up, reaching straight in front of you. Hold for a while: 3 seconds, 10 seconds, even longer if you can. Return to the starting position. Perform the movement with the other leg and arm. Do the exercise the same number of times on both sides.

Bridge Pose. The bridge pose can improve strength in your lower back, hips, and hamstrings. It provides a stretch to the neck, spine, and hips, and it improves blood flow and stimulation to the abdominal organs. Start by lying on your back with your knees bent and your feet flat on the floor. Gently thrust your hips toward the ceiling and clasp your hands beneath your buttocks. Hold for 30 to 60 seconds or as long as you can. Be sure to breathe freely throughout.

Plank Exercise. The plank is one of the best exercises you can do to strengthen your arms, shoulders, and abdominal muscles. It has even become an Internet phenomenon, with people posting pictures of their planks on their various social media platforms with hashtags such as #plank, #planking, and #plankqueens. Because it works isometrically (where muscles are static and don't stretch or contract), you are building strength through stability. There are many variations—resting on one arm at a time, resting on the elbows, turning to the side, etc. (look them all up!)— but doing the basic plank every day is a great way to gain strength and maintain a lean physique.

All these exercises have modifications and additional movements. There are several other exercises and poses for better posture, including single-leg

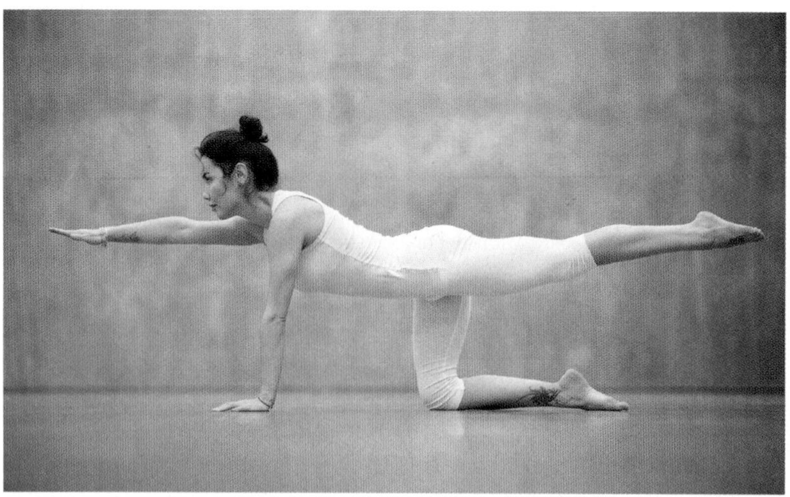

Advanced reach exercise (quadruped arm/leg raise).

© Fizkes/Shutterstock.

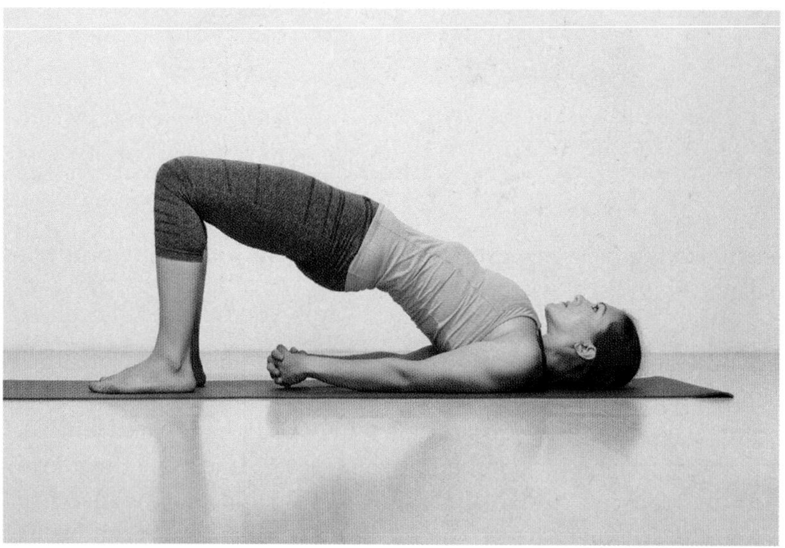

Bridge pose.

© DR Travel Photo and Video/Shutterstock.

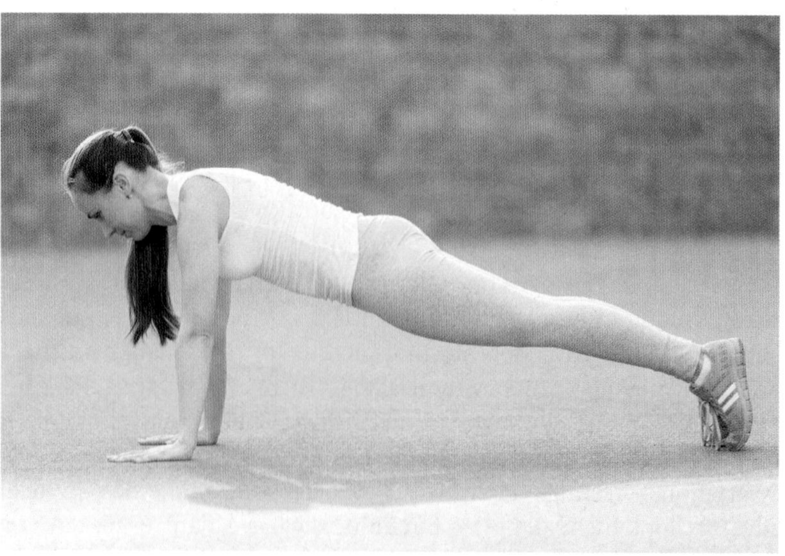

Plank exercise.

© fizkes/Shutterstock.

extensions, and back bends. Look these techniques up on the Internet; Doing any of them daily will help you improve posture and balance and performance in other sports.

Muscular Endurance

Muscular endurance is the ability of a muscle to exert force against resistance over repeated and prolonged periods. Compared to muscular strength, which draws on strength and power for activities requiring quick bursts, muscular endurance is the body's ability to perform activities of long duration but low intensity, such as doing repetitions of push-ups or sit-ups. Muscular endurance is important in nonathletic activities such as housework, yard work, construction—essentially any continuous physical effort.

muscular endurance The ability of a muscle to exert force against resistance over repeated and long periods. Compared to muscular strength, which draws on strength and power for short activities requiring quick bursts, muscular endurance is the body's ability to perform activities of long duration but low intensity, such as doing repetitions of push-ups or sit-ups.

While muscular strength is more specifically needed for sports requiring short bursts of energy such as lifting weights, muscular endurance is required for sports that require strength and power over time, such as hockey, soccer, tennis, boxing, swimming, cycling, downhill skiing, and long distance running. That "burn" you feel in your legs when you get to the top of a steep hill? You're feeling the limit of your muscular endurance.

Muscular endurance could involve a race from one end of the basketball court to the other, a 400-meter hurdle event, or a 100-mile bike ride. Using weights with several repetitions is often used to train for muscular endurance, but some physiologists and coaches rely on other, sometimes creative, ways to build more muscular endurance. Power endurance, a specific type of muscular endurance, is your ability to perform both types of power exercises (strength and speed) as long as possible and with the least amount of recovery time needed between movements. When you say, "Hold on a minute" before doing that next set of repetitions in the weight room, you are feeling the limits of your power endurance.

Power endurance training often relies on repeated bursts of activity, such as repeated basketball shots, football passes, or shots on a hockey goal. Squash, tennis, and racquetball, for example, require several shots made in succession, over and over, and power endurance is what you are tapping into by hitting the ball hard and accurately many times in a row. Martial arts and head-to-head sports such as wrestling also require quick bursts over and over to succeed.

There are two different types of muscle fibers, and they have different uses for different purposes. **Slow-twitch**, or type I, muscle fibers contract more slowly, are smaller, and have more oxidative (aerobic) capacity and less glycolytic (anaerobic) capacity than **fast-twitch** fibers, called type II. These are the muscle fibers needed for muscular endurance, as they can hold a steady paced twitch for long durations without fatigue. These fibers are most needed for endurance activities like long-distance running, cycling, and cross-country skiing. They can work for a longer time than fast-twitch muscles without getting tired. Fast-twitch muscles are effective for quick movements like jumping and sprinting. They contract quickly, but the fatigue is felt sooner than with the slow-twitch muscles.

slow-twitch Muscle fibers that contract more slowly, are smaller, and have more oxidative (aerobic) capacity, and less glycolytic (anaerobic) capacity than fast-twitch fibers. They are needed for endurance activities like long-distance running, cycling, and cross-country skiing. They can work for a longer time than fast-twitch muscles without getting tired.

fast-twitch Muscle fibers that are effective for quick movements like jumping and sprinting. They contract quickly, but fatigue is felt sooner than when using slow-twitch muscles.

Most of your muscles are made up of a mixture of both slow- and fast-twitch fibers. One exception is the soleus muscle in your lower leg and the muscles in your back used for posture, which are slow-twitch muscle fibers.

Many factors contribute to muscular endurance, including strength, fiber type, training, and even diet. All muscular activities produce greater levels of lactic acid. Larger muscles have greater muscle endurance than smaller muscles do, in part because they hold more glycogen, so these muscles will be able to sustain a series of contractions for a longer period.

TABLE 3-2 Sample Fitness Testing Norms

	Female	Male
1.5-Mile Run, Age 18–29 Years		
Superior	<12:34	<10:30
Good	12:34–13:45	8:26–10:30
Average	13:45–15:00	10:30–12:30
Fair	15:00–16:00	12:30–15:00
Low	>16:00	>15:00
3-Mile Bicycle Ride, Age 18–29 Years		
Superior	<9:30	<8:30
Good	9:30–10:15	8:24–10:12
Average	10:15–12:06	9:13–10:12
Fair	12:07–13:00	10:13–11:06
Low	>13:00	>12:00
1-Minute Push-Ups, Age 18–29 Years		
Superior	>35	>45
Good	21–35	30–44
Average	10–20	17–29
Fair	5–10	5–15
Low	<4	<4

Data from Keener, E. (1989). Undergraduate student physical fitness assessment. Muncie, IN: Ball State University.

Are you interested in measuring your own performance against norms of people within the 18- to 29-year-old category? **TABLE 3-2** shows norms from thousands of students conducted over several years at a large U.S. university and elsewhere.

What's the Right Order?

In general, it is probably best to perform strength training before a cardio workout. A strenuous aerobic workout can lead you to take shortcuts on ensuring the proper form for your weight training routine, which can cause injury. You will also have less energy to reach your strength and power objectives, which are a necessary component of strength training.

When exercising, the body draws on glycogen stores in both aerobic exercise and resistance training. To get the maximum benefits from your strength training workout, your body needs to tap into those glycogen stores to burn your stored fat as fuel for your exercise. Your body seeks glycogen as its primary source of energy during exercise, and if you have deprived it through a cardio workout, you won't have the strength to be as effective in the weight room as you would like. Insufficiency of glycogen leads to decreased performance and reduced chance of gaining strength and power in your muscles.

On the other hand, if you are primarily looking to lose fat through your workout, it makes sense to begin with cardio. Performing aerobic exercise first will deplete your supply of glycogen quickly, and then the body turns to its more long-term storage found in fat. This sequence will be more likely to result in a reduced chance of achieving your specific athletic goals and may increase the likelihood of injury, so be careful out there!

Flexibility

Flexibility refers to the range of motion of your joints, the ability of your joints to move freely, and the mobility of your muscles, which allows for more movement throughout your body.[54] Range of motion is the distance and direction your joints can move, while mobility is the ability to move without restriction.[55] Flexibility is essential for achieving smooth, efficient movement. It will improve your performance in any athletic pursuit, and it helps prevent muscle strains and injuries. Flexibility is closely associated with the prevention of lower-back pain and improved posture. Research has demonstrated that you can reduce your chances of having a heart attack by improving your ability to touch your toes through stretching.[56] Women generally have more flexibility than men because men have bulkier skeletal muscles.

Unfortunately, flexibility gets worse with age. As people get older, if they do not work on their flexibility, they begin to develop unhealthy postures and body movements. These postures, in turn, can make the health of their musculoskeletal system deteriorate. You may have seen this in middle-aged and older people—where they become stiff, with an uneven gait, or severely hunched over, which is why flexibility exercises are so important for older people.

Make sure you practice some basic regular stretching exercises throughout your life. There are several approaches to stretching, including picking up a basic routine of exercises or taking up fitness activities that place an emphasis on flexibility, such as yoga, tai chi, or qigong.

Flexibility is a great asset for high-performance athletes. A good example is multiple grand-slam tennis champion Novak Djokovic, for whom agility and flexibility always served as the cornerstone of his training, stretching for long periods, several times during the day. As his first coach, Jelena Gencic, once said, "We only worked on … only fitness on the court, not in the weight room."[57]

While much of your flexibility comes from genetics,[58] it is specific to each joint. You might have flexible knees and hamstrings, but your shoulders may be tight and stiff. It is important to get to know your body—your areas of strength, weakness, stiffness, and pliability—and to work on addressing your weak areas.

Methods to Improve Flexibility

Stretching. There are numerous ways to stretch your body to improve your flexibility (see **FIGURE 3-5** for some beginning ideas). The best way to start is by identifying (1) your personal goals—what activities you plan to do and what you seek to accomplish—and (2) your needs and limitations. For example, do

LENÔTRE
LENÔTRE
CÔTE D'AZUR
DUNLOP
SPORT
DUNLOP
SPORT
Façonnable
MIAMI
MONTE-CARLO
MASTERS
1000
ATP

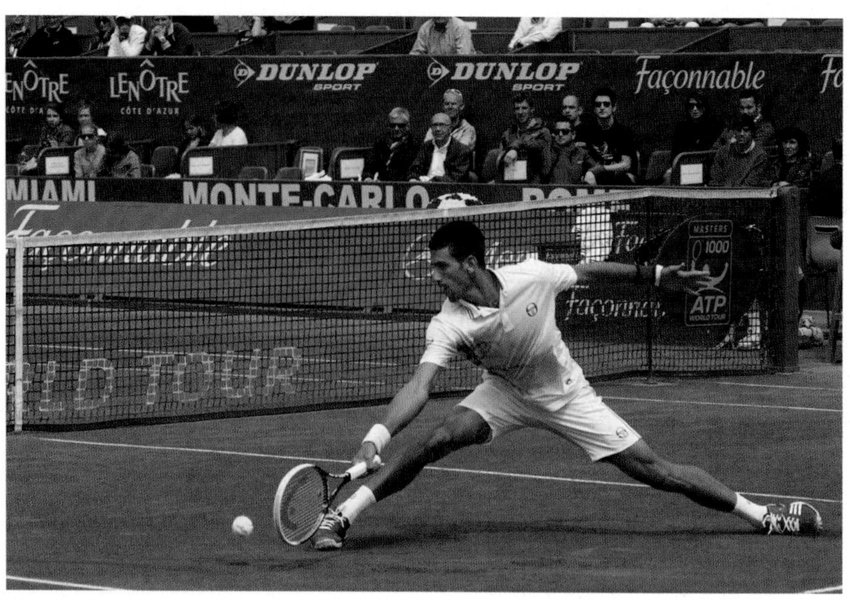

Flexibility: Essential for many high-performance athletes. Tennis star Novak Djokovic stretches several times per day as part of his fitness training.

1
Chest
2
Upper back
3
Back of upper arms
4
Calf
5
Back of thighs
6
Back of thighs
7
Front of thighs
8
Front of thighs
9
Outer thighs
10
Inner thighs
11
Inner thighs
12
Lower back
13
Lower back
14
Lower back
14
Torso

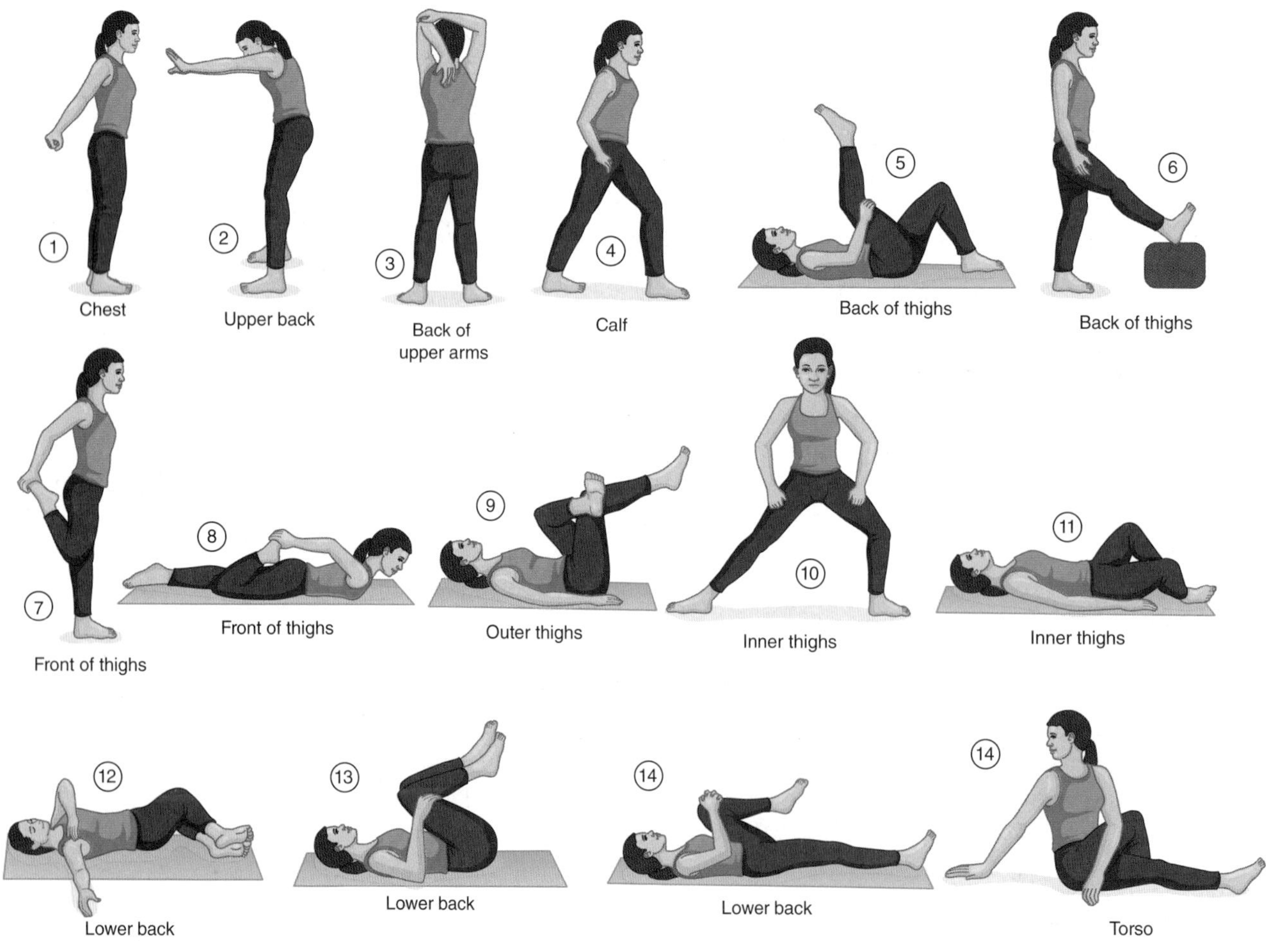

FIGURE 3-5 Sample stretching and flexibility exercises that can be done throughout your life. These stretches are examples of the many different possibilities available. Each can be done in short sets, holding for just a few seconds, or holding longer.

you have a hard time touching your toes when your legs are straight? You probably have tight hamstrings. If you feel your shoulders lack mobility, you should look into basic stretches to improve the flexibility in your shoulders.

While flexibility is clearly an important component of health-related fitness, stretching before exercise has not been shown to prevent injury. Despite what you may have been told in gym class or on your varsity sports team, studies have shown that "static stretching," or holding stretching poses for 15 seconds or more, does not specifically protect against injury. One study, conducted on runners, concluded that stretching "neither prevented nor induced injury when compared with not stretching before running."[59] There is also evidence that static stretching before a workout can actually *reduce* performance; one study, for example, showed that static stretching reduced vertical jump performance compared to not stretching.

When should you stretch, and what should you do before a workout, if anything? Recent research indicates that the best routine should consist of more of a warm-up than a stretch. You should start your workouts slowly and gradually increase the intensity, leading to some form of dynamic stretching where you are lightly bouncing to prepare for the movements you will be making later on. Going through your normal movements (shooting a basketball, swinging a racquet, lightly bounding a volleyball) warms up your brain and your flexibility. Instead of holding stretches for long periods, you walk, hop, and jog, increasing speed as you go, and performing repetitive motions that anticipate what you will soon be doing later on. If you are a competitive athlete, be sure to research the dynamic stretches that are commonly used for your sport.

Gentle stretching after exercising is good for recovery. Muscles tend to contract during exercise, and stretching is helpful to "reset" the muscles and the rest of the body to its relaxed and natural position.

Foam Rolling: Your Low-Tech Flexibility Tool. You have probably at least seen them, if you're not one of the increasing number of people who use them. A foam roller is a low-tech cylinder of foam, often 18 inches long and 3–6 inches wide (although it can be longer and thinner, and have bumps for a more penetrating effect).

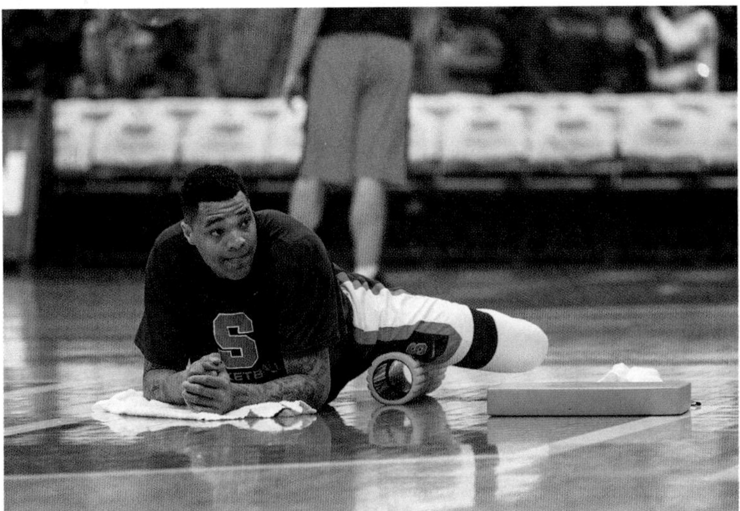

Foam rolling for flexibility. Foam rolling is increasingly recognized as an effective tool for flexibility. Here, DaJuan Coleman of the Syracuse Orange stretches with a foam roller before a 2016 game at the Carrier Dome in Syracuse, New York.

By applying your body weight back and forth onto the roller, you are smoothing and stretching your muscles and breaking up adhesions, knots, and muscular scar tissue. Recent scientific evidence recommends rollers as a post-workout recovery tool. Rollers effectively alleviate muscle soreness, relieve joint stress, improve range of motion, and promote optimal muscle functioning.[60,61] By activating the sensory receptors connecting your muscle fibers to your tendons, your muscles relax, which also helps improve blood circulation and speed up workout recovery.

Originally popularized by professional dancers,[61] foam rollers are now used by athletes everywhere and are an effective recovery component for any activity routine. Foam rollers can be painful, as bearing down your body's full weight onto one muscle takes some getting used to. But the evidence shows that with this simple apparatus, the short-term discomfort will pay off in the long term. Also foam rollers are inexpensive, and don't take up much room.

Yoga. Yoga is an ancient practice, originating approximately 2,500 years ago, in what is now India. It combines physical, mental, and spiritual elements and comes in numerous forms, through different schools, practices, and environments. It has numerous health benefits, including increased strength, improved blood flow, improved sleep, and decreased blood pressure.[62–64] It can be particularly effective, however, for improving flexibility and delivering all of the health benefits that are associated with that critical component of health-related fitness. Yoga is such a beneficial component of health that it is referenced in both Chapters 4 and 6.

Participants in yoga class notice that their body gradually becomes less stiff the more and more they learn yoga poses or attend classes. Many yoga poses and postures address the joints, such as loosening and opening the hips, thighs, and lower back. They also stretch major muscles such as hamstrings and arm and shoulder muscles. The "downward dog," a fundamental yoga pose, stretches several parts of the body.

Yoga is an excellent option for anyone wanting to improve flexibility. Getting started can be as simple as going to a local community center and taking a beginner class. It is an activity that you can do occasionally, or work on and study deeply for the rest of your life. By practicing yoga, you will become more limber and might discover a new passion to keep you healthy for the rest of your life.

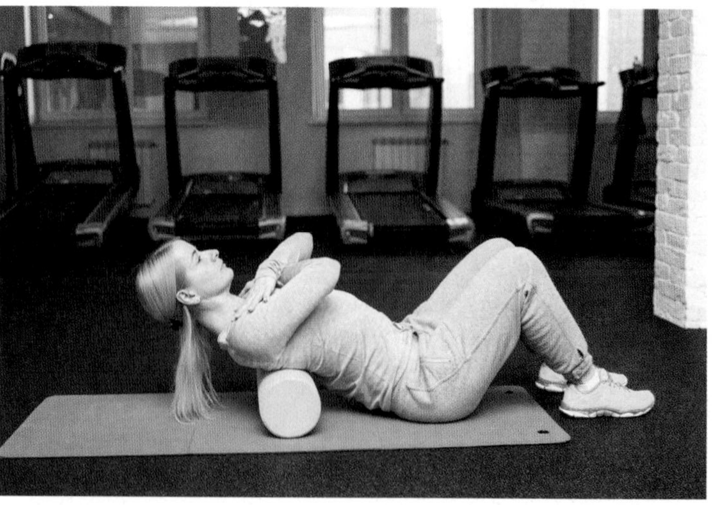

Example of a foam roller exercise.

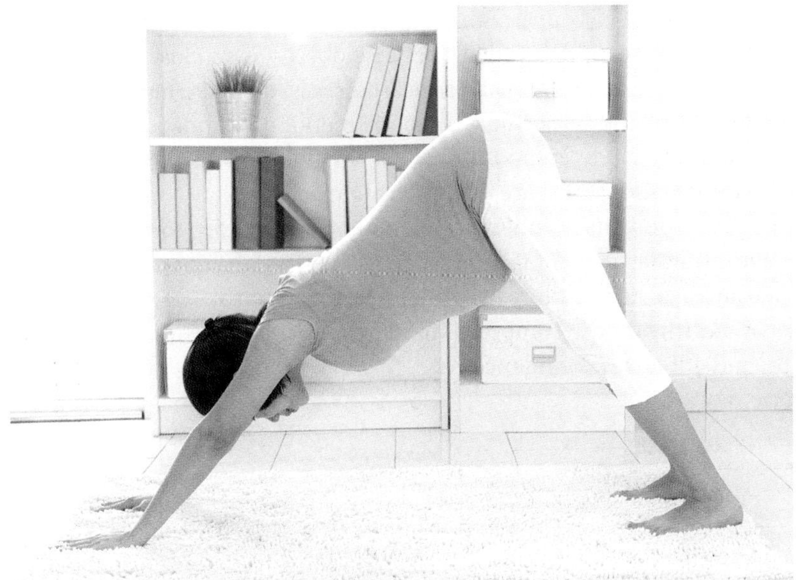

The downward dog yoga pose. Adho mukha svanasana pose, or "downward dog," is one of the fundamental yoga movements, and it provides the body with several stretch points.

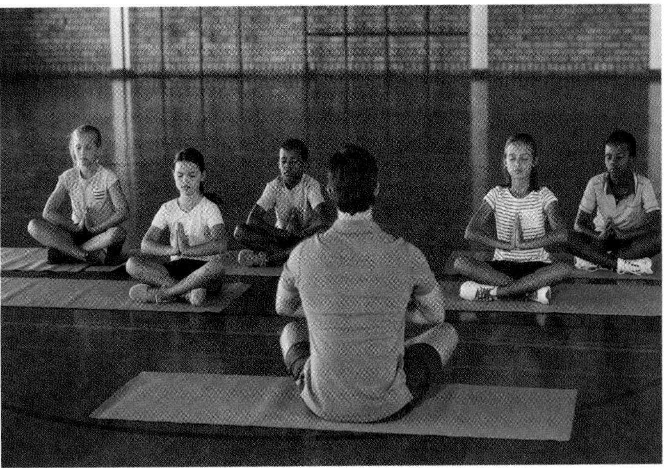

Yoga in elementary school.

Tai Chi and Qigong. Tai chi and qigong (pronounced *chee-gong*) are two fitness practices gaining popularity in the United States. Studies indicate that both activities can help improve balance, blood pressure, and flexibility. Both have been categorized, along with yoga, as "meditative movement,"[65] where grace and beauty are valued over power and speed, and where breathing is always considered an important component of the activity. Both have their origins in ancient China, and both are component activities to a larger martial arts practice; as well as being effective for those seeking improved flexibility. If you are interested in gaining strength and learning to move your body in a more fluid fashion, while learning to develop mental "mindfulness" and acuity, either of these activities may be for you.

Body Composition

The amount of body fat you have in proportion to your overall weight is sometimes called your body composition. The ratio between body fat and overall weight is a better assessment of your health than is body weight alone. Body composition is an important fitness component, because obesity is so closely associated with numerous health risk factors, such as heart disease, diabetes, high blood pressure, cancer, and knee and back injuries, not to mention confidence and well-being. You can improve body composition by losing fat, increasing lean muscle, or a combination of both. There are many ways to measure body composition, beyond the traditional body mass index (BMI) method (see the Up for Debate box).

High body fat percentage is associated with high blood pressure, cardiovascular disease, heart failure, irregular heartbeats, stroke, and diabetes. Meanwhile, a healthy body composition increases metabolism, supports overall health, and enhances confidence.

UP FOR DEBATE

Measuring Your Body Fat: Is There a Right Way?

How do you know if you are obese, overweight, underweight, or just about right? It turns out that answering this question is not as easy as you might think. Physiologists, and other health professionals often rely on the body mass index (BMI) to help determine if people are at a healthy weight, or to determine if someone is at risk for health problems such as heart disease, cancer, or musculoskeletal stress.

Your BMI is defined as your mass (weight) divided by the square of your height. It can be expressed in units of kg/m^2 (metric) or $lb/in.^2$ (in the United States). BMI calculators are easily available online, and you can input your height and weight (**TABLE 3-3**) to obtain your BMI. Once you determine your BMI, you can refer to the guidelines accepted by the World Health Organization.

TABLE 3-3 Body Mass Index Categories (Metric Units)

Category	BMI (kg/m^2)	
	from	to
Very severely underweight		15.0
Severely underweight	15	16
Underweight	16	18.5
Normal (healthy weight)	18.5	25
Overweight	25	30
Obese, class I (moderately obese)	30	35
Obese, class II (severely obese)	35	40
Obese, class III (very severely obese)	40	

Global Database on Body Mass Index, World Health Organization, 2006.

While BMI can provide helpful information, it is limited in its ability to tell you how healthy your weight really is. For one thing, it fails to distinguish between muscle and fat. A highly muscular frame will often tip the BMI measure to "obese" levels. This result can be frustrating for people who train hard to lose fat and increase muscle, only to see their BMI stay the same—or even get "worse."

The location of your fat deposits has a more clear connection to health condition than BMI alone. People whose fat is located primarily around the midsection of the body are at a greater risk of disease than people who have more of their weight in the legs and lower body. The circumference of the hips relative to height also may produce a more accurate measurement of overweight or obesity than BMI. The body adiposity index (BAI), for example, may be more useful than BMI in measuring health-threatening body fat deposits. More expensive dual-energy X-ray absorptiometry, or DXA scanning, measures body fat, muscle, and bone mineral using sophisticated scanning technology, but it can be expensive. All of these ways of measuring weight have benefits and limitations. But simply incorporating activity into your day-to-day living is a better use of your time than figuring out how best to measure your body fat.[66,67]

What do you think about the importance of body fat measurement and how it's done?

You're Good to Go! But What Does Our Population Data Show?

The ACSM's American Fitness Index®, a wide-scale research project conducted since 2007, measures the fitness levels of the 50 largest metropolitan areas in the United States (**TABLE 3-4**).

The rankings are based on such criteria as the percentage of the population who meet recommendations for physical activity, percentage diagnosed with heart disease and diabetes, percentage who live close to a park, amount each city spends on parks, and the percentage who walk or bike to work. Fitness is closely associated with wealth, and also education (the proportion of adults who hold a college degree). In general, fitter cities are more expensive cities to live in. Was your metropolitan area on the list? If not, why do you think it did not make it? What could be done to improve the ranking?

While our fitness is directly connected to our behavior, it is not just the result of individual choices. Physical fitness also results from how our culture

TABLE 3-4 American College of Sports Medicine's 10 Fittest Cities List, 2017 Edition

Rank	Metropolitan Area
1	Minneapolis-St. Paul-Bloomington, MN
2	Washington-Arlington-Alexandria, DC-VA-MD
3	San Francisco Bay Area, CA
4	Seattle Area, WA
5	San Jose Area, CA
6	Boston Area, MA
7	Denver Area, CO
8	Portland-Vancouver, OR-WA
9	Salt Lake City, UT
10	San Diego, CA

Data from 2017 American College of Sports Medicine American Fitness Index.

and society are structured. Fitness is still connected to affluence, jobs, education, and class position.

So what can we do? Years of research in health, human behavior, sociology, political science, and related fields tell us that making changes to our social and physical environment improves public health.[68] One way to do this is by revising laws and policies, such as the way that cigarette taxes and smoke-free workplace laws have reduced tobacco consumption. Cultural change is important too. Think of how bicycling to work and yoga saw big increases in popularity in recent years. Other improvements in population fitness can come from community mobilization, such as building and improving parks or recreation centers.

The following are examples of changes that have been shown to improve community fitness. As you read through them, think about where you live and what it would take to make it more conducive to physical activity and fitness.

Increasing Access to Places for Physical Activity

Adjusting and adapting a community so more people can be fit can mean creating new opportunities for activity or reducing the cost of fitness. This might mean building walking paths or installing exercise facilities in parks. It also might include cutting the daily fee for a community center with a gym and a pool. The more we can make these changes in low-income communities, the more effectively we can reduce the health and fitness inequities by income and race that are still seen in this country.

Exercise in Schools

Ensuring that schoolchildren have "active recess" can make significant differences in their overall health, particularly for kids under 10 years of age. When it comes to childhood fitness, the longer the recess time, the better.[69,70] Examples of making the most of recess include training teachers to better teach fitness, creating "activity zones," and making playground equipment more conducive to exercise.[71]

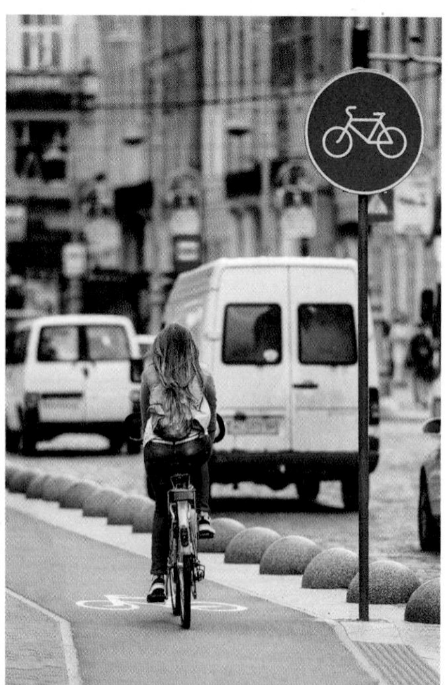

Bike lanes. Look what happens when a city constructs a protected bike lane downtown: People use it! That's what happened when Indianapolis installed the Indianapolis Cultural Trail, which now extends more than 10 miles in and around the city.

Incorporation of Bike and Pedestrian Paths into City Planning

When cities build more bicycle and pedestrian paths, people use them.[72] Bike lanes, bike racks, and walking trails all promote physical activity, especially when they are part of a comprehensive bicycle and pedestrian "master plan" conducted by cities. These plans, which coordinate these efforts into comprehensive city planning efforts, have been associated with improved health, and reduced injuries and accidents among pedestrians.[73]

Community Fitness Programs

Communities can reach better fitness by offering activity classes. Aerobic dance and cycle spinning classes have been shown to improve community health. Tai chi classes have been effective with elderly adults, improving balance, reducing falls, and improving cognitive function. Yoga classes can lower levels of blood pressure, cholesterol, and triglycerides. And pilates classes improve flexibility, balance, and endurance among participants. But it is not enough to just build it and assume people will come. Reaching out needs to be a part of the overall process to achieve success.[74,75] Do you know if your city or town has a plan to improve the fitness of its residents, and if so, do you know what it is? How are these classes promoted to the public?

Improving Our Built Environment

The "built environment" can have an enormous effect on community health. Are there sidewalks all around us, or do most people drive everywhere? Do our buildings make it easy to use the stairs, or are the stairs cold and dark—or locked behind an emergency exit with a threatening "alarm will sound" sign? Do we have to drive to get to all the places we need to go—school, grocery store, church? These are some of the questions public health advocates face as we try to structure our world so more people can be physically fit.

The idea of "mixed-use development" has received increased attention in recent years. Combining residential, commercial, recreational, and other types of construction within a single, walkable community, can also increase physical

TALES OF PUBLIC HEALTH

Let's Play the Stairs

What can we do to encourage more activity? One motivation is "fun," one of the reasons many of us engage in physical activity in the first place. While some of us exercise to lose weight, sleep better, or for the long-term health benefits, the immediate effect of exercise is often just for fun. Many people play sports like we play instruments.

So why not blend the two together—music and exercise? That's just what one effort did to create a built environment encouraging physical activity. The Fun Theory initiative is a community project supported by the Volkswagen Corporation. The project converted a set of steps at a subway station in Stockholm, Sweden, into working piano keys. People could choose the stairs or an adjacent escalator. After the intervention, the number of people using (or playing) the stairs increased by 66%. A video describing this project can be found online and now more "piano stairs" are being built all around the world.

We should never forget about creativity as a tool for solutions to our local and global public health problems.

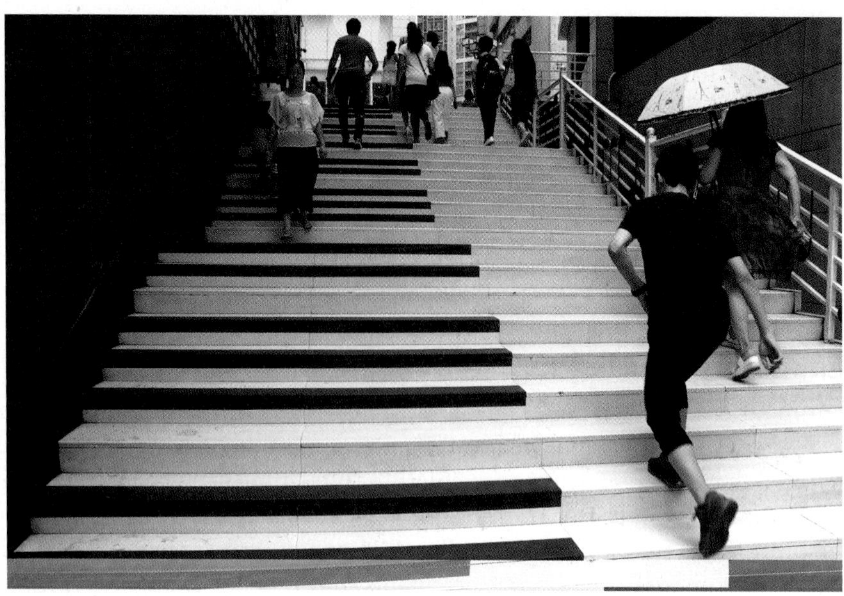

Piano stairs in Shanghai, China. A shopping mall in Shanghai features stairs that produce musical sounds of different notes when stepped on.

activity.[72] People walk and ride bicycles more often in mixed-use development areas, which has even been used in rural and suburban areas to sustain and promote active living.[76] Such environments help residents become more active, through increased playtime for children and more walking and biking opportunities for everyone.[77]

In Summary

Physical fitness is strongly connected to overall health, and should be an important priority for any individual, neighborhood, community, city, state, or country. This chapter has explored the five components of health-related fitness, to give us some guidelines about how we can examine and improve our own fitness levels. By better understanding the components of fitness, we can begin to envision what we need to do at the population level to improve our fitness. There are many paths to fitness—as individuals and communities. The most important thing is to get on the path . . . and get moving.

Key Terms

active living
aerobic exercise
anaerobic exercise
body composition
cardiac muscle
cardiorespiratory endurance
endorphins
exercise
fast-twitch
fitness
flexibility
glycogen
health-related fitness
metabolism
muscle protein myofibrils
muscular endurance
muscular strength
physical activity
skeletal muscle
skill-related fitness
slow-twitch

Student Discussion Questions and Activities

1. This chapter has discussed the decline in physical activity in the United States. Why do you think physical activity has declined over the past 100, 50, even 20 years in your country? Do you see environments, buildings, and roadways that actively discourage physical activity? What do they look like? Do you see policies that encourage activity, such as decisions giving more people access to physical activity, fitness, or exercise? What do they look like? What can be done to encourage those environments?
2. How much time should K-12 school children be required to spend on physical activity per week? What should constitute physical activity? Are there activities that were included in your school's gym class that you think should have been left out? Were there activities that were left out that you think should have been included?
3. The presence of parks in a town or a city has been shown to improve the health of the surrounding community, but these results can be variable. What can neighborhoods and communities do to help ensure that parks are used in ways that are most satisfying to residents and that are most likely to promote health?
4. Select one new fitness or exercise activity you can adopt for the next month, and document the following:
   - What is the activity?
   - Why did you select this activity?
   - How long does it take to complete the activity each time you do it?
   - How often did you do it?
   - Which component(s) of health-related fitness does this activity apply to?
   - How do you feel immediately after completing the activity?
   - Do you experience long-term changes 1 month after the activity?
     - Consider incorporating quantitative data: Take measurements such as weight, abdominal circumference, and BMI, both before initiating the exercise and 1 month later.
     - Incorporate other information, such as assessing your mood, sleep patterns, and even your academic performance.
   - Overall, what did you get out of adding this exercise? What did you get out of documenting the exercise using the recommended information?

References

1. Tremblay, M. S., Colley, R. C., Saunders, T. J., Healy, G. N., & Owen, N. (2010). Physiological and health implications of a sedentary lifestyle. *Applied Physiology, Nutrition, and Metabolism, 35*(6), 725–740.
2. Penedo, F. J., & Dahn, J. R. (2005). Exercise and well-being: A review of mental and physical health benefits associated with physical activity. *Current Opinion in Psychiatry, 18*(2), 189–193.
3. Evans, M. (2011, December 13). The single best thing you can do for your health [Online video clip]. *The Atlantic.* Retrieved from http://www.theatlantic.com/video/index/249913/the-single-best-thing-you-can-do-for-your-health/
4. Paddock, C. (2015, January 15). Lack of exercise "twice as deadly" as obesity. *Medical News Today.* Retrieved from http://www.medicalnewstoday.com/articles/288042.php
5. Voss, M. W., Nagamatsu, L. S., Liu-Ambrose, T., & Kramer, A. F. (2011). Exercise, brain, and cognition across the life span. *Journal of Applied Physiology, 111*(5), 1505–1513.
6. Cotman, C. W., & Engesser-Cesar, C. (2002). Exercise enhances and protects brain function. *Exercise and Sport Sciences Reviews, 30*(2), 75–79.
7. Ratey, J. J., & Loehr, J. E. (2011). The positive impact of physical activity on cognition during adulthood: A review of underlying mechanisms, evidence and recommendations. *Reviews in the Neurosciences, 22*(2), 171–185.
8. Lee, I.-M., Shiroma, E. J., Lobelo, F., Puska, P., Blair, S. N., Katzmarzyk, P. T., & Lancet Physical Activity Series Working Group. (2012). Effect of physical inactivity on major non-communicable diseases worldwide: An analysis of burden of disease and life expectancy. *The Lancet, 380*(9838), 219–229.

9. Lawlor, D. A., & Hopker, S. W. (2001). The effectiveness of exercise as an intervention in the management of depression: Systematic review and meta-regression analysis of randomized controlled trials. *BMJ, 322*(7289), 763–767.
10. Warburton, D., Nicol, C. W., & Bredin, S. (2006). Health benefits of physical activity: The evidence. *Canadian Medical Association Journal, 174*(6), 801–809.
11. Cauley, J. A., Lucas, F. L., Kuller, L. H., Stone, K., Browner, W., Cummings, S. R. (1999). Elevated serum estradiol and testosterone concentrations are associated with a high risk for breast cancer. *Annals of Internal Medicine, 130*(4), 270–277.
12. Peters, H. P. F., De Vries, W. R., Vanberge-Henegouw, G., & Akkermans, L. (2001). Potential benefits and hazards of physical activity and exercise on the gastrointestinal tract. *Gut, 48*(3), 435–439.
13. Kohl, H. W., Craig, C. L., Lambert, E. V., Inoue, S., Alkandari, J. R., Leetongin, G., & Kalmeier, S. (2012). The pandemic of physical inactivity: Global action for public health. *The Lancet, 380*(9838), 294–305.
14. Shalikashvili, J. M., & Shelton, H. (2010, August 6). The latest national security threat: Obesity. *The Washington Post.* Retrieved from http://www.washingtonpost.com/wp-dyn/content/article/2010/04/29/AR2010042903669.html
15. Costello, C. (2015, April 21). America: Too fat to fight. *CNN.com.* Retrieved from http://www.cnn.com/2015/04/21/opinions/costello-america-fat/
16. Colditz, G. A., & Wang, C. Y. (2008). Economic costs of obesity. *Obesity Epidemiology*, 261–274.
17. Carlson, S. A., Fulton, J. E., Pratt, M., Yang, Z., & Adams, E. K. (2015). Inadequate physical activity and health care expenditures in the United States. *Progress in Cardiovascular Disease, 57*(4), 315–323.
18. Caspersen, C. J., Powell, K. E., & Christenson, G. M. (1985). Physical activity, exercise, and physical fitness: Definitions and distinctions for health-related research. *Public Health Reports, 100*(2), 126–131.
19. Heath, C., & Heath, D. (2010). *Switch: How to change when change is hard.* New York, NY: Random House.
20. Turner, A., James, N., Dimitriou, L., Greenhalgh, A., Moody, J., Fulcher, D., . . . Kilduff, L. (2014). Determinants of Olympic fencing performance and implications for strength and conditioning training. *Journal of Strength and Conditioning Research, 28*(10), 3001–3011.
21. Centers for Disease Control and Prevention. (2014, September 3). Prevalence of childhood obesity in the United States, 2011–2012. *CDC Childhood Obesity Facts.* Retrieved from https://www.cdc.gov/healthyschools/obesity/facts.htm
22. American Heart Association. (2015, October 26). The price of inactivity. Retrieved from http://www.heart.org/HEARTORG/HealthyLiving/PhysicalActivity/FitnessBasics/The-Price-of-Inactivity_UCM_307974_Article.jsp#.WAEN7-ArKVM
23. Owen, N., Sparling, P. B., Healy, G. N., Dunstan, D. W., & Matthews, C. E. (2010). Sedentary behavior: Emerging evidence for a new health risk. *Mayo Clinic Proceedings, 85*(12), 1138–1141.
24. *The World Bank.* (2014, October 15). Sedentary lives, the other global epidemic. Retrieved from http://www.worldbank.org/en/news/feature/2014/10/15/vidas-sedentarias-la-otra-epidemia-global
25. Pratt, M., Norris, J., Lobelo, F., Roux, L., & Wang, G. (2014). The cost of physical inactivity: Moving into the 21st century. *British Journal of Sports Medicine, 48*(3), 171–173.
26. Sallis, J., & McKenzie, T. (1991). Physical education's role in public health. *Research Quarterly for Exercise and Sport, 62*(2), 124–137.
27. Rasberry, C., Lee, S. M., Robin, L., Laris, B. A., Russell, L. A., Coyle, K. K., & Nihiser, A. J. (2011). The association between school-based physical activity, including physical education, and academic performance: A systematic review of the literature. *Preventive Medicine, 52*(Suppl), S10–S20.
28. Ballard, W., & Chase, M. R. (2004). Nontraditional recreation activities: A catalyst for quality physical education. *Journal of Physical Education, Recreation & Dance, 75*(3), 40–45.
29. Sallis, J., Floyd, M. F., Rodríguez, D. A., & Saelens, B. E. (2012). Role of built environments in physical activity, obesity, and cardiovascular disease. *Circulation, 125*(5), 729–737.
30. Kuo, M. (2015). How might contact with nature promote human health? Promising mechanisms and a possible central pathway. *Frontiers in Psychology,* 6.
31. Cohen, D. A., McKenzie, T. L., Sehgal, A., Williamson, S., Golinelli, D., & Lurie, N. (2007). Contribution of public parks to physical activity. *American Journal of Public Health, 97*(3), 509–514.
32. Hallsmith, G. (2013). *The key to sustainable cities: Meeting human needs, transforming community systems.* Gabriola Island, British Columbia: New Society Publishers.
33. National Institute for Transportation and Communities. (2014). *The built environment, neighborhood safety, and physical activity among low income children.* Portland, OR: NITC.
34. Potwarka, L., Kaczynski, A. T., & Flack, A. L. (2008). Places to play: Association of park space and facilities with healthy weight status among children. *Journal of Community Health, 33*(5), 344–350.
35. Green, G., Henry, J., & Power, J. (2015). Physical fitness disparities in California school districts. *USC Price School of Public Policy.* Retrieved from http://www.cityprojectca.org/blog/wp-content/uploads/2015/06/FINAL-Physical-Education-Briefer-20150601.pdf
36. Gortmaker, S. L., Lee, R., Cradock, A. L., Sobol, A. M., Duncan, D. T., & Wang, Y. C. (2012). Disparities in youth physical activity in the United States: 2003–2006. *Medicine and Science in Sports and Exercise, 44*(5), 888–893.
37. Wilson-Frederick, S. M., Thorpe, R. J., Jr., Bell, C. N., Bleich, S. N., Ford, J. G., & LaVeist, T. A. (2014). Examination of race disparities in physical inactivity among adults of similar social context. *Ethnicity and Disease, 24*(3), 363–369.
38. U.S. Department of Health and Human Services. (1996). *Physical activity and health: A report of the Surgeon General.* Atlanta, GA: Diane Publishing.
39. U.S. Department of Health and Human Services, Office of Disease Prevention and Health Promotion. (2008). *Physical activity guidelines for Americans.* Washington, DC: The Secretary of Health and Human Services.
40. Vlahos, J. (2011, April 4). Is sitting a lethal activity? *New York Times.* Retrieved from http://www.nytimes.com/2011/04/17/magazine/mag-17sitting-t.html?_r=0
41. Harvard T. H. Chan School of Public Health. (n.d.) Examples of moderate and vigorous physical activity. *Obesity Prevention Source.* Retrieved from https://www.hsph.harvard.edu/obesity-prevention-source/moderate-and-vigorous-physical-activity/
42. Gerstacker, G. (2014, September 29). Sitting is the new smoking: Ways a sedentary lifestyle is killing you. *The Active Times. Huffington Post.* Retrieved from http://www.theactivetimes.com/sitting-new-smoking-7-ways-sedentary-lifestyle-killing-you
43. Haskell, W. L., Lee, I. M., Pate, R. R., Powell, K. E., Blair, S. N., Franklin, B. A., & Bauman, A. (2007). Physical activity and public health: Updated recommendation for adults from

the American College of Sports Medicine and the American Heart Association. *Circulation, 116*(9), 1081.

44. *Harvard Men's Health Watch*. (2016, January 5). Walking: Your steps to health. Retrieved from http://www.health.harvard.edu/newsletter_article/Walking-Your-steps-to-health
45. Reynolds, G. (2015, July 22). How walking in nature changes the brain. *The New York Times Well Blogs*. Retrieved from http://well.blogs.nytimes.com/2015/07/22/how-nature-changes-the-brain/
46. Reynolds, G. (2009, August 11). Phys ed: Can running actually help your knees? *The New York Times Well Blogs*. Retrieved from http://well.blogs.nytimes.com/2009/08/11/phys-ed-can-running-actually-help-your-knees/
47. Chakravarty, E. F., Hubert, H. B., Lingala, V. B., Zatarain, E., & Fries, J. F. (2008). Long distance running and knee osteoarthritis: A prospective study. *American Journal of Preventive Medicine, 35*(2), 133–138.
48. Lee, D.-C., Pate, R. R., Lavie, C. J., Sui, X., Church, T. S., & Blair, S. N. (2014). Leisure-time running reduces all-cause and cardiovascular mortality risk. *Journal of the American College of Cardiology, 64*(5), 472–481.
49. Fetters, A. K. (2014, April 25). How to achieve a runner's high. *Runner's World*. Retrieved from http://www.runnersworld.com/running-tips/how-to-achieve-a-runners-high
50. Tudor-Locke, C., & Bassett, D. R. (2004). How many steps/day are enough? Preliminary pedometer indices for public health. *Sports Medicine, 34*, 1–8.
51. Reynolds, G. (2013, December 16). Ask well: Benefits of swimming. *The New York Times Well Blogs*. Retrieved from http://well.blogs.nytimes.com/2013/12/16/ask-well-benefits-of-swimming/
52. Boston University Medical Campus. (2008, February 5). "Weight training" muscles reduce fat, improve metabolism in mice. *EurekAlert! Science News*. Retrieved from http://www.bumc.bu.edu/provost/bumcnews/%E2%80%9Cweight-training%E2%80%9D-muscles-shown-to-reduce-fat-improve-metabolism-in-obese-mice/
53. Layne, J. E., & Nelson, M. E. (1993). The effects of progressive resistance training on bone density: A review. *Medicine and Science in Sports and Exercise, 31*(1), 25–30.
54. Behringer, M., Vom Heede, A., Yue, Z., & Mester, J. (2010). Effects of resistance training in children and adolescents: A meta-analysis. *Pediatrics, 126*(5), e1199–e1210.
55. Study.com. (n.d.). Flexibility in fitness: definition, stretches and exercises. *Chapter 22, Lesson 16*. Retrieved from http://study.com/academy/lesson/flexibility-in-fitness-definition-stretches-exercises.html
56. Yamamoto, K., Kawano, H., Gando, Y., Iemitsu, M., Murakami, H., Sanada, K., . . . Miyachi, M. (2009). Poor trunk flexibility is associated with arterial stiffening. *American Journal of Physiology. Heart and Circulatory Physiology, 297*(4), H1314–H1318.
57. Clarey, C. (2016, July 2). Djokovic bends and twists, but doesn't break. *The New York Times Tennis*. Retrieved from http://www.nytimes.com/2013/07/03/sports/tennis/djokovic-bends-and-twists-but-doesnt-break.html
58. de Araujo, C. G. S. (2001). Flexitest: An office method for evaluation of flexibility. *Sports and Medicine Today*, 34–27. Retrieved from http://www.clinimex.com.br/Flexitest/Sport%20%26%20Medicine%20Today_Set01_flexitest%20office%20method.pdf
59. Reynolds, G. (2013, April 3). Reasons not to stretch. *The New York Times Well Blogs*. Retrieved from http://well.blogs.nytimes.com/2013/04/03/reasons-not-to-stretch/?mtrref=www.google.com&gwh=B615068D7A622C98DD4C F5 D2065A5F9C&gwt=pay
60. MacDonald, G. Z., Button, D. C., Drinkwater, E. J., & Behm, D. G. (2014). Foam rolling as a recovery tool after an intense bout of physical activity. *Medicine and Science in Sports and Exercise, 46*(1), 131–142.
61. Witkowski, K. R. (2012, September 3). The aesthetic athlete. *Rehab Management*. Retrieved from http://www.rehabpub.com/2012/09/the-aesthetic-athlete/
62. Ross, A., & Thomas, S. (2010). The health benefits of yoga and exercise: A review of comparison studies. *The Journal of Alternative and Complementary Medicine, 16*(1), 3–12.
63. Grossman, P., Niemann, L., Schmidt, S., & Walach, H. (2004). Mindfulness-based stress reduction and health benefits: A meta-analysis. *Journal of Psychosomatic Research 57*(1), 35–43.
64. Jayasinghe, S. (2004). Yoga in cardiac health (a review). *European Journal of Cardiovascular Prevention and Rehabilitation, 11*(5), 369–375.
65. Jahnke, R., Larkey, L., Rogers, C., Etnier, J., & Lin, F. (2010). A comprehensive review of health benefits of qigong and tai chi. *American Journal of Health Promotion, 24*(6), e1–e25.
66. Kravitz, L. (2010). Waist-to-hip ratio, waist circumference and BMI: What to use for health risk indication and why. *IDEA Fitness Journal, 7*(9), 18–21.
67. Bergman, R., Stefanovski, D., Buchanan, T. A., Sumner, A. E., Reynolds, J. C., Sebring, N. G., . . . Watanabe, R. M. (2011). A better index of body adiposity. *Obesity, 19*(5), 1083–1089.
68. Frieden, T. R. (2010). A framework for public health action: The health impact pyramid. *American Journal of Public Health, 100*(4), 590–595.
69. Erwin, H. E., Ickes, M., Ahn, S., & Fedewa, A. (2014). Impact of recess interventions on children's physical activity—a meta-analysis. *American Journal of Health Promotion, 28*(3), 159–167.
70. Larson, N., Ward, D. S., Neelon, S. B., & Story, M. (2011). What role can child-care settings play in obesity prevention? A review of the evidence and call for research efforts. *Journal of the American Dietetic Association, 111*(9), 1343–1362.
71. Escalante, Y., García-Hermoso, A., Backx, K., & Saavedra, J. M. (2014). Playground designs to increase physical activity levels during school recess: A systematic review. *Health Education and Behavior, 41*(2), 138–144.
72. Brownson, R. C., Hoehner, C. M., Day, K., Forsyth, A., & Sallis, J. F. (2009). Measuring the built environment for physical activity: State of the science. *American Journal of Preventive Medicine, 36*(4), S99–S123.
73. Steinman, L., Doescher, M., Levinger, D., Perry, C., Carter, L., Eyler, A., . . . Voorhees, C. (2010). Master plans for pedestrian and bicycle transportation: Community characteristics. *Journal of Physical Activity & Health, 7*(1), S60.
74. Holland, S. K., Greenberg, J., Tidwell, L., Malone, J., Mullan, J., Newcomer, R. (2005). Community-based health coaching, exercise, and health service utilization. *Journal of Aging and Health, 17*(6), 697–716.
75. Cruz-Ferreira, A., Fernandes, J., Laranjo, L., Bernardo, L. M., & Silva, A. (2011). A systematic review of the effects of pilates method of exercise in healthy people. *Archives of Physical Medicine and Rehabilitation, 92*(12), 2071–2081.
76. Dalbey, M. (2008). Implementing smart growth strategies in rural America: Development patterns that support public health goals. *Journal of Public Health Management and Practice, 14*(3), 238–243.
77. Heath, G. W., & Troped, P. J. (2012). The role of the built environment in shaping the health behaviors of physical activity and healthy eating for cardiovascular health. *Future Cardiology, 8*(5), 677–679.

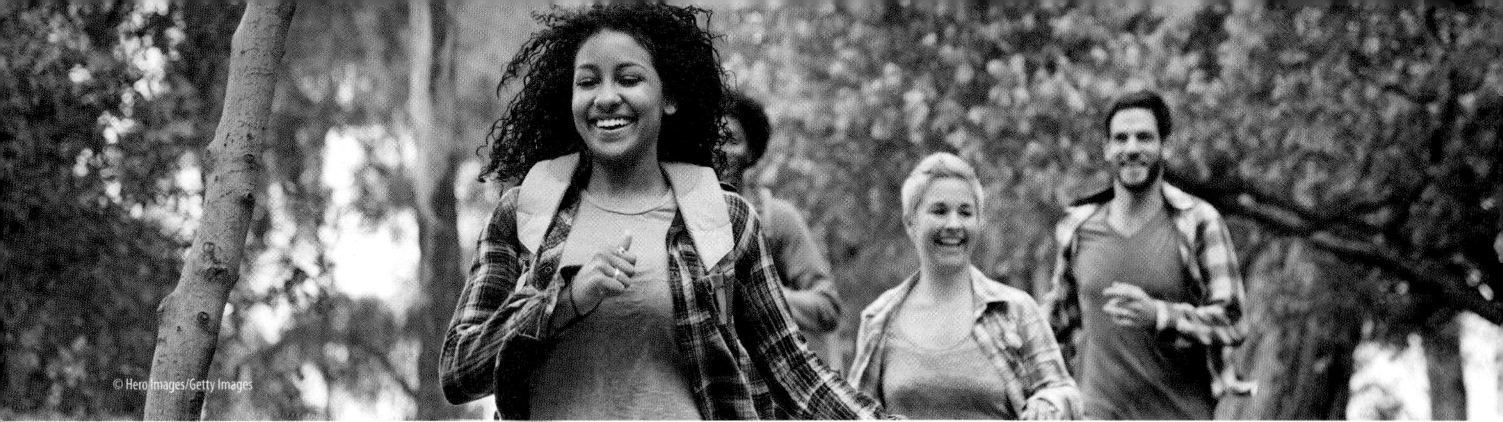

CHAPTER 4

Keep Calm and Carry On: Complementary, Alternative, and Spiritual Approaches to Health

CHAPTER OBJECTIVES

- Define common terms related to nontraditional health approaches.
- Describe nontraditional health approaches, discuss who uses them, and explain how these approaches affect health outcomes, for better or for worse.
- Explain who pays for complementary and alternative health therapies.
- Describe the current state of knowledge regarding how religion and spirituality may influence health.

A hot yoga class after your organic chemistry exam, taking echinacea to avoid getting whatever it is that has your roommate up coughing all night, a visit to the chiropractor to ease your back pain from volleyball practice—these complementary and alternative approaches to health have become increasingly popular in the last several decades. More and more, they are a regular part of how we think about and manage our health.

Understanding the Key Concepts

The definition of complementary health therapies is a "group of diverse medical and health care interventions, practices, products, or disciplines that are not generally considered part of conventional medicine."[1] A complementary approach refers to practices that are used *in conjunction with* conventional medicine, whereas an alternative health approach refers to nonmainstream practices that are used *instead of* traditional medicine.[2] These two approaches are often referred to together as **complementary and alternative medicine (CAM)**.

complementary and alternative medicine (CAM) An approach used in conjunction with conventional medicine or an approach that employs nonmainstream practices instead of traditional medicine.

You can seek these therapies from practitioners (such as chiropractors and massage therapists), or you can access them through self-care measures (such as the use of herbal dietary supplements, yoga, and meditation).[3] About 38% of adults and 12% of children use some form of complementary health therapy.[4] Each approach has its own potential health benefits and risks. For some approaches, the outcomes have been clearly demonstrated through research studies, whereas the evidence available for other approaches is limited or conflicting.

As we have learned more about evidence-based treatments and therapies, the definition of "conventional medicine" has changed drastically. "Evidence-based" means those treatments for which there are clear research findings that demonstrate effectiveness. Conventional medicine, also termed *biomedicine*, refers to medically approved and evidence-based screenings and treatments, such as getting a mammogram to detect breast cancer or taking insulin to treat diabetes.

integrative health An approach to health that seeks to bring together conventional and complementary treatments in a coordinated way.

Integrative health refers to efforts to bring together conventional and complementary treatments in a coordinated way.[2]

Because conventional treatments may be affected (positively or negatively) by a person's use of complementary practices, medical doctors and other healthcare providers have recently begun to ask their patients whether they engage in any complementary practices. Some have even started to recommend these therapies, in addition to conventional medications.

HOMEOPATHY

Homeopathy is one prominent alternative medical belief and practice system. Originating in Germany in the 1700s, it is based on the idea that the body heals itself. Homeopathic providers subscribe to the theory that diseases can be cured by treatments that create similar symptoms in people without the disease. They also believe that a lower dose of medication produces greater effectiveness. Homeopathic medicines are created from substances found in plants, minerals, and animals. These treatments are regulated by the U.S. Food and Drug Administration (FDA), but their safety and effectiveness are not evaluated, as prescription medications are. About 5 million adults and 1 million children report using some form of homeopathic treatment.[5] Homeopathy stands in contrast to the medical approach known as allopathic medicine. Allopathic medicine is practiced by medical doctors, who treat disease by using remedies that produce effects that differ from the effects of the disease.[6]

AYURVEDIC MEDICINE

Ayurveda is a medical system that originated in India over 3,000 years ago. Herbal supplements, diets, and other alternative health practices are promoted under this approach to health. Ayurvedic medicine includes concepts such as the belief in the interconnectedness of people, their health, and the universe; the body's make up (known as constitution); and life forces such as energy. Some Ayurveda treatments have been studied, but research is limited.[7]

Complementary and Alternative Health Approaches: Benefits and Risks

Many complementary and alternative therapies originated thousands of years ago in the Far East and South Asia, in countries such as China, Japan, and India. In modern times, some people have become increasingly frustrated with conventional medicine and treatments for myriad reasons. For instance, medications are sometimes prescribed and then retracted for their ill health effects. Also, medications are often expensive and unaffordable for many. Medical training is designed such that physicians and other healthcare providers choose a medical specialty, often focusing on one area, like the lungs, the heart, or the brain. Because of this specialized training, they may lack the holistic perspective of the interconnectedness of our body systems and treat only one system. These are just a few of the reasons why we as a society have begun to turn to complementary and alternative therapies for health.

The most popular reported complementary health approaches include supplements, chiropractic or osteopathic manipulation, yoga, massage, meditation, and special diets.[3]

Many of these approaches are used to help alleviate pain and improve emotional well-being. Even the federal government recognizes the impact of CAM and a national government institute, the National Center for Complementary and Integrative Health (NCCIH), funds research on these types of health approaches. The following discussion provides a brief overview of some of the more common approaches, including what they are, how they are used, and any known benefits or risks associated with their use (**FIGURE 4-1**).

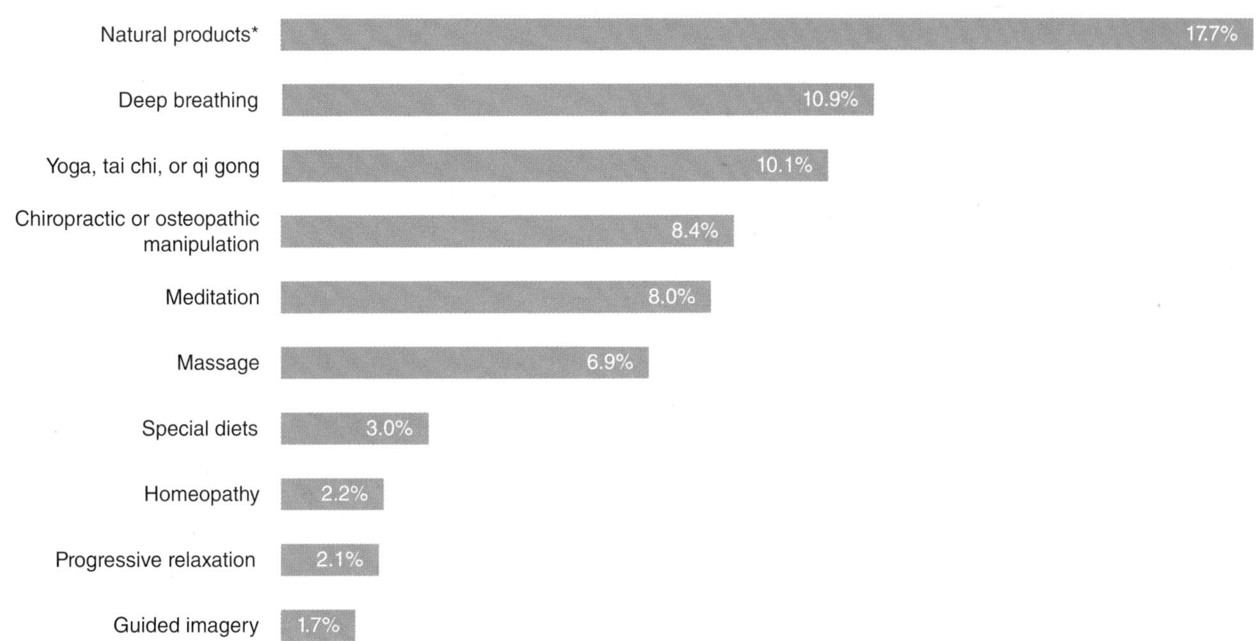

FIGURE 4-1 The 10 most common complementary health approaches among adults—2012.

Reproduced from Complementary, Alternative, or Integrative Health: What's In a Name?, National Center for Complementary and Integrative Health (NCCIH). Retrieved from https://nccih.nih.gov/health/integrative-health.

Supplements

complementary health approach A group of diverse medical and health care interventions, practices, products, or disciplines that are not generally considered part of conventional medicine.

In the United States, the most common **complementary health approach** is the use of nonvitamin, nonmineral (NVNM) supplements, with 18% of adults reporting that they use some form of NVNM supplement.[3]

These supplements are not required to have FDA approval for safety or effectiveness before they reach the market.[8] Dietary supplements are also often referred to as "herbal" or "natural" supplements. They include fish oils, amino acids, echinacea, and soy or flax products,[9] with fish oil being the most commonly used supplement.[10] Echinacea is a popular supplement that people use when they feel the beginnings of a cold, as it is thought to stimulate the immune system and increase its defense against infections. The science, however, is mixed on its ability to prevent or treat the common cold and other upper respiratory infections. Side effects are rare and include allergic reactions if the person taking it has allergies to plants related to the *Echinacea* family.[11]

If you plan to take echinacea, be mindful of the ingredients. An independent study found that only 4 of 11 brands of echinacea contained the stated ingredients on their labels, with 10% not containing any presence of the *Echinacea* plant. Try to choose these products from well-established companies that guarantee potency.[12] See Chapter 2 for more information on micronutrients and vitamins.

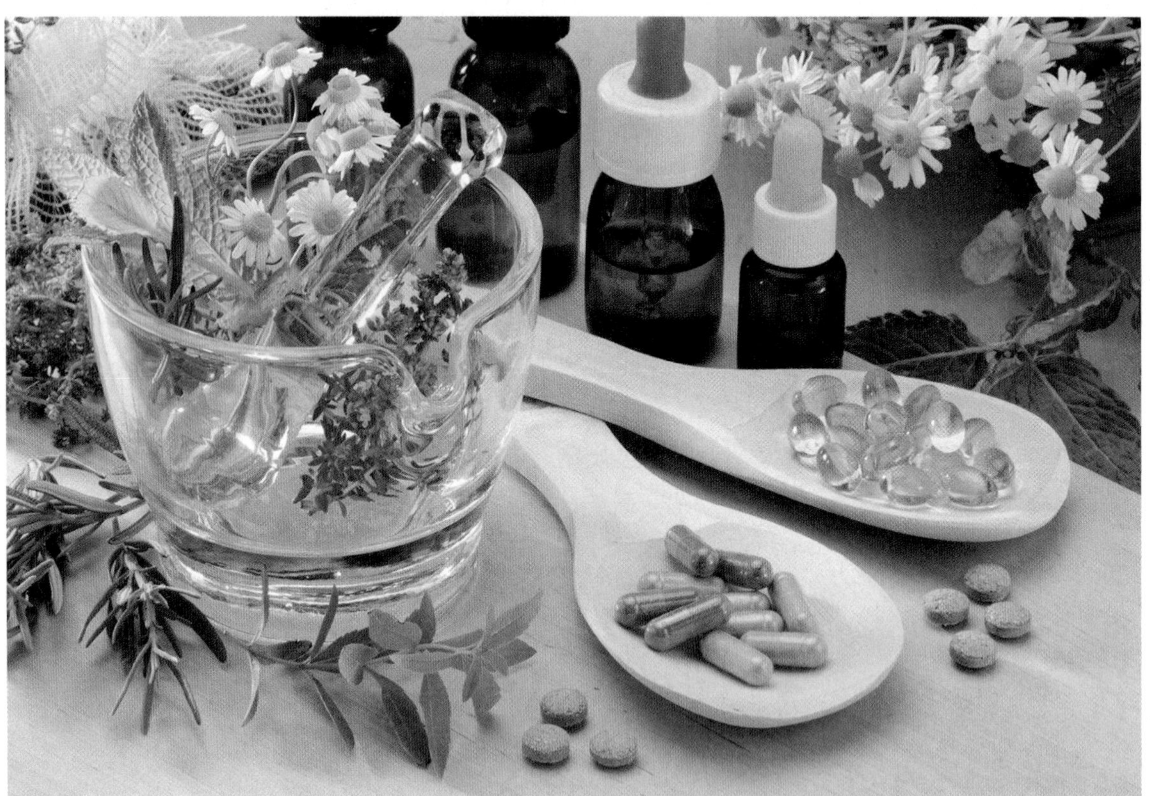

UP FOR DEBATE

When Is Marijuana Considered Medicine?

What do these movies have in common: *Ted, The Cabin in the Woods, Pineapple Express*, and *Neighbors*? They all feature actors smoking pot. But, when does smoking pot go from recreational use to legitimate health intervention? "Medical marijuana" refers to the use of the marijuana plant or its extracts to treat a health problem or symptom. The marijuana plant is not approved by the FDA to be medicinal, but the FDA has approved two medications that contain cannabinoids to treat some health problems.

Cannabinoids are the chemicals in marijuana. One type of cannabinoid is delta-9 tetrahydrocannabinol (THC). THC is the main ingredient in marijuana that alters the mind and has the potential to alleviate symptoms such as nausea and pain. The other is cannabidiol (CBD). CBD is not mind altering and has the potential to control epileptic seizures and possibly even help in treating mental illness and addiction.[13–15]

There is no federal law legalizing use of marijuana in the United States for medical reasons; however, the number of states passing laws to legalize medical marijuana is rapidly increasing. As of 2015, 23 states and the District of Columbia (DC) have enacted legislation to legalize medical marijuana in their states. Each state, however, has its own rules about what conditions it is approved to treat and the legal possession limit.[14] There is fairly good evidence that cannabinoids are effective in reducing chronic pain and spasticity. There is less evidence that it can improve chemotherapy-induced nausea, promote weight gain among those with HIV, or help alleviate sleep disorders or Tourette syndrome.[15]

A lot of research is exploring how THC and CBD can be used for medical purposes. As more research is conducted, positive results could prompt the FDA to approve the plant as medicine. There may even come a time when the federal government passes a law to legalize marijuana throughout the nation.

Special Diets

Every year it seems there is a new "fad" diet that is marketed as promoting health and facilitating weight loss. The diet industry makes billions of dollars marketing special foods, supplements, cookbooks, and other products to consumers. The specific diet trend (low carb, low fat, low calorie, high protein, gluten free, paleo, etc.) keeps changing as we learn more about how food is linked to health. These diets, used by millions of Americans every year, are considered a complementary or alternative health approach. See Chapter 2 for more specifics about special diets.

Chiropractic and Osteopathic Manipulation

How many times have you heard someone crack their back and say they should see the chiropractor? Truthfully, not everyone understands what chiropractic entails. **Chiropractic** and osteopathic manipulations involve physically adjusting the body, primarily the spine, to improve functioning, correct alignment problems, and alleviate pain.[16] Chiropractic manipulations are performed by chiropractors or osteopathic doctors using their hands or special devices designed specifically for adjustments.[17] Chiropractors are certified through a national agency and are trained through a doctor of chiropractic degree program. Chiropractors in the United States are required to be licensed through the passing of four board examinations.[18,19] Additional certifications are available in particular techniques. For example, a student can complete 300 to 400 hours of additional training in radiography (using electromagnetic radiation to view an internal structure).[20] Osteopathic physicians (or doctors of osteopathic medicine [DOs]) may also perform this type of manipulative therapy. DOs are medically trained (4 years of undergraduate, 4 years of medical school, and a minimum of 3 years of residency training), but they focus on the entire body and how various systems are interrelated to impact health.[21]

chiropractic A process that involves physically adjusting the body, primarily the spine, to improve functioning, correct alignment problems, and alleviate pain.

Chiropractic and osteopathic manipulations differ from physical therapy, which has distinct training requirements and focuses on exercises to gain or restore independence. Physical therapists diagnose movement dysfunction, prescribe exercises based on muscular imbalances or coordination deficits, and educate patients on modifications to promote ease of mobility, to reduce the risk of falls and other injuries.

Chiropractic may seem like a new therapy compared with meditation and other mind–body techniques, but writings from 2700 BC mention spinal

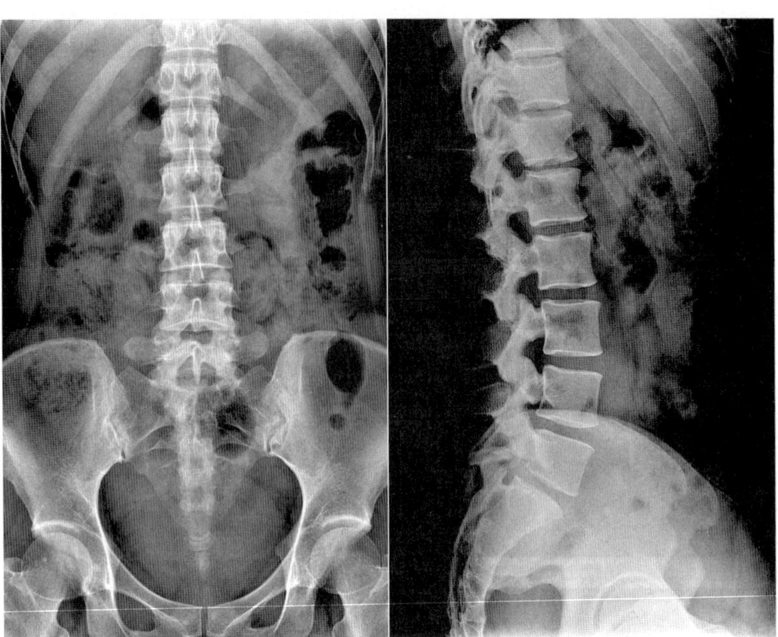

manipulations.[22] In the late 1800s the practice was named *chiropractic*, which means "done by hand." This concept of adjustments being made directly by hand (that is, *manually*) is why many chiropractic techniques are referred to as "manipulation."[23] Today, about 8% of adults (more than 18 million people) report using chiropractic care.[10] Many people start visiting a chiropractor to alleviate back pain or other musculoskeletal issues, especially if other medical treatments have failed. Some professional athletes rely on chiropractic care, such as Dana Torres and Tom Brady. Other celebrities on board with chiropractic are Cindy Crawford and Bill Murray. The initial visit with a chiropractor usually includes a physical examination, with particular emphasis on the spine. Some chiropractors use X-rays to learn more about the specific areas that require adjustment. If needed, a treatment plan is created with the patient that often involves more frequent initial visits that become less frequent as improvements are maintained. Sometimes other therapies, such as heat or ice, counseling about lifestyle changes in diet, or dietary supplements are used.[16]

The potential benefits of spinal manipulation include alleviation of low back and neck pain and improvement of joint conditions and whiplash injuries.[16,24] Chiropractic adjustments have been shown to be effective at alleviating some types of headaches, such as migraines, but not all.[25] Some people experience negative side effects of chiropractic adjustments, including discomfort, fatigue, and temporary headaches. There are a few reports of serious adverse events, but it remains unclear if spinal manipulations are responsible for those events.[16,24] What we do know is that more research is needed to fully understand any other benefits or risks of spinal manipulation. Chiropractors often view their role as not just healing neck and back pain, but increasing the quality of their patients' lives.[26]

Massage

massage Various types of movements utilized by trained therapists, usually with their hands, to apply pressure, rub, or manipulate muscle and other soft tissues.

When you think about health therapies, massage might not come to mind. It seems more like a luxury or an indulgence than a therapy. Yet, **massage** is among one of the oldest complementary approaches, appearing in ancient writings thousands of years ago.[27] Trained massage therapists use various types of movements, usually with their hands, to apply pressure, rub, or manipulate

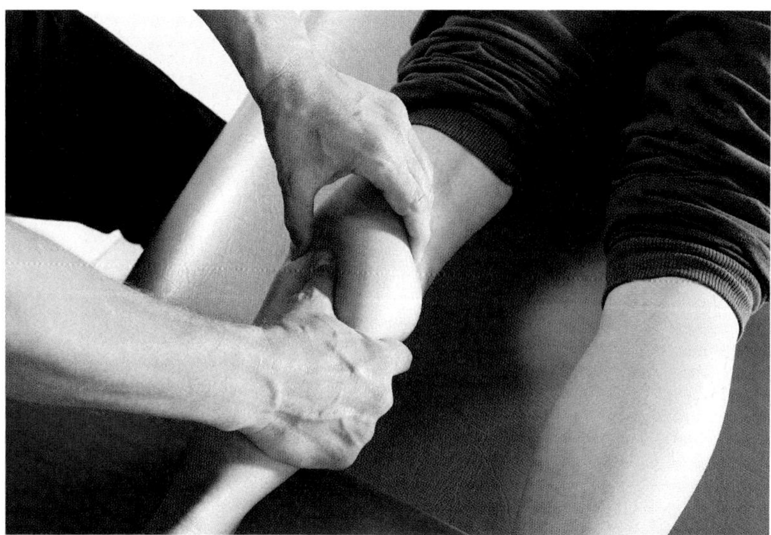

muscle and other soft tissues. There are almost 100 different types of massage, including hot stone, deep tissue, and reflexology.[28] Licensed massage therapy training usually involves at least 500 hours of practice through an accredited program. When performed by a trained practitioner, there are few risks associated with massage. As with other therapies, certain groups of people should not receive massages (some pregnant women and people with wounds or tumors, with bleeding disorders, or on blood thinners).[27] About 7% of adults use massage, which has increased in the last decade.[3,29]

A massage therapy session usually begins with the therapist asking you about any relevant medical history. The therapist then leaves the room while you undress to your comfort level and lie down on the massage table. The massage table is sometimes heated, and the room often has low lighting and music playing in the background. Depending on the visit, your massage may last 15 to 90 minutes. The therapist will usually begin by applying oil or lotion to reduce friction between his or her hands and your skin. The therapist will ask if the amount of pressure is too soft or hard and adjust according to your preferences.[28] Therapists recommend drinking a lot of water after a massage to compensate for the dehydration that can occur through perspiration and to assist the body in flushing out toxins released by the muscles through the massage process. However, there is insufficient evidence to indicate either that massage facilitates the body's release of toxins or that drinking water will help flush them out.[30]

Despite many studies, there is little evidence of the risks and benefits of massage. The strongest evidence supports its effectiveness in alleviating chronic low back and neck pain.[24] There is inconclusive evidence about its effect on depression, anxiety, fibromyalgia, headaches, quality of life for those with HIV/AIDS, and other professed health outcomes. Athletes often use massage to increase short-term flexibility and strength.[31] Massage is considered to be safe, with rare instances of reported adverse events.[32] Many people believe massage is a way to relax and ease tension in the body.

Acupuncture

Acupuncture is an ancient Chinese medicinal practice in which practitioners use thin needles to stimulate certain points on the body.

acupuncture An ancient Chinese medicinal practice where practitioners use thin needles to stimulate certain points on the body.

According to traditional Chinese medicine, acupuncture is a technique to aid in the balance and flow of energy, called qi (pronounced *chee*). This traditional

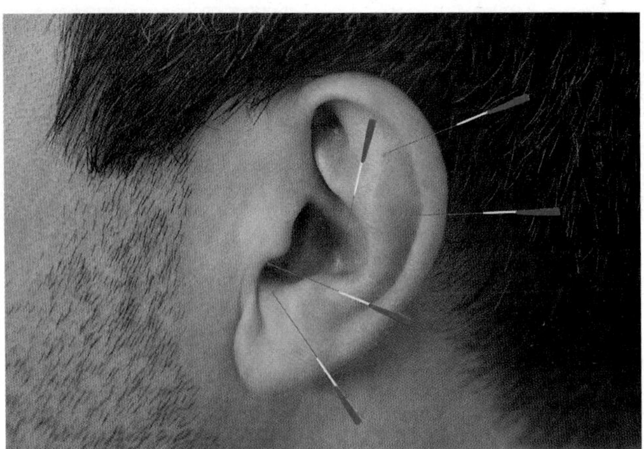

© Andrey_Popov/Shutterstock.

practice subscribes to the belief that the insertion of needles into certain points will balance one's flow of energy. In Western societies like the United States, however, practitioners believe the stimulation of certain body points triggers nerves and tissues to increase blood flow and prompt the body's natural pain management system.[33]

The effects of acupuncture on reducing pain appear promising, particularly for those with chronic pain or headaches. More research is needed to explain how it may impact other health outcomes, such as management of depression and smoking cessation. There is much debate about whether acupuncture itself works to alleviate pain or whether the recipients' expectations and other factors unrelated to acupuncture treatment affect their perceived benefits. As with other complementary and alternative therapies, acupuncture is relatively safe if conducted by a skilled practitioner. There is a risk of serious adverse effects only if needles are not sterile or are used incorrectly.[34]

Cupping

Remember the circles covering the back and chest of Michael Phelps during the 2016 Olympics? They were the result of a practice known as "cupping." Celebrities like Gwyneth Paltrow and Jennifer Aniston have been said to be fans of cupping, but what is it and does it work? Cupping is a form of CAM that has been around since ancient times, as early as 1550 BC in Egyptian, Chinese, and Middle Eastern cultures. Heated cups (in the form of glass, bamboo, or earthenware) are applied to the skin to create a vacuum or suction. The intent is to increase tissue blood flow to promote healing and alleviate pain.[35,36] There are 10 different types of cupping methods.[36]

Cupping has been shown to be effective in reducing pain. It has been tested for other indications such as high blood pressure and stroke, but without any clear, positive results.[37] There is some research to show that it is effective in the treatment of herpes zoster.[38] It can cause some adverse effects such as damage to the skin.[36] More research is needed to understand how cupping works and what conditions it can treat effectively.[39]

mind–body An approach that utilizes techniques, such as yoga and meditation, that seek to enhance health and well-being by living in the present moment.

Mind–Body Techniques

We live in a world of constant sensory and information overload: television, text messages, 24-hour news outlets, Facebook, Instagram, Twitter, and Snapchat. Because of this overload, many people feel the need to put down their phones, turn off their TVs, and engage in **mind–body** techniques, such as

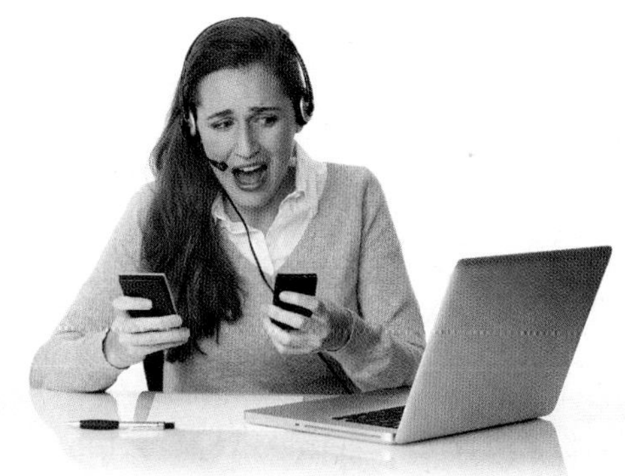

© STUDIO GRAND OUEST/Shutterstock.

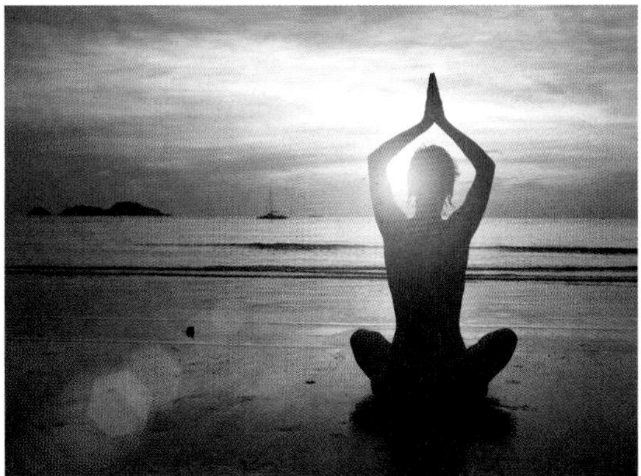

© De Visu/Shutterstock.

yoga and meditation, to enhance health and well-being by living in the present moment.

Many of these practices originated from Buddhism, a religion that began in India thousands of years ago. Buddhist practices such as meditation are intended to develop awareness, kindness, and wisdom.[40]

Mind–body techniques are popular and often used to promote physical and emotional health and well-being. Practicing these techniques promotes "mindfulness," or being continually present, with the hope that this translates into being more aware of thoughts and behaviors. The downstream effect is that it may positively impact the individual and others around him or her. These practices foster the relationship with oneself and the connection to others. Preliminary research suggests that use of mind–body techniques may even reduce healthcare utilization and save on healthcare spending.[41]

Yoga

Yoga practices began in India over 2,500 years ago and were first introduced in the United States in the 1920s. Yoga is not a religion; it is a discipline that involves physical postures and breathing exercises to promote health and well-being and balance of the mind, body, and spirit.[9] The word *yoga* is Sanskrit, meaning "to join" or "to yoke."[42] (A yoke is a wooden beam used to join oxen, forcing them to work together.)

yoga An ancient practice, originating approximately 2,500 years ago, in what is now India. It combines physical, mental, and spiritual elements, and comes in numerous forms, through different schools, practices, and environments.

It was not until the middle of the century that yoga gained popularity in the United States.[43] Currently, about 10% of adults report practicing yoga. This figure has almost doubled in the last 10 years.[10] Yoga is most popular among young and middle-aged adults, although more recently it has been employed in elementary school settings.[44] There are many different types of yoga (vinyasa, kundalini, Bikram, asana, hatha, Iyengar, and more). Each type of yoga has its own history, purpose, and practice; some focus more on breathing techniques and others on movement (**FIGURE 4-2**).

Yoga can be practiced individually or in a group class setting. Each person modifies and tailors the postures to his or her own abilities and comfort level. Training programs to become a certified yoga instructor vary depending on the type of yoga, but most require at least 500 hours of training.[45]

More and more research is being done to understand yoga's therapeutic influence on health (**FIGURE 4-3**). Yoga has been found to be effective for short-term chronic low back pain and moderately effective for long-term relief.[46] It also has the potential to reduce depressive symptoms and alleviate anxiety and stress without negative side effects.[45,47] For some people—such as women who are pregnant or people who have high blood pressure, glaucoma, or

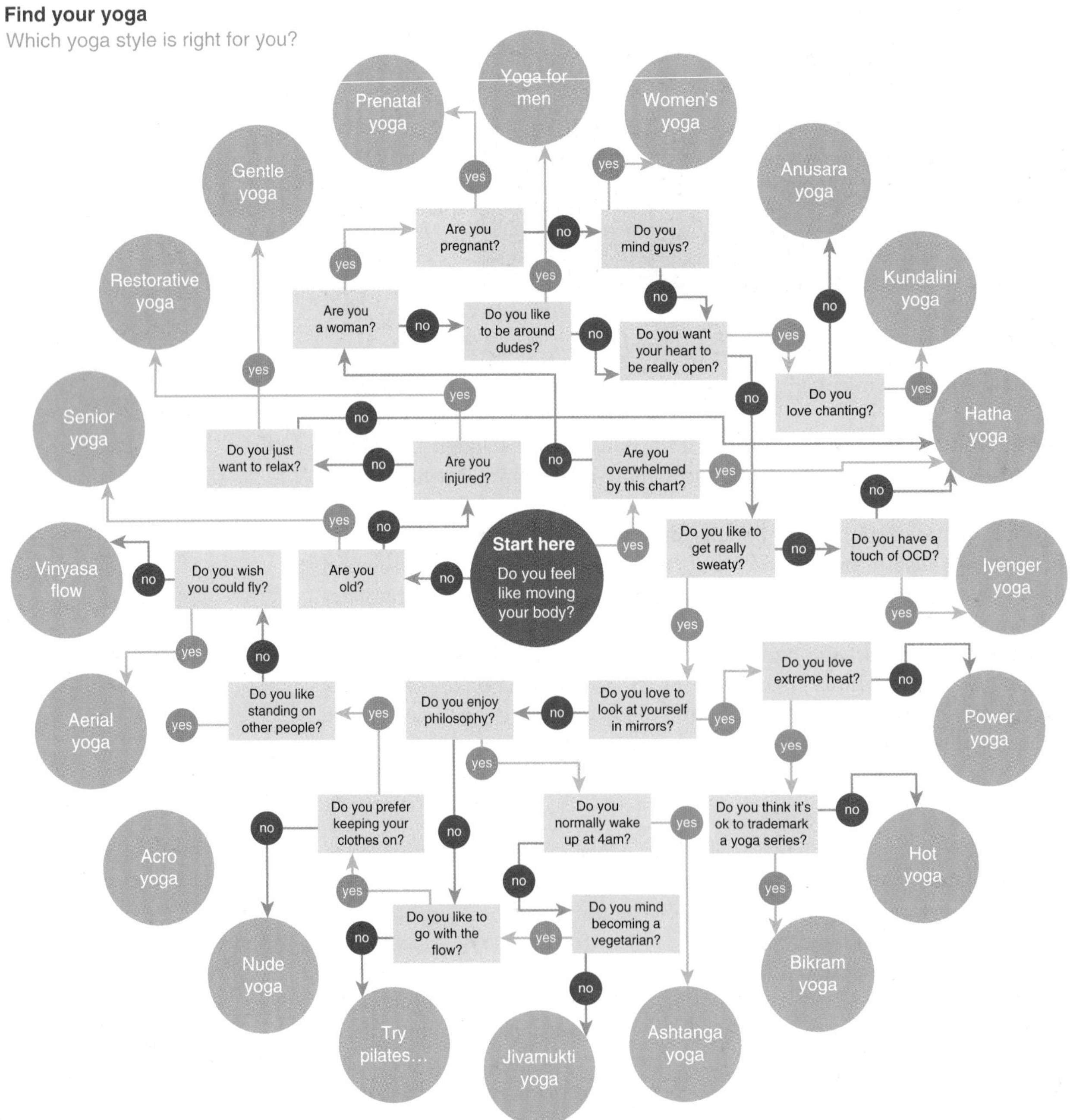

FIGURE 4-2 Find your yoga.

Yoga as a complementary health approach

Yoga is one of the top 10 complementary health approaches

More than **13 million adults** in the U.S. practiced yoga in the previous year.[1]

Yoga use increased from 5.1% to 6.1% between 2002 and 2007.[1]

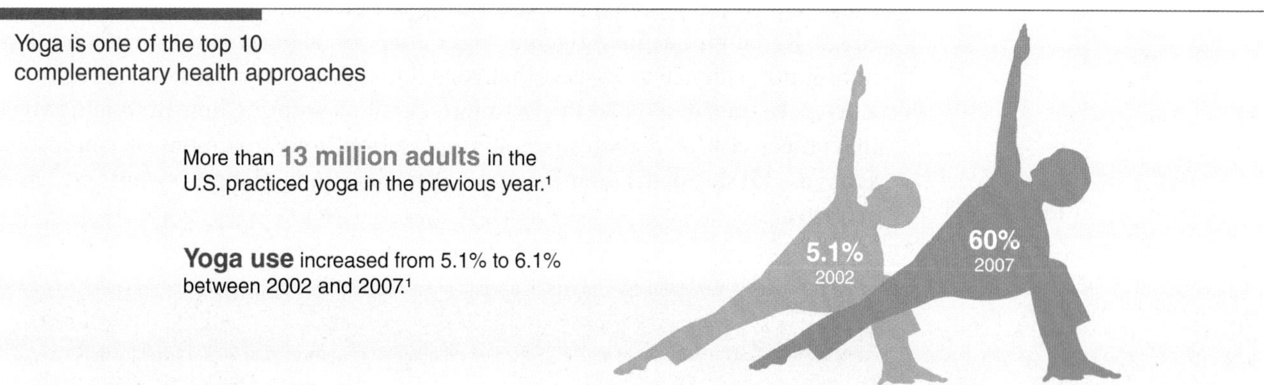

Why people practice yoga[2]

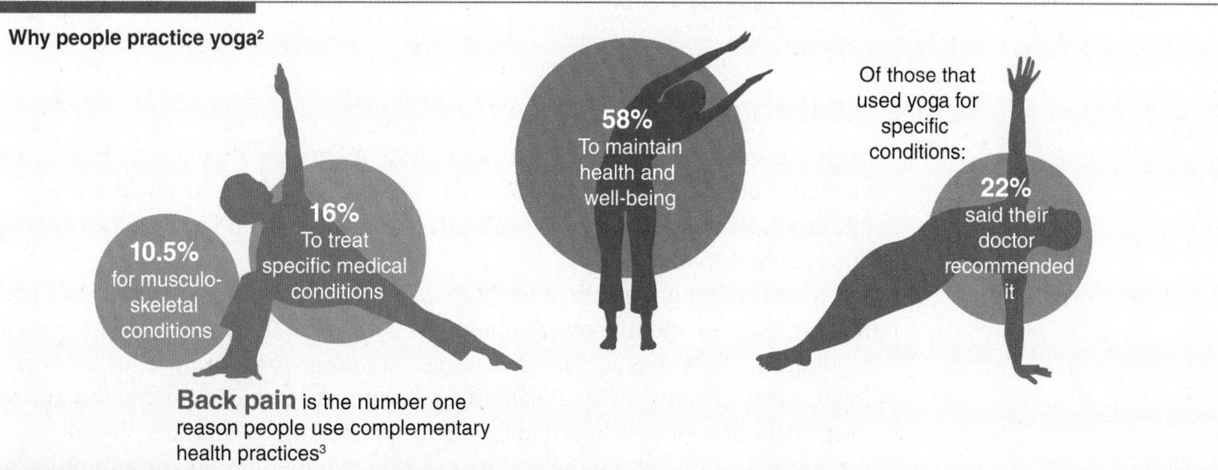

Back pain is the number one reason people use complementary health practices[3]

Yoga's impact on low-back pain

Back pain is the **number one reason** people use complementary health practices. Studies found people practicing yoga who experience low-back pain had:

Significantly **less disability, pain, and depression** after 6 months than patients in standard care.[4]

More pain relief than from a self-care book.[5]

Better function than usual medical care.[6]

Practice yoga safely

Follow these tips to minimize your risk of injury:

Talk to your care provider

Find a **trained and experienced** yoga practitioner

Adapt poses to your individual needs and abilities

FIGURE 4-3 Yoga as a complementary health approach.

Reproduced from Yoga as a Complementary Health Approach, National Center for Complementary and Integrative Health (NCCIH). Retrieved from https://nccih.nih.gov/news/multimedia/infographics/yoga

sciatica—yoga poses need to be modified or they will risk injury.[45] Yoga may even help to reduce high blood pressure, a risk factor for cardiovascular disease.[48] Research has investigated yoga's effect on asthma and arthritis but has not found evidence to suggest that yoga has an impact on either health issue.[49] Currently, the NCCIH is supporting research to examine how practicing yoga may affect risk of diabetes, smoking cessation, and treatment of conditions such as HIV, posttraumatic stress disorder, menopausal symptoms, and arthritis.[50]

TRY IT!

Interested in trying yoga out for yourself? You can watch this video to learn more. Search YouTube for "Yoga with Adriene Day 1 - Ease Into It - 30 days of Yoga."

Meditation

Yoga is considered to be a form of meditation because it integrates meditative elements into its practice. Meditation can also be practiced on its own. It is another technique to improve health that originated from Far Eastern religious and spiritual traditions.

Meditation is a group of techniques used to focus one's attention and promote relaxation and mental calmness.[9] As with yoga, there are different types of meditation. They may include repeating a calming word (or *mantra*), performing a series of movements during deep breathing, or having increased awareness. Visualization can be a helpful technique during meditation. Visualization is the practice of creating mental images. During meditation you can visualize your body relaxing, and can even say that as part of a mantra, such as "Breathing in, my body relaxes."

Regardless of the type, each form of meditation shares four necessary elements: a quiet location, a comfortable position, focused attention, and an open attitude.[51] Meditation is not about clearing your mind so you have absolutely no thoughts. It is about observing your thoughts and accepting, or letting go of them. About 2% of children 4 to 17 years of age engage in meditation, mostly as part of yoga, tai chi, or qigong,[52] and about 4% of adults report practicing meditation in the last year.[100]

There is wide regional variation in the use of yoga techniques and meditation; rates of use in the United States are highest in the Pacific and Mountain regions (**FIGURE 4-4**).[10]

Meditative practices have been studied for their effects on health outcomes, with largely mixed results. It is unclear, though, if the lack of conclusive results is because meditation does not have an effect or because the studies are of poor quality.[53] Yoga and meditation have been found to have potential positive effects on quitting smoking.[54] Meditation may also be associated with positive effects on various cardiovascular risk factors, including lowering blood pressure.[51,55] Meditation can moderately improve anxiety, depression, and pain.[56] Surprisingly, there is minimal evidence associating meditation with quality of life through reduced stress and improved mental health. There is insufficient evidence of its effect on attention, sleep, substance use, weight, or eating habits.

A lack of evidence does not mean that meditation has no effect on these health outcomes; it means we need more and better studies to understand the relationship. The NCCIH is currently funding studies to investigate meditation's impact on reducing or relieving stress, improving health in people with type 2 diabetes, enhancing weight management, improving sleep, and reducing the risk of heart disease.[51] Meditation has been shown to improve irritable bowel syndrome symptoms and may reduce stress-induced flare-ups from ulcerative colitis. Meditation is considered safe, with rare reports of exacerbated symptoms among individuals with psychiatric problems.[51]

meditation A group of techniques used to focus one's attention and promote relaxation and mental calmness.

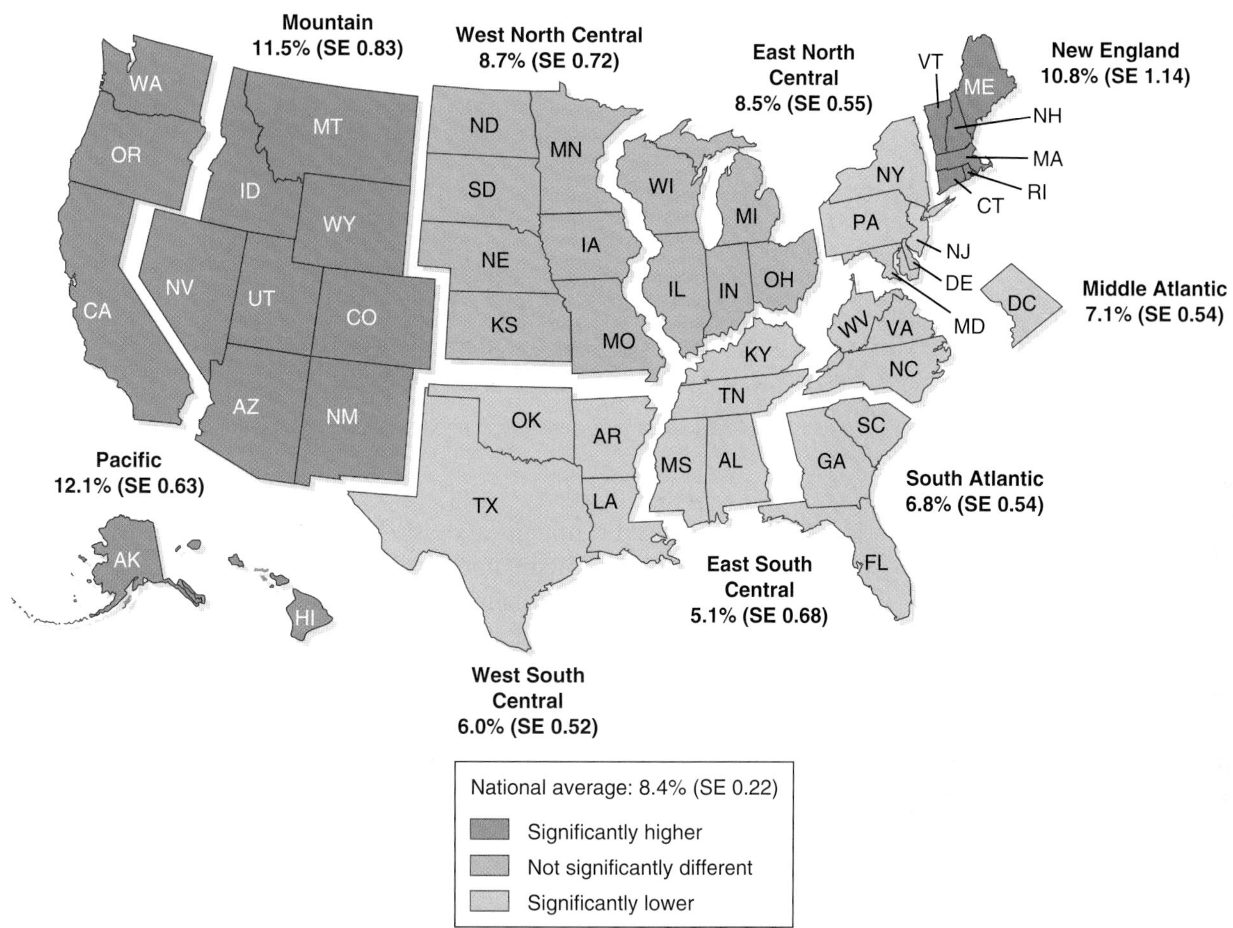

FIGURE 4-4 Map of regional variation in yoga and meditation.

Reproduced from CDC/NCHS, National Health Interview Survey, 2012. Retrieved from http://www.cdc.gov/nchs/data/databriefs/db146_fig4.png

TRY IT!

The One-Minute Meditation

Between class, activities, relationships, friends, and family, sometimes it's hard to find 25 minutes to just be still and meditate. One solution it to start with only 1 minute. Regardless of how busy you are, everyone can take 1 minute of their day when they're feeling stressed to meditate. Deepak Chopra, author and alternative medicine guru, suggests that you count your breaths (both your inhalations and exhalations) until you reach 30. In that simple 1-minute exercise, you can bring yourself back to your center.

To watch the 1-minute meditation with Deepak Chopra, visit this website: http://www.yogajournal.com/meditation/deepak-chopra-one-minute-meditation/.

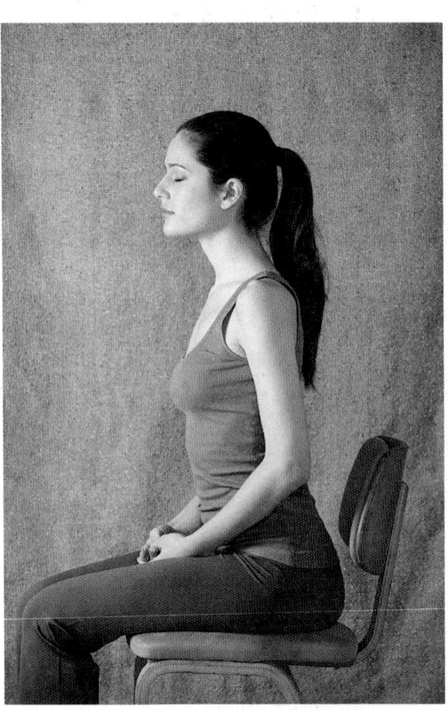

A quiet space and open attitude are all you need to start practicing meditation.

Calming the mind is not an easy task, but it becomes easier with practice. Once you find the type of meditation that is right for you, it is recommended to practice for about 25 minutes daily.[57,58] To learn more, check out this TED talk by searching www.TED.com for "the art of stillness."

Tai Chi and Qigong

tai chi A moving meditation that originated in China that is focused and grounded in martial art movement.

qigong A moving meditation that originated in China as a martial art that is designed to be a meditative, healing motion.

Tai chi (also known as tai chi chuan) and **qigong** are "moving meditations" that originated in China as a martial art.[59] Their principles are based on Taoism, an ancient Chinese philosophy that emphasizes balance and harmony with nature.[60] Tai chi and qigong are very similar practices, but tai chi is focused and grounded in martial art movement, whereas qigong is intended only as a meditative, healing motion.[61] People who practice tai chi and qigong breathe deeply while moving their bodies slowly. Practitioners believe that this practice supports a balance of *yin* and *yang*, thought to be opposing forces in one's body, to restore balance and energy flow.

Research is being conducted to understand more about how tai chi and qigong can influence health and well-being. Several studies have found that it can help to reduce blood pressure, improve the immune system and well-being in the elderly, and improve physical functioning in patients with chronic obstructive pulmonary disease.[59] Furthermore, there is some evidence that it helps prevent falls among older adults, helps manage depression, helps treat fibromyalgia, improves immune functioning among cancer patients, improves cognitive functioning, and more.[62–68] However, many of the existing studies that demonstrate how tai chi and qigong influence health outcomes have used insufficient methods to test and measure this relationship.[63,65-67,69,70] More research is currently underway to assess tai chi's effects on bone loss, arthritis, and depression. Tai chi and qigong have few risks, except the potential of strains

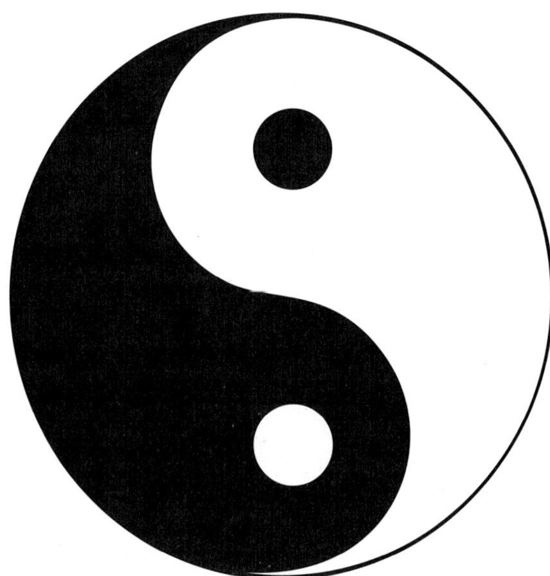

Yin and yang are thought to be two opposing but complementary forces that together bring balance.

"In meditation we discover our inherent restlessness. Sometimes we get up and leave. Sometimes we sit there but our bodies wiggle and squirm and our minds go far away. This can be so uncomfortable that we feel it's impossible to stay. Yet this feeling can teach us not just about ourselves but what it is to be human. . . . We really don't want to stay with the nakedness of our present experience. It goes against the grain to stay present. These are the times when only gentleness and a sense of humor can give us the strength to settle down. . . . So whenever we wander off, we gently encourage ourselves to "stay" and settle down. Are we experiencing restlessness? Stay! Are fear and loathing out of control? Stay! Aching knees and throbbing back? Stay! What's for lunch? Stay! I can't stand this another minute! Stay!"

—**Pema Chödrön**, *The Places That Scare You: A Guide to Fearlessness in Difficult Times*

or sprains. People with certain health issues will need to modify poses.[59] Currently, tai chi practitioners do not need to be licensed, so there is no standardized training. Traditionally, students of tai chi wishing to become an instructor need the approval of their "master" or teacher. See what tai chi looks like in action: nccih.nih.gov/video/taichidvd-full.

Reiki

Reiki is another complementary health approach, often classified as energy medicine, which practitioners use to help relieve stress and increase relaxation.

Reiki A subtle form of energy work where hands are placed gently on or above certain parts of the body used to help relieve stress and increase relaxation.

Reiki originated in Japan within the past century. In Reiki, the practitioner subtly controls energy by positioning his or her hands gently on or above certain parts of the body.[71] Very few studies have examined how Reiki can affect health. Some evidence suggests it may help to alleviate pain and anxiety,[72] whereas other studies have shown no impact of Reiki on anxiety or depression.[73] Reiki is not affiliated with any particular religion. However, the spiritual foundation of Reiki conflicts with some religions, such as Catholicism, which considers it to be an "occult practice" or "divination." Thus, Catholic healthcare facilities may not offer it.[74]

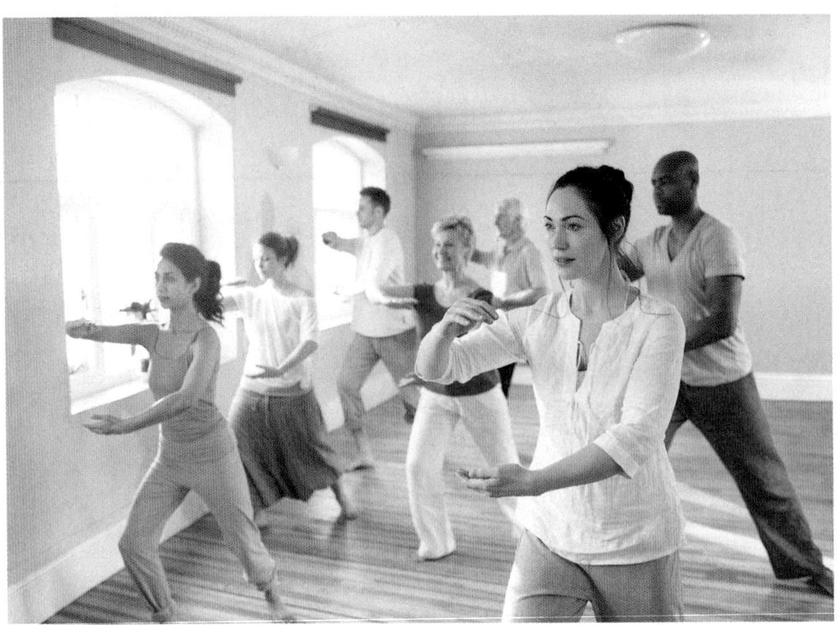

The slow body movements in tai chi and qigong lend themselves to easy participation for people of all ages.

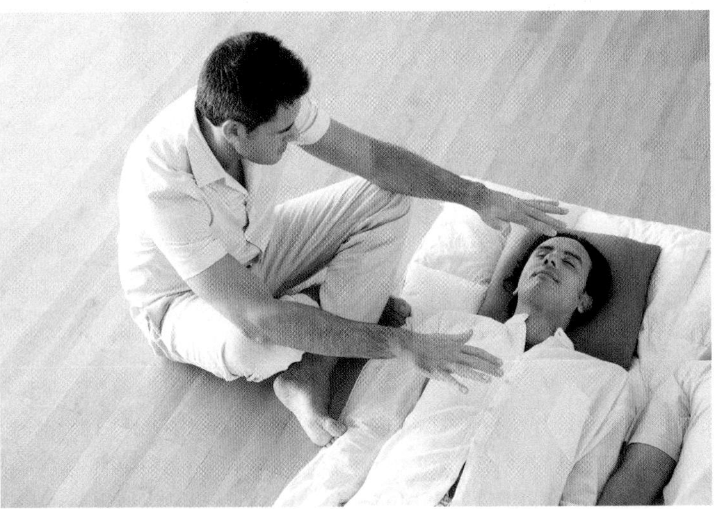

Reiki practitioners often do not even touch the patient, but instead hold their hands above certain body parts to help relieve stress.

Hypnotherapy

hypnotherapy A process by which trained clinicians guide clients into a relaxed state. While in this state, sometimes called a "trance," the person's sense of awareness is heightened, and this allows the person to focus attention on specific thoughts.

Hypnotherapy is a process by which trained clinicians guide clients into a relaxed, hypnotic state.

While in this state, sometimes called a "trance," the person's sense of awareness is heightened, allowing the person to focus attention on specific thoughts. It is often used in conjunction with psychotherapy (or counseling) to help clients change behavior or explore past, painful thoughts and experiences that the clients may have shielded from their current consciousness.[75] This practice was controversial for some time, but new evidence suggests it can be beneficial in relieving gastrointestinal symptoms associated with irritable bowel syndrome.[76] Hypnotherapy has been used most widely for helping clients quit smoking. Randomized controlled trials, however, do not provide evidence that hypnotherapy has lasting benefits on smoking cessation.[77]

How Do Mind–Body Techniques Affect Health?

Researchers have studied yoga, meditation, tai chi, and qigong for their effects on physical and mental health. But how would something like a breathing exercise alleviate pain or reduce blood pressure? Practices such as yoga, meditation, or prayer can incite a "relaxation response," defined as a physiologic state of deep rest that alters the physical and emotional response to stress; this state is thought to be the opposite of the body's fight-or-flight response.[78]

The fight-or-flight response to a stressor originated as a survival mechanism for mammals to quickly react to a potential danger such as being hunted as prey. Early humans, or cavemen, benefited from such a response mechanism when confronted by a saber-toothed tiger or other danger. During the fight-or-flight response, the sympathetic nervous system activates hormones (such as adrenaline and cortisol) and triggers physiological changes. The response instantaneously increases one's strength and speed to help fight off the danger or flee to safety.[79]

Thankfully we no longer live in a world where we are perpetually concerned about being hunted by tigers. However, our bodies' physiological response to stress has not evolved. Modern-day stressors that are not life threatening, such as work-related stress, a class presentation, or an argument, may trigger this fight-or-flight response. Having a prolonged stress response and exposure to cortisol and other hormones can adversely affect health, including such problems as heart disease, depression, and digestive issues.[80,81] The "relaxation

GOING UPSTREAM

Living in Stressful Environments

Although we may no longer live in an environment where we worry about being attacked by predatory animals, some of us do live in neighborhoods and homes where there are persistent stressors. For example, the United States has a deplorable history of racial discrimination and segregation. With the Civil Rights Movement and other subsequent political action, this discrimination has reduced over time, but it is clearly not gone. Because of this, people of color may live in a constant state of acute alertness. Although mind–body techniques would certainly benefit those of us who live in these types of stress-induced environments, such approaches merely treat the symptoms of discrimination without getting to the root cause of the stressors. What we really need are social policy reforms, such as universal access to high-quality education, and punishment of those who violate antidiscrimination laws.

Consider useful policy reforms that would address this issue: Why do you think people of color (racial/ethnic "minorities") might live in a state of chronic alertness? What are other examples of groups you think may live in such a state? What other social policies would help reduce this chronic stress?

response" initiated by mind–body therapies may help to shut off the body's fight-or-flight response to avoid the prolonged exposure to those hormones. See Chapter 6 for more specifics about stress.

Mind–body techniques can also change our brains. Practicing yoga increases brain wave activity,[82] and meditation alters regions of the brain associated with awareness, memory, and self-regulation.[83] Meditation has also been suggested to improve Alzheimer's disease symptoms because of its potential to reduce the impact of memory loss.[84] Similarly, studies of acupuncture found that it affects areas of the brain responsible for pain perception.[85] Through advances in neurologic science, we continually learn more about how these approaches positively affect brain activity and how that translates into better health and increased well-being (**FIGURE 4-5**).

CAM Across Cultures

The demographic characteristics of CAM users vary by health issue, gender, geography, income, and many other factors.[86] Cultural background plays an important role in the use of complementary and alternative approaches to health. A recent study using national survey data found that immigrants to the United States as a whole are less likely to use CAM (however this may not be the case for specific subpopulations of immigrants, who may use more). Lower rates of use may be because immigrants cannot afford or do not know about CAM therapies. As immigrants from various backgrounds stay longer in the United States or become more proficient in the English language, their likelihood of using CAM increases.[87] Interestingly, immigrants are usually healthier when they arrive in the United States, and their health declines over time.[88] As such, they may turn to other therapies and treatments to improve health as it declines.

CAM use also differs by race and ethnicity. In the United States, these approaches are more commonly used among Asian Americans.[90] For this group, using these methods is part of their spiritual beliefs.[91] Yoga is more common among non-Hispanic White adults.[10] This is likely related to the ability to pay for these services and availability in certain communities, as opposed to preferences or beliefs.

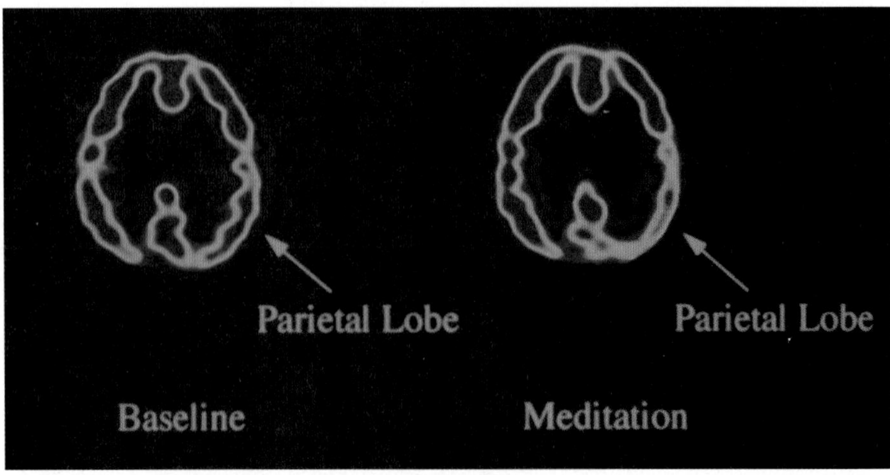

FIGURE 4-5 Meditation affects how our brain works.

GOING UPSTREAM

When Treatment Approaches Collide

In the book, *The Spirit Catches You and You Fall Down*, author Anne Fadiman presents the case of a young girl from Laos, Lia Lee, who was diagnosed with epilepsy while living in California. Her family's encounter with the U.S. medical system was fraught with miscommunication and struggles because they had distinct beliefs about how to treat her epilepsy—beliefs that did not align with the recommendations of U.S. medical doctors. Lia's family believed her epilepsy made her special, and their traditional Eastern practices influenced what they thought was appropriate care (including only partial compliance with the doctors' medication orders and efforts to "call her soul back"). The lack of understanding between Lia's doctors and her family resulted in Lia having a grand mal seizure that left her with permanent brain damage.[89]

Consider ways in which Lia Lee's condition could have been more effectively treated: How do you think medical professionals in the United States should handle a situation like this? Should they be respectful of the family's beliefs or promote the conventional Western medicine they were trained to use?

Paying for Integrative Health Approaches

Americans spend almost $34 billion per year on CAM therapies, of which about two-thirds is on self-care (products, classes, etc.) and one-third is on visits to specialized therapists/practitioners (**FIGURE 4-6**).[92] About one-quarter of users of these approaches account for 70% of the total out-of-pocket costs, meaning that a smaller group use a lot of these therapies (or are avid users of one or some of these therapies).[93] Who pays what (the users or their health insurance) for various therapies is complicated and depends on which therapy they are using, state laws, their specific health insurance coverage, the practitioner they see, and other factors. Out of all out-of-pocket spending in the

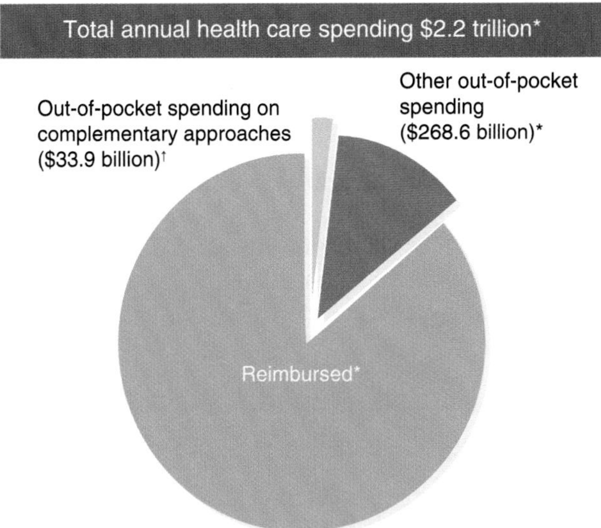

*National health expenditure data for 2007. Centers for Medicare & Medicaid Services web site. Accessed at www.cms.hhs.gov/NationalHealthExpendData/02_National-HealthAccountsHistorical.asp#TopOfPage on June 25, 2009.

†Nahin R. L. Barnes P. M. Stussman B. J. Bloom B. Costs of complementary and alternative medicine (CAM) and frequency of visits to CAM practitioners: United States, 2007. CDC national health statistics report #18. 2009.

FIGURE 4-6 Annual healthcare spending.

Reproduced from Paying for Complementary and Integrative Health Approaches, National Center for Complementary and Integrative Health (NCCIH). Retrieved from https://nccih.nih.gov/health/financial

UP FOR DEBATE

Should Complementary and Alternative Approaches to Health Be Covered by Health Insurance?

Formulate an argument in response to the question posed in this box's title. In your argument, consider the following:

- A variety of complementary approaches are used by about one-third of the U.S. population.
- If paid for out of pocket, these approaches are less accessible to low-income populations.
- The effectiveness of these approaches varies, with insufficient evidence for how they affect many health outcomes.
- Being covered under insurance allows patients to have more active participation in their treatment decision making.

SIX THINGS TO KNOW WHEN SELECTING A COMPLEMENTARY HEALTH PRACTITIONER

If you're looking for a complementary health practitioner to help treat a medical problem, it is important to be as careful and thorough in your search as you are when looking for conventional care. Here are six tips to help you in your search[96]:

1. **If you need names of practitioners in your area, first check with your doctor or other healthcare provider.** A nearby hospital or medical school, professional organizations, state regulatory agencies or licensing boards, or even your health insurance provider may be helpful.
2. **Find out as much as you can about any potential practitioner, including education, training, licensing, and certifications.** The credentials required for complementary health practitioners vary tremendously from state to state and from discipline to discipline.

Once you have found a possible practitioner, here are some tips about deciding whether he or she is right for you:

3. **Find out whether the practitioner is willing to work together with your conventional healthcare providers.** For safe, coordinated care, it is important for all of the professionals involved in your health to communicate and cooperate.
4. **Explain all of your health conditions to the practitioner, and find out about the practitioner's training and experience in working with people who have your conditions.** Choose a practitioner who understands how to work with people with your specific needs, even if general well-being is your goal. And, remember that health conditions can affect the safety of complementary approaches; for example, if you have glaucoma, some yoga poses may not be safe for you.
5. **Don't assume that your health insurance will cover the practitioner's services.** Contact your health insurance provider and ask. Insurance plans differ greatly in what complementary health approaches they cover, and even if they cover a particular approach, restrictions may apply.
6. **Tell all of your healthcare providers about all complementary approaches you use and about all practitioners who are treating you.** Keeping your healthcare providers fully informed helps you to stay in control and effectively manage your health.

Reproduced from National Center for Complementary and Integrative Health. (2016). 6 things to know when selecting a complementary health practitioner. National Institutes of Health. Retrieved from https://nccih.nih.gov/health/tips/selecting. Published 2015.

United States (meaning not covered under health insurance), complementary approaches comprise 11%.[92]

Do you know if your health insurance covers CAM? Why wouldn't health insurance companies cover these therapies? How do insurance companies decide whether they will pay for these alternative approaches? Consumer demand (how much people use them), the scientific evidence that the therapy works for the particular health issue, and the health insurance company's determination as to whether the therapy is cost-effective all factor into the decision.[94] An approach would be cost-effective if, for example, it prevents further low back pain and avoids the need for surgery. More scientific research with better methods would help insurance companies and patients understand what therapies work for which health issues.

The Patient Protection and Affordable Care Act of 2010 (ACA, or Obamacare) is a health insurance reform effort designed to expand insurance coverage to millions of previously uninsured Americans. Under this law, insurance companies are required to cover certain essential health approaches. Some states have included complementary and alternative therapies on the list of procedures covered by insurance companies.[95] As more research is conducted and users and practitioners advocate for the inclusion of complementary and alternative therapies as essential health care, more therapies may be covered under health insurance. See Chapter 13 for more about these issues.

Complementary and integrative health approaches are becoming increasingly popular in the United States. This may be due to an increase in the number of states that license practices, more media attention on benefits of therapies and treatments, or more exposure to techniques as travel to Eastern countries and virtual interconnectivity have become more popular.[29] The increase in use of CAM has transformed how we as a society think about our health. It has influenced our perceptions of illness and how we manage it. We have changed how we manage pain and stress and how we think about nutrition. The future popularity of these approaches in the United States will depend, in part, on cost and how much insurance companies are willing to pay for these services.

Keeping the Faith: How Do Religion and Spirituality Influence Our Health?

Some people think our religious beliefs and practices influence our health. **Religion** has been defined as involving "beliefs, practices and rituals related to the transcendent, where the transcendent is . . . a High Power."[97] Most religions include a set of beliefs and rituals designed to do two things: bring one closer to the High Power and clarify our responsibility to others in our society. The definition of **spirituality**, however, is debated and less well defined.[97]

Some people think of spirituality as being very similar to religion; others see it as more of a moral and individual experience of believing in something higher than themselves, though it may not be associated with an organized set of practices or beliefs. However, people who consider themselves to be spiritual may engage in practices such as meditation, prayer, or rituals.

In a review that synthesized findings of many studies, religion and spirituality were found to be associated with the ability to cope with adversity, hopefulness, optimism, having a sense of meaning or purpose, greater forgiveness, lower substance abuse rates, less crime/delinquency rates, and greater marital stability, social support, and social capital.[97] Social capital is the collective value

religion Beliefs, practices, and rituals related to the transcendent, where the transcendent is a High Power, designed to bring one closer to the High Power and clarify our responsibility to others in our society.

spirituality A concept similar to religion or a moral and individual experience of believing in something higher than oneself that may not be through an organized set of practices or beliefs.

of our social networks (the people we know). This concept is often used as a measure of community health, as opposed to individual health. The majority of studies found religion and spirituality to be associated with higher self-esteem and decreased levels of anxiety, depression, and suicide. However, a few studies found the opposite, suggesting that religion focuses on sins and humility and sets a high bar for expectations, thus increasing guilt and possibly lowering self-esteem. There are mixed results about how religion and spirituality may impact one's sense of control.[97] Many of these studies used self-reported survey data to ask participants if they were religious or spiritual, often without naming or studying a particular religion. Studying the specific religion itself may be more helpful in understanding how faith impacts health.[98]

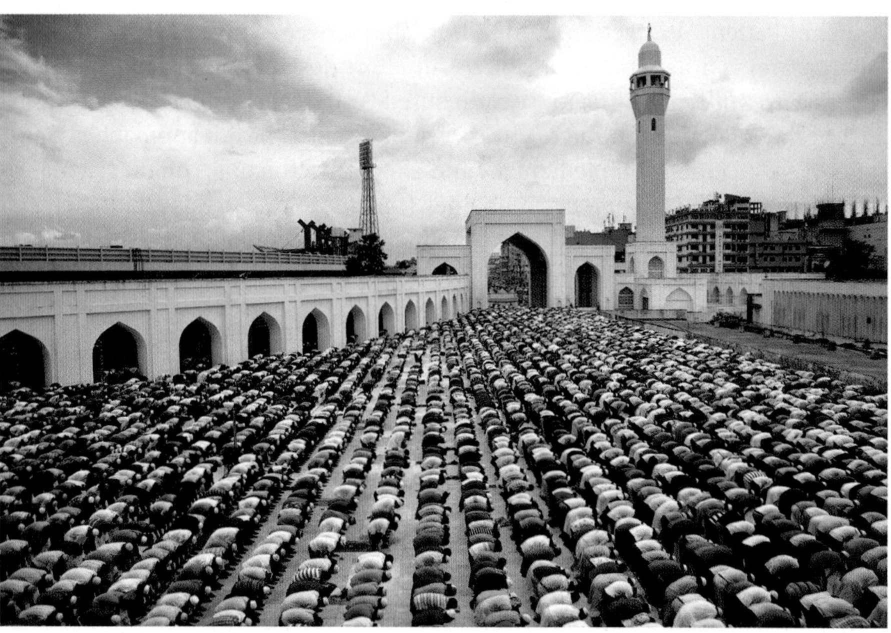

Practicing Muslims observe Ramadan, a month of holy fasting and prayer.

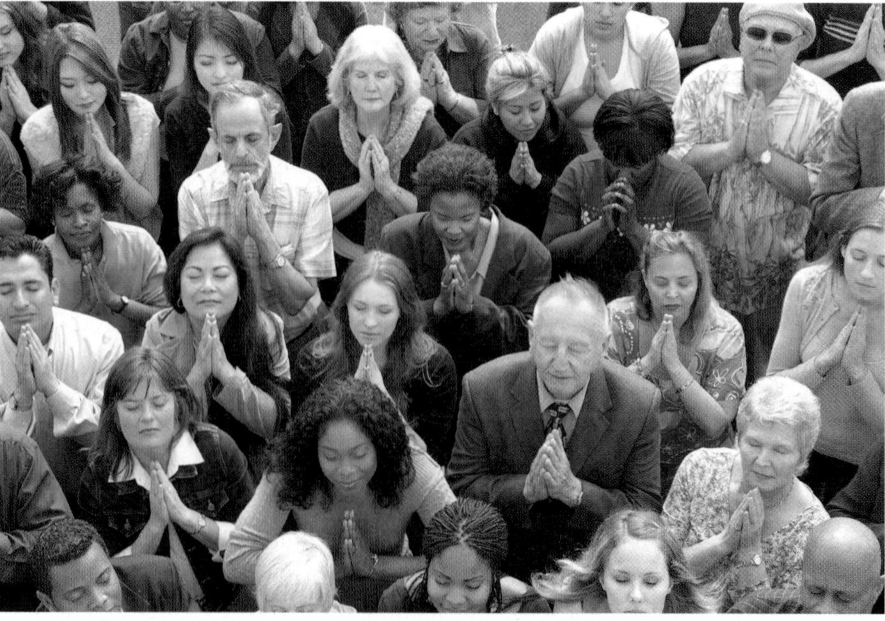

Religion and spirituality can affect one's health, but more research is needed to understand exactly what it can affect and how.

How do religion and spirituality affect health? The precise mechanism that links religion and spirituality to specific health outcomes is not known, but some hypothesize that religion and spirituality help provide a "social control mechanism" over the course of one's lifetime, which may promote health and impact health behaviors.[99] Some people believe that prayer has a powerful effect on health, but most of the research evidence is mixed on whether or not prayer can impact health outcomes.[3] Religion and spirituality may help to form social networks and promote community engagement.

Why Don't We Know More About How CAM Affects Health?

There are a host of reasons why we do not clearly understand if and how specific complementary and alternative therapies affect our health—individually and as a population. First, many of these approaches to health have only recently become popular, and some still are not popular at all. Thus, there may have been less interest and funding to conduct effectiveness research, or there may not be enough practitioners to conduct a study. Second, there are many potential problems in studying these techniques. For example, there are more than a dozen different types of yoga, there are many different techniques used for chiropractic care, there are almost 100 types of massage therapy, and so on. To add to this variety, providers who engage in these approaches may differ in how they deliver or practice them. They may have different approaches, for example, to adjusting a yoga posture to suit their clients' needs. At the individual level, one person may practice yoga 10 hours per week, whereas another may practice for 1 hour. All of this variation makes it difficult to rigorously study these therapies and answer a seemingly simple question such as "Does yoga reduce back pain?"

Thus, studying complementary and alternative therapies is different from studying whether a specific dosage of a pharmaceutical drug works, because there is virtually no variation from one pill to another. We would need to compare a random group of people using the same exact type of therapy, with the same provider, for the same length of time, and compare them to a control group who did not engage in those activities. To conduct the most rigorous kind of study, we would also need that control group to "look like" the group participating in the activity, meaning they may need to be similar in all important ways: have the same health problems (or lack of health problems) and be the same age, gender, race/ethnicity, education level, and so forth.

Also, study of complementary and alternative therapies can be affected by the "placebo effect," wherein a test participant has a response to a false (or inactive) treatment. This response is likely the result of the participant's belief about a medication and not the true effect of the medication itself. When researchers test medications in clinical trials, some participants may be given a sugar pill with no active medication in it; thus, none of the participants know whether they are receiving the treatment, meaning they do not know whether they are in the experimental or the control group. This method is called "blinding," and it helps researchers to understand if a reaction someone has is from the medication itself or from something else, such as psychological factors. ("Double blinding" is also used, wherein neither the participant nor the researcher knows who is in the experimental group and who is in the control group.) When studying complementary approaches to health, researchers cannot blind someone to the treatment because participants will know if they are doing yoga or doing nothing! Similarly, researchers cannot randomize someone into a group to be religious.

For these reasons, studying complementary and alternative health therapies has been difficult. Researchers, though, are starting to think more creatively about how to study different outcomes, and there is more interest in funding such projects. Some have included "sham" or "dummy" practices, whereby participants may think they are receiving the therapy when in fact they are not; for example, in a study of acupuncture, fake needles may be used to "pierce" the skin or needles may be inserted in nontherapeutic areas. We need more rigorous research to help us understand the health outcomes produced by each type of therapy, and how much of the therapy we should use to experience those outcomes.

TALES OF PUBLIC HEALTH

The American Medical Association Versus CAM

Historically, medical physicians and CAM providers have an uncomfortable, if not combative, relationship. The tension between CAM and conventional medicine has been evident since these communities first interacted. In 1910, Abraham Flexner wrote an evaluation of medical education in the United States and Canada. The report, known today as "The Flexner Report," highlighted the need for more rigorous medical training. Flexner questioned the validity of any medical practices not based on the scientific method, such as homeopathy and chiropractic methods. Thus, medical schools that provided training in these alternative methods were instructed to eliminate these courses from the medical training curriculum or risk losing their accreditation.[101,102] Today, there are only 7 accredited naturopathic medical programs, versus 141 medical schools granting medical doctorate (MD) degrees.[103,104]

These tensions culminated in a lawsuit, *Wilk v. American Medical Association*, in 1987. Chiropractic was under particular criticism from the American Medical Association (AMA), which sets standards and policies for the medical profession. In the 1960s, the Iowa Medical Society created a plan to conspire against chiropractic. They adopted a policy, including action items such as opposing chiropractors' participation in health insurance and unions, as a means to dissolve the profession. For this and other reasons, the AMA was found guilty of previously conspiring to destroy the chiropractic profession and was disallowed from restricting the freedom of its members in affiliating with chiropractors. The judge noted:

> They [the plaintiffs] want a judicial pronouncement that chiropractic is a valid, efficacious, even scientific health care service. I believe that the answer to that question can only be provided by a well-designed, controlled, scientific study. . . . No such study has ever been done. In the absence of such a study, the court is left to decide the issue on the basis of largely anecdotal evidence. I decline to pronounce chiropractic valid or invalid on anecdotal evidence.[105,106]

This sentiment remains today, with a call and increasing response to provide scientific evidence of the effectiveness of CAM therapies.

CAM and Population Health

With CAM's growing popularity, the field of population health has become more receptive to the idea of a truly integrative health approach, integrating CAM into our traditionally biomedical system.[107] One study found that health professionals themselves have high rates of CAM use and support more professional training to integrate CAM into their practice and research.[108] There has been a call for both conventional medical doctors and CAM providers to recognize the value each can bring to public health and integrate academic and clinical training into their respective programs that outline the benefits and risks of each.[109,110]

By definition, CAM health approaches are a complement or alternative to mainstream medicine, an approach formally more widely accepted as the gold standard or norm. If, over time, research evidence demonstrates the efficacy of CAM approaches, we may come to think more about truly "integrative health" where CAM and traditional therapies are used together to promote health.

In Summary

Complementary and alternative health approaches include supplements, special diets, chiropractic care, massage, acupuncture, and mind–body techniques, such as yoga and meditation. The demographics of people who use these therapies and treatments vary depending on cultural background, geographic area, ability to pay, and other factors. Religion and spirituality are also thought to influence health. Some of these approaches may impact health through physiological changes in the body. We need more rigorous research studies to fully understand how each of these practices may affect various health outcomes.

Key Terms

acupuncture
chiropractic
complementary and alternative medicine (CAM)
complementary health approach
hypnotherapy
integrative health
massage
meditation
mind–body
qigong
Reiki
religion
spirituality
tai chi
yoga

Student Discussion Questions and Activities

1. What factors could influence your decision to use a particular health approach?
2. What complementary and alternative approaches to health have you tried? What influenced your decision to use those approaches?
3. What are some reasons that CAM has become more popular in recent decades?
4. Why do you think variation in use of complementary health approaches exists by geographic region? By gender?
5. If everyone practiced mind–body techniques, how do you think it would change society?
6. Do you think CAM therapies should be more widely practiced, or should they be more regulated and limited? Why do you feel this way?

References

1. National Center for Complementary and Integrative Health. (2011). NCCAM third strategic plan 2011–2015: Exploring the sciences of complementary and alternative medicine. Retrieved from https://nccih.nih.gov/about/plans/2011
2. National Center for Complementary and Integrative Health. (2008). Complementary, alternative, or integrative health: What's in a name? Retrieved from https://nccih.nih.gov/health/integrative-health
3. Peregoy, J. A., Clarke, T. C., Jones, L. I., Stussman, B. J., & Nahin, R. L. (2014). Regional variation in use of complementary health approaches by U.S. adults. *NCHS Data Brief.* Retrieved from http://www.cdc.gov/nchs/products/databriefs/db146.htm
4. National Center for Complementary and Alternative Medicine. (2008, December). The use of complementary and alternative medicine in the United States. Retrieved from https://nccih.nih.gov/research/statistics/2007/camsurvey_fs1.htm
5. National Center for Complementary and Integrative Health. (2009). Homeopathy: An introduction. Retrieved from https://nccih.nih.gov/health/homeopathy
6. Johns Hopkins University. (2015). Allopathic medicine (M.D). Retrieved from http://studentaffairs.jhu.edu/preprofadvising/pre-medhealth/overview/allopathic-medicine/
7. National Center for Complementary and Integrative Health (NCCIH). (n.d.). Ayurvedic Medicine: In Depth. Retrieved from https://nccih.nih.gov/health/ayurveda/introduction.htm
8. U.S. Food and Drug Administration. (2015). Dietary supplements. Retrieved from http://www.fda.gov/Food/DietarySupplements/

9. National Center for Complementary and Integrative Health. (2015). Terms related to complementary and integrative health. Retrieved from https://nccih.nih.gov/health/providers/camterms.htm
10. Clarke, T. C., Black, L. I., Stussman, B. J., Barnes, P. M., & Nahin, R. L. (2015). Trends in the use of complementary health approaches among adults: United States, 2002–2012. *National Health Statistics Reports.* Retrieved from http://www.cdc.gov/nchs/data/nhsr/nhsr079.pdf
11. National Center for Complementary and Integrative Health. (2005). Herbs at a glance: Echinacea. Retrieved from https://nccih.nih.gov/health/echinacea/ataglance.htm
12. University of Maryland Medical Center. (2015). Echinacea. Retrieved from http://umm.edu/health/medical/altmed/herb/Echinacea
13. National Institute on Drug Abuse. (2015). DrugFacts: Is marijuana medical? Retrieved from http://www.drugabuse.gov/publications/drugfacts/marijuana-medicine
14. ProCon.org. (2015). 23 medical marijuana states and DC. Retrieved from http://medicalmarijuana.procon.org/view.resource.php?resourceID=000881
15. Whiting, P. F., Wolff, R. F., Deshpande, S., Di Nisio, M., Duffy, S., Hernandez, A. V., . . . Kleijnen, J. (2015). Cannabinoids for medical use: A systematic review and meta-analysis. *JAMA, 313*(24), 2456–2473.
16. National Center for Complementary and Integrative Health. (2012). Chiropractic: In depth. Retrieved from https://nccih.nih.gov/health/chiropractic/introduction.htm
17. National Center for Complementary and Integrative Health. (2015). Spinal manipulation. Retrieved from https://nccih.nih.gov/health/spinalmanipulation
18. Bureau of Labor Statistics. (2014). Chiropractors. *Occupational Outlook Handbook.* United States Department of Labor. Retrieved from http://www.bls.gov/ooh/healthcare/chiropractors.htm
19. National Board of Chiropractic Examiners. (2015). Examinations. Retrieved from http://www.nbce.org/examinations
20. Hildebrant, P. (2010, August). What is chiropractic radiology? *Radiology Today.* Retrieved from http://www.radiologytoday.net/archive/rt0810p20.shtml
21. Cleveland Clinic. (2013). Treatments and procedures: Osteopathic manipulation. Retrieved from http://my.clevelandclinic.org/health/treatments_and_procedures/hic_Osteopathic_Manipulation_for_Low_Back_Pain
22. American Chiropractic Association. (2015). Origins and history of chiropractic care. Retrieved from https://www.acatoday.org/About/History-of-Chiropractic
23. Novella, S. (2009). Chiropractic: A brief overview part I. Science Based Medicine. Retrieved from https://www.sciencebasedmedicine.org/chiropractic-a-brief-overview-part-i/
24. Bronfort, G., Haas, M., Evans, R., Leininger, B., & Triano, J. (2010). Effectiveness of manual therapies: The UK evidence report. *Chiropractic & Osteopathy, 18*, 3.
25. Bryans, R., Descarreaux, M. F., Duranleau, M. F., Marcoux, H., Potter, B., Ruegg, R., . . . White, E. (2011). Evidence-based guidelines for the chiropractic treatment of adults with headache. *Journal of Manipulative and Physiological Therapeutics, 34*(5), 274–289.
26. Robertson Chiropractic. (2015). NSA research. Robertson Chiropractic Network Spinal Analysis. Retrieved from http://www.robertsonnsa.com/nsa_research.shtml
27. National Center for Complementary and Integrative Health. (2006). Massage therapy for health purposes: What you need to know. National Institutes of Health. Retrieved from https://nccih.nih.gov/health/massage/massageintroduction.htm
28. University of Maryland Medical Center. (2011). Massage. Retrieved from http://umm.edu/health/medical/altmed/treatment/massage
29. Barnes, P. M., Bloom, B., & Nahin, R. L. (2008, December 10). Complementary and alternative medicine use among adults and children: United States, 2007. *National Health Statistics Reports,* 1–23.
30. Should you drink water after a massage? (2012, November 5). *Huffington Post.* Retrieved from http://www.huffingtonpost.com/2012/11/05/water-after-a-massage_n_2075604.html
31. Brummitt, J. (2008). The role of massage in sports performance and rehabilitation: Current evidence and future direction. *North American Journal of Sports Physical Therapy, 3*(1), 7–21.
32. Yin, P., Gao, N., Wu, J., Litscher. G. A., & Xu, S. (2014). Adverse events of massage therapy in pain-related conditions: A systematic review. *Evidence-Based Complementary and Alternative Medicine.* Retrieved from https://www.hindawi.com/journals/ecam/2014/480956/
33. Mayo Clinic. (2015). Acupuncture. Retrieved from http://www.mayoclinic.org/tests-procedures/acupuncture/basics/definition/prc-20020778
34. National Center for Complementary and Integrative Health. (2015). Acupuncture: What you need to know. Retrieved from https://nccih.nih.gov/health/acupuncture/introduction
35. WebMD.com. (2015). What is cupping therapy? Retrieved from http://www.webmd.com/balance/guide/cupping-therapy
36. Mehta, P., & Dhapte, V. (2014). Cupping therapy: A prudent remedy for a plethora of medical ailments. *Journal of Traditional and Complementary Medicine, 5*(3), 127–134.
37. Lee, M. S., Kim, J. I., & Ernst E. (2011). Is cupping an effective treatment? An overview of systematic reviews. *Journal of Acupuncture and Meridian Studies, 4*(1), 1–4.
38. Cao, H., Li, X. F., & Liu, J. (2012). An updated review of the efficacy of cupping therapy. *PloS One, 7*(2), e31793.
39. Kim, J. I., Lee, M. S., Lee, D. H., Boddy, K. F., & Ernst, E. (2011). Cupping for treating pain: A systematic review. *Evidence-Based Complementary and Alternative Medicine,* doi:10.1093/ecam/nep035
40. The Buddhist Centre. (2015). What is Buddhism? Retrieved from https://thebuddhistcentre.com/Buddhism
41. Stahl, J. E., Dossett, M. L., LaJoie, A. S., Denninger, J. W., Mehta, D. H., Goldman, R., . . . Benson, H. (2015). Relaxation response and resiliency training and its effect on healthcare resource utilization. *PLoS One, 10*(10), e0140212.
42. Yoga.org.nz. (2014). Definition of yoga. Retrieved from http://yoga.org.nz/what-is-yoga/yoga_definition.htm
43. Hammond, H. (2007). Yoga's trip to America. *Yoga Journal.* Retrieved from http://www.yogajournal.com/article/history-of-yoga/yogas-trip-america/
44. Khalsa, S. B. S., & Butzer, B. (2016, February 25). Yoga in school settings: A research review. *Annals of the New York Academy of Sciences.* Retrieved from http://onlinelibrary.wiley.com/doi/10.1111/nyas.13025/full
45. National Center for Complementary and Alternative Medicine. (2013). Get the facts: Yoga for health. Retrieved from https://nccih.nih.gov/sites/nccam.nih.gov/files/Get_The_Facts_Yoga_for_Health_06-04-2013%20%282%29.pdf

46. Cramer, H., Lauche, R. F., Haller, H. F., & Dobos, G. (2013). A systematic review and meta-analysis of yoga for low back pain. *The Clinical Journal of Pain, 29*(5), 450–460.
47. Skowronek, I. B., Mounsey, A. F., & Handler, L. (2014). Clinical inquiry: Can yoga reduce symptoms of anxiety and depression? *The Journal of Family Practice, 63*(7), 398–407.
48. Tyagi, A. F., & Cohen, M. (2014). Yoga and hypertension: A systematic review. *Alternative Therapies in Health and Medicine, 20*(2), 32–59.
49. National Center for Complementary and Integrative Health (2014, October). Yoga for health: What the science says. *NCCIH Clinical Digest*. Retrieved from https://nccih.nih.gov/health/providers/digest/yoga-science#lbpain
50. National Center for Complementary and Integrative Health. (2008). NCCIH-funded research. National Institutes of Health. Retrieved from https://nccih.nih.gov/health/yoga/introduction.htm
51. National Center for Complementary and Integrative Health. (2007). Meditiation: In depth. National Institutes of Health. Retrieved from https://nccih.nih.gov/health/meditation/overview.htm
52. Black, L. I., Clarke, T. C., Barnes, P. M., Stussman, B. J., & Nahin, R. L. (2015, February 10). Use of complementary health approaches among children aged 4–17 years in the United States: National health interview survey, 2007–2012. *National Health Statistics Reports,* 1–19.
53. Ospina, M. B., Bond, K., Karkhaneh, M., Tjosvold, L., Vandermeer, B., Liang, Y., . . . Klassen, T. P. (2007, June). Meditation practices for health: State of the research. *Evidence Report /Technology Assessment, 1-263.*
54. Carim-Todd, L., Mitchell, S. H., & Oken, B. S. (2013). Mind-body practices: An alternative, drug-free treatment for smoking cessation? A systematic review of the literature. *Drug and Alcohol Dependence, 132*(3), 399–410.
55. Ray, I. B., Menezes, A. R., Malur, P., Hiltbold, A. E., Reilly, J. P., & Lavie, C. J. (2014). Meditation and coronary heart disease: A review of the current clinical evidence. *The Ochsner Journal, 14*(4), 696–703.
56. Goyal, M., Singh, S., Sibinga, E. M., Gould, N. F., Rowland-Seymour, A., Sharma, R., . . . Haythornthwaite, J. A. (2014). Meditation programs for psychological stress and well-being: A systematic review and meta-analysis. *JAMA Internal Medicine, 174*(3), 357–368.
57. American Heart Association. (2014). Meditation and heart health. Retrieved from http://www.heart.org/HEARTORG/Conditions/More/MyHeartandStrokeNews/Meditation-and-Heart -Disease-Stroke_UCM_452930_Article.jsp
58. McGreevey, S. (2011, January 21). Eight weeks to a better brain. *Harvard Gazette*. Retrieved from http://news.harvard.edu/gazette/story/2011/01/eight-weeks-to-a-better-brain/
59. National Center for Complementary and Integrative Health. (2015). Tai chi and qi gong: In depth. National Institutes of Health. Retrieved from https://nccih.nih.gov/health/taichi/introduction.htm
60. Lam, P. (2007). History of tai chi. Tai Chi for Health Institute. Retrieved from http://taichiforhealthinstitute.org/history-of-tai-chi-2/
61. Wayne, J. (2013, October 13). Qi gong vs. tai chi. Livestrong.com. Retrieved from http://www.livestrong.com/article/359382-qi-gong-vs-tai-chi/
62. Lee, M. S., Pittler, M. H., & Ernst, E. (2009). Internal qigong for pain conditions: A systematic review. *The Journal of Pain, 10*(11), 1121–1127.
63. Wang, C. W., Chan, C. L., Ho, R. T., Chan, C. H., & Ng, S. M. (2013). The effect of qigong on depressive and anxiety symptoms: A systematic review and meta-analysis of randomized controlled trials. *Evidence-Based Complementary and Alternative Medicine,* doi:10.1155/2013/716094
64. Oh, B., Butow, P. F., Mullan, B. F., Hale, A., Lee, M. S., Guo, X., & Clarke, S. (2012). A critical review of the effects of medical qigong on quality of life, immune function, and survival in cancer patients. *Integrative Cancer Therapies, 11*(2), 101–110.
65. Zeng, Y., Luo, T., Xie, H., Huang, M., & Cheng, A. S. (2014). Health benefits of qigong or tai chi for cancer patients: A systematic review and meta-analyses. *Complementary Therapies in Medicine, 22*(1), 173–186.
66. Chan, C. L., Wang, C. W., Ho, R. T., Ng, S. M., Chan, J. S., Ziea, E. T., & Wong, V. C. (2012). A systematic review of the effectiveness of qigong exercise in supportive cancer care. *Supportive Care in Cancer, 20*(6), 1121–1133.
67. Chan, C. L., Wang, C. W., Ho, R. T., Ng, S. M., Ziea, E. T., & Wong, V. T. (2012). Qigong exercise for the treatment of fibromyalgia: A systematic review of randomized controlled trials. *Journal of Alternative and Complementary Medicine, 18*(7), 641–646.
68. Wayne, P. M., Walsh, J. N., Taylor-Piliae, R. E., Wells, R. E., Papp, K. V., Donovan, N. J., & Yeh, G. Y. (2014). Effect of tai chi on cognitive performance in older adults: Systematic review and meta-analysis. *Journal of the American Geriatrics Society, 62*(1), 25–39.
69. Wang, C. W., Ng, S. M., Ho, R. T., Ziea, E. T., Wong, V. C., & Chan, C. L. (2012). The effect of qigong exercise on immunity and infections: A systematic review of controlled trials. *The American Journal of Chinese Medicine, 40*(6), 1143–1156.
70. Guo, X., Zhou, B. F., Nishimura, T. F., Teramukai, S. F., & Fukushima, M. (2008). Clinical effect of qigong practice on essential hypertension: A meta-analysis of randomized controlled trials. *Journal of Alternative and Complementary Medicine, 14*(1), 27–37.
71. International Association of Reiki Professionals. (2015). What is Reiki? Retrieved from http://iarp.org/what-is-reiki/
72. Thrane, S., & Cohen, S. M. (2014). Effect of Reiki therapy on pain and anxiety in adults: An in-depth literature review of randomized trials with effect size calculations. *Pain Management Nursing, 15*(4), 897–908.
73. Joyce, J., & Herbison, G. P. (2015). Reiki for depression and anxiety. *The Cochrane Database of Systematic Reviews,* doi: 10.1002/14651858.CD006833.pub2
74. Arvonio, M. M. (2014). Cultural competency, autonomy, and spiritual conflicts related to Reiki/CAM therapies: Should patients be informed? *The Linacre Quarterly, 81*(1), 47–56.
75. Mental health and hypnosis. (2015). WebMD. Retrieved from http://www.webmd.com/anxiety-panic/guide/mental-health-hypnotherapy#3
76. Lee, H. H., Choi, Y. Y., & Choi, M. G. (2014). The efficacy of hypnotherapy in the treatment of irritable bowel syndrome: A systematic review and meta-analysis. *Journal of Neurogastroenterology and Motility, 20*(2), 152–162.
77. Barnes, J., Dong, C. Y., McRobbie, H. F., Walker, N. F., Mehta, M., & Stead, L. F. (2010). Hypnotherapy for smoking cessation. *The Cochrane Database of Systematic Reviews,* doi:10.1002/14651858.CD001008.pub2
78. Benson, H. (2002). Relaxation response. RelaxationResponse.org. Retrieved from http://www.relaxationresponse.org/
79. Harvard Health Publications. (2011). Understanding the stress response. Harvard Medical School. Retrieved from http://

www.health.harvard.edu/staying-healthy/understanding-the-stress-response

80. Gregoire, C. (2013, May 5). Relaxation gene response: What yoga, meditation and other stress busting activities do to the body. *Huffington Post*. Retrieved from http://www.huffingtonpost.com/2013/05/05/relaxation-gene-response-yoga-meditation-stress_n_3195257.html
81. Mayo Clinic. (2013). Chronic stress can wreak havoc on your mind and body. Take steps to control your stress. Stress Management. Retrieved from http://www.mayoclinic.org/stress/ART-20046037?p=1
82. Desai, R., Tailor, A., & Bhatt, T. (2015). Effects of yoga on brain waves and structural activation: A review. *Complementary Therapies in Clinical Practice, 21*(2), 112–118.
83. Fox, K. C., Nijeboer, S., Dixon, M. L., Floman, J. L., Ellamil, M., Rumak, S. P., . . . Christoff, K. (2014). Is meditation associated with altered brain structure? A systematic review and meta-analysis of morphometric neuroimaging in meditation practitioners. *Neuroscience and Biobehavioral Reviews, 43*, 48–73.
84. Innes, K. E., & Selfe, T. K. (2014). Meditation as a therapeutic intervention for adults at risk for Alzheimer's disease: Potential benefits and underlying mechanisms. *Frontiers in Psychiatry, 5*, 40.
85. Chae, Y., Chang, D. S., Lee, S. H., Jung, W. M., Lee, I. S., Jackson, S., . . . Wallraven, C. (2013). Inserting needles into the body: A meta-analysis of brain activity associated with acupuncture needle stimulation. *The Journal of Pain, 14*(3), 215–222.
86. Bishop, F. L., & Lewith, G. T. (2010). Who uses CAM? A narrative review of demographic characteristics and health factors associated with CAM use. *Evidence-Based Complementary and Alternative Medicine, 7*(1), 11–28.
87. Su, D., Li, L., & Pagan, J. A. (2008). Acculturation and the use of complementary and alternative medicine. *Social Science and Medicine, 66*(2), 439–453.
88. Antecol, H., & Bedard, K. (2006). Unhealthy assimilation: Why do immigrants converge to American health status levels? *Demography, 43*(2), 337–360.
89. Fadiman, A. (1997). *The spirit catches you and you fall down: A Hmong child, her American doctors, and the collision of two cultures*. New York, NY: Farrar, Straus and Giroux.
90. Mehta, D. H., Phillips, R. S., Davis, R. B., & McCarthy, E. P. (2007). Use of complementary and alternative therapies by Asian Americans. Results from the National Health Interview Survey. *Journal of General Internal Medicine, 22*(6), 762–767.
91. Hsiao, A. F., Wong, M. D., Goldstein, M. S., Becerra, L. S., Cheng, E. M., & Wenger, N. S. (2006). Complementary and alternative medicine use among Asian-American subgroups: Prevalence, predictors, and lack of relationship to acculturation and access to conventional health care. *Journal of Alternative and Complementary Medicine, 12*(10), 1003–1010.
92. National Center for Complementary and Integrative Health. (2013). Paying for complementary health approaches. National Institutes of Health. Retrieved from https://nccih.nih.gov/health/financial
93. Davis, M. A., & Weeks, W. B. (2012). The concentration of out-of-pocket expenditures on complementary and alternative medicine in the United States. *Alternative Therapies in Health and Medicine, 18*(5), 36–42.
94. Pelletier, K. R., & Astin, J. A. (2002). Integration and reimbursement of complementary and alternative medicine by managed care and insurance providers: 2000 update and cohort analysis. *Alternative Therapies in Health and Medicine, 8*(1), 38–39.
95. Fan, A. Y. (2014). "Obamacare" covers fifty-four million Americans for acupuncture as essential healthcare benefit. *Journal of Integrative Medicine, 12*(4), 390–393.
96. National Center for Complementary and Integrative Health. (2015). 6 things to know when selecting a complementary health practitioner. National Institutes of Health. Retrieved from https://nccih.nih.gov/health/tips/selecting
97. Koenig, H. G. (2012). Religion, spirituality, and health: The research and clinical implications. *ISRN Psychiatry*, 1–33.
98. Sullivan, A. R. (2010). Mortality differentials and religion in the U.S.: Religious affiliation and attendance. *Journal for the Scientific Study of Religion, 49*(4), 740–753.
99. Moeller, P. (2012, April 15). Why religion is linked with better health and well-being. *Huffington Post*. Retrieved from http://www.huffingtonpost.com/2012/04/15/religion-health-well-being_n_1423713.html
100. Roberts, L., Ahmed, I., Hall, S., & Davison, A. (2009). Intercessory prayer for the alleviation of ill health. *Cochrane Database of Systemic Reviews, 2009*(2), CD000368. doi: 10.1002/14651858.CD000368.pub3
101. Flexner, A. (1910). Medical education in the United States and Canada: A report to the Carnegie Foundation for the advancement of teaching. Retrieved from http://archive.carnegiefoundation.org/pdfs/elibrary/Carnegie_Flexner_Report.pdf
102. Stahnisch, F., & Verhoef, M. (2012). The Flexner Report of 1910 and its impact on complementary and alternative medicine and psychiatry in North America in the 20th century. *Evidence-Based Complementary and Alternative Medicine*, doi:10.1155/2012/647896
103. Association of Accredited Naturopathic Medical Colleges. (2015). Naturopathic medical school overview. Retrieved from https://aanmc.org/naturopathic-schools/
104. Glicksman, E. (2014). *AAMC annual report*. Association of American Medical Colleges. Retrieved from https://members.aamc.org/eweb/upload/2014%20Annual%20Report%20non-flash.pdf
105. Associated Press. (1987, August 29). U.S. judge finds medical group conspired against chiropractors. *The New York Times*. Retrieved from http://www.nytimes.com/1987/08/29/us/us-judge-finds-medical-group-conspired-against-chiropractors.html
106. Burkhart, L. A. (2012). *Wilk v. AMA* 25 years later: Why it still isn't over. American Chiropractic Association. Retrieved from https://www.acatoday.org/content_css.cfm?CID=4767
107. Silenzio, V. M. (2002). What is the role of complementary and alternative medicine in public health? *American Journal of Public Health, 92*(10), 1562–1564.
108. Burke, A., Ginzburg, K., Collie, K., Trachtenberg, D., & Muhammad, M. (2005). Exploring the role of complementary and alternative medicine in public health practice and training. *Journal of Alternative and Complementary Medicine, 11*(5), 931–936.
109. Giordano, J., Garcia, M. K., Boatwright, D., & Klein, K. (2003). Complementary and alternative medicine in mainstream public health: A role for research in fostering integration. *Journal of Alternative and Complementary Medicine, 9*(3), 441–445.
110. Park, C. M. (2002). Diversity, the individual, and proof of efficacy: Complementary and alternative medicine in medical education. *American Journal of Public Health, 92*(10), 1568–1572.

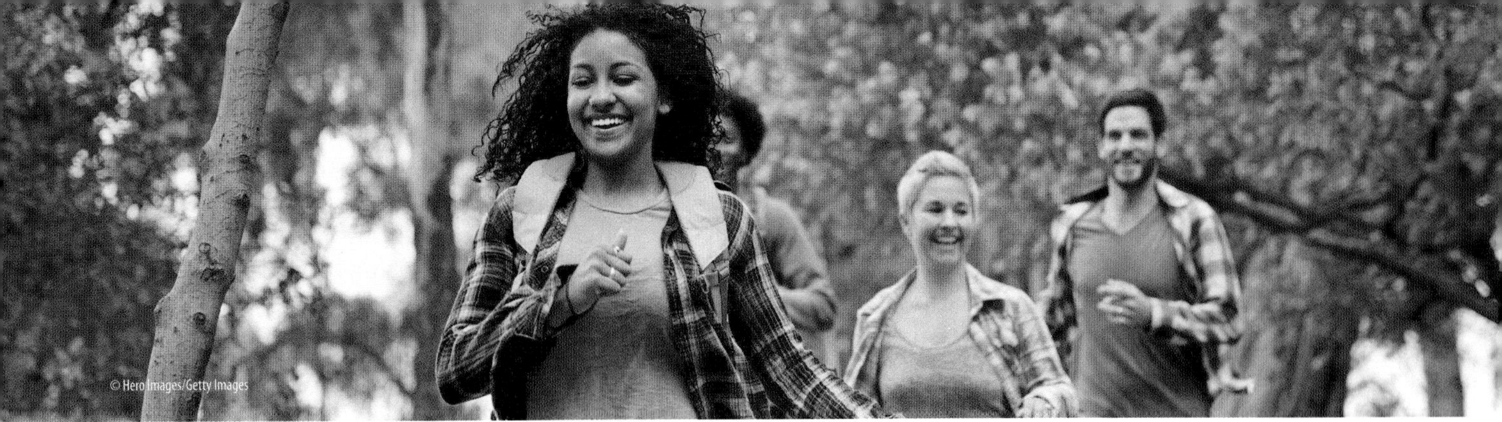

CHAPTER 5

Beyond the Birds and the Bees: Sexual and Reproductive Health

CHAPTER OBJECTIVES

- Describe reproductive anatomy, sexual intercourse, and conception.
- Discuss common sexually transmitted diseases and their prevention, screening, and treatment.
- Review contraceptive options for preventing pregnancy.
- Illustrate why reproductive and sexual health need to be understood in a broader context.

Sex on television, sex on social media, sex in books, sex in songs, actual sex in real life—the list goes on. Sex is seemingly everywhere. Yet in the United States, it continues to remain a taboo topic, often not discussed at home, in schools, with friends, or even with sexual partners!

Sexual intercourse, arousal, abuse, **sexually transmitted diseases (STDs)**, and pregnancy are all important health topics that warrant a comprehensive discussion informed by scientific evidence.

sexually transmitted diseases (STDs) Diseases that are transmitted through sexual contact; includes HIV/AIDS, human papilloma virus (HPV), chlamydia, gonorrhea, syphilis, genital herpes, hepatitis, and trichomoniasis.

Sexual and Reproductive Anatomy

Before we start talking about sex and its benefits and consequences, let's review the basics of the female and male sexual and reproductive anatomy. Our anatomy is a complex system of organs that each have a distinct purpose. When they function as intended, they are responsible for sexual arousal and reproduction.

Female Reproductive System

The female reproductive system is composed of internal (inside) and external (outside) parts. The main function of the external structure is to allow sperm to enter the body to fertilize an egg (for reproduction) and to protect against infections of the internal parts. The external structure is composed of the labia, the clitoris, a urinary opening (for urination), and a vaginal opening (**FIGURE 5-1**). The vaginal opening is the entry point for a man's penis during vaginal sex and also the exit point for unfertilized eggs being shed during menstruation.

The internal system consists of two ovaries connected to the fallopian tubes, the uterus, the cervix, and the vagina (**FIGURE 5-2**). After a female reaches puberty, the ovaries start to produce estrogen and create all sorts of changes in the body. (Exactly when this process will happen cannot be predicted, but these changes usually start when a girl is 10 to 14 years old. Some girls do not start menstruation, though, until several years later.) Ovulation, when the ovary releases an egg, occurs once a month. The egg moves through the fallopian tube and into the uterus, a journey that takes several days. During ovulation, the body is preparing for fertilization (pregnancy). In doing so, hormones thicken the lining of the uterus.

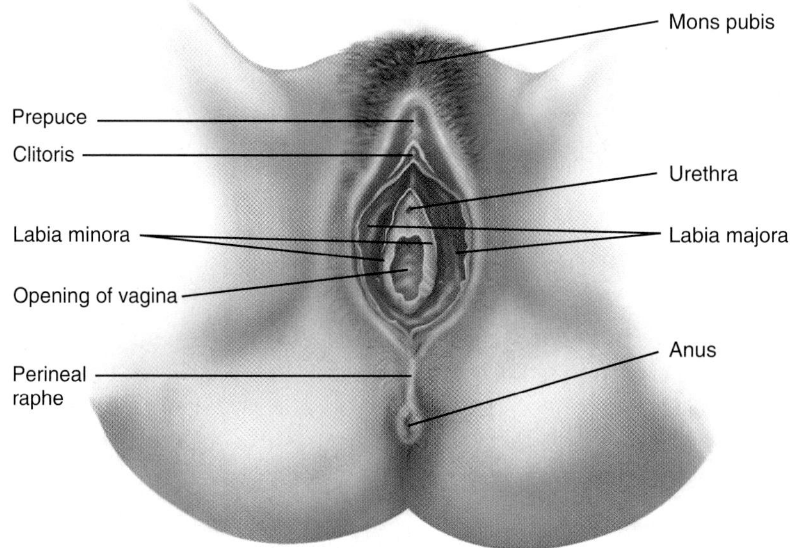

FIGURE 5-1 Female reproductive system (external).

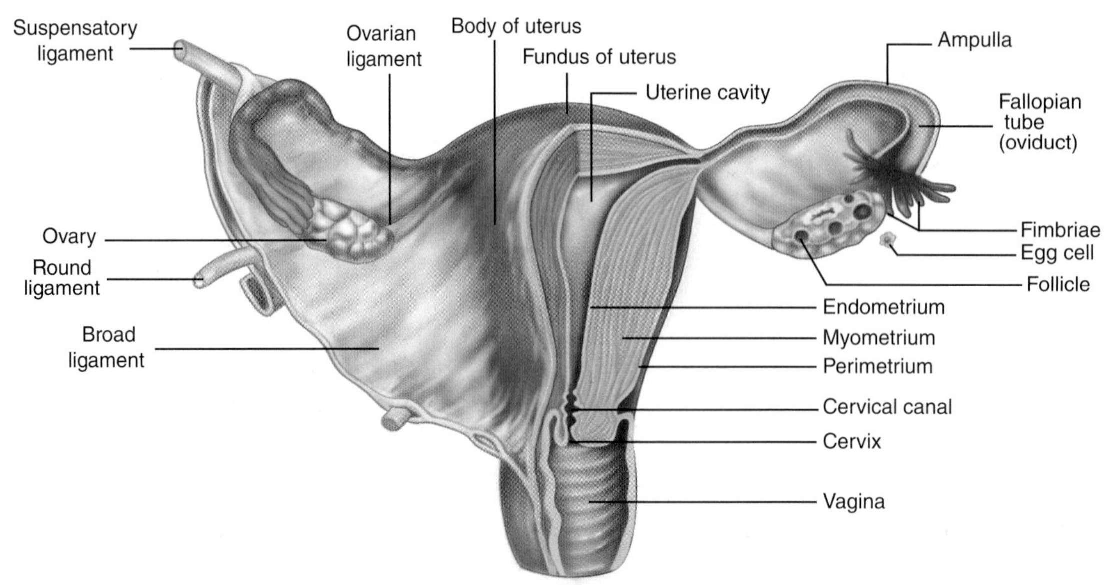

FIGURE 5-2 Female reproductive system (internal).

Of course, we're not always looking to get pregnant. If the egg is not fertilized by a sperm, it is shed along with the lining of the uterus. This blood and fluid passes through the cervix and out of the vagina. This process is menstruation, also called a "period." Although it sounds like something a person should be able to see, the shed egg is so small that it is not visible to the naked eye. To manage the bleeding and fluid discharge, women insert tampons or wear pads (also known as sanitary napkins) for the duration of their period, which is usually 3 to 7 days.

The first day of bleeding is considered day 1 of the menstrual cycle. Around day 12, the woman ovulates, releasing an egg. The actual timing of ovulation varies from person to person. It is around the time of the egg release that women can become pregnant. The released egg is awaiting fertilization by sperm. If fertilization does not occur, once again the egg is shed, resulting in menstrual bleeding. A period usually occurs once a month and lasts for several days. This monthly ovulation process starts during puberty and continues for decades until menopause. Menopause is a biological process, usually beginning in the woman's 40s to 50s, that ends this ovulation process.

Menstruation is an uncomfortable process and, for some women, can be painful. Often, women experience abdominal pain or cramps, changes in mood, headaches, and other symptoms. These symptoms are called premenstrual syndrome (PMS). When a young woman first begins menstruation, her periods are often irregular, meaning they may not occur once every month. Over time, a woman's periods become more regular. This regularity helps her understand her body's response to menstruation. Some symptoms can be treated with over-the-counter medication, such as pain relievers, but if symptoms are severe, the woman can consult with her healthcare provider.

Male Reproductive System

The male reproductive system is simpler (**FIGURE 5-3**). The penis and scrotum are the main external parts. The biological purpose of the male system is to produce

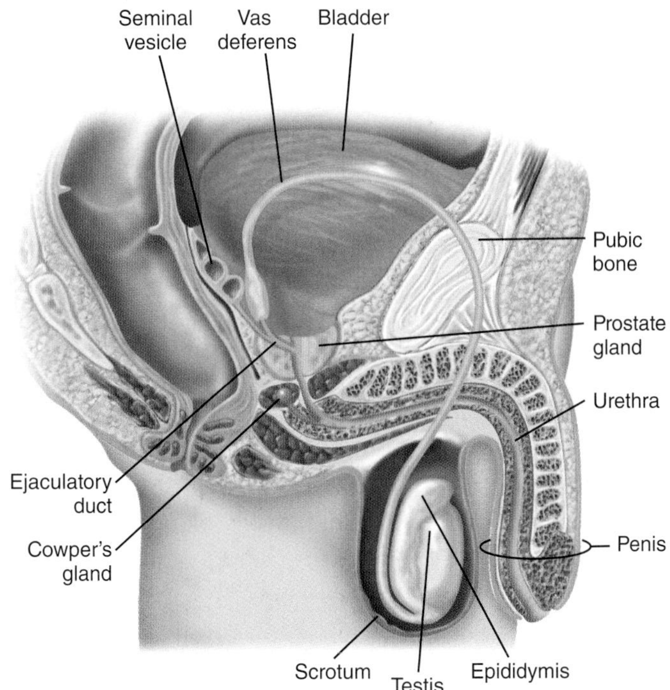

FIGURE 5-3 Male reproductive system.

and release sperm and to secrete male sex hormones. For males, puberty is characterized by the start of changes in the body caused by male hormones. The scrotum is a loose sac of skin that hangs behind the penis. The scrotum's function is to control the temperature of the testicles (or testes). Two testicles reside in the scrotum and are responsible for secreting testosterone (a male hormone) and producing sperm. The epididymis is a tube that rests behind each testicle. Its role is to mature the sperm and, once ready (during sexual arousal), release them into the vas deferens. The vas deferens is a tube that carries sperm to the urethra. The urethra runs through the center of the prostate gland, which produces fluid to nourish the sperm, creating the fluid referred to as semen. The urethra then transports the semen into the penis, from which it is ejaculated during orgasm. Note that the urethra is also attached to the bladder and is responsible for excreting urine.

At birth, parents may choose to have their male child circumcised. Circumcision is a surgical procedure that removes the skin covering the tip of the penis. It is a common procedure in the United States and around the globe. It is a ritual in certain religions and cultures. Circumcision facilitates hygiene. The long-term benefits of circumcision include reduced risk of sexually transmitted diseases, penile cancer, and urinary tract infections. Pediatricians acknowledge that the benefits of circumcision outweigh the risks, but it is ultimately the parents' decision if they want their son circumcised.[1]

Sexual Arousal and Pleasure

Biologically, the function of the female and male anatomy is to procreate. More often, however, people engage in sexual intercourse for pleasure without any intent to become pregnant. People do not think of their brain as part of their sexual anatomy, but it plays a significant role in controlling our sexual responses and by releasing sex hormones. Although men and women experience sexual **arousal** differently, the stages of physiological arousal are similar.

arousal The onset of sexual desire; it consists of four stages: excitement, plateau, orgasm and ejaculation, and resolution.

Sex researchers in the 1950s observed men and women performing sexual activities in their laboratory to develop models for sexual arousal. They found that sexual arousal has four stages: excitement, plateau, orgasm and ejaculation, and resolution. During the first stage, excitement can be triggered by any number of stimuli, including touch, images, and thoughts. Excitement prompts increased blood flow in the sexual organs, whereby the penis starts to become erect (for males) and the pelvic area produces fluid (for women). In the second stage, plateau, these sensations are intensified; the penis grows and the vagina becomes more sensitive. Ejaculation occurs in the third stage for men, in which semen is emitted through the urethra. Women may also experience orgasm, described as pleasurable muscle contractions and a full release of all tension. During the resolution stage, blood pressure decreases within the vagina and penis (and the erection subsides), and the body returns to normal.[2]

Sexual partners may engage in certain practices that they find mutually stimulating. One such example is sadomasochistic (S&M) activities. This practice involves bondage or inflicting pain or humiliation. As long as these practices are consensual and desired by those involved, they are perfectly normal.[3] Some people (often men) have fetishes, a reliance on nonliving objects for sexual stimulation. Fetishes are common and only become a problem if they interfere with intercourse or cause distress.[4]

Masturbation is touching one's own body for sexual pleasure. Despite myths and other misperceptions perpetuated over the years, it is natural activity and a common and healthy practice for men and women of all ages. In fact, masturbation has been found to be associated with stress relief, improved sleep, reduction of sexual tension, and other benefits. The four stages of sexual arousal may occur during masturbation. People masturbate by stimulating their vulva (for women) or penis (for men). Some may use lubricant to protect against irritation and increase stimulation. Sex toys (like vibrators) are also commonly used.[5]

What Is "Sex"?

We hear a lot about "sex," but exactly what are we talking about? There are many different ways to think about sex (and some people consider only some acts to be sex, while others hold a broader interpretation). Here is a brief description of some of the main types[6]:

- *Vaginal sex*: penis-in-vagina intercourse
- *Anal sex*: penis-in-anus intercourse (can be performed among heterosexual couples and gay men)
- *Oral sex*: mouth-to-genital contact (can be any combination of man or woman using his or her mouth on a partner's genitals)
- *Manual stimulation (fingering or hand jobs)*: hand-to-genital contact (fingering refers to female genitals and hand jobs to males; again, these actions can be performed by men or women)
- *Outercourse*: sexual stimulation that excludes any penetration (usually with clothing on)

The types most often discussed are vaginal, anal, and oral sex. These types also come with the greatest risk of transmitting diseases and pregnancy (in the case of vaginal sex). We will talk more about sexually transmitted diseases and pregnancy later in the chapter.

Gender Identity and Sexual Orientation

The language that we use to identify ourselves and others is important in creating an open and safe environment that is accepting of everyone. Using careful

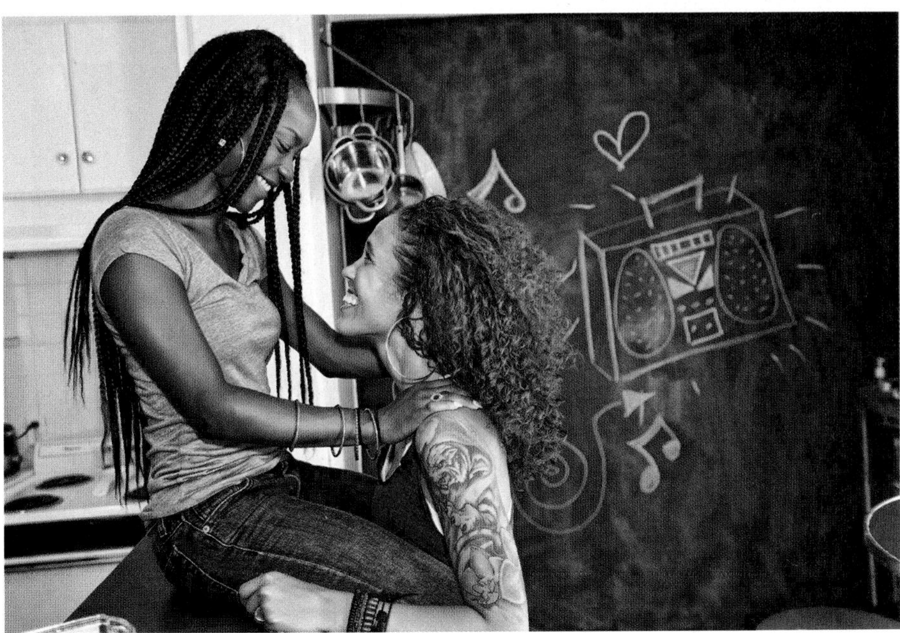

sexual orientation Refers to the gender or genders to which a person is sexually attracted; includes heterosexual, homosexual, and bisexual.

gender identity The attitudes, feelings, and behaviors a society associates with someone's biological sex; some people identify as transgender, which means that their identity does not conform to typical associations of their biological sex.

and appropriate language is needed when discussing our race, culture, religion, gender, and **sexual orientation**. When we talk about gender, we are referring to the attitudes, feelings, and behaviors a given society associates with someone's biological sex. Although someone may be born with anatomy for one biological sex (male or female), he or she may assume a **gender identity** or expression that does not conform to typical associations with sex assigned at birth. This gender identity is known as transgender (or "trans"). Those whom are not transgender, meaning their gender identity matches the sex assigned at birth, are referred to as cisgender.

Sexual orientation refers to a person's biological sex in relation to the biological sex of those to whom the person is sexually attracted. Here are the main terms used to describe sexual orientation:

- *Heterosexual*: attraction to members of the opposite sex
- *Homosexual* or *gay* (males or females), or *lesbian* (females): attraction to members of the same sex
    - *Queer*: attraction to members of the same sex. *Queer* was formerly a pejorative term but has since been "reclaimed" by people who wish to make it normal and mainstream. It is, however, still considered offensive to some so should be avoided unless someone refers to himself or herself in this manner.
- *Men who have sex with men (MSM)*: umbrella term for all men who engage in sexual activity with other men, regardless of how they identify themselves
- *Bisexual*: attraction to members of both sexes

Someone who is transgender may identify as any sexual orientation. Homosexuality and bisexuality can be stigmatized in our society. (See Chapters 6 and 10). Trying to change your own or someone else's sexual orientation because of stigma or shame can be futile and even harmful.[7] Regardless of sexual orientation or gender identity, everyone with female reproductive anatomy can get pregnant (female egg and male sperm are necessary for fertilization), and everyone (male, female, trans, or otherwise) is at risk for sexually transmitted diseases.

Note that throughout this chapter we may use the term *woman* or *female* when referring to conception and contraceptive options; these terms refer to those born with female anatomy, who can become pregnant. We do, however,

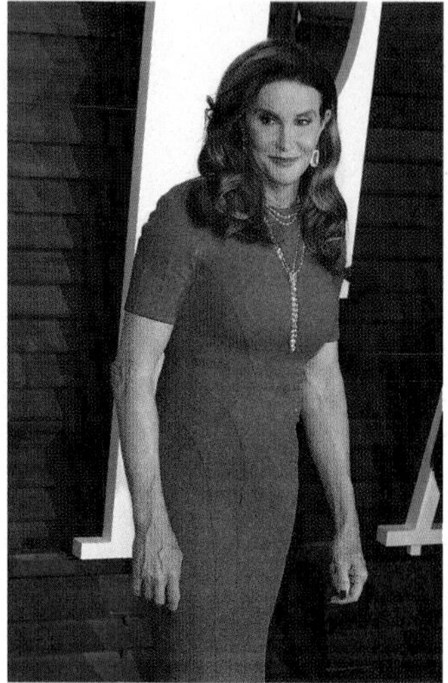

In 2015, Caitlyn Jenner, formerly Bruce Jenner, Olympic gold medal–winning decathlete, publicly announced her identity as a trans woman. Shortly before this public reveal, she said in an interview, "I'm not doing this to be interesting. I'm doing this to live."

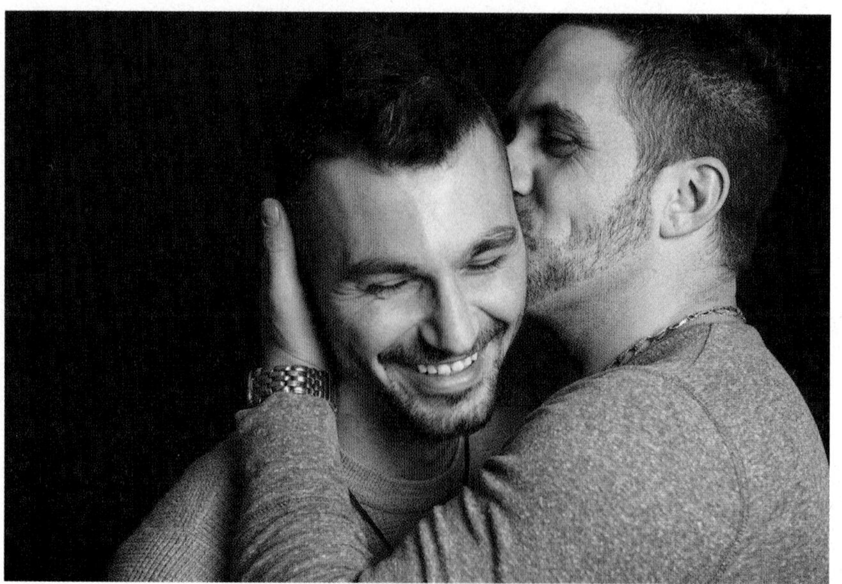

recognize that there are individuals who were not born with female anatomy who identify as women.

What Makes a Relationship "Healthy"?

What constitutes a "healthy" relationship may be different for different people. Generally, a healthy relationship is thought to be one in which there is mutual respect and support from both partners, without fear, pressure, or intimidation. Having open and honest communication, and sharing and respecting the boundaries each person has are two key components.[8]

Being clear about sexual consent is important and contributes to maintaining a healthy relationship. The best way to make sure your partner is on board or to communicate your consent is to say "yes." Silence should not be interpreted as consent. Consent (1) is given freely and without pressure, (2) is informed [sharing if either of you have any STDs and if/what birth control you are using], (3) can be taken back at any point, and (4) is enthusiastic. Consent applies to each and every instance of sexual activity—not just the first time.[9]

Intimate partner violence is a serious problem. Intimate partner violence refers to any physical or sexual violence, stalking, or psychological aggression of a current or former partner. It can vary in severity and affects millions of people in the United States. Its consequences include physical injuries, reproductive problems, psychological issues, and social and behavioral risks.[10] (See Chapter 10 for more information about unhealthy relationships and intimate partner violence.)

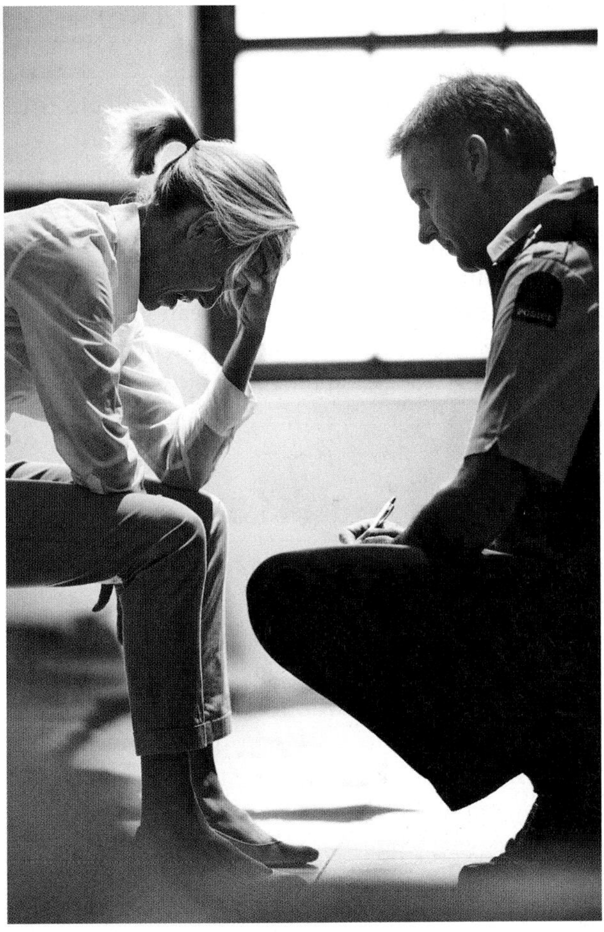

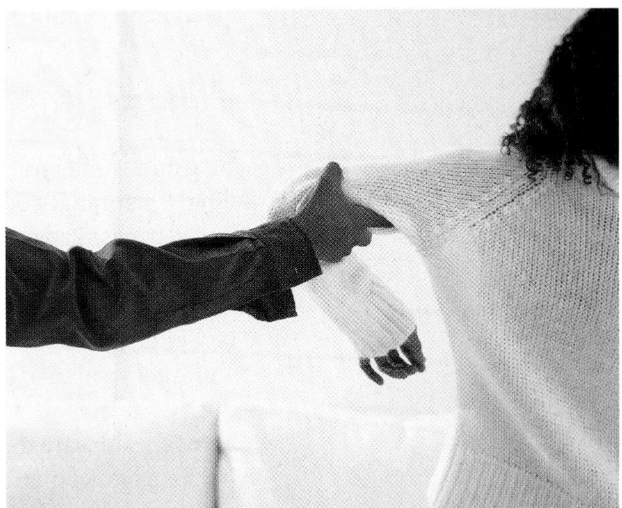

TALES OF PUBLIC HEALTH

The Catholic Church's Sex Abuse Scandal

It's a scandal that has stained the image of the Catholic Church. In recent decades, thousands of individuals have come forward with painful stories of being sexually abused by Catholic priests. The data are incomplete, but at least 16,000 men and women reported abuse, mainly after 1950. This figure includes only those who came forward. Likely there are many people who were abused but have not reported an incident. Most victims were young boys at the time of abuse but came forward as adults. As with most victims of sexual abuse, the children were told not to tell anyone.

Children or parents informed senior church leaders of these abuses, and the leaders chose to keep quiet. At the time, the leaders believed that priests could repent for their sins. They transferred the priests to other churches, putting more children at risk. In 2002, *The Boston Globe* newspaper printed a series of stories breaking the silence and uncovering this disgrace. (The 2015 Academy Award–winning film *Spotlight* portrays the journalists who broke this story at the *Globe*.) After this, church officials were forced to address the abuses that had plagued their community for decades. The church has spent over $2.5 billion in response to civil suits.

Pope Francis, who has held the position of the church's worldwide leader since 2013, has responded to the crisis, with mixed reaction from the public. He has established a committee to protect children, set guidelines to prevent abuse, established procedures for handling allegations, and publicly asked for forgiveness for the appalling abuses and gross mishandlings by the Catholic Church.[13,14] However, despite public promises to discipline church officials who protected priests who were guilty of molesting children, little action has been taken.[15]

Sexual Assault

Every person has the right to decide if and when to engage in any form of sexual activity. For some, that choice is violated by sexual offenders and rapists who coerce them into forced sexual acts. Victims of these perpetrators can be any gender or age. Any coerced sexual contact is considered sexual assault. Such violations have a substantial and negative impact on victims and can lead to addiction, depression, eating disorders, smoking, risky sexual behavior, and other adverse outcomes. Counseling and mental health providers can give ongoing support to help victims deal with feelings and trauma related to the abuse and can aid them on their road to healing.[11,12] (See Chapter 10 for more about sexual assault and childhood sexual abuse.)

Reproductive and Sexual Health Care

Men and women of all ages can seek counseling related to reproductive health, family planning, and sexually transmitted diseases from a variety of providers and settings. Providers of many different specialty backgrounds are tapped to deliver this type of care, including pediatricians, gynecologists, midwives, internists, and family medicine doctors and nurse practitioners. Some providers may be better trained, and thus better equipped, to engage in these conversations with their patients. Gynecologists, doctors who specialize in the female reproductive health system, play a fundamental role in delivering reproductive and sexual health care to women. Often, gynecologists are also certified in obstetrics (to manage women during pregnancy and birth) and referred to as Ob/Gyn providers. Women generally visit a gynecologist or family medicine physician to get screened for reproductive health issues and discuss contraceptive options or preconception care. Men can seek reproductive and sexual health counseling from primary care or family medicine providers.

College campus health services, community health clinics, hospitals, and private offices are all places where such health professionals may work. Title X clinics are federally funded clinics that offer comprehensive family planning and reproductive health services. These clinics provide subsidized care mostly to low income and uninsured individuals. They play a critical role in delivering quality reproductive health services to women and families.

Types of insurance coverage, location, office hours, and provider availability all play a role in influencing who may end up at what clinical site and what type of provider will deliver services. Under the Affordable Care Act (ACA or Obamacare), private health insurance plans are mandated to cover prescription contraceptives, without cost sharing by consumers. This requirement greatly increases access to contraceptive options. With this mandate, contraceptives are considered primary prevention. Early data indicate that the cost savings for consumers will be substantial and may help to reduce rates (and associated costs) of unintended pregnancy.[16] (For more on the ACA, see Chapter 12.)

Sexually Transmitted Diseases

A long time ago, sexually transmitted diseases (also known as sexually transmitted infections) were thought to be a result of poor hygiene or a punishment for an irreverent life. They were considered to be just one disease with varying symptoms. Eventually, scientists recognized the relationship of these symptoms to sexual interaction.[17] Today, we understand a lot more about the various STDs, how they are transmitted, and their physical and mental health consequences. Despite being preventable, STDs remain a prominent public health problem. **Abstinence** (not having vaginal, anal, or oral sex) is the only guaranteed method to prevent transmission of STDs. But because almost half of young people (students in grades 9 to 12) and over 90% of adult men and women have been sexually active, solely promoting or expecting abstinence would be an unrealistic public health approach.[18,19] Instead, barrier methods, such as using a **condom**, are often touted for their ability to prevent STDs during sexual intercourse. Condoms are considered a barrier method because they prohibit many infections from transferring from one person to another (and also prevent semen from entering a woman's vagina to prevent pregnancy).

abstinence In the context of sex, refers to the practice of abstaining (or not having) vaginal, anal, or oral sex.

condom Barrier device used during sexual intercourse to help prevent pregnancy or STDs.

A recent report by the Centers for Disease Control and Prevention (CDC) found that incidence of three STDs (chlamydia, gonorrhea, and syphilis) has increased for the first time in nearly a decade. The increases were largely among young people and men. Public health officials are still investigating what may have caused the increase.[20] Given that many people know about STD prevention, why do the rates remain so high, and, for some diseases, why have the rates increased over the last few years? The answer is complicated. Barrier methods need to be used correctly and consistently every single time a person has sex. Even when using condoms, though, people are not fully protected from all STDs. Transmission of certain STDs can occur because condoms do not completely cover the affected area. Inconsistent use may occur if people do not enjoy the feeling of sex with condoms and opt to not use them sometimes. Nonuse may also occur if someone is forced into having sex or has a partner who is controlling and insists on not using condoms. (See Chapter 10 for more information about sexual assault, unhealthy relationships, and intimate partner violence.)

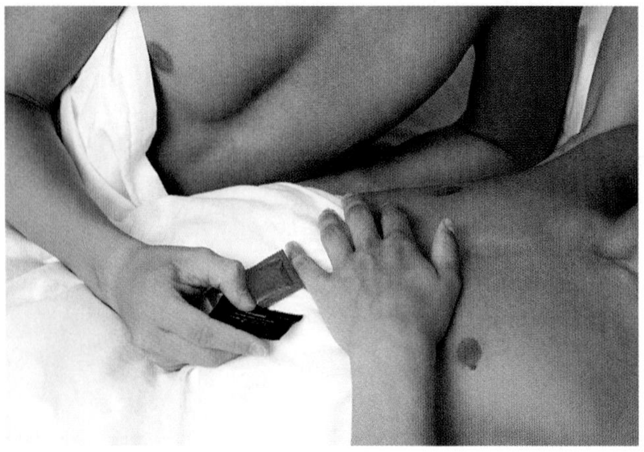

© Image Source/Gettyimages.

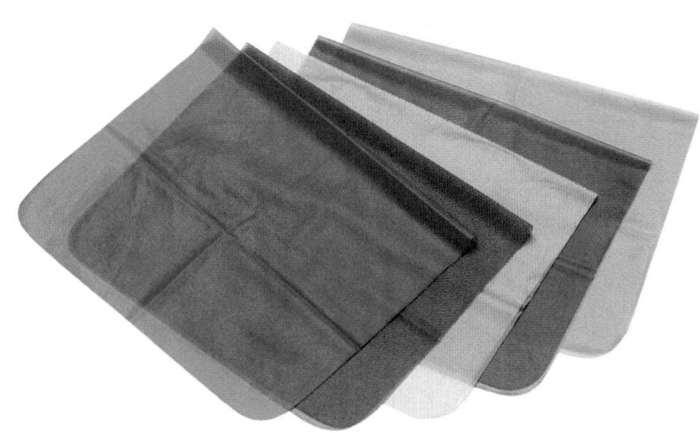

© WhiteJack/Shutterstock.

It is important for people to have open, honest, and continuing conversations with their partners about sex to know what their risks are. Many STDs are without symptoms and, thus, pose a problem for detection. Although some tests may sound (and sometimes are) uncomfortable, getting a diagnosis of an STD and proper treatment far outweighs the risk of letting an STD go untreated. If a person contracts an STD, he or she needs to make sure his or her partner is treated for STDs, too; otherwise the person risks being reinfected.

The best way to avoid STDs is abstinence, and the second best way is a mutually monogamous relationship in which sex does not occur until both partners test negative for STDs. If someone is sexually active, using condoms (along with a more effective method of birth control to avoid pregnancy) can help prevent most STDs. Dental dams (pictured below), small sheets of latex, can also be used as a protective barrier method during oral sex to prevent transmission of infections between the mouth and partner's vagina or anus.

The most common STDs are discussed in the next section; **TABLE 5-1** provides an overview of these diseases. Note that the images presented in this section are not intended to instill fear, but rather to increase awareness about how symptoms for various STDs may appear on the body.

Human Immunodeficiency Virus

Originally, the human immunodeficiency virus (HIV) was considered to be a disease occurring only among homosexual men (in 1982, its proposed name was "gay-related immunodeficiency"). Over the last several decades, with dedicated research and resources, we have learned much more about HIV and now know that anyone, regardless of sexual orientation, income, race, or any other factor, can become infected.

HIV is a virus that attacks the immune system by destroying cells that are needed to fight off infection (CD4-positive T cells) and leaves the body more susceptible to other diseases (**FIGURE 5-4**). If left untreated, HIV can destroy so many of these cells that the body is no longer able to fight off infections and can lead to death. HIV causes acquired immunodeficiency syndrome (AIDS), which is the last stage, when HIV is most severe. Not everyone with HIV progresses to having AIDS. Someone is considered to have AIDS when his or her CD4 count is below 200 cells per cubic milliliter of blood. At this stage, the body's immune system is weakened and susceptible to infection (**FIGURE 5-5**). Infections at this stage can be very dangerous. If not treated, the life expectancy for someone with AIDS is about 3 years.[21,22]

About 1.2 million people in the United States are living with HIV infection, including over 150,000 estimated people who do not know they are infected.

TABLE 5-1 Common Sexually Transmitted Diseases (STDs)

STD	Consequences	Screening Method	Treatment
Human immunodeficiency virus (HIV)	■ Causes acquired immunodeficiency syndrome (AIDS) ■ Can result in the body no longer being able to fight off infections and death	■ Blood test ■ Oral fluids and urine tests also possible	■ No cure, but antiretroviral therapy (ART) can help control the virus and allow for a longer life span.
Human papillomavirus (HPV)	■ Various strains that can cause genital warts or cervical and other cancers	■ Women: Pap test and sometimes HPV test ■ Men: no approved test for HPV; however, men with increased risk of anal cancer can get anal Pap test	■ No cure, but usually infections are harmless and go away on their own. ■ Persistent abnormal cells can be removed with clinical procedures if needed.
Chlamydia	■ Women: pelvic inflammatory disease, which can cause infertility; chronic pelvic pain; and ectopic pregnancy ■ Pregnant women: premature delivery and can transmit disease to baby, which can cause pneumonia or eye infections ■ Men: testicle pain or fever, rarely associated with long-term effects ■ Men and women: increased risk of HIV infection	■ Women: culture of the cervix or urine tests (Testing is mostly recommended for women, but also recommended for MSM.)	■ Antibiotics
Gonorrhea	■ Women: pelvic inflammatory disease ■ Men and women: disseminated gonococcal infection, which can cause arthritis and/or skin inflammation and can be life threatening ■ Pregnant women: can transmit disease to baby and cause blindness or infection	■ Testing of discharge from urethra, vagina, or anus, or urine test	■ Combination of two antimicrobial medications
Genital herpes	■ Herpetic lesions around the genitals, rectum, or mouth ■ Fever, aches, or swollen lymph nodes ■ Blindness and inflammation of the brain (rare) ■ Increased risk of HIV infection among those with outbreaks	■ Blood test, not recommended for people without symptoms	■ No cure, but outbreaks of lesions can be suppressed with antiviral medications.

(continues)

TABLE 5-1 Common Sexually Transmitted Diseases (STDs) *(continued)*

STD	Consequences	Screening Method	Treatment
Syphilis	▪ Long-term effects of untreated syphilis: heart problems, paralysis, blindness, trouble with muscle coordination, and dementia ▪ Increased risk of HIV infection ▪ Pregnant women: can transmit to fetus	▪ Testing of blood, tissue samples, or bodily fluid	▪ Antibiotics or penicillin
Trichomoniasis	▪ Genital itching, burning, or unusual discharge ▪ Increased risk of acquiring other STDs, including HIV ▪ Pregnant women: premature delivery and/or low birth weight	▪ Pelvic exam (for women) or urethra swab (for men)	▪ Oral antibiotics
Hepatitis A	▪ Fever, nausea, fatigue, and dark urine that can last up to a few months	▪ Blood test	▪ No treatment, but vaccine is available, which can be useful in preventing transmission if taken shortly after exposure. ▪ Most often the virus clears on its own.
Hepatitis B	▪ Can be acute or chronic ▪ Fever, fatigue, nausea, abdominal pain, dark urine, and other symptoms ▪ Serious liver problems, such as cirrhosis or cancer, which can lead to death	▪ Blood test; physical exam	▪ Vaccine is available. ▪ If a person receives an injection of hepatitis B immune globulin within 12 hours of exposure, it can help reduce the risk of transmission. ▪ Acute hepatitis B may not require treatment. ▪ Chronic hepatitis B can be treated with antiviral medications, an injection called Interferon, or, if severe, a liver transplant.
Hepatitis C	▪ Chronic ▪ Fever, fatigue, nausea, and abdominal pain ▪ Liver disease and cancer, which can lead to death	▪ Blood test	▪ No vaccine ▪ Antiviral medication

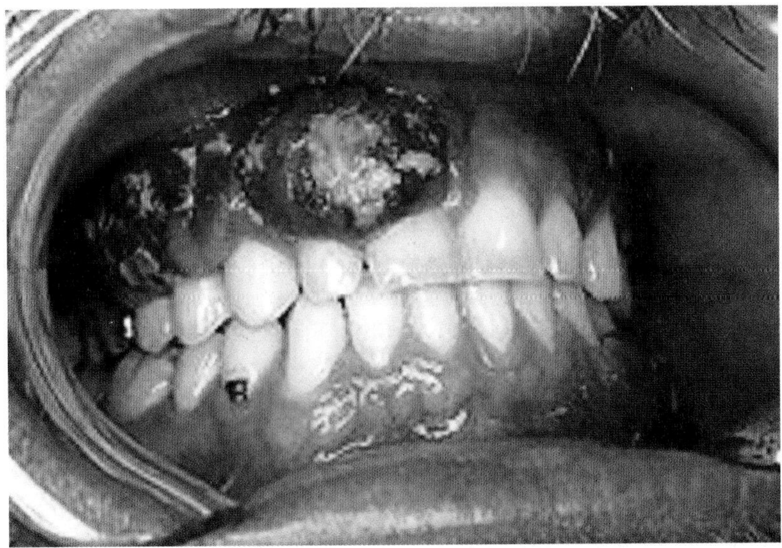

FIGURE 5-4 Kaposi's sarcoma is a common oral malignancy among patients who are HIV positive.

Iacovou, E., Vlastarakos, P. V., Papacharalampous, G., Kampessis, G., & Nikolopoulos, T. P. (2012). Diagnosis and treatment of HIV-associated manifestations in otolaryngology. *Infectious Disease Reports, 4*(1), e9. http://doi.org/10.4081/idr.2012.e9

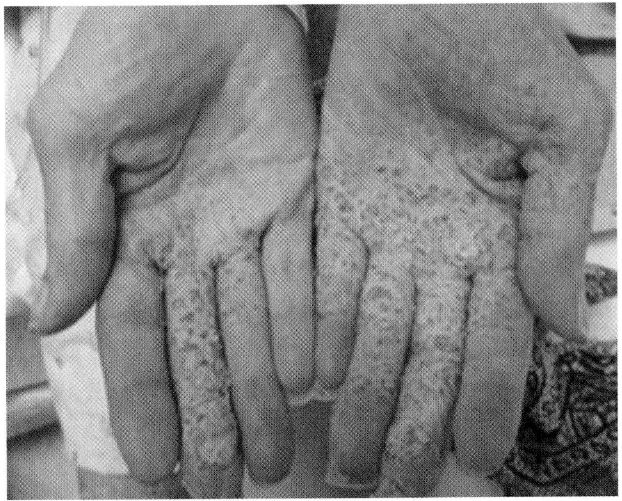

FIGURE 5-5 HIV skin infection.

Wang S., Basko-Plluska J., Tsoukas M. M. (2014). Generalized pruritic skin eruption in an immunocompromised patient. *Dermatol Pract Concept, 4*(4), 6. http://dx.doi.org/10.5826/dpc.0404a06

MSM have the highest rates of HIV, regardless of racial/ethnic background. There has been an alarming increase in new infections among MSM over the past decade, particularly among younger men (aged 13 to 24 years). Also, Black people account for over 40% of new HIV infections, despite representing only 12% of the U.S. population.[23]

For many, the latency period (time between exposure and having symptoms) may be long. Sometimes people exhibit symptoms shortly after infection. If HIV symptoms do occur, they can include flulike symptoms, fever, swollen lymph nodes, sore throat, or rash. The symptoms resolve even if the person is HIV positive. If you are sexually active and not consistently using protection, the only reliable way to know your HIV status is to be screened. HIV screening is generally a blood test for the presence of antibodies. Tests using oral fluids (not saliva) and urine are also available.[24,25]

HIV is transmitted through fluids (blood, semen, rectal fluids, vaginal fluids, or breast milk) coming into contact with a mucous membrane (the rectum, vagina, penis, or mouth) or damaged tissue, or through direct injection into the bloodstream. The most common ways HIV is spread in the United States are through anal or vaginal sex and through sharing of needles (a risk for those who inject drugs). Less commonly, it is spread from mother to child during birth or through breastfeeding, or by being stuck with a needle contaminated with the virus (a risk for healthcare workers). It is extremely rare to contract HIV through oral sex, blood transfusions (blood is now tested for HIV before donation), eating food chewed by someone with HIV, or kissing.[26] To reduce the risk of contracting HIV, people should use condoms consistently during every sexual encounter and avoid sharing needles. People at high risk of HIV (a partner of someone with HIV, someone who does not regularly wear condoms and does not know the HIV status of his or her previous partners, people who use drugs and share needles) can use preexposure prophylaxis (PrEP), a combination of two HIV medications. Using PreP consistently can reduce the risk of becoming infected. It is generally without side effects, with occasional nausea being the most commonly reported side effect.[27]

A diagnosis of HIV or AIDS used to be a death sentence. While there is no cure, HIV/AIDS is now managed with consistent monitoring and medication. A combination of medications, referred to as antiretroviral therapy (ART), can help control the virus and allow for a longer life span for those with HIV. A person recently exposed to HIV can take postexposure prophylaxis (PEP). To reduce the risk of acquiring HIV, an exposed person must take PEP within 2 to 3 days after exposure and continue the medication for a month. If someone is repeatedly at risk of acquiring HIV, PrEP may be a better option. For example, a person whose sexual partner is HIV positive should consider taking PrEP.[28] (See Chapter 8 for more information about the history and discovery of HIV.)

Human Papillomavirus

The most common STD is the human papillomavirus (HPV). Almost everyone who is sexually active (about 80%) will get HPV at some point in their lives.[29] Nearly 80 million people have HPV in the United States, with about 14 million new infections occurring every year.[30] Of sexually active women, the highest rate of infection is among 14- to 24-year-olds. (We do not have good data on the age group at greatest risk of HPV among men, but some research suggests that age is not as much of a risk factor for this group.)[31,32] HPV transmission happens by vaginal, anal, or oral sex. HPV has many different strains; some cause genital warts and others cause cervical and other cancers, including a type of cancer of the tongue and tonsils called oropharyngeal cancer. An HPV infection can take many years to develop into cancer (the rate at which it develops into cancer varies by individual). If someone has the strain of HPV that causes genital warts, small bumps may appear in the genital region. Other forms of HPV are asymptomatic (having no symptoms), which makes detection more difficult. Many times, HPV infections are harmless and go away on their own.

For women, a healthcare professional can test for abnormal cervical cells through a regular Pap test (**FIGURE 5-6**). During this test, the provider inserts an instrument called a speculum into the patient's vagina to widen it so the health practitioner can see her cervix. The health practitioner then takes a sample of the cervical cells to send to a laboratory to test for abnormalities that could lead to cervical cancer. Because HPV is not the only cause of cervical cancer, the Pap test is used to recognize any signs of abnormal cells. A Pap test can be combined with an HPV test, where the cells are also tested specifically for the HPV virus. Current recommendations are that women get a Pap test every 3 years, starting

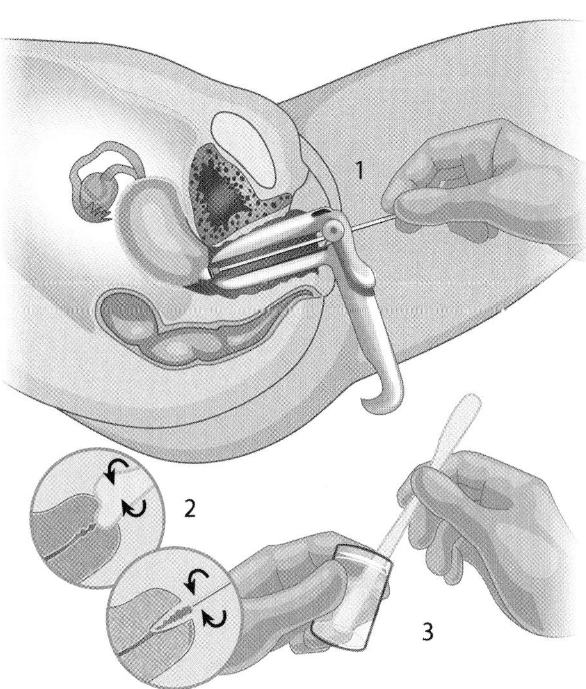

FIGURE 5-6 In a Pap test, the woman's doctor uses a vaginal speculum to hold the vaginal walls apart. Next, the doctor collects a sample of cells from the cervix using a small cone-shaped brush—or a cotton-tipped swab—and a tiny plastic spatula (1 and 2). The doctor then smears the cells onto a glass slide (3) or puts them into a bottle containing a solution to preserve the cells for examination under a microscope.

at age 21 years until age 29 years. (Because HPV at this younger age will usually resolve on its own, HPV tests are not recommended in addition to the Pap.) For women ages 30 to 65 years, the recommendation is to get a combined Pap and HPV test every 5 years.[33] If the test detects abnormal cells, doctors usually suggest monitoring and retesting within the year. If the abnormal cells do not resolve on their own, there are procedures to remove the cells.[34,35]

For a long time, there was no effective prevention method. Using condoms reduces risk, but because they do not cover the entire area that could be infected, there is still a risk of acquiring HPV even when using condoms correctly. In 2006, a vaccine was approved by the Food and Drug Administration (FDA) to prevent HPV infection.

The vaccine is recommended for boys and girls ages 11 or 12 years. If a person did not receive the vaccination when younger, he or she can get it through age 21 years for males and age 26 years for females or gay/bisexual men. The vaccine is a series of three shots given over a 6-month period.[34] The newest version of the vaccine prevents only 9 out of the 100 strains of HPV, but these include the most high-risk strains, that cause the majority of cervical cancers and genital warts.[35]

The discovery of a virus linked to cancer and the creation of an effective vaccination have constituted one of the major public health achievements in decades.[36] This vaccination provides the opportunity to significantly reduce certain types of cancer. About 11,000 women get cervical cancer each year. In addition, over 350,000 get genital warts. As use of the vaccination has increased, the prevalence of HPV has sharply declined, even beyond what public health experts expected.[37] One might assume that the opportunity to prevent such problems is welcomed with open arms. However, some parents have been vocally opposed to this vaccine, because they are worried about the side effects of giving it to a young child. Most people will not experience any side effects,

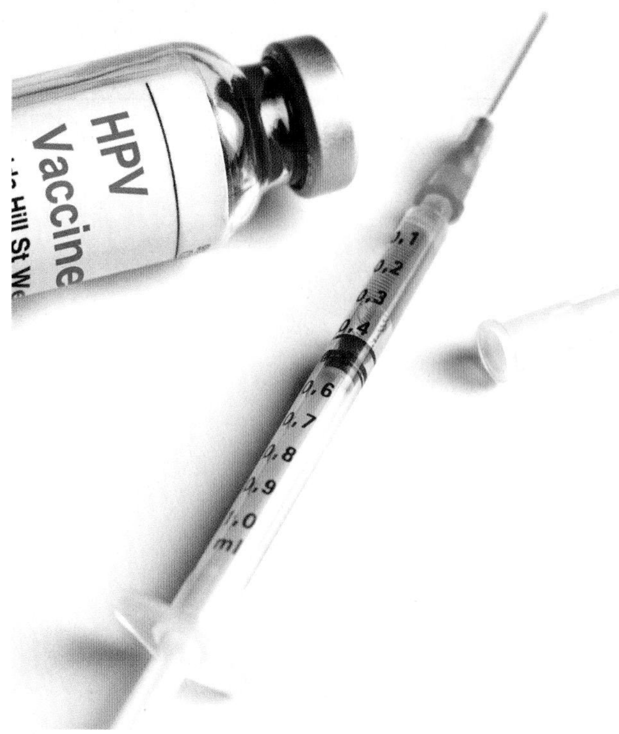

but with every vaccine comes some risk. Some of the more common side effects are pain at the site of the shot, fever, muscle pain, headache, and nausea. Very rarely have allergic reactions to the shot occurred. Parents should review those risks with their child's doctor. The benefits do need to be considered along with the low chances of adverse events. The vaccine is safe and effective at preventing four strains of HPV. Of course, remaining abstinent is one medication-free way to avoid STDs, but given that over 90% of people will become sexually active at some point in their lives, presumed abstinence rather than vaccination is not realistic.[19] Part of the worry is that the vaccine will prompt young people to engage in more sex. However, this is a false assumption; getting vaccinated for HPV does not increase sexual initiation.[38] When children reach 11 years of age, they are considered to be at an appropriate age for parents to talk with them about sex. Although it may be uncomfortable, having these discussions early and frequently can have a significant impact on the child's sexual behavior and future relationships.[34,39,40]

Chlamydia

In the United States, chlamydia is the most common bacterial STD, with almost 3 million cases occurring each year (**FIGURE 5-7**). People may not know if they have chlamydia because it is often asymptomatic. The lack of symptoms facilitates the spread of chlamydia between partners, who are likely unaware of their infection. If symptoms do occur, they may not show up until a few weeks after sexual contact. For women, symptoms can include vaginal discharge, abdominal pain, a burning or itching sensation around the vagina, and painful urination. Similarly, in men, chlamydia can cause penile discharge, burning or itching of the penis, and pain or swelling of the testicles. Individuals who contract chlamydia anally may experience rectal bleeding, discharge, or pain.

A health professional tests for chlamydia by taking a culture of the patient's cervix, penis, urethra, or anus. Urine tests also are available.[41] Chlamydia is

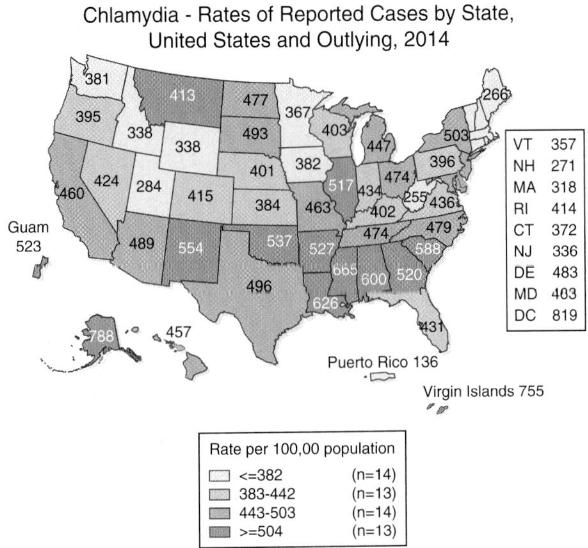

FIGURE 5-7 Rate of reported chlamydia cases by state, nationally in the United States, and in outlying areas, 2014.

Reproduced from Sexually Transmitted Disease Surveillance 2014, U.S. Department of Health and Human Services, Centers for Disease Control and Prevention. Retrieved from https://www.cdc.gov/std/stats14/surv-2014-print.pdf

most common among young people ages 15 to 24 years. It disproportionately affects Blacks and MSM. Chlamydia is spread through sexual contact with a partner's vagina, penis, mouth, or anus. Transmission can also occur from a pregnant woman passing it to her baby during childbirth, potentially causing pneumonia or eye infections in the newborn. Consistent use of condoms can help prevent chlamydia.

Men and women can both experience negative consequences associated with the infection. For women, if untreated, chlamydia can lead to pelvic inflammatory disease, which can cause infertility (inability to become pregnant), chronic pelvic pain, and possibly ectopic pregnancy (a pregnancy that occurs outside of the uterus). Ectopic pregnancy is life threatening to the mother, and the embryo will likely not survive. Women are also at risk of delivering babies prematurely. For men, chlamydia may cause fever or testicle pain but it is rarely associated with long-term effects. For both men and women, however, having chlamydia increases the risk of HIV infection, as any sores or breaks in the skin allow HIV to enter the body more easily. Fortunately, chlamydia is treatable with prescription antibiotics. Both the infected person and the person's partner need treatment to prevent reinfection. A gynecologist, internist, or family medicine provider can test for chlamydia.[41]

Gonorrhea

Transmission of gonorrhea occurs through sexual contact with the penis, vagina, mouth, or anus of someone infected with the bacterium *Neisseria gonorrhoeae*. It can be passed from mother to child during birth. It is a common STD, with over 800,000 new infections each year. The majority of these infections occur among people ages 15 to 24 years. Because, like chlamydia, it is often asymptomatic, less than half of these infections are detected and reported (**FIGURE 5-8**). If symptoms do occur, they are often mild and may include bleeding or discharge from or pain in the vagina, rectum, or urethra.

If left untreated, gonorrhea can lead to pelvic inflammatory disease in women. In both men and women, it can spread to the bloodstream, causing arthritis and/or skin inflammation and can be life threatening. If a child gets

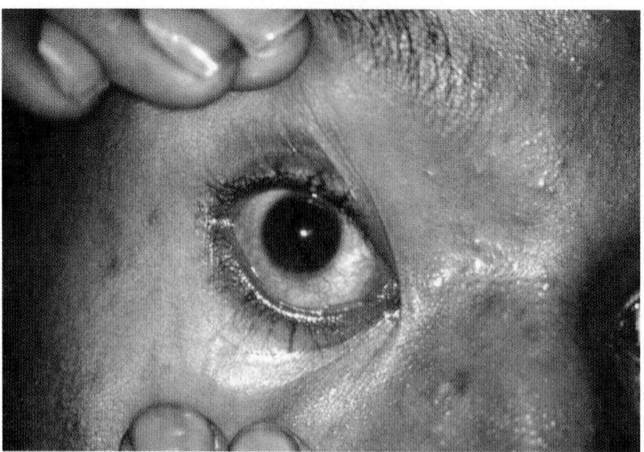

FIGURE 5-8 What looks like "pink eye" or an eye infection may actually be a sign of gonorrhea.
Courtesy of the CDC/Joe Miller, VD.

gonorrhea during birth, it can cause blindness or infection. Again, consistent use of condoms is the best method of prevention.

Healthcare providers screen for gonorrhea by testing discharge or swab samples from the urethra, vagina, or anus. A urine test may also be possible. Gonorrhea treatment includes two antimicrobial medications (an injection of cephalosporin ceftriaxone and either azithromycin or doxycycline), prescribed and administered by a health professional. Over time, though, gonorrhea has developed a resistance to the use of antibiotics, thus inhibiting successful treatment. This resistance is why the current treatment includes two medications. This type of resistance to medication is a major public health concern, as there are few other available, tested treatments for gonorrhea. Drug resistance complicates healthcare professionals' ability to effectively eliminate the bacteria and thus leaves infected individuals at higher risk of the health complications associated with this disease.[42,43]

Genital Herpes

Herpes simplex virus type 1 and type 2 cause genital herpes. Herpes is common; over 750,000 people get new herpes infections annually, and over 15% of individuals ages 14 to 49 years have herpes. The number of doctor visits for genital herpes has increased over the last several decades (FIGURE 5-9). Type 2 (HSV-2) is more common among women and non-Hispanic Blacks. Many people with herpes are not aware they are infected. Transmission of the herpes virus is through contact with mucosal surfaces, genital or oral secretions, or lesions. The usual way in which a person contracts HSV-2 is through sexual contact with an infected person.

Herpes can go undetected; many infected people do not experience symptoms. Symptoms, if they occur, include herpetic lesions around the genitals, rectum, or mouth (oral herpes). These ulcers can be painful. In some cases, someone with the infection may experience fever, aches, or swollen lymph nodes. Herpes cannot be "cured," but outbreaks of lesions can be suppressed with prescribed antiviral medications. In rare cases, both strains of herpes can lead to blindness and inflammation of the brain. The risk of acquiring HIV is also higher among those with genital herpes outbreaks. A blood test can confirm a herpes infection, but because there is no cure and the test can result in false positives, testing is not recommended for people without symptoms. Once again, consistent use of condoms during every sexual encounter can help

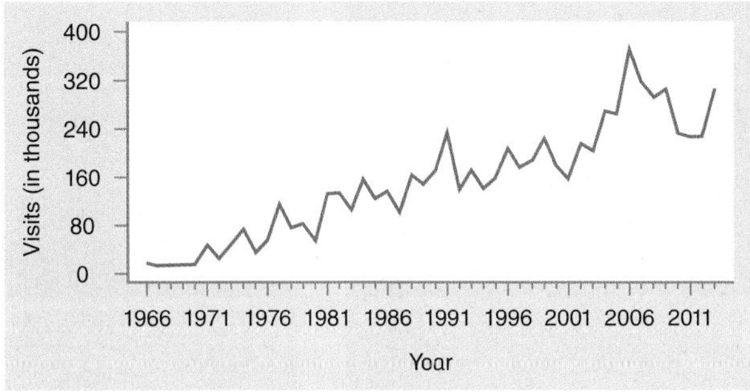

FIGURE 5-9 Physician office visits for genital herpes, 1966–2013.

Reproduced from Centers for Disease Control and Prevention. Genital Herpes Statistics.

prevent herpes, though the infected areas are not completely covered, so some risk remains.[44]

Syphilis

People often think of syphilis as an obsolete disease that only affected soldiers in World War II. Unfortunately, that is a myth, and syphilis is alive and well.

In fact, syphilis is one of the STDs that has increased in recent years, alarming public health officials. Despite reaching an all-time low in 2001, syphilis has been on the rise since then. Over 50,000 new infections were reported in 2013. There are about 6 cases per 100,000 population, the highest rate of syphilis since the early 1990s. The majority of new cases were among MSM. Why the increase among MSM? Researchers are investigating the answer to this question. It could be a combination of factors, including barriers to accessing STD services due to stigma, homophobia, or other reasons.[20] Syphilis also disproportionately affects Blacks and other communities of color.[45]

A person is at risk of contracting syphilis if he or she comes into contact with a syphilis sore through vaginal, anal, or oral sex. Pregnant women with syphilis can transmit the infection to the fetus. There are several tests doctors can use to detect syphilis, using blood, tissue samples, or bodily fluid. Syphilis can be treated with antibiotics or penicillin. If treated early, treatment will effectively eliminate the infection and prevent future damage. If left untreated, though, it can wreak havoc on the body (**FIGURE 5-10**). Symptoms start with sores. The sores are painless and thus often go undetected. After 3 to 6 weeks, the sores disappear, even if untreated, but the person still needs antibiotics for treatment. If the infection remains untreated, the person may develop a rash, but in some cases, the rash may go undetected because it could be faint and not itch.

A host of other potential symptoms could also arise, such as headache, fatigue, sore throat, and weight loss, and because these symptoms can be confused with so many other health issues, diagnosis of syphilis may not come easily. If syphilis continues to go untreated, it can remain latent, and decades later, the person could experience heart problems, paralysis, blindness, trouble with muscle coordination, and dementia.[46] Syphilis infection increases the risk of acquiring HIV.

Trichomoniasis

Trichomoniasis (often referred to as *trich*, pronounced "trick") is very common, affecting more than 3.5 million people. It is an infection caused by the protozoan parasite *Trichomonas vaginalis.* The parasite can be passed through sexual intercourse (or with the sharing of genital fluids), and there may be transmission to sexual partners of either gender. Over two-thirds of infections are asymptomatic. Those who do have symptoms may experience genital itching or burning or unusual

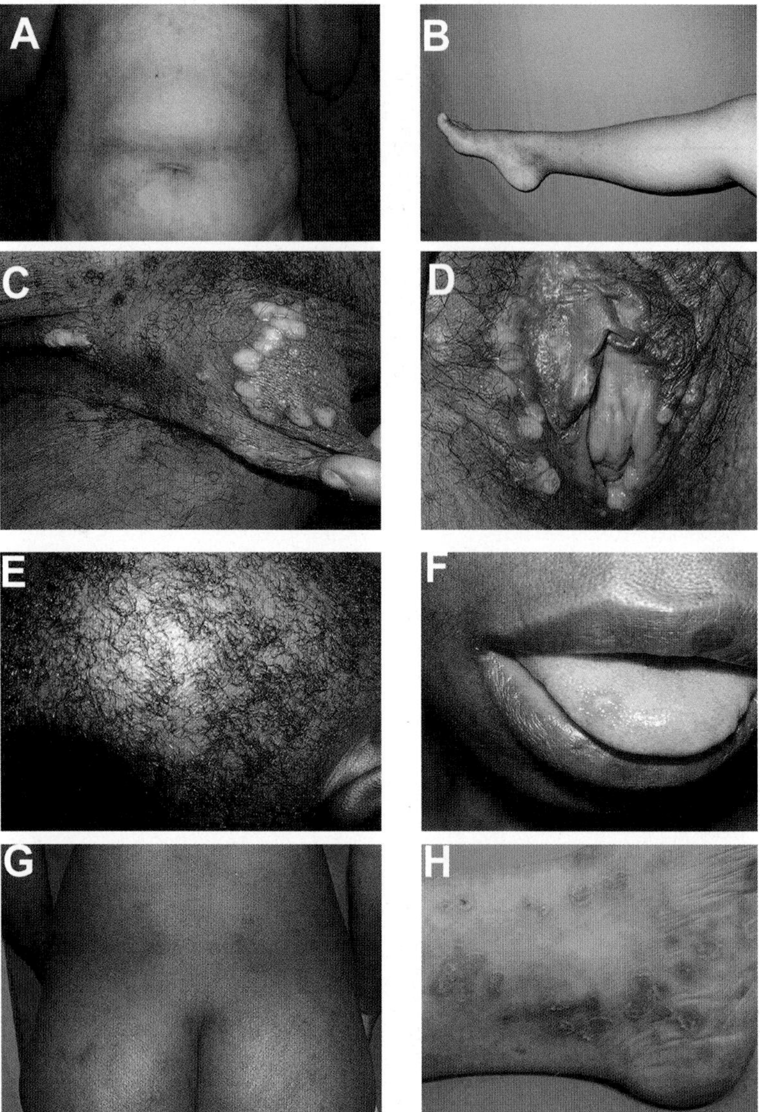

FIGURE 5-10 Syphilis can affect the whole body.

Cruz A. R., Pillay A, Zuluaga A. V., Ramirez L. G., Duque J. E., Aristizabal G. E., et al. (2010). Secondary syphilis in Cali, Colombia: New concepts in disease pathogenesis. *PLoS Negl Trop Dis 4*(5): e690. https://doi.org/10.1371/journal.pntd.0000690

discharge from the genitals. Even without symptoms, if someone is infected, he or she can pass on the parasite to a sexual partner. Using condoms consistently and effectively is the only way to prevent infection. However, because condoms do not always cover the entire areas at risk, a person can still acquire trichomoniasis while using a condom. As such, it is important for people to talk to their partners before having sex to be fully informed about their risk. Because people often do not have symptoms, they may be unaware that they are infected, and in the case of men, they may not recognize the added importance of wearing a condom.[48]

This infection is more common among women than among men. It is one of the few STDs that older women are more likely to have as compared to younger women. It is unclear why trichomoniasis is more common among older women. It could be that older women may become sexually active after divorce or death of a spouse and not think to use protection (since pregnancy is no longer a concern). Another hypothesis is that for women who became sexually active when they were young, they, by definition, would have more sexual partners and intercourse by later adulthood, which puts them at greater risk.[49] Trichomoniasis increases one's risk of acquiring other STDs, including HIV. A pregnant

TALES OF PUBLIC HEALTH

The Tuskegee Syphilis Experiment

The Tuskegee Study is widely recognized as one of the most egregious ethical violations in the history of public health. The study began in 1932 and lasted for 40 years. Its original intent was to understand more about the natural progression of syphilis before any treatment was known. The researchers enrolled rural, African American men but intentionally did not tell them about the purpose of the study. Participants found to have syphilis were not told of their diagnosis. Penicillin was discovered as a treatment in 1947, but knowledge of this breakthrough and the treatment was withheld from participants. Dozens of men died without access to this cure. Moreover, because the men were not informed of their disease and were not provided treatment, they continued to put their families at risk of transmission.

It was not until 1972 that a journalist broke the story. A panel of health experts was convened to investigate the study and found it was "ethically unjustified" because the men were not informed of the purpose of the study, their diagnoses, and treatment options. The settlement of a civil lawsuit gave participants and their families over $9 million. The revelations about the study led to the establishment of the "Belmont Report" in 1979, which summarized ethical principles and guidelines for research that involves human subjects, and the Office for Human Research Protections. In 1996, President Bill Clinton was the first president to acknowledge and apologize publicly for the gross maltreatment of the men in the study. The unfortunate legacy of Tuskegee lives on today, with lingering and understandable mistrust by some in the African American community about public health research and medicine.[47]

woman with trichomoniasis has a higher likelihood of giving birth prematurely or having a low-birth-weight baby. Both prematurity and low birth weight are associated with a host of neurologic impairments and developmental disabilities in a child. A doctor can test for trichomoniasis through a pelvic exam (for women) or urethra swab (for men). If a person tests positive, the infection can be easily treated with an oral antibiotic prescribed by a health professional.[48]

Hepatitis: The ABCs

Hepatitis types A, B, and C can be spread through sexual contact and therefore can be considered STDs, but they also have other forms of transmission. They are all contagious liver diseases often caused by a virus. In the United States, the most common forms are A, B, and C, though hepatitis types D and E (also forms of a liver infection) exist in other parts of the world. Laboratory tests can confirm if and what type of hepatitis a person may have.

There were about 3,500 cases of acute hepatitis A in the United States in 2013. In addition to sexual contact, hepatitis A is spread by the fecal–oral route. Transmission can occur through person-to-person contact or by consuming contaminated food or drinks. Not everyone gets symptoms of hepatitis A, but if they do occur, they include fever, nausea, fatigue, dark urine, and other symptoms. Hepatitis A can be prevented by getting a vaccine, which may also be useful in preventing transmission if taken shortly after exposure. Most often the virus clears on its own, and most people fully recover from hepatitis A without permanent liver damage.[50]

Unlike hepatitis A, hepatitis B can be acute (lasting for a short time) or chronic (a long-term illness that remains in the person's body). The risk of developing chronic hepatitis B decreases as the age of infection increases. Hepatitis B is more common than hepatitis A, with about 19,800 new cases occurring in

2013 and a total of between 700,000 and 1.4 million people living with chronic hepatitis B. The exact number is unknown because so many cases go unreported due to lack of awareness of being infected. Symptoms may not manifest for everyone infected with the hepatitis B virus. If they do exist, they can be similar to the symptoms of hepatitis A: fever, fatigue, nausea, abdominal pain, dark urine, and other symptoms. Hepatitis B is transmitted when blood, semen, or other bodily fluid from an infected person enters another person. The most common route of transmission is through sex, but transmission also occurs through needle sharing or exposure to blood, or during birth from an infected mother to her baby. Some people with chronic hepatitis B develop serious liver problems such as cirrhosis or cancer, which can lead to death. A vaccine exists to prevent hepatitis B. If a person is infected and receives an injection of hepatitis B immune globulin within 12 hours of exposure, it can help reduce the risk of transmission. Acute hepatitis B may not require treatment. Chronic hepatitis B requires treatment with antiviral medications, an injection called interferon, or, if severe, a liver transplant.[51]

Hepatitis C can also be an acute or chronic illness. For a minority of patients infected with the hepatitis C virus, the virus clears on its own, but most of those infected develop a chronic infection. It is transmitted by exposure to infected blood, with the most common route of infection being shared needles. It is less frequently spread through sex with someone infected with the hepatitis C virus. With about 30,000 estimated new infections in 2013 and about 3.5 million people currently infected, hepatitis C is the most common type of hepatitis in the United States. It may come as a surprise to learn that more than 75% of adults infected with the hepatitis C virus were born from 1945 to 1965. Many adults became infected during the height of transmission; in the 1970s and 1980s, there was less screening of blood and more needle sharing among intravenous drug users. Symptoms can be mild or may not appear; if they exist, they include fever, fatigue, nausea, abdominal pain, and other symptoms. Hepatitis C is associated with liver disease and cancer, which can lead to death. Unlike the other hepatitis viruses, there is no vaccination for the hepatitis C virus. Thus, the only way to prevent infection is to avoid risky behaviors. Antiviral medications can help treat hepatitis C. Historically, hepatitis C has been treated with injection medications, but oral pills to treat and cure hepatitis C with fewer side effects and discomfort than injections have recently been approved. The type of treatment regimen depends on various individual factors, so patients will discuss with their healthcare providers about their options.[52,53]

Preventing Pregnancy: What You Need to Know

Becoming pregnant and having a child can be a beautiful and welcome experience. Many individuals, though, may want to prevent pregnancy at a given time in their life. Worrying about getting pregnant should not be a concern for women only. It takes two people to get pregnant, and therefore both parties need to take action to prevent an unintended pregnancy.

What Makes Some People More Susceptible to STDs Than Others?

Although everyone who engages in sexual activity is at risk of contracting STDs, the following factors can increase the risk[54]:

- Early sexual initiation
- Having multiple sexual partners
- Having unprotected sex
- Substance use

We often talk about pregnancy as being unintended or intended. The definition of unintended pregnancy is a pregnancy that is reported by the parent (after birth) to have been mistimed (occurring sooner or later than desired) or unwanted, meaning the parent(s) did not want to have children at all or did not want additional children. According to this definition, an astounding half of all pregnancies are considered unintended (**FIGURE 5-11**).[55] There have been increasing critiques of this conceptualization of pregnancy, namely because it assumes all people can and should decide to have a child and plan their pregnancy.[55–58] Regardless of how we categorize pregnancy, an array of options exists to help women and men prevent pregnancy if they wish.

Contraception, also known as birth control, refers to medications, devices, and behaviors that can reduce the likelihood of becoming pregnant. Contraception works to prevent pregnancy in a variety of ways; for example, it can prevent

contraception Medications, devices, and behaviors that can reduce the risk of becoming pregnant by either preventing sperm from getting to an egg or preventing the ovaries from releasing an egg; also known as birth control.

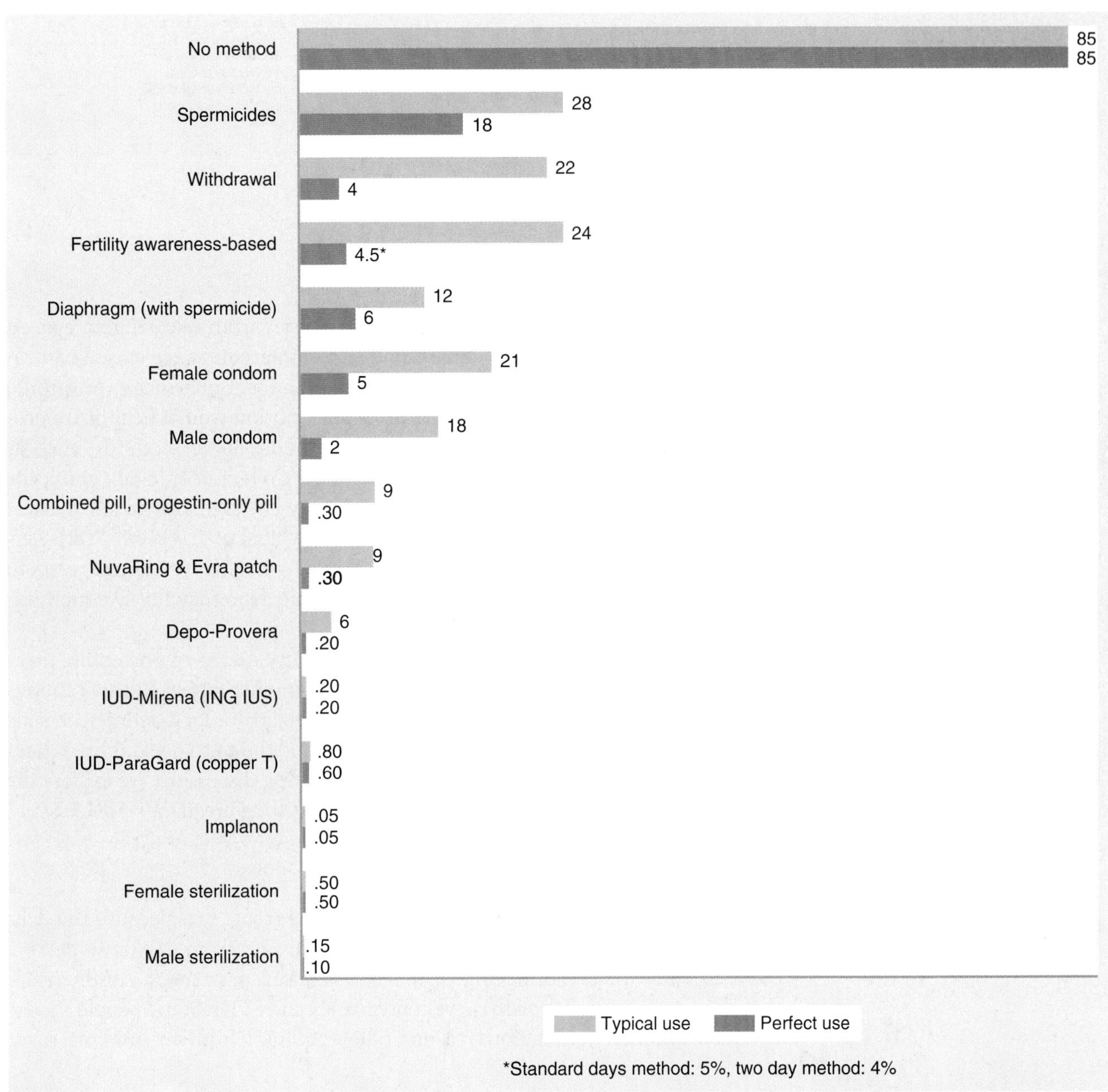

FIGURE 5-11 Percentage of women experiencing an unintended pregnancy during the first year of typical use and the first year of perfect use of contraception.

Reproduced from Association of Reproductive Health Professionals. (2008). Breaking the contraceptive barrier: Techniques for effective contraceptive consultations. Retrieved from https://www.arhp.org/Publications-and-Resources/Clinical-Proceedings/Breaking-the-Contraceptive-Barrier/Use-Knowledge

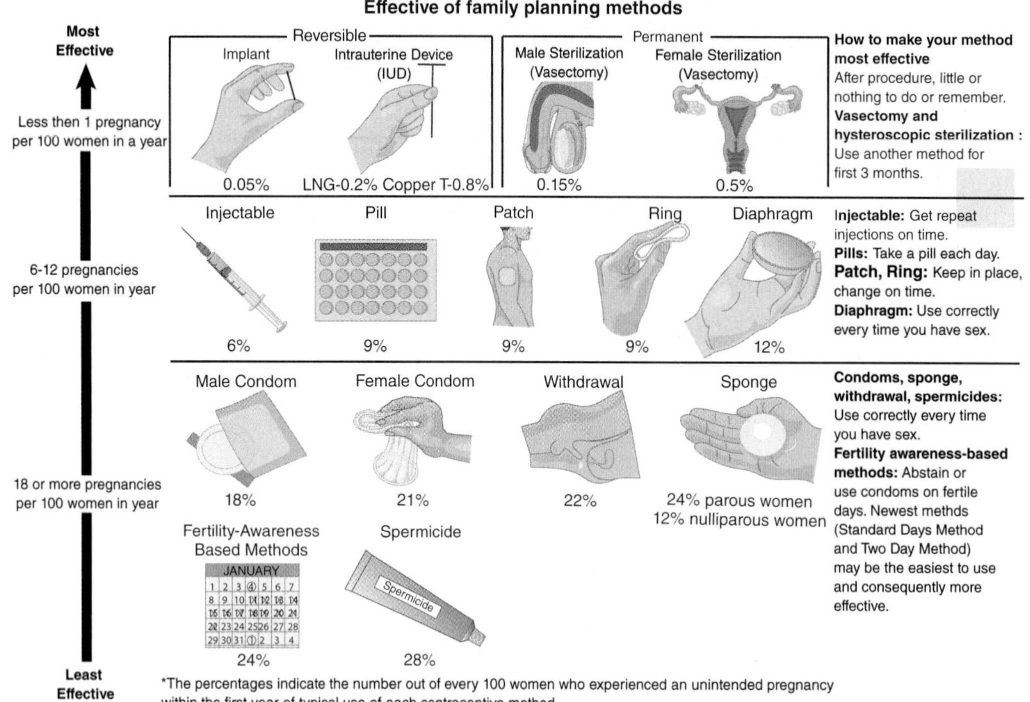

FIGURE 5-12 Graphic of contraceptive effectiveness.

Courtesy of Centers for Disease Control and Prevention. Retrieved from https://www.cdc.gov/reproductivehealth/unintendedpregnancy/pdf/contraceptive_methods_508.pdf

sperm from getting to an egg or prevent the ovaries from releasing an egg. At some point, 99% of women who have had sexual intercourse have used contraception.[59] Some contraceptives can be bought at a local pharmacy (or online) without a prescription, but others require a prescription from a healthcare professional. Insurance will often cover these methods. Some methods, such as condoms, are often given out free at local clinics.[60] When people talk about the effectiveness of different contraceptives, they may cite statistics called "perfect use," and others may use statistics that refer to "typical use" (**FIGURE 5-12**). Perfect use refers to how it worked in a clinical trial, whereas typical use refers to how that method is used in real life (by real people, who may not use methods consistently or correctly all of the time).

If a person chooses to have sex, the most effective means of preventing pregnancy and STDs is to use condoms in addition to another highly effective contraceptive method, such as birth control pills taken regularly or long-acting reversible contraception. Ultimately, the choice of which methods best fit a person's life, schedule, and needs belongs to that person. In the following discussion, we explore the most common contraceptive options to help avoid getting pregnant (**TABLE 5-2**).

Abstinence

Abstinence refers to not having (that is, abstaining from) sex. Because the definition of what constitutes sex is subjective and can vary from person to person, abstinence may mean not having vaginal sex, anal sex, or oral sex. Abstinence is the only guaranteed method to prevent pregnancy and STDs. Some people choose to remain abstinent for religious reasons, often refraining from sex until marriage.

Long-Acting Reversible Contraception

Intrauterine devices and contraceptive implants fall under the category called long-acting reversible contraception (LARC, pronounced "lark"). These methods function just as the name implies; they can be effective for a long time and

TABLE 5-2 Contraception Methods

Contraceptive Method	Description	Efficacy in Preventing Pregnancy	Prevents STDs?	Main Side Effects
Abstinence	Refraining from various forms of sex (vaginal, anal, oral)	100%	Yes	None
Intrauterine device (IUD)	Small plastic device shaped like a "T" inserted into the uterus	Less than 1 woman per 100 will get pregnant each year.	No	Ovarian cysts, ectopic pregnancy, cramps, heavy periods, and spotting between periods.
Implant	Implant, which releases progestin, implanted under the skin on the upper arm	About 1 in every 100 women will get pregnant each year.	No	Changes in menstrual bleeding, changes in mood, headache, acne, and depression.
Oral contraception	Hormones in pill form taken at the same time every day	With typical usage, about 9 out of 100 women will get pregnant each year.	No	Nausea, cramps, change in appetite, and acne. If a woman smokes and is over age 35 years, risk of heart attack, blood clots, and stroke increases.
Condom (male)	Thin sheath made of latex rubber, animal skin, or polyurethane designed to fit over a man's erect penis	With typical usage, 18 out of 100 women will get pregnant each year.	Yes (with the exception of animal skin condoms)	Allergic reaction to material used.
Condom (female)	Thin pouch that covers the vagina or anus made of polyurethane or nitrile	With typical usage, 21 out of 100 women will get pregnant each year.	Yes	Allergic reaction to material used.
Contraceptive ring	A hollow, flexible ring, about 2 inches in diameter, inserted into the vagina once a month (brand name NuvaRing)	With typical usage, 9 out of 100 women will get pregnant each year.	No	Bleeding between periods, breast tenderness, and nausea or vomiting. Heart attack, stroke, and blood clots (rare).
Transdermal patch	Two-inch square that sticks to skin and is applied to a woman's abdomen, buttock, upper arm, or torso (brand name Ortho Evra)	With typical usage, about 9 in 100 women will get pregnant each year.	No	Nausea, cramps, change in appetite, and acne. If a woman smokes and is over age 35 years, risk of heart attack, blood clots, and stroke increases.

(continues)

TABLE 5-2 Contraception Methods *(continued)*

Contraceptive Method	Description	Efficacy in Preventing Pregnancy	Prevents STDs?	Main Side Effects
Contraceptive injectable	Injection that is given in the arm once every 3 months that releases the hormone progestin (brand name Depo-Provera)	If injected in a timely fashion, less than 1 in 100 women will get pregnant each year. If not injected in a timely fashion, about 6 in 100 women will get pregnant each year.	No	Irregular bleeding, changes in sex drive and appetite, depression, and hair loss.
Emergency contraception	Comes in two forms: hormone pills or the copper IUD	Efficacy at preventing pregnancy is about 85–89% if used within 72 hours of sex.	No	Changes in period, headaches, and nausea or vomiting.
Fertility awareness-based methods	Tracking ovulation and abstaining from sexual intercourse at times most likely to get pregnant	With typical usage, 24 out of 100 women will get pregnant each year.	No	None
Withdrawal	Removal of penis from vagina before ejaculation (also known as coitus interruptus)	About 28 out of 100 women will get pregnant each year.	No	None
Sterilization	Women: tubal ligation, a surgical procedure whereby the fallopian tubes are closed, thereby blocking sperm from fertilizing the egg Men: vasectomy, which involves closing or blocking tubes that carry sperm	Women: About 1 out of 200 women may still become pregnant after tubal ligation. Men: Vasectomy is greater than 99% effective.	No	Women: Short term: bleeding from skin incision or internally, infection, organ damage, and anesthesia side effects. Long term: ectopic pregnancy or fallopian tube that does not close completely and results in pregnancy. Men: Short term: Bleeding and infection. Long term: pain and recanalization, in which a sperm is able to get across the vas deferens and cause pregnancy.

can be reversed at any time. After the initial one-time insertion by a health professional, these methods do not require any patient follow-up action (unlike taking a pill each day or remembering to get injections). LARC methods are the most effective means of preventing pregnancy. Keep in mind, however, that they

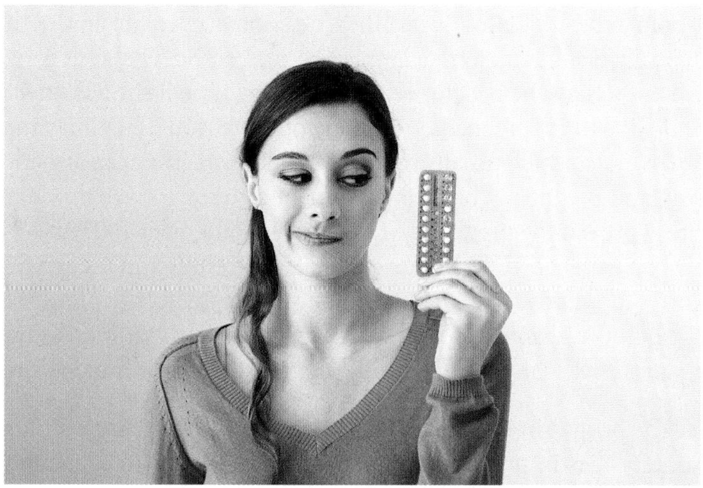

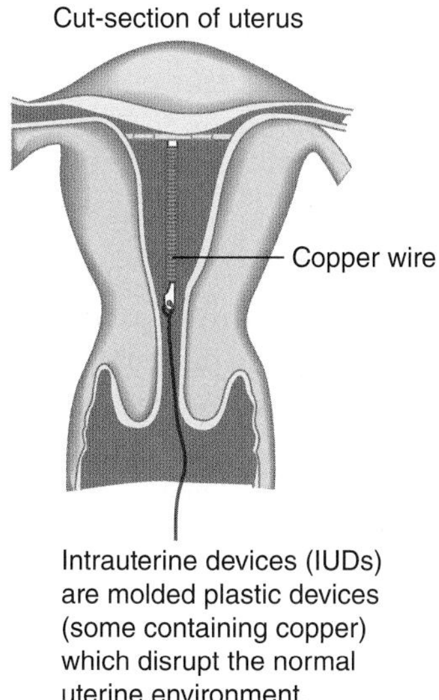

FIGURE 5-13 Intrauterine devices (IUDs) are one of the most effective types of contraception.

do not protect against STDs, so if a woman chooses a LARC method, she should also use condoms consistently to avoid infections.

Intrauterine Devices. An intrauterine device (IUD) is a small plastic device shaped like a "T" that is inserted into the uterus, where it remains for its life span (the amount of time the particular device has been proven effective) or until the woman wants it removed (**FIGURE 5-13**). There are two different types of IUDs that function to prevent pregnancy in distinct ways. The copper-releasing IUD (brand name ParaGard) releases copper ions, which are deadly to sperm. The shape of the device also blocks sperm from reaching an egg. It can stay in the uterus for up to 10 years. This type of IUD may cause cramps, heavy periods, or spotting between periods. Because it starts to work immediately, the copper IUD can also be used as emergency contraception (discussed later in the chapter). The other type of IUD releases progestin. Progestin is a hormone used in many birth control pills that prevents the release of an egg from the ovaries. Similar to the copper IUD, the progestin IUD is "T" shaped and thus helps to block sperm from reaching an egg. This IUD starts to work to prevent pregnancy a week after being inserted and can be left in the uterus for 3 to 5 years.

With both types of IUDs, a health professional needs to insert the device. Insertion usually occurs in a physician's office, and no hospital visit is required. A woman can opt to have her doctor remove it at any time if she has unwanted side effects, would like to get pregnant, or for any other reason. IUDs may increase the risk of ovarian cysts, which usually resolve on their own. They can also increase the risk for an ectopic pregnancy, but this may not be a concern given how highly effective they are at preventing pregnancy. Less than 1 woman per 100 will get pregnant each year when using an IUD. Because of its effectiveness and the freedom to not have to worry about doing any regular follow-up, many women find the IUD an appealing method of contraception. IUDs can be costly, but increasingly, insurance companies cover the cost, and unlike the pill, there is only a one-time fee.[61,62]

Implants. The progestin implant is another type of LARC. As previously noted, the hormone progestin prevents an ovary from releasing an egg, and thus prevents pregnancy. A health professional implants the device under the skin on the upper arm. The procedure takes only a few minutes, and the skin is numbed with medication. Like the IUD, about 1 in every 100 women will get pregnant each year while using the implant. Some side effects include changes in menstrual bleeding (sometimes stopping entirely), changes in mood, headache, acne, and depression. It is effective for up to 3 years, but a woman can have it removed whenever she wants.[63,64]

Oral Contraception (Birth Control Pills)

Oral contraception, commonly called "the pill," is a preparation of hormones (in pill form) taken at the same time every day to prevent pregnancy. This method works to prevent pregnancy in several different ways. Most birth control pills contain a combination of estrogen and progestin hormones. Some pills contain only progestin and are usually prescribed if a patient is sensitive to the combination hormone pill. The hormones work by preventing ovaries from releasing an egg and making the lining of the cervix thicker, to prevent sperm from getting to an egg.

The pill can be very effective at preventing pregnancy, with less than 1 in 100 women becoming pregnant each year (**FIGURE 5-14**). However, because it is difficult sometimes to remember to take the pill every day at the same time, many women accidentally miss a pill. The "typical" effectiveness rate, assuming the pill is not always taken each day, indicates that about 9 out of 100 women each year will get pregnant while on the pill. The more pills that are missed or taken at different times, the greater the risk of pregnancy. Different types of pills have different regimens; most come in packets of 21 or 28 pills. When using the 28-pill packet, a pill is taken every day. When using the 21-pill packet, a pill is taken for 3 weeks of the month; for the 4th week, no pills are taken, and the woman will have her period. The pill needs to be started on a certain day (the prescribing doctor will provide this detail) and needs to be taken at the same time each day.

Side effects of the pill may include nausea, cramps, change in appetite, acne, and other symptoms. If side effects persist, the woman should contact a medical professional. If a woman smokes cigarettes and is taking birth control pills, her risk of heart attack, blood clots, and stroke increases (especially if over the age of 35 years). If she has medical insurance, she often will have to pay a small co-pay each month for the pill. She will need a prescription from a healthcare professional for oral contraceptives.[65] As with LARC, oral contraceptives do not prevent STDs and need to be used in combination with a method such as latex condoms.

The Ring

The contraceptive ring (brand name NuvaRing) is a hollow, flexible ring, about 2 inches in diameter, that is inserted into the vagina once a month. It remains

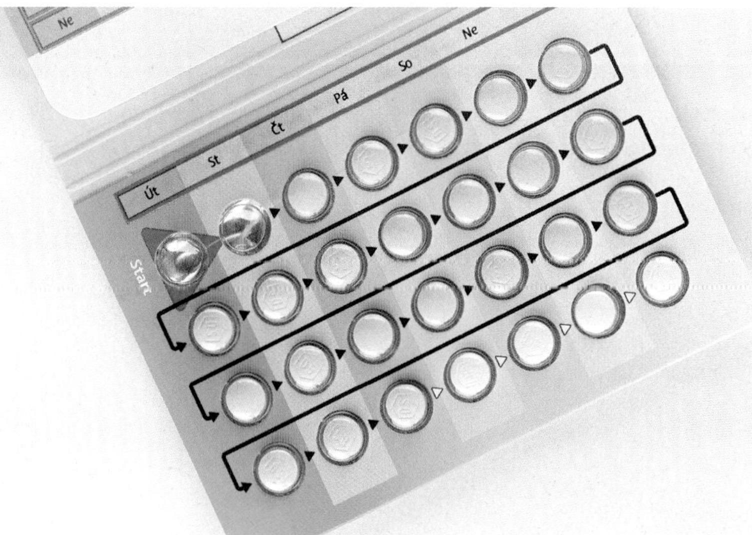

FIGURE 5-14 Oral contraceptives can be very effective if taken consistently.
© Calek/Shutterstock.

there for 3 weeks, releasing the same hormones found in oral contraceptives (estrogen and progestin) that prevent pregnancy. After 3 weeks, the woman removes it for 1 week and then inserts a new ring. She does not need a doctor to insert the ring; she can do it herself, but she does need a prescription (**FIGURE 5-15**). If used perfectly, less than 1 out of 100 women each year will get pregnant. The rate of pregnancy for typical use is 9 out of 100 women each year will get pregnant.

Some women find the ring to be a convenient and safe method of pregnancy prevention. The hormones in the ring, like the pill, may protect against acne, bone loss, iron deficiency, painful menstrual cramps, and other issues. The main side effects that some women experience are bleeding between periods, breast tenderness, and nausea or vomiting. Other, more serious risks associated with taking hormones are very rare but could include heart attack, stroke, blood clots, and other conditions.[70] The ring does not protect against STDs, so it needs to be used in combination with a method that does.

The Patch

The transdermal patch (brand name Ortho Evra) is a 2-inch square that sticks to skin and is applied to a woman's abdomen, buttock, upper arm, or torso (**FIGURE 5-16**). Once a week for 3 consecutive weeks a woman affixes a new patch. No patch is used during the 4th week. The patch releases the hormones estrogen and progestin to help prevent pregnancy, but it does not protect against STDs. If used as prescribed, fewer than 1 in 100 women each year will become pregnant. If not always used as directed, about 9 in 100 women each year will become pregnant. The patch is another safe and effective method of pregnancy prevention. The same potential benefits as the ring and pill exist with the patch because they all release a combination of the same hormones. Likewise, the side effects and risks are similar. A woman does need a prescription to start the patch, but she can apply the patch herself every week.[71]

The Shot

The contraceptive injectable (brand name Depo-Provera) is a shot that is given in the arm once every 3 months that releases the hormone progestin. When using an injectable contraceptive as prescribed (taken once every 12 weeks),

Are Hormones the Enemy?

For some women (and men), the idea of taking hormones for birth control feels "unnatural" or even dangerous. What type of birth control method you choose is up to you. Because many hormonal methods are more effective than just using condoms or fertility-based methods, before ruling them out, let's take a look at the scientific evidence (*real* evidence, not random claims made on the Internet)[66–68]:

According to the American College of Obstetricians and Gynecologists, hormonal methods of birth control, particularly combined hormone methods that have estrogen and progestin, have many benefits, including the following[69]:

- Reducing risk of cancer (in the uterus, ovaries, and colon)
- Regulating periods
- Reducing menstrual cramps
- Improving acne
- Treating fibroids or endometriosis
- Potentially reducing migraine headache frequency

For most women, hormonal methods are completely safe. A minority may experience some side effects, including the following:

- Deep vein thrombosis
- Stroke
- Heart attack

These risks are highest in women older than age 35 years who smoke regularly and in women with other risk factors for heart disease. A healthy woman who does not smoke will find hormonal methods to be a safe and effective way to prevent pregnancy. In making these decisions, a person must weigh the potential risks against the inherent risks that come with being pregnant and childbirth.

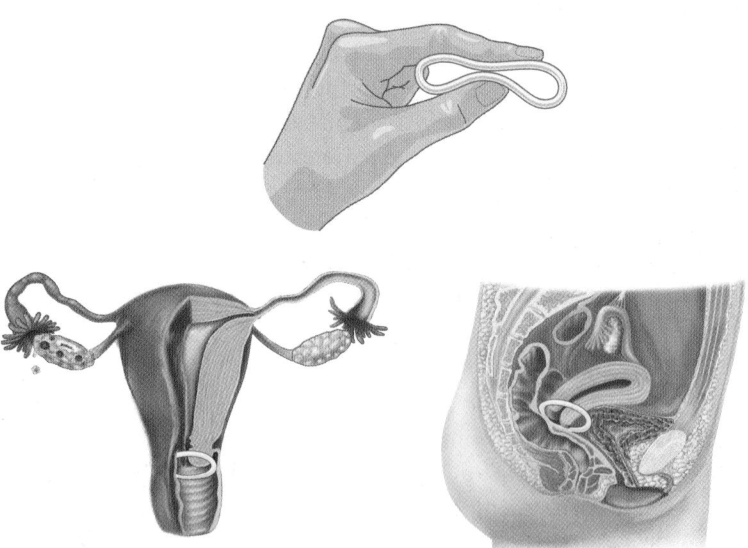

FIGURE 5-15 The vaginal ring can be inserted into the vagina on one's own. It slowly releases hormones into the body to prevent pregnancy.

fewer than 1 in 100 women will get pregnant each year. If they do not always get the shot every 12 weeks, about 6 in 100 women will get pregnant. The shot does not protect against STDs. It is considered a safe and effective contraceptive method. Although many women do not experience any symptoms, the most common complaint is irregular bleeding, especially during the first year of use. Other less common side effects include changes in sex drive and appetite,

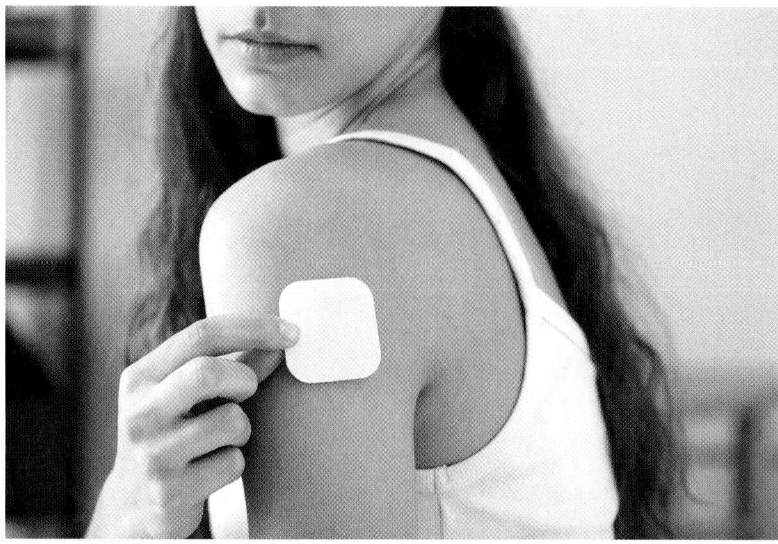

FIGURE 5-16 The contraceptive patch is a small patch that sticks to the skin to prevent pregnancy.

depression, and hair loss. A woman does need a prescription for the shot and a healthcare professional to administer it.[72]

Emergency Contraception

Emergency contraception (EC) is a method of *preventing* pregnancy *after* unprotected sexual intercourse. That may seem counterintuitive. How can something prevent a pregnancy after someone has sex? But that's just how EC works. It is *not* the abortion pill (**FIGURE 5-17**). If a woman has become pregnant and uses EC, it does not harm the existing pregnancy. EC used to be known as the "morning-after pill," but that name fell out of favor because it wrongly suggested that it can be taken only the morning after unprotected sex, and also because there is another form of EC that is not a pill. It is sometimes referred to by its brand name, Plan B.

EC comes in two forms: hormone pills or the copper IUD (not the hormone-releasing IUD because that takes too long to start working). Depending on the brand of pill, EC can be one or two pills. If it is two pills, the pills are taken 12 hours apart. Both types of EC can be used up to 5 days after unprotected sex, but they are most effective if used within 24 hours.

EC should not be the usual form of contraception (hence the name "emergency"). Think of it as a backup method, in the event the usual form of birth control fails, or if another method was not used. The copper IUD is a good choice of EC if a woman does not plan to get pregnant soon because, after insertion, it can function both as EC from the unprotected sexual encounter *and* as a regular form of birth control from then until whenever the woman chooses to have it removed.

EC is about 85–89% effective at preventing pregnancy if used within 72 hours after sex. Its effectiveness decreases as time passes. It does not protect against STDs. It is very safe; there are no reports of serious complications. Most women do not experience any side effects, but if they do, they can include changes in their period, headaches, and nausea or vomiting. Until recently, a person needed a prescription to obtain EC pills. Legislation was passed to allow people to get it over the counter without a prescription, but this legislation originally carried the restriction that only people of a certain age could buy it. The

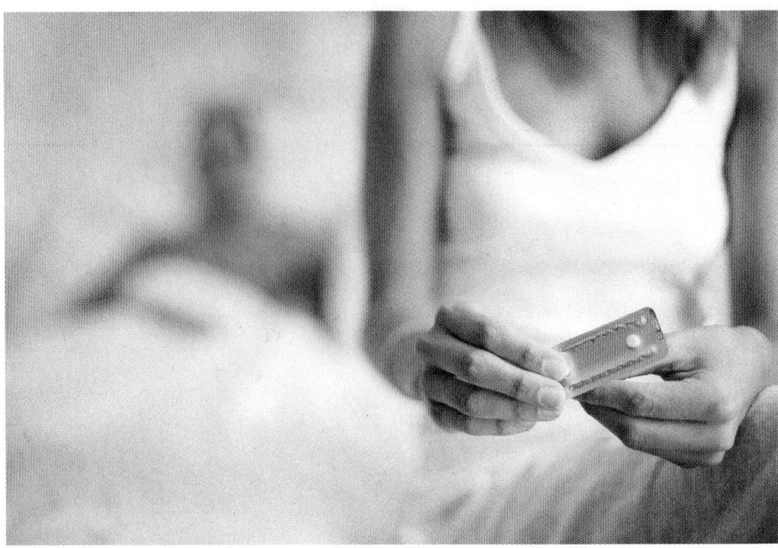

FIGURE 5-17 Emergency contraception is not the abortion pill. It is used to prevent a pregnancy after unprotected sex.

laws have changed and anyone—of any age—can now get the EC pill without a prescription at a local pharmacy. The copper IUD, however, does need to be inserted by a healthcare provider, so if a woman decides that is the best method of EC for her, she must see her doctor.[73]

Condoms

The male condom is a barrier device made of latex rubber, animal skin, or polyurethane that is designed to fit over a man's erect penis. If used correctly and consistently (every time someone has anal or vaginal sex), condoms can help to prevent pregnancy and most STDs (**FIGURE 5-18**). Note that condoms made of animal skin, however, do not protect against spreading infections. Latex is often the material most recommended because it is effective and widely available. If a latex allergy exists, polyurethane condoms are a good option that also provides protection from pregnancy and STDs. This material is thinner than latex and can transfer heat more easily so may increase pleasure. However, they are not as widely available so may be harder to find. There are rarely any side effects of using condoms, unless someone is allergic to the material from which they are made.

Condoms can be used only once; a new condom must be used every time a person has sex. Condoms are very effective at preventing pregnancy if used perfectly. The risk of pregnancy (and STDs), however, is increased if a condom falls off, breaks or tears, or is used incorrectly. If a man attempts to put a condom on before his penis is erect, it will not go on easily and semen may leak out. Because people are not always perfect and accidents can happen, the "typical" effectiveness is about 82%. This means that for 18 out of 100 people each year who have sex and use a condom as the *only* method of birth control, pregnancy will occur.[74,75] To learn more about how to use a male condom correctly, visit the learn/birth control/condom page of the Planned Parenthood website, and watch the video called "Condom."

A condom also exists that covers the woman's vagina (or anus). Despite its name of "female condom," it can also work for MSM to cover the anus during anal sex to prevent STDs. The female condom is made of polyurethane or nitrile. It works by inserting the condom into the vagina (or anus). It can also protect against STDs and pregnancy, but not as effectively as the male condom.

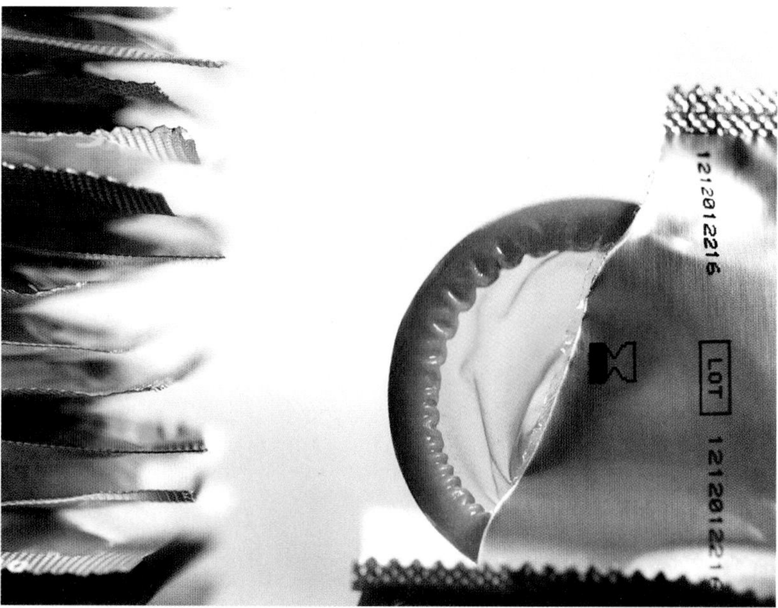

FIGURE 5-18 Condoms can help prevent both pregnancy and STDs.

Typically, 21 out of 100 women will become pregnant each year if using only the female condom. Similar to male condoms, the effectiveness is reduced if they are not worn consistently or accurately, break or tear, or are not worn before any contact with a man's penis, or if the semen spills into the vagina during removal. Again, the only side effect is a possible reaction to the condom material.[76,77]

Fertility Awareness-Based Methods

There are ways to track ovulation (specifically when an egg is released) and abstain from sexual intercourse during that period to prevent pregnancy. These approaches are known as fertility awareness-based methods (FAMs). Because they do not require any pills or devices, they are also sometimes referred to as "natural" family planning. In the absence of pills or devices, there are no side effects; FAMs are entirely safe. Be mindful, however, that FAMs do not protect against STDs.

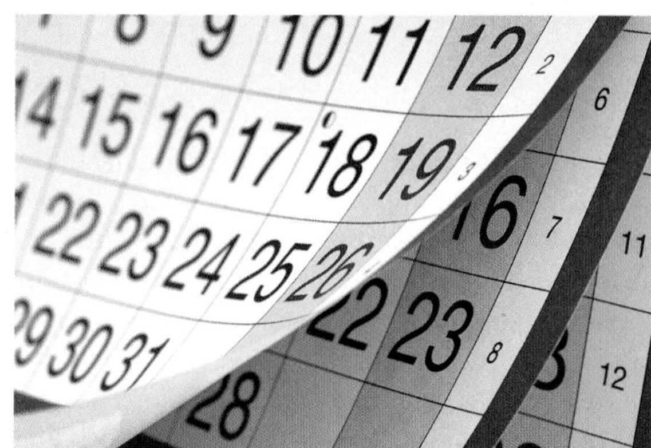

Following the fertility awareness-based methods may include tracking the woman's ovulation. These methods are safe and without side effects, but are among the least effective contraceptive options to prevent pregnancy.

How to Use a Condom

Putting a condom on (**FIGURE 5-19**):

1. First things first: Before using a condom, check the expiration date. Just like cheese, condoms can go bad. (Outdated condoms break more easily.)
2. Put the condom on before the penis touches the vulva or anus. Pre-ejaculate fluid ("pre-cum")—the fluid that leaks from the penis before ejaculation—can contain sperm from the last time the man ejaculated.
3. Use each condom for one erection only. (So stock up.)
4. Be careful not to tear the condom when unwrapping it. If it is torn, brittle, or stiff, toss it and use another.
5. You can put a drop or two of lubrication inside the condom to help the condom slide on and to increase pleasure for the man.
6. If the penis is not circumcised, pull back the foreskin before rolling on the condom.
7. Leave a half inch of extra space at the tip to collect the semen, then pinch the air out of the tip.
8. Unroll the condom over the penis as far as it will go.
9. Smooth out any air bubbles; they can cause condoms to break.

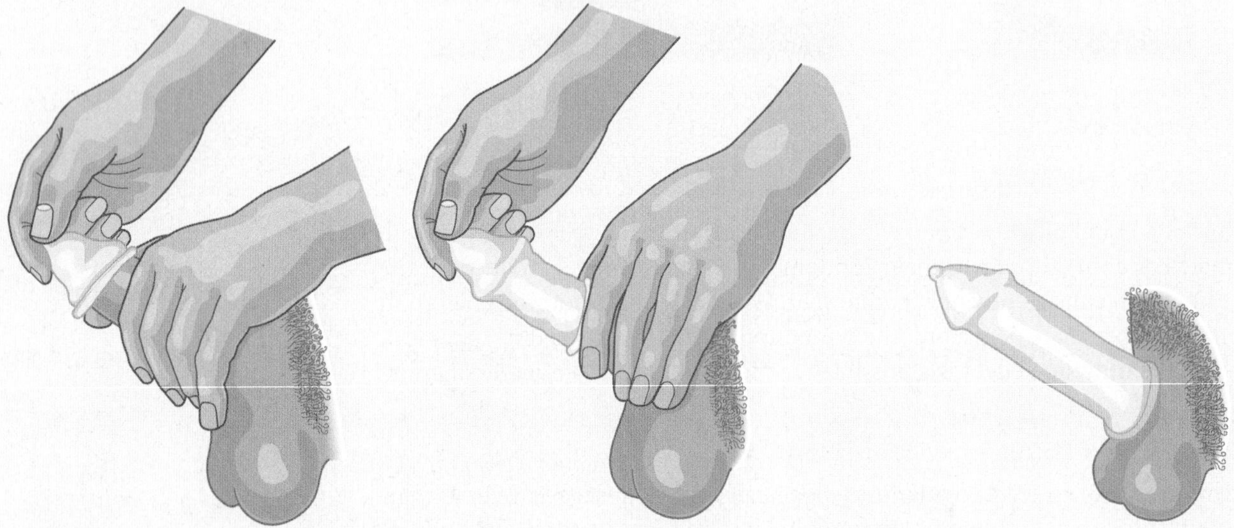

FIGURE 5-19 Putting on a condom correctly is crucial in making sure it prevents STDs and pregnancy.

Taking a condom off:

1. Remove the penis from the vagina/anus while it is still erect.
2. Hold the base of the condom while removing the penis so that semen doesn't spill out.
3. Throw the condom away in a trash can—preferably one that is out of the reach of children and pets. (Do not flush it down the toilet; condoms are bad for your plumbing.)
4. Wash the penis with soap and water before it gets near the vulva or anus again.

Adapted from www.bedsider.org

There are several ways to track ovulation and understand when a woman's most fertile days of the month happen. In one approach, the woman tracks her basal body temperature (which means the temperature when the body is at rest) daily. A woman's temperature usually rises right before ovulation and falls right before her next period. Using this method, she can assess which days to avoid sexual intercourse and to prevent pregnancy. The cervical mucus method is another FAM. Using this method, the woman checks daily for changes in her cervical mucus until she has ovulated for the month. She can check for mucus changes by assessing the color and texture of discharge in her underwear or by inserting her fingers into the vagina or opening the vagina before she urinates. Another FAM is the calendar method. There are several different ways to try to predict when a woman ovulates and track it on a calendar. The woman can also use an

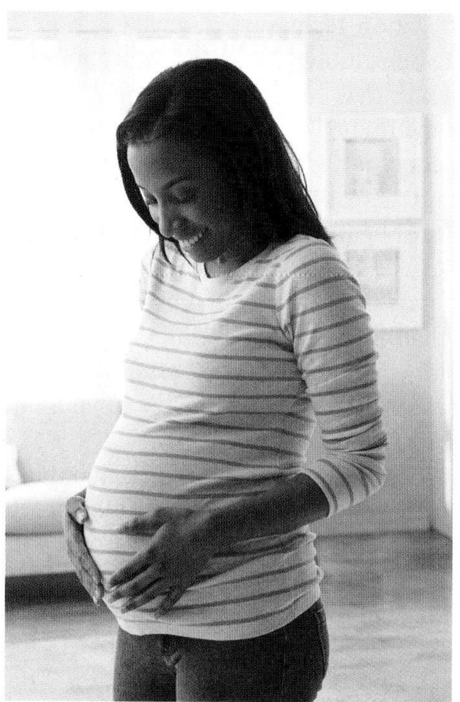

© KidStock/ Blend Images/Gettyimages.

ovulation kit (available on the shelves at local pharmacies) to help assess when she is most fertile. Finally, in the symptothermal method, two or more of the preceding methods are combined to increase the chances of predicting ovulation.[78]

While the safety and the affordability (often no or low cost) of FAMs are attractive, unfortunately, FAMs are among the least effective methods of preventing pregnancy. It is not clear how many women will get pregnant each year if they always practice these methods correctly. If FAMs are not practiced correctly all of the time, 24 out of 100 women will get pregnant annually. There are courses a woman can take and online information she can review to learn more about how to effectively use these methods.[78]

Withdrawal

Withdrawal (also known as coitus interruptus) is the withdrawal of the penis from the vagina before ejaculation occurs, as a method to prevent pregnancy. It does not prevent STDs. Although it is free, safe, and has no side effects, it is also one of the least effective methods of pregnancy prevention. About 28 out of 100 women who use withdrawal as the only birth control method will get pregnant annually. One of the reasons it does not work as well to prevent pregnancy is that men sometimes have difficulty anticipating when they are about to ejaculate. There is also mixed evidence about whether or not pre-ejaculate fluid (emitted from the man's penis before ejaculation) contains sperm. Because of this method's relative ineffectiveness, frequently couples will use withdrawal in combination with other birth control methods to better prevent pregnancy.[79]

Sterilization

Sterilization is a surgical procedure intended to be a permanent method of preventing pregnancy. Sterilization methods should be chosen only if someone or a couple is certain they do not want to become pregnant (again or ever).[80] There are two options for sterilization, one for women and one for men. Neither male nor female sterilization protects against STDs.

The female sterilization technique is tubal ligation. Tubal ligation, often referred to as "having one's tubes tied," is a surgical procedure whereby the fallopian tubes are blocked, tied, or cut, blocking sperm from fertilizing the egg. This is a permanent method of birth control and thus only a good option if a woman is certain she does not want to become pregnant. Trying to reverse this procedure is costly, and there is no guarantee the tubes can be rejoined. As it is a surgical procedure, tubal ligation can be costly and does come with some risks. One main risk is that tubes will rejoin on their own and cause an ectopic pregnancy (fertilized egg stays in the fallopian tube instead of moving to the uterus). Another procedure that makes a woman infertile is a hysterectomy. A hysterectomy is a major surgery that removes the uterus. It is generally performed for medical reasons other than sterilization, but it will nonetheless result in the inability to become pregnant.[80]

Male sterilization, or vasectomy, involves closing or blocking tubes that carry sperm. Like female sterilization, it can be costly but is highly effective. It is fairly safe, but as it is a medical procedure, a vasectomy does come with some risks, namely infection. After the procedure, men should rest for a few days. Again, reversal is at least a theoretical option, but there is no guarantee that it will be a success.

Selecting the Right Contraceptive Method

The best way for individuals to go about finding the contraceptive method that works best for them is to review information on various methods provided by reputable websites or provided by a healthcare provider, talk to people who have used various methods, and discuss options with a healthcare provider. A person may want to consider factors such as effectiveness (how well it prevents pregnancy), STD prevention, cost, and schedule. Individuals may need to try out a method or two before they find the one (or combination) that is best for them.

Abortion

abortion A procedure that a woman undergoes to end a pregnancy; there are two types of abortion: the "abortion pill" and clinical procedures, which include aspiration, and dilation and evacuation (D&E).

Sometimes contraception fails or isn't used at all and a woman becomes pregnant. She may decide to have an **abortion** because it is not the right time for her to have a child, to protect her life, or for other medically indicated reasons. Abortion is a procedure that a woman undergoes to terminate (end) a pregnancy. Although the rate of abortion has declined, abortions are more common than one may think. Almost one-third of women will have an abortion by the age of 45 years.[81]

Each year, about 2% of women have an abortion. Many women have more than one abortion in their lifetime. However, because of stigma, and sometimes shame or fear, abortion is rarely discussed publicly. With the advent of social media, and in reaction to laws that are increasingly restrictive of access to abortion, more and more women and couples are becoming vocal about having had abortions.

Women seek abortion when they have an unwanted pregnancy (where birth control may not have been used or failed). Or a woman may have wanted a pregnancy initially, but some circumstance changed after becoming pregnant (medically, in her relationship, or otherwise). In the United States, abortions are legal when performed by a licensed clinician. However, different states have different laws regarding what types of abortion procedures can be used and at what stage in pregnancy (**FIGURE 5-20** and **TABLE 5-3**).[82] Given upcoming changes to the Supreme Court (at the time this book was published), state laws around abortion may drastically change. For the most recent overview of abortion laws by state visit the website for the Guttmacher Institute.

There are two types of abortion: the "abortion pill" and clinical procedures. The abortion pill is a combination of two medications (mifepristone and misoprostol)

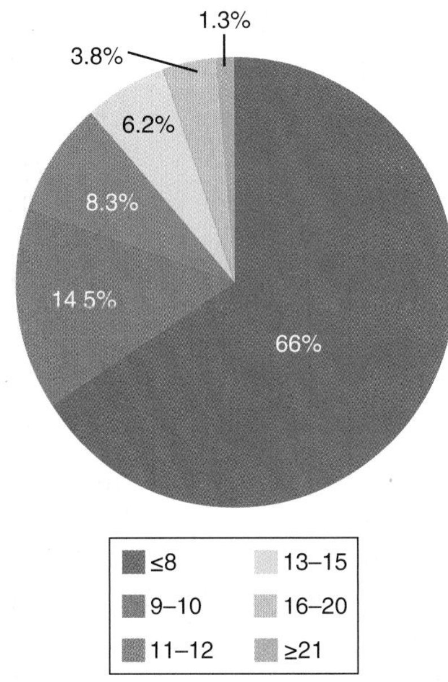

FIGURE 5-20 One-third of abortions occur at 6 weeks of pregnancy or earlier; 89% occur in the first 12 weeks, 2010.

Guttmacher Institute. Induced Abortion in the United States (as of January 1, 2018), 218, https://www.guttmacher.org/fact-sheet/induced-abortion-united-states

that can terminate a pregnancy. The abortion pill is available through some healthcare providers, such as Planned Parenthood clinics. The pill can be taken up to 10 weeks after the first day of a woman's last period. Women may choose this option because it can be done at home and without any medical intervention. The provider administers the first medication, mifepristone, and sends the woman home with the misoprostol to take 1 to 2 days later. Women experience cramping and bleeding during this time. It usually takes about 5 hours after taking the second medication for the abortion to be complete. After this, patients follow up with their healthcare provider within 2 weeks (or earlier if there are side effects) to ensure the abortion is complete. New FDA regulations have reduced the dosage needed (to reflect current medical practice) and reduced the number of needed doctor visits from three to two. This change has minimized some of the burden on women to travel to their doctor more than needed.[83] Medication abortion is safe and effective; it works 97 out of 100 times in completing an abortion. As with any medication, there may be some side effects. In rare cases, the abortion may be incomplete. Women may experience infection or have a reaction to the pill. Any side effects should be discussed with the provider immediately.

There are two types of clinical abortive procedures: aspiration, and dilation and evacuation (D&E). Clinical procedures are administered by a licensed clinician and can be done within a hygienic clinic setting, much like other outpatient procedures.[83] An aspiration is the most common and can be done up to 16 weeks after a woman's last period; after that time, the health provider performs a D&E. The procedure is similar for both types of abortion. The patient is given medication to numb the pain (and sometimes a sedative). The cervix is opened and a suction device is used to empty out the uterus. The procedure usually takes less than 20 minutes, but the preparation takes longer. Antibiotics are given to prevent an infection.

For most women, the procedure feels similar to having menstrual cramps. Bleeding is also common and normal after the procedure. These procedures are safe, but as with all medical procedures, they do come with some potential risks, such as infection, heavy bleeding, and incomplete abortion. The procedures,

TABLE 5-3 Overview of State Abortion Laws

State	Must Be Performed by a Licensed Physician	Must Be Performed in a Hospital if at:	Second Physician Must Participate if at:	Prohibited Except in Cases of Life or Health Endangerment if at:	"Partial-Birth" Abortion Banned	Public Funding of Abortion		Private Insurance Coverage Limited	Providers May Refuse to Participate		Mandated Counseling Includes Information on:			Waiting Period (in hours) after Counseling	Parental Involvement Required for Minors
						Funds All or Most Medically Necessary Abortions	Funds Limited to Life Endangerment, Rape and Incest		Individual	Institution	Breast Cancer Link	Fetal Pain	Negative Psychological Effects		
AL	X	Viability	Viability	20 weeks*	▼		X							48	Consent
AK	X				▼	X			X	Private	X	X			▼
AZ	X	Viability	Viability	Viability	X	X		X	X	X				24	Consent
AR	X		Viability	20 weeks†	X		X		X	X		XΦ		48	Consent
CA				Viability		X			X	Religious					▼
CO							X								Notice
CT		Viability		Viability		X			X						
DE	X			ViabilityΩ			X		X	X					Notice§
DC							X								
FL	X	Viability	24 weeks	24 weeks	▼		X		X	X				▼	Notice
GA	X			20 weeks*	Post viability		X		X	X		X		24	Notice
HI	X§			Viability		X			X	X					
ID	X	Viability	3rd trimester	Viability	▼		X	X	X	X				24	Consent

IL	X[ξ]		Viability	Viability	▼	X			X	Private					Notice
IN	X	20 weeks	20 weeks	20 weeks*	X		X*	X	X	Private		X		18	Consent
IA	X			20 weeks*	▼		X		X	Private				§	Notice
KS	X		Viability	20 weeks*	X		X	X	X	X	X	X	X	24	Consent
KY	X	2nd trimester		20 weeks*	▼		X	X	X	X				24	Consent
LA	X		Viability	20 weeks*	X		X		X	X		X	X	24	Consent
ME	X			Viability			X		X	X					
MD	X			Viability[Ω]		X			X	X					Notice
MA	X[ξ]			24 weeks		X			X	X				▼	Consent
MI	X			Viability[‡]	X		X	X	X	X			X	24	Consent
MN	X		20 weeks	Viability		X			X	Private		X[Φ]		24	Notice[þ]
MS	X[Φ]			20 weeks*,[€]	X		X[Ω]		X	X	X			24	Consent[þ]
MO	X	Viability	Viability	Viability	▼		X	X	X	X		X[Φ]		72	Consent
MT			Viability	Viability*	Post viability	X			X	Private				▼	▼
NE	X			20 weeks*	▼		X	X	X	X			X	24	Consent
NV	X	24 weeks		24 weeks			X		X	Private					▼
NH					X		X								Notice

(continues)

TABLE 5-3 Overview of State Abortion Laws *(continued)*

State	Must Be Performed by a Licensed Physician	Must Be Performed in a Hospital if at:	Second Physician Must Participate if at:	Prohibited Except in Cases of Life or Health Endangerment if at:	"Partial-Birth" Abortion Banned	Public Funding of Abortion		Private Insurance Coverage Limited	Providers May Refuse to Participate		Mandated Counseling Includes Information on:			Waiting Period (in hours) after Counseling	Parental Involvement Required for Minors
						Funds All or Most Medically Necessary Abortions	Funds Limited to Life Endangerment, Rape and Incest		Individual	Institution	Breast Cancer Link	Fetal Pain	Negative Psychological Effects		
NJ	X[ξ]	14 weeks			▼	X			X	Private					▼
NM	X[ξ]				Post viability	X			X	X					▼
NY	X[ξ]		24 weeks	24 weeks[‡]		X			X						
NC	X	20 weeks		20 weeks			X		X	X			X	72	Consent
ND	X			20 weeks[*]	X		X	X	X	X				24	Consent[b]
OH	X	20 weeks	20 weeks	20 weeks[*]	X		X		X	X				24	Consent
OK	X	2nd trimester	Viability	20 weeks[*]	X		X	X	X	Private	X	X[Φ]		72	Consent and Notice
OR						X			X	Private					
PA	X	Viability	Viability	24 weeks[*]			X		X	Private				24	Consent
RI				24 weeks[‡]	▼		X	▼	X						Consent
SC	X	3rd trimester	3rd trimester	20 weeks*	X		X		X	Private				24	Consent
SD	X	24 weeks		20 weeks*	X		Life Only		X	X		X	X	72◊	Notice
TN	X	Viability	Viability	Viability*	X		X		X	X				48	Consent

TX	X			20 weeks*	X		X		X	Private	X	X	X	24	Consent and Notice
UT	X			Viability[†,Ω]	X		X*	X	X	Private		X[Φ]		72[◊]	Consent and Notice
VT						X									
VA	X	2nd trimester	Viability	3rd trimester	X		X[Ω]		X	X				24	Consent and Notice
WA	X[ξ]			Viability		X			X	X					
WV				20 weeks*	▼	X							X	24	Notice[ξ]
WI	X	Viability		20 weeks*	▼		X*		X	X		X		24	Consent[ξ]
WY	X			Viability			X		X	Private					Consent and Notice
TOTAL	**41**	**19**	**19**	**43**	**20**	**17**	**32+DC**	**11**	**45**	**42**	**5**	**13**	**8**	**27**	**37**

Guttmacher Institute, An Overview of Abortion Laws, State Laws and Policies (as of April 1, 2018). (2018). https://www.guttmacher.org/state-policy/explore/overview-abortion-laws

▼ Permanently enjoined; law not in effect.
* Exception in case of threat to the woman's physical health.
† Exception in case of rape or incest.
‡ Exception in case of life endangerment only. A 2016 New York Attorney General opinion determined that the state's law conflicts with U.S. Supreme Court rulings on abortion, and that abortion care is permissible under the U.S. Constitution to protect a woman's health, or when the fetus is not viable.
Ω Exception in case of fetal abnormality.
ξ Only applies to surgical abortion. In New Mexico, some but not all advanced practice clinicians may provide medication abortion.
Φ Law limits abortion provision to OB/GYNs.
€ A court has temporarily blocked enforcement of a Mississippi law that would have banned abortion at 15 weeks after the patient's last menstrual period.

http://www.guttmacher.org/statecenter/spibs/spib_OAL.pdf

▼ Permanently enjoined; law not in effect.
§ Enforcement temporarily enjoined by court order; policy not in effect.
Φ Fetal pain information is given only to women who are at least 20 weeks gestation; in Missouri at 22 weeks gestation.
Þ Both parents must consent to the abortion.
ξ Specified health professionals may waive parental involvement in certain circumstances.
◊ In South Dakota, the waiting period excludes weekends or annual holidays and in Utah the waiting period is waived in cases of rape, incest, fetal defect or if the patient is younger than 15.

however, are almost 100% effective at completing an abortion. After an abortion, the woman may be asked to schedule a follow-up clinic visit within a few weeks. It is often recommended to avoid vaginal sex for a few weeks to allow for healing. Having an abortion can provoke a variety of feelings, such as relief, guilt, or sadness. Serious long-term psychological problems (similar to those of childbirth), however, are very rare.

An abortion can be prohibitively expensive, costing as much as $800. Most clinics, though, offer the pill for less. As noted earlier, the abortion pill is different from EC. EC *prevents* a pregnancy, whereas the abortion pill aborts an existing pregnancy.

Abortion has been around since ancient times. It was illegal in many states as of the late 1800s. Despite being illegal, abortions were still sought by women who did not want to be pregnant. Illegal abortions were called "back alley" abortions. Untrained laypeople often performed the abortion in unhygienic conditions that put the patient's life at risk. In 1973, a landmark Supreme Court ruling was decided in the case of *Roe v. Wade*. The Court struck down state laws that made abortion illegal, citing constitutional rights to make one's own decision about pregnancy. This ruling made abortion legal throughout the country. Despite this victory for those who support access to abortion, over time, states have slowly integrated policies that make having an abortion more challenging. These laws include conditions relating to where the procedures can occur, what week in pregnancy they are allowed, what kind of funding can be used to pay for the procedures, parental requirements for minors, mandatory waiting periods, and other factors. Some laws are ambiguous regarding what is legal and at what stage of pregnancy, resulting in greater physician reluctance to perform abortions due to fear of lawsuits and losing their medical license. Though abortion is still technically legal, these legislative restrictions have made abortion less available.[82]

Despite clearly being a health issue, abortion has become a politically divisive topic, with people who support access to abortion (pro choice) often aligning with Democratic or liberal views and those who support restrictions to or even illegalization of abortion (pro life) often aligning with Republican or conservative views. Many conservative groups and people with religious beliefs that oppose abortion have initiated legislative actions to increase restrictions. They believe life starts at conception and, thus, that abortion is a crime. They view abortion restrictions as an effort to protect the life of the fetus. Both sides of the debate are passionate about their cause.

Public health scientists have found that abortion is safe and effective, and its availability has many positive benefits for families and society as a whole. Without safe and legal access, abortions will still continue, but they will occur in much less safe conditions that may risk a woman's life.[84–87]

Getting Pregnant: Reproductive and Maternal Health

Preconception Health

Bringing a new life into the world can be a wonderful experience. Even before thinking about conceiving, however, a woman needs to start considering her physical and mental health, even years in advance. Making sure the expectant mother's health is in optimal condition is a critical component of having a

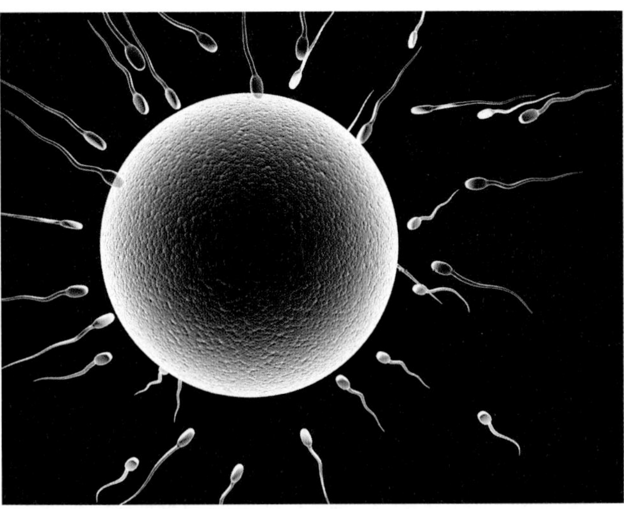

About 250 million sperm cells are released when a man ejaculates, but only one may enter the woman's egg and start the fertilization process.

healthy pregnancy and healthy baby. Because many pregnancies are not planned, it is important for a woman to keep the preconception health recommendations in mind well before she hopes to get pregnant. Even if a woman plans never to get pregnant, the following recommendations are things that most people should do anyway to maintain optimal health.

The CDC recommends that women take 400 micrograms of folic acid (a B vitamin found on pharmacy shelves) daily before becoming pregnant. Having enough folic acid in a woman's body before and during early pregnancy can help prevent neural tube defects in the child (a birth defect of the brain and spine).[88]

If a woman has any medical conditions, such as high blood pressure, diabetes, STDs, eating disorders, or other chronic diseases, she should make sure they are under control before pregnancy. Some medications are contraindicated during pregnancy because they may harm the fetus. The safest approach is to talk to a healthcare provider about which medications to continue and, if the recommendation is to discontinue any medication, what alternatives are available. Even some herbal supplements that do not require a prescription may be harmful. Be sure to take an inventory of every medication and supplement regularly consumed to review with your healthcare professional. The full effects of drug use during pregnancy are not clear, but research indicates that drugs such as cocaine, nicotine, heroine, methamphetamine, inhalants, and marijuana may all have adverse prenatal effects such as miscarriage, premature birth, and cognitive problems in the child.

There are several things one can do to increase the likelihood of a healthy pregnancy (**FIGURE 5-21**). Maintaining a healthy weight before pregnancy is important. Being overweight or obese increases the risk of pregnancy complications. Exposure to toxic substances can alter both men's and women's reproductive systems, making it difficult to conceive. Limiting exposure to toxic substances is a smart idea regardless of whether someone ever plans to conceive. Also, women should eliminate exposure to violence, which can be harmful during pregnancy and to children; if a woman is in a violent relationship, there are steps she can take to minimize her danger. (See Chapter 10) A woman considering having a baby should make sure she is mentally healthy; if she does have any mental health disorders, before getting pregnant is a great time to make sure they are under control, so she is feeling ready to go!

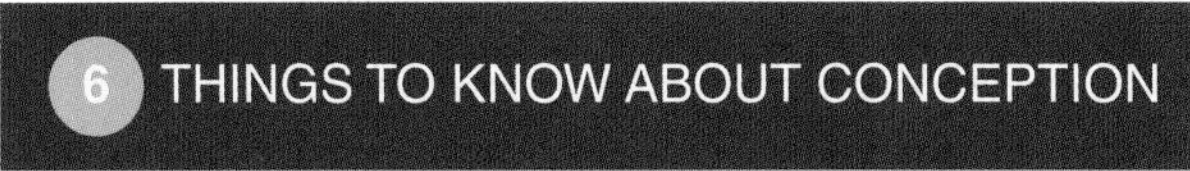

90% **of women** don't know that **2 days before through the day of ovulation** is the best time to try to get pregnant.

40% **of women** don't know that **a woman is born with all of the eggs she will ever have.**

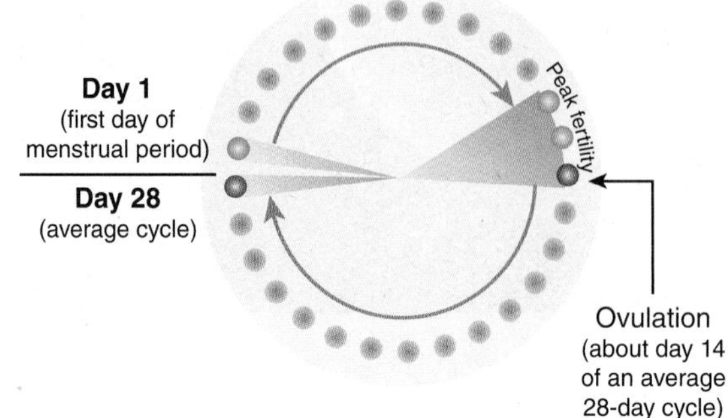

The science behind Conception

Normal ovulation leaves only a small window for conception.

Conception can occur only in the 6 days before ovulation through the day of ovulation. **Here's what it takes for conception to occur:**

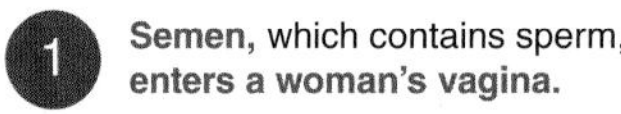

1. **Semen,** which contains sperm, **enters a woman's vagina.**

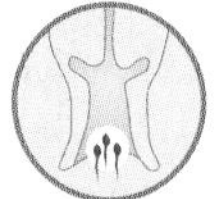

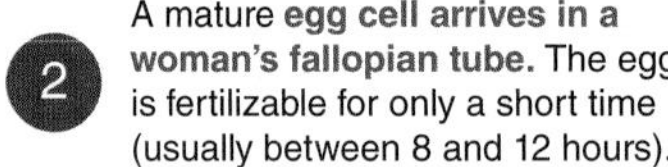

2. A mature **egg cell arrives in a woman's fallopian tube.** The egg is fertilizable for only a short time (usually between 8 and 12 hours).

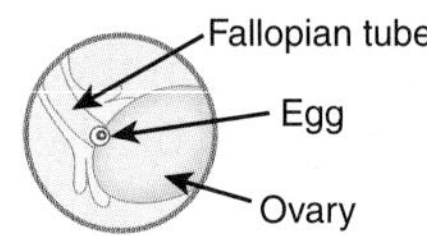

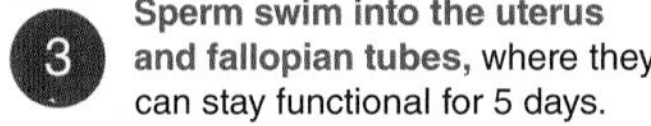

3. **Sperm swim into the uterus and fallopian tubes,** where they can stay functional for 5 days.

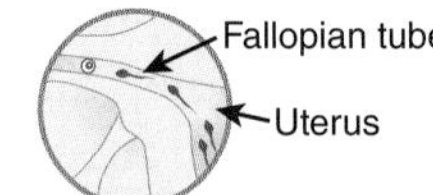

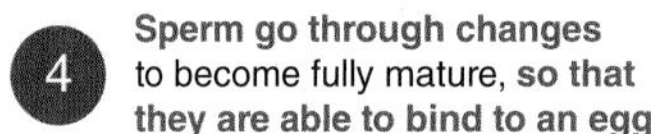

4. **Sperm go through changes** to become fully mature, **so that they are able to bind to an egg.**

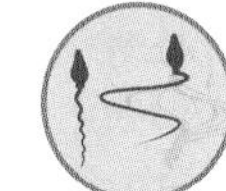

5. In the fallopian tube, **one sperm fertilizes the egg** to form an embryo.

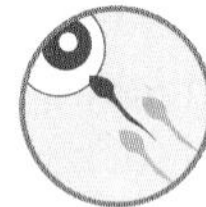

6. After several days, the **developing embryo moves to the uterus.** There, it attaches to the uterine lining, where the pregnancy can progress.

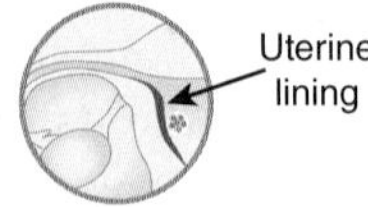

Women's and men's health conditions and behaviors, genetics, and age all influence the chance of conception.
To learn more, visit http://go.usa.gov/8rZ3.

FIGURE 5-21 Six things to know about conception.

Courtesy of National Institutes of Health. Women's Health Infographic: Conception, National Institute of Child Health and Human Development. Retrieved from https://www.nichd.nih.gov/news/resources/links/infographics/Pages/conception.aspx

Conception and Pregnancy

Previously, we reviewed the initial stage of reproduction: A woman's body ovulates an egg each month into the fallopian tubes. For someone who is trying to become pregnant, fertility awareness-based methods are often used to gauge when a woman

Preconception Health: Things a Woman Should Do Before Trying to Get Pregnant[89]

- Get any chronic medical conditions under control.
- Check with her healthcare professional regarding whether her medications are safe during pregnancy.
- Take 400 micrograms of folic acid daily.
- Maintain a healthy weight.
- Eliminate exposure to toxic substances.
- Get help for violence.
- Manage and maintain mental health.

Planning for Pregnancy, Centers for Disease Control and Prevention, Retrieved from http://www.cdc.gov/preconception/planning.html

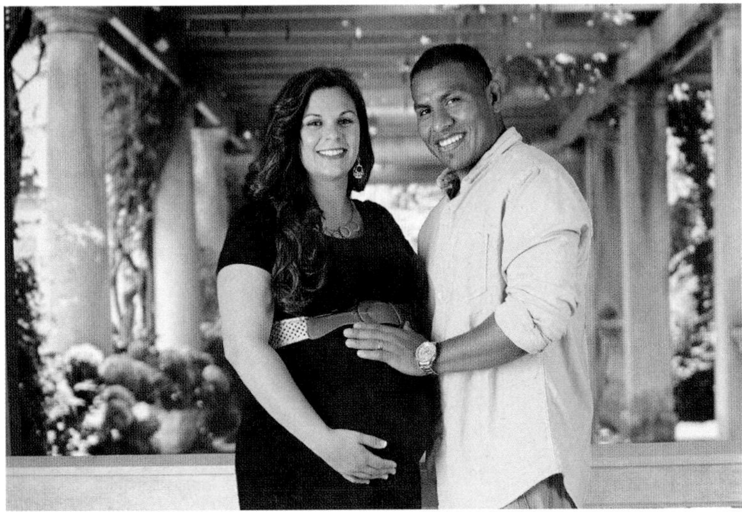

is ovulating. During vaginal intercourse between a man and a woman, a man inserts his erect penis into the woman's vagina. When the man ejaculates, about 250 million (!) sperm cells in his semen are released into the vagina. Those sperm swim through the cervix, into the uterus, and up to the fallopian tubes, all in a quest to find and fertilize the woman's egg. They can survive for up to 5 days on this journey. Only one sperm will reach and enter the egg, a process known as fertilization (**FIGURE 5-22**). The resulting cell formed from this process is called a zygote. (In some cases, such as for those who have fertility problems or individuals with same-sex partners, this process of egg fertilization is facilitated in a laboratory instead of through vaginal intercourse.) Once the egg is fertilized, no other sperm can enter the egg.

During the next stage of development, the fertilized egg is known as an embryo. The embryo moves down toward the uterus over the course of several days, where it attaches to the lining and stays for the next 9 months during pregnancy. A tissue called the placenta develops between the uterus and the embryo and provides the embryo, and later the fetus, with oxygen and nutrients.[89] The baby develops over the next 40 weeks, at which time a woman gives birth. We describe pregnancy as divided into trimesters, with different milestones for fetal development at each stage.

First Trimester (Weeks 1 to 12)

Many women first realize they are pregnant because they don't get their period. Recall that a period occurs when the egg is not fertilized and is therefore shed. If the egg is fertilized, then a period does not happen. A woman can buy a home pregnancy test at the pharmacy to test whether she is pregnant. If the test is

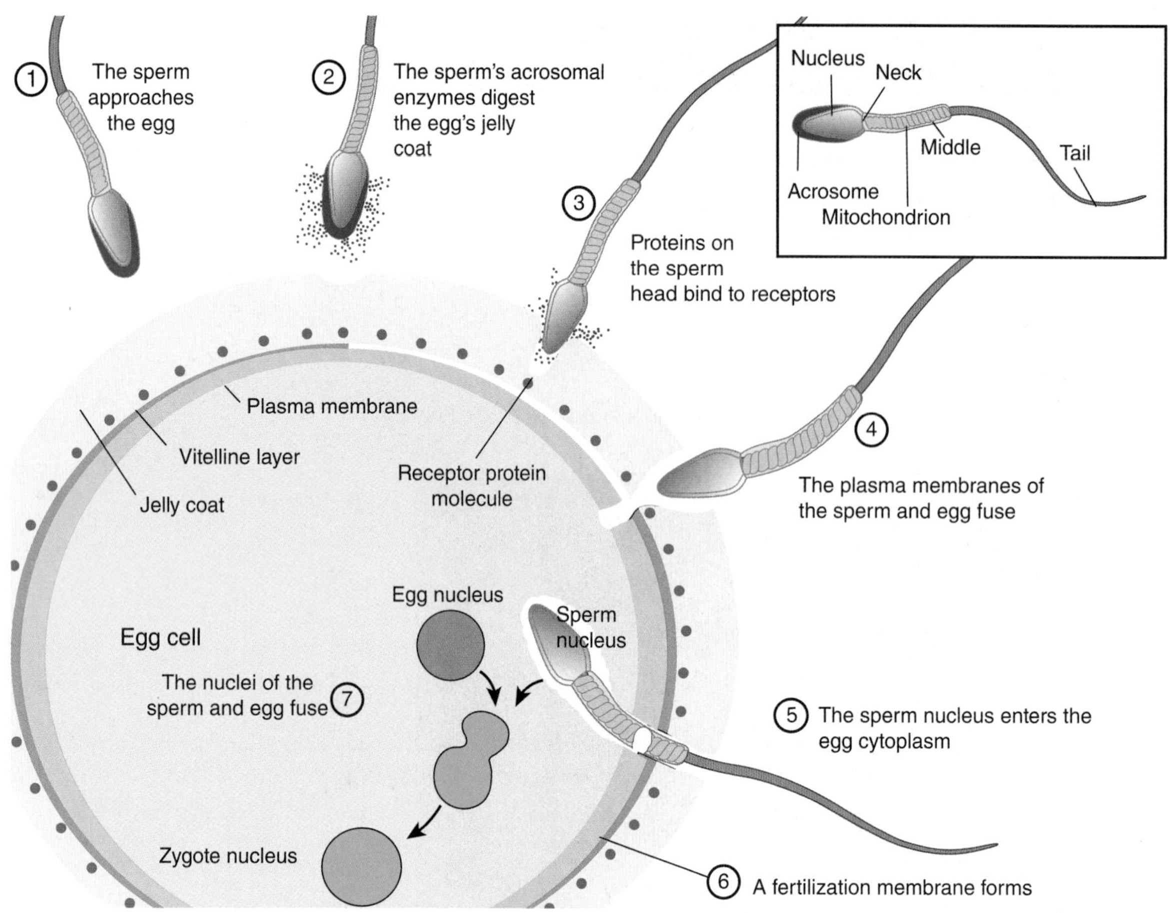

FIGURE 5-22 The stages of fertilization.

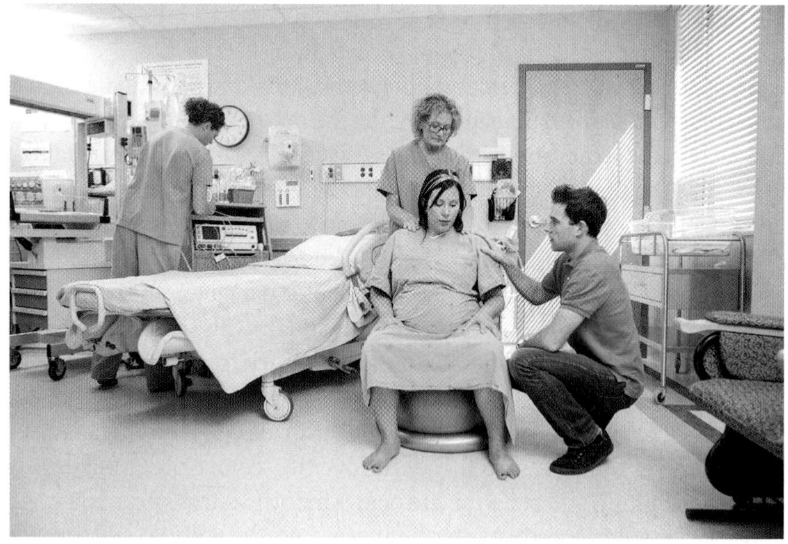

positive, she can schedule a visit with her practitioner, who can confirm she is pregnant, counsel her about medications and other things she may need to avoid, and set up a schedule for visits throughout the pregnancy.

The first trimester is an exciting time. Even before the pregnancy becomes evident, there's a lot happening. The embryo's major organs are developed by the 8th week of pregnancy; thus, early pregnancy is the time when the embryo is most vulnerable to toxic substances, such as alcohol, and infections. There

What Kind of Practitioner Is Right for Me?

Determining what kind of health practitioner a woman would like to manage her pregnancy and birth is a big decision. There are several options that can be used alone or in combination with one another:

- *Obstetrician*. An obstetrician is a medical doctor who deals with women's health needs related to pregnancy, birth, and delivery. Obstetricians receive specialized training in surgery and the female reproductive system.
- *Family physician*. A family physician is a medical doctor who provides comprehensive care for men, women, and children of all ages.
- *Midwife*. There are several types of midwives, with different levels of education and training[90–92]:
  - A certified nurse-midwife is a registered nurse who has graduated from an accredited nurse-midwifery program with a minimum of a master's degree, has passed a national certification examination, and is licensed to work in all states.
  - A certified midwife has a background in a health-related field, has graduated from an accredited midwifery program with a minimum of a master's degree, and has passed a national certification examination. Twenty-eight states regulate certified midwives.
  - A certified professional midwife has a minimum of a high school diploma, has undergone apprenticeship or formal education, has passed written exams and skill evaluations, and is licensed to work in 28 states.
  - A direct-entry or lay midwife has no educational requirements. These individuals may or may not have had an apprenticeship or formal instruction. Not all states allow direct-entry or lay midwives to practice or regulate them.
  - A doula is a trained professional who offers physical, emotional, and informational support to a mother before, during, and shortly after birth; a doula may also offer practical and emotional support to a mother during the postpartum period.

Ultimately, the decision is up to the mother. She may want to consider where she wants to give birth and what kind of training she would like the birth attendant to have based on whether she is at high risk of needing any medical intervention that requires a certain level of training and her comfort level.

are certain foods that may contain harmful bacteria, viruses, or chemicals that pregnant women should avoid (**TABLE 5-4**).

Initially, the embryo resembles a small seed, and it then grows into what looks more like a tadpole. Toward the end of the first trimester, the embryo becomes a fetus. By the end of week 12 (marking the end of trimester 1), the fetus is the size of a plum and starts to take the shape of a human body.

Second Trimester (Weeks 13 to 28)

The fetus starts moving in the second trimester, and the mother starts to gain weight (usually about 1 pound per week). Around 20 weeks, the fetal sex can be determined by ultrasound (a blood test is also available to determine the sex in the first trimester). The fetus starts to develop its bones and hair. By the end of the second trimester, the fetus is about 14 inches long.

Third Trimester (Weeks 29 to 40)

In the third trimester, the mother continues to gain weight. The fetus grows to be about the size of a pumpkin. It usually settles itself head down in the uterus, preparing for birth. Delivery usually occurs between 37 and 40 weeks of pregnancy.

Birth

Every birth delivery experience is different. It is impossible to predict exactly when a pregnant woman will go into labor. What usually happens (at around 37 to 40 weeks of pregnancy) is the mother will experience contractions. Contractions are the tightening of the uterine muscles and can be painful. They start to open up the cervix (dilation) to prepare for childbirth. Contractions gradually become longer and longer. This process can take hours. Once the mother

TABLE 5-4 Checklist of Foods to Avoid During Pregnancy

Don't Eat These Foods	Why	What to Do
Soft CHEESES made from unpasteurized milk, including Brie, feta, Camembert, Roquefort, queso blanco, and queso fresco	May contain *E. coli* or *Listeria*.	Eat hard cheeses, such as cheddar or Swiss. Or, check the label and make sure that the cheese is made from pasteurized milk.
Raw COOKIE DOUGH or CAKE BATTER	May contain *Salmonella*.	Bake the cookies and cake. Don't lick the spoon!
Certain kinds of FISH, such as shark, swordfish, king mackerel, and tilefish (golden or white snapper)	Contains high levels of mercury.	Eat up to 12 ounces a week of fish and shellfish that are lower in mercury, such as shrimp, salmon, pollock, and catfish. Limit consumption of albacore tuna to 6 ounces per week.
Raw or undercooked FISH (sushi)	May contain parasites or bacteria.	Cook fish to 145° F.
Unpasteurized JUICE or cider (including fresh squeezed)	May contain *E. coli*.	Drink pasteurized juice. Bring unpasteurized juice or cider to a rolling boil and boil for at least 1 minute before drinking.
Unpasteurized MILK	May contain bacteria such as *Campylobacter*, *E. coli*, *Listeria*, or *Salmonella*.	Drink pasteurized milk.
SALADS made in a store, such as ham salad, chicken salad, and seafood salad	May contain *Listeria*.	Make salads at home, following the food safety basics: clean, separate, cook, and chill.
Raw SHELLFISH, such as oysters and clams	May contain *Vibrio* bacteria.	Cook shellfish to 145° F.
Raw or undercooked SPROUTS, such as alfalfa, clover, mung bean, and radish	May contain *E. coli* or *Salmonella*.	Cook sprouts thoroughly.
Be Careful With These Foods	**Why**	**What to Do**
Hot dogs, luncheon meats, cold cuts, fermented or dry sausage, and other deli-style meat and poultry	May contain *Listeria*.	Even if the label says that the meat is precooked, reheat these meats to steaming hot or 165° F before eating.
Eggs and pasteurized egg products	Undercooked eggs may contain *Salmonella*.	Cook eggs until yolks are firm. Cook casseroles and other dishes containing eggs or egg products to 160° F.
Eggnog	Homemade eggnog may contain uncooked eggs, which may contain *Salmonella*.	Make eggnog with a pasteurized egg product or buy pasteurized eggnog. When you make eggnog or other egg-fortified beverages, cook to 160°F.

Be Careful With These Foods	Why	What to Do
Fish	May contain parasites or bacteria.	Cook fish to 145° F.
Ice cream	Homemade ice cream may contain uncooked eggs, which may contain *Salmonella*.	Make ice cream with a pasteurized egg product safer by adding the eggs to the amount of liquid called for in the recipe, then heating the mixture thoroughly.
Meat: Beef, veal, lamb, and pork (including ground meat)	Undercooked meat may contain *E. coli*.	Cook beef, veal, and lamb steaks and roasts to 145° F. Cook pork to 160° F. Cook all ground meats to 160° F.
Meat spread or pate	Unpasteurized refrigerated pates or meat spreads may contain *Listeria*.	Eat canned versions, which are safe.
Poultry and stuffing (including ground poultry)	Undercooked meat may contain bacteria such as *Campylobacteror Salmonella*.	Cook poultry to 165° F. If the poultry is stuffed, cook the stuffing to 165° F. Better yet, cook the stuffing separately.
Smoked seafood	Refrigerated versions are not safe, unless they have been cooked to 165° F.	Eat canned versions, which are safe, or cook to 165° F.

Courtesy of U.S. Department of Health and Human Services. Checklist of Foods to Avoid During Pregnancy. Retrieved from: http://www.foodsafety.gov/risk/pregnant/chklist_pregnancy.html

dilates to about 10 centimeters, she will start to push the baby through the birth canal (vagina) and into the world. Many women choose to manage the pain of the childbirth process by getting an epidural. An epidural is an injection delivered into the spine that numbs the patient from the waist down. An epidural is one of the safest methods of pain management. About 1 in 3,000 women experience serious complications with an epidural. Managing pain is entirely optional and a decision made by the woman giving birth. Some women choose a "natural" birth and deliver without any medication or other interventions.

Where and how a woman chooses to give birth is up to her, her partner, and the birth attendant. Many women choose to deliver in a hospital or a birthing center, but others may choose to give birth in their home. Other practices such as walking, meditation, immersion in water, massage, or listening to music may be used during the birthing process to help manage pain.[93]

Some women may medically require a cesarean section (C-section). A C-section is a surgery to deliver the baby through the mother's abdomen. Most of the time, C-sections occur if there is an unanticipated problem during labor. Because having a C-section is surgery, it carries some risks such as infection, blood loss or clots, and injuries to the bladder or bowel. Vaginal births, if possible, are recommended instead of a scheduled C-section. For most babies, vaginal births come with less risk. During a vaginal birth, infants come in contact with bacteria or microbes from the mother that help in immune system development. The lack of exposure to these helpful elements may partly explain why babies born via C-section can have a higher risk of allergies, obesity, asthma, and other health problems.[94-96] Thus, it is recommended that women try to avoid a C-section unless it is medically necessary.[97]

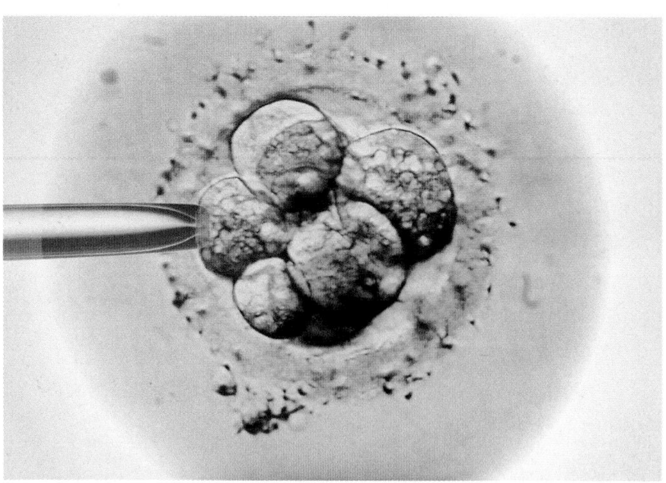

If a woman is not able to get pregnant, she may choose to undergo in vitro fertilization (IVF), in which an egg and sperm are manually combined in a laboratory dish and then moved to the uterus.

Delivering a baby too early in its development can lead to health complications. The fetus can be viable (able to survive outside of the uterus) at around 24 weeks. The chances that the baby will survive increase with each passing week of pregnancy. Delivering a baby before 37 weeks is considered preterm or premature. Because they have not spent as much time in the womb growing, babies who are born early are also likely to be low birth weight (defined as less than 2,500 grams). Low birth weight and prematurity put a baby at higher risk of neurologic impairments and developmental disabilities. The smaller the baby is at birth, the higher the risk is. Low-birth-weight or preterm babies are more likely to have lower academic achievement and attention and behavioral problems as they transition into young adulthood, even after adjusting for sociodemographic characteristics, including low socioeconomic status.[98]

Low birth weight, preterm births, and infant mortality all affect non-White women, specifically Black women,[99,100] more frequently than they affect White women, even after adjusting for parental education.[101,102] Studies have begun to assess the impact of social and structural determinants of health (neighborhood, racism, availability of healthy foods, income inequality, etc.).[103] More recently, research has examined how these social determinants, specifically racism, may impact birth outcomes.[104–106] The cumulative implications of these stressors over the life course may partly explain racial disparities in low birth weight, preterm births, and infant mortality. The United States ranks 30th in the world in infant mortality rate (IMR).[107] The current IMR of 6.2 deaths per 1,000 live births is higher than the rates in some countries with severely limited resources, including Bosnia, Serbia, and Cuba.[108,109]

After Birth: Postpartum

Having a newborn can be a life-altering and wonderful experience. Some women (10–15%), regardless of how much they are excited about having a baby and love their child, experience postpartum depression. Postpartum depression is when depressive symptoms—such as loss of interest in things previously enjoyed, feelings of worthlessness, and sad mood—occur after giving birth. In addition to the regular depressive symptoms, women with postpartum depression may experience feeling disconnected from the baby, having scary thoughts about the baby, and feeling ashamed about not being able to care for the baby. There are many effective treatments (medication and/or psychotherapy) that can help to alleviate these symptoms.[110] (See Chapter 6 for more information about treatment for depression.)

The best choice for feeding newborns is breastfeeding, if the mother is able. It has many benefits for the mother and child. Breast milk contains nutrients and antibodies that protect infants from illnesses such as asthma, infections, and diabetes.[111,112] The benefits do not end there. Breastfeeding also lowers the risk in mothers for certain types of breast cancer, ovarian cancer, and diabetes. Many women lose weight if they breastfeed. It can also save money and provide a unique bonding experience between mother and child. Breastfeeding is recommended for at least the first 6 months after birth. The decision to breastfeed is a personal choice. In rare circumstances, where mothers have health issues, they may be advised not to breastfeed. Some women may not produce enough breast milk, may not be comfortable breastfeeding, or may have a schedule that is not conducive to 6 months of exclusive breastfeeding; these mothers can supplement breast milk with formula.[113]

Infertility

Some people spend a lot of time and effort preventing pregnancy, and then when they are ready to conceive, learn that they may not be able to do it on their own. Someone is thought to be "infertile" after a year of trying to conceive without success. About 15% of couples have fertility issues. Infertility is caused by different factors for men and women. For men, things like toxins in the environment, some medical conditions, smoking, heavy substance use, and overheating of the testicles may cause problems in the number of sperm that can be produced and their movement and shape—all which can affect their ability to fertilize an egg. In women, medical conditions that affect the functioning of the ovaries, fallopian tubes, or uterus can cause infertility. Other risks include advanced age, smoking, heavy alcohol use, or absent periods (sometimes caused by physical or emotional stress). When a couple is unable to conceive, the first test is often a

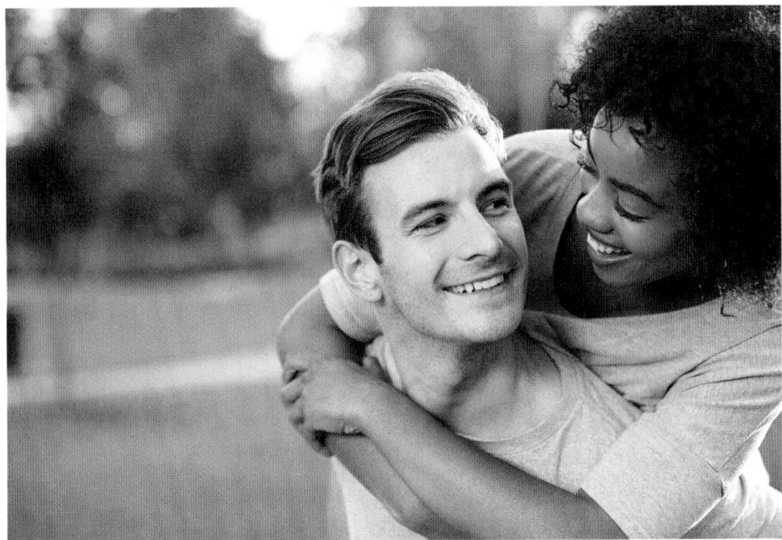

semen analysis for the man. There are a series of medical tests that can evaluate infertility in women as well. For both sexes, there are medications, surgeries, and procedures to assist couples in having a child.[114]

Sex and Politics

Despite sexual health and health care being critical issues related to our health and well-being, they have become widely politicized. We have enacted policies related to sexual education in schools, access to reproductive health care, and abortion based on politicians' partisanship and religious or philosophical beliefs rather than on scientific evidence. One example in recent decades is the debate over how and what to teach our children in school about sex and sexuality (**FIGURE 5-23**). Comprehensive sexual education is effective, but it has been

Hey, can I borrow your laptop to look something up?
Sure!

What are you doing here?
You said I could borrow your laptop.

I let you borrow it last week. You can't just use my laptop whenever you want!
That's crap! You said I could borrow it once, so I should be able to use it anytime I want!

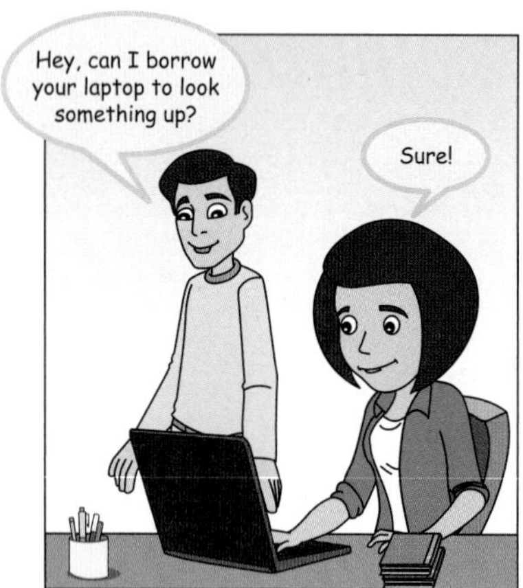

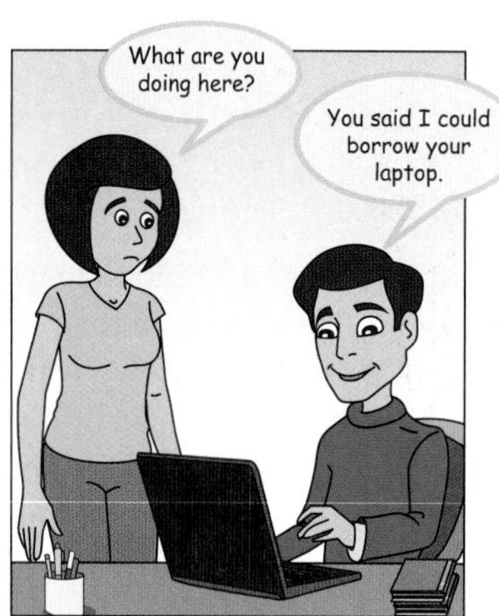

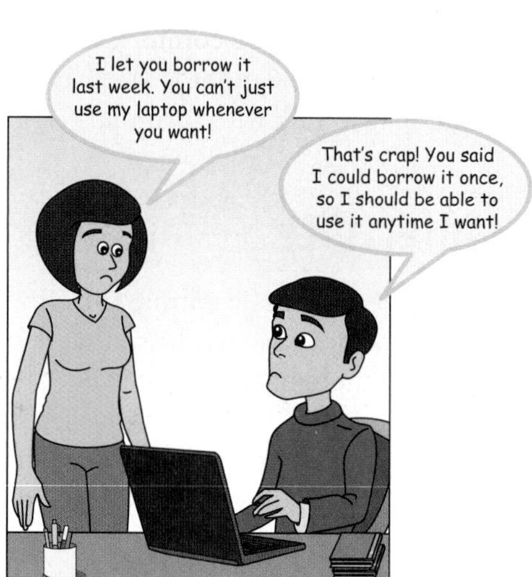

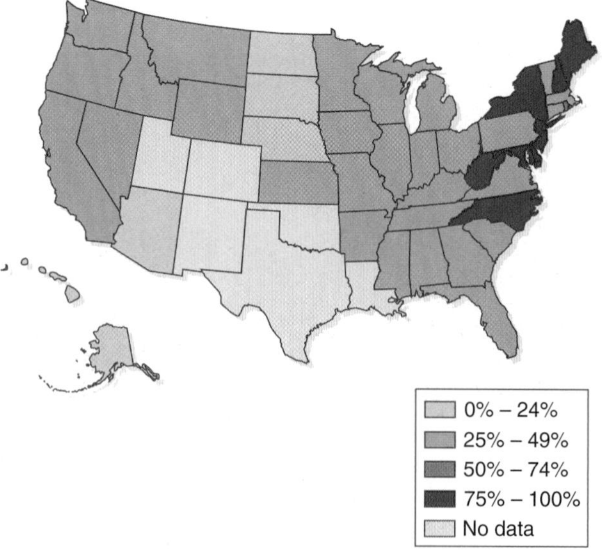

FIGURE 5-23 Sex education in the United States.

Courtesy of Centers for Disease Control and Prevention. School Health Profiles 2014 State Results. Retrieved from http://www.cdc.gov/healthyyouth/data/profiles/pdf/2014/2014_profiles_state_maps.pdf

impeded by politicization. Some support the provision of comprehensive, scientific information about these issues—referred to as "comprehensive" sexual education—to aid in young people's awareness and the reduction of certain sexual risk-taking behaviors based on scientific evidence. Others believe that the provision of such information will increase risky sexual activity among youth and thus support programs in schools that only review and advocate for abstinence (not engaging in sexual activity), referred to as "abstinence-only" sexual education. The abstinence-only movement took off in 1996 after money was specifically allocated for these programs, and over $1.5 billion has been spent since then on these efforts.[115] These programs support abstaining from sexual activity until marriage.

To meet the federal definition of abstinence-only education, a program must meet the following eight requirements[116]:

1. Has as its exclusive purpose teaching the social, psychological, and health gains to be realized by abstaining from sexual activity
2. Teaches abstinence from sexual activity outside marriage as the expected standard for all school-age children
3. Teaches that abstinence from sexual activity is the only certain way to avoid out-of-wedlock pregnancy, STDs, and other associated health problems
4. Teaches that a mutually faithful monogamous relationship in the context of marriage is the expected standard of human sexual activity
5. Teaches that sexual activity outside the context of marriage is likely to have harmful psychological and physical effects
6. Teaches that bearing children out of wedlock is likely to have harmful consequences for the child, the child's parents, and society
7. Teaches young people how to reject sexual advances and how alcohol and drug use increase vulnerability to sexual advances
8. Teaches the importance of attaining self-sufficiency before engaging in sexual activity

Unfortunately, this definition was determined without the consultation or application of the available public health evidence at the time, and it was more geared toward the views of policy makers. Abstinence-only programs have been found not only to have no impact on delaying sexual initiation but also to be potentially harmful to youth. In some cases, youths who complete such a program are less likely to use condoms or get tested for STDs once they do initiate sexual activity. Abstinence-only programs also have been found to have erroneous or misleading information about the risks of sex, abortion, and contraception, and often lack basic information on human biology and reproductive health systems.[117] In contrast, well-designed comprehensive sexual education programs can reduce risky sexual behaviors, such as decreasing the number of sexual partners, delaying first sexual contact, and reducing unprotected sex.[118] Currently, states determine if and what type of sexual health education should be taught in schools. Note that many differences can be found among states (**TABLE 5-5**).[119]

Because many young people are not receiving information about sex and sexual risks in school, almost by default, the media ends up playing an integral role in sexual education. Unfortunately, television shows, movies, magazines, and other media outlets do not display a comprehensive picture of medically accurate information. Ensuring access to accurate and complete sexual and reproductive health information is a vital public health goal.

TABLE 5-5 Sex and HIV Education by State

State	Sex Education* Mandated	HIV Education Mandated	When Provided, Sex or HIV Education Must				Parental Role		
			Be Medically Accurate	Be Age Appropriate	Be Culturally Appropriate and Unbiased	Cannot Promote Religion	Notice	Consent	Opt-Out
Alabama		X		X					X
Arizona				X			HIV	Sex	HIV
California	X	X	X	X	X	X	X		X
Colorado			X	X	X		X		X
Connecticut		X							X
Delaware	X	X							
Dist. of Columbia	X	X		X			X		X
Florida				X					X
Georgia	X	X					X		X
Hawaii	X	X	X	X					X
Idaho									X
Illinois†		X	X	X					X
Indiana		X							
Iowa	X	X	X	X	X		X		X
Kentucky	X	X							

Louisiana				X		X	X		X
Maine	X	X	X	X					X
Maryland	X	X							X
Massachusetts							X		X
Michigan		X	X‡	X			X		X
Minnesota	X	X							X
Mississippi[Ω]	X			X			X		X
Missouri		X		X			X		X
Montana	X	X							
Nevada	X	X		X			X	X	
New Hampshire		X							X
New Jersey	X	X	X	X	X		X		X
New Mexico	X	X							X
New York		X		HIV					HIV
North Carolina	X	X	X	X					
North Dakota	X								
Ohio	X	X							X
Oklahoma		X					X		X
Oregon	X	X	X	X	X		X		X

(continues)

TABLE 5-5 Sex and HIV Education by State *(continued)*

State	Sex Education[*] Mandated	HIV Education Mandated	When Provided, Sex or HIV Education Must				Parental Role		
			Be Medically Accurate	Be Age Appropriate	Be Culturally Appropriate and Unbiased	Cannot Promote Religion	Notice	Consent	Opt-Out
Pennsylvania		X		HIV			X		HIV
Rhode Island	X	X	X	X	X				X
South Carolina	X	X		X			X		X
Tennessee	X[Ψ]	X		HIV					X
Texas				X			X		X
Utah[ξ]	X	X	X		X		X	X	
Vermont	X	X		X					X
Virginia				X			X		X
Washington		X	X	X	X		X		X
West Virginia	X	X					X		X
Wisconsin		X					X		X
TOTAL	**24 + DC**	**34 + DC**	**13**	**26 + DC**	**8**	**2**	**22 + DC**	**3**	**36 + DC**

Guttmacher Institute, Sex and HIV Education, State Laws and Policies (as of April 1, 2018). (2018). https://www.guttmacher.org/state-policy/explore/sex-and-hiv-education

[*] Sex education typically includes discussion of STIs.

[†] Sex education is not mandatory, but health education is required and it includes medically accurate information on abstinence.

[‡] Sex education "shall not be medically inaccurate."

[Ω] Localities may include topics such as contraception or STIs only with permission from the State Department of Education.

[Ψ] Sex education is required if the pregnancy rate for 15–17 teen women is at least 19.5% or higher.

[ξ] State also prohibits teachers from responding to students' spontaneous questions in ways that conflict with the law's requirements.

http://www.guttmacher.org/statecenter/spibs/spib_SE.pdf

The Bigger Picture: Public Health Campaigns and Reproductive Justice

Because we know that individual behavior, such as using a consistent and effective method of birth control, can substantially reduce unintended pregnancy, public health efforts have historically promoted such behavior in campaigns, policies, and programs. Don't have sex when you're young! Use condoms! Even better, use a condom plus another method of birth control! Don't sleep around! Have a plan for getting pregnant! Of course, this is sound advice that most of us try to follow. But only focusing on individual behavior ignores a fundamental understanding of other influences on pregnancy, such as those outlined in the socioecological model (families, communities, policies, etc.).

Thinking focused on individual behaviors continues to assume that deciding to have a child is a universally rational decision, in which an individual or couple weighs the benefits and drawbacks of childbearing, comes to a decision, and then acts upon it. Among other things, there is an assumption that individuals of all socioeconomic and racial backgrounds possess the ability to establish a career, gain financial stability, and start a family, in that particular order. This assumption, though, fails to consider the dynamic social, economic, and other contextual variables, such as discrimination, that may affect those living at the lower end of the socioeconomic spectrum.[120,121] We need to keep this perspective in mind as we develop campaigns and policies to advocate for increased access to contraception. Looking "upstream" to the larger social determinants of health and pregnancy, if we want to reduce unintended pregnancy, we also need to think about the bigger picture—universal access to a quality education, increased job availability, antidiscrimination laws, and more.

There is a shameful and disconcerting history in the United States regarding controlling the reproductive rights of women of color, from the time of slavery until as recently as the 1970s.[122] Practices such as coercive sterilization were common and mostly forced on low-income women of color and individuals with limited mental capacity. The **reproductive justice** movement has grown in response to the inequities experienced by such women.[123] Reproductive justice is "the human right to have children, not have children, and parent the children we have in safe and healthy environments [and] . . . to bodily autonomy from any form of reproductive oppression."[124]

reproductive justice A movement dedicated to the human right to have children, not have children, and parent the children people already have in safe and healthy environments and to bodily autonomy from any form of reproductive oppression.

This movement recognizes the intersection of race, gender, and class in reproductive health and calls for a new framework that focuses on the ultimate health and well-being of women and their families. The historic and persistent ill effects of reproductive oppression and the awareness that unequal opportunities for social mobility play a key role in health, inform reproductive justice. Health services and advocacy for equality are fundamental tenets to the continued promotion and achievement of reproductive justice.[124]

Such egregious acts of reproductive coercion contributed to a long-lasting and deserved mistrust of the government and medical community and of their efforts to promote contraceptive and abortion access. Only recently have the medical and public health communities begun to understand that efforts to promote certain methods of contraception may engender distrust and suspicion (**FIGURE 5-24**). Engaging communities in the process to ensure they are using a reproductive justice framework helps build trust. Campaigns and programs to increase contraceptive use need to both be sensitive and respectful of women's autonomy to choose a method that best suits her needs and recognize that promoting contraceptive use is

Got a good job? I cost thousands of dollars each year.
THINK BEING A TEEN PARENT WON'T COST YOU?
EXPECT TO SPEND MORE THAN $10,000 A YEAR TO RAISE A CHILD.
Text 'NOTNOW' to 877877 for the real price of teen pregnancy.
Standard text messaging rates may apply. Check with your service provider.
NYC
Dad, you'll be paying to support me for the next 20 years.
THINK BEING A TEEN PARENT WON'T COST YOU?
NY STATE LAW REQUIRES A PARENT TO PAY CHILD SUPPORT UNTIL A CHILD IS 21.
Text 'NOTNOW' to 877877 for the real price of teen pregnancy.
NYC
Honestly Mom... chances are he won't stay with you. What happens to me?
ARE YOU READY TO RAISE A CHILD BY YOURSELF?
90% OF TEEN PARENTS DON'T MARRY EACH OTHER.
Text 'NOTNOW' to 877877 for the real price of teen pregnancy.
NYC
I'm twice as likely not to graduate high school because you had me as a teen.
KIDS OF TEEN MOMS ARE TWICE AS LIKELY NOT TO GRADUATE THAN KIDS WHOSE MOMS WERE OVER AGE 22.
Text 'NOTNOW' to 877877 for the real price of teen pregnancy.
NYC

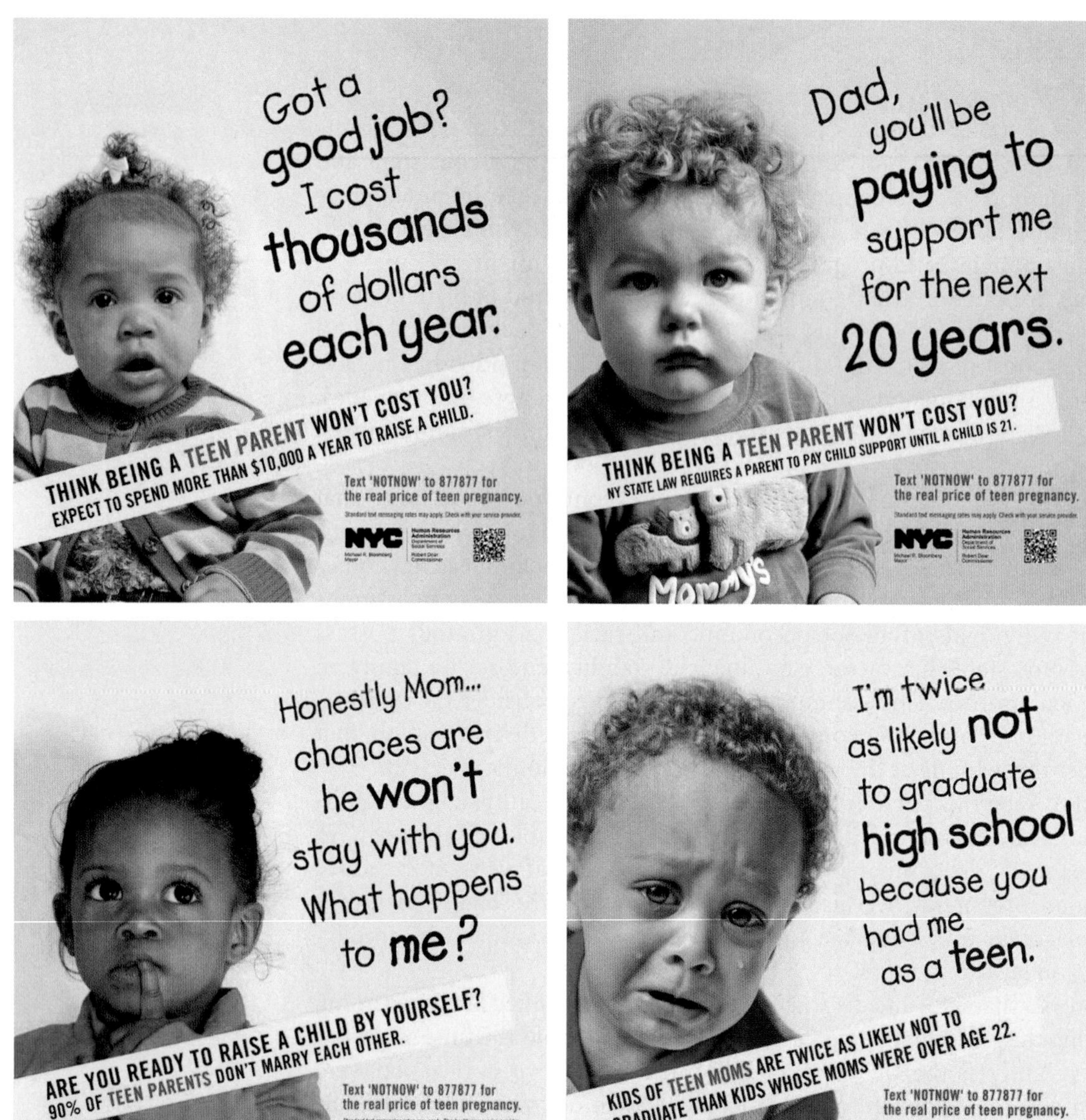

FIGURE 5-24 This public health campaign garnered criticism among reproductive health advocates for stigmatizing teen parents without offering support or information.

only one way to help women and families have kids on their own terms. We need to continue to promote access to and use of contraception, but also think more broadly about what different communities may need to plan their reproductive lives.

In Summary

Despite being a main facet of public health, how we inform people about and give access to sexual and reproductive health in the United States is often politicized. Understanding our sexual anatomy, how conception works, and how to prevent pregnancy and STDs is vitally important to maintaining health. Promotion of reproductive justice in policies and health care for all women and men is a key public health goal.

Key Terms

abortion
abstinence
arousal
condom
contraception
gender identity
reproductive justice
sexual orientation
sexually transmitted diseases (STDs)

Student Discussion Questions and Activities

1. Do you think comprehensive sexual education should be mandatory in all schools? Why or why not? Investigate your justification to understand more about evidence to support the inclusion or exclusion.
2. Why do you think people who do not want to get pregnant don't always use contraception?
3. Abortion is a very sensitive topic. Many people view abortion through the lens of their religious beliefs (i.e., that life starts at conception and therefore abortion should be illegal). Do you think there is a solution to the legality of abortion that most people could agree on?
4. Do you think violation of human rights, such as the Tuskegee Experiment and forced sterilization of people of color, have an impact on how people in those communities trust medical professionals in general? Research studies? Contraception?

Resources

Contraception: https://bedsider.org/
Abortion, understanding the procedures: https://www.plannedparenthood.org/learn/abortion/in-clinic-abortion-procedures
Abortion, finding a provider: http://prochoice.org/think-youre-pregnant/find-a-provider/

References

1. American Academy of Pediatrics Task Force on Circumcision. (2012). Circumcision policy statement. *Pediatrics, 130*(3), 585–586.
2. Our Bodies Ourselves. (2011). Models of sexual response. Retrieved from http://www.ourbodiesourselves.org/health-info/models-sexual-response/
3. Go Ask Alice! (2014). S/M role-playing. Columbia University. Retrieved from http://goaskalice.columbia.edu/answered-questions/sm-role-playing
4. World Health Organization. (1992). *The ICD-10 classification of mental and behavioural disorders: Clinical descriptions and diagnostic guidelines.* Retrieved from http://www.who.int/classifications/icd/en/bluebook.pdf
5. Go Ask Alice! (1995). Masturbation healthy? Columbia University. Retrieved from http://goaskalice.columbia.edu/answered-questions/masturbation-healthy
6. Planned Parenthood. (2016). What's sex? Retrieved from https://www.plannedparenthood.org/teens/sex/whats-sex
7. American Psychological Association (APA). (n.d.). Report of the APA task force on appropriate therapeutic responses to sexual orientation. Retrieved from http://www.apa.org/pi/lgbt/resources/sexual-orientation.aspx
8. The National Domestic Violence Hotline. (2013). What is a healthy relationship? Retrieved from http://www.thehotline.org/2013/01/what-is-a-healthy-relationship/
9. Planned Parenthood. (n.d.). Consent and rape. Retrieved from https://www.plannedparenthood.org/teens/relationships/consent-and-rape
10. Centers for Disease Control and Prevention. (2016). Intimate partner violence. National Center for Injury Prevention and Control: Division of Violence Prevention. Retrieved from http://www.cdc.gov/violenceprevention/intimatepartnerviolence/index.html
11. Centers for Disease Control and Prevention. (2015). Child abuse prevention. Retrieved from http://www.cdc.gov/features/healthychildren/
12. Womenshealth.gov. (2015). Sexual assault ePublication. U.S. Department of Health and Human Services. Retrieved from http://www.womenshealth.gov/publications/our-publications/fact-sheet/sexual-assault.html
13. Childress, S. (2014, February 25). What's the state of the Church's child abuse crisis? *Frontline.* Retrieved from http://www.pbs.org/wgbh/frontline/article/whats-the-state-of-the-churchs-child-abuse-crisis/

14. The Vatican's child abuse response. (2014, April 24). *BBC News*. Retrieved from http://www.bbc.com/news/world-europe-25757218
15. Editorial Board. (2017, July 7). The Vatican's failure in the abuse scandal. Retrieved from https://www.nytimes.com/2017/07/07/opinion/pope-francis-catholic-church-sexual-abuse.html
16. Becker, N. V., & Polsky, D. (2015). Women saw large decrease in out-of-pocket spending for contraceptives after ACA mandate removed cost sharing. *Health Affairs (Millwood), 34*(7), 1204–1211.
17. Burg, G. (2012). History of sexually transmitted infections (STI). *Giornale Italiano Di Dermatologia e Venereologia, 147*(4), 329–340.
18. Centers for Disease Control and Prevention. (2014). Youth risk behavior surveillance—United States, 2013. *Morbidity and Mortality Weekly Reports, 63*(4).
19. Copen, C., Chandra, A., & Febo-Vazquez, I. (2016). National health statistics reports: Sexual behavior, sexual attraction, and sexual orientation among adults aged 18–44 in the United States: Data from the 2011–2013 National Survey of Family Growth. Retrieved from http://www.cdc.gov/nchs/data/nhsr/nhsr088.pdf
20. Centers for Disease Control and Prevention. (2015). Reported cases of STDs on the rise in the U.S. National Center for HIV/AIDS, Viral Hepatitis, STD, and TB Prevention. Retrieved from http://www.cdc.gov/nchhstp/newsroom/2015/std-surveillance-report-press-release.html
21. AIDS.gov. (2015). What is HIV/AIDS? Retrieved from https://www.aids.gov/hiv-aids-basics/hiv-aids-101/what-is-hiv-aids/
22. Centers for Disease Control and Prevention. (2015). About HIV/AIDS. National Center for HIV/AIDS, Viral Hepatitis, STD, and TB Prevention: Division of HIV/AIDS Prevention. Retrieved from http://www.cdc.gov/hiv/basics/whatishiv.html
23. Centers for Disease Control and Prevention. (2015). Basic statistics. National Center for HIV/AIDS, Viral Hepatitis, STD, and TB Prevention: Division of HIV/AIDS Prevention. Retrieved from http://www.cdc.gov/hiv/basics/statistics.html
24. Centers for Disease Control and Prevention. (2015). HIV in the United States: At a glance. National Center for HIV/AIDS, Viral Hepatitis, STD, and TB Prevention: Division of HIV/AIDS Prevention. Retrieved from http://www.cdc.gov/hiv/statistics/overview/ataglance.html
25. UCSF Center for HIV Information. (2011). What kinds of HIV screening tests are available in the United States? HIV InSite. Retrieved from http://hivinsite.ucsf.edu/insite?page=basics-01-01
26. Centers for Disease Control and Prevention. (2015). HIV transmission. National Center for HIV/AIDS, Viral Hepatitis, STD, and TB Prevention: Division of HIV/AIDS Prevention. Retrieved from http://www.cdc.gov/hiv/basics/transmission.html
27. Centers for Disease Control and Prevention. (2016). PrEP. National Center for HIV/AIDS, Viral Hepatitis, STD, and TB Prevention: Division of HIV/AIDS Prevention. Retrieved from http://www.cdc.gov/hiv/basics/prep.html
28. Centers for Disease Control and Prevention. (2016). PEP. National Center for HIV/AIDS, Viral Hepatitis, STD, and TB Prevention: Division of HIV/AIDS Prevention. Retrieved from http://www.cdc.gov/hiv/basics/pep.html
29. American Sexual Health Association. (2016). Fast facts. Retrieved from http://www.ashasexualhealth.org/stdsstis/hpv/fast-facts/
30. Centers for Disease Control and Prevention. (2007). QuickStats: Prevalence of HPV infection among sexually active females aged 14–59 years, by age group—National Health and Nutrition Examination Survey, United States, 2003–2004. Retrieved from http://www.cdc.gov/mmwr/preview/mmwrhtml/mm5633a5.htm
31. Dunne, E. F., Nielson, C. M., Stone, K. M., Markowitz, L. E., & Giuliano, A. R. (2006). Prevalence of HPV infection among men: A systematic review of the literature. *Journal of Infectious Diseases, 194*(8), 1044–1057.
32. Giuliano, A. R., Tortolero-Luna, G., Ferrer, E., Burchell, A. N., de Sanjose, S., Kjaer, S., K., . . . Bosch, F. X. (2008). Epidemiology of human papillomavirus infection in men, cancers other than cervical and benign conditions. *Vaccine, 26*(Suppl 10), K17–K28.
33. American Cancer Society. (2014). Cervical cancer prevention and early detection. Retrieved from http://www.cancer.org/cancer/cervicalcancer/moreinformation/cervicalcancerpreventionandearlydetection/cervical-cancer-prevention-and-early-detection-cervical-cancer-screening-guidelines
34. Centers for Disease Control and Prevention. (2016). Genital HPV infection—fact sheet. National Center for HIV/AIDS, Viral Hepatitis, STD, and TB Prevention: Division of STD Prevention. Retrieved from http://www.cdc.gov/STD/HPV/STDFact-HPV.htm
35. National Cancer Institute. (2014). Pap and HPV testing. U.S. Department of Health and Human Services, National Institutes of Health. Retrieved from http://www.cancer.gov/types/cervical/pap-hpv-testing-fact-sheet
36. Centers for Disease Control and Prevention. (1999). Achievements in public health, 1900–1999 impact of vaccines universally recommended for children—United States, 1990–1998. Retrieved from https://www.cdc.gov/mmwr/preview/mmwrhtml/00056803.htm
37. Markowitz, L. E., Liu, G., Hariri, S., Steinau, M., Dunne, E. F., & Unger, E. R. (2016). Prevalence of HPV after introduction of the vaccination program in the United States. *Pediatrics*. Retrieved from http://pediatrics.aappublications.org/content/early/2016/02/19/peds.2015-1968
38. Bednarczyk, R. A., Davis, R., Ault, K., Orenstein, W., & Omer, S. B. (2012). Sexual activity-related outcomes after human papillomavirus vaccination of 11- to 12-year-olds. *Pediatrics, 130*(5), 798–805.
39. Centers for Disease Control and Prevention. (2015). Human papillomavirus (HPV) vaccine safety. National Center for Emerging and Zoonotic Infectious Diseases: Division of Healthcare Quality Promotion. Retrieved from http://www.cdc.gov/vaccinesafety/vaccines/hpv-vaccine.html
40. Centers for Disease Control and Prevention. (2014). Talking with your teens about sex: Going beyond "the talk." National Center for HIV/AIDS, Viral Hepatitis, STD, and TB Prevention: Division of Adolescent and School Health. Retrieved from http://www.cdc.gov/healthyyouth/protective/pdf/talking_teens.pdf
41. Centers for Disease Control and Prevention. (2015). Chlamydia—CDC fact sheet (detailed). National Center for HIV/AIDS, Viral Hepatitis, STD, and TB Prevention: Division of STD Prevention. Retrieved from http://www.cdc.gov/std/chlamydia/stdfact-chlamydia-detailed.htm

42. Centers for Disease Control and Prevention. (2015). Gonococcal infections. National Center for HIV/AIDS, Viral Hepatitis, STD, and TB Prevention: Division of STD Prevention. Retrieved from http://www.cdc.gov/std/tg2015/gonorrhea.htm
43. Centers for Disease Control and Prevention. (2015). Gonorrhea—CDC fact sheet (detailed version). National Center for HIV/AIDS, Viral Hepatitis, STD, and TB Prevention: Division of STD Prevention. Retrieved from http://www.cdc.gov/std/gonorrhea/stdfact-gonorrhea-detailed.htm
44. Centers for Disease Control and Prevention. (2015). Genital herpes—CDC fact sheet (detailed). National Center for HIV/AIDS, Viral Hepatitis, STD, and TB Prevention: Division of STD Prevention. Retrieved from http://www.cdc.gov/std/herpes/stdfact-herpes-detailed.htm
45. Centers for Disease Control and Prevention. (2015). Syphilis. National Center for HIV/AIDS, Viral Hepatitis, STD, and TB Prevention: Division of STD Prevention. Retrieved from http://www.cdc.gov/std/stats14/syphilis.htm
46. Centers for Disease Control and Prevention. (2016). Syphilis—CDC fact sheet. National Center for HIV/AIDS, Viral Hepatitis, STD, and TB Prevention: Division of STD Prevention. Retrieved from http://www.cdc.gov/std/syphilis/stdfact-syphilis.htm
47. Tuskegee University. (n.d.). About the USPHS syphilis study. Retrieved from http://www.tuskegee.edu/about_us/centers_of_excellence/bioethics_center/about_the_usphs_syphilis_study.aspx
48. Centers for Disease Control and Prevention. (2015). Trichomoniasis—CDC fact sheet. National Center for HIV/AIDS, Viral Hepatitis, STD, and TB: Division of STD Prevention. Retrieved from http://www.cdc.gov/std/trichomonas/stdfact-trichomoniasis.htm
49. Pearson, C. (2011, July 12). Trichomoniasis: An STI most common in women over 40? *Huffington Post*. Retrieved from http://www.huffingtonpost.com/2011/07/12/an-std-most-common-in-wom_n_895707.html
50. Centers for Disease Control and Prevention. (2015). Hepatitis A questions and answers for the public. National Center for HIV/AIDS, Viral Hepatitis, STD, and TB Prevention: Division of Viral Hepatitis. Retrieved from http://www.cdc.gov/hepatitis/hav/afaq.htm
51. Centers for Disease Control and Prevention. (2015). Hepatitis B FAQs for the public. National Center for HIV/AIDS, Viral Hepatitis, STD, and TB Prevention: Division of Viral Hepatitis. Retrieved from http://www.cdc.gov/hepatitis/hbv/bfaq.htm
52. Centers for Disease Control and Prevention. (2015). Hepatitis C: Why people born from 1945–1965 should get tested. Retrieved from http://www.cdc.gov/knowmorehepatitis/Media/PDFs/FactSheet-Boomers.pdf
53. Centers for Disease Control and Prevention. (2015). Viral hepatitis—hepatitis C information. National Center for HIV/AIDS, Viral Hepatitis, STD, and TB Prevention: Division of Viral Hepatitis. Retrieved from http://www.cdc.gov/hepatitis/hcv/
54. Mayo Clinic. (2016). Sexually transmitted diseases (STDs): Symptoms and causes. Retrieved from http://www.mayoclinic.org/diseases-conditions/sexually-transmitted-diseases-stds/symptoms-causes/dxc-20180596
55. Centers for Disease Control and Prevention. (2015). Unintended pregnancy prevention. National Center for Chronic Disease Prevention and Health Promotion: Division of Reproductive Health. Retrieved from http://www.cdc.gov/reproductivehealth/unintendedpregnancy/
56. Santelli, J., Rochat, R., Hatfield-Timajchy, K., Gilbert, B. C., Curtis, K., Cabral, R., . . . Unintended Pregnancy Working Group. (2003). The measurement and meaning of unintended pregnancy. *Perspectives on Sexual and Reproductive Health, 35*(2), 94–101.
57. Kearney, M. S., & Levine, P. B. (2012). Why is the teen birth rate in the United States so high and why does it matter? *Journal of Economic Perspectives, 26*(2), 141–166.
58. Geronimus, A. T., & Korenman, S. (1992). The socioeconomic consequences of teen childbearing reconsidered. *The Quarterly Journal of Economics, 107*(4), 1187.
59. Guttmacher Institute. (2015). Contraceptive use in the United States. Retrieved from http://www.guttmacher.org/pubs/fb_contr_use.html
60. U.S. Department of Health and Human Services, National Institutes of Health, U.S. National Library of Medicine. (2016). Birth control. MedlinePlus. Retrieved from https://www.nlm.nih.gov/medlineplus/birthcontrol.html
61. U.S. Department of Health and Human Services, National Institutes of Health, U.S. National Library of Medicine. (2016). Deciding about an IUD. MedlinePlus. Retrieved from https://www.nlm.nih.gov/medlineplus/ency/patientinstructions/000774.htm
62. Planned Parenthood. (2016). IUD. Retrieved from https://www.plannedparenthood.org/learn/birth-control/iud
63. U.S. Department of Health and Human Services, National Institutes of Health, U.S. National Library of Medicine. (2016). Birth control—slow release methods. MedlinePlus. Retrieved from https://www.nlm.nih.gov/medlineplus/ency/article/007555.htm
64. American College of Obstetricians and Gynecologists. (2014). Long-acting reversible contraception (LARC): IUD and implant. Retrieved from http://www.acog.org/Patients/FAQs/Long-Acting-Reversible-Contraception-LARC-IUD-and-Implant#implant
65. U.S. National Library of Medicine. (2015). Estrogen and progestin (oral contraceptives). MedlinePlus. Retrieved from https://www.nlm.nih.gov/medlineplus/druginfo/meds/a601050.html
66. Hannaford, P. C., Iversen, L., Macfarlane, T. V., Elliott, A. M., Angus, V., & Lee, A. J. (2010). Mortality among contraceptive pill users: Cohort evidence from Royal College of General Practitioners' Oral Contraception Study. *BMJ, 340*, c927.
67. University of Maryland Medical Center. (2012). Birth control options for women. Retrieved from http://umm.edu/health/medical/reports/articles/birth-control-options-for-women
68. Cerel-Suhl, S. L., & Yeager, B. F. (1999). Update on oral contraceptive pills. *American Family Physician, 60*(7), 2073–2084.
69. American College of Obstetricians and Gynecologists. (2014). Combined hormonal birth control: Pill, patch, and ring. Retrieved from http://www.acog.org/Patients/FAQs/Combined-Hormonal-Birth-Control-Pill-Patch-and-Ring
70. Planned Parenthood. (2016). How effective are condoms? Retrieved from https://www.plannedparenthood.org/learn/birth-control/condom/how-effective-are-condoms
71. Association of Reproductive Health Professionals. (2014). Choosing a birth control method: Vaginal ring. Retrieved from https://www.arhp.org/Publications-and-Resources/Quick-Reference-Guide-for-Clinicians/choosing/Vaginal-Ring

72. Association of Reproductive Health Professionals. (2014). Choosing a birth control method: Transdermal contraceptive patch. Retrieved from https://www.arhp.org/Publications-and-Resources/Quick-Reference-Guide-for-Clinicians/choosing/Transdermal-Patch
73. Association of Reproductive Health Professionals. (2014). Choosing a birth control method: Injectable. Retrieved from https://www.arhp.org/Publications-and-Resources/Quick-Reference-Guide-for-Clinicians/choosing/Injec
74. Association of Reproductive Health Professionals. (2014). Choosing a birth control method: Emergency contraception. Retrieved from http://www.arhp.org/Publications-and-Resources/Quick-Reference-Guide-for-Clinicians/choosing/Emergency-contraception
75. U.S. Department of Health and Human Services, National Institutes of Health, U.S. National Library of Medicine. Condoms—male. MedlinePlus. Retrieved from https://www.nlm.nih.gov/medlineplus/ency/article/004001.htm
76. U.S. Department of Health and Human Services, National Institutes of Health, U.S. National Library of Medicine. (2016). Female condoms. MedlinePlus. Retrieved from https://www.nlm.nih.gov/medlineplus/ency/article/004002.htm
77. Planned Parenthood. (2016). Female condom. Retrieved from https://www.plannedparenthood.org/learn/birth-control/female-condom
78. Planned Parenthood. (2016). Fertility awareness-based methods (FAMs). Retrieved from https://www.plannedparenthood.org/learn/birth-control/fertility-awareness
79. Mayo Clinic. (2015). Withdrawal method (coitus interruptus). Retrieved from http://www.mayoclinic.org/tests-procedures/withdrawal-method/basics/definition/PRC-20020661?p=1
80. American College of Obstetricians and Gynecologists. (2015). Sterilization for women and men. Retrieved from http://www.acog.org/Patients/FAQs/Sterilization-for-Women-and-Men
81. Guttmacher Institute. (2016). Fact sheet: Induced abortion in the United States. Retrieved from https://www.guttmacher.org/pubs/fb_induced_abortion.html
82. Guttmacher Institute. (2016). State policies in brief: An overview of abortion laws. Retrieved from http://www.guttmacher.org/statecenter/spibs/spib_OAL.pdf
83. U.S. Food and Drug Administration (FDA). (2016). Mifeprex (mifepristone) information. Retrieved from http://www.fda.gov/Drugs/DrugSafety/PostmarketDrugSafetyInformation-forPatientsandProviders/ucm111323.htm
84. Guttmacher Institute. (2016). United States: Abortion. Retrieved from http://www.guttmacher.org/in-the-know/abortion-safety.html
85. Khazan, O. (2015, November 17). Texas women are inducing their own abortions. *The Atlantic*. Retrieved from http://www.theatlantic.com/health/archive/2015/11/texas-self-abort/416229/
86. World Health Organization. (2016). Unsafe abortion: Global and regional estimates of the incidence of unsafe abortion and associated mortality in 2003. Retrieved from http://apps.who.int/iris/bitstream/10665/43798/1/9789241596121_eng.pdf
87. Planned Parenthood. (2016). Medical and social health benefits since abortion was made legal in the U.S. Retrieved from https://www.plannedparenthood.org/files/4713/9611/5762/Abortion_Medical_and_Social_Benefits.pdf
88. Centers for Disease Control and Prevention. (2016). Preconception health and health care. Retrieved from http://www.cdc.gov/preconception/planning.html
89. Centers for Disease Control and Prevention. (2015). Reproductive health and the workplace—what you should know about the female reproductive system. National Institute for Occupational Safety and Health: Division of Surveillance, Hazard Evaluations and Field Studies. Retrieved from http://www.cdc.gov/niosh/topics/repro/femalereproductivesystem.html
90. American College of Nurse-Midwives. (2016). The credentials CNM and CM. Retrieved from http://www.midwife.org/The-Credential-CNM-and-CM
91. American College of Nurse-Midwives. (2016). Comparison of certified nurse-midwives, certified midwives, and certified professional midwives. Retrieved from http://www.midwife.org/acnm/files/ccLibraryFiles/Filename/000000005543/CNM-CM-CPM-Comparison-Chart-2-25-14.pdf
92. The Nemours Foundation. (2016). Midwives. KidsHealth. Retrieved from http://kidshealth.org/en/parents/midwives.html
93. March of Dimes. (2016). Stages of labor. March of Dimes. Retrieved from http://www.marchofdimes.org/pregnancy/stages-of-labor.aspx#
94. Renz-Polster, H., David, M. R., Buist, A. S., Vollmer, W. M., O'Connor, E. A., Frazier, E. A., & Wall, M. A. (2005). Caesarean section delivery and the risk of allergic disorders in childhood. *Clinical and Experimental Allergy, 35*(11), 1466–1472.
95. Darmasseelane, K., Hyde, M. J., Santhakumaran, S., Gale, C., & Modi, N. (2014). Mode of delivery and offspring body mass index, overweight and obesity in adult life: A systematic review and meta-analysis. *PLoS One, 9*(2), e87896.
96. Blustein, J., & Liu, J. (2015). Time to consider the risks of caesarean delivery for long term child health. *BMJ*, 350, h2410. doi:10.1136/bmj.h2410
97. American College of Obstetricians and Gynecologists. (2013). Vaginal delivery recommended over maternal-request cesarean. Retrieved from http://www.acog.org/About-ACOG/News-Room/News-Releases/2013/Vaginal-Delivery-Recommended-Over-Maternal-Request-Cesarean
98. Aarnoudse-Moens, C. S., Weisglas-Kuperus, N., van Goudoever, J. B., & Oosterlaan, J. (2009). Meta-analysis of neurobehavioral outcomes in very preterm and/or very low birth weight children. *Pediatrics, 124*(2), 717–728.
99. Matthews, T. J., MacDorman, M. F., & Division of Vital Statistics. (2013, January 24). Infant mortality statistics from the 2009 period linked birth/infant death data set. *National Vital Statistics Reports, 61*(8), 2–10.
100. Martin, J. A., Hamilton, B. E., Ventura, S. J., Osterman, M. J. K., Wilson, E. C., & Mathews, T J. (2012, August 28). Births: Final data for 2010. *National Vital Statistics Reports, 61*(1), 1–72.
101. Centers for Disease Control and Prevention, National Center for Health Statistics. (2009). Health, 2008, United States. Retrieved from http://www.cdc.gov/nchs/data/hus/hus09.pdf
102. U.S. Institute of Medicine, Committee on Understanding Premature Birth and Assuring Healthy Outcomes. (2007). *Preterm birth: Causes, consequences, and prevention.* Washington, DC: National Academies Press.
103. Marmot, M. (2006). *Social determinants of health* (2nd ed.). New York, NY: Oxford University Press.
104. Hogue, C. J., & Bremner, J. D. (2005). Stress model for research into preterm delivery among black women. *American Journal of Obstetrics and Gynecology, 192*(Suppl 5), S47–S55.
105. Krieger, N., Chen, J. T., Coull, B., Waterman, P. D., & Beckfield, J. (2013). The unique impact of abolition of Jim Crow laws on

reducing inequities in infant death rates and implications for choice of comparison groups in analyzing societal determinants of health. *American Journal of Public Health, 103*(12), 2234–2244.
106. Dominguez, T. P. (2008). Race, racism, and racial disparities in adverse birth outcomes. *Clinical Obstetrics and Gynecology, 51*(2), 360–370.
107. Centers for Disease Control and Prevention. (2009). NCHS data brief: Behind international rankings of infant mortality: How the United States compares with Europe. National Center for Health Statistics, Division of Vital Statistics, Reproductive Statistics Branch. Retrieved from http://www.cdc.gov/nchs/data/databriefs/db23.htm#ranking
108. Centers for Disease Control and Prevention. (2014). Infant health. Retrieved from http://www.cdc.gov/nchs/fastats/infant-health.htm
109. Central Intelligence Agency. (2014). Country comparison: Infant mortality rate. *The World Factbook.* Retrieved from https://www.cia.gov/library/publications/the-world-factbook/rankorder/2091rank.html
110. Centers for Disease Control and Prevention. (2016). Depression among women. National Center for Chronic Disease Prevention and Health Promotion: Division of Reproductive Health. Retrieved from http://www.cdc.gov/reproductivehealth/depression/index.htm
111. Dogaru, C. M., Nyffenegger, D., Pescatore, A. M., Spycher, B. D., & Kuehni, C. E. (2014). Breastfeeding and childhood asthma: Systematic review and meta-analysis. *American Journal of Epidemiology, 179*(10), 1153–1167.
112. Dieterich, C. M., Felice, J. P., O'Sullivan, E., & Rasmussen, K. M. (2013). Breastfeeding and health outcomes for the mother–infant dyad. *Pediatric Clinics of North America, 60*(1), 31–48.
113. Womenshealth.gov. (2014). Breastfeeding. U.S. Department of Health and Human Services, Office on Women's Health. Retrieved from http://www.womenshealth.gov/breastfeeding/
114. Centers for Disease Control and Prevention. (2015). Infertility FAQs. National Center for Chronic Disease Prevention and Health Promotion, Division of Reproductive Health. Retrieved from http://www.cdc.gov/reproductivehealth/Infertility/
115. Sexuality Information and Education Council of the United States (SIECUS). (2016). A history of federal abstinence-only-until-marriage funding FY10. Sexuality Information and Education Council of the United States (SIECUS). Retrieved from http://www.siecus.org/index.cfm?fuseaction=page.viewpage&pageid=1340&nodeid=1
116. Social Security Administration. (2016). U.S. Social Security Act, §510(b)(2). Retrieved from https://www.ssa.gov/OP_Home/ssact/title05/0510.htm#ft23
117. Kay, J., & Jackson, A. (2008). Sex, lies and stereotypes: How abstinence-only programs harm women and girls. Human Rights at Harvard Law. Retrieved from http://hrp.law.harvard.edu/wp-content/uploads/2013/03/sexlies_stereotypes2008.pdf
118. Centers for Disease Control and Prevention. (2016). Effective HIV and STD prevention programs for youth: A summary of scientific evidence. National Center for HIV/AIDS, Viral Hepatitis, STD, and TB Prevention: Division of Adolescent and School Health. Retrieved from http://www.cdc.gov/healthyyouth/sexualbehaviors/pdf/effective_hiv.pdf
119. Guttmacher Institute. (2016). State policies in brief: Sex and HIV education. Retrieved from http://www.guttmacher.org/statecenter/spibs/spib_SE.pdf
120. Marmot, M., & Wilkinson, R. G. (2006). *Social determinants of health* (2nd ed.). New York, NY: Oxford University Press.
121. Kendall, C., Afable-Munsuz, A., Speizer, I., Avery, A., Schmidt, N., & Santelli, J. (2005). Understanding pregnancy in a population of inner-city women in New Orleans—results of qualitative research. *Social Science and Medicine, 60*(2), 297–311.
122. Roberts, D. (1998). *Killing the Black body: Race, reproduction and the meaning of liberty.* New York, NY: Vintage.
123. SisterSong. (2015). What is reproductive justice? Retrieved from http://sistersong.net/reproductive-justice/
124. Ross, L. (2006). Understanding reproductive justice: Transforming the pro-choice movement. *Off Our Backs, 36*(4), 14–19.

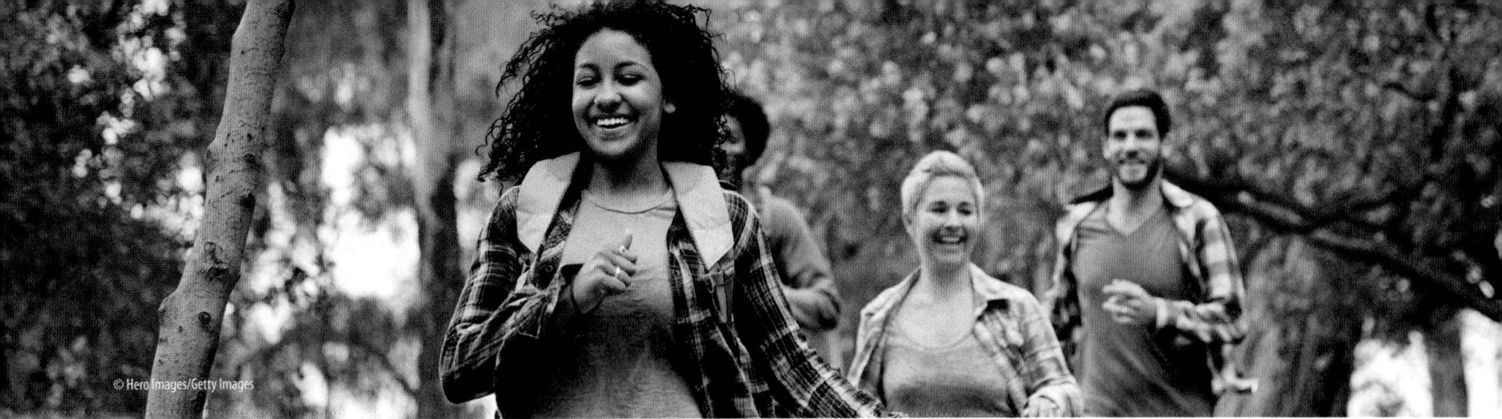

CHAPTER 6

Minding Your Mental Health

CHAPTER OBJECTIVES

- Define well-being, mental health, and mental illness.
- Recognize the roles of stress and sleep in mental health.
- Describe the causes, symptoms, and prevalence of mental disorders.
- Discuss the treatments for mental disorders.
- Discuss the problems with the mental healthcare system.
- Explain how some communities are disproportionately affected by mental illness.

What comes to mind when you hear the word "health"? Most people first think about efforts to maintain their physical health, such as treating chronic illnesses, exercising to stay fit, or avoiding a cold. Health, though, is not just the absence of disease; it encompasses much more. The World Health Organization defines health as "a state of complete physical, mental and social well-being and not merely the absence of disease or infirmity."[1]

But what does it mean to be in a state of physical, mental, and social well-being? Who gets to decide? These terms are subjective, meaning they are interpreted and defined differently by different people. Well-being is a broad term that includes being physically healthy; having positive emotions, such as being happy and content; being absent of negative emotions, such as anxiety; and feeling satisfied with one's life.[2] It is essentially being without any physical or **mental health** issues and feeling good. Well-being is often dependent on having access to basic resources such as shelter and food, maintaining positive relationships, and being in good health.[3]

mental health A component of well-being in which the individual realizes his or her abilities, copes with the normal stresses of life, works productively and fruitfully, and makes a contribution to the community; also defined as having emotional, psychological, and social well-being.

The notion that physical and mental health are two separate states is not quite accurate. Your physical health often affects your mental well-being, and, vice versa, your mental health can influence your physical health. For example, being diagnosed with cancer might trigger feelings of stress and anxiety. Conversely, if you have anxiety, you may smoke cigarettes to relieve tension, which can lead to cancer and other physical health problems. Mental and physical health are interconnected. (See Chapter 3 for more about the relationship between exercise and well-being.)

Understanding Mental Health

Mental health can be thought of as one part of "well-being" and defined as "a state of well-being in which the individual realizes his or her abilities, can cope with the normal stresses of life, can work productively and fruitfully, and is able to make a contribution to his or her community."[4] Mental health has also been defined as having emotional, psychological, and social well-being.[5] Good mental health may sound like a tall order, and indeed only an estimated 17% of adults in the United States report meeting this definition of being mentally healthy.[6] You may not feel like you meet this definition of mental health, but at the same time you may not meet the criteria of having a **mental illness**. Despite the importance of mental health, researchers have dedicated resources to the detection and treatment of mental *illness*, as opposed to helping to maintain the mental health of those without a particular diagnosable mental illness.[5]

mental illness The collective group of mental disorders or health conditions that are characterized by alterations in thinking, mood, or behavior (or some combination thereof) associated with distress and/or impaired functioning.

Mental illness refers to the collective group of mental disorders or "health conditions that are characterized by alterations in thinking, mood, or behavior (or some combination thereof) associated with distress and/or impaired functioning."[6] Mental disorders are classified and defined in the *Diagnostic and Statistical Manual of Mental Disorders* (*DSM*).[9] The current version of the *DSM* includes over 150 psychiatric disorders.[10]

The effects of mental disorders can include disruption to daily functioning or abnormal alterations in thinking, mood, or behavior.[13] Genetic predisposition, social factors, and environment can all play a role in causing or exacerbating mental illness. The environment refers to anything outside of one's body (the food we eat, the medicines we take, the air we breathe, etc.).

Mental illness does not discriminate. People of all different ages, genders, and racial, ethnic, and socioeconomic backgrounds are at risk of mental illness. About 20% of adults in the United States reported having a mental illness.[14] This figure may be significantly lower than the actual prevalence. Some people may be reluctant to share their diagnosis of a mental disorder for fear of being stigmatized. It is not uncommon for people to have more than one mental illness. Mental illness and its effects are pervasive in our society; it costs an astonishing $300 billion per year, including lost wages, disability benefits, and healthcare expenditures.[14]

The mental health field is in its infancy compared to what we know about the causes, tests, and treatments for many other illnesses, such as breast cancer

TIPS FOR MAINTAINING MENTAL HEALTH

The following are practices that can contribute positively to mental health[7,8]:

- Talk about your feelings—to loved ones, friends, or a therapist
- Respect yourself
- Stay active
- Eat well
- Limit alcohol, drugs, and nicotine
- Stay in touch with friends and loved ones
- Ask for help when you need it
- Try meditating
- Be grateful and kind
- Get enough sleep
- Manage your stress

WHAT IS THE *DSM*?

The *Diagnostic and Statistical Manual of Mental Disorders*, or *DSM*, is a comprehensive resource used in clinical practice (among medical doctors, psychiatrists, and psychologists) to diagnose mental disorders.[9,10–12] What can be considered the first version of the *DSM* was written in 1952. In 2013, the most recent version of the *DSM*, the fifth edition (abbreviated *DSM-5*), was published.[11] With each version comes updates, refinements, additions, and removals of the diagnostic criteria for mental disorders.

Who decides what is considered a mental disorder, and who defines the diagnostic criteria? Criteria used to diagnose a person with a mental disorder are continually refined by experts in the field with each new version of the *DSM*. These experts often include leaders of the National Institute of Mental Health (NIMH) and the American Psychiatric Association (APA). Over the course of 13 years, experts from the United States and around the world used their clinical expertise and evidence-based literature to develop the *DSM-5*.[12] From the previous version, the number of mental disorders in *DSM-5* decreased from 172 to 152.

As with most aspects of the medical field, debates and criticisms have arisen about the most recent version, with claims that evidence is lacking to support some conditions being considered a mental disorder versus a "normal" struggle that happens every day. Psychiatry is a science but, at the moment, not a perfect science. As the field continues to evolve and research is conducted, our knowledge of the causes, symptoms, and treatments of mental illness will improve, as will our understanding of how to diagnose mental disorders.[10]

American Psychological Association. (2014). Incarceration nation. Retrieved from http://www.apa.org/monitor/2014/10/incarceration.aspx; James, D. J., Glaze, L. E., & BJS Statisticians. (2006). Mental health problems of prison and jail inmates. U.S. Department of Justice. Retrieved from http://www.bjs.gov/content/pub/pdf/mhppji.pdf; Torrey, E. F., Kennard, A. D., Eslinger, S., Lamb, R., & Pavle, J. (2010). More mentally ill persons are in jails and prisons than hospitals: A survey of the states. Retrieved from http://www.treatmentadvocacycenter.org/storage/documents/final_jails_v_hospitals_study.pdf; Treatment Advocacy Center. (n.d.). TACReports. Retrieved from http://www.tacreports.org/bed-study

TALES OF PUBLIC HEALTH

History of Mental Illness in the United States

The treatment of the "mentally ill" was, until fairly recently, a dark spot in America's history. Insane asylums were established around the 1700s. The earliest version of these "hospitals" often kept patients thought to be mentally ill in shackles in a basement. Dorothea Dix, an American activist, uncovered the cruel treatment of those kept in horrific conditions in the mid-1850s and advocated for more humane treatment of people with mental illness. She lobbied for state-run mental hospitals, and by the end of the 19th century, each state had one. Eventually, they became overcrowded.

In the 1930s, those with serious and persistent mental disorders such as schizophrenia were treated with electroconvulsive therapy and lobotomies, where doctors removed part of the patient's brain. Through the 1950s, patients with schizophrenia, obsessive disorders, severe depression, and anxiety were treated by being given lobotomies.

Around that time, President Harry Truman called for more research into mental illness. An Australian psychiatrist had recently discovered lithium as a treatment. Other successful antipsychotic drugs were discovered in the 1950s. With the advent of these new medications and treatments that allowed individuals to be fully functioning members of society, mental hospitals began to decrease in size around this time. The 1990s brought newer and better versions of antipsychotic drugs that treat schizophrenia more effectively and with fewer side effects. However, some of those who were de-institutionalized from state mental hospitals lacked appropriate follow-up care and became homeless.[15,16]

Psychiatric hospitals still exist today to treat serious mental illness, as do psych "wards" or sections of larger hospitals. Treatment of patients is much more humane than it was previously, and there are laws protecting patient rights. Quality mental health care, however, is not widely available. The unfortunate outcome is that today U.S. prisons house many people with mental illness.

and diabetes. There is no blood test or radiologic scan we can do to diagnose mental disorders, such as depression or schizophrenia.

Trained medical professionals often make a diagnosis by observing a person's behavior or by evaluating the person's (or loved ones') responses to questions about his or her feelings and behavior. The treatments for various mental disorders have gained popularity since around the 1950s.[15] Treatment of mental illness can be complicated by the **stigma**, or perceived disgrace, of being on medication for a mental health issue or being in denial about having a disorder.

stigma A mark of disgrace; can manifest as either public stigma or self-stigma.

Treatment of Mental Illness

Perhaps someone in your life has been treated for a mental illness. If so, you may realize that science has a long way to go in understanding the causes of mental illness. As such, scientists continue to study the illnesses in hopes of developing more effective treatments. Treatment for mental illness is usually a combination of medication and psychotherapy. The type of pharmaceutical medication depends on the particular mental illness. Some of the more common types of medications for mental disorders include antidepressants, antipsychotics, mood stabilizers, and antianxiety medications.[17] These medications help people manage their symptoms so they may function fully in society. Despite being successful at managing symptoms, some medications come with side effects, some of which can be severe. Specifically, antidepressants come with a "black box" warning that they may cause suicidal thoughts or attempts in adolescents taking these medications.[18] (A black box warning appears on a prescription drug label to highlight any serious or life-threatening risks.)[19] Developing effective treatments with minimal side effects continues to be a goal of scientists in the mental health field. If you are taking medication to manage a mental illness, a medical doctor should be overseeing your treatment to monitor side effects.

In psychotherapy, often known as "talk therapy" or behavioral counseling, individuals with an illness talk with a trained professional to understand more about their mental disorder, and the professional, in turn, offers tools to help manage various situations and symptoms. Cognitive behavioral therapy (CBT) is a type of psychotherapy that helps people to learn new ways of thinking, behaving, and reacting to various situations. The therapist learns to identify the ways in which the patient has distorted thinking and behaviors and then tries to help the patient change this process and adopt healthier patterns and behaviors.[20] Sometimes people without a diagnosed mental disorder may seek counseling, such as those experiencing grief or a problem they need help to address. Group therapy is one example, in which a group of about 10 people, along with a therapist to facilitate, meet to discuss a shared problem or experience. Relationship counseling is another example, during which couples talk to a therapist about problems in the relationship and learn how to change how they communicate and behave in order to improve their relationship.

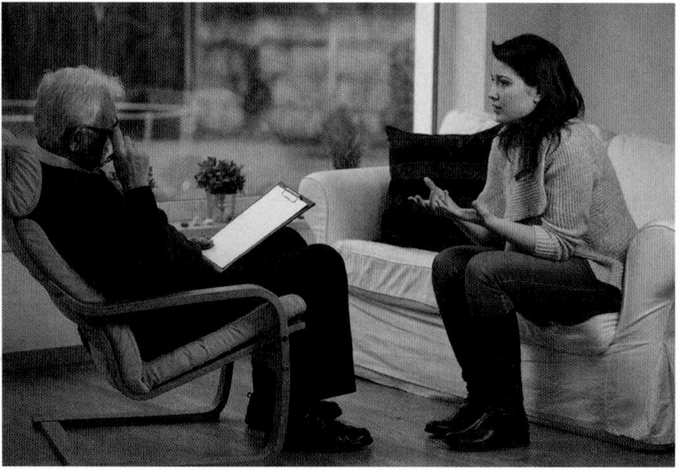

Psychotherapy, or "talk therapy," involves talking to a trained professional one on one.

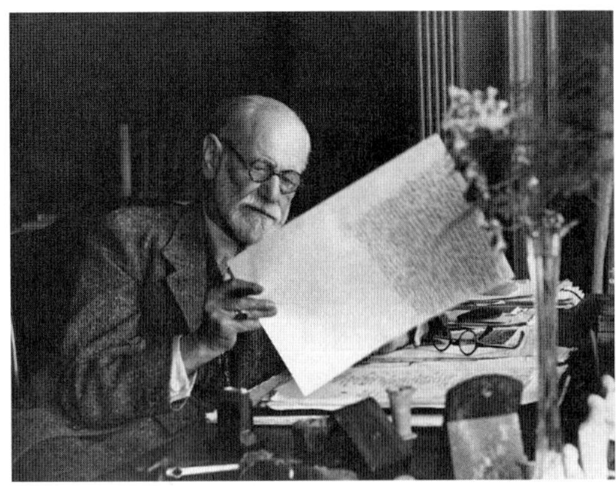

Sigmund Freud, a neurologist known as the father of psychoanalysis, developed the earliest version of psychotherapy.

RESOURCES

Looking for more information, support, or help? Here are a few resources to check out:

- National Suicide Prevention Lifeline (free and confidential): www.suicidepreventionlifeline.org or 1–800-273-TALK (8255)
- National Institute of Mental Health (a source of information about mental illness): www.nimh.nih.gov
- National Alliance on Mental Illness (a resource for family and friends of someone with a mental illness): www.nami.org

There are several types of mental health professionals, and they serve related but distinct functions. The two most common are psychiatrists and psychologists. A psychiatrist is a medical doctor who specializes in mental health. Psychiatrists can diagnose, counsel, and prescribe medication. Because of their medical training, psychiatrists are able to determine what may be a physical or psychological cause of what appears to be a mental health issue. A psychologist has a doctoral degree (PhD) in psychology. Psychologists can diagnose a mental health disorder and provide psychotherapy but not prescribe medication. They are trained to help people manage mental health issues, such as overcoming anxiety, dealing with grief, or combatting addiction.[21]

For some people, psychotherapy alone is enough to allow them to manage their symptoms. For most mental disorders, however, a combination of medication and psychotherapy is often recommended and the most successful treatment. How quickly or effectively a treatment works varies by person. For each of the mental disorders reviewed in this chapter, we include the standard recommended treatment. Scientists in the field of mental health continue to study how genetics, the brain, and the environment all contribute to mental illness, in order to develop more effective interventions and treatments.[22] If you, a friend, or a loved one needs help finding treatment for a mental illness, consult a doctor or other healthcare provider and review the resources online as a starting point to get care. If you are a college student, contact your campus's wellness services to get connected to care.

FINDING A THERAPIST

Navigating the mental health system to find a therapist can be daunting. Here are some tips to help you find one that's right for you:

- Call your medical insurance company to get a list of providers in your area who are covered by your insurance plan. You can ask them to restrict the search based on certain criteria you may have, such as provider gender, credentials, number of miles from your house, etc. Not all therapists accept new patients, so be sure to get information on several providers to find one who has an opening that works with your schedule. (Often patients meet weekly with therapists, at the same time and day of the week.)
- Ask your insurance company if there are any restrictions on the number of visits per year that will be covered and learn what your co-payment will be for each visit.
- Not all therapists are the same. There are many different types of training and credentials. Search for information online or by calling therapists to learn more about their type of credentials and licensing. The most common ones are master of social work (MSW); licensed clinical social worker (LCSW); licensed marriage and family therapist (LMFT); psychiatrist (MD); doctor of psychology (PsyD); doctor of social work (DSW). Providers with a doctorate have had more advanced training in their field. Professional licenses are issued to mental health providers with a master's degree. Licensing requirements vary by state, but all include passing a licensing examination.
- Psychiatrists have a doctorate and can prescribe medication, but often do not engage in psychotherapy. If you need medication *and* talk therapy, you may want to explore having a psychiatrist (for medication purposes) as well as a social worker or other type of therapist (for talk therapy).
- Often therapists have training in a specific area, such as addiction, eating orders, anxiety, etc. Be sure to search online or call to find therapists who have expertise in the area of counseling you may need.

Prison and Mental Illness

The United States has one of the world's highest incarceration rates.[23-26] There is an ongoing debate in the United States regarding whether prisons serve as a form of punishment or means for reform and rehabilitation for people who have committed crimes. What is clear, though, is that prisons have become home to many of those in our society with a serious mental illness, and prison is being viewed as America's new "asylum." In 2005, more than half of inmates in prison or jail had a mental health diagnosis.[24] This means that there are more people with a mental illness in prison and jail than there are in hospitals.[25] The most common mental health issues that inmates suffer from include depression, bipolar disorder, and other psychotic disorders.[24]

These individuals have higher rates of homelessness, foster care involvement as youths, substance dependence, physical and sexual abuse, engagement in illegal sources of income, and unemployment compared to inmates without a mental health issue.[24]

To resolve the issue of pervasive mental illness in our prisons, we need to figure out a better system for providing access to quality and continued mental health care for all people.

Stigma: An Undue Burden

Given the history of how people with mental illness have been treated in this country, it is easy to understand why many people are reluctant to accept a mental illness diagnosis and their need to manage both the illness and the stigma associated with having a disorder. Two forms of stigma exist: public stigma and self-stigma. The general public holds stereotypes and prejudices (agreeing with those stereotypes) about people with mental illness. Ultimately, society as a whole discriminates against people with mental disorders. This is public stigma. Self-stigma is when an individual with a mental illness holds negative beliefs about himself or herself (because of the illness).[27] Perceived stigma is one of the top five barriers that people with a mental illness report regarding why they did not want to seek treatment.[28] Also, public stigma often prevents people with a mental illness from having all of the opportunities, such as stable employment and quality health care, for a quality life. For example, a doctor who knows you have schizophrenia may not trust that you will follow certain treatment regimens for a health problem and only offer you limited options for treatment.

Part of what perpetuates this stigma is how we talk about these disorders. Sometimes we joke about them in film, in songs, and on social media. When we talk about these illnesses as "mental" or "behavioral" disorders, we may be perpetuating the notion that these conditions are personal faults, within one's control. But many of these disorders are caused by differences in brain chemistry or neuronal connections, genetics, or the environment.[29] Combating stigma helps reduce the barriers that people with mental illness face to get treatment, manage their symptoms, and live a full, quality life. It is difficult to change society's perception, and it will likely take many years to fully overcome the damage that stigma has done to mental health.

UP FOR DEBATE

Patient Privacy: A Help or Hindrance?

Many of us feel as though information about our personal health is private and should be protected. The Health Insurance Portability and Accountability Act (HIPAA) was passed in 1996 to do just that—help protect the privacy of patients' health information. It provides legal assurance that you are able to access your own medical records, edit erroneous information in your record, and know who has seen your medical records. Although your records are sometimes shared for specific and legitimate reasons, like assessing quality of care, you can ask your provider to not share information with certain people or groups.[30–32]

On the surface, this law seems like a positive step to help reduce potential stigma by protecting patient health information, particularly for those with a mental illness. On the other side of the debate, however, are family members, such as parents or spouses of someone with a serious mental illness. They are often restricted from accessing information about their loved one's care, unless explicit consent has been granted by the patient.[31] Consider the following scenarios:

- A 27-year-old airline pilot with a history of depression intentionally crashes a plane, killing himself, the crew, and over 100 passengers. The pilot had sought mental health care and his doctors believed he was unfit to fly, but because of privacy laws, they were restricted from notifying his employer. (This account, involving a Germanwings copilot, happened in March 2015.[32])
- A 24-year-old woman with a history of schizophrenia has stopped taking her medication. She becomes delusional and paranoid while at work, and her employer contacts her doctor, who discloses her diagnosis. Despite immediately restarting treatment and having her symptoms stabilize, she returns to work to find that her coworkers all know about her illness. She experiences increased stress and shame surrounding her disclosed diagnosis.

Consider the two sides of this debate: Do you think patient privacy laws are too strict when it comes to mental illness? Do you think they do more harm than good, or vice versa?

Stress and Mental Health

Stress is how our brains respond to a demand or stimulus.[33] Stress is hard to define because the same stressor can cause different reactions in different people. For example, two people may attend the same concert; one may be excited to see the band and experience live music, whereas the other may be claustrophobic and worried about being stuck in the crowd. Stress can be acute (meaning short term) or chronic (lasting a long time). Sometimes stress can be positive, like helping you finish a paper on time. But when stress endures for a long time, it can damage your health and wreak havoc on your body.[34] Having a prolonged stress response can adversely affect health, contributing to conditions like headaches, digestive disorders, and heart disease. Also, stress can worsen symptoms of a mental disorder, such as depression.[35]

Not all stress is equal. People of color are more often victims of discrimination. Gender-based and sexual orientation–based discrimination are also common. This discrimination may manifest in ways such as not getting hired for a job despite being the most qualified candidate, people making negative assumptions about one's character without knowing that person, or being bullied or threatened. Discrimination is linked to chronic stress, as is living in poverty. This stress, in turn, can contribute to health disparities in cardiovascular disease, diabetes, poor birth outcomes, increased substance use, and mental health disorders.[36] Broader policies and antidiscrimination laws are one way to help stop discrimination and reduce health disparities.

Mind–body techniques such as meditation can help manage stress (**FIGURE 6-1**). Other recommendations for coping with stress include exercising regularly, not dwelling on problems, recognizing the symptoms of stress, and seeking professional care when needed.[33] (See Chapter 4 for more information on how stress can affect well-being and for tips on controlling stress.)

defense mechanisms
Subconscious thoughts that we use to avoid feeling anxious or guilty when we are confronted with situations in which we feel threatened.

HOW WE COPE

Sigmund Freud, the father of psychoanalysis, was one of the first to propose that humans employ **defense mechanisms** in order to deal with conflict, or problems. Defense mechanisms are subconscious thoughts that we use to avoid feeling anxious or guilty when we are confronted with situations in which we feel threatened. A few of the most common defense mechanisms are as follows:

- *Repression*: disturbing or threatening thoughts are repressed, or quieted
- *Denial*: refusing to experience or believe something, so you are not actively aware of it
- *Projection*: attributing your own unacceptable or inappropriate thoughts and feelings to another person
- *Displacement*: redirecting an aggressive or inappropriate impulse instead to a powerless target
- *Regression*: moving back in time to engage in behaviors that are childish
- *Sublimation*: displacing emotions, but in a constructive or socially acceptable way

We use these mechanisms to avoid feelings of guilt or anxiety. Often they do not work effectively, especially as long-term coping strategies. More effective and positive strategies to cope with stressful situations include the following[37]:

- Meditation
- Physical activity
- Being social and talking to friends
- Having a creative outlet like reading, writing, or other hobbies
- Getting enough sleep
- Eating healthfully
- Seeking out a therapist if other strategies don't work

HOW TO DEAL WITH STRESS AND ANXIETY

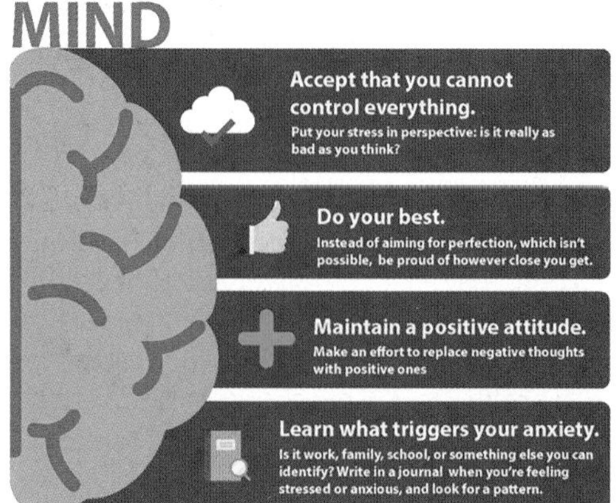

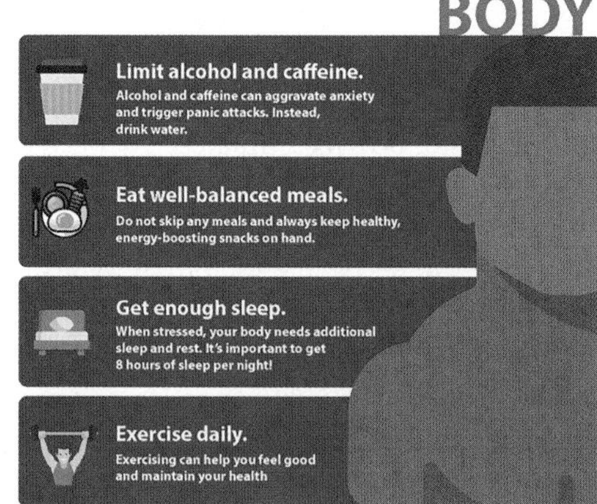

ACTION
Take deep breaths.
Inhale and exhale slowly throughout the day when you are feeling stressed.
10
Slowly count to 10.
Repeat, and count to 20 if necessary.
Give back to your community.
Volunteer or find another way to be active in your community, which creates a support network and gives you a break from everyday stress.
Take a time out.
Practice yoga, listen to music, meditate, get a massage, or learn relaxation techniques. Stepping back from problems helps clear your head.
Get help online.
If you are struggling with stress and anxiety in your life, consider taking a mental health screen. Screening is an anonymous, free, and private way to learn about your mental health.
www. mhascreening.org
Talk to someone.
Tell friends and family you're feeling overwhelmed, and let them know how they can help you. Talk to a physician or therapist for professional help.

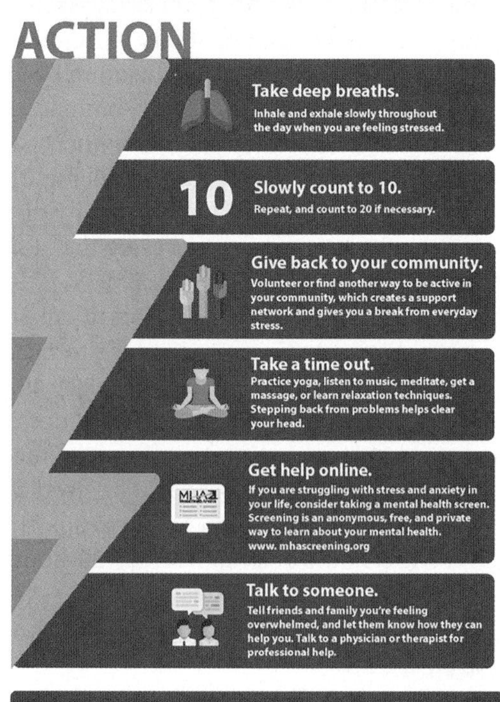

To access webinars, blogs, and other tools to help you manage stress and anxiety visit: www.adaa.org

MHA Mental Health America

ADAA

FIGURE 6-1 How to deal with stress and anxiety.

Anxiety and Depression Association of America. (n.d.). Tips to Manage Anxiety and Stress. Retrieved from https://adaa.org/tips-manage-anxiety-and-stress#

STUDENT LOANS AND MENTAL HEALTH

The burden of student loans can obviously affect your wallet, but can it impact your health? As the price of higher education continues to climb, average family income has plateaued or declined. Thus, the need for students to borrow money to attend college has increased. On average, students carry about $23,000 in loans and collectively borrow about $1 trillion in the United States.

Research indicates that student loan debt is associated with poorer psychological function. How would debt affect mental health? Stress is a logical culprit. Carrying such debt may affect other aspects of one's livelihood in terms of not being able to live on your own, taking a higher paid but less-fulfilling job, or delaying marriage or having kids. All of these things can contribute to stress and affect your mental health. Do you have student loan debt? Will you when you graduate? What type of policies, if any, would you like to see implemented to help ease the burden of student loan debt?

The Importance of Sleep

The importance of sleep cannot be overestimated. We need sleep to survive just like we need food and water. We all know that we need a good night's sleep to feel rested and function the next day, but only recently have scientists discovered why that is.[38] Sleep is necessary for our nervous system to function properly. It contributes to memory performance, emotional resistance, optimal growth in children, and many other beneficial functions. Lack of sufficient sleep is associated with a host of health problems.[39]

There are many types of sleep disorders, and they have symptoms ranging from excessive tiredness to difficulty sleeping. Insomnia is a common type of sleep disorder, affecting 30% of adults, and it is characterized by difficulty falling asleep or staying asleep, thus affecting one's ability to function during the day.[40] CBT is one nonpharmacological treatment for insomnia. Several medications are available to assist with periodic or persistent insomnia.[41]

In terms of mental health, lack of sleep could be either a symptom of a mental disorder or a potential cause. Problems getting a full night's rest are common among people with anxiety, attention deficit hyperactivity disorder, bipolar disorder, and other disorders. Scientists are discovering that a sleep disorder may also put the person at risk of some mental illnesses.[42]

Experts recommend techniques and behaviors to maintain good "sleep hygiene," which refers to measures a person can take to maintain a consistent sleeping pattern. The recommendation for healthy sleep is a combination of lifestyle changes (like reducing caffeine and other substance use), exercise, psychotherapy, and engagement in relaxation practices like meditation. One key tip is to use the bedroom only for being intimate or sleeping (no television!), although this can be difficult in a dorm room or studio apartment.[42] It is recommended that adults get 7 to 9 hours of sleep within a 24-hour period.

Anxiety Disorders

We have all felt anxious at some point—our heart beating rapidly right before an exam or our breathing coming in rapid bursts at the start of an oral presentation. But when anxiety and fear are persistent and affect your daily life, it may be a clinical anxiety disorder. Nearly 30% of adults will have an anxiety disorder at some point in their lives.[43] There are several anxiety disorders classified in the *DSM*. Here we will discuss two of the more common ones: **generalized anxiety disorder** and **panic disorder**. Anxiety disorders, in general, can begin in childhood and occur twice as frequently among women compared to men.[44]

generalized anxiety disorder A disorder that includes excessive anxiety and worry for at least 6 months that causes significant distress and impedes social or occupational functioning.

panic disorder A disorder that causes a person to experience panic attacks, that is, an abrupt surge of intense fear or intense discomfort that reaches a peak within minutes.

Generalized Anxiety Disorder

Anxiety that becomes excessive and causes a person to persistently worry that something bad will happen to an extent that is out of proportion with the likelihood of it happening is a sign of generalized anxiety disorder. This level of anxiety demands a lot of time and energy and interferes with daily life, including one's ability to perform at work and to maintain a healthy social life. It is not clear why some people develop this disorder. Researchers are studying differences in the region of the brain associated with fear and anxiety, as well as how physical and social environments can impact mental health. The main features of the *DSM* criteria for generalized anxiety disorder are excessive anxiety and worry for at least 6 months that causes significant distress and impedes social or occupational functioning.[44]

About 2% of adults in the United States have generalized anxiety disorder, affecting females almost twice as often as males.[45] The average age of onset is 31 years.[46] Individuals with generalized anxiety may experience other conditions associated with stress, such as headaches, irritable bowel syndrome, muscle tension, and/or become startled easily.[44] Psychotherapy, particularly CBT, is the recommended treatment for generalized anxiety disorder. A physician may also recommend medication, such as an antianxiety or antidepressant medication.[46]

Panic Disorder

Panic disorder can influence every aspect of a person's life—employment, social life, physical health, and finances. It is unclear what causes a panic disorder. It can run in families but may also be influenced by differences in the brain and how it processes stress.[18] Panic attacks are "an abrupt surge of intense fear or intense discomfort that reaches a peak within minutes."[44] To be classified as a panic disorder, panic attacks need to be accompanied by several specific symptoms, including accelerated heart rate and shortness of breath.[44]

Panic attacks can occur in other mental disorders as well as in anxiety disorder. People having a panic attack may mistakenly believe they are having a heart attack because it often entails shortness of breath and feeling dizzy. Of all the anxiety disorders, panic disorder is associated with the most medical visits.[44]

About 5% of adults have a panic disorder.[47] It is much less common among children, and it generally starts to increase in adolescence, particularly among females.[48] Older individuals are less likely to have a panic disorder.[42] Interestingly, compared to non-Hispanic Whites, individuals identified as Latino, African American, Caribbean Black, and Asian American have lower rates of panic disorder, while American Indians have significantly higher rates. It is unclear why this disparity exists; possibly because the criteria for panic disorder do not include culturally specific symptoms.[47]

You should seek treatment if you experience a panic attack. Treatments can help manage and prevent future panic attacks. Effective treatment for panic disorder can vary but often includes medication and psychotherapy. Antidepressant medications can reduce the frequency and severity of panic attacks and related symptoms. CBT has been successful in managing panic disorder.[49] Relaxation techniques, such as meditation and yoga, are also recommended for people with anxiety disorders.[50] (See Chapter 4 for more about these therapies.)

Posttraumatic Stress Disorder

posttraumatic stress disorder (PTSD) The development of specific symptoms after being exposed to one or more traumatic events.

Posttraumatic stress disorder (PTSD) is the development of specific symptoms after being exposed to one or more traumatic events. Scientists are studying how many different factors may cause PTSD and in what ways.

Genetics may play a role in creating "fear memories," which may predispose someone who has experienced a traumatic event to have PTSD. Differences in the brain—particularly the amygdala, which deals with emotion, learning, and memory—may be part of the cause. People exposed to environmental factors, such as childhood trauma or head injury, may be predisposed to PTSD.[51] Sexual abuse in childhood or sexual assault are also traumatic events that can lead to PTSD.[52]

Different people have different PTSD symptoms; some may have distressing dreams about the traumatic event, and others may show psychological distress, such as being paranoid or hearing their thoughts spoken in different voices. PTSD first appeared in the *DSM* in 1980, largely associated with veterans returning from the Vietnam War.[53] In the most recent version of the *DSM*, PTSD was moved from being an anxiety disorder to a new category of trauma and stressor-related disorders. The criteria were also refined to clarify what exposures constitute a trigger for PTSD.[54] The new criteria (for individuals age 6 years and over) include having been exposed to actual or threatened death and serious injury or sexual violence that subsequently causes intrusive symptoms such as distressing memories.[44]

About 7% of adults have experienced PTSD—4% of men and 10% of women.[55,56] For men, co-occurring substance use disorder is more common than among women. The rates of PTSD among military personnel deployed in recent wars and those whose work revolves around exposure to trauma (e.g., police and emergency medical personnel) are much higher compared to the general population.[44]

Given the nature of PTSD, it can cause significant distress and affect one's ability to have positive social interactions and maintain interpersonal relationships. Individuals with PTSD may have trouble working and in other areas of daily functioning.[54] They may act out with verbal or physical aggression and have problems sleeping. This has been portrayed in films like *Born on the Fourth of July* or *The Hurt Locker*. As with other mental disorders, psychotherapy and medication are often recommended to treat PTSD. There is one common type of CBT used for PTSD called exposure therapy. In exposure therapy,

TALES OF PUBLIC HEALTH

Homosexuality: Mental Illness No More

As noted earlier in this chapter, the *DSM* that is used to diagnosis mental disorders has been revised four times over the last 70 years. It may surprise you to learn of some diagnoses that used to be considered mental health problems. Homosexuality (a sexual preference for members of one's own sex) is one example of these obsolete diagnoses. It is included in the first version of the *DSM* as a mental illness.

This information may be more than just surprising, but, in fact, insulting. Homosexuality was listed as a sociopathic personality disturbance, because it was then considered to be a pathological fear of the opposite sex. This categorization helped lay the groundwork for persistent discrimination against gay men and women in the United States. After Dr. Evelyn Hooker debunked the myth that homosexuality was associated with psychological maladjustment, the diagnosis was subsequently removed in 1973 in the *DSM*'s second edition.[58] Today we have a much more holistic and comprehensive understanding about sexuality and sexual preferences.

the therapist uses mental imagery, writing, or visits to safely expose patients with PTSD to their trauma, as a means of helping them cope with their feelings.[51] Eye movement desensitization and reprocessing (EMDR), developed by Dr. Francine Shapiro, is another type of therapy used to treat PTSD. This therapy consists of eight phases that take place over 3 months. The main goal is for patients to process a trauma so it is no longer distressing. After learning the patient's history, preparing them for the treatment and assessing which trauma is to be the main focal point, a trained therapist leads a patient to focus on a traumatic memory. The patient then follows the therapist's hand as it moves back and forth to produce the effects of rapid eye movements that occur during the REM phase of sleep, all while thinking of the trauma. If successful, over the course of several sessions, EMDR can help the patient to process the trauma.[57] Watch these videos to learn about PTSD and effective treatments: http://www.ptsd.va.gov/public/materials/videos/whiteboards.asp.

Depression

We sometimes casually use the word "depressed" to describe feeling upset about something. We all get upset or sad sometimes, but clinical depression is a serious mental health issue. It can impair one's ability to work and maintain social relationships and can lead to suicidal ideation (thinking about killing oneself) or attempts (trying to kill oneself). **Depression** is a brain disorder, likely caused by a combination of genetic, biological, environmental, and psychosocial factors.[59] There are several disorders classified as "depressive." Here we will discuss the most well-known—major depressive disorder. The criteria for major depressive disorder in adults include having persistent symptoms such as depressed mood most of the day, diminished pleasure in activities, and feelings of worthlessness that interfere with daily functioning.[44]

depression Mood disorder characterized by symptoms that include feelings of sadness, worthlessness, or hopelessness; diminished pleasure in activities; and thoughts of death or suicide.

Everyone is different in terms of how long they may go without any depressive episodes; some people can have years without symptoms while for others the symptoms are chronic. Diagnosing depression can be complicated if someone is also suffering from a medical condition, such as cancer or pregnancy, that may cause some of the same symptoms—for example, weight loss (for cancer), insomnia, low energy, or fatigue. If someone's symptoms are not completely attributed to their medical condition, then the symptoms can be considered as part of the assessment by a trained professional to determine a depressive diagnosis. Misdiagnosis can also occur in someone who presents with major depressive symptoms. For example, it may be determined that the person has bipolar disorder, of which depression is one component (see the section on bipolar disorder). Depression is also different from grieving over the loss of someone important. Grieving and bereavement are marked by feelings of loss, whereas depression is characterized by a persistently depressed mood.[44] See Chapter 12 for more information.

Worldwide, major depression is ranked as the highest cause of disability and is associated with having other chronic conditions.[60] So, in addition to the personal suffering produced by the disorder itself, the person also is burdened by a great deal of healthcare costs associated with this illness. About 16% of people have experienced major depressive disorder in their lifetime, with about 7% to 8% of adults having a current diagnosis. It can arise at any age but peaks during the 20s, and women are at higher risk than men (**FIGURES 6-2** and **6-3**).[61]

Antidepressant medications are commonly prescribed to manage symptoms. Selective serotonin reuptake inhibitors (SSRIs) are the newest class of antidepressants and are popular because they have fewer side effects than older antidepressants.[59] Psychotherapy is also a common treatment for depression.

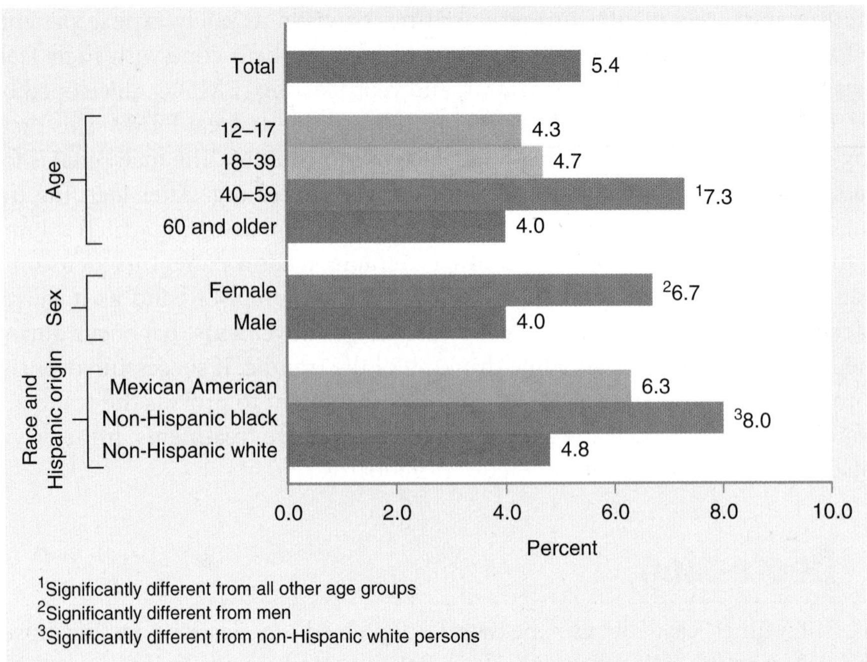

FIGURE 6-2 Percentage of persons 12 years of age and older with depression by demographic characteristics: United States, 2005–2006.

Centers for Disease Control and Prevention. (n.d.). Anxiety and Depression Optional Module—Behavioral Risk Factor Surveillance System (BRFSS). Retrieved from http://www.cdc.gov/mentalhealth/data_stats/depression.htm

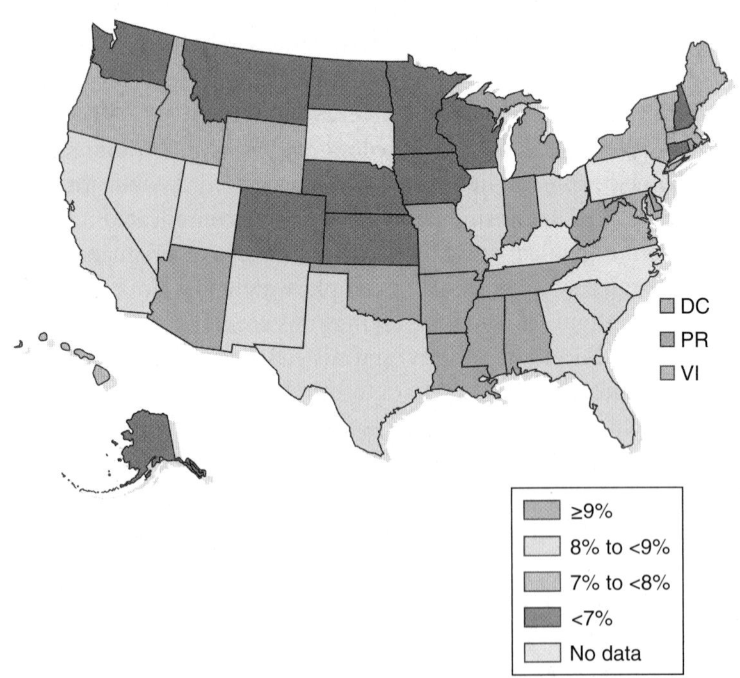

FIGURE 6-3 Prevalence of current depression among adults 18 years of age and older by state quartile: Behavioral Risk Factor Surveillance System—United States, 2006. Depression estimates generally are highest in the southeastern states (e.g., 13.7% in Mississippi and West Virginia vs. 4.3% in North Dakota).

Centers for Disease Control and Prevention. (2011). CDC Report: Mental Illness Surveillance Among Adults in the United States. Retrieved from http://www.cdc.gov/mentalhealthsurveillance/fact_sheet.html

Learn more about this mental disorder by viewing this collection of TED Talks about depression: www.ted.com/topics/depression.

Bipolar Disorder

We are learning more and more each year about bipolar disorder, previously known as manic depression. **Bipolar disorder** is a brain disorder that causes extreme changes in mood. The word "bipolar" means having two poles, and as it relates to the mental disorder, those poles are mania and depression. We all experience periods of being happy and sad. But for someone with bipolar disorder, those moods are extreme. Bipolar disorder runs in families, which means there is a genetic predisposition that may be passed down from parents to children. However this predisposition does not mean that all children with a family history of bipolar disorder will develop the illness; in fact, most will not. In addition to genes, some environmental factors can contribute to a person developing bipolar disorder. What are those environmental factors? Scientists are still exploring the causes, specifically trying to understand more about differences in brain functioning.[62]

bipolar disorder A disorder that causes extreme changes in mood and includes mania or hypomania, and sometimes depression as well; formerly known as manic depression.

A manic episode may come before or after a hypomanic or major depressive episode (each of which has its own criteria). During a manic episode, individuals often do not feel as though anything is wrong or that they need treatment. Someone in a manic episode usually feels euphoric, but there can be rapid changes in mood from excessively elated to irritable. They usually have a lot of energy, talk fast, get distracted easily, and engage in impulsive behaviors, such as gambling, spending a lot of money, using substances, or engaging in risky sexual behaviors. Their behavior often becomes disruptive and unpredictable, and it can affect their ability to work and maintain relationships. Because of this behavior, the individual may be involuntarily hospitalized or encounter problems with the law. In some cases, the condition can lead to **suicide**. In a "mixed episode," some symptoms of depression may be integrated into a manic episode.

suicide The act of killing oneself; the desire to commit suicide is often expressed first by suicidal ideation (thinking about killing oneself) and then attempts (trying to kill oneself).

There are two types of bipolar disorder, type I and type II, which have distinct criteria for their manic and depressive episodes. For bipolar type I, a person

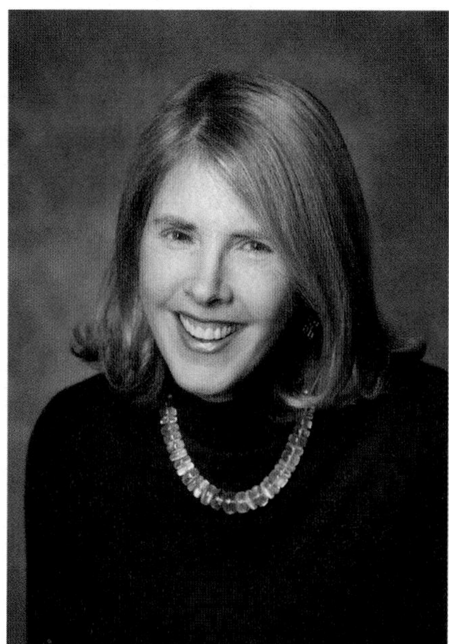

Kay Jamison is a clinical psychologist who has written extensively and spoken publicly about her own bipolar disorder.

From Eric Vohr, Media Relations, Johns Hopkins Medical Institutions.

needs to have at least one manic episode, marked by abnormal and persistently elevated or irritable mood and energy that lasts at least 1 week. During this episode, the person often has an inflated self-esteem, is easily distracted, and has a diminished need for sleep.[44] Less than 1% of adults have bipolar type I, with no significant differences in males versus females. The first full-blown episodes usually occur in late adolescence, before 25 years of age, but it can occur in children. Bipolar type II has less-frequent and less-extreme features.[44] Bipolar disorder is often accompanied by other mental health issues, such as substance use and anxiety disorders. People with bipolar disorder are also at higher risk for certain physical health problems, including diabetes and migraine headaches. It is unclear if the coexistence of these conditions is a result of the treatment for bipolar disorder or if those problems cause bipolar symptoms.[44,62]

Bipolar disorder is a chronic condition, but it can be well managed with proper treatment. The standard first line of treatment usually includes medications, such as mood stabilizers, atypical antipsychotics, or antidepressants. People react differently, however, to certain medications and even different doses of the same medication, so they need to work closely with their care provider to determine the best type of treatment to manage their symptoms. An individual may experience symptoms even after being on medication that had been managing the illness well for years. In addition to the stigma of having bipolar disorder, some people stop taking medication because the initial feelings of mania (euphoria, grandiosity, only needing a few hours of sleep) are enjoyable. It is of key importance, however, for individuals diagnosed with this disorder to continue taking their medication and to work with their healthcare provider to adjust the treatment plan as needed.[62]

Schizophrenia

schizophrenia A disorder that affects how people think and behave and may include delusions, hallucinations, disorganized speech, grossly disorganized or catatonic behavior, and negative symptoms.

Schizophrenia is a brain disorder that affects how people think and behave.[63] Like bipolar disorder, we are still learning about the causes of and developing more effective treatment for schizophrenia. Genes play a role in the development of schizophrenia, but there is no one specific gene that causes it, nor are genes the only determinant. Brain chemistry may play a role. Environment may be another contributing factor, such as exposure to certain viruses in utero (in the womb).[64] Scientists are studying other ways in which the physical and social environment may cause schizophrenia.

Although there are several disorders along the schizophrenia spectrum, the most well-known is schizophrenia. The main features of schizophrenia[44] include delusions (false beliefs held despite strong evidence to the contrary), hallucinations (sensory perceptions not based in reality), disorganized speech (such as sequences of unrelated ideas or words), grossly disorganized or catatonic behavior (such as stupor, mania, and rigidity or extreme flexibility of the limbs), and negative symptoms (disruptions to normal emotions and behaviors such as a flat affect and lack of drive to perform purposeful activities). Schizophrenia-like symptoms may be caused by schizoaffective disorder, depressive or bipolar disorder with psychotic features, drug abuse, medication, or autism spectrum disorder, so proper diagnosis by a trained professional is important.

About 1% of adults are diagnosed with schizophrenia, with no significant differences by gender. Men, however, may experience the onset of symptoms earlier than women do.[64] Onset can occur in mid- to late-teenage years; it is less common in children.[65] This disorder is difficult to diagnose because individuals with schizophrenia can vary dramatically in their symptoms, so there is no one particular sign for which to look. Some characteristics of individuals with

GUNS AND MENTAL ILLNESS

Random acts of violence committed by people with serious mental illness are rare. But when they do occur, they can be devastating for families, communities, and the nation. Several mass killings in recent years have been committed by individuals with a history of mental health issues. As just one example, on December 14, 2012, a 20-year-old man fatally shot 20 children and 6 adults at an elementary school in Newtown, Connecticut, before killing himself. Experts have cited a failed system for the lack of proper treatment for the shooter's mental health problems and as the main impetus for these attacks.[66–68] This tragedy struck the residents of the community of Newtown but was felt around the United States.

The Newton shootings and similar incidents have led to a call for more restrictive gun laws, particularly for those with a history of mental illness. Both professionals in the field of public health and people living in our society worry about gun violence. But we must be mindful not to perpetuate the stigma that all individuals with mental illness are dangerous and should be treated differently in their rights as citizens. Public health experts suggest reframing the issue of guns and mental illness. Their policy recommendations, supported by the evidence of gun violence, are to enact laws prohibiting access to firearms based on a person's history of certain dangerous behaviors, not based simply on whether the person has been diagnosed with a mental illness.[68]

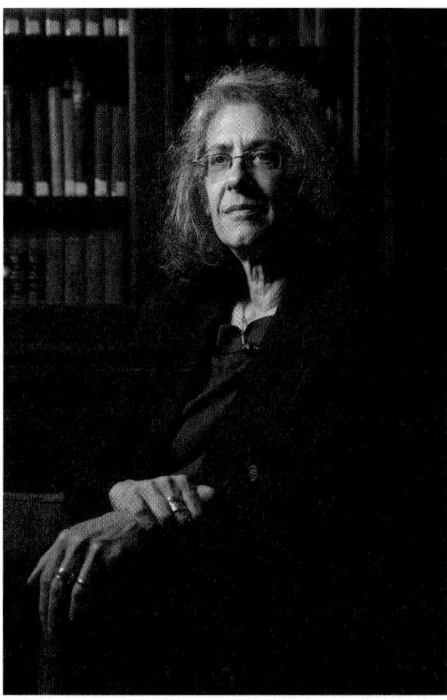

Elyn Saks is a law professor who has spoken publicly about her schizophrenia, helping to reduce the stigma that this disorder prevents people from working and living a quality, fulfilling life.

schizophrenia, such as worsening academic performance, sleep problems, and changing friends, are also common among teenagers without this disorder.[64]

People with schizophrenia might express inappropriate behaviors, disturbed sleep patterns, anxiety, or cognitive deficits. Being aggressive or hostile can be common, but random acts of assault or violence toward strangers are not.

The effects of schizophrenia may limit a person's ability to maintain a steady job and social relationships. Because of these difficulties, people with schizophrenia often need to rely on family or friends.

Without knowing the exact cause of schizophrenia, scientists have more work to do to figure out the most effective treatments and to understand whether this disorder can be "cured." Thus far, the use of antipsychotic medications for managing symptoms is the first line of treatment. As with other medications, different people react differently. These medications can be effective at managing symptoms but come with side effects such as dizziness and vision problems. In addition to medication, psychotherapy has been effective in helping to manage this illness.[64] Lacking insight into this illness is a common symptom of schizophrenia and also partly responsible for why people with schizophrenia may not take their prescribed medication or maintain other recommended treatment.[44]

Personality Disorders

How we think, feel, and behave are part of our individual personalities—it is what makes each of us unique. Everyone's personality is different, but each culture has a socially acceptable way of acting. When how one thinks, feels, or behaves is not in line with what our culture expects or causes some distress, it may be a personality disorder. About 9% of people have a personality disorder in the United States.[69] Features of personality disorders include distorted thinking, problematic emotional responses, problems with impulse control, and interpersonal problems. There are 10 types of personality disorders, categorized into three clusters: (A) odd or eccentric behavior, (B) dramatic, emotional, or erratic behavior, and (C) anxious or fearful behavior.[70] Two of the most common types are borderline and paranoid personality disorder.

Borderline Personality Disorder

borderline personality disorder A personality disorder characterized by a pervasive pattern of instability of interpersonal relationships, self-image, and affect, with marked impulsivity.

Borderline personality disorder is a Cluster B disorder and characterized by unstable moods and behaviors. It is not well known what causes borderline personality disorder, but research indicates it is likely a combination of genetics and environment. Living in a community, for example, where unstable family relationships are common might contribute to borderline personality disorder.[71] It is defined as a pervasive pattern of instability of interpersonal relationships, self-image, and affect, with marked impulsivity.

To diagnose borderline personality disorder, symptoms must be present by early adulthood and in a variety of contexts. According to *DSM* criteria, people with borderline personality disorder often engage in frantic efforts to avoid real or imagined abandonment as well as relationships where they alternate between extremes of idealization (intense love) and devaluation (intense dislike). They may have an unstable sense of self and engage in impulsive, self-damaging behaviors in areas such as sex, spending, substance abuse, reckless driving, and binge eating. Recurrent suicidal or self-mutilating behavior is common, as well as paranoid ideation or severe dissociative symptoms. They may suffer from rapid and abrupt mood shifts, feelings of emptiness, and inappropriate or difficult-to-control anger.[44]

Borderline personality disorder can be serious, and it is marked by unstable moods and relationships and impulsive behavior. Some may even have short-term psychotic episodes during stressful times. Another feature is a pattern of undermining themselves at a point just before a goal is reached, like dropping out of school right before graduation. Borderline personality disorder is associated with self-harming behavior, such as cutting, hitting, and hair pulling. Up to 80% of people with this diagnosis have suicidal behavior, with about 4% to 9% committing suicide. Often, people who have borderline personality disorder were traumatized in their childhood by physical or sexual abuse or neglect. It can occur in conjunction with other mental illnesses such as depression and bipolar disorder. Because of the difficulty of diagnosis, the prevalence of borderline personality disorder is unclear but has been estimated at 1.6% of adults.[71]

Psychotherapy is often recommended for borderline personality disorder. Dialectical behavior therapy is a type of CBT that focuses on mindfulness and has been shown to reduce suicide attempts among women with borderline personality disorder. There are no approved medications to treat borderline personality disorder, but individuals often are prescribed medications to manage symptoms of depression or anxiety.[71]

Paranoid Personality Disorder

Paranoid personality disorder is characterized by having excessive distrust and suspicion of others, and falls under the Cluster A disorders. Those with paranoid personality disorder assume others' actions are threatening or demeaning, and often refrain from confiding in others.[70] It is not known what causes paranoid personality disorder, but, like borderline, a combination of genes and environment are likely. Medications and therapy can also successfully control paranoia—as long as the patient's suspicion of the doctor administering the treatment does not get in the way.[72]

paranoid personality disorder A personality disorder characterized by excessive distrust and suspicion.

Self-Injury: Cutting and Other Self-Injurious Behaviors and Suicide

Self-injury, also called self-harm, is the act of deliberately harming one's own body. Usually, this behavior is an unhealthy way to cope with emotional pain, intense anger, and frustration (not a suicide attempt).

self-injury The act of deliberately harming one's body; also called self-harm.

Self-injury is a complex yet poorly understood behavior. For some, self-injury may bring a momentary sense of calm and a release of tension; however, it is followed by guilt and the return of painful emotions. Self-injury may be linked to a variety of mental disorders, such as depression and eating disorders.[73] It occurs in both adolescents and adults.[74]

Cutting is the most common form of self-injury. People use a sharp object to cut or severely scratch themselves. The usual "targets" are the arms, legs, and torso. These areas are not only easily reachable but can be hidden under clothing. Other forms of self-injury include burning (using matches, cigarettes, or hot, sharp objects), carving words or symbols into the skin, hitting or punching, head-banging, biting, or pulling out hair.[73] Regardless of the method, the conscious intention is to harm oneself.

Self-injurious behaviors are considered a sign of increased risk for suicide.[75] Because human behavior is often unpredictable, it is impossible to determine the level of suicide risk of any individual. Research has divided individuals into three levels of suicide risk—lowest, moderate to higher, and highest suicide risk—depending on the frequency of self-injurious behavior, psychosocial behaviors, and suicidal ideation. Over two-thirds of young adults with self-injurious behavior fit the low-risk profile.[75] Even though not everyone who engages in self-injury is at moderate or high risk for suicide, all self-injury includes the risk of infection and possibly permanent damage. Even infrequent self-harm indicates underlying problems related to belonging, self-esteem, anxiety, or other issues that can and should be addressed.

There is no simple explanation for why people self-injure. As suggested by the Mayo Clinic, people may choose to self-injure because of psychological pain

SELF-INJURY: IT'S NOTHING TO BE ASHAMED OF

You may feel embarrassed or ashamed by your behavior. Put that aside and get help. If you have injured yourself severely or feel suicidal, call 9-1-1 or your local emergency service. If you discover that a friend or family member is self-injuring, you may be concerned and scared. Take all talk of self-injury seriously. Even if you have promised not to share the information, your friend or family member needs professional help. Self-injury is too big a problem for you to deal with alone. Encourage the person to self-disclose to a parent, teacher, or counselor and to seek medical and psychological treatment.[73]

related to issues of personal identity. These individuals may have a hard time understanding and expressing their emotions. They may experience feelings of loneliness, anger, guilt, rejection, or self-hatred.[73]

A recent study reviewed 40 self-injury first aid videos on YouTube.[76] At the time the study was published, the videos had been viewed more than 157,000 times. There were few messages to encourage people to seek help. Several of the videos provided "safe" instructions. Such messages are problematic because they may lead to the belief that professional medical and psychological help is not necessary, which is untrue.[76]

If you (or a friend or family member) self-injure, it is very important to get the appropriate treatment so that you can learn healthier ways to cope. Even if your self-injury is minor, or if you are having thoughts about harming yourself, reach out for help. These thoughts are often a sign of bigger issues. Talk to someone you trust, such as a friend, family member, healthcare provider, religious leader, or school official. Even if you feel isolated, there are people around you who will help you.

Suicide: At the Edge of the Abyss

Societies' attitudes toward suicide have varied across cultures and over time. From ancient cultures that were accepting of suicide to modern cultures that now understand suicide is a preventable and unnecessary way for someone to die.[77,78] Until it was banned in 1829 by the British, Hindu widows would throw themselves onto their husband's funeral pyre in order to "enter the next life with him," in a practice called *sati* or *suttee*.[78]

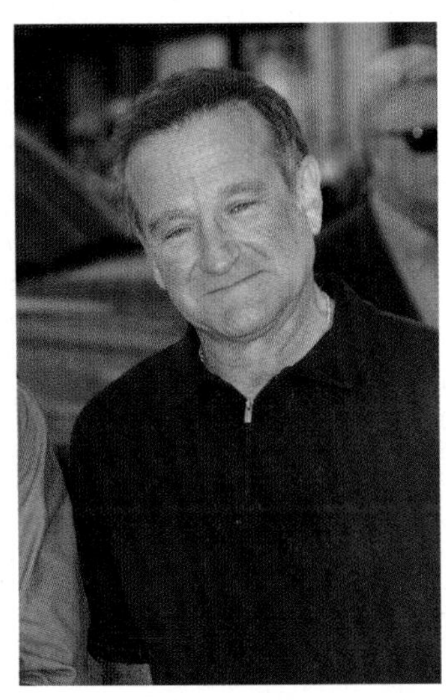

Actor and comedian Robin Williams committed suicide in August of 2014.

Because of the stigma, family members of people who may have committed suicide questioned whether the death was actually a suicide. Famous individuals whose death is considered a suicide or suspected suicide include the painter Vincent van Gogh (1890); the composer Pyotr Tchaikovsky (1893); the writers Virginia Woolf (1941), Ernest Hemingway (1961), and Sylvia Plath (1963); musician Kurt Cobain (1994); and actor Robin Williams (2014).

Why do people commit suicide? Although we can only make educated guesses, it is likely that a suicidal person feels alone and without hope. Predictors of suicide are diagnosable mental conditions, substance abuse, loss of social support, and access to a firearm.[79] Additionally, suicidality may run in families, through shared genetic and environmental factors.[80] For example, in the family of Ernest Hemingway, a Nobel Laureate and Pulitzer Prize winning author, not only did he commit suicide, but his father, two siblings, and a granddaughter all did as well.

BY THE NUMBERS

Suicide Rates

In 2013, suicide was the second leading cause of death among persons 15 to 24 years of age and persons 25 to 34 years of age, and the fourth leading cause among persons 35 to 44 years of age.[81] About 78% of the deaths were male, and 22% were female. The highest suicide rates were among Whites, American Indians, and Alaska Natives. More than half of all people who committed suicide in 2013 used firearms.[82] Advocates for gun laws cite recent research that limiting access to guns may help reduce suicides.[67]

It is important to recognize signs of suicidal behavior in yourself or someone else. According to the Department of Health and Human Services, the warning signs of suicide include the following[83]:

- Talking about killing oneself
- Researching ways to kill oneself
- Expressing feelings of hopelessness or having no reason to live
- Talking about being in pain, being trapped, or being a burden to others
- Sleeping too much or too little
- Using alcohol or drugs in excess
- Engaging in reckless behavior
- Withdrawing from social engagement or feeling isolated
- Having extreme mood swings
- Displaying rage or seeking revenge

Suicide affects not only the victim but others as well. When people die by suicide, their family and friends often experience shock, anger, guilt, and depression. If you or someone you know is showing any of these warning signs and may be at risk of suicide, get help immediately from a parent, teacher, or trusted adult. If you think someone is in immediate danger of harming himself or herself, do not leave the person alone. The National Suicide Prevention Lifeline is a free and confidential hotline where you can call for help at 1–800-273-TALK (8255). Learn more about the lifeline by watching the videos offered on their website: http://suicidepreventionlifeline.org/stories/.

Obsessive-Compulsive and Related Disorders

Obsessive-Compulsive Disorder

Everyone has routines, and we often double-check that we did something we were supposed to, like going back to make sure we locked our car or sent out an email. People who feel the need to check things or repeatedly engage in certain routines may have **obsessive-compulsive disorder (OCD)**.

obsessive-compulsive disorder (OCD) A disorder in which an individual has either obsessions, compulsions, or both; obsessions are recurrent and persistent thoughts, urges, or images that are intrusive and unwanted and cause anxiety and distress. In an attempt to reduce distress, an individual may perform compulsions, which consist of repetitive behaviors that are clearly excessive.

You may have seen characters on television, such as the main character in *Monk*, who exhibit these features. We still are not sure what causes OCD, but like other mental disorders, it is likely a combination of genetics, differences in the brain, and the environment. To be diagnosed with OCD, an individual must have either obsessions, compulsions, or both.[44] According to the *DSM*, obsessions are recurrent and persistent thoughts, urges, or images that are intrusive and unwanted and cause anxiety and distress. In an attempt to reduce distress, an individual may perform compulsions, which consist of repetitive behaviors (e.g., hand washing, ordering, checking) or mental acts (e.g., praying, counting, repeating words silently) that are clearly excessive. To meet the diagnosis, obsessions and compulsions must be time-consuming or cause significant distress or impairment in functioning. Other causes of obsessive-compulsive symptoms, such as drug abuse, medication, medical conditions, or other mental disorders, must be ruled out in order to give a proper diagnosis.

People with OCD try to avoid triggers for their compulsions, such as staying away from public places to avoid germs. The time spent on obsessive thinking or engaging in routines creates a reduced quality of life. If OCD develops at a young age, children may experience developmental problems, such as not having an active social life. About 1.2% of adults have OCD; the condition affects females slightly more often than males. Psychotherapy and medication, most commonly antianxiety medications and antidepressants, are prescribed as treatment.[84]

Body Dysmorphic Disorder

Think about the last time you looked in a mirror and thought, "Damn, I look fabulous!" Turn on the television, open a magazine, or pull up almost any social media site. You don't have to go far to be inundated with messages promoting weight loss. Our society's obsession with skinny began at the turn of the 20th century and continues today. Despite these messages, there has been a

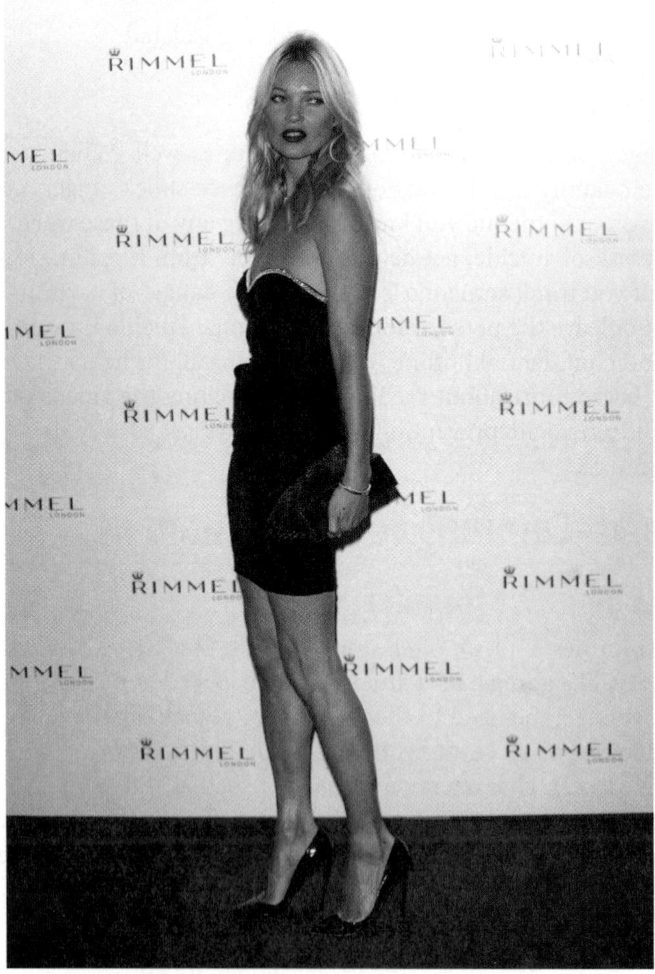

Kate Moss, an English model who rose to fame in the 1990s, has been quoted as saying, "Nothing tastes as good as skinny feels."

© Featureflash Photo Agency/Shutterstock.

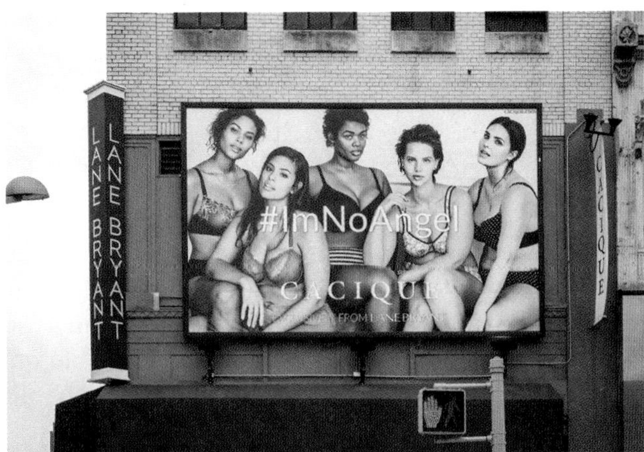

Lane Bryant, a retailer for "plus-size" clothing, took on Victoria's Secret "Angel" advertisements with their "I'm No Angel" campaign.

© Richard Levine/Alamy Stock Photo.

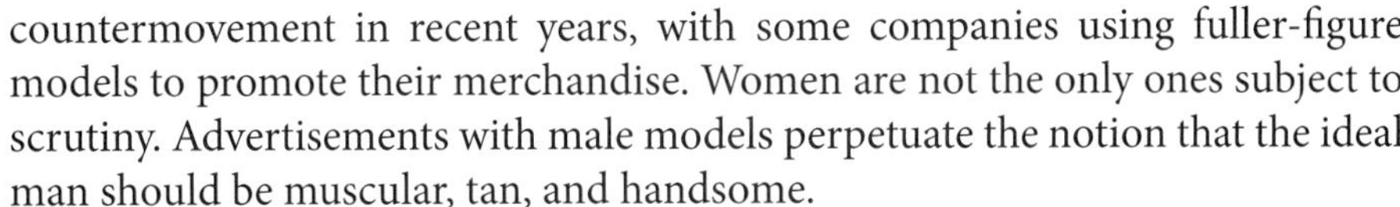

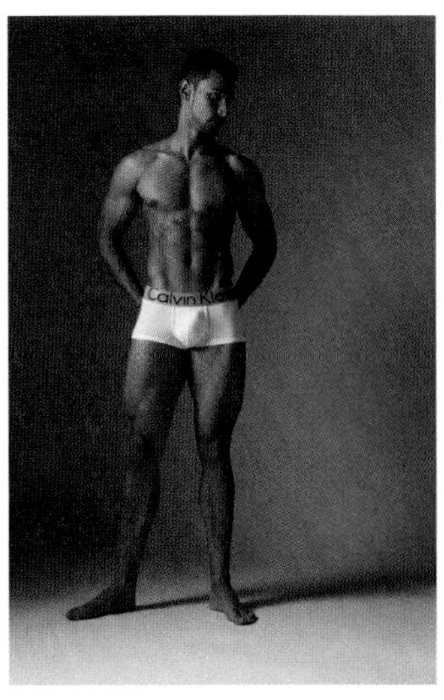

An example of a photo found in a Calvin Klein ad.

© Dan Galic / Alamy Stock

countermovement in recent years, with some companies using fuller-figure models to promote their merchandise. Women are not the only ones subject to scrutiny. Advertisements with male models perpetuate the notion that the ideal man should be muscular, tan, and handsome.

Many of us struggle with having a healthy body image and are overly critical of our bodies and appearance. For some people, however, their appearance is an obsession that significantly impacts their daily lives. The most extreme form of obsession about one's appearance and perceived flaws is called **body dysmorphic disorder**, also called "imagined ugliness."[85] Despite being prevalent for a long time, research on body dysmorphic disorder has only gained traction in the last few decades. The causes of body dysmorphic disorder are unknown.

body dysmorphic disorder A disorder in which a person becomes preoccupied with perceived flaws in physical appearance that other people may not notice or consider to be an issue, which escalates to a point that the individual performs repetitive behaviors or mental acts that cause distress or impairment in functioning.

DSM criteria state that people with body dysmorphic disorder are preoccupied with perceived flaws in physical appearance that other people may not notice or consider to be an issue. The preoccupation escalates to a point that the individual performs repetitive behaviors or mental acts (similar to OCD) that cause distress or impairment in functioning. This preoccupation is not better explained by concerns with body fat or weight in an individual whose symptoms meet the criteria for an eating disorder.[44] The most common areas of focus are the skin, hair, and nose.

About 2.4% of adults in the United States have body dysmorphic disorder, with little difference by gender. One form of body dysmorphic disorder is muscle dysmorphia, which is the preoccupation with the perception that one's body is too small or not sufficiently muscular. Muscle dysmorphia occurs almost entirely in men and may lead to excessive dieting and exercise, and, in some cases, taking steroids or other dangerous substances to enhance muscle building.[44]

It is common for individuals with body dysmorphic disorder to have delusions that other people are mocking their appearance or taking special notice of how they look. It is associated with anxiety, social avoidance, depression, and other mental health issues. People with this disorder seldom express their obsessions or worry over their appearance to others.

Not surprisingly, people with body dysmorphia have abnormalities in their visual processing, tending to process details but not the more holistic aspects of something.[44] The primary treatment is CBT. No medications are approved for treating body dysmorphic disorder, but antidepressants are sometimes used to manage symptoms. In extreme cases, people with body dysmorphic disorder can become a danger to themselves and must be hospitalized in a psychiatric facility.[86]

Eating Disorders

People "diet" all of the time to lose weight and feel better. (See Chapter 2 to learn about why strict "dieting" [versus eating healthy] isn't the best approach to a healthy lifestyle.) For some people, though, eating can become a serious problem. An eating disorder may exist when regular disruptions to one's everyday eating occur, such as eating very small amounts of food or extreme overeating. Science is still not clear on what causes eating disorders, but researchers are investigating how genes, the environment, and differences in brain activity may all play a role. Treatment involves psychotherapy, usually CBT. No medication is designed specifically to treat an eating disorder, but use of fluoxetine (brand name Prozac) has been successful in some patients.[87] Often dentists are the first to notice signs of eating disorders because of oral health complications, such as erosion and lesions due to frequent vomiting or deficiencies in key nutrients.[88] Here we discuss three of the most common types of eating disorders: anorexia, bulimia, and binge eating. Learn more about diagnosis and treatment of eating disorders by viewing this documentary: http://www.pbs.org/wgbh/nova/body/dying-to-be-thin.html.

anorexia nervosa An eating disorder characterized by restriction of energy intake to the point of resulting in significantly low body weight; fear of gaining weight; and inability to recognize that perceptions of their body are out of touch with reality and that they are putting themselves in danger due to their low body weight.

Anorexia Nervosa

Anorexia nervosa, often referred to simply as anorexia, is an eating disorder in which individuals restrict energy (i.e., food) intake to the point of having significantly low body weight, fear gaining weight, and are unable to recognize that their perceptions of their bodies are out of touch with reality and that they are putting themselves in danger due to their low body weight.[44]

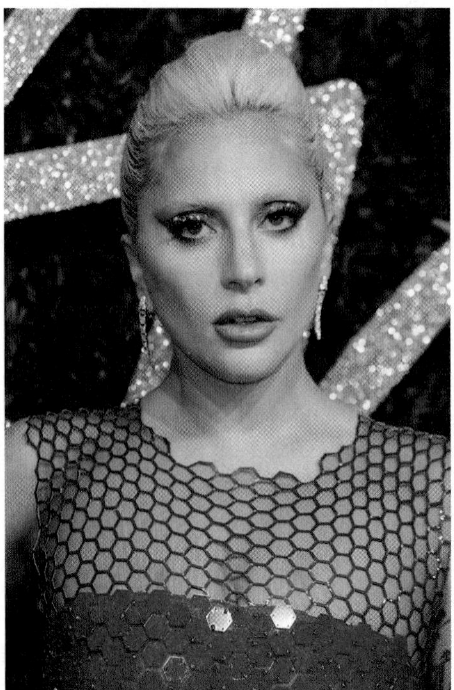

Pop star and singer Lady Gaga has spoken publicly about her struggles with anorexia and bulimia.

Most people with anorexia do not think they have a problem. In fact, they perceive themselves as overweight even though they may be dangerously thin. It is usually their family or friends who seek professional help out of concern for the individual. Some features of anorexia include a strong desire to control one's environment, avoiding eating in public, and excessive physical activity. Anorexia can lead to many physical problems, including malnutrition, heart problems, bone density loss, and kidney problems. Women may experience amenorrhea (absence of a menstrual period), and men may experience decreased testosterone.[44,89] In severe cases, anorexia can lead to cardiac arrest and sudden death (**FIGURE 6-4**).[90] Many of these problems can be largely (but not entirely) reversed with proper treatment and restoration of healthy eating habits. People with anorexia often exhibit signs of other mental health issues, such as depression, obsessive-compulsive features, and insomnia.

Some people think of anorexia as a "rich White girl's disease." However, this disease afflicts females and males of all racial backgrounds, ages, and income levels.[91] Among adolescents 13 to 18 years of age, the lifetime prevalence is about 0.3% for both males and females.[92] Among adults 18 years and older, about 1% of women and 0.3% of men report ever having anorexia in their lifetime.[93]

The priority in treating someone with anorexia is restoring the person to a healthy weight with adequate nutrition. Doing so involves treating the underlying psychological issues related to the disorder and trying to eliminate the behaviors associated with restricted eating. This is often done with

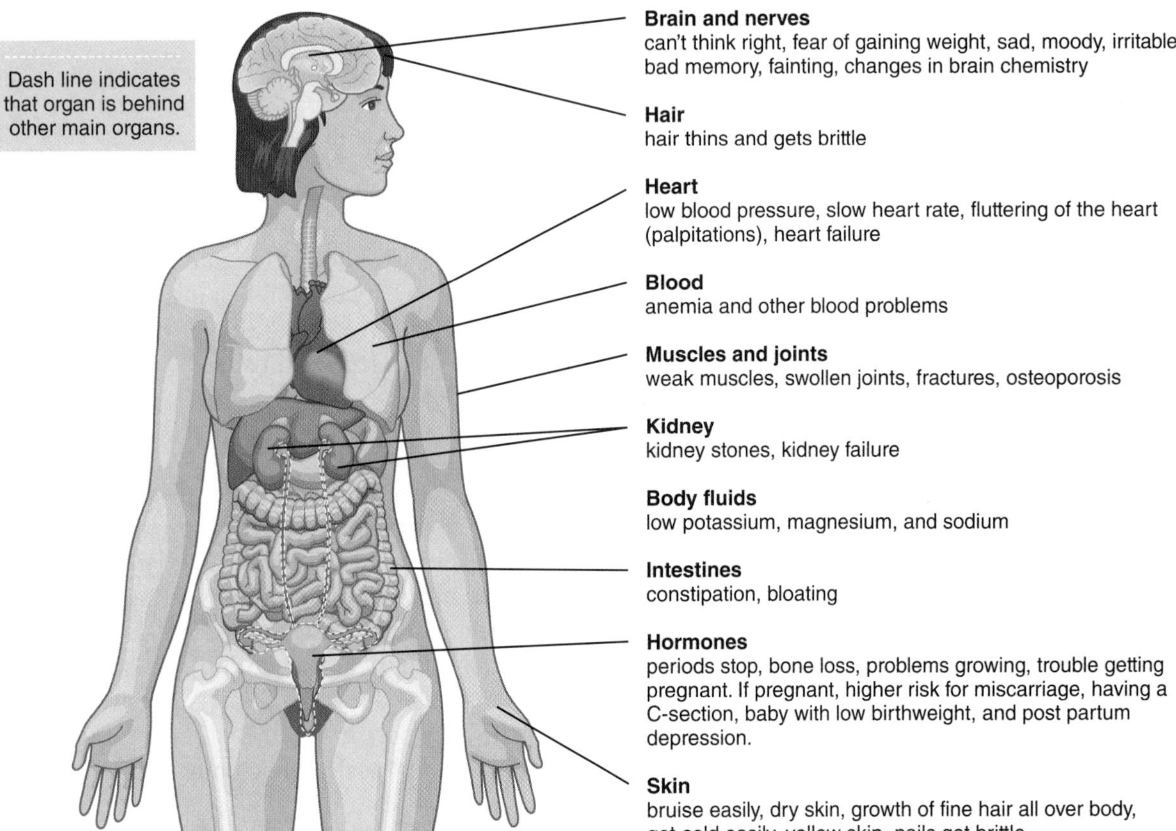

FIGURE 6-4 Anorexia affects every part of a person's life.

Smith, M., & Segal J. (2018). Anorexia nervosa: Signs, symptoms, causes, and treatment. Helpguide.org. Retrieved from http://www.helpguide.org/articles/eating-disorders/anorexia-nervosa.htm

psychotherapy. Medications, such as antidepressants, are sometimes prescribed, but no specific medication is approved to treat anorexia.[94] Current research is studying brain function, genetics, behavior, and environment to understand more about what causes eating disorders, to develop more effective treatment.[95]

bulimia nervosa An eating disorder characterized by binging and purging (inappropriate compensatory behavior designed to prevent weight gain from the excessive eating).

Bulimia Nervosa

Bulimia nervosa—or simply, bulimia—is another eating disorder and is characterized by two behaviors: binging and purging.

According to the *DSM* criteria, binging refers to eating large quantities of food in a discrete period, exceeding what most people would eat under similar circumstances, and feeling a lack of control with respect to eating during that episode. Purging consists of inappropriate compensatory behavior designed to prevent weight gain from the excessive eating, such as self-induced vomiting; misuse of laxatives, diuretics, or other medications; fasting; or excessive exercise.[44]

There is a spectrum from mild to extreme bulimia, characterized by how often one engages in "inappropriate compensatory behavior" such as self-induced vomiting. Bulimia is sometimes thought of as the opposite of anorexia because the person binge eats and then engages in self-induced vomiting or overuse of laxatives or diuretics. Like anorexia, bulimia has serious health consequences, including amenorrhea, gastrointestinal problems, and heart problems.[44]

BY THE NUMBERS

Bulimia

Bulimia is more common than anorexia among adults age 18 years and older, with 1.5% of women and 0.5% of men reporting ever having bulimia.[93] The lifetime prevalence of bulimia in adolescents 13 to 18 years of age is 0.9%, with rates of 0.5% among males and 1.3% among females.[92]

Like anorexia, bulimia is treated by psychotherapy and sometimes prescription medication, such as an SSRI. CBT focuses on helping people identify distorted beliefs related to their weight and replacing this pattern with more productive ways of thinking, to promote healthier eating habits.[94]

binge eating disorder An eating disorder characterized by binging (eating large quantities of food, in a discrete period of time, without having control over one's eating during that episode).

Binge Eating Disorder

Even more common than anorexia or bulimia is **binge eating disorder**. Unlike those disorders, however, purging or control of body weight are not features of binge eating. Similar to bulimia, binge eating consists of eating large quantities of food in a discrete period, without having control over one's eating during that episode. In addition, binge eating includes eating faster than normal, until feeling uncomfortably full, when not physically hungry, and alone due to embarrassment. Binge eaters feel disgusted with themselves, depressed, or guilty afterward.[44]

Binge eaters often conceal their behaviors from others. Binge eating disorder can run in families and occurs in individuals of any body weight (normal, overweight, and obese). Triggers of binge eating include stress, negative feelings about one's body weight, and boredom. Binge eating may indicate an early phase of another eating disorder. It is associated with lower reported health-related quality of life and satisfaction and with weight gain.[44]

BY THE NUMBERS

Binge Eating Disorder

Of adolescents age 13 to 18 years, 1.6% have binge eating disorder. It is significantly more prevalent among females.[86] Among adults 18 years and older, the lifetime prevalence is 2.8%.[93] As with the other eating disorders discussed, treatment involves CBT and sometimes medication.[94]

Neurodevelopmental Disorders

Neurodevelopmental disorders are those that arise during the developmental stage of life (early childhood through adolescence). There are over a dozen neurodevelopmental disorders, ranging from specific to broad impairments, but they all affect one's ability to function socially, in school, or at work. Here we will discuss two of the more common neurodevelopmental disorders—autism and attention deficit hyperactivity disorder.[44]

Autism Spectrum Disorder

The features of **autism spectrum disorder (ASD)** include a continued deficiency in social interaction and restricted patterns of behavior that occur early (often in the first 2 years of life). The spectrum refers to the range of symptoms and impairments that a child with ASD may exhibit (**FIGURE 6-5**). What causes autism? This question has plagued scientists since autism was first identified. It is still not exactly clear, but genetics and environment both seem to play a role. Most likely there are many genetic and environmental factors that contribute to ASD, not just one. Scientists are studying how factors such as parental age and complications during pregnancy may affect ASD. (See Chapter 8 to learn about a fabricated study that scared parents into thinking vaccines caused autism.)

autism spectrum disorder (ASD) A spectrum of disorders that includes a continued deficiency in social interaction and restricted patterns of behavior that occur early in life.

In the most recent version of the *DSM*, previous diagnoses of autistic disorder, Asperger disorder, childhood integrative disorder, and pervasive development disorder not otherwise specified are now grouped under ASD.[96] A person with ASD has persistent deficits in social communication and social interaction

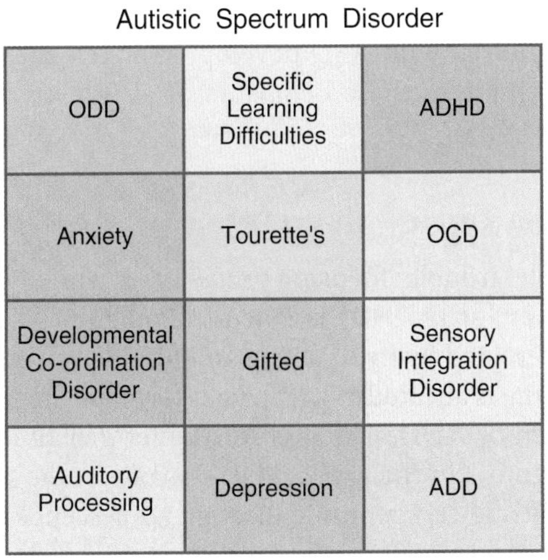

Autistic Spectrum Disorder

ODD	Specific Learning Difficulties	ADHD
Anxiety	Tourette's	OCD
Developmental Co-ordination Disorder	Gifted	Sensory Integration Disorder
Auditory Processing	Depression	ADD

FIGURE 6-5 Autism spectrum disorder is a brain disorder that consists of a range of various symptoms.

Data from Hanselman, J. (2014, August 14). Exploring autism spectrum disorders. Retrieved from http://wvxu.org/post/exploring-autism-spectrum-disorders#stream/0

across multiple contexts. Some examples of these deficits include inability to hold normal back-and-forth conversations, failure to initiate or respond to social interactions, lack of eye contact, inability to understand or use body language or gestures, lack of facial expressions, absence of interest in peers, and difficulty adjusting behavior to suit the social context.

Another prominent symptom of ASD has to do with restricted, repetitive patterns of behavior, interests, or activities. These patterns may include stereotyped or repetitive motor movements, use of objects, or speech; insistence on sameness, inflexible adherence to routines, or ritualized patterns of verbal or nonverbal behavior; highly restricted, fixated interests that are abnormal in intensity or focus; and hyper- or hyporeactivity to sensory input or unusual interest in sensory aspects of the environment. Symptoms of ASD begin to manifest in the early developmental period and cause significant impairment in social, occupational, or other important areas of current functioning. It is important to rule out other potential causes, such as intellectual disability or global developmental delay.

BY THE NUMBERS

Autism Spectrum Disorder

About 1% of children have autism spectrum disorder. The prevalence has increased over time, but it is not clear whether this finding represents an actual increase in the disorder's prevalence or reflects changes in how we define ASD or an increased awareness of the disorder.[44] Boys are 4 to 5 times more likely to be diagnosed with ASD than are girls. A diagnosis of ASD can be made as early as 2 years of age.[22]

There is currently no approved medication specifically to treat ASD. Medications, though, are sometimes used to manage related symptoms, such as depression or anxiety. Two antipsychotics are approved to manage some of the symptoms of ASD, such as aggression. Because children are often young at the time of diagnosis and may be nonverbal, traditional psychotherapy does not make sense as a treatment. Instead, "early intervention" programs that include intensive behavioral therapy are recommended. The most popular type of behavioral therapy is applied behavior analysis. Applied behavior analysis is an intensive therapy, usually one-on-one sessions with the teacher and child, that helps children with ASD develop positive behaviors like speaking and playing and reinforces these behaviors; it also helps to reduce negative behaviors.[22]

Attention Deficit Hyperactivity Disorder

It's normal to have trouble focusing once in a while. **Attention deficit hyperactivity disorder (ADHD)** is when the inability to pay attention persists, possibly exacerbated by hyperactive and impulsive behavior, to the point that daily functioning is affected.[44] The former term for this disorder was attention deficit disorder, or ADD, which is still sometimes used today despite no longer being a diagnosis in the *DSM*. ADHD is one of the most common disorders in childhood and can continue through adolescence and adulthood. As with other mental disorders, it is not entirely clear what causes ADHD, but it appears to run in families. Scientists are studying other potential contributing factors such as nutrition, maternal behaviors during pregnancy (like smoking and drinking alcohol), and brain injuries. The newest research is studying the

attention deficit hyperactivity disorder (ADHD) A disorder in which the inability to pay attention and/or hyperactive and impulsive behavior is persistent and affects daily functioning.

potential of food additives causing ADHD. Despite popular beliefs that sugar consumption contributes to ADHD, thus far study results have not supported this notion.[97]

People with ADHD have a persistent pattern of inattention and/or hyperactivity and impulsivity that interferes with functioning or development. The *DSM* specifies that inattentive behavior can include failure to notice details, difficulty remaining focused and being easily distracted, lack of attention when being spoken to directly, inability to follow through on instructions or complete tasks and forgetfulness, difficulty organizing tasks and activities and poor time management, and tendency to lose things. Hyperactive and impulsive behavior can include fidgeting or squirming, inability to stay in one place for extended periods, inability to play or engage in leisure activities quietly, excessive talking, tendency to interrupt people, and inability to wait one's turn. To be diagnosed with ADHD, the symptoms must have presented prior to 12 years of age in multiple settings and interfere with functioning. Again, it is important to rule out other mental disorders that can cause similar symptoms, such as schizophrenia, mood disorders, personality disorders, and substance abuse.[44] Pharmaceutical companies and even some doctors have been accused of promoting ADHD diagnosis and treatment when all of the diagnostic criteria are not met.[98]

About 5% of children have ADHD, and 2.5% of adults.[44] ADHD is commonly treated with a class of medications called stimulants. It sounds counterintuitive, but stimulants actually can have a calming effect in children with ADHD. Psychotherapy is also recommended.[97]

Addiction and Substance Use

Substance-related disorders are also considered mental illnesses and have specific *DSM* criteria for diagnosis. They encompass 10 distinct classes of drugs, including alcohol, cannabis, caffeine, and tobacco. Substance use often co-occurs with other mental illnesses, as the substance is often used as a mechanism to self-medicate. (See Chapter 7 for more information.)

Mental Illness Affects You, Your Family, Your Community, and Beyond

Even though individuals with a mental disorder sometimes may have trouble appreciating it, having a mental disorder does not affect only the person with the disorder. Often those afflicted need to rely on their families, particularly for serious mental disorders that impair daily functioning. As such, the weight of managing the disorder may be borne by a person's entire household or support system.

Recently, professionals have recognized that entire communities can be thought of as at risk for mental health problems. Research suggests that being displaced can impact one's health. *Root shock* is "the traumatic stress reaction to the loss of some or all of one's emotional ecosystem."[99] When communities are forced out of where they live, to allow for wealthier individuals to move in, and lose their social capital, jobs, and livelihood, it causes stress and adversely affects health.[99,100] In addition to community-level displacement, persistent exposure to violence may predispose entire communities to ill health effects, including mental health disorders, such as depression, PTSD, and anxiety.

We mentioned earlier that mental illness does not discriminate, and that's true. Any person of any background can have a mental disorder. But certain disorders, like PTSD, may be more influenced by the environment, and certain communities may be at greater risk. Gang violence is more common in low-income neighborhoods, as is displacement due to gentrification (when wealthier people arrive in an urban area and the cost of living subsequently increases). Chronic stress is another problem in communities of color and low-income communities. When it is difficult to make ends meet, medical bills pile up, and when a person is persistently discriminated against because of the color of his or her skin, stress endures. As noted previously, stress can trigger or worsen symptoms of a mental disorder. When entire groups of people are at disproportionate risk for an adverse health outcome, it becomes a real public health problem. Policies to alleviate the root causes of health disparities, such as violence within a community, are needed to produce a lasting impact on mental health and well-being at the population level.

The Trouble With Mental Health Care

People with a serious mental health illness die 25 years earlier than the general population. These premature deaths are not a result of mental illness itself but of preventable and treatable medical conditions like smoking, access to care, and substance use.[101] The mental healthcare system in the United States has been plagued with problems throughout history. Almost $130 billion is allocated from the federal government to be applied to mental health care, but only a small portion of that actually benefits those with mental health disorders.[102] Mental health care was expanded under the Patient Protection and Affordable Care Act (ACA), also known as "Obamacare," which now requires that most individual and small employer insurance plans cover mental health care and substance use services (**FIGURE 6-6**).[103] (See Chapter 13 for more information about the ACA.) In addition, under the Mental Health Parity and Addiction Equity Act of 2008, the money paid out of pocket and treatment limitations, like number of visits, must be the same for mental health or substance use services as they are for any other medical benefits offered by that plan.[104]

This recent legislation is a good start in helping more people obtain access to quality mental health care, but many barriers to care remain. Being allowed to get treatment is not the same as actually getting treatment. There may be a limited number of mental health providers accepting new patients, and those who are may not accept the person's type of insurance. Finding quality mental health providers, even with what is considered "good" insurance, is difficult. The stigma associated with having a mental illness also prevents some people from seeking treatment to help manage their illness. In addition, a significant challenge in managing brain disorders like schizophrenia or bipolar disorder is that some people do not believe they have a problem. This situation is known as anosognosia (lack of insight), which is thought to be one of the biggest reasons why many of the people with these illnesses do not seek out or comply with treatment.[105] To protect those with serious mental disorders, the criteria for involuntary treatment are very stringent. Thus, it is exceedingly difficult to get treatment for someone who refuses it. For those who do want help, they may experience problems of insufficient number of available beds and other issues with access to quality mental health care. Hopefully, future policies can address these barriers and provide people seeking treatment with the high-quality mental health care they deserve.

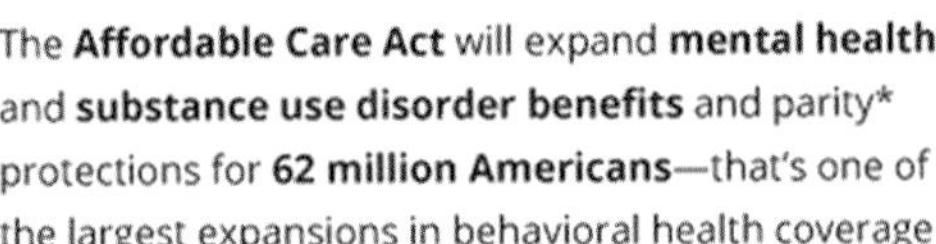
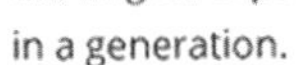

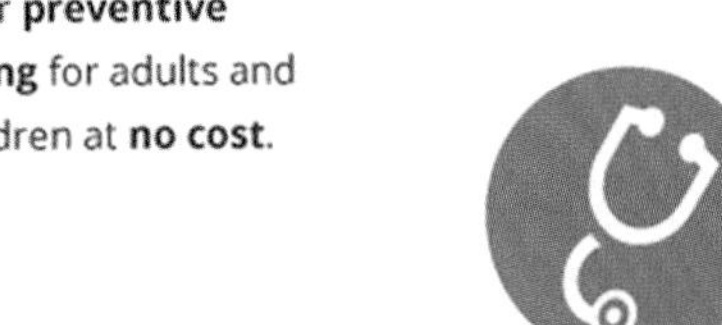
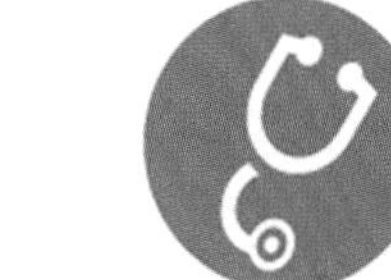

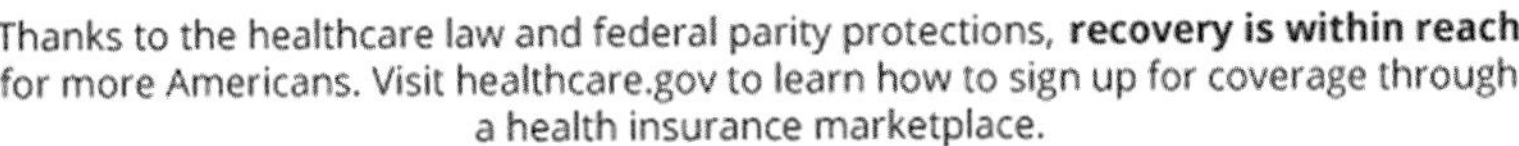

FIGURE 6-6 How does the Affordable Care Act help mental health services?

Health Insurance and Mental Health Services. (n.d.). Retrieved April 02, 2018, from https://www.mentalhealth.gov/get-help/health-insurance

In Summary

Scientists still have much to learn about the causes of mental disorders. We know that a combination of brain activity, genetics, and the environment may play a role. Currently, most mental disorders are treated with a combination of medication and psychotherapy. As science advances, hopefully we will understand more about how the brain works, to develop methods for early detection and intervention before behavioral symptoms begin and start to affect someone's life. In the meantime, continued successes to advance access to quality mental health care are needed.

Key Terms

anorexia nervosa
attention deficit hyperactivity disorder (ADHD)
autism spectrum disorder (ASD)
binge eating disorder
bipolar disorder
body dysmorphic disorder
borderline personality disorder
bulimia nervosa
defense mechanisms
depression
generalized anxiety disorder
mental health
mental illness
obsessive-compulsive disorder (OCD)
panic disorder
paranoid personality disorder
posttraumatic stress disorder (PTSD)
schizophrenia
self-injury
stigma
suicide

Student Discussion Questions and Activities

1. What are some of the barriers to seeking (and maintaining) treatment for a mental disorder?
2. Why do you think women have twice the risk of having an anxiety disorder compared to men?
3. What are some of the ways (including those that may not be thought of as healthy) in which you manage stress in your own life?
4. What are some ways we can work to reduce stigma associated with having a mental disorder? Should we change the language we use to refer to mental illness?
5. Why are certain communities at higher risk of developing mental health problems?

Resources

National Suicide Prevention Lifeline (free and confidential): www.suicidepreventionlifeline.org, 1–800-273-TALK (8255)

National Institute of Mental Health (a source of information about mental illness): www.nimh.nih.gov

National Alliance on Mental Illness (a resource for family and friends of someone with a mental illness): www.nami.org

References

1. World Health Organization. (2003). WHO definition of health. Retrieved from http://www.who.int/about/definition/en/print.html
2. Centers for Disease Control and Prevention. (2013). Well-being concepts: How is well-being defined? Health Related Quality of life (HRQOL). Retrieved from http://www.cdc.gov/hrqol/wellbeing.htm#three
3. Centers for Disease Control and Prevention. (2013). Well-being concepts: Why is well-being useful for public health? Health Related Quality of Life (HRQOL). Retrieved from http://www.cdc.gov/hrqol/wellbeing.htm#two
4. World Health Organization. (2014). Mental health: Strengthening our response. Fact sheet no. 220. Retrieved from http://www.who.int/mediacentre/factsheets/fs220/en/
5. Centers for Disease Control and Prevention. (2011). Mental health basics. Retrieved from http://www.cdc.gov/mentalhealth/basics.htm
6. Department of Health and Human Services, Substance Abuse and Mental Health Services Administration. (1999). Mental health: A report of the Surgeon General. Retrieved from https://profiles.nlm.nih.gov/ps/retrieve/ResourceMetadata/NNBBHS

7. Mental Health Foundation. (n.d.). How to look after your mental health. Retrieved from https://www.mentalhealth.org.uk/publications/how-to-mental-health
8. Holmes, L. (2015, December 17). Sixteen ways to improve your mental health in 2016. *Health Living*. Retrieved from http://www.huffingtonpost.com/entry/how-to-improve-mental-health_us_56684e10e4b0f290e52154ba
9. American Psychiatric Association. (2015). *Diagnostic and statistical manual of mental disorders (DSM-5): Explore the DSM-5*. Retrieved from http://www.psychiatry.org/practice/dsm
10. McCarron, R. M. (2013). The *DSM-5* and the art of medicine: Certainly uncertain. *Annals of Internal Medicine, 159*(5), 360–361.
11. American Psychiatric Association. (2015). *DSM* history. Retrieved from http://www.psychiatry.org/psychiatrists/practice/dsm/history
12. American Psychiatric Association. (2014). *DSM-5* overview: The future manual. Retrieved from http://www.dsm5.org/about/Pages/DSMVOverview.aspx
13. Centers for Disease Control and Prevention. (2011). CDC report: Mental illness surveillance among adults in the United States. Retrieved from http://www.cdc.gov/mentalhealthsurveillance/fact_sheet.html
14. Centers for Disease Control and Prevention. (2011). Mental illness surveillance among adults in the United States. *Morbidity and Mortality Weekly Reports, 60*(3), 1–32.
15. PBS. (1999). Timeline: Treatments for mental illness. Retrieved from http://www.pbs.org/wgbh/amex/nash/timeline
16. U.S. National Library of Medicine. (2006). Diseases of the mind: Highlights of American psychiatry through 1900. National Institutes of Health. Retrieved from http://www.nlm.nih.gov/hmd/diseases/early.html
17. National Institute of Mental Health. (2015). Mental health medications. National Institutes of Health. Retrieved from http://www.nimh.nih.gov/health/topics/mental-health-medications/mental-health-medications.shtml
18. National Institute of Mental Health. (2015). Anxiety disorders. National Institutes of Health. Retrieved from http://www.nimh.nih.gov/health/topics/panic-disorder/index.shtml
19. Food and Drug Administration. (2012). A guide to drug safety terms at FDA. Retrieved from http://www.fda.gov/downloads/ForConsumers/ConsumerUpdates/UCM107976.pdf
20. National Institute of Mental Health. (2015). Psychotherapies. National Institutes of Health. Retrieved from http://www.nimh.nih.gov/health/topics/psychotherapies/index.shtml
21. Mayo Clinic. (2014). Mental health providers: Tips on finding one. Retrieved from http://www.mayoclinic.org/diseases-conditions/mental-illness/in-depth/mental-health-providers/art-20045530?pg=1
22. National Institute of Mental Health. (2015). Autism spectrum disorder. National Institutes of Health. Retrieved from http://www.nimh.nih.gov/health/topics/autism-spectrum-disorders-asd/index.shtml
23. American Psychological Association. (2014). Incarceration nation. Retrieved from http://www.apa.org/monitor/2014/10/incarceration.aspx
24. James, D. J., & Glaze, L. E. (2006). Mental health problems of prison and jail inmates. Bureau of Justice Statistics. Retrieved from http://www.bjs.gov/content/pub/pdf/mhppji.pdf
25. Torrey, E. F., Kennard, A. D., Eslinger, D., Lamb, R., & Pavle, J. (2010). More mentally ill persons are in jails and prisons than hospitals: A survey of the states. Treatment Advocacy Center. Retrieved from http://www.treatmentadvocacycenter.org/storage/documents/final_jails_v_hospitals_study.pdf
26. Treatment Advocacy Center. (2012). No room at the inn: Trends and consequences of closing public psychiatric hospitals. Retrieved from http://www.treatmentadvocacycenter.org/storage/documents/no_room_at_the_inn-2012.pdf
27. Corrigan, P. W., & Watson, A. C. (2002). Understanding the impact of stigma on people with mental illness. *World Psychiatry, 1*(1), 16–20.
28. Clement, S., Schauman, O., Graham, T., Maggioni, F., Evans-Lacko, S., Bezborodovs, N., Thornicroft, G. (2015). What is the impact of mental health-related stigma on help-seeking? A systematic review of quantitative and qualitative studies. *Psychological Medicine, 45*(1), 11–27.
29. National Institute of Mental Health. (2013). Director's update: Mental disorders as brain disorders: Thomas Insel at TEDx-Caltech. National Institutes of Health. Retrieved from https://content.govdelivery.com/accounts/USNIMH/bulletins/77d777
30. Department of Health and Human Services, Office for Civil Rights. (2015). Your health information privacy rights. Department of Health and Human Services. Retrieved from https://www.hhs.gov/sites/default/files/ocr/privacy/hipaa/understanding/consumers/consumer_rights.pdf
31. Gold, J. (2014). Privacy law frustrates parents of mentally ill adult children. National Public Radio. Retrieved from http://www.npr.org/sections/health-shots/2014/06/04/318765929/privacy-law-frustrates-parents-of-mentally-ill-adult-children
32. Keaten, J. (2015, June 11). Prosecutor: Co-pilot who crashed Germanwings jet feared blindness, sought doctors' help. *U.S. News and World Report*. Retrieved from http://www.huffingtonpost.com/2015/06/11/germanwings-copilot-blindness-health-lubitz_n_7562258.html
33. National Institute of Mental Health. (2015). Adult stress: Frequently asked questions. National Institutes of Health. Retrieved from https://www.nimh.nih.gov/health/publications/stress/Stress_Factsheet_LN_142898.pdf
34. National Institute of Mental Health. (2015). Stress and your health. National Institutes of Health. Retrieved from http://www.nlm.nih.gov/medlineplus/ency/article/003211.htm
35. Hall-Flavin, D. K. (2014). Can chronic stress cause depression? Mayo Clinic. Retrieved from http://www.mayoclinic.org/healthy-lifestyle/stress-management/expert-answers/stress/faq-20058233
36. American Psychological Association. (n.d.). Fact sheet: Health disparities and stress. Retrieved from http://www.apa.org/topics/health-disparities/fact-sheet-stress.aspx
37. McLeod, S. (2009). Defense mechanisms. SimplyPsychology website. Retrieved from https://www.simplypsychology.org/defense-mechanisms.html
38. National Institute of Mental Health. (2008). A night's sleep gives emotional memories their staying power. National Institutes of Health. Retrieved from http://www.nimh.nih.gov/news/science-news/2008/a-nights-sleep-gives-emotional-memories-their-staying-power.shtml
39. National Institute of Mental Health. (2014). Brain basics: Understanding sleep. National Institutes of Health. Retrieved from http://www.ninds.nih.gov/disorders/brain_basics/understanding_sleep.htm
40. Roth, T. (2007). Insomnia: Definition, prevalence, etiology, and consequences. *Journal of Clinical Sleep Medicine*, 3(5

Suppl), S7–S10. Retrieved from https://www.ncbi.nlm.nih.gov/pmc/articles/PMC1978319/

41. Stanford Health Care. (n.d.). Treating insomnia with medications. Retrieved from https://stanfordhealthcare.org/medical-conditions/sleep/insomnia/treatments/treating-insomnia-with-medications.html
42. Harvard Health Publications. (2009). Sleep and mental health. Harvard Medical School. Retrieved from http://www.health.harvard.edu/newsletter_article/Sleep-and-mental-health
43. Kessler, R. C., Berglund, P. F., Demler, O. F., Jin, R., Merikangas, K. R., & Walters, E. E. (2005). Lifetime prevalence and age-of-onset distributions of *DSM-IV* disorders in the National Comorbidity Survey Replication. *Archives of General Psychiatry, 62*(6), 593–602.
44. American Psychiatric Association. (2013). *Diagnostic and statistical manual of mental disorder* (5th ed.). Washington, DC: Author.
45. Kessler, R. C., Petukhova M., Sampson, N. A., Zaslavsky, A. M., & Wittchen, H.-U. (2012). Twelve-month and lifetime prevalence and lifetime morbid risk of anxiety and mood disorders in the United States. *International Journal of Methods in Psychiatric Research, 21*(3), 169–184.
46. National Institute of Mental Health. (2015). Anxiety disorder. National Institutes of Health. Retrieved from http://www.nimh.nih.gov/health/topics/generalized-anxiety-disorder-gad/index.shtml
47. Lewis-Fernandez, R., Hinton, D. E., Laria, A. J., Patterson, E. H., Hofmann, S. G., Craske M. G.,... Liao, B. (2010). Culture and the anxiety disorders: Recommendations for *DSM-V*. *Depression and Anxiety, 27*(2), 212–219.
48. Craske, M. G., Kircanski, K. F., Epstein, A. F., Wittchen, H.-U., Pine, D. S., Lewis-Fernandez, R., . . . *DSM-V* Anxiety, OC Spectrum, Posttraumatic and Dissociative Disorder Work Group. (2010). Panic disorder: A review of *DSM-IV* panic disorder and proposals for *DSM-V*. *Depression and Anxiety,* 1–20.
49. Ham, P., Waters, D. B., & Oliver, M. N. (2005). Treatment of panic disorder. *American Family Physician, 71*(4), 733–739.
50. Anxiety and Depression Association of America. (2010). Treatment. Retrieved from http://www.adaa.org/finding-help/treatment
51. National Institute of Mental Health. (2015). Post-traumatic stress disorder (PTSD). National Institutes of Health. Retrieved from http://www.nimh.nih.gov/health/topics/post-traumatic-stress-disorder-ptsd/index.shtml
52. Babbel, S. (2013, March 12). Trauma: Childhood sexual abuse. Sexual abuse can lead to post-traumatic stress disorder (PTSD). *Psychology Today*. Retrieved from https://www.psychologytoday.com/blog/somatic-psychology/201303/trauma-childhood-sexual-abuse
53. Crocq, M. A., & Crocq, L. (2000). From shell shock and war neurosis to posttraumatic stress disorder: A history of psychotraumatology. *Dialogues in Clinical Neuroscience, 2*(1), 47–55.
54. American Psychiatric Association. (2013). Posttraumatic stress disorder. Retrieved from http://www.dsm5.org/Documents/PTSD%20Fact%20Sheet.pdf
55. Kilpatrick, D. G., Resnick, H. S., Milanak, M. E., Miller, M. W., Keyes, K. M., & Friedman, M. J. (2013). National estimates of exposure to traumatic events and PTSD prevalence using *DSM-IV* and *DSM-5* criteria. *Journal of Traumatic Stress, 26*(5), 537–547.
56. Gradus, J. L. (2014). Epidemiology of PTSD. U.S. Department of Veterans Affairs. Retrieved from http://www.ptsd.va.gov/professional/PTSD-overview/epidemiological-facts-ptsd.asp
57. American Psychological Association. (2018). Eye movement desensitization and reprocessing (EMDR) therapy. Retrieved from http://www.apa.org/ptsd-guideline/treatments/eye-movement-reprocessing.aspx
58. Milar, K. S. (2011). The myth buster. American Psychological Association. Retrieved from http://www.apa.org/monitor/2011/02/myth-buster.aspx
59. National Institute of Mental Health. (2015). Depression. National Institutes of Health. Retrieved from http://www.nimh.nih.gov/health/topics/depression/index.shtml
60. Pratt, L. A., & Brody, D. J. (2008). Depression in the United States household population, 2005–2006. Centers for Disease Control and Prevention. Retrieved from http://www.cdc.gov/nchs/data/databriefs/db07.pdf
61. Kessler, R. C., Berglund, P. F., Demler, O. F., Jin, R., Koretz, D., Merikangas, K. R.,... National Comorbidity Survey Replication. (2003). The epidemiology of major depressive disorder: Results from the National Comorbidity Survey Replication (NCS-R). *JAMA, 289*(23), 3095–3105.
62. National Institute of Mental Health. (2015). Bipolar disorder. National Institutes of Health. Retrieved from http://www.nimh.nih.gov/health/topics/bipolar-disorder/index.shtml
63. Substance Abuse and Mental Health Services Administration. (2015). Mental disorders. Retrieved from http://www.samhsa.gov/disorders/mental
64. National Institute of Mental Health. (2015). Schizophrenia. National Institutes of Health. Retrieved from http://www.nimh.nih.gov/health/statistics/prevalence/schizophrenia.shtml
65. National Alliance on Mental Illness. (1998). Facts on schizophrenia. Retrieved from http://www.nami.org/Press-Media/Press-Releases/1998/Facts-On-Schizophrenia
66. Cowan, A. L. (2014, November 21). Adam Lanza's mental problems "completely untreated" before Newtown shooting, report says. *New York Times*. Retrieved from http://www.nytimes.com/2014/11/22/nyregion/before-newtown-shootings-adam-lanzas-mental-problems-completely-untreated-report-says.html?_r=1
67. Crifasi, C. K., Meyers, J. S., Vernick, J. S., & Webster, D. W. (2015). Effects of changes in permit-to-purchase handgun laws in Connecticut and Missouri on suicide rates. *Preventive Medicine, 79*, 43–49.
68. McGinty, E. E., Frattaroli, S., Appelbaum, P. S., Bonnie, R. J., Grilley, A., Horwitz, J., . . . Webster, D. W. (2014). Using research evidence to reframe the policy debate around mental illness and guns: Process and recommendations. *American Journal of Public Health, 104*(11), e22–e26.
69. National Institute of Mental Health. (2007). National survey tracks prevalence of personality disorders in U.S. population. National Institutes of Health. Retrieved from https://www.nimh.nih.gov/news/science-news/2007/national-survey-tracks-prevalence-of-personality-disorders-in-us-population.shtml
70. American Psychiatric Association. (2016). What are personality disorders? Retrieved from https://www.psychiatry.org/patients-families/personality-disorders/what-are-personality-disorders
71. National Institute of Mental Health. (2015). Borderline personality disorder. National Institutes of Health. Retrieved from http://www.nimh.nih.gov/health/topics/borderline-personality-disorder/index.shtml
72. *Psychology Today*. (2018). Paranoid personality disorder. Retrieved from https://www.psychologytoday.com/conditions/paranoid-personality-disorder
73. Mayo Clinic. (2012). Self-injury/cutting. Retrieved from http://www.mayoclinic.org/diseases-conditions/self-injury/basics/definition/con-20025897

74. Favazza, A. R. (1996). *Bodies under siege: Self-mutilation and body modification in culture and psychiatry* (2nd ed.). Baltimore, MD: The Johns Hopkins University Press.
75. Hamza, C. A., & Willoughby, T. (2013). Nonsuicidal self-injury and suicidal behavior: A latent class analysis among young adults. *PloS One, 8*(3), e59955.
76. Lewis, S. P., & Knoll, A. K. (2015). Do it yourself: Examination of self-injury first aid tips on YouTube. *Cyberpsychology, Behavior and Social Networking, 18*(5), 301–304.
77. Joiner, T. (2007). *Why people die by suicide.* Cambridge, MA: Harvard University Press.
78. Evans, G., & Farberow, N. L. (2003). *The encyclopedia of suicide (facts on file library of health and living)* (2nd ed.). New York, NY: Facts on File.
79. U.S. Department of Veterans Affairs. (2015). Suicide risk assessment guide. Retrieved from www.mentalhealth.va.gov/docs/suicide_risk_assessment_reference_guide.pdf
80. Tidemalm, D. F., Runeson, B. F., Waern, M. F., Frisell, T., Carlstrom, E., Lichtenstein, P., & Langstrom, N. (2011). Familial clustering of suicide risk: A total population study of 11.4 million individuals. *Psychological Medicine, 41*(12), 2527–2534.
81. American Foundation for Suicide Prevention. (2015). Facts and figures. Retrieved from http://www.afsp.org/understanding-suicide/facts-and-figures
82. Centers for Disease Control and Prevention. (2012). Suicide facts at a glance. Retrieved from http://www.cdc.gov/violenceprevention/pdf/Suicide-DataSheet-a.pdf
83. MentalHealth.gov. (n.d.). Suicidal behavior. Retrieved from https://www.mentalhealth.gov/what-to-look-for/suicidal-behavior/
84. National Institute of Mental Health. (2015). Obsessive-compulsive disorder. National Institutes of Health. Retrieved from http://www.nimh.nih.gov/health/topics/obsessive-compulsive- disorder-ocd/index.shtml
85. Phillips, K. A. (2004). Body dysmorphic disorder: Recognizing and treating imagined ugliness. *World Psychiatry, 3*(1), 12–17.
86. Mayo Clinic. (2013). Body dysmorphic disorder. Retrieved from http://www.mayoclinic.org/diseases-conditions/body-dysmorphic-disorder/basics/treatment/con-20029953
87. Fluoxetine Bulimia Nervosa Collaborative Study Group. (1992). Fluoxetine in the treatment of bulimia nervosa. A multicenter, placebo-controlled, double-blind trial. Fluoxetine Bulimia Nervosa Collaborative Study Group. *Archives of General Psychiatry, 49*(2),139–147. Retrieved from https://www.ncbi.nlm.nih.gov/pubmed/1550466
88. American Dental Association. (2015). Anorexia nervosa. Retrieved from http://www.ada.org/en/member-center/oral-health-topics/anorexia-nervosa
89. Mayo Clinic. (2014). Diseases and conditions: Anorexia nervosa. Retrieved from http://www.mayoclinic.org/diseases-conditions/anorexia/basics/complications/con-20033002
90. Jauregui-Garrido, B., & Jauregui-Lobera, I. (2012). Sudden death in eating disorders. *Vascular Health and Risk Management, 8*, 91–98.
91. National Institute of Mental Health. (2014). 9 eating disorders myths busted. National Institutes of Health. Retrieved from https://www.nimh.nih.gov/news/science-news/2014/9-eating-disorders-myths-busted.shtml
92. Swanson, S. A., Crow, S. J., Le Grange, D. F., Swendsen, J., & Merikangas, K. R. (2011). Prevalence and correlates of eating disorders in adolescents. Results from the National Comorbidity Survey Replication adolescent supplement. *Archives of General Psychiatry, 68*(7), 714–723.
93. Hudson, J. I., Hiripi, E., Pope, H. G., Jr., & Kessler, R. C. (2007). The prevalence and correlates of eating disorders in the National Comorbidity Survey Replication. *Biological Psychiatry, 61*(3), 348–358.
94. National Institute of Mental Health. (2015). Eating disorders. National Institutes of Health. Retrieved from http://www.nimh.nih.gov/health/topics/eating-disorders/index.shtml
95. National Institute of Mental Health. (2014). Eating disorders: About more than food. National Institutes of Health. Retrieved from http://www.nimh.nih.gov/health/publications/eating-disorders-new-trifold/index.shtml
96. Autism Speaks. (2015). Answers to frequently asked questions about *DSM-5*. Retrieved from https://www.autismspeaks.org/dsm-5/faq#why
97. National Institute of Mental Health. (2015). Attention deficit hyperactivity disorder. National Institutes of Health. Retrieved from http://www.nimh.nih.gov/health/topics/attention-deficit-hyperactivity-disorder-adhd/index.shtml
98. Schwarz, A. (2013, December 14). The selling of attention deficit disorder. *New York Times*. Retrieved from http://www.nytimes.com/2013/12/15/health/the-selling-of-attention-deficit-disorder.html?pagewanted=all
99. Root Shock. (2015). What is root shock? Retrieved from http://www.rootshock.org
100. Fullilove, M. T. (2001). Root shock: The consequences of African American dispossession. *Journal of Urban Health, 78*(1), 72–80.
101. Mauer, B. (2006). Morbidity and mortality in people with serious mental illness. National Association of State Mental Health Program Directors (NASMHPD) Medical Directors Council. Retrieved from http://www.nasmhpd.org/sites/default/files/Mortality%20and%20Morbidity%20Final%20Report%208.18.08.pdf
102. National Alliance on Mental Illness. (2015). How do we fix America's mental health care system? Retrieved from http://www.nami.org/Blogs/NAMI-Blog/March-2015/How-Do-We-Fix-America%E2%80%99s-Mental-Health-Care-System#
103. U.S. Department of Health and Human Services. (2015). Health insurance and mental health services. Retrieved from http://www.mentalhealth.gov/get-help/health-insurance
104. U.S Department of Labor. (2010). The Mental Health Parity and Addiction Equity Act of 2008 (MHPAEA). Retrieved from http://www.dol.gov/ebsa/newsroom/fsmhpaea.html
105. National Alliance on Mental Illness. (2016). Anosognosia. Retrieved from https://www.nami.org/Learn-More/Mental-Health-Conditions/Related-Conditions/Anosognosia

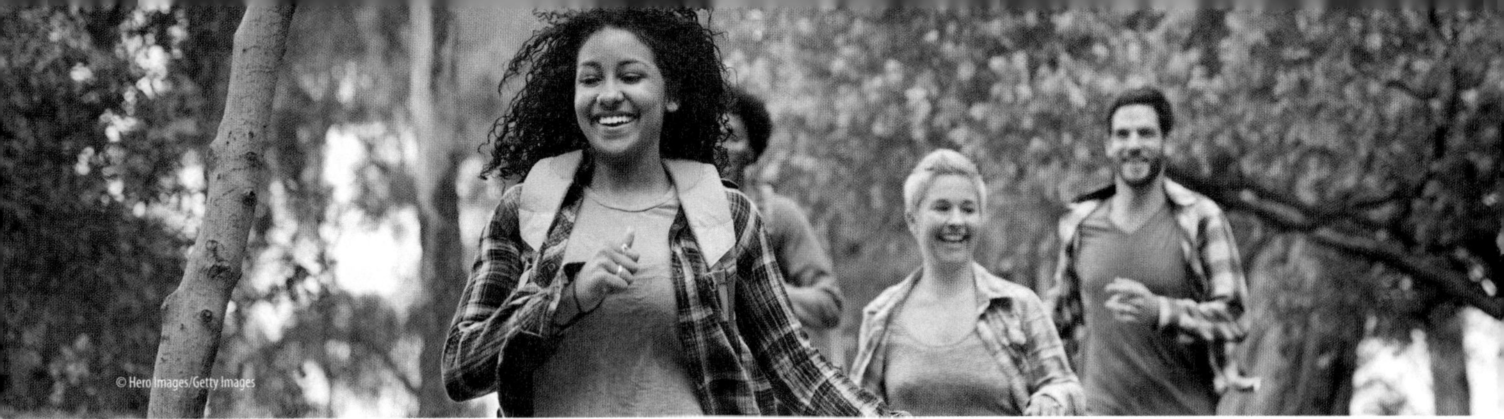

CHAPTER 7

This Is Your Brain on Addiction: Substance Use and Addictive Behaviors

CHAPTER OBJECTIVES

- Describe how substances can affect the brain and behavior.
- Explain reasons why people engage in substance use.
- Recognize the role of the tobacco industry in promoting tobacco use.
- Review chemical drugs (both legal and illegal) and addictive behaviors, including what they are, who is affected, and the short- and long-term health consequences.
- Explain what the harm reduction movement entails and identify its guiding principles and strategies.

The What, How, and Why of Substance Use

Over the last century, we have learned much about how substances affect both behavior and the brain. Specifically, we have learned that the use of addictive substances is based on a problem with how the brain becomes wired with repeated use of a substance.[1]

You may hear people use various terms like *substance use*, *substance abuse*, *substance dependence*, and *addiction* when referring to problems with drugs and other substances. The *Diagnostic and Statistical Manual of Mental Disorders*, 5th edition (*DSM-5*) now uses the term **substance use disorder** (instead of abuse or dependence) to characterize and diagnose problems with substance use. Whatever the term used, however, the point is that using substances such as alcohol and cocaine can be dangerous and harmful to one's health. When substance use becomes problematic, it is often characterized by behavioral, cognitive, and physiological issues. Together, these dynamics make it difficult to

substance use disorder A term used by the *Diagnostic and Statistical Manual of Mental Disorders* to characterize and diagnose problems with substance use. This term is used rather than terms such as *abuse* or *dependence*.

control use, increase the desire for using the substance, and make people prioritize the substance over other obligations.[2,3]

Most people understand that drug use is dangerous and can have serious implications for one's health and mortality. Why, then, do people use substances? There are many reasons. Some people may enjoy the feeling of euphoria (happiness, excitement) found when using certain substances. Others may be self-medicating to reduce feelings related to stress, anxiety, or trauma, or possibly symptoms of serious mental health disorders such as schizophrenia. Some people may take substances to improve performance, such as in athletics, or to help them focus. Others may use a substance due to peer pressure, boredom, or curiosity—to see what being under the influence feels like. In some cases, people take prescription medications to treat pain and then become addicted. Whatever the reason, because substances affect the brain, occasional use can turn into a serious problem for women and men (**FIGURE 7-1**).[4–7]

Most substances contain chemicals that affect the brain's communication and reward circuit (**FIGURE 7-2**). Drugs like marijuana and heroin trick the brain

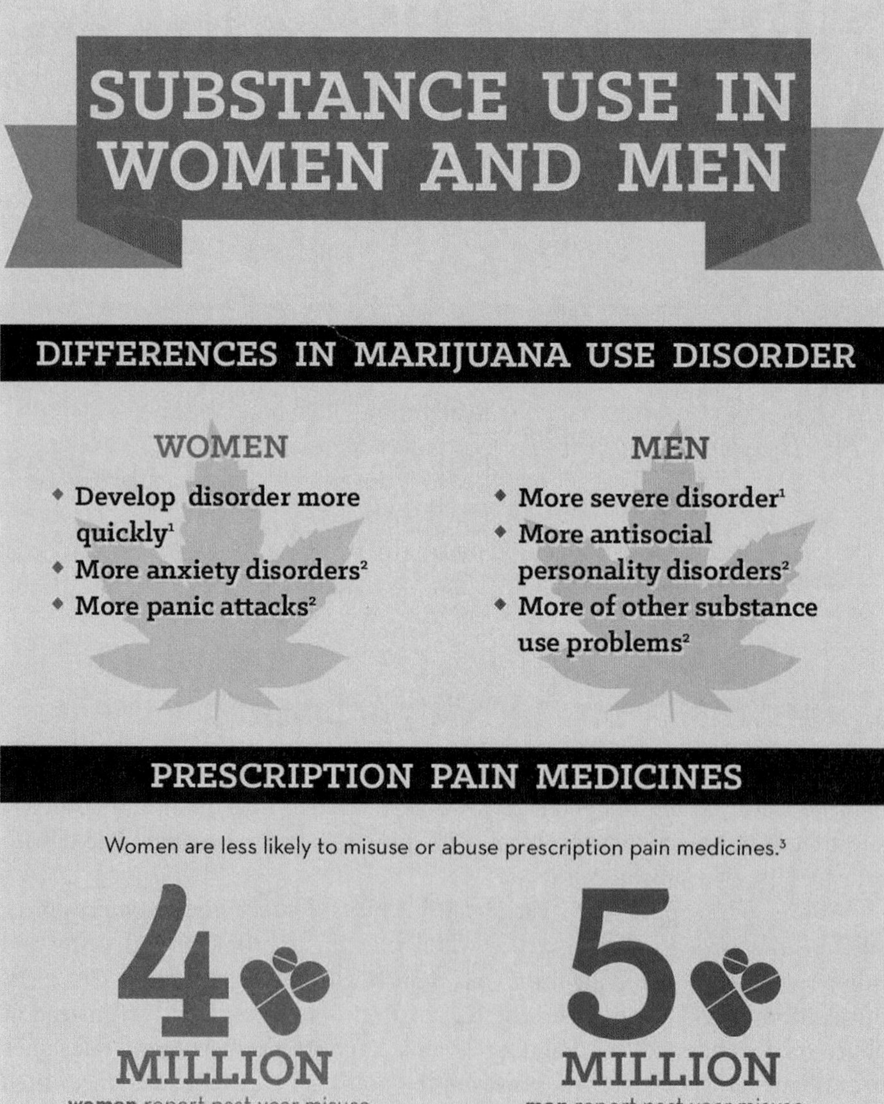

FIGURE 7-1 Substance use and gender.

National Institute on Drug Abuse. (2016). Substance Use in Women and Men. Retrieved from https://www.drugabuse.gov/related-topics/trends-statistics/infographics/substance-use-in-women-men

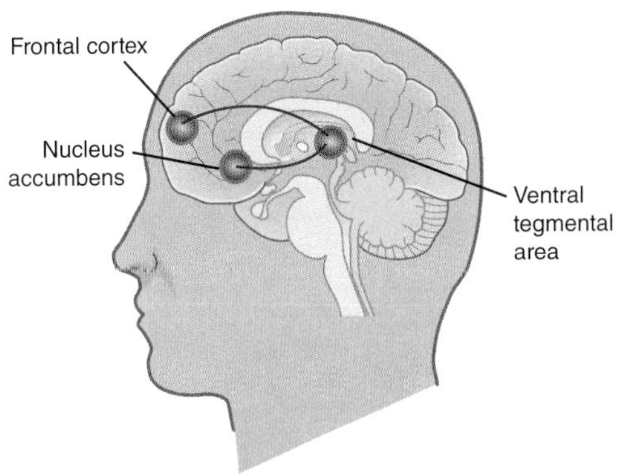

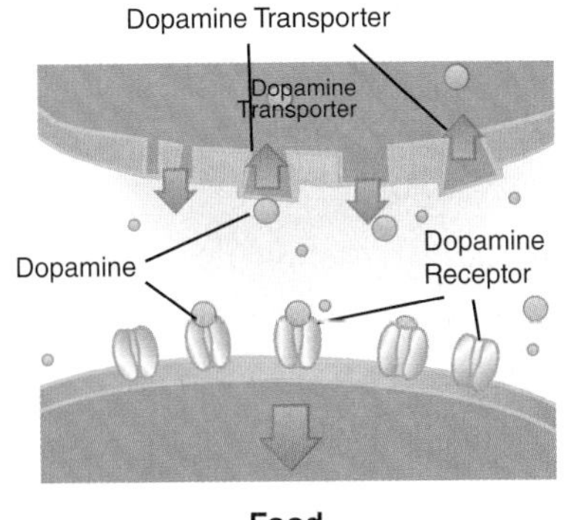

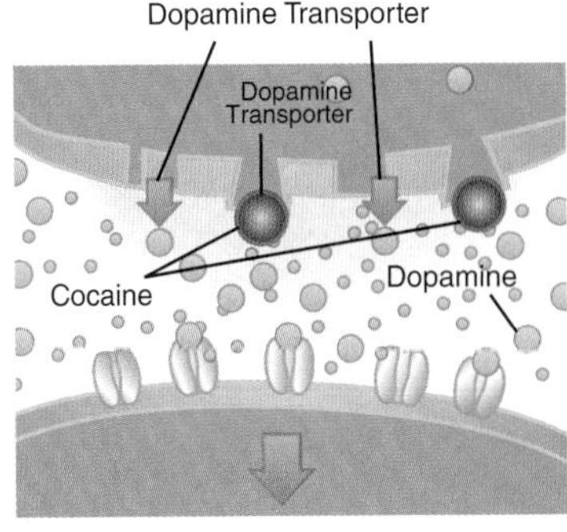

FIGURE 7-2 Drugs of abuse target the brain's pleasure center.

National Institute on Drug Abuse. (2014). Drugs, brains, and behavior: The science of addiction: Drugs and the brain. Retrieved from https://www.drugabuse.gov/publications/drugs-brains-behavior-science-addiction/drugs-brain

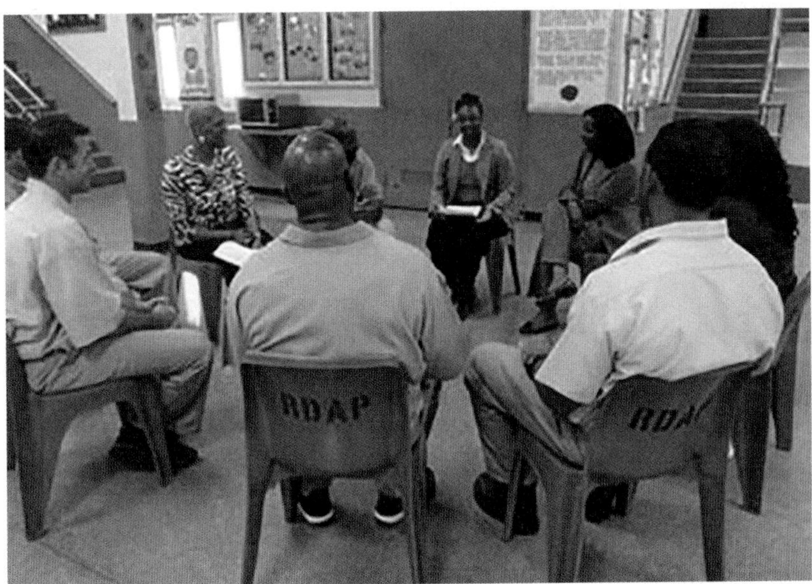

Because drug use before entering prison is so prevalent among people who are incarcerated, substance use treatment programs can be incorporated into these settings to aid in rehabilitation.

Federal Bureau of Prisons. (n.d.). Custody and care: Substance abuse treatment. Retrieved from https://www.bop.gov/inmates/custody_and_care/substance_abuse_treatment.jsp

into thinking they are naturally occurring neurotransmitters (mainly dopamine), thus allowing the drugs to send abnormal messages to the brain. Drugs like cocaine and methamphetamine also stimulate nerve cells to release large quantities of neurotransmitters. These excess neurotransmitters overstimulate the brain's reward system and cause a feeling of euphoria. This feeling creates a cycle in which the brain learns that the drug will provide this reward, thus potentially making the drug's use a repeated behavior.[1] Some behaviors, such as gambling and eating, can also affect the brain's reward system and become addictive. Unfortunately, despite our understanding of the effect of substances on the brain's reward center, substance use—or misuse—is still often considered to be a matter of willpower, not a true addiction.

The fact that substance use and addictive behaviors affect one's brain, however, does not mean someone becomes powerless over an addiction; it just means that the repeated use of a drug causes the brain to become wired differently.

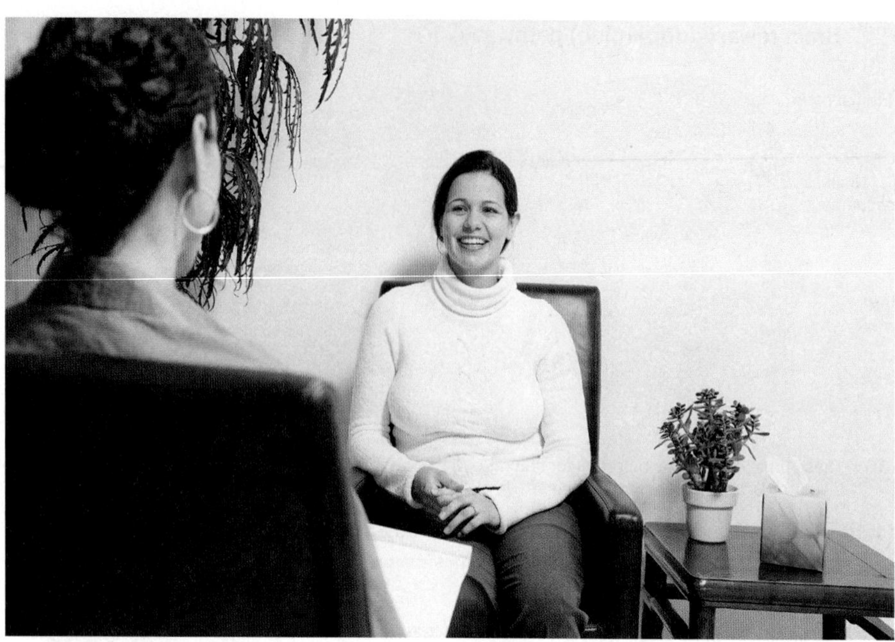

Behavioral counseling by a social worker, psychologist, or psychiatrist is recommended to treat substance use disorder and addictive behaviors.

Supportive and empowering therapies (along with medication, if available) can foster one's ability to change behavior.

Various treatment options are available for people who become dependent on certain substances or behaviors. For substance use disorders, the main focus of treatment is to manage withdrawal symptoms and prevent relapses (using the substance again). For certain drug addictions, there are approved medications for treatment. Some people, however, feel that becoming dependent on an approved (and perhaps more socially acceptable) medication is still problematic. Behavioral therapies and counseling are also appropriate for managing all kinds of substance use disorders and addictive behaviors. One popular form of therapy for substance use is cognitive behavioral therapy (CBT), a type of psychotherapy in which the therapist and patient work to understand how thoughts can affect one's mood and behavior.[8] (See Chapter 6 for more on cognitive behavioral therapy.)

The *DSM-5* lists four groups of criteria that apply to all substance use disorders:

- *Impaired control*: for example, craving and using the substance more than intended; unsuccessful attempts to discontinue use
- *Social impairment*: failure to fulfill work or school obligations due to substance use; interpersonal problems due to substance use; continued use despite effects at work or home
- *Risky use*: using the substance in physically hazardous situations; recurrent use despite associated physical or psychological problems
- *Pharmacological*: tolerance; withdrawal[9]

People can become dependent on many different types of substances and behaviors. In this chapter, we'll explore chemical drugs, both legal (e.g., nicotine, caffeine, alcohol, pharmaceutical drugs, and marijuana) and illegal (e.g., heroin, cocaine, methamphetamine, certain hallucinogens), and behavioral addictions (e.g., sex, eating, gambling, exercise).

▸ Legal (but Dangerous) Drugs

Stimulants and Depressants

Nicotine and alcohol are unusual because they can function as both a stimulant *and* a depressant. Nicotine can produce a stimulating effect immediately after exposure, especially if someone smokes a cigarette slowly. It can also have a sedative effect, depending on the dose and how quickly it is absorbed. Smoking a cigarette quickly can produce a depressant effect. Similarly, alcohol can have a stimulating effect. If too much alcohol is consumed, however, it can produce a depressant effect in which the user can lose coordination. See **TABLE 7-1** for a list of many substances and their health effects.

Tobacco

Tobacco companies have their sights set on you—yes, you. The tobacco industry is like any other business: Its goal is to make money by selling a product. Companies market to groups they believe are likely to adopt their product, and one key group tobacco companies focus on is young adults.[10]

tobacco A product that contains the addictive substance nicotine used for cigarettes, cigars, pipes, and smokeless tobacco; consists of dried leaves from the tobacco plant.

Historically, tobacco companies have used advertising tactics such as portraying good-looking people smoking cigarettes as "macho" or "cool." For the most part, these efforts have been successful in getting young people to start smoking, and the addictive agent nicotine keeps these individuals smoking for many years to come.[11] Take a look at how tobacco companies have used advertising strategies to encourage use of their products: http://tobacco.stanford.edu/tobacco_main/main.php.

TALES OF PUBLIC HEALTH

The "Dilemma" of Selling Cigarettes in the 1980s

Read how one marketing consultant described the "dilemma" of selling cigarettes in the 1980s:

> The problem is, how do you sell death? How do you sell a poison that kills 350,000 people per year, 1,000 people a day? You do it with the great open spaces ... the mountains, the open places, the lakes coming up to the shore. They do it with healthy young people. They do it with athletes. How could a whiff of a cigarette be of any harm in a situation like that? It couldn't be—there's too much fresh air, too much health—too much absolute exuding of youth and vitality—that's the way they do it.[12]

Public health campaigns have attempted to counteract the tobacco industry's promotion of tobacco products. The Truth Initiative is one of the most well-known of these efforts; it is a nonprofit dedicated to spreading the truth about tobacco use through education, research, and activism.[13] The Truth Initiative uses powerful advertisements to expose tobacco company tactics and the downsides of using tobacco. To watch one example of the Truth Initiative's influential media campaigns, search for "The Truth - 1200" on YouTube.

What Is Tobacco and Why Is It So Bad? The tobacco leaf, which is grown around the world, can be dried and used for cigarettes, cigars, pipes, chewing tobacco, and snuff (powdered tobacco that is sniffed through one's nose) (**FIGURE 7-3**). Tobacco contains the chemical nicotine, which is an addictive substance. Nicotine is the main reason that it is difficult to quit after starting to

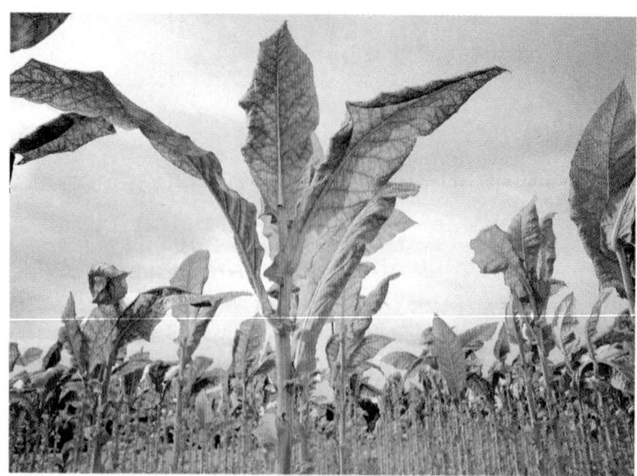

Tobacco leaf plantation in Poland.
© Zbigniew Guzowski/Shutterstock.

A TIP FROM A
FORMER SMOKER
RECORD YOUR VOICE FOR LOVED ONES WHILE YOU STILL CAN.
Terrie, Age 52
North Carolina
Smoking causes immediate damage to your body.
For Terrie, it gave her throat cancer. You can quit.
For free help, call 1-800-QUIT-NOW.
#CDCTips
CDC
U.S. Department of Health and Human Services
Centers for Disease Control and Prevention
CDC.gov/tips

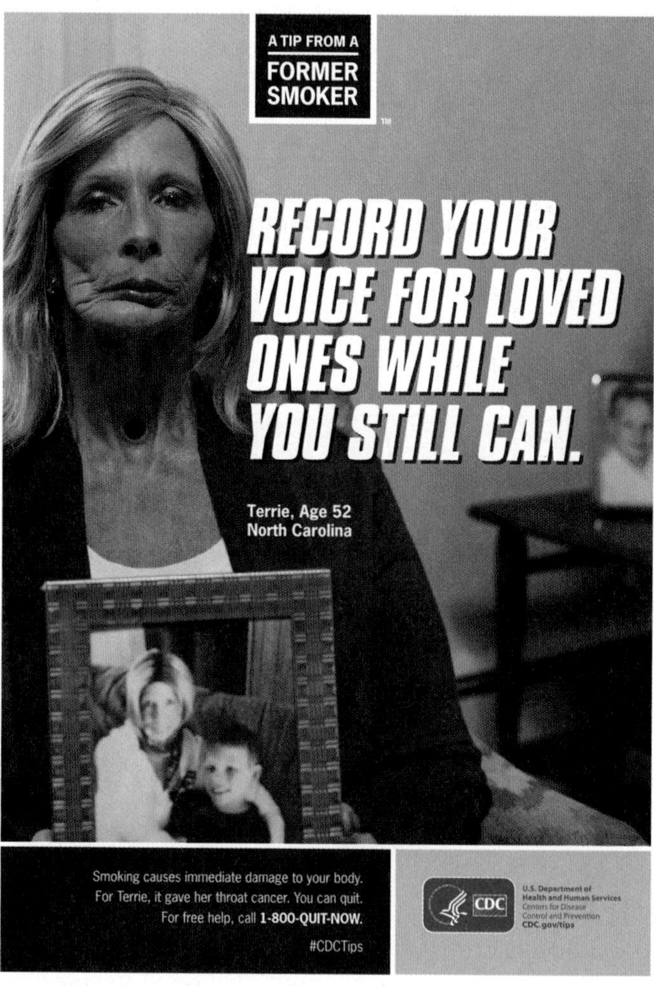

FIGURE 7-3 What is tobacco and why is it so bad?
Reproduced from CDC. A Tip from a Former Smoker Campaign. Retrieved from http://www.cdc.gov/tobacco/campaign/tips/resources/social/index.html

smoke, chew, or sniff tobacco.[14] Researchers suspect there may be other addictive chemicals in tobacco as well. Many people who use tobacco express a desire to quit, but nicotine is so powerful that over 85% of people who try to quit relapse within a week.[15] As with other addictive substances, nicotine increases levels of the neurotransmitter dopamine, causing a pleasurable feeling. Because these effects don't last very long, the smoker continues to crave nicotine to maintain that pleasurable feeling. People can experience withdrawal if they stop smoking, symptoms of which include anxiety, depression, irritability, sleep disruptions,

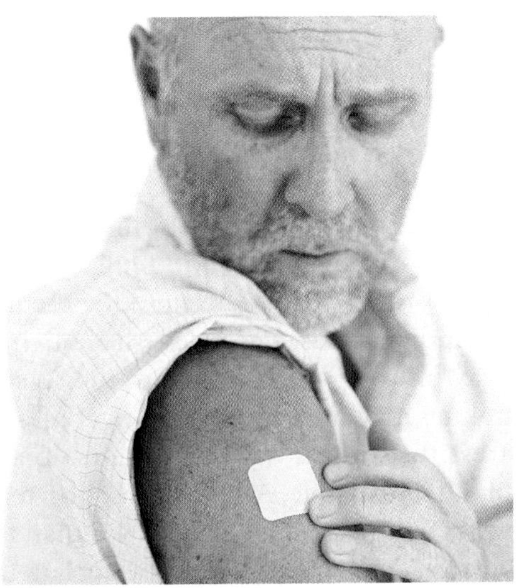

The nicotine patch can help smokers wean off of cigarettes.

and more. Withdrawal symptoms are at their worst during the first few days of quitting; however, some symptoms may linger for several months, making quitting altogether very difficult.[15] Clearly, it is very hard for someone to stop smoking once they have started, so it's better not to start smoking in the first place.

If you (or someone close to you) have already started using tobacco, there are treatment options and resources available to help you quit. Nicotine replacement therapies can help alleviate the withdrawal symptoms and come in the forms of gum, lozenges, prescription patches, nasal sprays, and inhalers. Prescription medications are also available. Because the urge to use tobacco may persist, there are also behavioral therapies to help smokers manage these cravings. Using counseling strategies and medication together is the most effective means of cessation. Often it will take several attempts before someone can successfully quit tobacco.[16] Some tobacco users have found relief in nonmedicinal, alternative methods of tobacco cessation, such as hypnosis, acupuncture, herbal supplements, yoga, and meditation, despite there being little scientific evidence as to their effectiveness.

Cigarettes. Smoking cigarettes is the most common method of tobacco use and is responsible for the greatest number of preventable deaths in the United States, with over 400,000 deaths each year attributed to tobacco use. It is the number one cause of cancer for men and women. Cigarette smoking wreaks havoc on almost all bodily systems. Smoking is associated with 90% of lung cancer cases as well as other cancers of the stomach, pancreas, cervix, and bladder. The negative effects of smoking do not stop at cancer; cigarettes affect the health of your teeth, eyes, immune system, and other bodily organs and systems and cause other health problems such as emphysema and heart disease. Smoking can affect a woman's ability to become pregnant and the health of her baby, and it can reduce men's fertility by affecting sperm.[17]

Smoking puts more than just the smoker at risk; secondhand smoke (the smoke that is emitted from burning tobacco products such as cigarettes) can cause lung cancer and other health problems, such as childhood asthma, among those who live in the same home as a smoker or who have sustained exposure. Even brief exposure to secondhand smoke can be harmful. Unfortunately, using air filters or opening windows does not prevent others near you from inhaling secondhand smoke. Over 2.5 million people have died from problems related to exposure to secondhand smoke.[18] And as if all of these health risks that come with smoking are not bad enough, cigarettes are also a main cause of home fires and associated deaths.[19]

About 40 million adults (17% of the adult population) in the United States smoke cigarettes. The good news is that this is down from about 21% of adults who smoked a decade ago. This reduction is, in part, thanks to public health efforts that spread the word about the detriments of cigarette smoking.[20] The groups with the highest rates of cigarette smoking are men, people age 18 to 24 years, American Indians/Alaska Natives, those living below the poverty level, and lesbian/gay/bisexual adults.[21] Part of the reason these groups have higher rates of smoking may be due to using cigarettes as a means of easing psychological distress that results from discrimination.[22] There may also be cultural issues at play. For example, American Indians tend to value not interfering in the behaviors of others, even those of youth; it is not socially acceptable to tell others not to smoke. This may partly explain the higher prevalence among this group.[23]

BY THE NUMBERS

Purchasing Cigarettes

Depending on the city or state, cigarettes can be legally purchased at ages 18 to 21 years. There is growing public support for increasing the age of tobacco sales from 18 to 21 years. This change would reduce the number of young people who start smoking by about 12% and thus reduce the number of related fatalities by about 10%.[24] A 1986 report written by the tobacco company Philip Morris noted that "Raising the legal minimum age for cigarette purchaser to 21 could gut our key young adult market (17–21) where we sell about 25 billion cigarettes and enjoy a 70% market share."[24]

Another major public health effort to reduce tobacco sales has been to increase the sales tax. In 2009, as part of President Obama's health initiative, the federal tax rate increased from $0.39 to $1.01 per pack of cigarettes, along with similar increases for other forms of tobacco. This tax increase reduced the number of youth who smoked cigarettes or used smokeless tobacco by 355,000 within the first 2 months.[25] States also have a tobacco tax, but the rates are highly variable from state to state.

At this point, thanks to public health research and education, most people know that using tobacco and smoking cigarettes is bad for their health. The question, then, becomes, why do so many people still do it? Some people, especially young people, say they do it to relieve boredom or to "fit in." Some smoke to self-medicate preexisting mental health disorders (over 40% of the cigarettes smoked are by people with a mental health disorder).[26] However, smoking can also cause mental health disorders; heavy smoking in adolescence is associated with increased likelihood of developing agoraphobia, generalized anxiety disorder, and panic disorder.[27]

Some people use smoking as a weight management tool, as smoking functions as an appetite suppressant.[28] Some people experience a short-term feeling of being relaxed after smoking cigarettes; however, evidence suggests that nicotine has been found to increase stress for those who are dependent, causing people to become irritable and tense between cigarettes.[29] Many people start smoking under the illusion that their cigarette use is beneficial, but the truth is that despite any perceived benefits, using tobacco has lasting and detrimental effects on health, well-being, and mortality.

Hookah Smoking. Tobacco comes in other forms besides cigarettes. Sometimes these methods are thought of as "safer" alternatives to smoking cigarettes, but they all come with equal, if not greater, health risks.

Hookah smoking is one of these methods. A hookah is a water pipe. Burning charcoal heats tobacco inside of the water pipe, and the user inhales the tobacco smoke, which passes through a water basin and through a mouthpiece. The tobacco often comes in flavors, such as mint, cherry, or bubble gum, meant to appeal to younger smokers. Heavy marketing by tobacco companies is one reason hookah smoking has increased in popularity among young adults.

A hookah can be shared by several users at one time. Businesses have capitalized on this shared experience, creating hookah bars and lounges in which groups of people (over 18 years of age) can come to share a hookah pipe. Don't be fooled by this party atmosphere; just because someone isn't smoking does not mean the person isn't inhaling toxic agents. Hookah tobacco contains many of the toxins known to cause a variety of cancers. Hookah smoking increases the risk of oral cancer and has also been associated with heart disease, infections (from sharing the same hookah with others), and respiratory diseases. Hookah smoking is just as harmful as smoking cigarettes; the inhaled smoke still contains nicotine and toxic agents. Because hookahs use burning charcoal, which contains high levels of carbon monoxide, metals, and toxic chemicals, research indicates that they may be even more dangerous than cigarettes.[30,31]

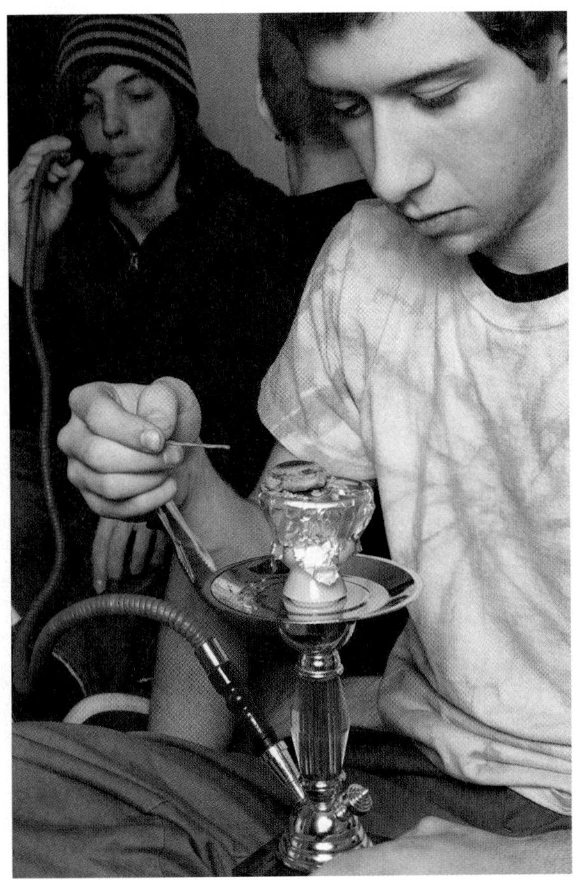

At hookah lounges, several people can smoke from the hoses at once, increasing the risk of spreading infections along with other health issues.

Smokeless Tobacco. Smokeless tobacco is a tobacco blend that is chewed, sucked, or sniffed. More men (7%) use chewing tobacco compared to women (less than 1%), and it is most popular among American Indians/Alaska Natives (9%). Even though chewing tobacco is not inhaled, it still has harmful side effects. Chewing tobacco contains nicotine and is associated with esophageal and oral cancers (of the mouth, throat, cheek, gums, lips, and tongue), tooth decay (from the added sugar and other particles), gum disease, heart disease, and mouth lesions.[32,33]

Cigars and Pipes. Cigars and pipes are additional means of inhaling tobacco. Cigars are tobacco rolled in a casing (leaf) made of tobacco, and they lack a filter. Pipes are usually made of an acrylic stem that has a bowl at the end where the tobacco is placed and lit. Some pipes have filters. About 5% of adults in the United States smoke cigars. It is most prevalent among men, African Americans, and American Indian/Alaska Natives. Due to expanded marketing efforts, young people are also increasingly using cigars; 8% of high school students report using cigars. Some people do not inhale cigar or pipe smoke, but even without inhaling, using these products increases the risk of mouth and throat cancers. Cigars and pipes are associated with lung cancer, heart disease, and complications related to childbearing and birth.[34]

electronic cigarettes Battery-powered devices that deliver nicotine via a vaporizer. Also known as e-cigarettes, e-cigs, or electronic nicotine delivery systems.

Electronic Cigarettes. **Electronic cigarettes** (known as e-cigarettes, e-cigs, or electronic nicotine delivery systems) are the most recent addition to the "cigarette alternative" market. Over 250 brands are currently available. E-cigarettes are battery-operated devices. Some are designed to resemble cigarettes (**FIGURE 7-4**). E-hookahs are also on the market. Through these devices, nicotine is delivered to the user via vapor (instead of the traditional smoke of cigarettes, hookahs, cigars, and pipes). An e-cigarette consists of a cartridge, heating

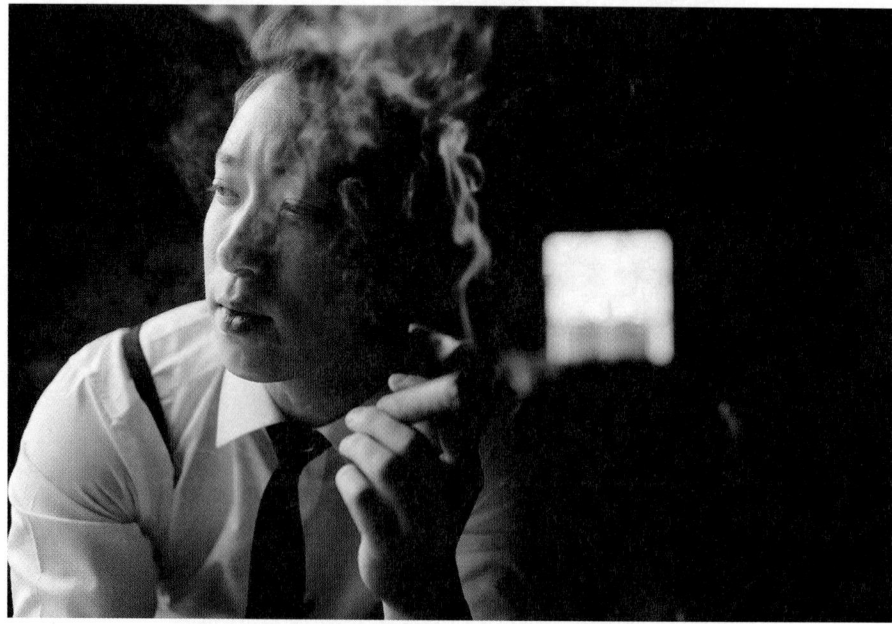

Because of magazines like *Cigar Aficionado*, cigars have gained popularity among young people.

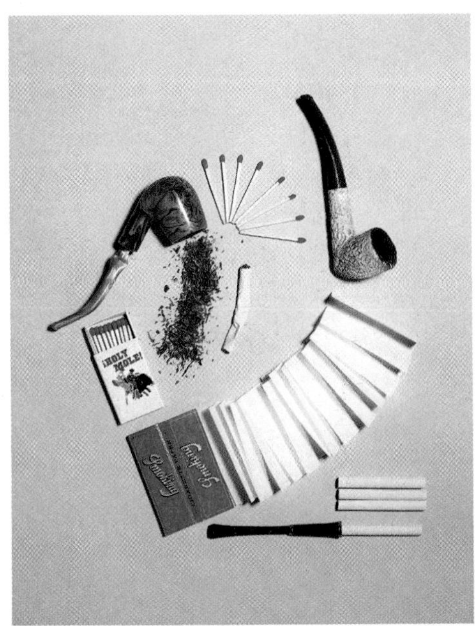

Even if pipe smoke is not inhaled, users still have an increased risk of mouth and throat cancers.

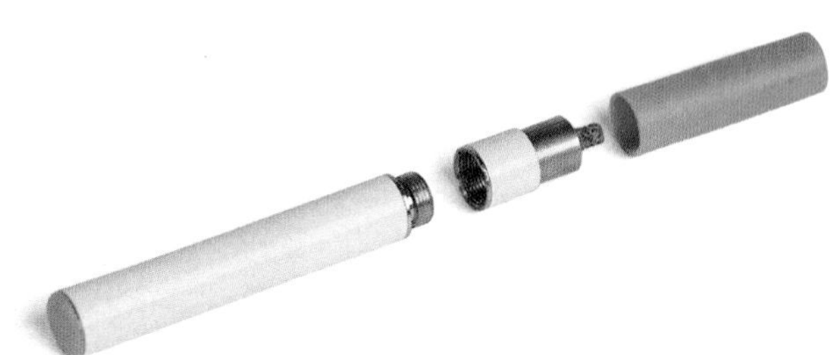

FIGURE 7-4 An e-cigarette, designed to resemble a real cigarette.

device, and power source. The cartridge holds a liquid solution containing nicotine, flavoring, and other chemicals. The heating device is a vaporizer, and it is usually powered by a battery. As the user "puffs" on the e-cigarette, the heating device activates and vaporizes the liquid contained in the cartridge, creating a vapor to be inhaled. This process is known as "vaping."[35]

So, is vaping a safe alternative to smoking? Often, when there is no evidence to demonstrate that something is harmful, we are tempted to assume it is safe; surely a company would not be allowed to manufacture and sell a product that is harmful without comprehensive testing, right? In fact, e-cigarettes have not been thoroughly tested in scientific studies to understand the effects of vaping. Very little is known about e-cigarette safety, but preliminary evidence suggests that e-cigarette vapor may contain, in addition to nicotine, carcinogens and unsafe chemicals such as heavy metals. The inhalation of these substances into the lungs is of concern to public health experts. In addition, secondhand inhalation of these vapors may be harmful. More testing is underway, but it will take time to determine the results so that consumers can be fully informed of the health risks they are exposing themselves to when they use these products.[35,36] The novelty of e-cigarettes and the presumption that they are "safer" than cigarettes has made them attractive. In 2014, about 13% of adults and high school students had ever tried e-cigarettes.[36,37]

A 2016 ruling confirmed that the Food and Drug Administration's (FDA) regulatory authority now includes oversight of electronic cigarettes, and e-cigarettes are banned from being sold to individuals under 18 years of age. This ruling was welcomed by public health experts, who have been stating since the early 2000s that e-cigarettes need more oversight and scientific testing. Producers of electronic nicotine delivery systems now must apply to the FDA for permission to sell their products and must provide detailed information on their products' ingredients.[38]

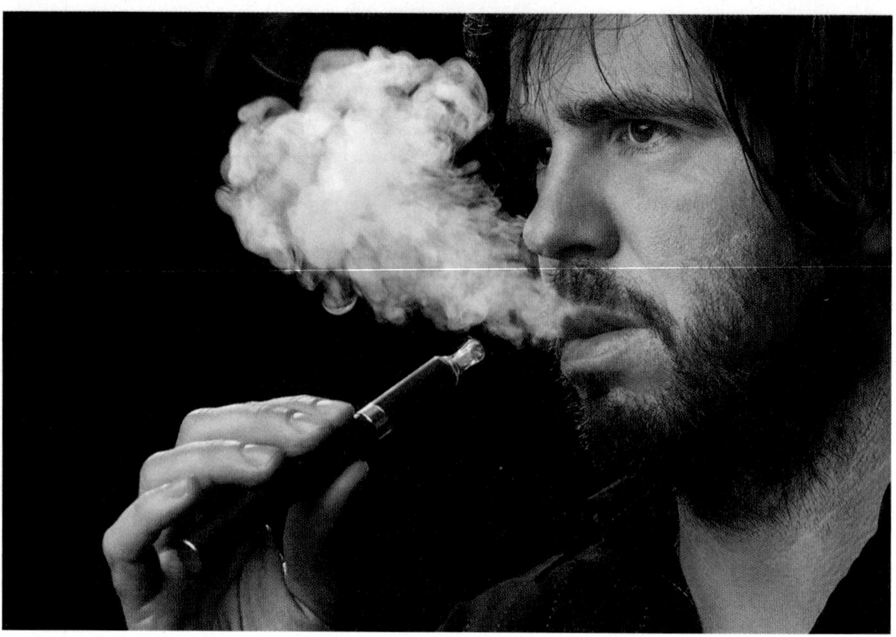

Unlike for cigarettes, there are no widespread current regulations on using e-cigarettes in public, despite a lack of evidence about the potential dangers of the secondhand vapor.

Alcohol

alcohol A substance that results from the fermentation of yeasts, sugars, and starches that is an ingredient in beer, wine, and other liquors.

Alcohol (also known as ethyl alcohol or ethanol) is a substance that results from the fermentation or distillation of yeasts, sugars, and starches. When consumed, it is quickly absorbed into the bloodstream and functions as a central nervous system depressant.[39] Each person has a different alcohol metabolism, which is the way alcohol is broken down and eliminated by your body. This depends on genetic and environmental factors, such as personal nutrition.[40]

Drinking alcohol is socially acceptable and part of many celebrations. So, when does drinking alcohol become problematic? There are different definitions, depending on the amount of alcohol consumed. Moderate alcohol consumption is up to one drink per day for women and two drinks for men. There are several definitions of binge drinking. The Substance Abuse and Mental Health Services Administration defines binge drinking as drinking five or more alcoholic drinks on the same occasion on at least 1 day in the past 30 days. Heavy drinking, the most extreme, is defined as drinking five or more drinks on the same occasion on 5 days or more in the past 30 days.[41] Regardless of how much an individual drinks, he or she can still have a problem with alcohol, known as alcohol use disorder (AUD), which a healthcare provider can diagnose. A person receives a medical diagnosis of AUD when his or her drinking meets a set of specific criteria outlined in the *DSM-5* (see the Diagnosing Alcohol Use Disorder box).

The effects of alcohol are different for men than for women. Men tend to drink more than women; however, because the female body takes longer to break down alcohol, the effects of alcohol occur more rapidly and last longer in women.[45]

What constitutes "one drink"? It might be surprising to learn that the following are considered one drink: 12 fluid ounces (fl. oz.) of regular beer, 8 to 9 fl. oz. of malt liquor, 5 fl. oz. of table wine, and 1.5 fl. oz. of 90-proof distilled spirits (tequila, vodka, etc.) (**FIGURE 7-5**). The amount of alcohol in each of these drinks can vary greatly. Don't be fooled by "light" beers; many contain the same amount of alcohol as regular beer (just fewer calories).[46] If someone is pregnant,

12 fl oz of **regular beer**	=	8–9 fl oz of **malt liquor** (shown in a 12 oz glass)	=	5 fl oz of **table wine**	=	3–4 oz of **fortified wine** (such as sherry or port; 3.5 oz shown)	=	2–3 oz of **cordial, liqueur, or aperitif** (2.5 oz shown)	=	1.5 oz of **brandy** (a single jigger or shot)	=	1.5 fl oz shot of **80-proof spirits** ("hard liquor")
about 5% alcohol		about 7% alcohol		about 12% alcohol		about 17% alcohol		about 24% alcohol		about 40% alcohol		about 40% alcohol

The percentage of "pure" alcohol, expressed here as alcohol by volume (alc/vol), varies by beverage.

FIGURE 7-5 This infographic depicts the equivalent of what is considered to be one drink.

National Institute on Alcohol Abuse and Alcoholism. (n.d.). What is a standard drink? Retrieved from https://www.niaaa.nih.gov/alcohol-health/overview-alcohol-consumption/what-standard-drink

DIAGNOSING ALCOHOL USE DISORDER

A healthcare provider may use the following questions developed by the National Institute on Alcohol Abuse and Alcoholism to determine whether someone has AUD:[42–44]

In the past year, have you

- Had times when you ended up drinking more, or longer, than you intended?
- More than once wanted to cut down or stop drinking, or tried to, but couldn't?
- Spent a lot of time drinking? Or being sick or getting over the aftereffects?
- Experienced craving—a strong need, or urge, to drink?
- Found that drinking—or being sick from drinking—often interfered with taking care of your home or family? Or caused job troubles? Or school problems?
- Continued to drink even though it was causing trouble with your family or friends?
- Given up or cut back on activities that were important or interesting to you, or gave you pleasure, in order to drink?
- More than once gotten into situations while or after drinking that increased your chances of getting hurt (such as driving, swimming, using machinery, walking in a dangerous area, or having unsafe sex)?
- Continued to drink even though it was making you feel depressed or anxious or adding to another health problem? Or after having had a memory blackout?
- Had to drink much more than you once did to get the effect you want? Or found that your usual number of drinks had much less effect than before?
- Found that when the effects of alcohol were wearing off, you had withdrawal symptoms, such as trouble sleeping, shakiness, irritability, anxiety, depression, restlessness, nausea, or sweating? Or sensed things that were not there?

Depending on the person's responses, AUD may be diagnosed as mild, moderate, or severe. About 7% of adults age 18 years and older (16 million people) had a diagnosis of AUD in 2014. Whites and Native Americans have the greatest risk of having AUD compared to other racial/ethnic groups.

Modified from Niaaa.nih.gov. (2018). Alcohol Use Disorder | National Institute on Alcohol Abuse and Alcoholism (NIAAA). [online] Available at: https://www.niaaa.nih.gov/alcohol-health/overview-alcohol-consumption/alcohol-use-disorders and Mayo Clinic. (2018). Alcohol use disorder - Symptoms & causes. [online] Available at: http://www.mayoclinic.org/diseases-conditions/alcohol-use-disorder/basics/definition/con-20020866.

takes medication that may interact with alcohol, or has a medical condition that can be exacerbated by alcohol, then it is recommended that the person avoid alcohol entirely. It is also recommended that a person avoid consuming alcohol if he or she may have to drive a vehicle or operate machinery.[41]

Blood alcohol concentration (BAC) levels are often used as an indicator of intoxication and to determine your ability to drive safely (**FIGURE 7-6**). It is commonly calculated as a percentage of ethanol in the bloodstream per volume of blood. Different countries have different legal BAC limits for

Blood Alcohol Concentration (BAC) Levels	Effects
0.15% About 7 beers	• Serious difficulty controlling the car and focusing on driving
0.10% About 5 beers	• Markedly slower reaction time • Difficulty staying in lane and braking when needed
0.08% About 4 beers	• Trouble controlling speed • Difficulty processing information and reasoning
0.05% About 3 beers	• Reduced coordination and ability to track moving objects • Difficulty steering
0.02% About 2 beers	• Loss of judgment • Trouble doing two tasks at the same time

FIGURE 7-6 This figure shows the effects of driving at various blood alcohol concentration levels.

Centers for Disease Control and Prevention, National Center for Injury Prevention and Control, Division of Unintentional Injury Prevention.

BY THE NUMBERS

Alcohol Use by Age

Most adults older than age 18 years (87%) report having consumed alcohol in their lifetime at least once. Within this population, 25% reported binge drinking and 7% engaged in heavy drinking in the last month. Despite alcohol being legal only for adults 21 years of age and older, 23% of 12- to 20-year-olds reported drinking alcohol in the last month. About 14% were categorized as binge drinkers and 3% as heavy drinkers.[48]

These figures increase dramatically when we talk about college students. About 60% of college students 18 to 22 years of age drank alcohol in the past month. This statistic is compared to about 52% of the same age group who are not in college. Binge drinking and heavy drinking are also much more prevalent among college students; about 38% of college students engaged in binge drinking and 12% in heavy drinking in the last month.[48]

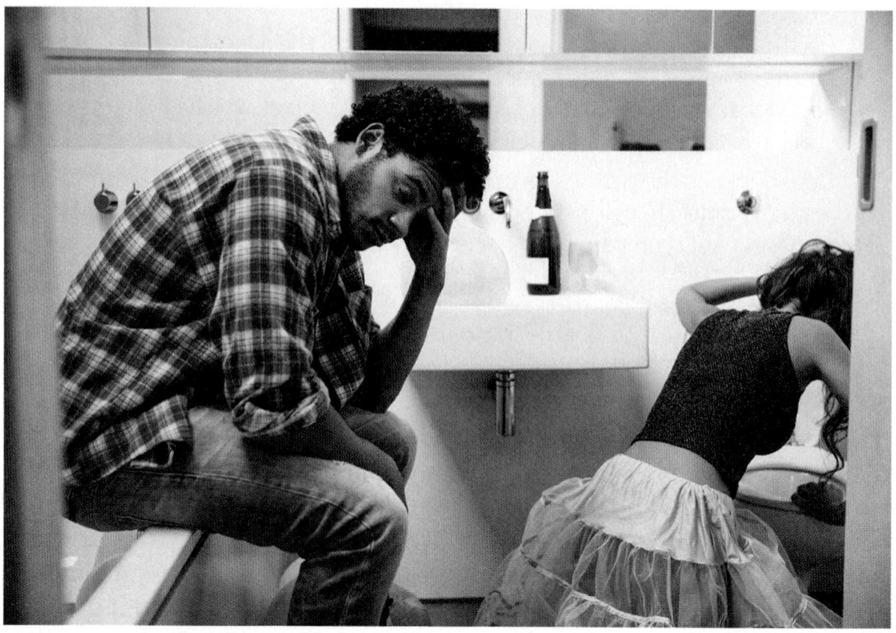

Over 600,000 people visit the emergency department each year because of alcohol.

driving; in countries such as Brazil, it is illegal to have almost any alcohol measured in your bloodstream if you are driving, while in others, such as the United States, the BAC limit is 0.08%.[47] Although Figure 7-6 depicts about how many beers will result in a 0.08% BAC level, because everyone's alcohol metabolism is different, it is hard to say exactly how many drinks is too many.

Drinking alcohol leads to intoxication (usually referred to as being "drunk"), which can impair judgment, perception, and behavior. Undoubtedly, everyone has seen someone who has drunk too much (in real life or on television). An intoxicated person may have slurred speech, be unable to walk straight, and act strangely. If you drink too much alcohol, you may experience a "hangover" the next day, usually characterized by headache, nausea, decreased ability to concentrate, sensitivity to light and sound, and fatigue. Why, then, do so many people drink alcohol and often drink too much of it? The reasons are multifaceted. Research suggests that alcohol use among college students has to do with being at a developmental stage of exploring one's identity (and using alcohol as a coping mechanism for not yet having a clear identity), self-medication, and desire to be social. People in this age group may not be able to fully recognize the negative consequences of drinking. This explanation introduces a neurodevelopmental component, as not all parts of the brain become fully mature until the mid-20s. The part of the brain that controls impulses may mature faster than another region that helps people assess long-term consequences of behavior. Thus, young people may choose to drink alcohol for its short-term "rewards" (or feelings of intoxication) without thinking about the long-term consequences.[49]

However, the legal drinking age in Europe ranges from 16 to 18 years, and many young people, here and abroad, are able to drink responsibly.

If you decide to drink alcohol, here are some tips for drinking responsibly:

- *Food first.* Eating before you drink will help slow down absorption.
- *Sip and enjoy.* Enjoy your drink like "the most interesting man in the world" (from the Dos Equis beer commercials), who sips drinks to enjoy the taste and experience.
- *Size matters.* If you're pouring drinks at home, try to estimate the same amount of alcohol as you would get in a bar.
- *Switch it up.* Try alternating nonalcoholic drinks in between those with alcohol.
- *You decide.* If you're not in the mood to drink, don't feel pressured. It's always your choice. If you're worried about fitting in, offer to buy a round for those who do want to drink to still feel like part of the group. By the same token, if you do want to drink but someone else doesn't want to, respect that person's decision.
- *Stick together.* Don't go to parties solo. Stick with friends who look out for one another and whom you trust.
- *Track.* Keep track of how much you're drinking in a given week. Take a break from drinking if you've had a big night out.
- *No driving.* Always designate a driver and have a clear discussion about how much (if any) that person will drink.
- *Mind your medicine.* Be mindful of alcohol interacting with other medications you may be taking.

The allure of mixing energy drinks with alcohol may seem appealing. But studies show that those who combine energy drinks with alcohol are more likely to binge drink and report unwanted or unprotected sex, being injured, or driving drunk. Drinks that are premixed with alcohol and caffeine are also

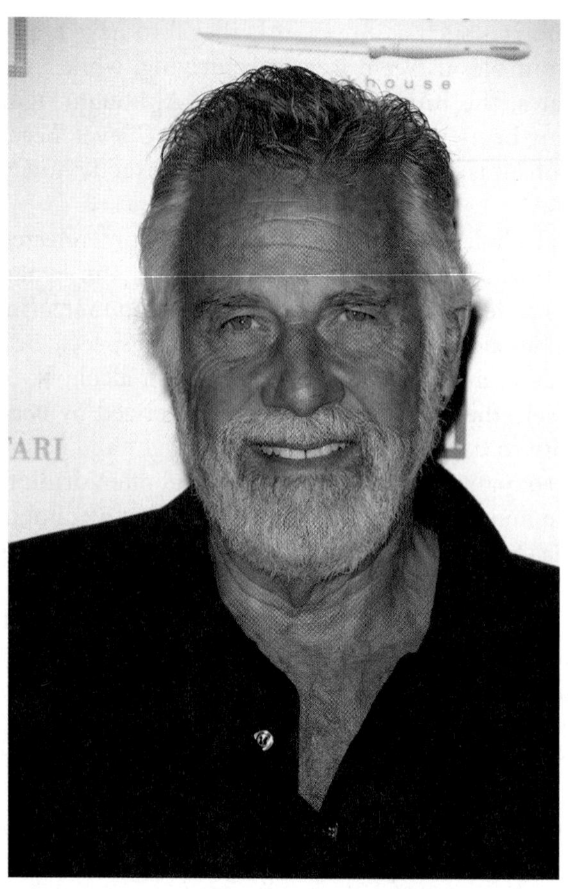

The most interesting man in the world.

dangerous because they often have a high alcohol content. In 2010 the FDA restricted manufacturers from allowing these drinks to stay on the market because the addition of caffeine was not "generally recognized as safe." In response, some removed caffeine but some continue to produce and sell caffeinated alcoholic beverages.[50]

Why does drinking alcohol matter to your health? Drinking alcohol is legal (at age 21 years) but is associated with a host of short- and long-term negative outcomes. Many of these involve violent and risky behaviors. The main consequences include academic problems, physical and sexual assaults, unintentional injuries, car accidents, memory loss (blackouts), unprotected sexual activity (resulting in sexually transmitted diseases and pregnancy), and, in some cases, death. (See Chapter 9 for more information about alcohol-related car crashes.) About half of sexual assaults involve alcohol, either by the victim, perpetrator, or both. Why might alcohol contribute to sexual assault? Research suggests that alcohol consumption by perpetrators may enhance misperceptions of cues from a victim, prompt aggressive behavior, and be used as an excuse for socially unacceptable behavior. A victim's drinking may impair his or her ability to assess being at risk of sexual assault and the ability to fight a perpetrator.[51]

Persistent heavy drinking also takes its toll on the body, causing problems such as a weakened immune system, heart disease, liver inflammation, pancreatitis, and many types of cancer (**FIGURE 7-7**).[49,52]

AUD does not affect just the person who is intoxicated, but others as well; children of parents with AUD are at increased risk of being abused and/or neglected, having emotional problems, and developing AUD themselves later in life.

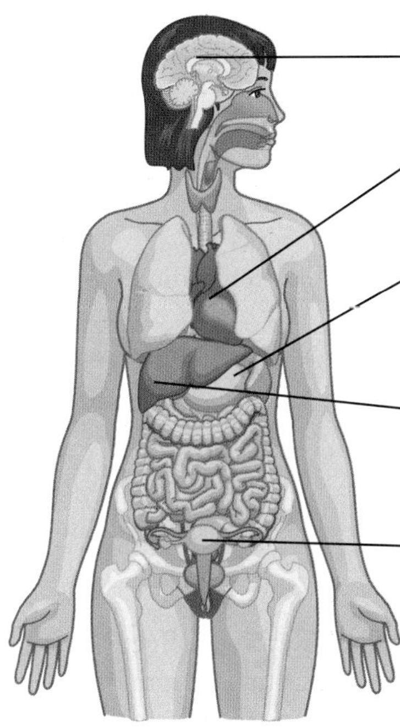

FIGURE 7-7 How alcohol affects your body.

Girlshealth.gov. (2013). Straight talk about alcohol. Retrieved from http://www.girlshealth.gov/substance/alcohol/

Alcohol has been a prominent part of Greek life on college campuses. Students who are a part of these organizations are more likely to engage in heavy drinking.[53] "Hazing" is a practice that fraternities and sororities use to initiate new members (students) into their chapters. This often involves pressure to drink heavily, in some cases causing death due to alcohol poisoning or fatal injuries. Hazing was formerly considered an accepted part of college life, but in recent years it has gained negative media attention. Families of those who died from hazing rituals have pushed for reform on campuses. Some colleges have suspended Greek life or increased the severity of hazing and alcohol violations in hopes of reducing what has proven to be dangerous behavior.

For people who have a problem with alcohol, there are treatment options. One of the most popular approaches to help individuals stop drinking and prevent relapse is support groups such as Alcoholics Anonymous (AA). AA follows a 12-step program that encourages participants to admit they are powerless over alcohol, believe in a higher power, and make amends to people they have harmed.

Twelve-step programs have been successful for some and criticized by others. Critics argue that being faith-based excludes individuals who do not believe in the existence of God. AA has been accused of "moralizing" addiction—alcoholism being the only disease whose treatment requires that individuals apologize for their actions. Additionally, there is a lack of scientific consensus regarding the impact of these programs on drinking cessation.[54] Twelve-step programs often encourage family and friends to alienate the "addicts" if they do not agree to enter treatment. This approach has been challenged by people who believe that loving support is needed to nurture a willingness to change.[55,56]

Other treatments include medication and behavioral therapy. There are currently three medications approved in the United States to assist individuals with AUD. These medications require a prescription and monitoring from a medical professional. Counseling, often from a social worker, psychologist, or psychiatrist, to help change behavior, is also a popular method to treat problematic drinking. The National Institute on Alcohol Abuse and Alcoholism suggests strategies for quitting drinking, including[57]:

- Seek medical attention to plan a safe recovery.
- Find alternatives—such as filling your time with hobbies.
- Avoid triggers—such as avoiding any places or people that make you want to drink.
- Create a plan to handle your urges—such as reminding yourself why you are changing.
- Know your "no"—giving a fast "no" response when offered a drink.

You can find interactive worksheets to help by searching "NIAAA Rethinking Drinking" and clicking on "Tools."

Stimulants

Caffeine

When we think about substances that can be addictive, caffeine may not readily come to mind. However, caffeine is one of the most commonly used mind-altering drugs. Its widespread use has made it one of the more socially acceptable substances. In North America, an astounding 80% to 90% of adults *and* children regularly consume some form of caffeine. This intake largely comes from drinking coffee, tea, and soft drinks, with coffee having the highest levels of caffeine. Four cups of coffee or five soft drinks or cups of tea per day are considered a moderate amount of caffeine. (But keep in mind the amount of calories in drinking five soft drinks a day!)

Most adults drink caffeine in the morning to increase mental alertness and help them wake up. Caffeine stimulates the central nervous system, heart, and muscles. There is some evidence that caffeine could increase blood pressure, but this may not be the case for those who use caffeine regularly. There has been mixed evidence over the last several decades about caffeine's association with cancer. The World Health Organization (WHO) reviewed the recent literature and declared that caffeine was not associated with cancer, and in some cases may even reduce the risk of certain cancers.[58] Caffeine is not recommended for people with anxiety disorders or acid reflux and during pregnancy.

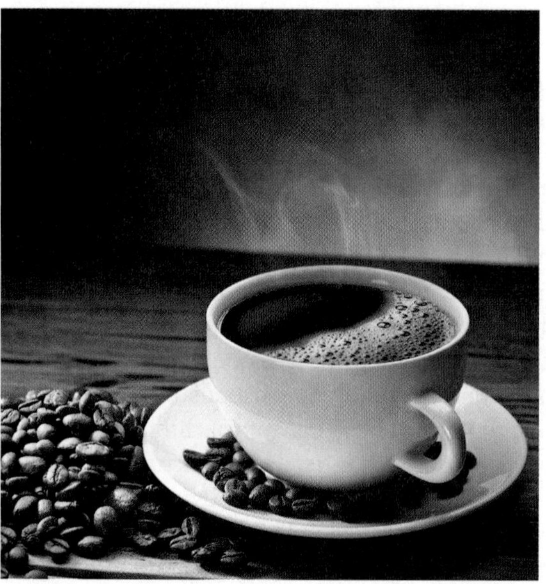

In North America, 80% to 90% of adults and children regularly consume caffeine.

People can become physically dependent on caffeine, as evidenced by the unpleasant withdrawal symptoms experienced by those who try to stop. These symptoms include distress, headache, fatigue, and anxiety.[59] However, caffeine dependence is not found in the *DSM-5,* nor is it considered a substance use disorder.

Pharmaceutical Drugs

Many pharmaceutical drugs, both prescription and nonprescription, are abused. Pharmaceutical drug abuse refers to taking medications for reasons or at doses for which they are not intended. The most commonly abused prescription drugs are opioids (to alleviate pain), depressants (for anxiety and sleep disorders), and stimulants (for attention deficit hyperactivity disorder).[60] The most commonly abused nonprescription medications (over-the-counter medications) are cough and cold remedies.

People of all ages, genders, races/ethnicities, and backgrounds abuse pharmaceutical drugs. About 52 million people (20%) have reported taking a prescription medication for a nonmedical reason at least once. Young people in particular have a higher prevalence of misusing these drugs.[61] Why would someone take a drug that is not needed? Many of the commonly abused drugs have mind-altering properties that can produce a temporary pleasurable feeling, or "high."

TABLE 7-1 Types of Substances and Their Health Effects

Substance	What Is It?	Selected List of Health Effects
Tobacco	■ Contains the addictive chemical nicotine as well as carcinogens and other toxic substances ■ Most popular method of using tobacco is via cigarettes	Cigarettes ■ Cancer, in particular lung cancer ■ Lung diseases, such as chronic bronchitis and emphysema ■ Increased risk of heart disease, including stroke, heart attack, vascular disease, and aneurysm ■ Leukemia ■ Cataracts ■ Pneumonia ■ On average, adults who smoke die 10 years earlier than nonsmokers
Alcohol	■ Substance that results from the fermentation of yeasts, sugars, and starches ■ Ingredient in beer, wine, and other liquors ■ Functions as a central nervous system depressant and is quickly absorbed into the bloodstream	Short term ■ Injuries ■ Violence ■ Alcohol poisoning ■ Risky sexual behavior ■ Miscarriage, stillbirth, or fetal alcohol spectrum disorder Long term ■ High blood pressure, heart disease, stroke, liver disease, and digestive problems ■ Cancer ■ Learning and memory problems ■ Mental health problems ■ Social problems ■ Alcoholism

(continues)

TABLE 7-1 Types of Substances and Their Health Effects *(continued)*

Substance	What Is It?	Selected List of Health Effects
Caffeine	■ Found in coffee, tea, and soft drinks ■ Most adults drink caffeine in the morning to increase mental alertness and help them wake up ■ Stimulates the central nervous system, heart, and muscles	Excessive consumption ■ Insomnia ■ Nervousness ■ Restlessness ■ Irritability ■ Stomach upset ■ Fast heartbeat ■ Muscle tremors
Pharmaceutical drugs	■ Includes both prescription and nonprescription drugs ■ Abuse is taking these drugs for reasons other than intended purpose or in a different manner than prescribed ■ Most commonly abused prescription drugs are opioids (to alleviate pain), depressants (for anxiety and sleep disorders), and stimulants (for attention deficit hyperactivity disorder) ■ Most commonly abused nonprescription medications are cough and cold remedies	Opioids ■ Constipation ■ Nausea ■ Slowed breathing ■ Hypoxia ■ Coma ■ Brain damage ■ Death Stimulants ■ Increased blood pressure ■ Seizures ■ Heart failure Depressants ■ Movement issues ■ Memory issues ■ Lowered blood pressure ■ Slowed breathing Nonprescription drugs ■ Increased heart rate ■ Increased blood pressure ■ Seizures ■ Hypoxia
Marijuana	■ Dried leaves, flowers, stems, and seeds of the plant *Cannabis sativa* ■ Contains the chemical delta-9-tetrahydrocannabinol (THC)	Short term ■ Panic ■ Paranoia ■ Impaired cognitive development and psychomotor performance Long term ■ Prolonged cognitive impairment ■ Frequent respiratory infections ■ Coughing ■ Problems with fetal development ■ Development of mental disorders
Synthetic cannabinoids	■ Most notably known as K2 or Spice ■ Portrayed as similar to marijuana but more dangerous and potent	■ Paranoia ■ Hallucinations ■ Seizures ■ Anxiety ■ Changes in blood flow to heart

Cocaine	■ White powdery substance derived from leaves of coca plant ■ Also comes in freebase form known as crack	Short term ■ Bizarre, erratic, and violent behavior ■ Restlessness, irritability, anxiety, panic, and paranoia ■ Tremors, vertigo, muscle twitches ■ Increased heart rate and blood pressure ■ Heart attacks ■ Strokes ■ Coma ■ Seizures Long term ■ Loss of smell, nosebleeds, problems with swallowing, hoarseness, chronically inflamed, runny nose ■ Lung damage and exacerbation of asthma ■ Allergic reactions ■ Tears and ulcerations in gastrointestinal tract ■ Weight loss and malnutrition ■ Chest pain ■ Stroke ■ Aortic rupture ■ Movement disorders ■ Impaired cognitive function ■ Bleeding in the brain
Methamphetamine	■ Synthetic white powder made from nonprescription medicines, solvents, and chemical products	Short term ■ Cardiovascular problems ■ Hyperthermia ■ Convulsions Long term ■ Psychosis ■ Anxiety and confusion ■ Insomnia ■ Violent behavior ■ Weight loss ■ Severe dental problems ■ Skin sores ■ Deficits in thinking and motor skills ■ Memory loss
Heroin	■ Powder or tarlike substance derived from opium poppy plant	Short term ■ Nausea and vomiting ■ Severe itching ■ Miscarriage ■ Slowed breathing and heart function ■ Clouded mental functions ■ Coma ■ Permanent brain damage

(continues)

TABLE 7-1 Types of Substances and Their Health Effects *(continued)*

Substance	What Is It?	Selected List of Health Effects
		Long term ■ Insomnia ■ Constipation ■ Lung complications ■ Mental health disorders ■ Sexual dysfunction ■ Collapsed veins ■ Bacterial infections ■ Abscesses ■ Infection of heart lining and valves ■ Arthritis and other rheumatologic problems ■ Liver and kidney disease
Hallucinogens and dissociative drugs	■ Drugs that distort perceptions of reality ■ Include LSD and PCP	■ Disorientation, confusion, and loss of coordination ■ Changes in sensory perceptions ■ Nausea ■ Hallucinations ■ Increase in blood pressure, heart rate, respiration, and body temperature ■ Memory loss ■ Psychological distress ■ Seizures ■ Amnesia ■ Mood swings ■ Speech difficulties ■ Flashbacks ■ Psychosis

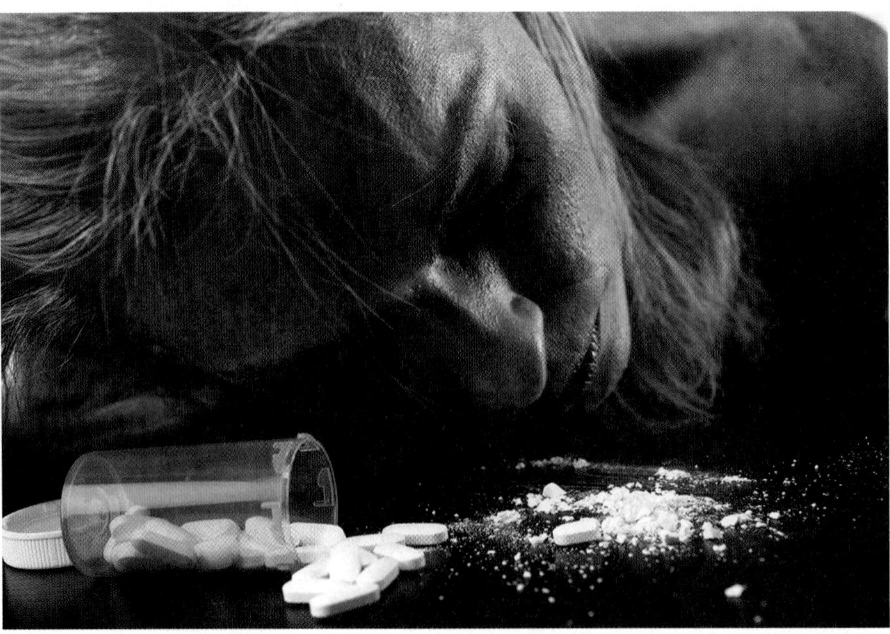

Prescription drug abuse and overdose have become a national crisis.

Prescription medications can be safe when taken according to a doctor's instructions for specific symptoms. However, when they are taken for reasons other than their intended purpose, in higher doses, or in a manner other than how they were prescribed, they can be extremely dangerous (**FIGURE 7-8**). Opioids include oxycodone and fentanyl, medications that are both used to manage pain. Prescriptions for these medications have increased dramatically, from 76 million in 1991 to 207 million in 2013 globally. The United States is the biggest consumer of opioids, for things like postsurgical pain and severe backaches. When medications are prescribed by a doctor, there is an assumption by patients that they will not be harmful. But opioids function in the same way that some illicit drugs do, by prompting a "high," or feeling of euphoria. If used chronically or not as prescribed, patients can become dependent on these medications and experience withdrawal symptoms.[62]

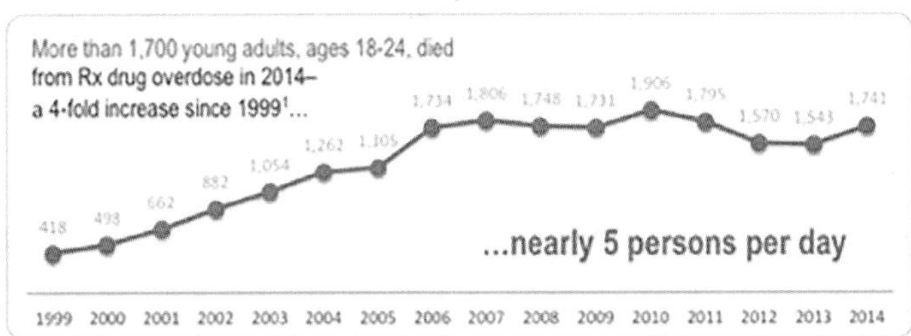

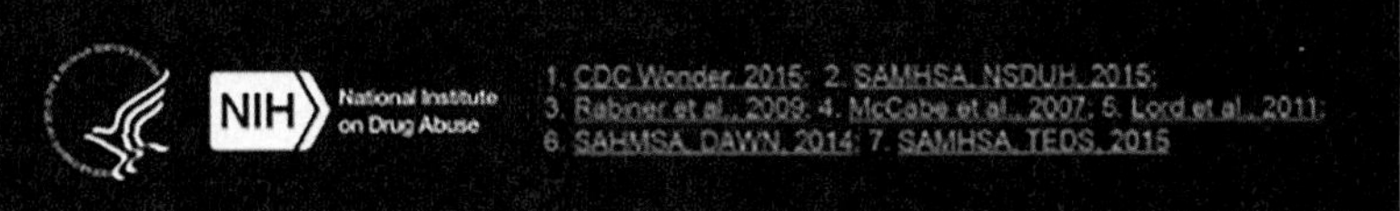

FIGURE 7-8 Consequences of prescription drug overdose.

National Institute on Drug Abuse. (2016). Abuse of prescription (Rx) drugs affects young adults most. Retrieved from https://www.drugabuse.gov/related-topics/trends-statistics/infographics/abuse-prescription-rx-drugs-affects-young-adults-most

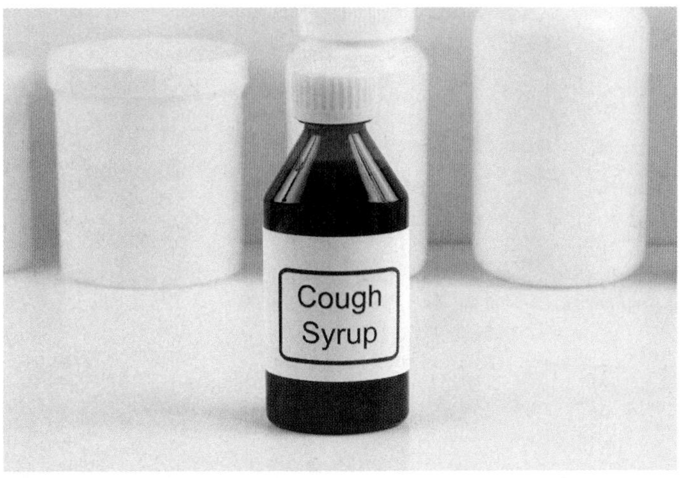

Over-the-counter cough and cold medicines are the most commonly abused nonprescription drugs.

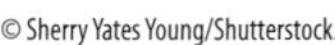
© Sherry Yates Young/Shutterstock.

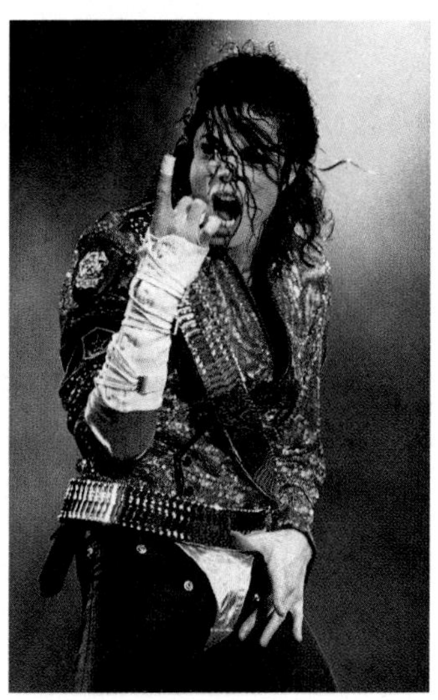

Michael Jackson performing on the Dangerous World Tour, 1992–1993. He died of prescription drug overdose in 2009.

© John Gunion/Redferns/Getty images.

Abusing opioids can result in minor side effects such as constipation and nausea, but can result in more serious conditions. They can slow down breathing, for example, which can cause reduced oxygen to the brain (hypoxia) and induce a coma or cause brain damage. Hence, opioid abuse can be fatal. Because opioid overdose has been responsible for so many deaths in recent years (165,000 from 1999 to 2014), and because these drugs can be addictive even when taken as prescribed, the Centers for Disease Control and Prevention released new guidelines in 2016 for primary care physicians regarding prescribing opioids for chronic pain (**FIGURE 7-9**).[63,64] To curb abuse, the guidelines suggest that doctors start with less habit-forming pain medications such as ibuprofen, and, if needed, prescribe opioids only for a few days at a time.

Stimulant abuse also has serious consequences; it can cause increased blood pressure and lead to seizures and heart failure. When used improperly, depressants can reduce brain activity and cause problems with movement, memory, lowered blood pressure, and slowed breathing. Abuse of dextromethorphan (found in cough and cold medicines) can increase heart rate and blood pressure and cause seizures. In severe cases, it can cause hypoxia.[7,64]

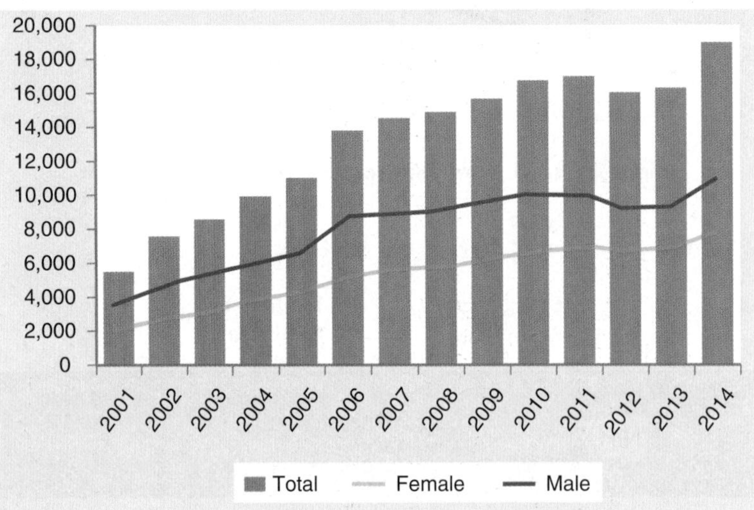

FIGURE 7-9 National Overdose Deaths: Number of Deaths from Prescription Opioid Pain Relievers.

National Institute on Drug Abuse. (2017). Overdose death rates. Retrieved from https://www.drugabuse.gov/related-topics/trends-statistics/overdose-death-rates

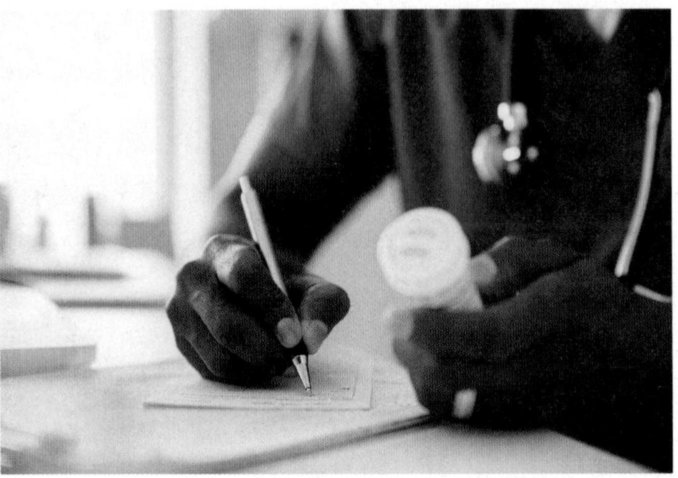

The FDA provides guidelines for safely disposing of unused medication.

For those who have become dependent on prescription medication, treatments are available. Three medications are approved for use to treat opioid addiction. In addition, behavioral therapies such as counseling or Narcotics Anonymous (similar to the 12-step program used to help those with AUD) can be used. There are no approved medications for those who abuse stimulants, depressants, or over-the-counter medications. Often, behavioral therapy is the first line of treatment.[64]

Marijuana

Marijuana, or cannabis, is made from dried leaves and flowers of the plant, *Cannabis sativa*. People smoke or ingest marijuana for its mind-altering effects, primarily a result of the chemical delta-9-tetrahydrocannabinol (THC) (**FIGURE 7-10**). It is the most commonly used illegal drug—almost 10% of Americans report using it.[65] The prevalence among young people is even higher; about 12% of eighth graders and 35% of high school seniors reported using marijuana in the past year.[66]

marijuana A psychoactive drug used recreationally and in some medical contexts. It is the most commonly used illegal drug in the United States. It consists of dried leaves, flowers, stems, and seeds of the plant, *Cannabis sativa*.

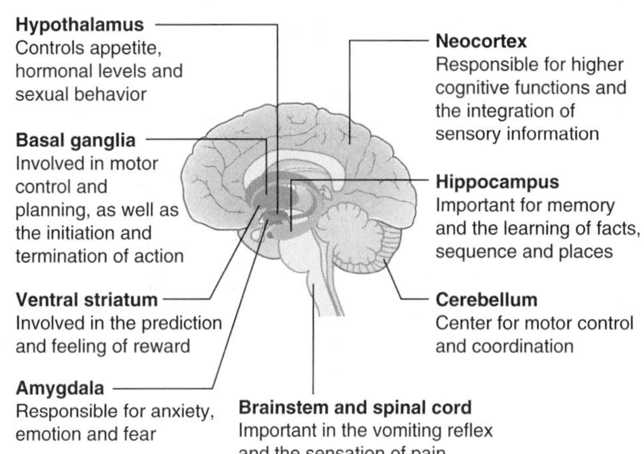

FIGURE 7-10 Marijuana's effects on the brain.

Drugabuse.gov. (n.d.). Marijuana's effects on the brain. Retrieved from https://www.drugabuse.gov/sites/default/files/images/colorbox/brain2.jpg

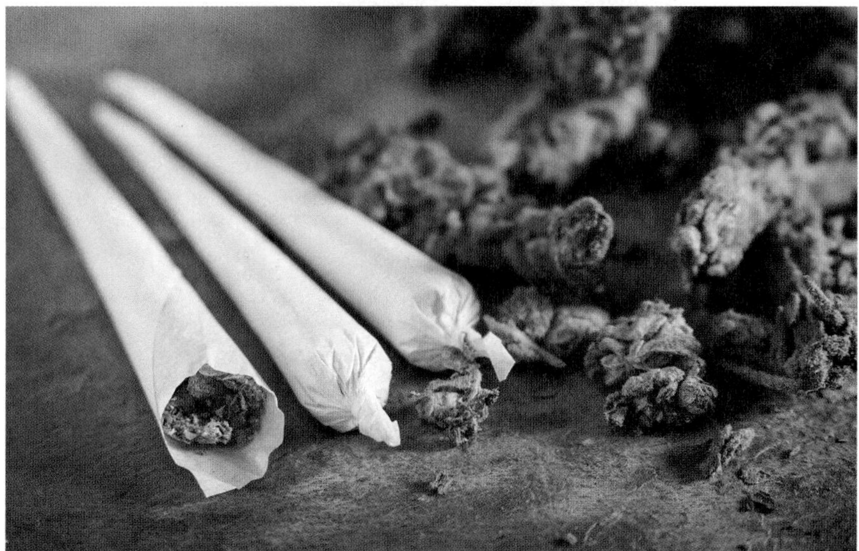

Marijuana plants being prepared for sale.

SYNTHETIC CANNABINOIDS

Synthetic cannabinoids (most commonly known as K2 and Spice, although there are dozens of other names) are man-made, mind-altering chemicals (not derived from the *Cannabis* plant). Although they have similar properties to cannabis, they are not the same. Synthetic cannabinoids are more dangerous than marijuana because they can be extremely potent. Poison control centers across the United States received 2,668 calls about K2 exposure in 2013, 3,682 calls in 2014, and 7,794 calls in 2015.[67] K2 has been shown to cause severe paranoia, seizures, anxiety, hallucinations, and changes in blood flow to the heart.

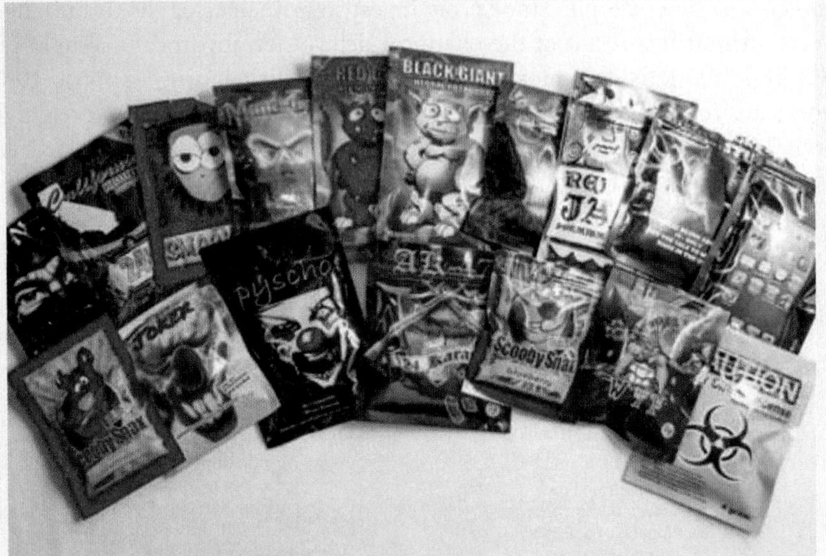

Synthetic cannabinoids are sold in packages like these.

Retrieved from NY State Department of Health.

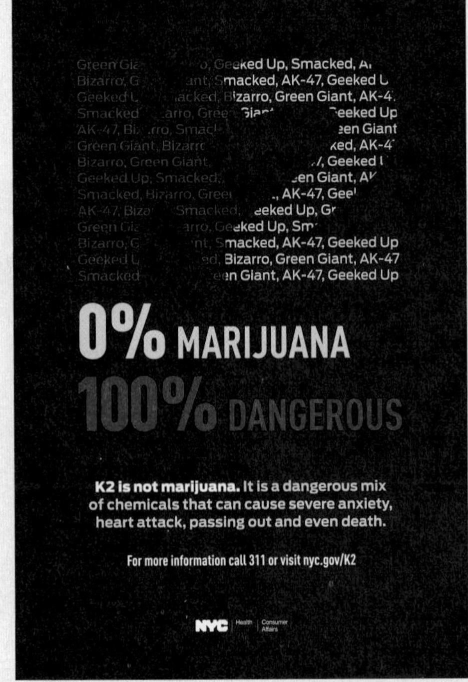

© New York City Department of Health and Mental Hygiene and New York City Department of Consumer Affairs. Reprinted with permission. http://www1.nyc.gov/site/doh/health/health-topics/k2.page

Marijuana is not legal in the United States according to federal law; however, the legality of marijuana is rapidly changing at the state level. As of November 2017, eight states (Alaska, California, Colorado, Maine, Massachusetts, Nevada, Oregon, and Washington) and the District of Columbia had legalized the purchase of marijuana for personal use by adults. The use of marijuana for medical purposes is approved in over half of U.S. states. (See Chapter 4 for more information about medical marijuana.)

The marijuana legalization debate has been going on for decades. Those who support legalizing marijuana believe that it is less dangerous than alcohol, and, given that it is already so widespread, regulating its use and taxing it could benefit both users and states that can use the revenue. The opposition feels that legalizing marijuana would increase its availability and thus its use, especially among adolescents.

GOING UPSTREAM

Marijuana Arrests and Communities of Color

Many people who support legalizing marijuana do so not just on the basis of how marijuana compares to other legal drugs, but also as a social justice issue.[68] Possession, use, and sale of marijuana are considered crimes in most states. About $3.5 billion are spent each year to enforce laws related to marijuana possession.

Aside from the issue of whether this money could be spent in more useful ways, there is a significant racial issue at play; namely, communities of color are disproportionately targeted for marijuana violations. Despite the fact that White individuals and Black individuals have similar rates of marijuana use, Blacks are nearly four times as likely to be arrested for possessing marijuana.

These arrests lead to entry into the criminal justice system, which can have lasting negative effects. Having a criminal record can impact a person's ability to gain employment, financial aid, housing, and more. Thus, for some, supporting the legalization of marijuana is an effort to reduce racial disparity in criminal justice.

FACT VERSUS FICTION

Is Marijuana Addictive?

So is marijuana harmful? Addictive? A "gateway drug"? Let's take a closer look at the evidence. For many people, the mind-altering effects of marijuana include feeling relaxed and euphoric; however, some people experience panic or paranoia, especially depending on the dosage. The short-term effects of marijuana include impaired cognitive and psychomotor performance. These effects can result in increased risk of motor vehicle accidents and memory problems.

Chronic marijuana use also has long-term effects, including prolonged cognitive impairment, frequent respiratory infections, coughing, and problems with fetal development if smoked during pregnancy. Chronic use is also associated with increased risk of developing mental disorders.[3,64,69] "Overdosing" on marijuana is unlikely to be fatal.

For a long time, marijuana was not viewed as addictive, but now chronic marijuana use is recognized as problematic. Regular use of marijuana at a young age is a risk factor for developing cannabis use disorder, which is defined as use of cannabis that causes impairment or distress, and has specific criteria a medical professional would consider for diagnosis.[9]

Six million people aged 12 years and older meet the criteria for cannabis use disorder, with men almost twice as likely to meet the criteria as women.[70] Most people with this disorder are considered dependent on marijuana. Symptoms of withdrawal for those who are dependent may not be as severe as those from a substance like heroin, but they can be uncomfortable. Withdrawal symptoms include difficulty sleeping, irritability, anxiety, and changes in appetite. This disorder is considered to be an addiction when someone cannot stop using marijuana despite its interference in his or her daily life.[64,71,72]

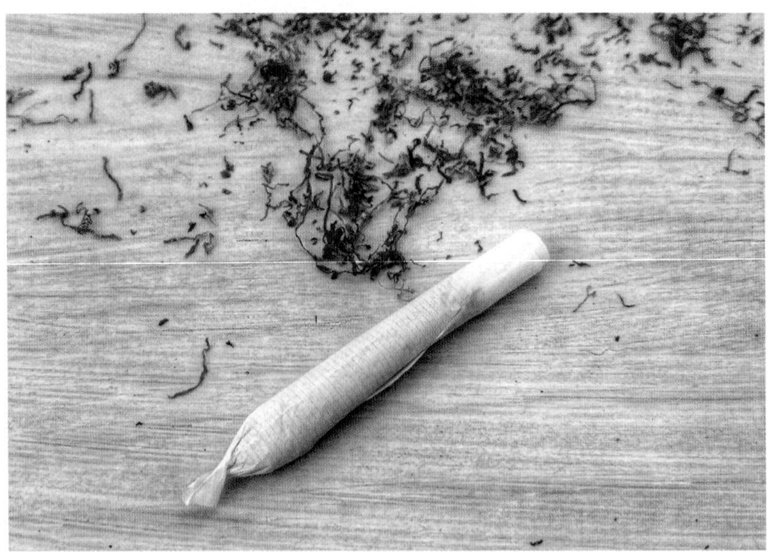

Marijuana is often rolled into a paper (or placed in a handheld device) to be smoked.

People who are against the legalization of marijuana are concerned that marijuana is a gateway drug—one that "opens the door" for the user to get involved with other illicit substances. There is some research that suggests marijuana users are more likely to develop AUD later in life. Some studies done on rats suggest that exposure to cannabis at an early age can affect the brain in a way that makes one susceptible to using other substances. However, most people who use marijuana do not use other illicit substances.[73]

UP FOR DEBATE

Legalize It?

Think about everything that you have ever read about marijuana, specifically its health effects, how it compares to other drugs, and how arrests affect communities of color. Do you think that marijuana possession, sale, and/or use should be made legal in the United States? Why or why not?

Like other substance use problems, behavioral support and counseling can be beneficial for those dependent on marijuana. No medications have yet been approved specifically for this purpose.

Food

With the rise of obesity and other food-related health problems in the last few decades, we have begun to understand the profound effect food can have on our health. Research has demonstrated that "food addiction" is a real phenomenon. Highly palatable foods, namely those high in sugar, salt, or fat, are everywhere in our society and appear to function similarly to drugs. Consumption of these types of foods can alter a person's brain chemistry and cause behavioral changes such as compulsive overeating, or a person may use food to self-medicate as a means of dealing with negative emotions, trauma, or anxiety. Food companies have worked hard to make their products taste good, often by carefully calibrating ingredients such as sugar, salt, and fat. They have dedicated considerable amounts of money and resources to try to get people hooked on these foods.[74–77]

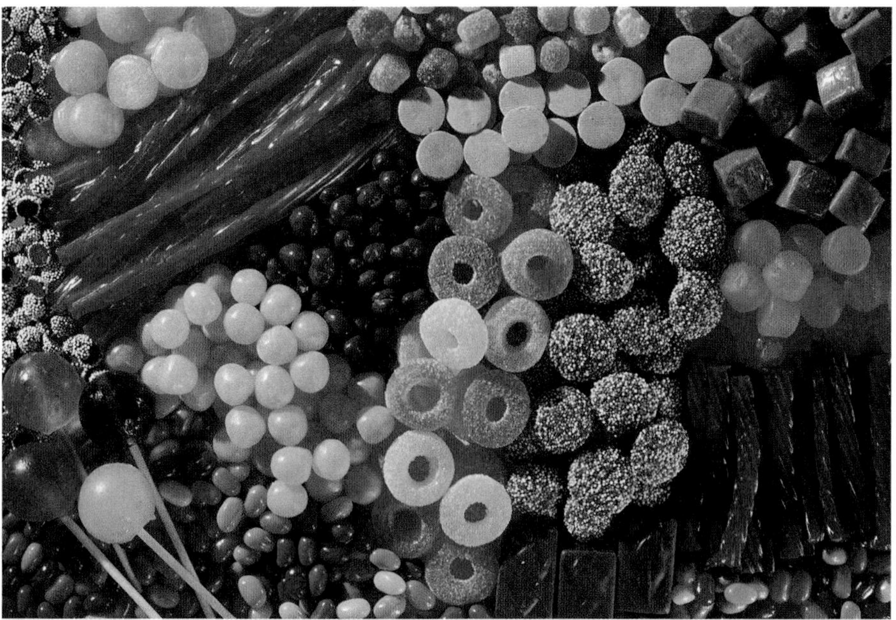

Highly palatable foods are often engineered with large amounts of sugar, salt, and fat.

Unlike other addictive substances, food is needed to sustain life. Thus, someone with a "food addiction" must face this issue on a daily basis. (See Chapters 2 and 6 for more on food and eating disorders.)

Illegal Drugs

Stimulants

Cocaine

Cocaine became a popular drug in the 1980s and 1990s, but it has been around much longer; it is actually one of the oldest psychoactive drugs.[78] Cocaine, also known as "coke," "blow," or "snow," is a white powdery substance derived from the leaves of the coca plant, which primarily grows in South America. A century ago, the purified cocaine (cocaine hydrochloride) was used in medicinal treatments for a variety of health problems. It is an illegal substance that is snorted or injected to obtain a feeling of euphoria. Freebase cocaine (cocaine that has been heated; known as "crack") can also be smoked.[79]

cocaine A white powdery or crystalline stimulant derived from the leaves of the coca plant. Also known as coke, blow, snow, or crack.

In a 2008 survey, almost 2 million people reported using cocaine in the past month. Almost 1.5 million people meet the criteria for cocaine dependence or abuse. The highest rates of use are among 18- to 25-year-olds. It is more common among Whites and males.[80,81]

Cocaine is extremely addictive and dangerous. It can increase heart rate and blood pressure and cause anxiety, violent behavior, paranoia, heart attacks, strokes, seizures, organ damage, and other problems. Over 5,000 people died of cocaine overdose in 2014, a 42% increase from 2001.[82] People under the influence of cocaine appear to have a lot of energy, are very talkative, and seem restless. Stopping cocaine after regular use can result in withdrawal symptoms, including depression, fatigue, insomnia, and slower cognitive abilities. No medications exist to treat cocaine addiction, and therapeutic approaches to recovery include CBT.[64,83]

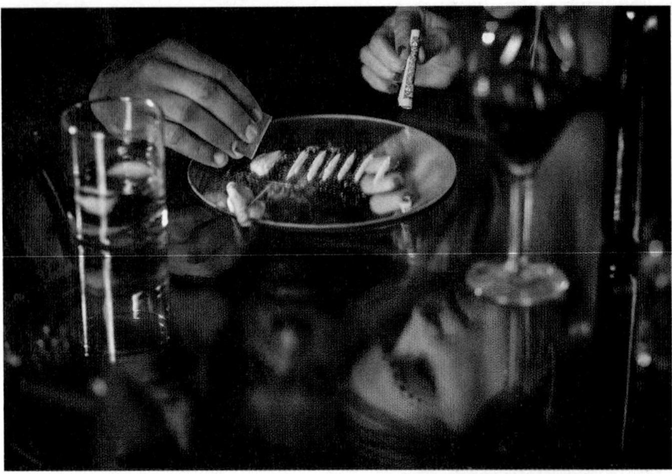

Cocaine became a popular "party" drug in the 1980s and 1990s.

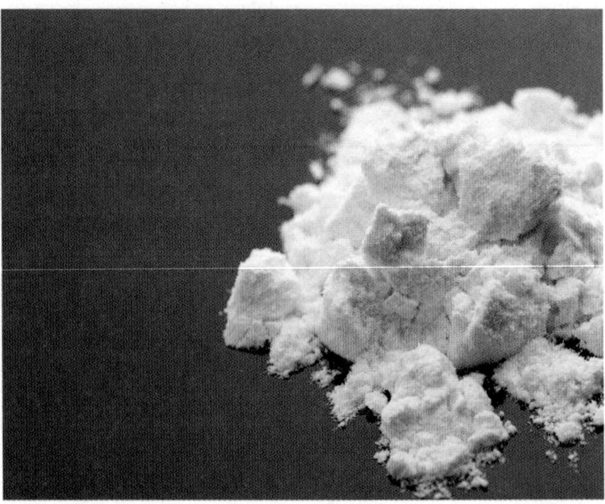

Crack cocaine.

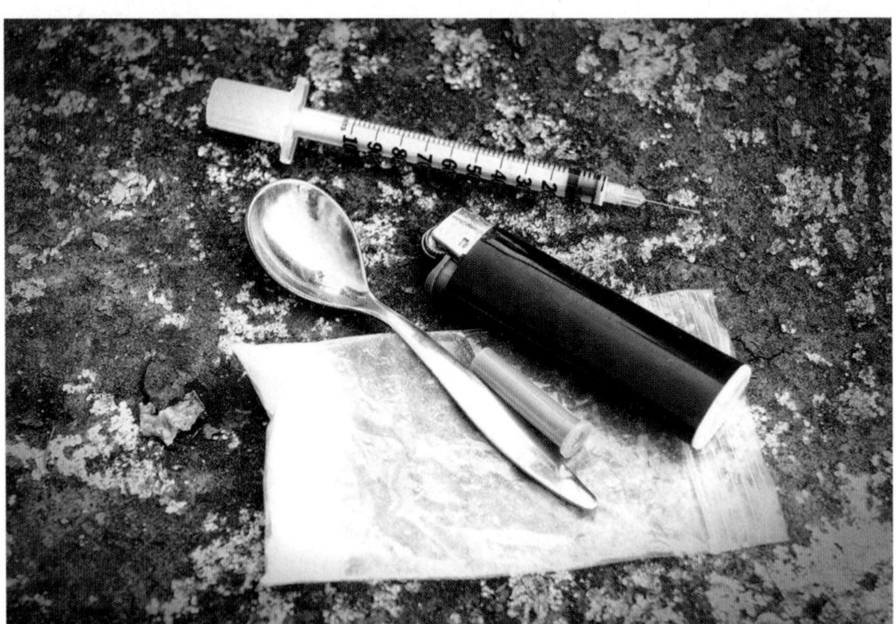

Crack cocaine is sometimes heated on a spoon and then injected.

Methamphetamines

methamphetamine An extremely addictive stimulant chemically similar to amphetamine. Also known as meth, crystal, chalk, and ice.

Methamphetamine (commonly known as "meth") is another highly addictive substance. It is a white powder that can be snorted, smoked, injected, or taken orally. Crystal methamphetamine comes in the form of a rock that is blue-white in color, and it can be smoked, snorted, swallowed, or injected. It is a stimulant that affects the central nervous system. Methamphetamine was originally developed as a nasal decongestant. In rare cases, methamphetamine is prescribed to treat attention deficit hyperactivity disorder, but the prescribed dose is very low.[84]

Methamphetamine produces a sense of euphoria and increased talkativeness in the user. In the short term, it can also induce hyperthermia, increased heart rate, and respiratory problems. Taking a large dose of the drug is extremely dangerous and can cause seizures, heart attack, breathing problems, kidney damage, and other problems. Users may appear psychotic, engage in violent behavior, or seem anxious or confused. Skin sores and tooth loss (known as "meth mouth") are common among regular users.[85,86]

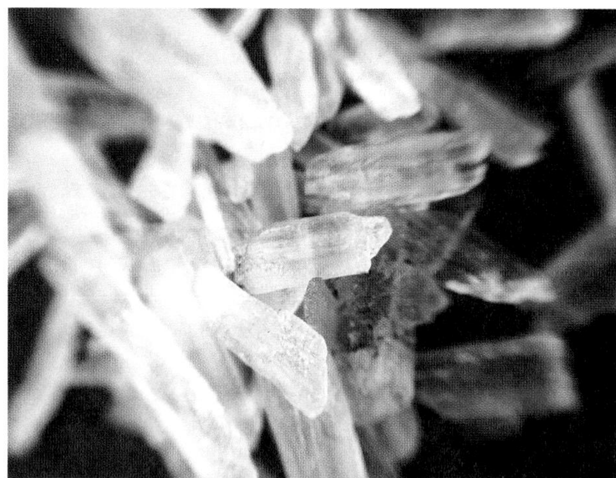

Users vaporize and smoke methamphetamine crystals.

METHAMPHETAMINE LABS

"Meth labs," where people make methamphetamine from readily available substances such as over-the-counter medications, solvents, and chemical products, have been popping up across the United States. These clandestine labs, like the one popularized in the TV series, "Breaking Bad," have consequences not only in terms of increasing the drug supply, but also in terms of environmental pollution.

Cooking (producing) meth often involves hazardous chemicals; as a result of the meth-making process, labs have exploded, caught on fire, or released toxic gases, injuring innocent bystanders who unknowingly were in close proximity. The hazardous waste left over from meth cooking can contaminate the building, surrounding areas, or places where the waste was dumped. If a meth lab is discovered by the authorities, specific guidelines are set forth by the Environmental Protection Agency that detail how to clean up the site without further endangering workers or the environment.

FIGURE 7-11 provides a 2014 map of the locations of methamphetamine laboratory incidents.[87] Note the high rates in states like Indiana and Missouri.

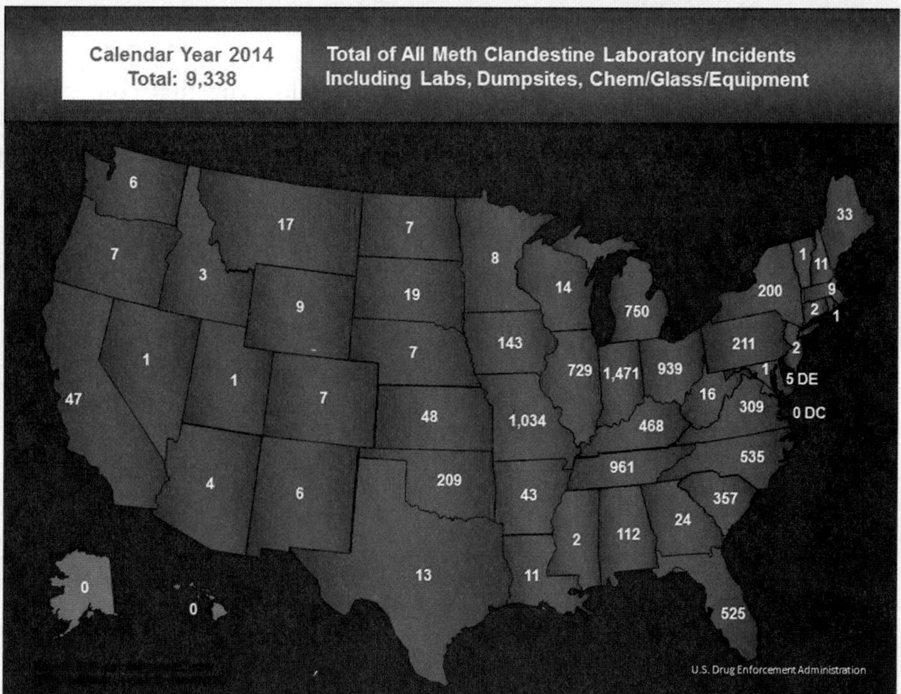

FIGURE 7-11 Locations of methamphetamine lab incidents.

Drug Enforcement Administration. (2014). Methamphetamine lab incidents, 2004-2014. Retrieved from https://www.dea.gov/resource-center/meth-lab-maps.shtml

RESOURCES

If you or a loved one needs help, here are some resources:

- National Institute on Alcohol Abuse and Alcoholism: http://www.niaaa.nih.gov/alcohol-health/support-treatment
- Rethinking Drinking: http://rethinkingdrinking.niaaa.nih.gov/Tools/Default.aspx
- National Institute on Drug Abuse, brief description of treatment approaches to drug addiction: https://www.drugabuse.gov/related-topics/treatment
- National Institute on Drug Abuse, overview of behavioral therapies relevant to drug addiction: https://www.drugabuse.gov/publications/principles-drug-addiction-treatment/evidence-based-approaches-to-drug-addiction-treatment/behavioral-therapies

Over one million people reported that they have used meth in the last year. Methamphetamine use is more common among men, Whites, and residents of rural areas. However, as drug availability has spread, its use is increasing among other populations.[88]

When the drug is used frequently, it depletes the brain's stores of dopamine and destroys dopamine receptors, leaving methamphetamine as the only way for the user to experience pleasure and euphoria. Thus, once the user stops, there is a high risk of depression. There are no medical treatments approved for methamphetamine addiction. Recovery is difficult because it takes many months for dopamine receptors to regrow. However, recovery is possible with behavioral therapies, and medication that may be needed to treat depression.[88]

Opioids

Heroin

heroin An opioid drug that is synthesized from morphine, a powder or tar-like substance extracted from the seed pod of the Asian opium poppy plant.

Heroin is a highly addictive opioid drug that comes in a powder or as a tar-like substance that is derived from the opium poppy plant. Almost one-quarter of people who use heroin will become addicted to it. Heroin can be injected, inhaled, or smoked. Regardless of the way it is administered, heroin goes to the brain very quickly. Initially, it gives the user a euphoric feeling. It can also initially cause nausea, vomiting, or itchiness. After a few hours, the user feels as if his or her surroundings are in slow motion. Heroin is illegal and not indicated for any medical conditions. Heroin use is less common than the drugs discussed so far. About 2% of people have ever tried heroin. However, this number has increased over the last decade, especially among young people 18 to 25 years of age. Many people who use heroin have mental health disorders. Use is more common among Whites, men, and those who are poor.[64,89,90] A heroin epidemic has emerged in recent years in rural areas such as Vermont.[91]

Heroin can have a serious impact on one's health (**TABLE 7-2**). Abuse is associated with increased risk of infectious diseases, breathing problems, and liver or kidney disease. The toxic agents in heroin can clog blood vessels and permanently damage organs. People use heroin to experience a euphoric feeling, but when people overdose, they can lose consciousness and stop breathing, which can cause permanent brain damage or death. Some signs of an overdose include

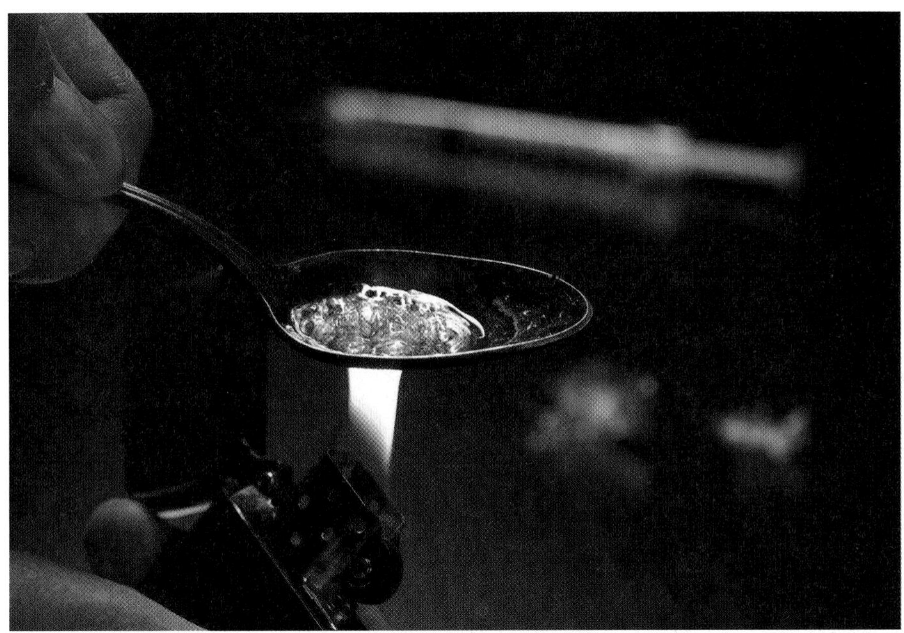

TABLE 7-2 Entertainers Who Died of Substance Overdoses

Name	Occupation	Primary substance(s) implicated in death	Birth–Death
John Belushi[a]	Comedian, actor, and musician	Heroin and cocaine	1949–1982
Kurt Cobain[b]	Lead singer, songwriter, and primary guitarist of band Nirvana	Heroin and diazepam	1967–1994
Chris Farley[c]	Comedian and actor	Morphine and cocaine	1964–1997
Jimi Hendrix[d]	Rock guitarist, singer, and songwriter	Barbiturates	1942–1970
Whitney Houston[e]	Singer, actress, producer, and model	Cocaine	1963–2012
Michael Jackson[f]	Singer, songwriter, record producer, dancer, and actor	Propofol and lorazepam	1958–2009
Janis Joplin[g]	Singer	Heroin	1943–1970
Chris Kelly[h]	Member of hip-hop duo Kris Kross	Cocaine and heroin	1978–2013
Heath Ledger[i]	Actor and director	Oxycodone, hydrocodone, diazepam, temazepam, alprazolam, and doxylamine	1979–2008
Cory Monteith[j]	Actor and musician	Heroin and alcohol	1982–2013

(continues)

TABLE 7-2 Entertainers Who Died of Substance Overdoses *(continued)*

Name	Occupation	Primary substance(s) implicated in death	Birth–Death
River Phoenix[k]	Actor, musician, and activist	Morphine and cocaine	1970–1993
Philip Seymour Hoffman[l]	Actor, director, and producer	Heroin, cocaine, benzodiazepines, and amphetamine	1967–2014
Amy Winehouse[m]	Singer and songwriter	Alcohol	1983–2011

[a] Stewart, R. W. (1985, September 19). Heroin killed Belushi, pathologist asserts. *Los Angeles Times*. Retrieved from http://articles.latimes.com/1985-09-19/local/me-1899_1_heroin
[b] *Seattle Post-Intelligencer*. (1994, April 15). Nirvana's Kurt Cobain was high when he shot himself. Retrieved from http://articles.baltimoresun.com/1994-04-15/features/1994105028_1_kurt-cobain-cobain-suicide-heroin
[c] Associated Press. (1998, January 3). Accidental drug overdose killed Farley, autopsy shows. *Los Angeles Times*. Retrieved from http://articles.latimes.com/1998/jan/03/entertainment/ca-4431
[d] *Rolling Stone*. (1970, October 29). Hendrix inquest inconclusive. Retrieved from http://www.rollingstone.com/music/news/hendrix-inquest-inconclusive-19701029
[e] Blankstein, A. (2012, April 4). Whitney Houston: Final coroner's report. *Los Angeles Times*. Retrieved from http://documents.latimes.com/whitney-houston-coroners-report-final/
[f] Tourtellotte, B. (2009, August 28). Jackson death ruled homicide, focus on doctor. *Entertainment News*. Retrieved from http://www.reuters.com/article/us-jackson-idUSTRE57R4EY20090828
[g] Gent, G. (1970, October 6). Death of Janis Joplin attributed to accidental heroin overdose. Retrieved from http://www.nytimes.com/books/99/05/02/specials/joplin-obit2.html
[h] Duke, A. (2013, July 3). Kris Kross' Chris Kelly died from overdose, autopsy says. *CNN entertainment*. Retrieved from http://www.cnn.com/2013/07/03/showbiz/chris-kelly-autopsy/
[i] Leiberman, P. (2008, February 7). 6-drug combo blamed. *Los Angeles Times*. Retrieved from http://articles.latimes.com/2008/feb/07/entertainment/et-ledger7
[j] D'Zurrilla, C. (2013, October 2). Cory Monteith's death ruled accidental; heroin-alcohol mix blamed. *Los Angeles Times*. Retrieved from http://www.latimes.com/entertainment/gossip/la-et-mg-cory-monteith-death-heroin-alcohol-20131002-story.html
[k] Connell, R., & Hall, C. (1993, November 13). Drug overdose killed Phoenix, coroner says. *Los Angeles Times*. Retrieved from http://articles.latimes.com/1993-11-13/news/mn-56484_1_drug-overdose
[l] Sanchez, R. (2014, February 28). Coroner: Philip Seymour Hoffman died of acute mixed drug intoxication. *CNN entertainment*. Retrieved from http://www.cnn.com/2014/02/28/showbiz/philip-seymour-hoffman-autopsy/
[m] Ministry of Gossip. (2011, October 26). Amy Winehouse: "Death by misadventure"—alcohol—coroner says. *Los Angeles Times*. Retrieved from http://latimesblogs.latimes.com/gossip/2011/10/amy-winehouse-death-alcohol-poisoning-amy-winehouse.html

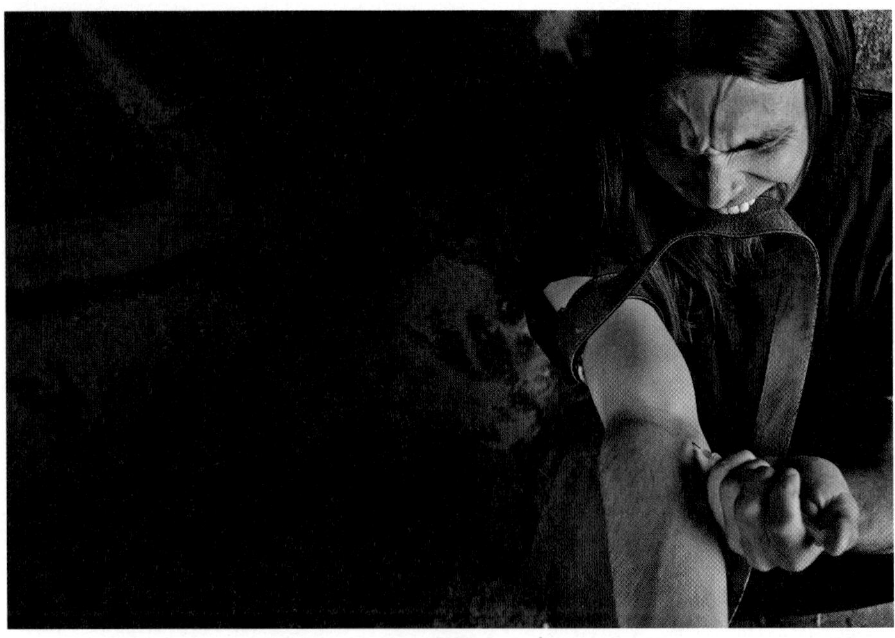

Like crack cocaine, heroin can be heated ("cooked") and then injected.

difficulty breathing, small pupils, low blood pressure, and uncontrolled muscle movements.[83,92]

If people who are dependent on heroin try to stop using it, they may experience withdrawal symptoms, including insomnia, cold flashes, muscle pain, and heroin craving (leading to relapse). As with other substance

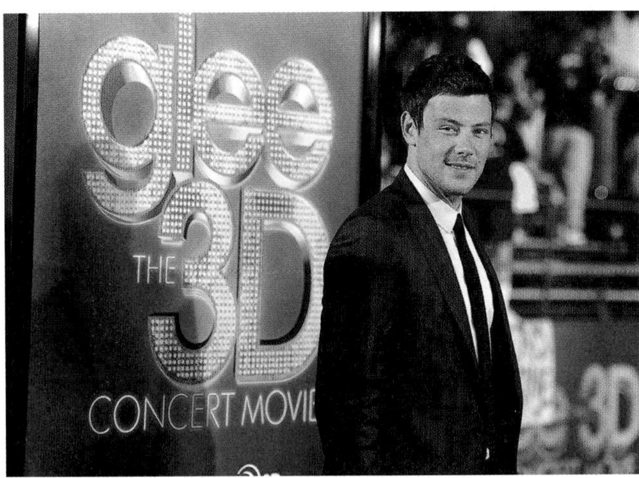

Actor and musician Cory Monteith was a star of the hit television show "Glee" before his death from heroin and alcohol in 2013.

dependence, heroin addiction can be treated with behavioral therapies and medications. Three prescription medications are approved to treat heroin addiction: methadone, buprenorphine, and naltrexone. They affect the same receptors as heroin, but without the harmful side effects or behavioral changes.[90]

Naloxone (brand name Narcan) is a medication that can help victims in the middle of an overdose episode. It can be injected into a muscle or given intravenously or as a nasal spray and works within minutes. Emergency medical personnel have naloxone on hand in case they need to treat a patient in the midst of an overdose. Physicians can prescribe the drug to patients at risk of heroin overdose. Heroin users can show friends and family how to administer the drug in case of an emergency. Having access to this medication has not been shown to increase the likelihood of using opiates; instead, it provides a lifesaving treatment in the event of a critical emergency.[93]

hallucinogens A class of drugs that causes hallucinations—profound distortions in a person's perceptions of reality; can be found in some plants and mushrooms (or their extracts) or can be man-made.

dissociative drugs A class of drugs that can distort one's perception of reality. The sensations experienced when taking these types of drugs are referred to as "tripping."

Hallucinogens and Dissociative Drugs

Hallucinogens and **dissociative drugs** are distinct from the drugs described previously in how they can distort one's perception of reality. The sensations experienced when taking these types of drugs are referred to as "tripping." Certain hallucinogens are highly addictive. Other hallucinogens, like LSD, do not cause users to seek repeated use in a way that is uncontrollable and thus are not considered addictive; however, they do produce tolerance, which means higher doses are needed to attain the same effect.[94]

An estimated 15% of people have tried hallucinogens at some point in their lifetime. Compared to other countries, the United States has one of the highest proportions of high school students who have ever tried LSD or other hallucinogens (6%).[95,96]

Hallucinogens can alter perceptions of time, motion, and color, and drugs like LSD can also cause unpredictable mood swings. Dissociative drugs like phencyclidine (PCP) can cause a feeling of being outside of one's own body. These sensations, sometimes referred to as a "bad trip," can be frightening and cause erratic and sometimes dangerous behavior. Other short-term effects of hallucinogens include increased heart rate and blood pressure, excessive sweating, panic, paranoia, and psychosis. Another mood-altering drug

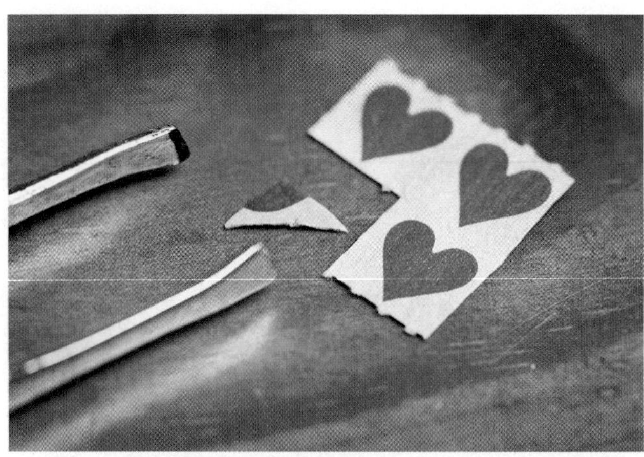

A blotter sheet of LSD-soaked paper. Users ingest the squares by mouth.

is 3,4-Methylenedioxy-methamphetamine (MDMA; also called Ecstasy or Molly)—a synthetic drug usually sold in powder or capsules. It functions in much the same manner as a stimulant and hallucinogen, increasing one's energy and providing a sense of pleasure.[94,97,98]

The long-term effects of using these drugs are unclear. Research suggests that in rare cases, repeated hallucinogen use can result in persistent psychosis and flashbacks. Chronic PCP use may cause problems with speech, memory, anxiety, and depression. Trying to quit using drugs like PCP may cause withdrawal symptoms such as cravings and headaches. There is no approved medical treatment for hallucinogen addiction. Behavioral therapy may be helpful, but more research is needed.[94]

Hallucinogens and dissociative drugs have no approved medical indication; however, in the 1970s, some hallucinogens were used to supplement talk therapy. Researchers have explored the use of small doses of hallucinogens in a controlled environment to treat mental health disorders such as end-of-life anxiety, posttraumatic stress disorder, and depression.[98-100] More research is needed to understand if these drugs have a place in treating mental health disorders.

Harm Reduction

The typical 12-step program and counseling for substance use are based on a model of promoting complete abstinence (not using the drug of choice at all). However, there is a distinct, parallel movement, one based in social justice and respect for those with substance use disorders, that employs approaches to reduce harm and consequences associated with drug use rather than promote abstinence. This philosophy is called **harm reduction**. The Harm Reduction Coalition developed a set of guiding principles for proponents of this philosophy, which include understanding drug use as a continuum of behaviors, and encouragement of resource provision to help users reduce drug use as desired.[73]

harm reduction A movement based in social justice and respect for those with substance use disorder that employs approaches to reduce harm and consequences associated with drug use rather than promote abstinence; includes tactics such as needle exchange and safe injection sites.

Harm reduction encompasses supervised injection facilities, needle-exchange programs that provide clean hypodermic needles to users, and access to methadone maintenance programs. These harm reduction strategies are controversial in the United States; however, they are supported by public health and human rights advocates for their realistic and considerate approach. In addition, harm-reduction strategies have been shown to reduce morbidity and mortality among substance users.[101]

Behavioral Addictions

Many people think about addiction only in terms of drug abuse, but the truth is that people can also become addicted to behaviors—even ones that may be considered healthy or harmless. Gambling, exercise, sex, and even technology use can be problematic behaviors under certain circumstances.

Gambling

Have you ever made a bet with a friend about which team would win the Super Bowl, or bought a scratch-off ticket in hopes of winning a few bucks? This type of social or casual gambling can be harmless and even fun. For some, however, these behaviors can progress into compulsive gambling. Compulsive gambling is a disorder characterized by continued gambling despite the negative consequences it has on one's life and relationships. Like substance use, gambling can affect the brain's chemical reward system and cause a pattern of addictive and destructive behavior. Compulsive gambling is not about money as much as it is about the thrill and excitement of winning. Compulsive gamblers can accrue debt, hide gambling from loved ones, become preoccupied with gambling, take increasingly bigger risks, prioritize gambling over work or family, and use gambling as a means of dealing with depression or stress. Those who gamble casually can set limits and stop when they lose a certain amount, compared

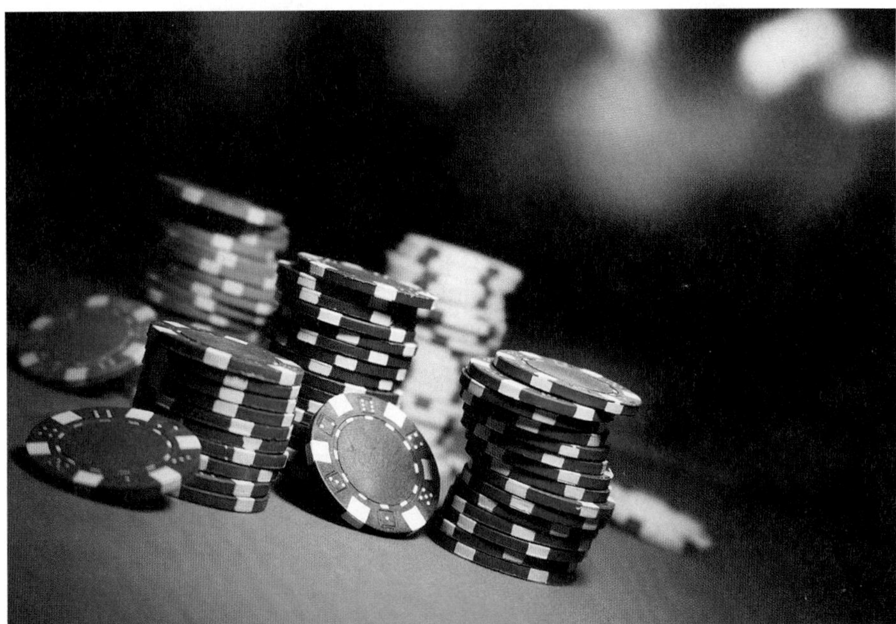

Compulsive gambling is more about the thrill of winning than the actual money.

BY THE NUMBERS

Gambling

Most states allow legalized gambling, such as casinos or race tracks, for those over age 18 years. About 1% of adults and 6% to 9% of younger people have a gambling disorder. Over 95% of people with a gambling problem also have (or have had) another mental health disorder. [103]

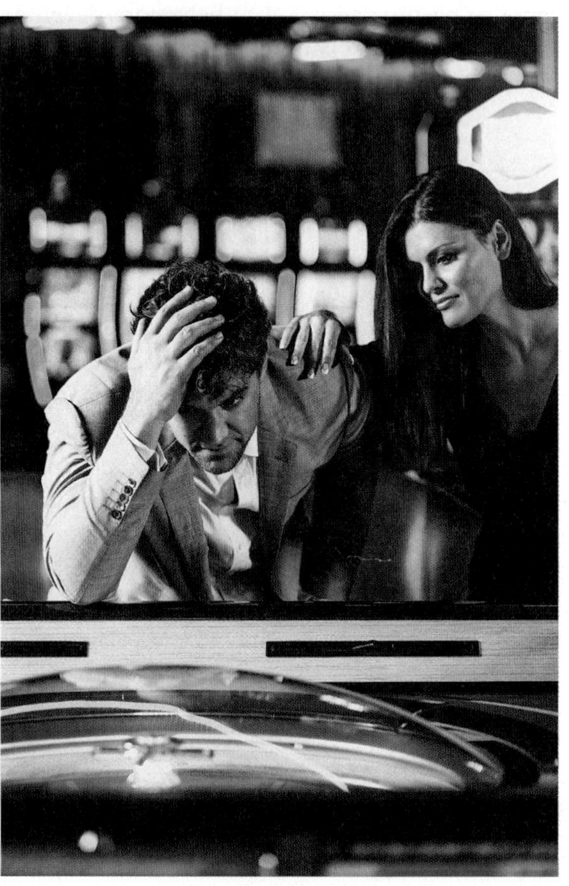

to compulsive gamblers, who will keep betting or playing no matter what.[102] Treatment for a gambling disorder is promising. About one-third of people who try to quit gambling are successful. For those who are unable to quit on their own, behavioral therapy and counseling are recommended.[103]

Exercise

Exercising is one of the single most important things individuals can do to maintain their health. (See Chapter 3.) It's normal and even encouraged to be committed to routine physical activity. But exercise can become an addictive behavior if one continues to engage in it frequently despite reaching one's stated goals, physical injury, or disruption to one's life. Much like other addictions, not being able to control this behavior is indicative of dependence. Exercise addiction can start to affect relationships and other commitments, such as work, and often results in psychological, social, and financial problems. Someone who is addicted to exercise experiences withdrawal symptoms when he or she is not able to engage in activity.[104]

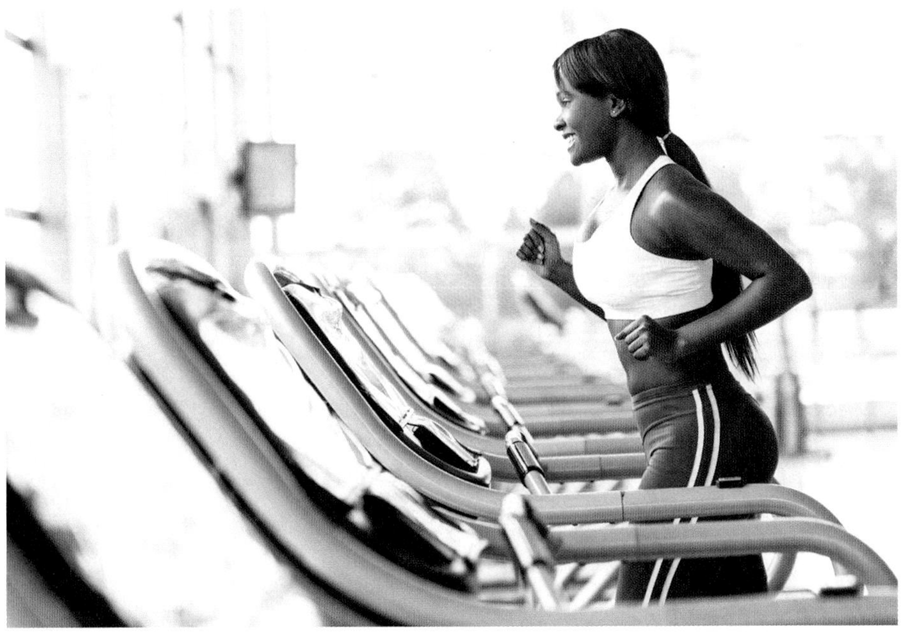

Exercise is a fundamental part of staying healthy. For some, however, it can become an addictive behavior.

It is not known exactly how many people suffer from exercise addiction, but incidence is estimated at 3% of adults. Preliminary research suggests that exercise addicts are also at higher risk of other addictive behaviors, substance use, and eating disorders.[105]

Because exercise addiction is a relatively new phenomenon, more research is needed to understand the best treatment approach. Treatment for substance use disorders often entails completely abstaining from using any mind-altering substance, but exercise is a special case, as moderate exercise is considered healthy. One suggestion has been for those addicted to a certain form of exercise to switch to an alternative form. Behavioral counseling is also recommended.[106]

Sex

Sexual intimacy among consenting adults is normal and healthy. (See Chapter 5.) But can someone become addicted to sex? Sexual addiction is not considered a mental health disorder according to the *DSM-5*, but preliminary research suggests that it exists and can be problematic.

Sexual addiction is characterized as "continued engagement in sexual activities despite the negative consequences created by these activities."[107] These consequences can be physical, social, and psychological. Risk of sexually transmitted diseases increases with repeated unsafe sexual behavior. Sex may interfere with one's relationships and work. Sexual addiction can also create a distorted view of sex and intimacy and incite shame and guilt.[107]

It is estimated that about 12 million people have an addiction to sex.[108] Sex addiction is not just about liking sex; like drugs, sex can affect the brain's reward system and create the urge for continued engagement to seek pleasurable effects. Sexual addiction is associated with such behaviors as excessive watching of pornography, engaging in compulsive masturbation, and soliciting prostitutes.[108]

Health professionals debate if and how sex addiction should be classified and defined. Some have argued it falls under obsessive-compulsive or

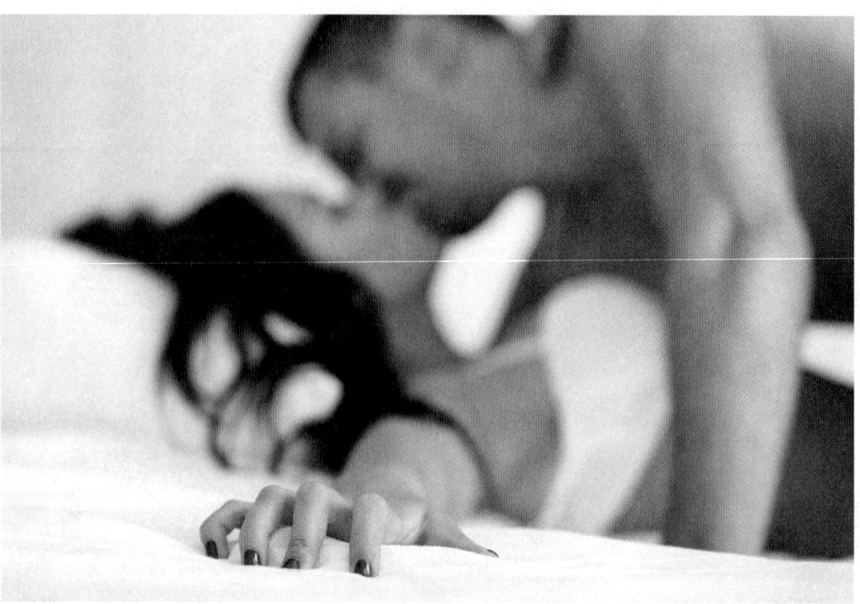

Can someone be addicted to sex?

impulse-control disorder, while others believe it is its own addictive disorder. Large-scale research studies are needed to better understand sex addiction.

Technology

Think about how many times a day you check your phones, tablets, or computers for emails, text messages, and social media updates. How often do you stream videos, listen to music, do homework on laptops, or play video games? The average person spends a large amount of time each day engaged with some sort of technology. On average, teenagers spend a whopping 9 hours per day using media. This is a relatively new phenomenon. In 2000, about 50% of Americans owned a cell phone, compared with 90% of Americans in 2014. Similarly, only 8% of Internet-using adults used a social networking site in 2005, compared with over 75% in 2015 (**FIGURE 7-12**).[109,110]

One large-scale study found that one in eight Americans exhibited signs of problematic Internet use. Almost 14% found it hard to stay away from the Internet for several days, and 12% saw a need to cut back on time spent online.[111]

Is our ever-increasing use of technology considered addictive? That's up for debate. Like sex addiction, "technology addiction" is not listed in the *DSM-5*; some argue that it is a manifestation of another disorder (like anxiety, depression, or impulse control). Early research suggests the signs of excessive technology use (not for work purposes) include the following[88]:

- Changes in mood
- Preoccupation with the Internet and digital media
- The inability to control the amount of time spent interfacing with digital technology
- The need for more time or a new game to achieve a desired mood
- Withdrawal symptoms when not engaged
- A continuation of the behavior despite family conflict, a diminishing social life, and adverse work or academic consequences

More research is needed to understand what technology addiction entails and if and what the diagnostic criteria should be.

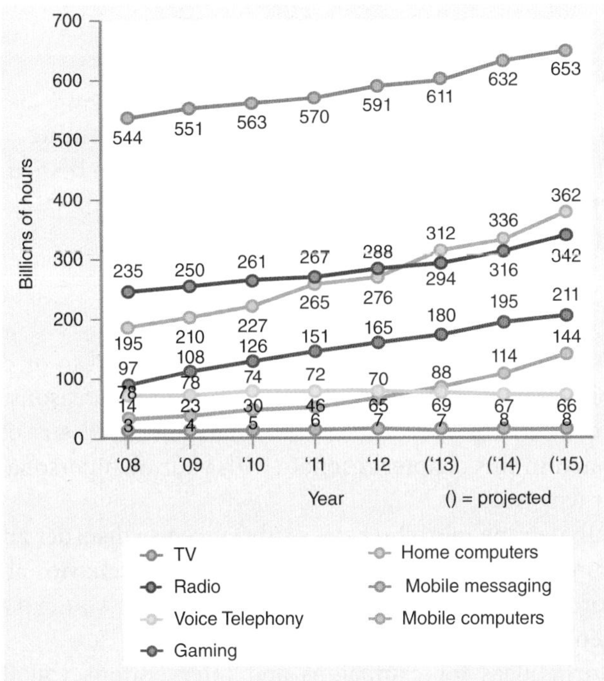

FIGURE 7-12 The number of hours Americans spend watching television and using computers or phones has increased steadily in the last few years.

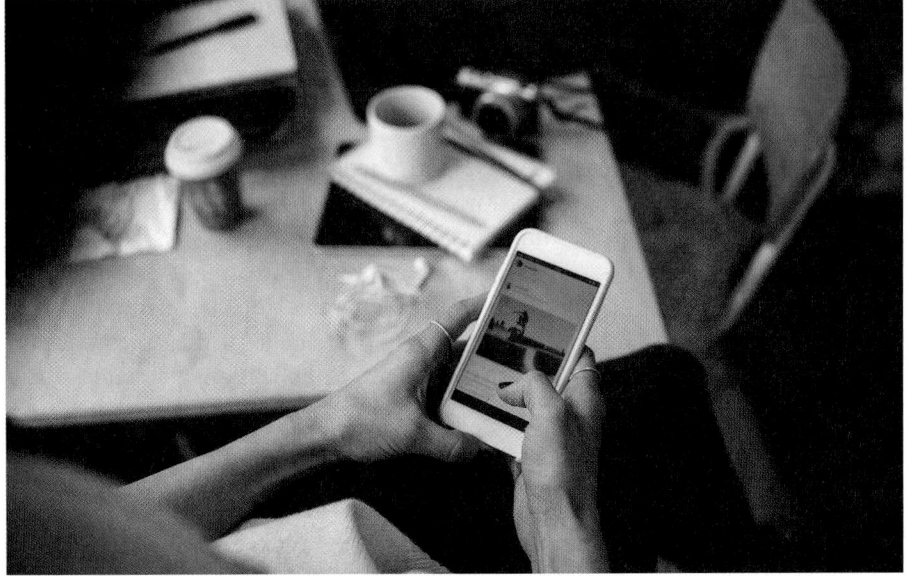

Are we becoming addicted to technology?

In Summary

Our understanding of substance use and addictive behaviors has grown tremendously over the last century and continues to expand as we learn more about the prominent role that the brain and body play in addiction. In this chapter, we reviewed the more widely used legal and illegal drugs and behaviors that affect health. Behavioral counseling and medication (if available) are recommended to treat substance use disorders and addictive behavioral problems.

Key Terms

alcohol
cocaine
dissociative drugs
electronic cigarettes
hallucinogens
harm reduction
heroin
marijuana
methamphetamine
substance use disorder
tobacco

Student Discussion Questions and Activities

1. Think about a time when you were either tempted to or did use drugs or alcohol. What do you think were some of the reasons behind your desire or decision? If you did use a substance, did any of the reasons mentioned in this chapter resonate with your own personal experience? Why or why not?
2. Unfortunately, people who have a substance use disorder are stigmatized and blamed for not being able to control their behavior and stop using drugs or alcohol. With this in mind, how would you explain addiction to someone?
3. Brainstorm ideas for campaigns and interventions you think may be relevant and effective in preventing drug use. Why do you think these approaches would be successful?
4. What do you think of the harm reduction concept, which seeks to move from a criminalization approach to drugs to one of treatment and counseling? Why do you think harm-reduction strategies are so controversial in the United States, compared to other countries?

Resources for Treatment

National Institute on Alcohol Abuse and Alcoholism: http://www.niaaa.nih.gov/alcohol-health/support-treatment

Rethinking Drinking: http://rethinkingdrinking.niaaa.nih.gov/Tools/Default.aspx

National Institute on Drug Abuse, brief description of treatment approaches to drug addiction: https://www.drugabuse.gov/related-topics/treatment

National Institute on Drug Abuse, overview of behavioral therapies relevant to drug addiction: https://www.drugabuse.gov/publications/principles-drug-addiction-treatment/evidence-based-approaches-to-drug-addiction-treatment/behavioral-therapies

References

1. National Institute on Drug Abuse. (2016). Retrieved from https://www.drugabuse.gov/
2. World Health Organization. (2016). Substance abuse. Retrieved from http://www.who.int/topics/substance_abuse/en/
3. Substance Abuse and Mental Health Services Administration. (2015). Substance use disorders. Retrieved from http://www.samhsa.gov/disorders/substance-use
4. The Partnership. (2017, February 13). Top 8 reasons why teens try alcohol and drugs. Partnership for Drug-Free Kids. Retrieved from http://www.drugfree.org/resources/top-8-reasons-why-teens-try-alcohol-and-drugs/2016
5. National Institute on Drug Abuse. (2014, July). Drugs, brains, and behavior: The science of addiction: Drug abuse and addiction. Retrieved from https://www.drugabuse.gov/publications/drugs-brains-behavior-science-addiction/drug-abuse-addiction
6. National Institute on Drug Abuse. (2010, September). Comorbidity: Addiction and other mental illnesses: Why do drug use disorders often co-occur with other mental illnesses? Retrieved from https://www.drugabuse.gov/publications/research-reports/comorbidity-addiction-other-mental-illnesses/why-do-drug-use-disorders-often-co-occur-other-men
7. National Institute on Drug Abuse. (2015, November). Prescription and over-the-counter medications. Retrieved from https://www.drugabuse.gov/publications/drugfacts/prescription-over-counter-medications
8. National Alliance on Mental Illness. (2016). Psychotherapy. Retrieved from https://www.nami.org/Learn-More/Treatment/Psychotherapy
9. American Psychiatric Association. (2013). *Diagnostic and statistical manual of mental disorders* (5th ed.). Washington, DC: American Psychiatric Association.

10. King, C., III, & Siegel, M. (2001). The master settlement agreement with the tobacco industry and cigarette advertising in magazines. *New England Journal of Medicine, 345*(7), 504–511.
11. Bach, L. (2016). Trends in tobacco industry marketing. Campaign for Tobacco-Free Kids. Retrieved from https://www.tobaccofreekids.org/research/factsheets/pdf/0156.pdf
12. TobaccoTactics. (2012). Advertising strategy. Retrieved from http://www.tobaccotactics.org/index.php/Advertising_Strategy
13. Truth Initiative. (2016). Who we are and what we do. Retrieved from http://truthinitiative.org/about-us
14. BeTobaccoFree.gov. (2016). Tobacco and nicotine. U.S. Department of Health and Human Services. Retrieved from http://betobaccofree.hhs.gov/about-tobacco/tobacco-and-nicotine/index.html
15. National Institute on Drug Abuse. (2012, July). Tobacco/nicotine: Is nicotine addictive? Retrieved from https://www.drugabuse.gov/publications/research-reports/tobacco/nicotine-addictive
16. National Center for Chronic Disease Prevention and Health Promotion, Office on Smoking and Health. (2016). Quitting smoking. Centers for Disease Control and Prevention. Retrieved from http://www.cdc.gov/tobacco/data_statistics/fact_sheets/cessation/quitting/
17. National Center for Chronic Disease Prevention and Health Promotion, Office on Smoking and Health. (2015). Health effects of cigarette smoking. Centers for Disease Control and Prevention. Retrieved from http://www.cdc.gov/tobacco/data_statistics/fact_sheets/health_effects/effects_cig_smoking/
18. Centers for Disease Control and Prevention. (n.d.) Smoking and tobacco use: Secondhand smoke (SHS) facts. Retrieved from https://www.cdc.gov/tobacco/data_statistics/fact_sheets/secondhand_smoke/general_facts/index.htm
19. National Institute on Drug Abuse. (2012, July). Tobacco/nicotine: What are the medical consequences of tobacco use? Retrieved from https://www.drugabuse.gov/publications/research-reports/tobacco/what-are-medical-consequences-tobacco-use
20. Centers for Disease Control and Prevention. (1999). Achievements in public health, 1900–1999: Tobacco use—United States, 1900–1999. Retrieved from https://www.cdc.gov/mmwr/preview/mmwrhtml/mm4843a2.htm
21. National Center for Chronic Disease Prevention and Health Promotion, Office on Smoking and Health. (2016). Current cigarette smoking among adults in the United States. Centers for Disease Control and Prevention. Retrieved from http://www.cdc.gov/tobacco/data_statistics/fact_sheets/adult_data/cig_smoking/
22. Purnell, J. Q., Peppone, L. J., Alcaraz, K., McQueen, A., Guido, J. J., Carroll, J. K., . . . Morrow, G. R. (2012). Perceived discrimination, psychological distress, and current smoking status: Results from the Behavioral Risk Factor Surveillance System Reactions to Race module, 2004–2008. *American Journal of Public Health, 102*(5), 844–851.
23. Hodge, F. S. (Ed.). (2012). American Indian and Alaska Native teen cigarette smoking: A review. *Smoking and tobacco control monograph no. 14.* U.S. Department of Health and Human Services. Retrieved from http://cancercontrol.cancer.gov/brp/tcrb/monographs/14/m14_17.pdf
24. Knox, B. (2016). Increasing the minimum legal sale age for tobacco products to 21. Campaign for Tobacco-Free Kids. Retrieved from https://www.tobaccofreekids.org/research/factsheets/pdf/0376.pdf
25. Huang, J., & Chaloupka, F. J., IV. (2012). The impact of the 2009 federal tobacco excise tax increase on youth tobacco use. National Bureau of Economic Research. Retrieved from http://www.nber.org/papers/w18026
26. Lasser, K., Boyd, J. W., Woolhandler, S., Himmelstein, D. U., McCormick, D., & Bor, D. H. (2000). Smoking and mental illness: A population-based prevalence study. *JAMA, 284*(20), 2606–2610.
27. Johnson, J. G., Cohen, P., Pine, D. S., Klein, D. F., Kasen, S., & Brook, J. S. (2000). Association between cigarette smoking and anxiety disorders during adolescence and early adulthood. *JAMA, 284*(18), 2348–2351.
28. Audrain-McGovern, J., & Benowitz, N. (2011). Cigarette smoking, nicotine, and body weight. *Clinical Pharmacology and Therapeutics, 90*(1), 164–168.
29. Parrott, A. C. (1999). Does cigarette smoking cause stress? *American Psychologist, 54*(10), 817–820.
30. American Lung Association. (2016). Hookah smoking: A growing threat to public health. American Lung Association. Retrieved from http://www.lung.org/assets/documents/tobacco/hookah-policy-brief-updated.pdf
31. National Center for Chronic Disease Prevention and Health Promotion, Office on Smoking and Health. (2015). Hookahs. Centers for Disease Control and Prevention. Retrieved from http://www.cdc.gov/tobacco/data_statistics/fact_sheets/tobacco_industry/hookahs/index.htm
32. National Center for Chronic Disease Prevention and Health Promotion, Office on Smoking and Health. (2015). Smokeless tobacco use in the United States. Centers for Disease Control and Prevention. Retrieved from http://www.cdc.gov/tobacco/data_statistics/fact_sheets/smokeless/use_us/
33. Mayo Clinic. (2016). Chewing tobacco: Not a safe product. Retrieved from http://www.mayoclinic.org/healthy-lifestyle/quit-smoking/in-depth/chewing-tobacco/art-20047428
34. National Center for Chronic Disease Prevention and Health Promotion, Office on Smoking and Health. (2015). Cigars. Centers for Disease Control and Prevention. Retrieved from http://www.cdc.gov/tobacco/data_statistics/fact_sheets/tobacco_industry/cigars/index.htm
35. National Institute on Drug Abuse. (2016, May). Electronic cigarettes (e-cigarettes). Retrieved from https://www.drugabuse.gov/publications/drugfacts/electronic-cigarettes-e-cigarettes
36. National Center for Chronic Disease Prevention and Health Promotion, Office on Smoking and Health. (2015). E-cigarette information. Centers for Disease Control and Prevention. Retrieved from http://www.cdc.gov/tobacco/stateandcommunity/pdfs/cdc-osh-information-on-e-cigarettes-november-2015.pdf
37. Centers for Disease Control and Prevention. (2015). E-cigarette use triples among middle and high school students in just one year. Retrieved from http://www.cdc.gov/media/releases/2015/p0416-e-cigarette-use.html
38. U.S. Food and Drug Administration. (2016). Vaporizers, e-cigarettes, and other electronic nicotine delivery systems (ENDS). Retrieved from http://www.fda.gov/TobaccoProducts/Labeling/ProductsIngredientsComponents/ucm456610.htm
39. National Institute on Drug Abuse. (2016, September). Alcohol. Retrieved from https://www.drugabuse.gov/drugs-abuse/alcohol
40. National Institute on Alcohol Abuse and Alcoholism. (2007). Alcohol metabolism: An update. Retrieved from https://pubs.niaaa.nih.gov/publications/AA72/AA72.htm
41. National Institute on Alcohol Abuse and Alcoholism. (2016). Drinking levels defined. Retrieved from http://www.niaaa.nih.gov/alcohol-health/overview-alcohol-consumption/moderate-binge-drinking
42. National Institute on Alcohol Abuse and Alcoholism. (2016). Alcohol use disorder. Retrieved from http://www.niaaa

.nih.gov/alcohol-health/overview-alcohol-consumption/alcohol-use-disorders

43. Chartier, K., & Caetano, R. (2016). Ethnicity and health disparities in alcohol research. National Institute on Alcohol Abuse and Alcoholism. Retrieved from http://pubs.niaaa.nih.gov/publications/arh40/152-160.htm
44. Mayo Clinic. (2015). Alcohol use disorder. Retrieved from http://www.mayoclinic.org/diseases-conditions/alcohol-use-disorder/basics/definition/con-20020866
45. National Center for Chronic Disease Prevention and Health Promotion, Division of Population Health. (2016). Fact sheets—excessive alcohol use and risks to women's health. Centers for Disease Control and Prevention. Retrieved from http://www.cdc.gov/alcohol/fact-sheets/womens-health.htm
46. National Institute on Alcohol Abuse and Alcoholism. (2016). What is a standard drink? Retrieved from http://www.niaaa.nih.gov/alcohol-health/overview-alcohol-consumption/what-standard-drink
47. Library of Congress. (2013, January 31). Global legal monitor: Brazil: zero tolerance of drunk driving. Retrieved from http://www.loc.gov/law/foreign-news/article/brazil-zero-tolerance-of-drunk-driving/
48. National Institute on Alcohol Abuse and Alcoholism. (2016). Alcohol facts and statistics. Retrieved from http://www.niaaa.nih.gov/alcohol-health/overview-alcohol-consumption/alcohol-facts-and-statistics
49. Merrill, J. E., & Carey, K. B. (2016). Drinking over the lifespan: Focus on college ages. *Alcohol Research, 38*(1), 103–114.
50. Centers for Disease Control and Prevention. (2017). Alcohol and public health: Fact sheets—alcohol and caffeine. Retrieved from https://www.cdc.gov/alcohol/fact-sheets/caffeine-and-alcohol.htm
51. Abbey, A., Zawacki, T., Buck, P. O., Clinton, A. M., & McAuslan, P. (n.d.). Alcohol and sexual assault. National Institute on Alcohol Abuse and Alcoholism. Retrieved from https://pubs.niaaa.nih.gov/publications/arh25-1/43-51.htm
52. National Institute on Alcohol Abuse and Alcoholism. (2016). Alcohol's effects on the body. Retrieved from http://www.niaaa.nih.gov/alcohol-health/alcohols-effects-body
53. Turrisi, R., Mallett, K. A., Mastroleo, N. R., & Larimer, M. E. (2006). Heavy drinking in college students: Who is at risk and what is being done about it? *Journal of General Psychology, 133*(4), 104–420. Retrieved from https://www.ncbi.nlm.nih.gov/pmc/articles/PMC2238801/
54. Glaser, G. (2015, April). The irrationality of alcoholics anonymous. *The Atlantic.* Retrieved from http://www.theatlantic.com/magazine/archive/2015/04/the-irrationality-of-alcoholics-anonymous/386255/
55. Szalavitz, M. (2016, June 25). Can you get over an addiction? *New York Times.* Retrieved from http://www.nytimes.com/2016/06/26/opinion/sunday/can-you-get-over-an-addiction.html?_r=0
56. Hari, J. (2015). Everything you think you know about addiction is wrong. TED: Ideas Worth Spreading. Retrieved from http://www.ted.com/talks/johann_hari_everything_you_think_you_know_about_addiction_is_wrong
57. National Institute on Alcohol Abuse and Alcoholism. (n.d.). Self-help strategies for quitting drinking. Retrieved from https://www.rethinkingdrinking.niaaa.nih.gov/Thinking-about-a-change/Support-for-quitting/Self-Help-Strategies-For-Quitting.aspx
58. Loomis, D., Guyton, K. Z., Grosse, Y., Lauby-Secretan, B., El Ghissassi, F., Bouvard, V., . . . International Agency for Research on Cancer Monograph Working Group. (2016). Carcinogenicity of drinking coffee, mate, and very hot beverages. *Lancet Oncology, 17*(7), 877–878.
59. Behavioral Biology Research Center. (2016). Caffeine dependence. Johns Hopkins Medicine. Retrieved from https://www.hopkinsmedicine.org/psychiatry/research/bpru/docs/caffeine_dependence_fact_sheet.pdf
60. National Institute on Drug Abuse. (2016, May). Prescription drugs and cold medicines. Retrieved from https://www.drugabuse.gov/drugs-abuse/prescription-drugs-cold-medicines
61. National Institute on Drug Abuse. (2016, August). Misuse of prescription drugs. Retrieved from https://www.drugabuse.gov/publications/misuse-prescription-drugs/summary
62. Volkow, N. D. (2014, May 14). America's addiction to opioids: Heroin and prescription drug abuse. National Institute on Drug Abuse. Retrieved from https://www.drugabuse.gov/about-nida/legislative-activities/testimony-to-congress/2016/americas-addiction-to-opioids-heroin-prescription-drug-abuse
63. Centers for Disease Control and Prevention, National Center for Injury Prevention and Control, Division of Unintentional Injury Prevention. (2017, April 16). Injury prevention and control: Opioid overdose. Retrieved from https://www.cdc.gov/drugoverdose/
64. National Institute on Drug Abuse. (2016, January). Commonly abused drugs charts. Retrieved from https://www.drugabuse.gov/drugs-abuse/commonly-abused-drugs-charts. Updated 20162016.
65. National Institutes of Health. (2015). Prevalence of marijuana use among U.S. adults doubles over past decade. Retrieved from https://www.nih.gov/news-events/news-releases/prevalence-marijuana-use-among-us-adults-doubles-over-past-decade
66. National Institute on Drug Abuse. (2017, April). Marijuana: What is the scope of marijuana use in the United States? Retrieved from https://www.drugabuse.gov/publications/research-reports/marijuana/what-scope-marijuana-use-in-united-states. Updated 2016.
67. American Association of Poison Control Centers. (n.d.). Synthetic cannabinoids. Retrieved from http://www.aapcc.org/alerts/synthetic-cannabinoids/
68. American Civil Liberties Union. (2013). The war on marijuana in black and white. Retrieved from https://www.aclu.org/sites/default/files/field_document/1114413-mj-report-rfs-rel1.pdf
69. World Health Organization. (2016). Management of substance abuse: Cannabis. Retrieved from http://www.who.int/substance_abuse/facts/cannabis/en/
70. National Institutes of Health. (2016). Marijuana use disorder is common and often untreated. Retrieved from https://www.nih.gov/news-events/news-releases/marijuana-use-disorder-common-often-untreated
71. National Institute on Drug Abuse. (2017, February). DrugFacts—marijuana. Retrieved from https://www.drugabuse.gov/publications/drugfacts/marijuana
72. National Institute on Drug Abuse for Teachers. (2017). Drug facts chat day: Marijuana. Retrieved from https://teens.drugabuse.gov/national-drug-alcohol-facts-week/drug-facts-chat-day-marijuana
73. National Institute on Drug Abuse. (2017, April). Marijuana: Is marijuana a gateway drug? Retrieved from https://www

.drugabuse.gov/publications/research-reports/marijuana/marijuana-gateway-drug
74. Ahmed, S. H., Guillem, K., & Vandaele, Y. (2013). Sugar addiction: Pushing the drug-sugar analogy to the limit. *Current Opinion in Clinical Nutrition and Metabolic Care, 16*(4), 434–439.
75. Avena, N. M., Rada, P., & Hoebel, B. G. (2008). Evidence for sugar addiction: Behavioral and neurochemical effects of intermittent, excessive sugar intake. *Neuroscience and Biobehavioral Reviews, 32*(1), 20–39.
76. Corsica, J. A., & Pelchat, M. L. (2010). Food addiction: True or false? *Current Opinions in Gastroenterology, 26*(2), 165–169.
77. Moss, M. (2013, February 20). The extraordinary science of addictive junk food. *New York Times*. Retrieved from http://www.nytimes.com/2013/02/24/magazine/the-extraordinary-science-of-junk-food.html
78. Foundation for a Drug-Free World. (2016). Cocaine: A short history. Retrieved from http://www.drugfreeworld.org/drugfacts/cocaine/a-short-history.html
79. National Institute on Drug Abuse. (2016, May). Cocaine: What is cocaine? Retrieved from https://www.drugabuse.gov/publications/research-reports/cocaine/what-cocaine
80. Center for Behavioral Health Statistics and Quality. (2015). Results from the 2014 National Survey on Drug Use and Health: Detailed tables. Substance Abuse and Mental Health Services Administration. Retrieved from http://www.samhsa.gov/data/sites/default/files/NSDUH-DetTabs2014/NSDUH-DetTabs2014.htm
81. National Institute on Drug Abuse. (2016, May). Cocaine: What is the scope of cocaine use in the United States? Retrieved from https://www.drugabuse.gov/publications/research-reports/cocaine/what-scope-cocaine-use-in-united-states
82. National Institute on Drug Abuse. (2017, January). Overdose death rates. Retrieved from https://www.drugabuse.gov/related-topics/trends-statistics/overdose-death-rates
83. U.S. National Library of Medicine. (2015). Cocaine intoxication. National Institutes of Health. MedlinePlus. Retrieved from https://www.nlm.nih.gov/medlineplus/ency/article/000946.htm
84. National Institute on Drug Abuse. (2013 September). Methamphetamine: What is methamphetamine? Retrieved from https://www.drugabuse.gov/publications/research-reports/methamphetamine/what-methamphetamine
85. National Institute on Drug Abuse. (2013, September). Methamphetamine: What are the long-term effects of methamphetamine abuse? Retrieved from https://www.drugabuse.gov/publications/research-reports/methamphetamine/what-are-long-term-effects-methamphetamine-abuse
86. National Institute on Drug Abuse. (2013, September). Methamphetamine: What are the immediate (short-term) effects of methamphetamine abuse? Retrieved from https://www.drugabuse.gov/publications/research-reports/methamphetamine/what-are-immediate-short-term-effects-methamphetamine-abuse
87. U.S. Drug Enforcement Administration. (2016). Methamphetamine lab incidents, 2004–2014. Retrieved from https://www.dea.gov/resource-center/meth-lab-maps.shtml
88. *Frontline*. (2016). Frequently asked questions. PBS. Retrieved from http://www.pbs.org/wgbh/pages/frontline/meth/faqs/
89. Centers for Disease Control and Prevention. (2015). New research reveals the trends and risk factors behind America's growing heroin epidemic. Retrieved from http://www.cdc.gov/media/releases/2015/p0707-heroin-epidemic.html
90. National Institute on Drug Abuse. (2017, January). DrugFacts—Heroin. Retrieved from https://www.drugabuse.gov/publications/drugfacts/heroin
91. Seelye, K. Q. (2014, February 27). A call to arms on a Vermont heroin epidemic. *New York Times*. Retrieved from http://www.nytimes.com/2014/02/28/us/a-call-to-arms-on-a-vermont-heroin-epidemic.html
92. U.S. National Library of Medicine. (2015). Heroin overdose. National Institutes of Health. MedlinePlus. Retrieved from https://www.nlm.nih.gov/medlineplus/ency/article/002861.htm
93. UW Alcohol and Drug Abuse Institute. (n.d.). Learn about naloxone. StopOverdose.org. Retrieved from http://stopoverdose.org/section/learn-about-naloxone/
94. National Institute on Drug Abuse. (2016, January). DrugFacts—Hallucinogens. Retrieved from https://www.drugabuse.gov/publications/drugfacts/hallucinogens
95. National Institute on Drug Abuse. (2014, May). Hallucinogens. Retrieved from https://www.drugabuse.gov/drugs-abuse/hallucinogens
96. National Institute on Drug Abuse. (2015, February). Hallucinogens and dissociative drugs: How widespread is the abuse of hallucinogens and dissociative drugs? Retrieved from https://www.drugabuse.gov/publications/research-reports/hallucinogens-dissociative-drugs/why-do-people-take-hallucinogens
97. National Institute on Drug Abuse. (2015, February). Hallucinogens and dissociative drugs: From the director. Retrieved from https://www.drugabuse.gov/publications/research-reports/hallucinogens-dissociative-drugs/director
98. National Institute on Drug Abuse. (2016, October). DrugFacts—MDMA (Ecstasy/Molly). Retrieved from https://www.drugabuse.gov/publications/drugfacts/mdma-ecstasymolly
99. Gasser, P., Holstein, D., Michel, Y., Doblin, R., Yazar-Klosinski, B., Passie, T., & Brenneisen, R. (2014). Safety and efficacy of lysergic acid diethylamide-assisted psychotherapy for anxiety associated with life-threatening diseases. *Journal of Nervous and Mental Disease, 202*(7), 513–520.
100. Join Together Staff Writer. (2010, April 14). Research revived on using hallucinogens to treat mental illness, addiction. Partnership for Drug-Free Kids. Retrieved from http://www.drugfree.org/join-together/research-revived-on-using-hallucinogens-to-treat-mental-illness-addiction-2/
101. Harm reduction: An approach to reducing risky health behaviours in adolescents. (2008). *Paediatrics and Child Health, 13*(1), 53–56.
102. Mayo Clinic. (2014). Compulsive gambling. Retrieved from http://www.mayoclinic.org/diseases-conditions/compulsive-gambling/basics/definition/con-20023242
103. National Center for Responsible Gambling. (2016). Gambling disorders. Retrieved from http://www.ncrg.org/sites/default/files/oec/pdfs/ncrg_fact_sheet_gambling_disorders.pdf
104. Landolfi, E. (2013). Exercise addiction. *Sports Medicine, 43*(2), 111–119.
105. Sussman, S., Lisha, N., & Griffiths, M. (2011). Prevalence of the addictions: A problem of the majority or the minority? *Evaluation and Health Professions, 34*(1), 3–56.
106. Freimuth, M., Moniz, S., & Kim, S. R. (2011). Clarifying exercise addiction: Differential diagnosis, co-occurring disorders, and phases of addiction. *International Journal of Environmental Research and Public Health, 8*(10), 4069–4081.

107. Fong, T. W. (2006). Understanding and managing compulsive sexual behaviors. *Psychiatry (Edgmont), 3*(11), 51–58.
108. Bailey, C. E., & Case, B. (2016). Sexual addiction. American Association for Marriage and Family Therapy. Retrieved from http://aamft4-imisupg2.aamft.org/iMIS15/AAMFT/About/Therapy-Topics/Content/Consumer_Updates/Sexual_Addiction.aspx
109. Pew Research Center. (2016). Retrieved from http://www.pewinternet.org/
110. Common Sense Media. (2015). The common sense census: Media use by tweens and teens. Retrieved from https://www.commonsensemedia.org/research/the-common-sense-census-media-use-by-tweens-and-teens
111. Stanford Medicine. (2006, October 17). Internet addiction: Stanford study seeks to define whether it's a problem. Stanford Medicine News Center. Retrieved from https://med.stanford.edu/news/all-news/2006/10/internet-addiction-stanford-study-seeks-to-define-whether-its-a-problem.html

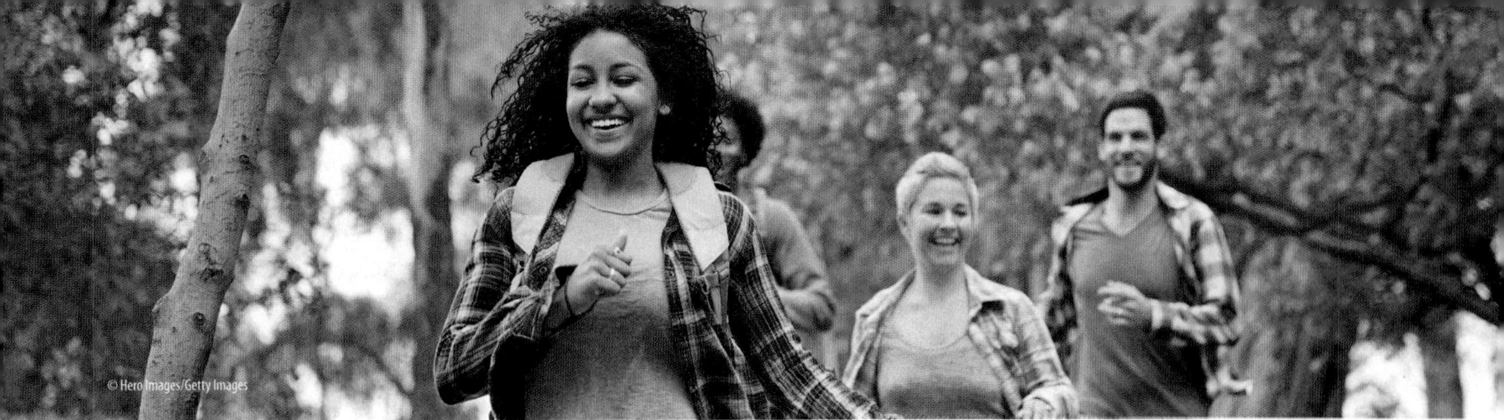

CHAPTER 8

Don't Share These With Your Friends: Infectious Diseases

CHAPTER OBJECTIVES

- Describe how diseases spread.
- Distinguish the different causes of infectious diseases.
- Explain the steps you can take to prevent getting infectious diseases.
- Describe important infectious diseases in the world.
- Recognize some of the past and current pandemics.

Do you realize that *everybody* reading this book has had an infectious disease? Yes, even you! Everyone has experienced at least one infectious disease, even if it is only a cold or an ear infection. We don't even think much about those examples of infectious disease today. But there was a time not so long ago when most people died of infectious diseases. Have you ever thought about why and how people catch diseases that are contagious? In this chapter, you will learn about how you (and others) catch diseases and what it means for your family, your community, and the world at large when pandemics strike.

EPIDEMICS VERSUS PANDEMICS

An **epidemic** is when new cases of a disease over a period of time substantially exceed what is expected, based on the recent past. Epidemics usually occur in a particular place. Zika is an example of a recent epidemic (that some already consider a pandemic).

A **pandemic** is an epidemic that spreads across a large geographic region, such as a continent or worldwide. Before Zika, the most recent example of a pandemic is the 2009 H1N1 flu virus.

epidemic A widespread occurrence of an infectious disease in a community at a particular time.

pandemic An epidemic occurring over a very wide area (several countries or continents) and usually affecting a large proportion of the population.

Knowingly or not, we have all been in a room with someone who has an infectious disease. Why do you sometimes catch it and sometimes not? Or, it might seem like you catch every infectious disease that comes along, but your friends don't. In some ways, answering the overarching question of "How do I stay healthy?" is easy, and the changes needed to protect ourselves are easy to implement. Other parts of the answer may be easy to figure out, but the necessary changes may be either very difficult or something over which we have no control. First, we need to understand the ways that infections spread and the means of transmission.

Transmission of Infections

There are a number of ways to classify how diseases spread from a **host** (the person or animal that has the disease) to a susceptible individual (**FIGURE 8-1**). Here, we start with contact versus noncontact transmission. **Contact transmission** includes **direct transmission**, indirect transmission, and droplet transmission. **Noncontact transmission** includes airborne, vehicle-borne, and vector-borne methods. Some diseases have multiple modes of transmission. Just because a disease is usually transmitted one way, does not mean that is the only way to catch it.

host A person or other living organism that can be infected by an infectious agent under natural conditions.

contact transmission A transmission mechanism in which the infectious agent is transferred via direct transmission, indirect transmission, or droplet transmission.

direct transmission A transmission mechanism in which the infectious agent is transferred directly into the body via touching, biting, kissing, or sexual intercourse or by droplets entering the eye, nose, or mouth.

noncontact transmission A transmission mechanism in which the infectious agent is transferred indirectly into the body; includes airborne, vehicle-borne, and vector-borne methods.

Contact Transmission

Direct transmission means there is an immediate transfer of the infectious agent from the host, which can be a person or an animal, to a susceptible individual. Examples of direct transmission include kissing, sexual intercourse, and biting. Among the diseases transmitted directly are infectious mononucleosis (sharing saliva), chlamydia and gonorrhea (sexual contact), human immunodeficiency virus/acquired immunodeficiency syndrome (HIV/AIDS; sexual contact or through breast milk), and rabies (bite).

Indirect transmission means that a person is infected by touching a surface on which the infectious material has been deposited and that the infectious material survives long enough to be picked up. Examples of indirect transmission are rhinoviruses (the common cold) and Norwalk or norovirus (made famous by cruise ship outbreaks). Items we touch every day can be a source of indirect transmission, including, but not limited to, doorknobs, faucet handles, cell phones, and computer keyboards. But how long do viruses and bacteria live outside the body? If an infected person touches your laptop, how long until it is safe to touch it again without becoming infected? That depends on the specific bug, the surface on which the **virus** or **bacteria** are deposited, the temperature, and the amount of moisture the particular organism needs to survive.

virus An organism that relies on a host organism to replicate and survive.

bacteria Microscopic living organisms, usually one-celled, that can be found everywhere. Bacteria can be dangerous, such as when they cause infection, or beneficial, as in the process of fermentation (such as in wine) or decomposition.

Cold viruses can last more than 7 days, with the virus living longer on non-porous or water-resistant surfaces, although the virus's ability to cause infection decreases after 24 hours. Respiratory syncytial virus (RSV) can live for up to 6 hours on countertops, 30 to 45 minutes on cloth or paper, and 20 minutes on skin. Flu viruses can live on hard surfaces for 24 hours, tissues for 15 minutes, and skin for 5 minutes. When the virus is released into the air through coughs or sneezes (see droplet transmission), the virus can live for several hours. Survival time increases in low temperatures, which helps to explain why people get more colds in the winter. Noroviruses can live for days to weeks on hard surfaces.[1]

Droplet transmission means that the disease is spread through coughing, sneezing, or even talking. There is a long list of diseases that can be spread by droplet transmission, including upper respiratory infections, the common cold,

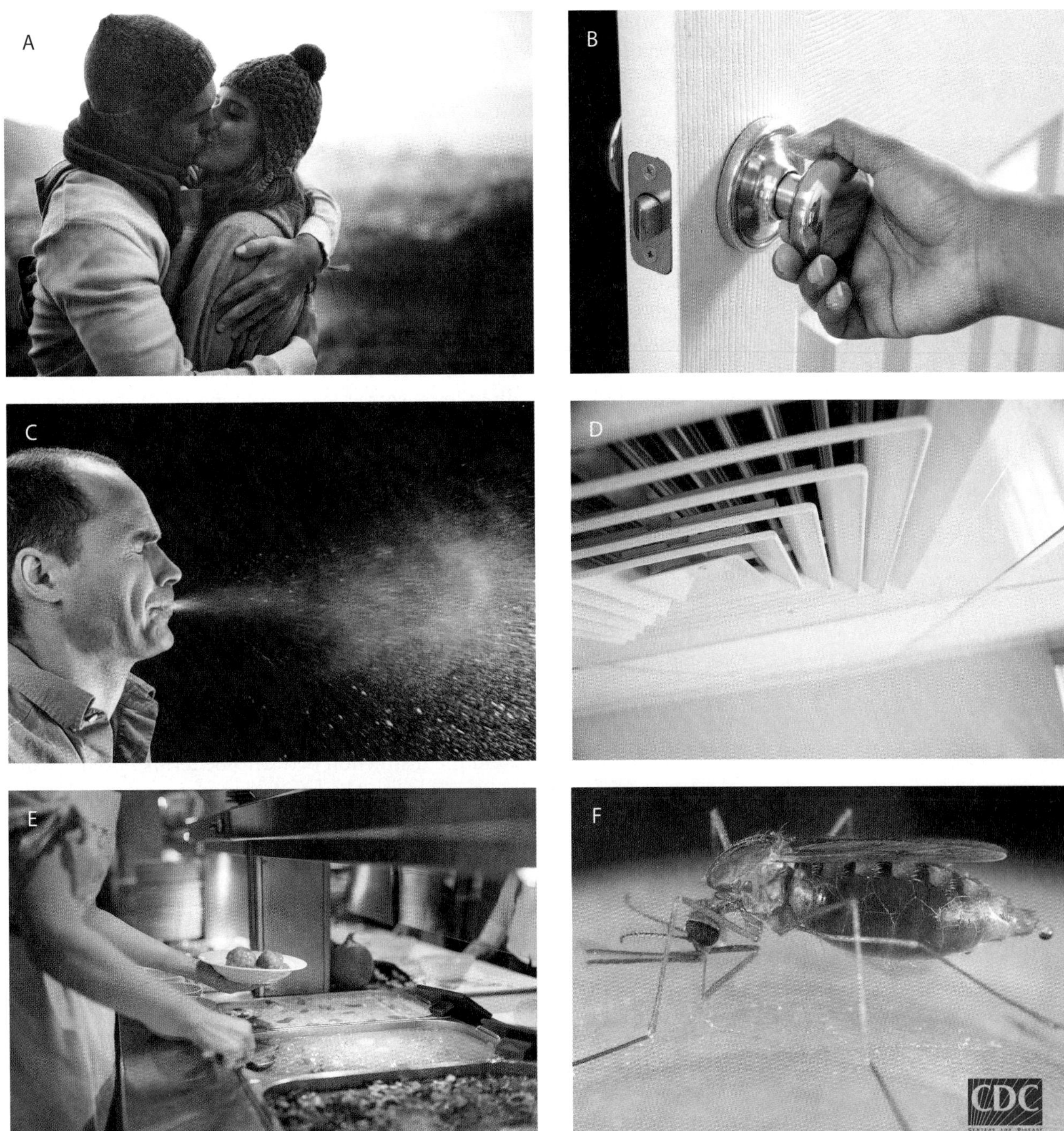

FIGURE 8-1 Contact transmission: A) direct transmission, B) indirect transmission, and C) droplet transmission; and non-contact transmission: D) airborne transmission, E) vehicle transmission, and F) vector-borne transmission.

the flu, bacterial and pneumococcal meningitis, leprosy, pneumococcal pneumonia, pneumonic plague, psittacosis, rubella (German measles), severe acute respiratory syndrome (SARS), strep throat, tuberculosis, and whooping cough.

Noncontact Transmission

Just as you might imagine, noncontact transmission means that a person can catch a disease without direct contact with the person who is ill. Airborne transmission occurs through what we call "aerosols." Because the particles are small, they can easily travel longer distances. If you are in a building with a poor ventilation system, you may catch a disease this way. Diseases transmitted this way must be resistant to drying out and must be capable of living a long time outside a host. Fortunately, there are not too many diseases that are transmitted this way, but ones that are include tuberculosis, chickenpox, and measles.

Vehicle transmission occurs when an inanimate object or vehicle (fomite) transmits the infection via touch, ingestion of food, or intravenous fluid administration. Vehicle transmission means germs disperse by many sources, including cooking or eating utensils, bedding or clothing, toys, surgical or medical instruments (like catheters), or dressings. Other vehicles include water, food, drinks (such as milk), and biological products, including blood, serum, plasma, tissues, and organs. Diseases that can be transmitted by this mode are cholera, dysentery, enteric fever, diphtheria, scarlet fever, and typhoid. If those are diseases you have never heard of, you should consider yourself fortunate to live in a society that has come to understand the importance of cleanliness and that has the means to maintain, by and large, living conditions that limit the spread of these germs.

Vector-borne transmission means that an animal or insect transmits the disease to the susceptible person. The insect may simply be the transporter of the infection. Examples of vector-borne diseases are malaria (a serious and sometimes fatal illness), West Nile Virus, and Zika, all transmitted by mosquitoes, and Lyme disease, transmitted by ticks.

Infections Versus Contagious Diseases

It is important to understand the distinction between the terms *infectious* and *contagious*. Infectious diseases are caused by bacteria or viruses that infect the body, causing disease. As noted in **TABLE 8-1**, some infectious diseases spread directly from one person to another. Infectious diseases that are spread from person to person, such as measles or rhinoviruses, are referred to as contagious. Vector-borne diseases (such as Lyme disease) are not contagious because one person cannot directly transmit them to another person.

What Can Infect You?

Infectious diseases have been around for a very, very long time. In fact, some 3,000-year-old Egyptian mummies have evidence of smallpox.[2] Egyptian paintings include pictures of people with polio (**FIGURE 8-2**).[3] Hippocrates (about 460 BC to about 370 BC), the "Father of Medicine," proposed that disease was spread by air, water, and places. This approach to thinking about diseases changed when Antonie van Leeuwenhoek (1632–1723) made and used the first real compound microscope. The microscope allowed him and other scientists to view microorganisms, which at the time were referred to as animalcules (little animals).[4]

Disease is defined as any deviation from or interruption of the normal structure or function of any body part, organ, or system that is manifested by a characteristic set of symptoms and signs and whose **etiology** (the cause or causes of a disease), **pathology** (the way a disease works), and **prognosis** (the prediction of the future course of a disease and how likely a person is to recover) may be known or unknown. While there are certainly other causes of disease, such as vitamin deficiency, infectious diseases are caused by the entrance, growth, and multiplication of microorganisms in the body. The microorganisms that cause disease can be bacteria, viruses, fungi, or parasites.

etiology The study of the cause or causes of a disease.

pathology The study of diseases and the changes that they cause; the way a disease works.

prognosis The prediction of the future course of a disease and how likely a person is to recover.

TABLE 8-1 Transmission of Diseases

Contact Transmission		Noncontact Transmission	
Mechanism of Transmission	**Examples of Diseases**	**Mechanism of Transmission**	**Examples of Diseases**
Direct transmission	Athlete's foot Chlamydia Genital warts Gonorrhea HIV/AIDS Infectious mononucleosis Influenza Rabies Syphilis Tetanus Trichomoniasis	Airborne transmission	Tuberculosis Chickenpox Measles Smallpox
Indirect transmission	Athlete's foot Norovirus Norwalk virus Rhinoviruses	Vehicle transmission	Cholera Diphtheria Dysentery Enteric fever Hantavirus Listeriosis Scarlet fever Typhoid
Droplet transmission	Upper respiratory infections Rhinoviruses Influenza Bacterial meningitis Chickenpox Coronavirus Pneumococcal meningitis Leprosy Measles Mumps Pneumococcal pneumonia Pneumonic plague Psittacosis Rubella Strep throat Tuberculosis Whooping cough	Vector-borne transmission	Dengue fever Malaria Leishmaniasis Lyme disease Plague Rickettsial diseases Schistosomiasis Sleeping sickness West Nile virus Yellow fever Zika

Bacteria

Bacteria (singular: *bacterium*) are all around us. Not all bacteria are bad; in fact, some bacteria are necessary to our survival. While it might seem strange to think about, we have bacteria in our gut that help us digest food and protect us from diseases. "Good" bacteria are used to make many of the foods we eat: yogurt, cheese, beer, wine, sauerkraut, sourdough bread, olives, soy sauce, coffee, and chocolate. The creation of some medicines, such as penicillin, involves good bacteria.

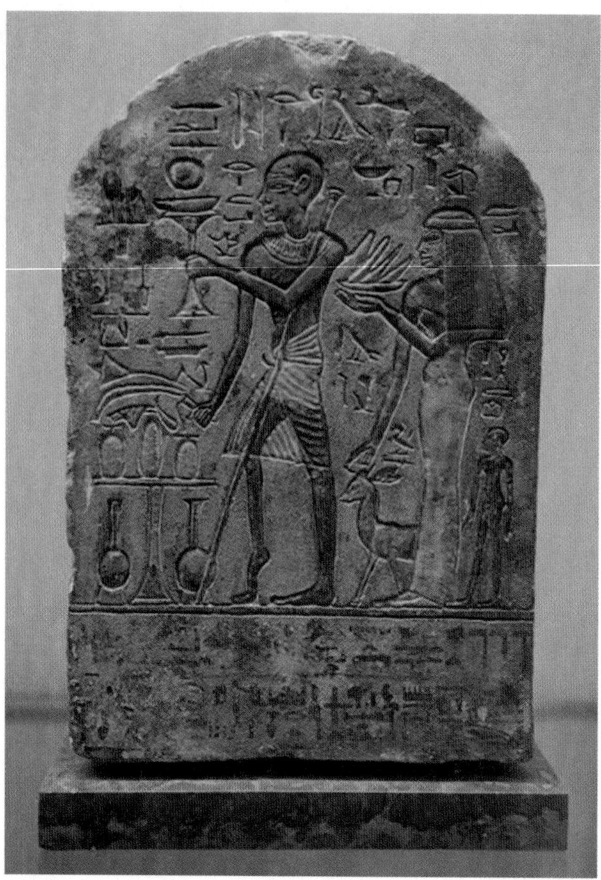

FIGURE 8-2 An Egyptian stele thought to represent a polio victim—18th dynasty (1403–1365 BC).

Bacteria are single-celled organisms and are classified by shape. There are three basic shapes: spherical (cocci), rod-shaped (bacilli), and spiral (**FIGURE 8-3**). Spiral-shaped bacteria can further be classified depending on the amount of spiraling: vibrio, spirilla, and spirochete. Because there are thousands of species of bacteria, knowing the shape is not necessarily a way to definitively identify the type of bacterium.[5] A laboratory test is needed to classify the type of bacterium correctly.

Cocci

Cocci are round bacteria that are found as a single microbe, a pair of microbes (diplococci), a chain of microbes (streptococci), or a cluster of microbes (staphylococci). *Neisseria gonorrhoeae* (which causes gonorrhea) is an example of diplococci. Another example of diplococci is *Neisseria meningitidis*, which causes meningococcal meningitis. Although it is rare, because of the seriousness of meningococcal meningitis, almost every college requires or strongly recommends that students be vaccinated for this disease, especially if they plan to live in the dorms (**FIGURE 8-4**). *Staphylococcus aureus* (referred to as *Staph aureus*) is a common type of cocci, frequently found in the nose or skin without causing disease. Many bacteria are part of the normal flora that lives on our bodies. Some strains of bacteria can live on our bodies without causing disease and at other times make us ill. As noted in a microbiology textbook, "the central problem in understanding the link between colonization and disease is that although we know some strains clearly have enhanced potential to produce disease, we

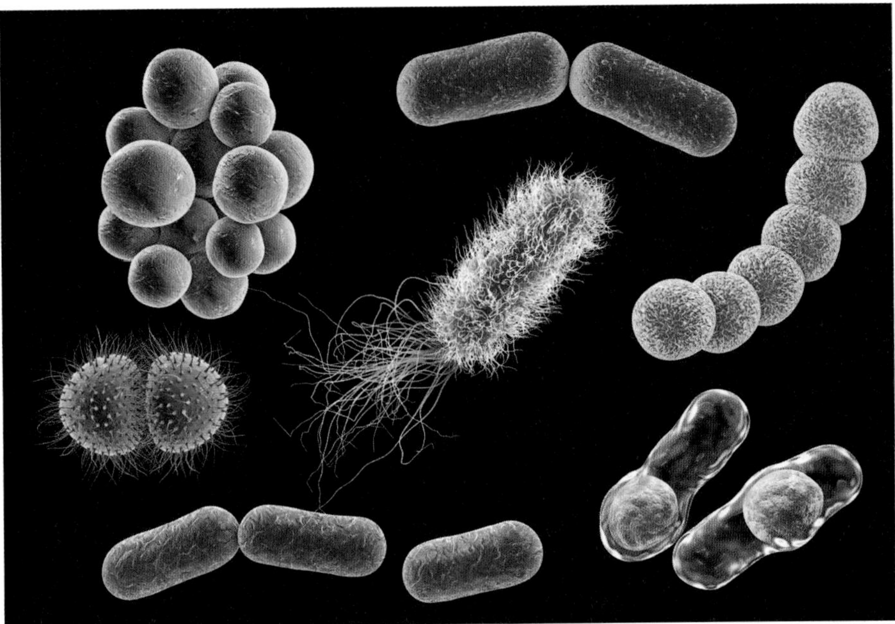

FIGURE 8-3 Bacteria of different shapes: staphylococci, streptococci, *Neisseria*, *Clostridium*, rod-shaped, *Escherichia coli*, *Klebsiella*.

Meningococcal Disease on U.S. College Campuses, 2013-2017
While this graph only includes college students, all young adults ages 16-21 years old are at increased risk of getting meningococcal disease.
States where campus outbreak occurred
States where single cases occurred on a campus
Confirmed serogroup B cases
Non-serogroup B cases or unknown type
Cases not covered by media, reported directly to NMA
University of Wisconsin-Madison: 1 case, 1 death (2014) 3 cases, survived (2016)
Penn State University: 2 cases, survived
Providence College: 2 cases, survived (outbreak)
Northeastern University: 1 case, 1 death
University of North Carolina, Charlotte: 1 case, 1 death
Yale University: 2 cases, survived
St. Ambrose University: 1 case, survived
Marquette University: 1 case, survived
University of Rochester: 1 case, survived
University of Idaho: 1 case, survived
Dakota Wesleyan University: 1 case, 1 death
Kalamazoo College: 1 case, 1 death
State University College at Oswego: 1 case, survived
University of Oregon: 7 cases, 1 death (outbreak)
University of Hartford: 1 case, 1 death
West Chester University: 1 case, 1 death
Humbolt State University: 1 case, survived
St. Mary's College: 1 case, survived
Loyola University: 1 case, survived
Northern Arizona University: 1 case, survived
John Tyler Community College: 1 case, survived
University of California, Davis: 1 case, survived
Rutgers Uninversity: 2 cases, survived
Santa Clara University: 3 cases, survived
Princeton University: 8 cases, survived (outbreak)
Georgia Tech: 1 case, survived
University of California, Long Beach: 1 case, outcome unknown
Drexel University: 1 case, 1 death
Seminole State College: 1 case, survived
Palomar Community College: 1 case, survived
Georgetown University: 1 case, 1 death
San Diego State University: 1 case, 1 death
Missouri University: 1 case, survived
Auburn University: 1 case, survived
University of California, Santa Barbara: 4 cases, survived (outbreak)
Kutztown University: 1 case, survived
• Of those who survived, it is not known how many suffer long-term complications. In general, as many as 20 percent of survivors live with permanent disabilities, such as brain damage, hearing loss, loss of kidney function or limb amputations.
• This data is based on media reports and cases reported directly to NMA. Additional cases that were not featured in the news may be missing. If you know of any cases not reported on this map, please contact NMA.
NMA
NATIONAL MENINGITIS ASSOCIATION
© 2015 National Meningitis Association, please credit NMA for any use.

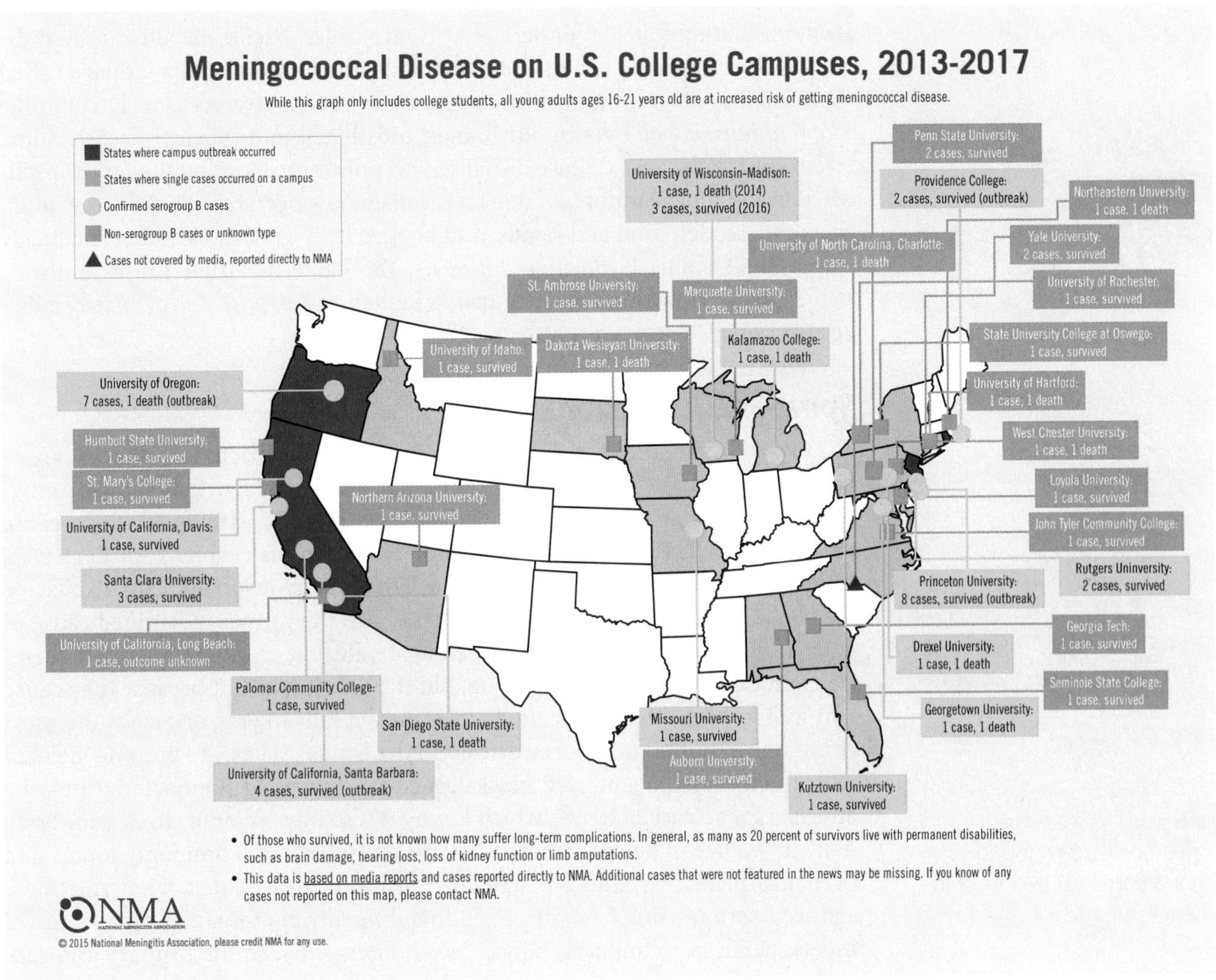

FIGURE 8-4 Case map of meningococcal meningitis.

National Meningitis Foundation. (2015). Meningococcal disease on U.S. college campuses, 2013–2017. Retrieved from http://www.nmaus.org/wp-content/uploads/2017/01/College-Cases-Map.pdf

have no way to predict which they are."[5] *Staph aureus* is also a cause of pneumonia. One common infection, *Streptococcus* infection (usually called strep throat), is caused by a chain of cocci.

FACT VS. FICTION

Meningococcal Meningitis

Myth: Most healthy adolescents and young adults don't need to worry about getting meningococcal meningitis.

Facts: While the disease is rare, the risk of getting it increases in adolescents and young adults. The disease progresses rapidly; an otherwise healthy person can die within 24 to 48 hours. For this reason, almost every college requires or strongly recommends that students be vaccinated for meningococcal meningitis. Schools have good reason for taking such precautions! Five college campuses—Santa Clara University, University of Oregon, Providence College, Princeton University, and University of California, Santa Barbara—experienced outbreaks of meningococcal disease between 2013 and 2016.[6]

Does your school have this requirement? Did you receive a vaccination? Were other vaccinations recommended by your school before starting there?

Bacilli

Bacteria that look like cylinders or rods are called bacilli. Bacilli can be individual or arranged as chains. Bacilli can also be found in pairs and are called diplobacilli. A common bacillus is *Escherichia coli*, referred to as *E. coli*. Like *Staph aureus*, *E. coli* lives in our bodies, mostly without causing disease. Some strains of *E. coli* cause disease, usually food poisoning. Among the foods implicated in foodborne outbreaks due to *E. coli* are raw beef, raw chicken, raw milk, mayonnaise, deli food and salads, and bagged leafy greens.[7] Another medically important bacillus is *Bacillus anthracis*, the bacterium that causes anthrax. While people may think of anthrax as a biological weapon, it is primarily a disease of horses, sheep, and cattle.[5]

Spiral-Shaped Bacteria

As noted, there are three types of spiral-shaped bacteria. Vibrios are a comma-shaped rod with a partial twist. Vibrios usually live in an aquatic environment. The most notable example is *Vibrio cholerae*, strains of which cause cholera. (We will review more about cholera later in the chapter.) Spirilla have a more rigid spiral shape. One spirillum is *Helicobacter pylori*, a major risk factor for peptic ulcers. Infection with *H. pylori* is also the primary identified cause of gastric cancer. Spirochetes are thin, elongate, flexible, corkscrew-shaped bacteria. Spirochetes are not a large group, but they are important because they cause two well-known diseases: Lyme disease and syphilis.[5] Lyme disease is the most commonly reported tick-borne disease in the United States.[5] To become infected with the disease, an infected black-legged tick carrying the bacteria must be attached for at least 24 hours, which is why it is so important to check your body daily if you live in an area where ticks are **endemic** (i.e., commonly found in a particular place).[8] Syphilis is a sexually transmitted disease that, if left untreated, can have serious complications, including difficulty coordinating muscle movements, paralysis, numbness, blindness, and dementia. In the primary and secondary phases of the disease, it is simple to cure with the right treatment.[9]

endemic A disease or condition regularly found among particular people or in a certain area.

Viruses

Viruses are small infectious organisms that are smaller than bacteria and smaller than fungi. They replicate by attaching to a living cell, entering it, and releasing their DNA or RNA (the genetic material) inside the cell. The viral DNA or RNA then hijacks the cell and forces it to replicate. The cell dies, releasing new viruses. Viruses are usually specific in that they infect only one type of cell.[5]

Viruses spread in a number of ways, similar to bacteria. They may be swallowed, inhaled, spread through sexual transmission, or transferred through a contaminated blood transfusion. The last method of transmission is much less common, as medical science has improved methods of screening blood donors and testing blood. Insects can also transmit viruses.

Sometimes viruses cause illness, not by killing the cells they infect but by changing the cells' functions. An example of this process is when viruses disrupt normal cell division so that the cells become cancerous. The human papillomavirus (HPV), for example, can affect cells of the cervix, causing cervical cancer. (See Chapter 5 for more information on HPV.) Viruses can also leave their genetic material in the host cell. The material is initially dormant, but when it is disturbed, the virus can begin replication and cause disease. The herpes viruses, for example, function in this manner.

More on Bacteria and Viruses

Regarding health, the most important difference between viruses and bacteria is that viruses must have a living host (like you!) to multiply; they cannot survive on their own. Bacteria can grow and multiply on nonliving surfaces. Antibiotics can kill bacteria but cannot be used to treat viruses. While bacteria are complex, viruses are simple (**FIGURE 8-5**). Viruses are tiny compared to bacteria. In fact, the largest virus is smaller than the smallest bacteria.

Bacteria and viruses are similar in many ways. Both types of microbes cause infections and are spread in similar ways (kissing, having sex, coughing, sneezing, consuming contaminated food or water, or having contact with an infected animal or insect). Depending on the microbe in question, bacteria and viruses can cause mild, moderate, or severe disease. The symptoms they cause can be

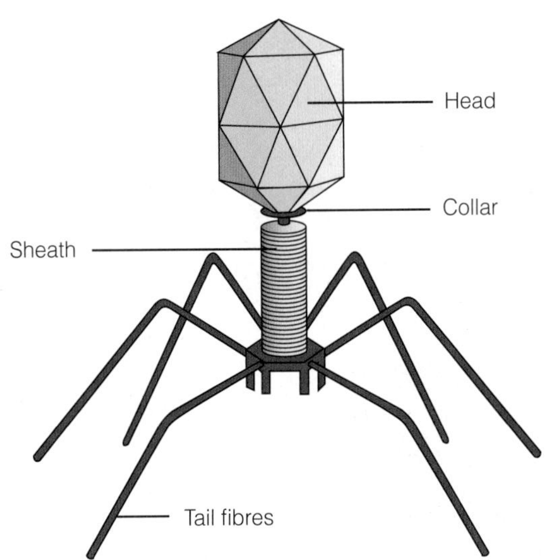

FIGURE 8-5 A virus has a simple structure.

similar. Sometimes the disease in question can be caused by a bacterium *or* by a virus. Pneumonia, for example, is a lung condition that can begin with either a viral or a bacterial infection (among other causes). Bacteria and viruses also differ: More than 99% of bacteria do not cause disease in people. In fact, as mentioned previously, we need bacteria to help digest food, and they provide both anti-inflammatory and immune system benefits.

Fungi

fungi Simple, aerobic organisms (such as mildews, molds, mushrooms, smuts, toadstools, and yeast) that can grow in low moisture and low pH environments and that have their genetic material bound in a membrane.

While there are over a million different species of fungi, only about 300 of them make people sick. **Fungi** live outdoors in the soil (you might have noticed them springing up in your lawn as mushrooms after it rains), on plants, on trees, and on human skin. Most fungi do not cause diseases, but the ones that do are common in the environment.[5]

A common fungus that infects people is tinea. There are three common types of tinea, depending on where on the body the infection occurs: ringworm, which can be on the skin or scalp (tinea corporis or capitis, respectively); athlete's foot (tinea pedis); and jock itch (tinea cruris). These infections are not serious, but because they can cause burning and itching, they are uncomfortable. Ringworm can cause a circular rash that is red and itchy, and, despite its name, ringworm is neither a worm nor caused by a worm (**FIGURE 8-6**). While these rashes may be unattractive, they are usually not painful or life threatening. You can get tinea from touching an infected person, from damp surfaces like shower floors, and from wearing socks or shoes of someone who has athlete's foot. Often, over-the-counter (OTC) creams and powders will get rid of tinea, particularly athlete's foot and jock itch. Other times antifungal medication requires a prescription.[5]

Parasites

parasite An organism that lives in or on another organism (its host) and benefits by deriving nutrients at the host's expense.

A **parasite** is an organism that lives in or on another organism (its host) and benefits by drawing nutrients from the host. Because many parasites thrive in warm, moist climates, they are a large problem in tropical and subtropical regions. However, there are parasites in the United States, including *Trichomonas* (causing trichomoniasis), *Giardia* (causing giardiasis), *Cryptosporidium* (causing cryptosporidiosis), and *Toxoplasma* (causing toxoplasmosis).[5]

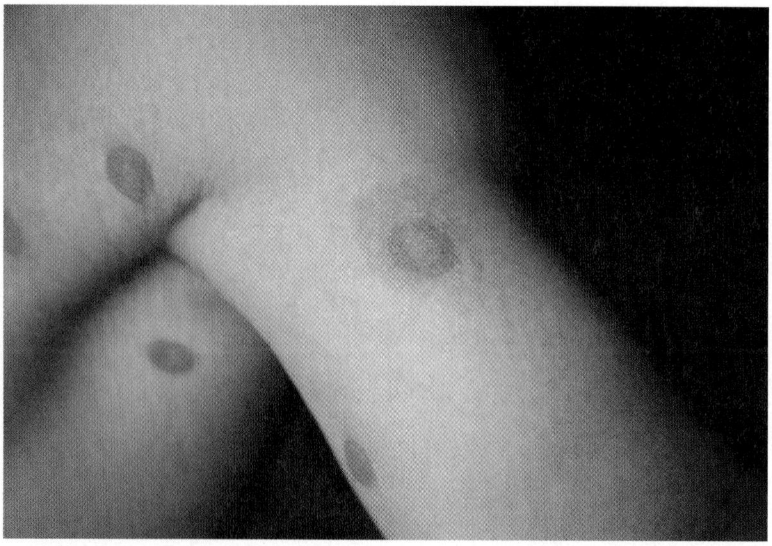

FIGURE 8-6 Tinea is called ringworm because it can cause a circular rash that is red and itchy.

Trichomoniasis is a sexually transmitted disease (STD) of the vagina or urethra caused by the protozoan *Trichomonas vaginalis*. It is important to consider because many people with trichomoniasis also have gonorrhea or other STDs. Thus, if you test positive for trichomoniasis, you should also be tested for other STDs. Women are much more likely to develop symptoms than men are. Although men usually have either no symptoms or only mild ones, they can still infect their sexual partners. There are two other *Trichomonas* parasites, but only *Trichomonas vaginalis* is an established pathogen (the agent that causes disease).[5] (Learn more about trichomoniasis in Chapter 5.)

Giardia occurs worldwide and is the most common parasitic intestinal infection in the United States. Most people get infected by drinking contaminated water. People who backpack or hike need to boil untreated water taken from streams and lakes before drinking. The main symptoms of giardiasis are abdominal cramping and diarrhea. If untreated, the symptoms may persist for weeks.[5]

Toxoplasma occurs around the world wherever there are cats. It has been referred to as "the most cosmopolitan of parasites." Most warm-blooded animals, both domestic and wild, have toxoplasmosis, with approximately 50% of adults in the United States having toxoplasmosis. While many people in the United States have toxoplasmosis, for most people it is self-limiting and asymptomatic. Only people with weakened immune systems are likely to develop

INFECTIOUS DISEASES AFTER DISASTERS

After a natural disaster, such as a hurricane, earthquake, tornado, or tsunami, there are often infectious disease outbreaks. The reason for these outbreaks is population displacement, lack of water and sanitation facilities, crowding, and the lack of available healthcare services.[10,11]

When a natural disaster does not result in population displacement, it rarely results in infectious disease outbreaks.

Water-Related Communicable Diseases

Water-related diseases occur with flooding, as happens after a hurricane or tsunami. In addition to parasitic infections, including cryptosporidiosis and giardiasis, both of which cause diarrhea, bacterial infections (*E. coli, Shigella, Salmonella, Vibrio*, or leptospirosis) and viral infections (hepatitis A, norovirus, or rotavirus) also occur. Flood waters may also be contaminated by sewage or toxic chemicals.

Diseases Associated With Crowding

Diseases like measles, which are highly contagious, can spread if there are not enough vaccinated people in the population. (See the explanation in this chapter on herd immunity.) Outbreaks of measles occurred following natural disasters in the Philippines,[12] Indonesia,[13] and Pakistan.[14] Other diseases associated with crowding which occurs after a disaster include *Neisseria meningitidis* and acute respiratory infections.[13,14]

Vector-Borne Diseases

Standing water after flooding provides breeding sites for mosquitos, including those that carry diseases, including malaria and Dengue fever.

Injuries

Wading through flood waters or rubble from buildings increases the risk of puncture wounds and cuts from hidden objects. Depending on the bacteria or virus, wounds and cuts can become infected.

(continues)

INFECTIOUS DISEASES AFTER DISASTERS *(Continued)*

Other Services

When power is lost (as in the 2017 hurricane season, when all of Puerto Rico lost power) over an entire geographic area, water treatment and supply plants may be offline, increasing the risk for waterborne infections.[15] It may also disrupt health facilities, such as workers' ability to get to the facility and things like refrigeration for vaccines.

Helpful advice: After a natural disaster, water may not be safe to drink. Ideally you want to keep a 2-week supply, but as a minimum, at least a 3-day supply (figure 1 gallon per person and per pet for each day.) Replace every 6 months. Also keep a bottle of unscented chlorine bleach (between 5% or 6% and 8.25% sodium hypochlorite) for purifying water and general sanitizing.[16]

If you don't have a supply of bottled water, a source of clean water is from your hot water tank. The best way to treat water is to boil it to kill viruses, bacteria, and parasites. If you have a way to boil water, bring it to a rolling boil for 1 full minute. (If you are above 6,500 feet elevation, boil for 3 minutes.) If the water is cloudy, filter it through a clean cloth, paper towel, or coffee filter before boiling. Make sure you have clean, sanitized containers with tight covers to store your boiled water.

To treat water: If the water is cloudy, use ¼ teaspoon of unscented liquid bleach to 1 gallon of water. If the water is clear, use 1/8 teaspoon of bleach. Allow it to sit for 30 minutes before drinking.

symptoms. Women who get toxoplasmosis when they are pregnant can pass the disease on to their fetus. This is why pregnant women are recommended to avoid contact with cats. If avoiding cats is impossible, pregnant women should preferably not clean cat litter boxes or should wear gloves when doing so.[5]

Three types of organisms cause parasitic infections in humans: protozoa, helminths, and ectoparasites. Protozoa are single-celled organisms that can live and multiply inside the body. Helminths (worms) are multicelled organisms that can live alone or in humans. Helminths include flatworms, tapeworms, ringworms (different from the tinea-related ringworm), and roundworms (**FIGURE 8-7**).

Ectoparasites, such as mosquitoes, fleas, ticks, and mites, live outside the human body. Parasitic infections spread through contaminated water, waste, fecal matter (which is why you should always wash your hands with soap, scrubbing for 20 seconds after going to the bathroom!), and food that has not been properly handled. Malaria is a serious parasitic infection spread by mosquitoes.

More on How Are Diseases Spread: Or, Your Mother Was Right, Wash Your Hands!

Diseases spread when bacteria, viruses, or other germs transfer from one person or animal to another. As you read earlier in the chapter, this can happen when you kiss someone who is infected, when you have sex with an infected person, when you touch someone who is infected, or when an infected person coughs or sneezes near you. You can also get sick from being bitten or scratched by an infected animal or from eating contaminated food. A pregnant woman can pass some diseases on to her unborn baby.

Before the discovery of pathogens, many people believed that diseases resulted from evil spirits. To be healthy, a person needed the proper balance of the four humors. Medical theory postulated that a person's illness was the result of his or her humors being out of balance. Each person's balance was different,

Parasitic Helminths

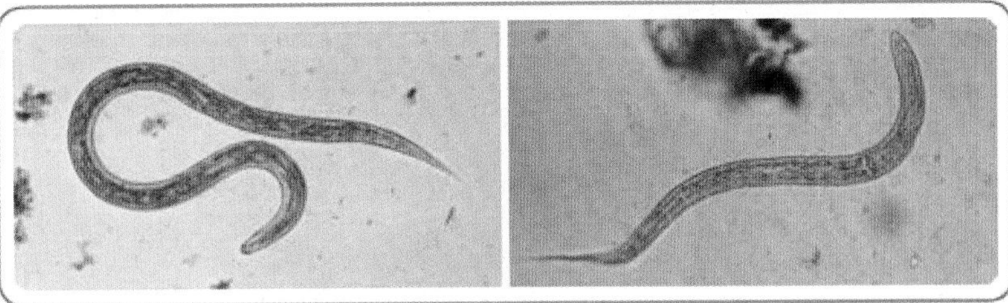

Hookworms are known as soil-transmitted helminths.

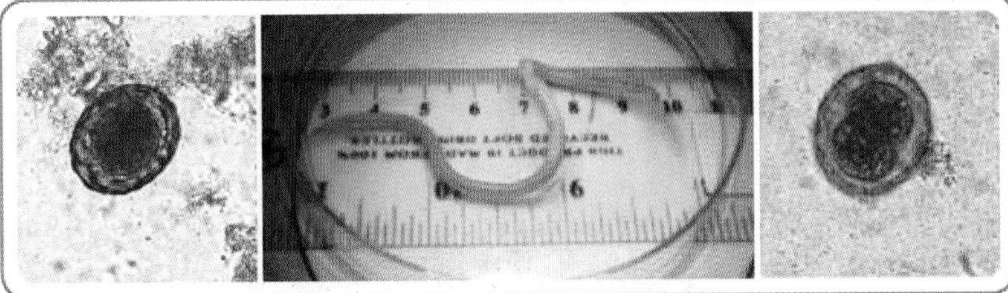

Ascacaris (a round worm) are also a soil-transmitted helminths.

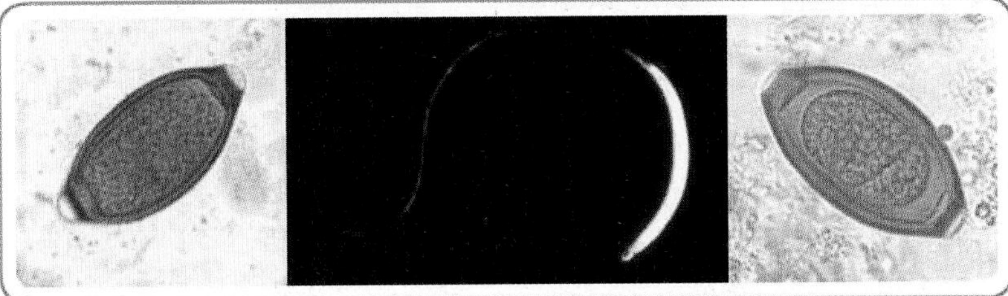

Whipworm, a soil-transmitted helminth, live in the large intestine.

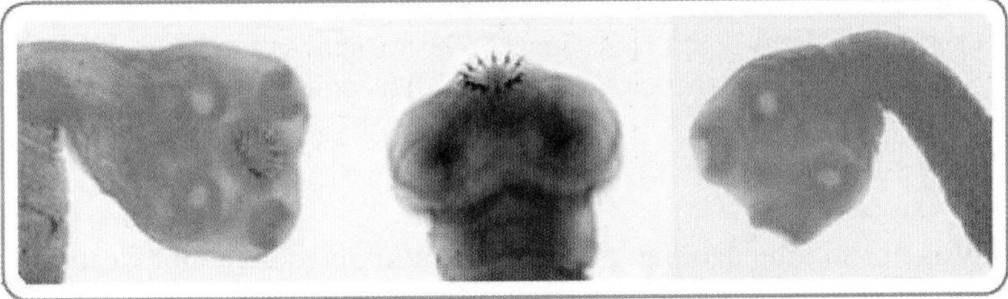

Taeniasis in humans is a parasitic infection caused by the tapeworm (flat segmented worms) species.

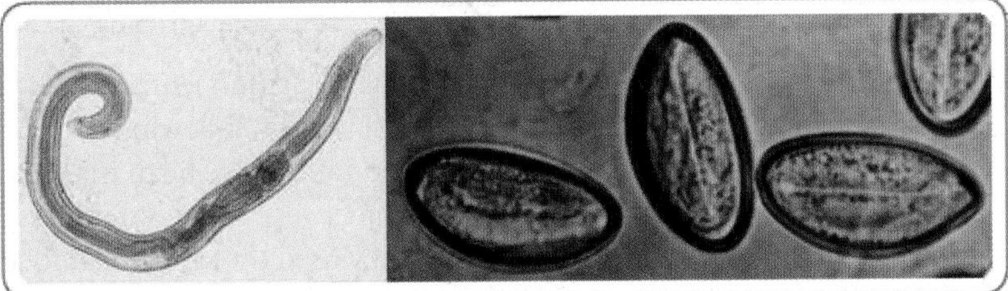

Pinworm infection is caused by a small, thin, white roundworm. Pinworms most commonly affect children.

FIGURE 8-7 From top to bottom: Hookworms are a soil-transmitted helminth. *Ascaris* (a roundworm) is also a soil-transmitted helminth. Whipworms, a soil-transmitted helminth, live in the large intestine. Taeniasis in humans is a parasitic infection caused by the tapeworm (flat segmented worms) species. Pinworm infection is caused by a small, thin, white roundworm. Pinworms most commonly affect children.

Courtesy Centers for Disease Control and Prevention.

but it was the physician's job to diagnose the humoral imbalance and correct it (see **FIGURE 8-8**). Besides vaccines (discussed later in this chapter), several concepts changed the course of human history because they had such a profound effect on people's health.

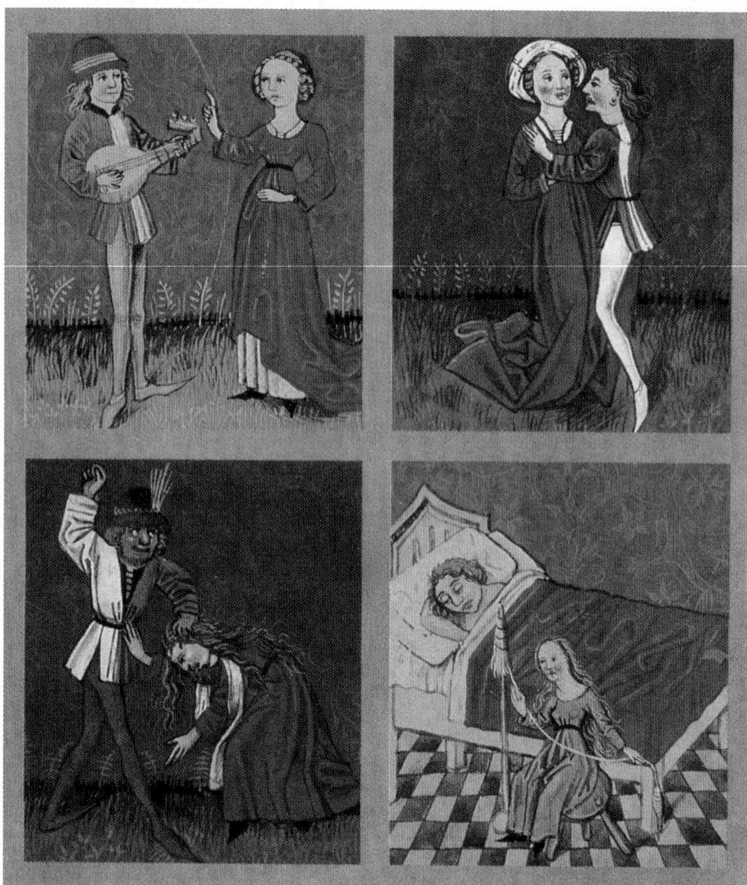

FIGURE 8-8 Images from Deutsche Kalendar, 1498. The images are (from left to right) Choleric (hot and dry), Melancholic (cold and dry), Phlegmatic (cold and moist) and Sanguine (hot and moist).

It was not so long ago that people did not understand about cleanliness or the necessity of washing their hands. Before the mid-1800s even surgeons did not wash their hands before performing surgery. The person who introduced the importance of hand washing was Ignaz Semmelweis, a Hungarian-born physician, who specialized in obstetrics.

Semmelweis noted that two maternity clinics at the same Vienna hospital had significantly different rates of fatal childbed fever (infection following childbirth). Even pregnant women knew about this and would rather give birth in the street than at the clinic with the higher fatality rate. Semmelweis wanted to understand why the rates were different, especially because they used the same techniques.

The only difference between the clinics was that the first clinic was for teaching medical students and the second was for the instruction of midwives. Semmelweis's scientific breakthrough came when his good friend Jakob Kolletschka died after being poked with a medical student's scalpel that had been used in a postmortem examination. Kolletschka's autopsy showed pathology similar to that of the women who died of childbed fever. Semmelweis noticed that medical students went directly from the dissecting room to the maternity clinic. Most physicians didn't believe in washing their hands.

Despite being ridiculed for his ideas, Semmelweis made hand washing compulsory for everyone entering the maternity clinics. Even though the rates of death for both mothers and newborns dropped precipitously, the Royal Society of Medicine refused to follow his advice because Semmelweis's scientific observations conflicted with the scientific and medical establishment.[17] To promote his theory, Semmelweis took to his version of social media: He lectured, published papers, wrote a book, and even handed out pamphlets about the importance of hand washing.[17] Imagine if he'd had access to Twitter or Instagram!

When you get a drink of water from the water fountain or the kitchen sink, do you ever stop to wonder what it was like before houses had running water? Imagine if you had to go to a neighborhood pump to get your water and there was no bottled water available. Such an inconvenience is hard to imagine. We now move to London, years after Ignaz Semmelweis was forced to resign from the Vienna hospital.

In the mid-1800s the Soho district of London was crowded and filthy. Although other parts of London had a sewer system, Soho did not. Most houses had cesspools (an underground container for sewage from a building or house) that were overflowing. In 1854, the London government decided to deal with the problem by dumping the waste into the River Thames. The government's choice was unfortunate because this action contaminated the water supply, leading to a severe cholera outbreak. Cholera is an acute diarrheal disease caused by ingesting contaminated food or water. Because cholera has a short incubation period (2 hours to 5 days), large outbreaks of the disease can occur quite quickly. If left untreated, cholera can be deadly. The World Health Organization estimates that there are 3 million to 5 million cholera cases every year and 100,000 to 120,000 deaths.[18]

At the end of August 1854, 127 people on or near Broad Street in Soho had died. By September 10, another 500 people had died. By the time the outbreak was over, 616 people had died. Enter John Snow, a physician who is now considered the father of epidemiology. By studying the disease's distribution pattern, Snow identified the source of the outbreak as the public water pump on Broad Street. Although he could not explain why the water was causing the illness, he correctly figured out that the people who were using that pump were getting cholera. The authorities removed the pump handle, but the epidemic was already waning. Interestingly, there was a monastery near the Broad Street pump, but none of the monks got cholera because they drank only the beer they brewed. The beer was safer to drink than the water from the pump.[19]

Although John Snow published his theory about the spread of disease, doctors and scientists thought he was wrong. They believed that breathing bad vapors caused cholera. There are two important messages to understand from this story. One is that by studying the distribution of the disease, the source of the infection was identified. The other message is how important clean water is to health.

Host Susceptibility

Our review of the reasons people get sick from infectious diseases still does not explain why you can get sick when your friend doesn't, even if you have been exposed to the same illness at the exact same time and place. There are many reasons people get sick, and they may be due to the individual or their environment. Babies who are too young to build **immunity** (the body's ability to resist a particular infection) or people who are old or not in good health may be more likely to get a disease. Some people just have strong immune systems.

immunity Resistance developed in response to stimulus by an antigen (infecting agent or vaccine) and usually characterized by the presence of antibodies produced by the host.

There are easy things that you can do to help your body fight illness, starting with nourishing your body. Eating a well-rounded, balanced diet with lots of fresh fruits and vegetables is important. Foods rich in antioxidants, such as beets, blueberries, broccoli, green tea, garlic, ginger, and turmeric, boost immunity. Your body cannot function at its best when the food you eat is not healthy. A poor diet also increases the risk of various illnesses. (See Chapter 2.) Your

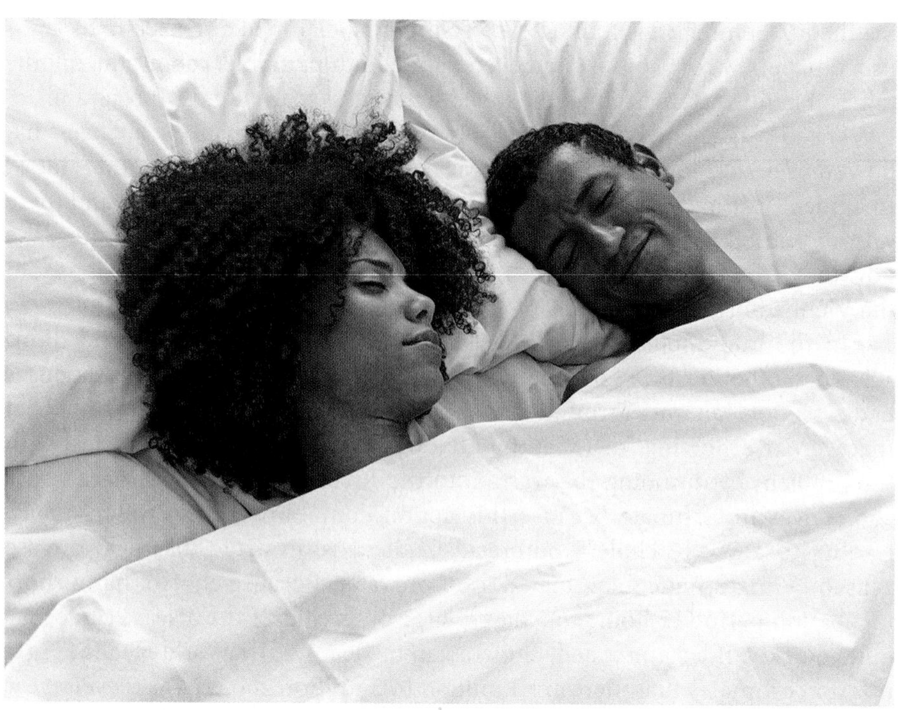

body is 60% water, but you lose some of that water when you sweat, when you urinate, and even when you breathe. Being mildly to moderately dehydrated can make you sick. Drinking enough water is essential for staying healthy.

People underestimate the importance of a good night's sleep. Many people, particularly college students, do not get enough sleep. When you sleep, your body's immune system releases cytokines that help your body fight inflammation and disease.[20] If you are sleep deprived, your body cannot produce enough cytokines. Sleep deprivation is one reason that some people get sick more often.

Regular physical activity and moderate, rather than strenuous exercise, helps prevent disease.[21]

Oral hygiene, too, is often underappreciated. Taking good care of your teeth and gums is an important and easy way to help ensure good health. Our mouths are full of bacteria all the time and contain the sorts of organisms that can cause oral infection(s). When you are healthy, your body's natural defenses help ensure that you have more of the good bacteria. Brushing your teeth at least twice a day and flossing every day helps keep the harmful bacteria under control. An infection in your mouth is an infection in your whole body. Medical studies have shown that poor oral health is related to heart disease,[22] type 2 diabetes,[23] strokes,[24] and, for pregnant women, premature delivery.[25]

Your body comes with many built-in defenses (**FIGURE 8-9**). In fact, the job of many of your body parts is to help protect you from diseases. Your skin provides a very effective obstacle to germs unless something happens that breaches that barrier. If you get a cut or a burn, the sore provides a place for germs to enter your body. Nose hair may not be terribly attractive, but it is very important. It traps dirt and germs until we sneeze, blow our noses, or swallow them. One study from Turkey found that having more nasal hair protected people from asthma.[32]

Many parts of your body have mucous membranes: your mouth, lungs, nasal passages, and genital area. Although they may feel delicate, the mucus they secrete is protective. Your eyes tear and help eliminate foreign objects from your eyes. When you cough and sneeze, your body is doing its job to rid you of germs. If the germs still get through, your saliva has many enzymes and your stomach has acid, which helps prevent you from getting sick.

FACT VS. FICTION

Myths About Oral Health

Myth 1: The main cause of tooth decay is sugar. The corollary is that if I drink diet soda, I don't need to worry about my teeth because diet soda does not have sugar.

Facts: Sugar definitely plays a part in tooth decay. Even nutritious foods contain surprising amounts of natural sugars that are just as damaging to young mouths as sugar-added treats, soda, and sports drinks. The bacteria in your mouth need processed sugar to survive, but even if you don't eat sugar and have poor oral hygiene habits, you will experience the same kind of decay as a heavy sugar eater. Ultimately, the real cause of tooth decay comes from a combination of sugar, acid, and bacteria. Diet soda is highly acidic and can weaken the surface of the enamel, raising the risk for cavities, so while it does not contain sugar, it still is bad for your teeth. The best choice is to eat a balanced diet and adhere to dietary guidelines.[26]

Myth 2: Whiter teeth are healthier teeth.

Facts: Healthy teeth come in a wide range of natural shades. You can have bright white teeth and still have cavities. Teeth naturally discolor as you get older, and certain foods stain your teeth, including coffee, tea, wine, blueberries, blackberries, balsamic vinegar, citrus, and acidic foods. It is important to understand that color does not necessarily mean healthier teeth. The effects of whitening your teeth may be temporary.[27]

Myth 3: A harder toothbrush is better.

Facts: There are many choices in toothbrushes: electric or manual; hard, medium, soft, and very soft. We do know that electric (or battery operated) toothbrushes do a better job of removing plaque and bacteria than do manual toothbrushes.[28] Research suggests that hard toothbrushes may traumatize the gum margin.[29] Although not studied directly, it appears that it is a better choice to brush longer with a soft brush than to use a hard brush.

Myth 4: Flossing isn't necessary.

Facts: Flossing in addition to tooth brushing reduces gum disease compared to tooth brushing alone. Flossing will not prevent cavities.[30] If your gums bleed after flossing or brushing, it usually means you need to floss and brush those areas more. By choosing not to floss you miss one-third of the tooth surface.

Myth 5: Gum disease is not common.

Facts: Gum disease is surprisingly common. A study from the Centers for Disease Control and Prevention found that 47.2% of adults aged 30 years and older have some form of periodontal disease and that periodontal disease increases with age. Of adults 65 years and older, 70.1% have periodontal disease. The condition occurs more frequently in men than women, among those who are poor, current smokers, and those with less than a high school education.[31]

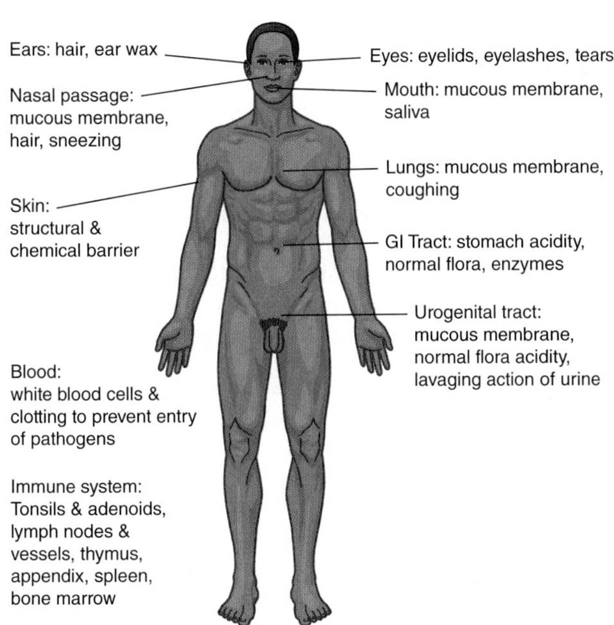

FIGURE 8-9 Your body's built-in defenses.

IMMUNE SYSTEM

Your body's immune system is your defense! The immune system's job is to defend you against microbes, bacteria, toxins, viruses, and parasites. It protects you from environmental assaults and is essential to your survival. It is the most complex system in your body.[33]

As long as your body's defense system is working well, you don't notice it. Think of it like a medieval city. There is a wall around the city. As long as it does its job, nobody pays attention to it. But when the enemy breaks down the wall and enters the city, everybody pays attention.

The immune system is made up of various body parts. These include, but are not limited to, the following:

- *Bone marrow*: Every cell that is part of your immune system originates from bone marrow. These stem cells become either the mature cells of the immune system or they migrate to other parts of the body and develop into red blood cells (carry oxygen through your body), white blood cells (fight infections), platelets (help with blood clotting), granulocytes (remove parasites and bacteria), T cells (help identify and destroy damaged, cancerous, and infected cells), B cells (produce antibodies), and natural killer cells (protect against pathogens and tumor development).
- *Thymus*: Organ within the immune system where T cells mature.
- *Spleen*: Organ within the immune system that filters blood. The spleen activates B cells and produces antibodies. It also destroys old red blood cells.
- *Lymph nodes*: Occur throughout the body (neck, armpits, groin, thorax, knees, and elbows) and filter the bodily fluids. When you are sick they become swollen.

The skin is the first barrier the microbe must pass. This usually happens when you get a cut or an abrasion. Microbes can also enter through your digestive system or your respiratory system. Those systems have their own lines of defense against microbes. Underneath the skin, there are cells (macrophages, B cells, and T cells) waiting to attack germs that get through the skin. Microbes that pass that barrier are attacked by general defenses. Microbes that get across the general defenses find weapons the body created specifically to attack those particular germs. These weapons, antibodies and T cells, are prepared to recognize and attack designated targets.[34]

Finally, there is your immune system. Your immune system is a team made up of cells, tissues, and organs that work together to make sure you stay healthy by protecting your body. These factors all contribute to your ability to resist illness when you are exposed to an infectious agent.

Preventing and Treating Infectious Diseases

Considerable progress has been made in treating infectious diseases with **antibiotics** and preventing infectious diseases with vaccines. Many diseases that once spread fear among the population are either eradicated or manageable.

antibiotics Substances, such as penicillin, that are capable of destroying or weakening certain microorganisms, especially bacteria or fungi, that cause infections or infectious diseases.

Antibiotics

The word *antibiotic* means "against life." In practice, *antibiotic* means against microbes. There are antibacterial medicines, antiviral medicines, antifungal medicines, and antiparasitic medicines. These are all antimicrobials. Although all the types of medications just mentioned are antibiotics, in general use, *antibiotic* is taken to mean antibacterial. Other drugs are referred to specifically as antivirals, antifungals, and antiparasitics.

Some drugs, such as penicillin, are called broad-spectrum antibiotics because they are used to treat many different bacterial infections. Medicines that treat just a few organisms—for example, erythromycin—are called narrow-spectrum antibiotics. Broad-spectrum antibiotics can kill many different types of bacteria, so when a healthcare provider prescribes one of those, it is likely to kill whatever is making you sick. The disadvantage is that they also kill beneficial organisms that we need. Narrow-spectrum antibiotics are prescribed only when the clinician knows the organism that is causing the disease. If the provider chooses incorrectly, the medicine may not cure the infection. The advantage of narrow-spectrum antibiotics is that they do not kill as many of the good organisms as broad-spectrum antibiotics do.

When people take too many antibiotics or take only part of a prescription, the bacteria may develop resistance to the medicine. Two common scenarios exacerbate this problem. In the first scenario, a healthcare provider gives you a prescription for antibiotics, and you start taking the medication. When you feel better, you stop taking the antibiotics, or you share your antibiotics with someone else, meaning that you both take less than the full prescription. In the second scenario, you get sick and assume that you need antibiotics, which your healthcare provider agrees to prescribe, though your sickness cannot be treated by antibiotics. Today, public health professionals are concerned about the overuse of antibiotics, which occurs because clinicians prescribe medication when patients do not need it.[35] In fact, an estimated 30% to 50% of antibiotics are prescribed inappropriately.[36] Taking antibacterial medicine will not cure a cold or the flu (**TABLE 8-2**). It will not make you feel better and

TABLE 8-2 When You Need an Antibiotic and When You Don't[39]

Illness	Usual Cause: Virus	Usual Cause: Bacteria	Antibiotic Needed?
Bacterial vaginosis		√	Yes
Chlamydia		√	Yes
Cold/runny nose	√		**NO**
Genital herpes	√		**NO**
Gonorrhea		√	Yes
Hepatitis	√		**NO**
Human papillomavirus	√		**NO**
Influenza (flu)	√		**NO**
Mononucleosis	√		**NO**
Pneumonia (bacterial)		√	Yes
Pneumonia (viral)	√		**NO**

(continues)

TABLE 8-2 When You Need an Antibiotic and When You Don't[39] *(continued)*

Illness	Usual Cause		Antibiotic Needed?
	Virus	Bacteria	
Sore throat (except strep)	√		**NO**
Strep throat		√	Yes
Syphilis		√	Yes
Trichomoniasis		√	Yes
Urinary tract infection		√	Yes
Whooping cough		√	Yes

Antibiotics aren't always the answer | features | CDC. http://www.cdc.gov/Features/GetSmart/

keep you from giving your disease to other people. This practice of misusing antibiotics is a big problem for individuals and communities and has led to "superbugs"—bacteria that are resistant to several types of antibiotics. Even using antibiotics correctly drives antibiotic resistance,[37] although misusing antibiotics makes the problem worse. Approximately 23,000 people die each year because of antibiotic-resistant germs.[36] **FIGURE 8-10** depicts how antibiotic resistance spreads.[39]

For some infections, it is difficult even for healthcare providers to know whether bacteria or viruses are the cause. There are other times when you have a viral disease and that leads to a bacterial infection. There are also many diseases, such as pneumonia, meningitis, and diarrhea, that can be caused by either bacteria or a virus.

Sometimes you may be given an antibiotic, and you use it exactly as prescribed. In addition to killing the organisms that are making you sick, it kills good bacteria, leaving you more vulnerable to other infections. A typical example of this is when a woman gets a urinary tract infection; the antibiotics kill the good bacteria, but she ends up with a yeast infection afterward because the good bacteria that control the fungus that causes yeast infections have been killed. If you are prone to getting yeast infections, be sure to ask your healthcare provider for antifungal medicine to follow your regimen of antibiotics.

FACT VS. FICTION

Does Cranberry Juice Prevent Urinary Tract Infections?

Myth: Drinking cranberry juice can prevent and cure urinary tract infections.

Facts: Because this idea has existed for a long time, there is actually a lot of research on the relationship. The results of studies have been mixed, with some finding that cranberry juice or cranberry pills prevent urinary tract infections and others that conclude that it does not work. A systematic review of the medical literature concluded that individuals cannot rely on cranberry juice to prevent urinary tract infections.[40] There is no evidence to suggest that cranberry juice effectively treats urinary tract infections.[41]

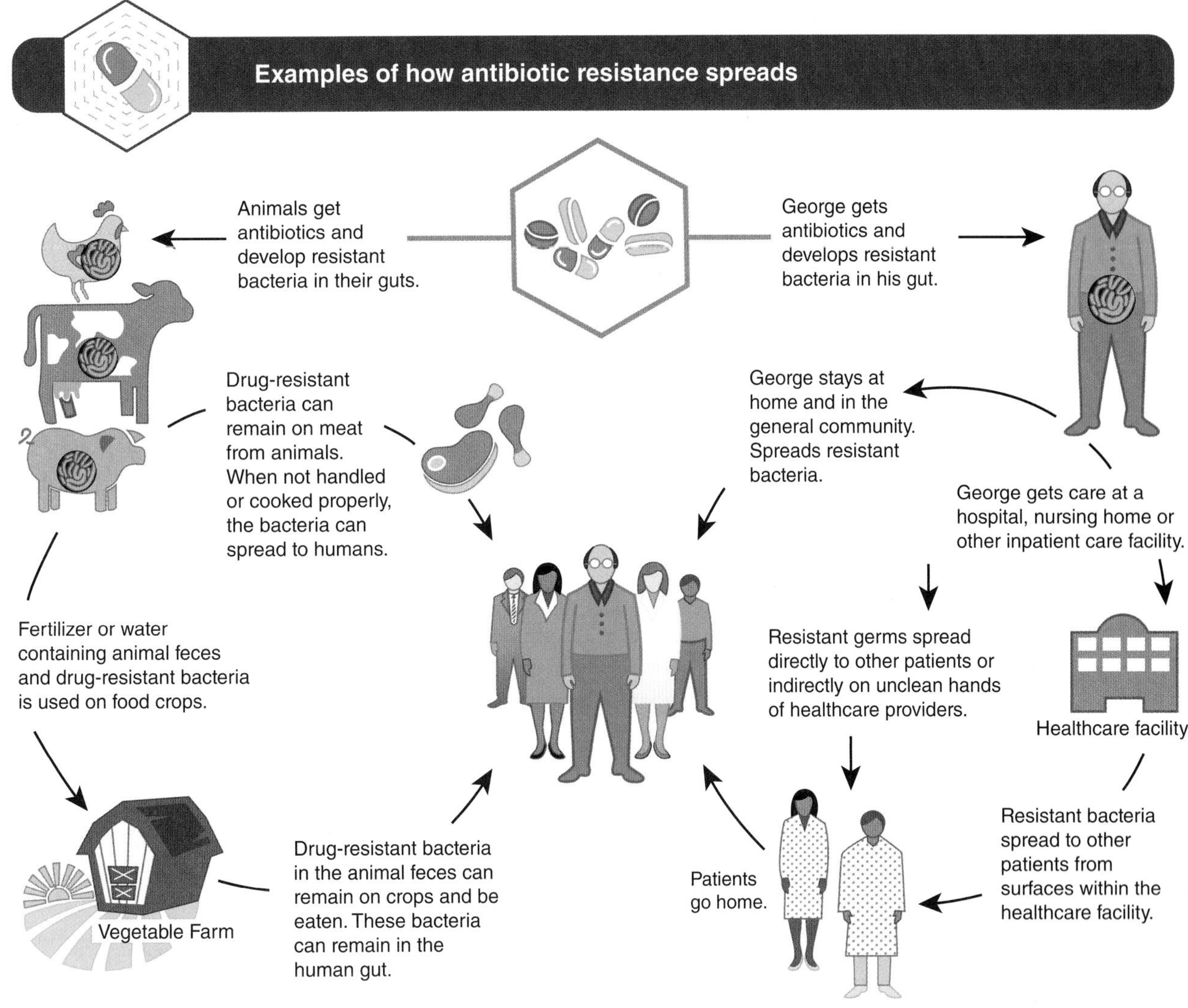

FIGURE 8-10 Examples of how antibiotic resistance spreads.

Centers for Disease Control and Prevention. (2017). Antibiotic/antimicrobial resistance: About antimicrobial resistance. Retrieved from https://www.cdc.gov/drugresistance/about.html

FACT VS. FICTION

Does Eating Yogurt Prevent Yeast Infections?

Myth: Eating yogurt can prevent and cure yeast infections.

Facts: The ways to prevent yeast infection include wearing breathable underwear, wearing clothing on the bottom that is a little loose, not douching, not using scented feminine products, changing out of wet clothing, wiping from front to back after using the toilet, changing tampons, pads, and panty liners often, and using antibiotics only when you have a bacterial infection.[42] Eating yogurt? Not so much. Data do not support yogurt therapy or oral lactobacillus treatment.[43]

Vaccines and Vaccine-Preventable Diseases

The world has a long history of attempts at creating vaccinations. Indian Buddhists in the seventh century consumed snake venom in hopes of becoming immune to snake bites.[44] Although uncertain, there are authors who describe inoculation and variolation (the deliberate inoculation of an uninfected person with the smallpox virus to produce immunity to the disease) in 10th-century China.[45] What is certain is that since 1695, well before Edward Jenner is credited with creating the first vaccination, the Chinese practiced inoculation against smallpox.[45]

Vaccines prevent more than 2.5 million deaths each year.[46] According to the United Nations, since 2000, inoculation with the measles vaccine has averted over 14 million deaths.[47] Clearly, vaccines play a significant role in the health of the world. There are several different types of vaccines (**FIGURE 8-11**).

Live, attenuated vaccines are made from living microbes that have been weakened in the lab so you cannot get the disease. Because they are live, however, your body will have a strong response to them. Usually, one or two doses of a live, attenuated vaccine will provide lifelong immunity.

Live vaccines are relatively easy to create for viruses such as measles, mumps, and chickenpox.[48] Inactivated vaccines are made by killing the disease-causing microbe. Inactivated vaccines are more stable than live vaccines but do not elicit as strong a response in your body as a live vaccine.[48] The polio vaccine is an example of an inactivated vaccine.

Toxoid vaccines are made from toxins produced by bacteria. Toxoid vaccines work because the immune system responds to them and learns to respond to the natural toxin. The vaccines for diphtheria and tetanus are toxoid vaccines.

A conjugate vaccine is created by joining an antigen (a substance that when introduced into the body stimulates the production of an antibody) to a protein molecule. Conjugated vaccines are usually used to immunize babies and children against certain bacterial infections.[48] Given how immature infants' immune

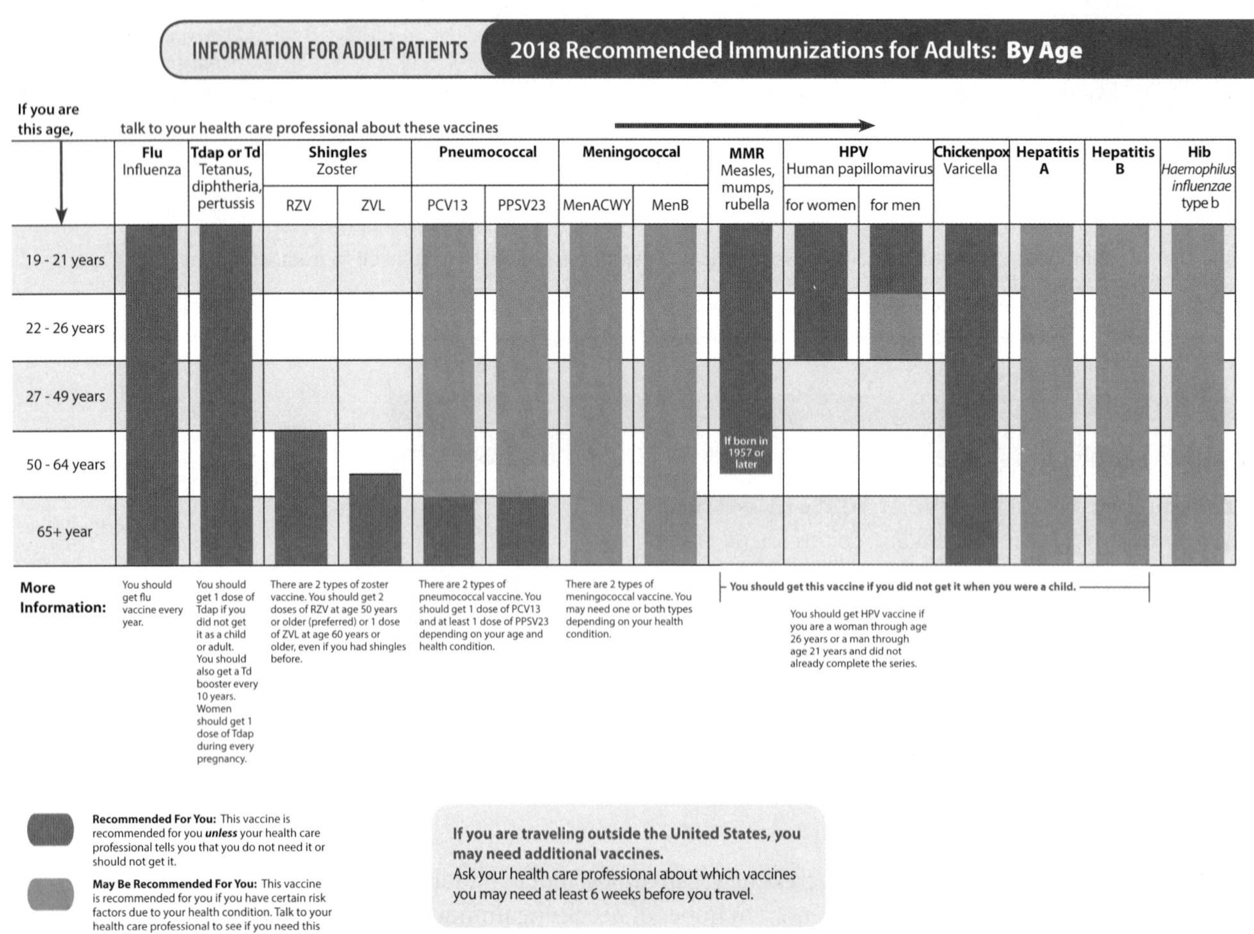

FIGURE 8-11 CDC Recommended Adult Vaccination Schedule (*continues*)

systems are, ordinary vaccines are not effective. The vaccine for *Haemophilus influenzae* type B (Hib) is a conjugate vaccine. The hepatitis B vaccine is administered to newborns because of the seriousness of the disease, although it does require multiple doses. Other types of vaccines include subunit vaccines, DNA vaccines, and recombinant vector vaccines.[49]

Each year, the Advisory Committee on Immunization Practices reviews the recommended immunization schedules for children and adults. Figures 8–11a and 11b provide a general guide to the immunizations that you and your teen or adult family members should have. It is based on the Centers for Disease Control and Prevention (CDC) schedules.[50–52] Sometimes the schedule changes as new vaccines are developed, but your physician or other healthcare professional will have the most updated version. Or, if you are interested, you can look at the CDC's website. If you miss a needed vaccination, your healthcare professional will know the catch-up schedule. Some people are at high risk for infection and need a different immunization schedule. If you plan to travel outside the United States, you may need additional vaccinations not listed on this schedule. Allow at least 6 weeks before your travel date to get the needed vaccinations.[53]

The CDC's website (wwwnc.cdc.gov/travel/destinations/list) provides recommendations about vaccinations for travelers for every country around the globe, even ones you probably don't want to visit. Before you travel to any country you should be up-to-date on routine vaccines. Routine vaccines include measles-mumps-rubella (MMR) vaccine, diphtheria-tetanus-pertussis vaccine,

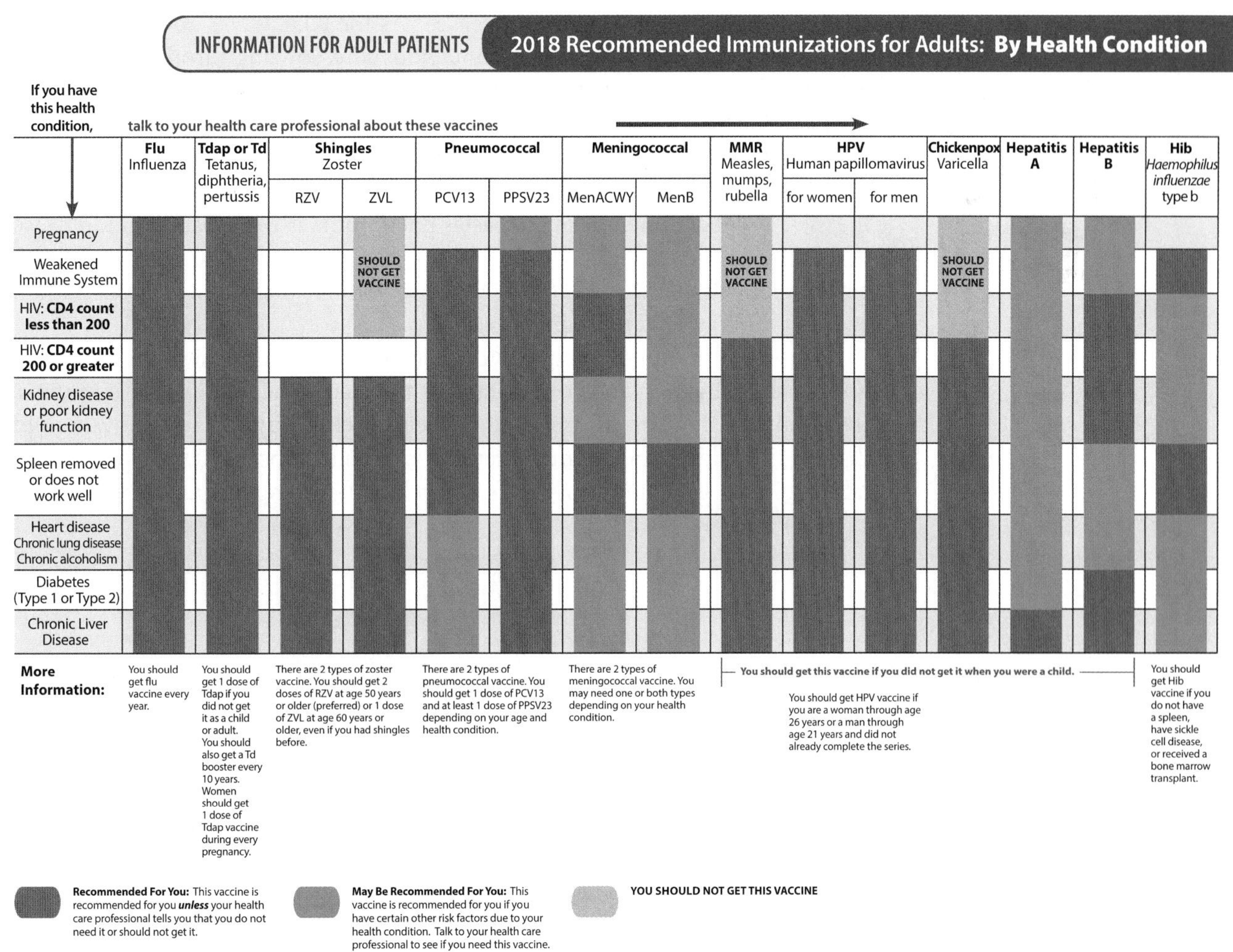

FIGURE 8-11 (CONTINUED) CDC Recommended Adult Vaccination Schedule

Reproduced from Centers for Disease Control and Prevention. (2018). Recommended Immunizations for Adults by Age in Easy-to-read Format United States, 2018. Accessed at, https://www.cdc.gov/vaccines/schedules/easy-to-read/adult-shell-easyread.html

varicella (chickenpox) vaccine, polio vaccine, and your yearly flu shot. If you are traveling to Western Europe, your routine vaccinations are sufficient. If you are traveling to the former Soviet bloc countries, you need routine plus the hepatitis A vaccination. For most other countries you need routine plus hepatitis A and typhoid vaccinations. Other vaccinations you may need include yellow fever, malaria, and polio. Always ask your healthcare provider what vaccines and medicines you need based on your own medical history, where you are going, how long you are staying, what you will be doing, and if you are traveling from a country other than the United States.

Many diseases can be prevented by vaccines,[48] and many of us have gotten these vaccines. Most people born before 1957 got a series of childhood illnesses at some point in their lives, including measles, mumps, rubella (German measles), and chickenpox. There are other diseases (e.g., polio) against which people are now vaccinated that, before the vaccine, caused disabling illness to many people. Vaccines also have enabled us to eradicate at least one disease (smallpox).[48]

For most people, rubella (German measles) is a relatively mild disease, but for pregnant women, rubella is dangerous. Before the vaccine (1969), there were epidemics of rubella every 6 to 9 years.[54] Most of the cases affected children in elementary schools, but there were also cases among pregnant women. Congenital rubella is a syndrome that occurs when a fetus has been infected with the rubella virus while in the uterus. When a child has congenital rubella syndrome, the disease may cause mental retardation, defects of the heart and eyes, deafness, and other medical problems.

Measles can be a dangerous disease.[54] As the CDC says, "Measles isn't just a little rash."[55] Measles is highly contagious and spreads through the air via coughing and sneezing. If someone has measles, 9 out 10 people in contact with the person who are not vaccinated or have not had the disease will get it. Measles is a serious illness and can have severe consequences. One out of four people who get measles will end up in the hospital. Out of every 20 children with measles, 1 will get pneumonia. Measles pneumonia is the most common cause of death from measles in young children. One to 2 out of 1,000 individuals who get measles will die. One out of 1,000 people who get measles will develop brain swelling that can lead to brain damage.[44]

Mumps is another contagious disease characterized by swelling of one or both of the salivary glands on the side of the face. When people have mumps, they look like they are storing food in their cheeks. Mumps is a relatively mild disease in children but is more serious in adults. About 10% of postpubertal males who get mumps suffer from orchitis (swelling of one or both of the

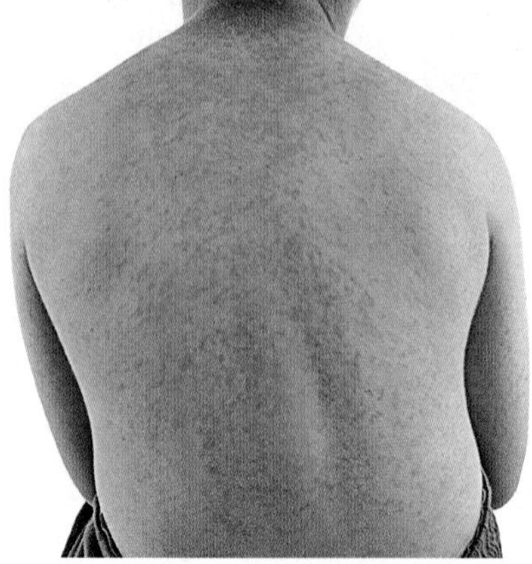

Child with measles.

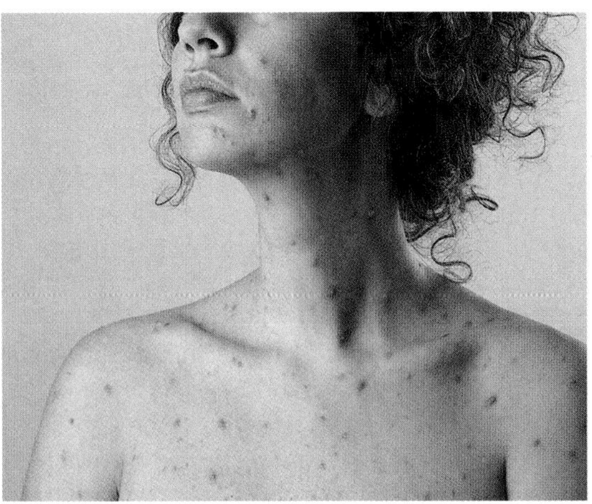

Chickenpox.

testicles). About half of males who get orchitis from mumps will experience some degree of testicular atrophy.[54]

The varicella-zoster virus causes chickenpox.[54] Mostly it is young children who get chickenpox, but older children and adults can get it too, as it is very contagious. Chickenpox produces an uncomfortable, itchy rash. One of the treatments for chickenpox is colloidal oatmeal, which is made by grinding whole oats into a fine powder and then dissolving the powder in bath water. It is important not to give aspirin to someone with chickenpox as it may cause a serious disease called Reye syndrome. When you have had chickenpox, the varicella-zoster virus stays in your body. Although you likely will not get chickenpox again, you may get a disease called shingles. While shingles is not life threatening, it is very painful. The risk of shingles increases with age, although the current recommendation for the shingles vaccine is after age 50 years. This vaccine may be important for your older relatives because people whose immunity to the varicella-zoster virus is derived from having had chickenpox (as opposed to having been vaccinated against it) are at much higher risk for getting shingles.[56]

Some people choose not to vaccinate their children, and after reading about these diseases, you may wonder why. There are many reasons why people make this decision. Some people have religious reasons, and some children may have medical conditions that make getting vaccinations dangerous for them. Unfortunately, some children do not get vaccinated because their parents believe that vaccines are dangerous, or at least, more dangerous than getting the disease. For some parents who have not experienced how bad childhood diseases can be, the necessity of vaccines may be less clear. In 1998, a British surgeon and medical researcher published a paper in *The Lancet*,[57] one of the most prestigious medical journals in the world. The paper raised the possibility that there was a link between autism and the vaccine for measles, mumps, and rubella. Subsequent research failed to prove his hypothesis or replicate his results; moreover, his data were found to be fraudulent. The doctor was forced to resign his position at the hospital and his medical license was revoked. The journal retracted the paper in 2010. (It may not seem important that the journal retracted the paper, but for such a prestigious journal to have to admit that an author duped them is very critical in the scientific world.) Nonetheless, the idea had been planted in many parents' minds, and they chose not to vaccinate their children.

Before you were born, maybe before even your parents were born, virtually all children got the measles. In 1963, a measles vaccine was created. In 2000, measles was declared eliminated in the United States. But measles is still

TALES OF PUBLIC HEALTH (VACCINATION PART 1)

Outbreak of Measles at Disneyland

Sometime between December 15 and December 20, 2014, an unidentified person who had measles (even though they likely didn't know it) visited Disneyland. Within 2½ weeks, there were nine cases of measles linked to Disneyland. Of the nine, only one person was vaccinated. By January 9, there were five more cases. By a week after the first announcement, there were 42 cases of measles linked to Disneyland. A California high school told its unvaccinated students to stay home. On January 21, Disneyland announced that five employees had the measles.

By the end of March 2015, there were at least 146 confirmed cases linked to the California outbreak, including 130 cases in California, 7 in Arizona, 3 in Utah, 2 each in Washington and Nebraska, and 1 each in Colorado and Oregon. The measles outbreak spread to Mexico (2 cases) and Canada (10 cases) as tourists returned home.

In mid-February, a news website reported that most of the patients in the outbreak were unvaccinated. Of the then 63 patients from California with vaccination records, 49 were completely unvaccinated. As stated in the report: "Twenty-eight were intentionally unvaccinated due to a parent's personal beliefs, one was on an 'alternative plan for vaccination,' and 12 were too young to be immunized, state officials said."[58]

It is likely that the person who started the outbreak was from the Philippines, although the genotype was also found in 14 different countries and six states in the 6-month period around the time of the epidemic.[59] The measles virus from this outbreak shares the same genetic material as the type most commonly found in the Philippines, including an outbreak there in 2014. This incident shows how contagious measles is and how even one infected traveler from a country where measles is endemic can cause a significant outbreak. This risk is increasing because vaccination levels are declining in the United States.[59] To protect everyone in a community, 92% to 95% of people need to be vaccinated against measles.

A Different Point of View: A Conversation in Cuba

The most recent data on childhood (19 to 35 months) vaccination rates show that only 70% of children in the United States have received all their recommended vaccines. In Cuba, the vaccination rate is greater than 99%. Cuba has a different approach. Their philosophy is that vaccination is so important that physician/nurse teams will undertake home visits to ensure complete vaccination. A visiting group's translator noted about her child, "I am obligated to do this for the good of the community."[61]

TALES OF PUBLIC HEALTH (VACCINATION PART 2)

Cubans do not experience the same realities that we do in the United States. Cubans do not understand our healthcare system because it is so different from theirs. In Cuba, medicine and public health are a united whole. This is, in part, because education and medical care are free to all. Thus, the social determinants of health, as evident in the United States, do not exist in Cuba.[61]

Given their resources, Cuba has achieved remarkable health outcomes. Save the Children ranks Cuba as the best country in Latin America in which to be a mother and has among the world's highest doctor-to-patient ratios. Additionally, a higher percentage of pregnant women in Cuba have four or more prenatal care visits than women in the United States. The infant mortality rate in the United States is 1.3 times higher than in Cuba. These statistics are particularly remarkable given that their technology is far behind that of the United States.[61]

common in other countries. When visitors infected with the measles virus come to the United States, given how contagious measles is and how rapidly it can spread where people are unvaccinated, outbreaks can easily happen (see Tales of Public Health box).

In the United States, some parents choose not to vaccinate their children. The rise in the number of these parents has been termed the "anti-vaxxers movement." A quote from the Internet summarizes how some parents feel about the pressure they feel to follow standardized immunization practices: "I also don't appreciate being told that I'm supposed to set aside what I believe is in the best interest of my child in an effort to help you do what you feel is the most important for yours."[60] Even celebrities can't contain their thoughts on vaccines, with Jim Carey, Jenny McCarthy, Alicia Silverstone, Jenna Elfman,

Rob Schneider, and even President Donald Trump making comments that support anti-vaccination sentiments. On the flip side, Salma Hayek, Kristen Bell, John Oliver, Kim Kardashian, Jennifer Lopez, and Bill Gates have all publicly weighed in with their support of vaccines.

One disease for which you should get vaccinated every year is influenza (the flu).[54] The vaccine is based on which viruses are most likely to spread and cause illness in the current year. Flu viruses constantly mutate (change), so a new vaccine must be created each year. Annually, the World Health Organization consults their collaborators, reviews the data, and makes recommendations for the seasonal flu vaccine. Although there are many different flu viruses, the vaccine will protect you from the three or four that are likely to be the ones most commonly circulating. How well an individual year's vaccine works partially depends on how little the viruses change from the time of vaccine production and the time you are exposed. If you have a healthy immune system, your body is likely to do a good job of making protective antibodies, so that vaccine's effectiveness is partially individual. People who are elderly or have weakened immune systems may not have as strong of a response as someone who is very healthy. Sometimes you get vaccinated and still get the flu. This may be because the virus causing the infection was not part of the year's vaccine. If your illness is caused by a virus that has mutated, but is still similar to the one in the vaccine, your symptoms will likely be milder than if you had opted not to get vaccinated.

Herd Immunity

Herd immunity occurs when enough people in the population cannot get a disease (because they are vaccinated or have natural immunity from having previously had the disease) to protect people who are susceptible. If enough people are vaccinated, the disease cannot spread from person to person. It is indirect protection. The chain of infection from one person to another is interrupted, which slows the spread of infection.[62] Vaccinating many members of a population makes it more difficult for a virus to spread.

herd immunity A form of immunity that occurs when the vaccination of a significant portion of a population (or herd) provides a measure of protection for individuals who have not developed immunity.

Some people have to depend on herd immunity to prevent getting a disease. Very young babies are too young to be vaccinated. Babies rely on the immunity of their family members and other adults to protect them. Other people may have cancer or another condition that makes vaccines contraindicated. Women who are pregnant should not be vaccinated with live, attenuated vaccines. If you are allergic to eggs, the only vaccines that may be problematic for you are the influenza vaccine and the yellow fever vaccine. The measles, mumps, and rubella vaccine has a very small amount of egg protein but is not harmful even if you have an egg allergy.

▸ Important Infectious Diseases

Looking at the world as a whole, infectious diseases are the leading cause of death for children and adolescents and one of the leading causes in adults. These causes of death are diseases that can be prevented or treated. In low- and middle-income countries, 16% of deaths are due to infectious diseases, including diarrhea, lower respiratory infections, HIV/AIDS, tuberculosis, and malaria. Even though the cure may seem simple, the interventions are, unfortunately, often unavailable to those who need them most. Diarrhea and respiratory infections are the two most common causes of pediatric deaths.[63] AIDS is addressed later in this chapter under epidemics. (For more on AIDS, see Chapter 5.)

Malaria

Malaria was once the world's most serious endemic disease. Although no longer a problem in the United States, malaria is still a significant infectious disease to know about and understand. In 2016, according to the CDC, there were an estimated 216 million cases of malaria around the world, and 445,000 people, mostly children, died from the disease, mostly in Africa.[64] In societies such as the United States and Europe, population health measures and economic development have successfully eliminated malaria.

The bite of *Anopheles* mosquitoes that carry the *Plasmodium* parasite transmits malaria. Usually, it is a serious disease, although it can be mild. When people get malaria, they are typically very sick with high fevers, shaking chills, sweating, headaches, body aches, nausea, and vomiting. If treated, malaria is a curable disease. If left untreated, people with malaria may develop severe complications and die.

The incubation period between being bitten and developing symptoms is between 1 week and 1 month. Because the incubation period can be so long, people traveling in countries where malaria is endemic can return home seemingly healthy. There are about 1,700 cases of malaria diagnosed annually in the United States. Most of these cases are from travelers and immigrants. In many parts of the world, the parasites have developed resistance to the medicines used to treat malaria. The main interventions that are used to control malaria include insecticidal nets and spraying homes with insecticides.[64,65]

If you plan to travel to a country where malaria is endemic (**FIGURE 8-12**), it is important to take medicine to help prevent malaria. The medicine you are given depends on where you are traveling. Because no antimalarial drug is 100% protective, it is important to use protective measures like wearing long pants and long-sleeved shirts and using an insecticidal net when sleeping.

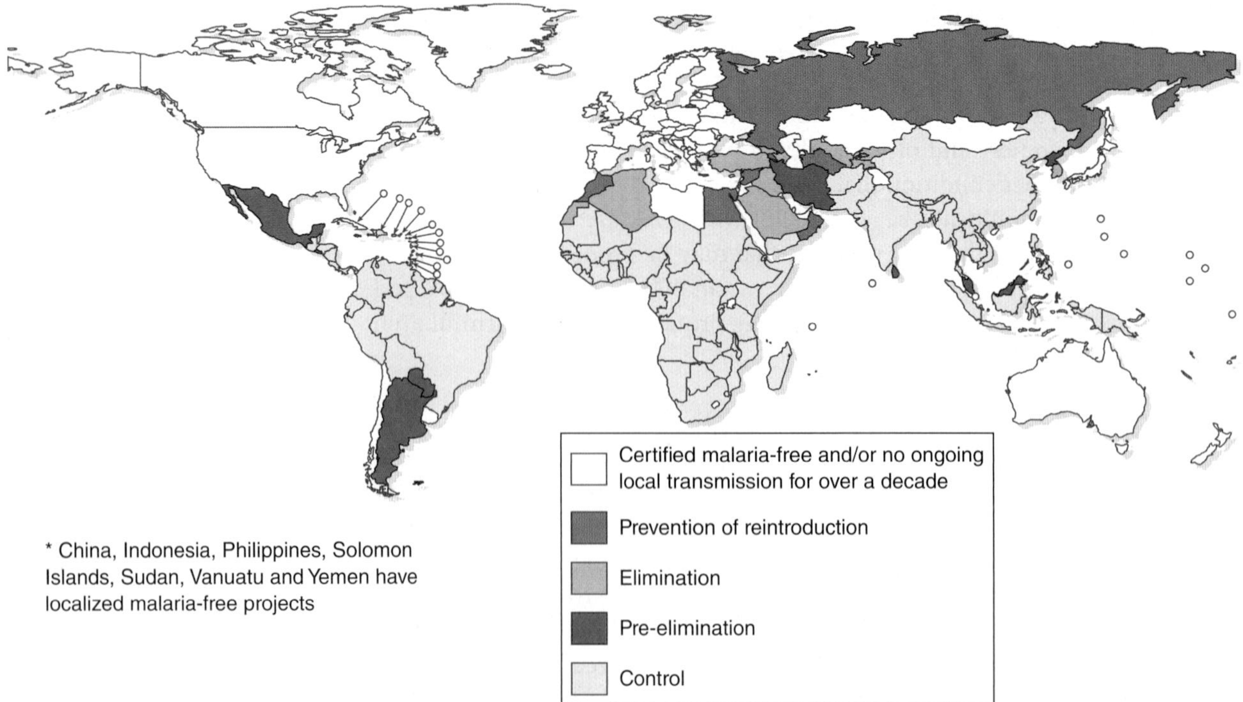

FIGURE 8-12 Map showing the distribution of malaria worldwide and the malaria burden stages of countries and adapted interventions deployed toward malaria control and elimination.

World Malaria Report 2016. Geneva: World Health Organization; 2016.

Tuberculosis

The bacterium *Mycobacterium tuberculosis* causes tuberculosis (TB). The bacteria usually attack the lungs, but other body parts, such as the kidney, spine, and brain, can also be infected. If not treated, TB disease can kill you. TB is spread by droplet transmission (see Table 8-1) when a person with the disease releases germs into the air by coughing, sneezing, or speaking. Not everyone infected with the TB-causing bacterium gets the disease. Thus there are two TB conditions: latent TB infection and TB disease.[66]

Latent TB Infection

When you have latent TB infection, the bacteria live in your body without making you sick, as your body prevents the bacteria from multiplying. When you have latent TB, you do not have symptoms and do not feel ill; nor can you spread the infection to other people. If the bacteria become active and multiply, you go from having latent TB to having TB disease.[66]

TB Disease

TB disease occurs when the TB bacteria are active (multiplying in your body), and your immune system cannot stop the bacteria from growing. People with TB disease are sick. They may also be able to spread the bacteria to people with whom they spend time every day. When you are infected with the bacteria, you can develop TB disease within weeks, or it may take years. If you have a weak immune system because of another illness, such as HIV, you are at higher risk of developing TB disease than if you have a healthy or strong immune system. Symptoms of TB disease include a bad cough that lasts 3 weeks or longer, chest pain, coughing up blood or sputum, weakness or fatigue, weight loss, no appetite, chills, fever, and night sweats.[66]

The CDC recommends that certain groups of people get tested for TB because they are more likely to develop TB disease. These groups include individuals who have spent time with someone who has the disease, people with weakened immune systems (such as a person who is HIV positive), people having symptoms consistent with TB disease, individuals who are from countries where TB is common (most countries in Latin America, the Caribbean, Africa, Asia, Eastern Europe, and Russia), people who work or live in homeless shelters or jails, and people who use illegal drugs.[66]

Many people born outside of the United States have had the BCG, or bacillus Calmette-Guérin vaccine, for TB disease. Having been vaccinated may cause a positive skin test for TB, even if the person is not infected. A person's healthcare provider will choose the most appropriate test to use after considering the reason for the test, test availability, and cost.[66]

Zika Virus

What we know about the Zika virus, as of August 2017, is that it was discovered in 1947 in the Zika Forest in Uganda. The first human cases were documented in 1952. Zika is spread primarily through the bite of an infected *Aedes aegypti* or *Aedes albopictus* mosquito.[67]

A Zika infection is usually mild, and symptoms last for several days to a week. The most common Zika symptoms are fever, rash, joint pain, and conjunctivitis ("pinkeye"). Sometimes people get muscle pain and headache. The virus usually stays in the blood for about a week, but it can be longer. The CDC believes that once you have had Zika, you are unlikely to get it again.[68]

There is no vaccine to prevent Zika. If you become ill, treat the symptoms: Get plenty of rest and stay hydrated. If you have fever or pain, take acetaminophen or paracetamol.[68]

Mosquitoes that spread Zika virus bite during the day and night. The best way to prevent the spread of Zika is to avoid mosquito bites. The Environmental Protection Agency recommends insect repellents with one of the following active ingredients: DEET, picaridin, IR3535, oil of lemon eucalyptus, or para-menthane-diol.[69]

If a pregnant woman gets Zika, the virus can infect her fetus. Zika is a cause of microcephaly and other severe fetal brain defects. Currently we do not know if there is a safe time during pregnancy to travel in an area where there is a risk of getting Zika. Nor do we know how likely it is that Zika will affect a pregnancy. There is no evidence that infants can get Zika from breastfeeding. Keep in mind that anyone who is infected can spread Zika to his or her sex partners, even if the person does not have symptoms. The virus is present in semen longer than in blood, vaginal secretions, or urine.[70]

If you are thinking about getting pregnant and need to travel to an area with a risk of Zika, the CDC has some timing guidelines (**TABLE 8-3**).

At the CDC's website, maps are available to help you decide where it is safe to travel if you are concerned about Zika infection (www.cdc.gov/zika/geo/index.html). Some areas within the United States have previously been considered cautionary. Because what we know about Zika is still evolving, if you have concerns, check at the CDC's website before you make travel plans.

West Nile Virus

Of all people who get West Nile virus infection, 70% to 80% have no symptoms. About 20% of individuals will develop a fever and may have other symptoms, such as a headache, body aches, joint pains, vomiting, diarrhea, or rash. Most people who develop symptoms of West Nile virus disease recover completely. The fatigue that comes with the illness can last for weeks or months. Less than 1% of people with West Nile virus infection will become seriously ill.

BY THE NUMBERS

Where is Zika?

By March 2018, there were reports of locally-transmitted Zika cases from 50 countries and territories in the Americas, including U.S. and U.S. territories, 14 countries and territories in Asia, Oceania, and Pacific islands, and 29 countries in Africa.[71]

TABLE 8-3 Couples Who Are Not Pregnant and Concerned About Zika: Travel and Sexual Transmission

Who is traveling?	How long to wait before trying to conceive
Only the male	Wait at least 6 months before trying to conceive. Use condoms or abstain from sex for at least 6 months after returning from the trip but having no symptoms, or after diagnosis of Zika.
Only the female	Use condoms or abstain from sex for at least 2 months after returning from the trip but having no symptoms, or after diagnosis of Zika.
Both partners	Use condoms or abstain from sex for at least 6 months after returning from the trip but neither partner has symptoms, or after the male partner has a diagnosis of Zika.

The serious illness is usually encephalitis (inflammation of the brain) or meningitis (inflammation of the lining of the brain and spinal cord). Approximately 10% of people who develop neurologic infection due to West Nile virus die.[72] Infected mosquitoes spread West Nile virus. Currently, there are neither medications available to treat the disease nor vaccines to prevent infection. The best way to reduce your risk of infection is to use insect repellant containing DEET, picaridin, IR3535, oil of lemon eucalyptus, or para-menthane-diol when you go outdoors. From dawn until dusk, wear long sleeve shirts and long pants. Make sure to use window and door screens. Reduce standing water around your apartment or house by emptying flower pots, pet water dishes, discarded tires, and other items that collect water.[73]

Mosquitoes become infected by biting infected birds. Infected mosquitoes then transmit the disease to other birds and humans. Some birds (hawks, owls, crows) can also become infected from eating sick or dead birds that have West Nile virus. Most birds do not die of infection, although crows and jays frequently do. There is no evidence that humans can get West Nile virus directly from handling live or dead birds. Even so, you should avoid picking up dead birds with your bare hands! Check with your state health department or state wildlife agency for information about reporting dead birds in your area.[74]

Lyme Disease

Infected ticks spread Lyme disease. In the northeast, mid-Atlantic, and north-central United States, Lyme disease is transmitted by the black-legged tick (also called deer tick), and on the Pacific Coast, Lyme disease is spread by the Western black-legged tick. The infected tick must be attached to your body for 36 or more hours before the Lyme disease bacterium can be transmitted. Most of the time, Lyme disease is spread by immature ticks which are very tiny (less than 2 mm or 0.079 inch). Because these immature ticks are so small, they are difficult to see. Adult ticks can also spread disease, but they are much larger and more likely to be found and removed before they have time to transmit the bacteria.[75]

Between 3 and 30 days after being infected, a person may experience fever, chills, headache, fatigue, muscle and joint aches, and swollen lymph nodes. About 70% to 80% of people get an erythema migrans rash that gradually spreads. Sometimes the rash clears as it spreads, giving it a bull's eye appearance. People whose disease is not treated can get severe headaches, neck stiffness, severe joint pain, facial palsy (loss of muscle tone on one or both sides of the face), irregular heartbeat, dizziness, shortness of breath, nerve pain, and problems with short-term memory.[76] Patients who receive early antibiotic treatment usually recover quickly and completely.

Most of the cases in the United States occur in the Northeast and upper Midwest. Ninety-five percent of 28,453 confirmed cases in 2015 were from the following states: Connecticut, Delaware, Maine, Maryland, Massachusetts, Minnesota, New Hampshire, New Jersey, New York, Pennsylvania, Rhode Island, Vermont, Virginia, and Wisconsin. The incidence in 2015 was 8.9 confirmed cases/100,000 population.[77]

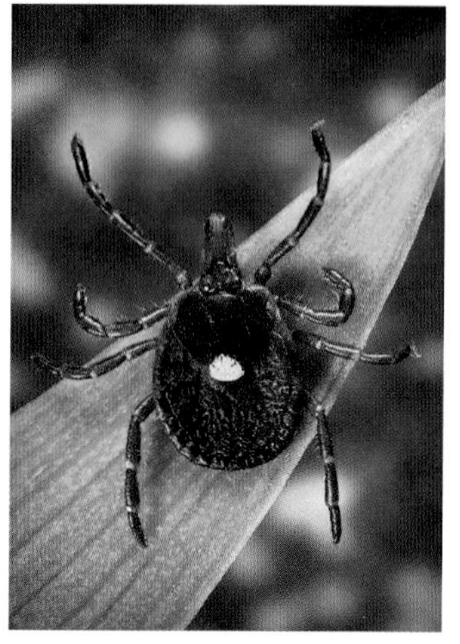

Black-legged tick (*Ixodes scapularis*)

Centers for Disease Control and Prevention/Jim Gathany.

▸ Infectious Diseases on College Campuses

Health isn't a topic that is always on the top of a student's agenda. But living on a college campus may increase the likelihood of getting an infectious disease. Even if you don't live on campus, in classes and at social events you interact with a large number of people. When you are growing up, your body builds immunity to the germs you commonly encounter. Most colleges are diverse places with large numbers of individuals from all over. This diversity is good and important because it helps students learn about other cultures. But it also increases the likelihood that students will get sick because of exposure to germs they haven't encountered before. Often, college students live in confined spaces, share bathrooms with many people, and touch classroom equipment handled by many others who may have contracted the flu or colds. Students share personal items with friends and may not take the necessary preventive measures to protect themselves.

TABLE 8-4 provides a summary of infectious diseases that are common among college-aged people. By following the recommendations in this book, you can minimize the chances or at least the number of times you get sick. While preventing a disease is better than getting sick, if you do get sick, many times it is important to see a healthcare provider. This table is intended to be a general guideline, not to replace a healthcare provider's examination and advice.

Is It a Cold or the Flu?

Both the flu and the common cold are respiratory infections, but the viruses that cause them are different. As can be seen in **TABLE 8-5**, they share many symptoms. Colds are usually milder than the flu and complications are less common. The young, the elderly, women who are pregnant, and people with some chronic medical conditions are at higher risk of developing complications from the flu.[78]

Healthy adults usually get two to three colds every year. Colds are contagious for the first two to three days, so it is best to stay home during this period. Colds usually last from 7 to 10 days but may last longer in people who smoke.[79]

STDs

STD means sexually transmitted disease and STI means sexually transmitted infections. People often use the terms interchangeably. STI is broader and more encompassing than STDs because some infections may not cause any symptoms. If the infection results in altering the typical function of the body, it is then called a disease. However, in this book, we use STD because that is how the CDC refers to them.

Eradication of Infectious Diseases

Eradication of infectious diseases means that there are no cases of the disease in the population. It would be great to imagine that we had the technology to eradicate many diseases. But, for eradication to be a possible goal, it must be biologically and technically feasible. There must also be broad support, and measures must be cost effective. Smallpox (*Variola major* and *Variola minor*) is the only disease in humans that has been eradicated. Many famous people had smallpox, including Chief Sitting Bull, Ramses V of Egypt, Emperor Peter II of Russia, George Washington, and Abraham Lincoln. Some of those people died, and some survived. In Europe, the many deaths from smallpox changed the succession of rulers.

With his creation of a vaccine for smallpox, Edward Jenner changed the history of infectious diseases by demonstrating the first successful vaccine (see Tales of Public Health box). In the 1960s, smallpox was still endemic in Africa and Asia. The strategies to prevent its spread included performing mass

TABLE 8-4 Common Infectious Diseases Among College-Aged People

Illness	Bacterial or Viral?	Prevention	Symptoms	Home Remedy	When to Call or See a Medical Professional
Bacterial vaginosis	Bacterial	Limit the number of sex partners or do not have sex; do not douche.	Many women don't have symptoms. A thin white or gray vaginal discharge, odor, pain, itching, or burning in the vagina may occur. Some women have a strong fish-like odor, especially after sex.	There are no effective OTC medications or home remedies for bacterial vaginosis, although sometimes it may resolve on its own.	See a doctor f you have symptoms of bacterial vaginosis. Male sex partners do not need to be treated, but female sex partners do need treatment.
Bronchitis/chest cold	Viral	Reduce risk and complications by not smoking and by getting flu shots and following cold and flu prevention.	Coughing spells that may be accompanied by phlegm and breathlessness. Lasts from 1 to 3 weeks.	Humidify the air using a vaporizer or humidifier or stand in or near a hot shower. Drink hot tea or soup. If you have a fever, take aspirin (only if you are 20 years or older), ibuprofen, or acetaminophen to reduce fever.	If you have severe or persistent symptoms or a high fever, or if you cough up blcod, you should see your doctor right away.
Common cold	Viral	Wash your hands often with soap and water for 20 seconds. Avoid touching your eyes, nose, and mouth with unwashed hands. Stay away from people who are sick.	Runny nose and sometimes a sore throat, followed by coughing and sneezing	Get lots of rest and drink fluids. OTC remedies may help symptoms but won't cure the infection.	See a doctor if your symptoms last longer than 10 days or are severe or unusual; if your symptoms get worse after 3 days; or if you are unable to swallow or have difficulty breathing or a stiff neck.

(continues)

TABLE 8-4 Common Infectious Diseases Among College-Aged People *(continued)*

Foodborne illness	Bacterial or viral	Wash produce well. Cook meat, poultry, and eggs thoroughly. Refrigerate leftovers promptly.	Diarrhea, abdominal cramps, nausea	Approach depends on the symptom(s). Replace lost fluids and electrolytes. (CDC recommends oral rehydration solutions rather than sports drinks.) Bismuth subsalicylates can reduce duration and severity of simple diarrhea.	See a doctor if you have a high fever (over 101.5°F, measured orally), blood in stools, prolonged vomiting, signs of dehydration (decrease in urination, dry mouth and throat, and feeling dizzy when standing up), or diarrhea for more than 3 days.
Influenza (flu)	Viral	Get vaccinated annually in the fall. Wash hands well and avoid contact with people who have the flu. Avoid crowds and people who are sick.	Fever over 100°F, aching muscles (especially in your back, arms, and legs), chills and sweats, headache, dry cough, fatigue and weakness, nasal congestion	Rest, drink plenty of fluids, and avoid smoking or secondhand smoke. Use OTC medications to treat symptoms. Avoid antihistamines.	If you have flu symptoms and are high risk (pregnant, have asthma, have chronic medical condition), see your doctor right away. See a doctor if your symptoms get worse after a few days. If you have difficulty breathing, call 9-1-1.
Meningococcal meningitis	Bacteria	Get immunized. Don't share drinks, foods, straws, eating utensils, or toothbrushes with anyone else. Stay healthy.	Symptoms of bacterial meningitis usually appear suddenly. The most common symptoms are fever, severe and persistent headache, stiff and painful neck, especially when trying to touch the chin to the chest, vomiting, confusion, and decreased level of consciousness and seizures.	None	Call your doctor right away if you have symptoms of meningitis, such as severe and persistent headache, stiff neck, fever, rash, nausea, and vomiting. Acute bacterial meningitis requires prompt treatment with intravenous antibiotics and cortisone medications to ensure recovery and reduce the risk of complications, such as brain swelling and seizures.

Mononucleosis (mono)	Viral	Don't kiss or share dishes or eating utensils with someone who has mono. Mono is spread thru sharing saliva.	Fever, from 101°F to 104°F, and chills; sore throat, often with white patches on the tonsils; swollen lymph nodes, especially in the neck; swollen tonsils; head or body aches; fatigue and a lack of energy; loss of appetite and pain in the upper left part of the abdomen, which can be due to an inflamed spleen	Rest as needed; take acetaminophen or ibuprofen to reduce fever and to treat a headache or sore throat. Drink plenty of fluids, especially if you have a fever. Gargle with salt water. Avoid contact sports and heavy lifting for several weeks after you become ill to prevent rupture of the spleen.	Most cases of mono do not require treatment. If you have fatigue, body aches, or swollen lymph nodes for 7 to 10 days, call your doctor. If you have been diagnosed with mono and have severe pain in the upper left side of your abdomen or you have difficulty breathing or swallowing, call your doctor immediately.
Strep throat	Bacterial	Wash your hands often with soap and water for 20 seconds. Avoid sharing eating utensils.	Sore throat that usually starts quickly; a fever of 101°F or higher; red, swollen tonsils, sometimes with white patches; tiny red spots on back of the roof of the mouth; headache, nausea, or vomiting; swollen lymph nodes in the neck; body ache	Gargle with salt water (½ to ¾ tsp salt dissolved in 1 cup warm dechlorinated water); use analgesics and throat lozenges as needed.	If you think you have a strep infection (your symptoms are consistent with a strep infection), it is important to see a doctor. Antibiotics will reduce the duration of symptoms and reduce the risk of complications.
Urinary tract infection (UTI)	Bacterial	Women should wipe from front to back (not back to front) after both urination and bowel movements. Empty the bladder regularly and completely, especially after sexual intercourse. Drink lots of fluids.	Painful urination and urinary urgency. Your urine may be cloudy, bad smelling, or bloody. You may also feel lower abdominal pain or pelvic pressure.	Home remedies should be used in addition to medicine prescribed by your physician. Drink lots of fluids.	If you have symptoms of a UTI, a medical professional should evaluate you, preferably within 24 hours.

(continues)

TABLE 8-4 Common Infectious Diseases Among College-Aged People *(continued)*

Sexually Transmitted Disease (STDs)—Bacterial				
Bacterial STD—includes chlamydia, gonorrhea, and trichomoniasis	The only way to prevent is to not have vaginal, anal, or oral sex. If you are sexually active, risk is reduced by being in a long-term mutually monogamous relationship with a partner who has been tested and found not to have an STD. Use a latex condom correctly every time you have sex. It is possible to spread trichomoniasis even when using a condom.	Many people don't have symptoms. Women may have an abnormal vaginal discharge and/or a burning sensation when urinating. Men can have a discharge from their penis and/or a burning sensation when urinating.	There are no effective OTC medications or home remedies for bacterial STDs.	See a doctor if you have any of the symptoms, if your partner has symptoms, or if your partner tests positive for an STD.
Syphilis	Condoms prevent transmission of syphilis by preventing contact with a sore. Sometimes sores occur in areas not covered by a condom. Contact with these sores can still transmit syphilis.	Syphilis symptoms are divided into stages. The primary stage includes a firm, round, painless sore.	There are no effective OTC medications or home remedies for bacterial STDs.	See a doctor if you have any of the symptoms, if your partner has symptoms, or if your partner tests positive for an STD.
STDs—Viral				
Genital herpes	The only way to prevent is to not have vaginal, anal, or oral sex. If you are sexually active, risk is reduced by being in a long-term mutually monogamous relationship with a partner who has been tested and found not to have genital herpes. Use a latex condom	Most people have no, or very mild, symptoms. Sores usually appear as one or more blisters on or around the genitals, rectum, or mouth. The blisters break and leave painful sores that may take weeks to heal. The first outbreak may also include flu-like symptoms such as fever, body aches, or swollen	Hygiene is important. Avoid touching the sores. Keep blisters or sores clean and dry. Avoid tight-fitting clothing, and wear cotton underwear. Avoid sex during both outbreaks and prodromes (early symptoms) of herpes. OTC medications can be used	You should be examined by your doctor if you notice any of these symptoms or if your partner has an STD or symptoms of an STD, such as an unusual sore, a smelly discharge, burning when urinating, or, for women specifically, bleeding between periods.

	correctly every time you have sex. Outbreaks can also occur in areas that are not covered by a condom, so condoms may not fully protect you from getting herpes.	glands. Repeat outbreaks are common, especially during the first year after infection. Repeat outbreaks are usually shorter and less severe. Herpes can stay in the body for the rest of the person's life; outbreaks tend to decrease over a period of years.	to treat pain and reduce fever.	
Hepatitis A and B	Vaccination	Some people have no symptoms. If symptoms occur, they may include fever, fatigue, loss of appetite, nausea, vomiting, abdominal pain, dark urine, clay-colored bowel movements, joint pain, or jaundice (a yellowing of the skin or eyes).	Rest, and ensure adequate nutrition and fluids.	If you have symptoms or know you were exposed, you should go see a doctor.
Human immunodeficiency virus (HIV)	Choose less risky sexual behaviors, limit your number of sex partners, use condoms, use medicines to prevent HIV if appropriate, and get checked for STDs. If you are at high risk, consider preexposure prophylaxis.	Many people infected with HIV do not have any symptoms at all for 10 years or more. Some people report having flu-like symptoms 2 to 4 weeks after exposure. People who have been recently exposed are the most contagious even though they test negative for HIV.	There are no effective OTC medications or home remedies for HIV.	Post-exposure prophylaxis (PrEP) must be started as soon as possible to be effective—and always within 3 days of a possible exposure. If you think you may have been exposed to HIV, see a doctor as soon as possible. PrEP should be used only right after an uncommon situation. If you are at ongoing risk for HIV, speak to your doctor about preexposure prophylaxis.
Human papillomavirus (HPV)	Vaccination	Most people have no symptoms, but they can develop years after being infected, making it hard to know when the person first became infected.	There are no effective OTC medications or home remedies for HPV.	Women over 30 years old should be screened for cervical precancer. If you develop genital warts, see a doctor.

TABLE 8-5 Comparison of Colds and the Flu[78,80]

Symptoms	Cold	Flu
Onset	Usually begins with a sore throat	Sudden
Fever	Occasionally, but if there is a fever it is usually only a slight fever	Common; higher (100–102°F; may be higher in young children); lasts 3 to 4 days; feeling feverish/chills
Headache	Occasionally	Common
General aches, pains	Slight	Common; often very achy
Fatigue, weakness	Sometimes	Common; can last 2 to 3 weeks
Extreme exhaustion	Never	Usual; particularly at the beginning of the illness
Stuffy nose	Common	Sometimes
Sneezing	Common	Sometimes
Sore throat	Common, particularly at the beginning	Sometimes
Chest discomfort, cough	Mild to moderate	Common; can become severe
Complications	Sinus congestion; middle ear infection	Sinusitis, bronchitis, ear infection, pneumonia; can be life-threatening; can make chronic medical problems worse
Prevention	Wash hands often; avoid close contact with anyone with a cold	Wash hands often; avoid close contact with anyone who has flu symptoms; get annual flu vaccine
Treatment	Decongestants; pain reliever/fever reducer medicines	Decongestants, pain relievers, or fever reducers are available over the counter; OTC cough and cold medicines should not be given to young children; prescription antiviral drugs for flu may be given in some cases; call your doctor for more information about treatment.

vaccination, finding and quickly vaccinating anyone who had close contact with a person with smallpox as well as other face-to-face contacts of known smallpox patients, and maintaining frequent surveillance of contacts. The last naturally occurring case of smallpox was in Somalia in 1977.[81] In 1980, the World Health Organization officially declared smallpox eradicated.[82]

Successful eradication of a disease requires the following conditions[82]:

- An effective vaccine that produces long-lasting immunity
- A large portion of the population is already vaccinated

TALES OF PUBLIC HEALTH

Creation of the Smallpox Vaccine

Edward Anthony Jenner was an English scientist famous for his discovery of the smallpox vaccine. His discovery has saved many, many lives.

As a doctor, Jenner worked in rural Gloucestershire, where most of his patients were farmers or worked on farms with cattle. At the time, smallpox was considered the most deadly disease. In 1788, there was an epidemic of smallpox. During this epidemic, Jenner noticed that his patients who worked with cattle never got smallpox. To prove his theory, on May 14, 1796, Jenner selected a healthy young boy whom he inoculated with cowpox, a mild disease. After a week, the boy developed a mild disease but recovered well. Six weeks later, Jenner vaccinated the boy with smallpox matter. Because he did not get sick, Jenner concluded that the boy's inoculation with cowpox completely protected him from smallpox.[83]

After doing more successful tests, Jenner published his findings, and the smallpox vaccination was born. We have been so successful at eradicating smallpox that currently no one gets vaccinated for it.

- The virus is both stable and genetically simple
- Only humans get the disease (no animals)
- The disease is only moderately contagious, with subclinical cases being rare

Subclinical Infections

A **subclinical infection** occurs when the person with the illness (the host) shows no evidence of being ill. Unless this person is explicitly tested for the infectious agent, no one would know he or she has the infection. For the person, this lack of awareness may or may not be a problem, depending on the disease. If the infected person with subclinical disease spreads the disease to others, it can be a major problem. Probably the most infamous case in history is a woman called Typhoid Mary, who worked as a cook and unknowingly transmitted typhoid to many people.

subclinical infection An infection that is nearly or completely asymptomatic (no signs or symptoms).

Diseases that are asymptomatic still occur. Among young adults who are sexually active, some STDs can be asymptomatic and transmitted to a sexual partner. These include chlamydia,[84] genital herpes,[85] gonorrhea,[86] and syphilis[87] (see Table 8-4). (See also Chapter 5.)

Slow Viruses and Atypical Slow Viruses

A slow virus is a virus or virus-like agent that has a very long incubation period, ranging from a few months to several years. There is an initial infection without symptoms, so an infected person is unaware of being ill, much like an asymptomatic carrier. Unlike the asymptomatic carrier, however, a person with a slow virus eventually will become ill. Slow viruses frequently involve the central nervous system and follow a slow but relentless course to death. Rabies is considered a slow virus, despite having an incubation period of 3 to 12 weeks. The most well-known slow virus is HIV, the virus that causes AIDS, with an incubation period of 5 to 10 years.

Diseases caused by prions used to be considered atypical slow viruses. Although they have similar features, they are not actually viruses because they do not contain DNA or RNA. **Prions** are misfolded proteins that are considered

prions Misfolded proteins that are considered "infectious" because they cause normal proteins to misfold.

"infectious" because they cause normal proteins to misfold. Proteins are what make up the cells in your body. Different proteins have different jobs. Each protein in your body has its own three-dimensional shape that it requires to do its job correctly. Usually, when your body has a protein that is not the right shape, it disposes of the protein, but this is not true of prions. Animal diseases caused by prions include bovine spongiform encephalopathy (commonly called mad cow disease) and scrapie in sheep. Human diseases caused by prions are Creutzfeldt-Jakob disease and kuru (see Tales of Public Health box).[87] According to the National Institute of Neurological Disorders and Stroke, kuru belongs to a group of infectious diseases called transmissible spongiform encephalopathies, also called prion diseases. [88]

TALES OF PUBLIC HEALTH

Kuru: An Unusual Way to Get Sick

In the 1950s and 1960s, a disease called kuru was endemic among the South Fore people of Papua New Guinea. It is now rare, but it is still a fatal brain disorder. The disease name comes from the word *kuria* or *guria* (to shake) because people who have kuru have body tremors. It is also known as the laughing sickness because people with kuru have fits of uncontrollable laughter. Individuals with kuru have difficulty walking, talking, chewing, and swallowing. There is a long incubation period, and decades can pass between exposure and the appearance of symptoms. There is no cure, and the time between the beginning of symptoms and death is between 6 months and 1 year.[88]

Kuru was transmitted from generation to generation because the South Fore ate the brains of their dead relatives as a way to honor them. The majority of the victims were women. It was women who prepared the body and ate the brains of dead family members. Upon dying, the maternal relatives would remove the arms and feet, strip the muscles, and remove the brain and internal organs. Children also participated in the ritualistic cannibalism. As a researcher into the disease notes, "Kuru victims were highly regarded as sources of food."[89]

Epidemics and Pandemics

An epidemic is a disease outbreak in which the number of cases of disease exceeds the expected number based on past experience in a given population or community. At one time, the term epidemic was limited to infectious diseases, but there can be epidemics of chronic, noninfectious diseases as well. Pandemics occur when the epidemic is prevalent over an entire country or around the world.

We live in an increasingly globalized world, making it easy for contagious diseases to spread quickly. Pandemics are not a new development, however. There are many examples of pandemics throughout much of recorded history. Diseases spread quickly from place to place—in part because no one understood the mechanism of infection, and in part because they had no way to treat the disease.

Epidemics and Pandemics in the Past

Smallpox

You have already read about the creation of a smallpox vaccine. Smallpox has been called the most devastating disease in human history—because for most of human history, there was no treatment for the disease. Until the creation of a vaccine for smallpox, there was little people could do but hope not to get the disease. The last case in the United States occurred in 1949, and the last case in the world was in Somalia in 1977.[81]

Smallpox has been around for a very long time. Because the disease has such a characteristic presentation, there is no doubt that historical records are describing this disease. Descriptions of smallpox are available from fourth-century China, seventh-century India and the Mediterranean region, and tenth-century Asia. As vaccinations for the disease became available, there were fewer epidemics, but even as recently as the 1950s there were an estimated 50 million cases of smallpox each year.

The Plague

One of the most infamous pandemics in history was caused by the bubonic plague. Between 1336 and 1353, the Black Death killed approximately 50 million people, or between 30% to 50% of the population of Europe.[90] Imagine a disease killing that much of the population today! What is the plague? There are three forms of plague: bubonic, septicemic, and pneumonic. *Yersinia pestis* bacteria cause all three forms.

The most common form of plague is the bubonic plague. The usual source is a bite from an infected flea or rodent. The bubonic plague is rarely spread from person to person. Three to 7 days after infection, a person develops a fever and swollen lymph nodes, called buboes. They usually occur in the groin, in the underarm area, or on the neck. Septicemic plague occurs when the bacteria multiply in a person's blood. The symptoms of the septicemic plague are similar to the bubonic plague, but without buboes. The usual source is a bite from an infected flea or rodent. A person can develop septicemic plague from untreated bubonic or pneumonic plague. Like the bubonic plague, it is rarely spread from person to person. The most serious form is pneumonic plague, which occurs when the bacteria infect the lungs. Unlike the other forms, the pneumonic plague is contagious and spreads when an infected person coughs and bacteria are released into the air. Although it is still a serious disease, antibiotics are available that can treat plague. Two antibiotics—gentamicin and doxycycline—are effective for treating plague. There is a high fatality rate if the disease is untreated.[91,92]

When the plague arrived from the East in the 1340s, people had no understanding of how diseases spread and no way to treat them. The plague terrified people because it had such a high fatality rate (the proportion of deaths among people with the disease) and it killed so quickly, usually 2 to 7 days after initial infection. One way the plague reached Europe was on ships. As ships left

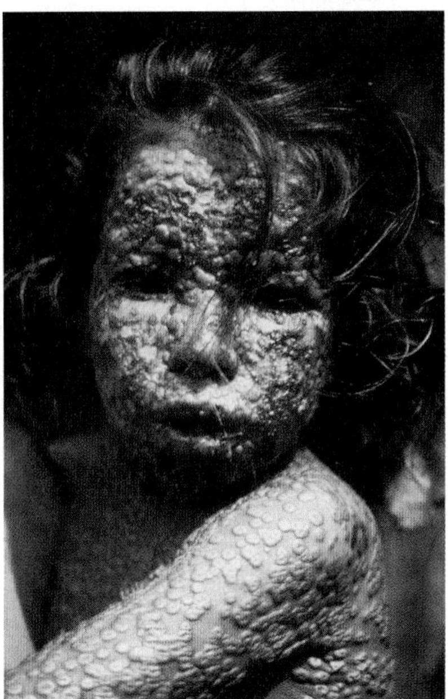

A young girl in Bangladesh infected with smallpox in 1973.

Centers for Disease Control and Prevention/James Hicks.

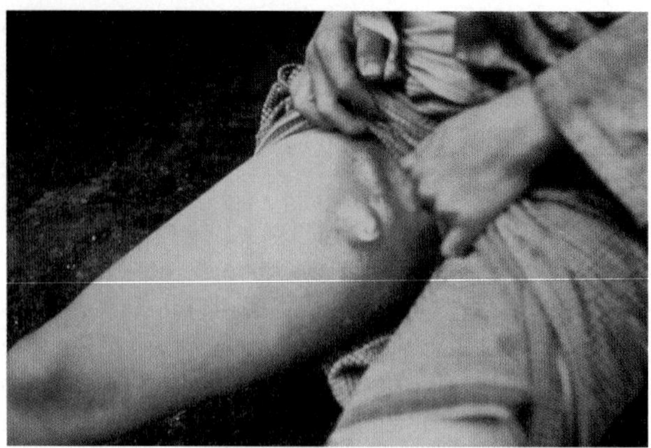

An inguinal bubo on the upper thigh of person infected with bubonic plague.

one port, they took the disease with them to another. Ships from Italy spread the disease to France, Spain, Portugal, and England. People who were exposed also fled from one place to another. Because they did not understand about the spread of disease, they could not and did not go far enough away. Also, by the time people fled an area of contagion, they generally took the disease with them.

1918 Spanish Flu

Just as World War I was beginning to wind down, the influenza pandemic of 1918 to 1919 spread around the world. No one is exactly sure how many people died. The disease was unusual because normally the flu is most dangerous for the very young and the very old. For this flu, however, individuals 20 to 40 years of age were at highest risk of dying. In 1918, there were no vaccines to prevent or effective drugs to treat the flu. To maintain morale during World War I, early reports of the flu were censored. Spain, however, was neutral during this war, so censorship was not in place. Because newspapers there were free to report on the illness, the pandemic received more press attention there than elsewhere. Although the evidence suggests that this pandemic did not originate in Spain, it will always be called the Spanish flu.[93]

Because influenza is endemic, it is hard to be certain exactly where the Spanish flu pandemic began. Historians suggest that the most likely answer is Fort Riley, Kansas. In 18 months, the flu circled the globe, infecting 500 million people and killing, depending on the source, 20 to 100 million people,[94] including about 675,000 Americans. It waned almost as suddenly as it had begun.

Modern Pandemics

We are certainly better at treating diseases, have more medicines in our arsenals, and are more aware of how diseases spread than in the past. But it is also true that the world is ever-more interconnected, increasing the potential for the spread of infectious diseases. Pandemics that have occurred in more recent times include HIV/AIDS, mad cow disease, and Ebola.

HIV/AIDS

HIV destroys the body's immune system. AIDS is the advanced stage of an HIV infection. The main mode of HIV transmission is unprotected sex with an infected person, but HIV can also be spread by sharing drug needles with an infected person or by coming into contact with the blood of an infected person; also, if untreated, an infected pregnant woman can pass HIV on to her

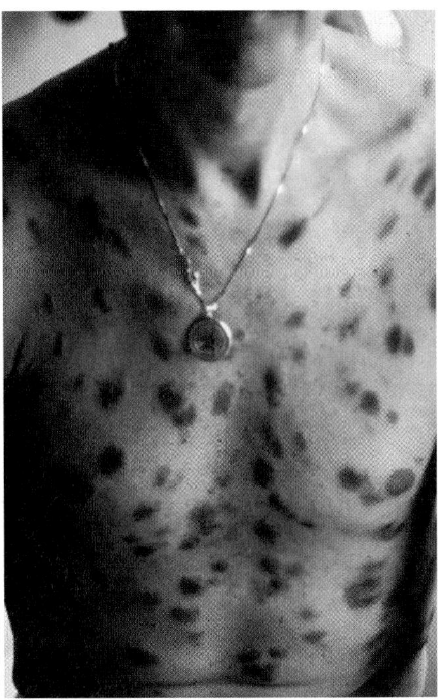

Kaposi's sarcoma.
Paul A. Volberding, MD, University of California San Francisco.

fetus. Here we will talk about the history and current rates of HIV/AIDS. (For more on HIV transmission, see Chapter 5.)

What helped define HIV/AIDS were two diseases with unusual presentations. Kaposi sarcoma was a relatively benign and rare cancer, usually seen in older people. However doctors in New York were diagnosing a more aggressive form of Kaposi sarcoma among young gay men. At the same time, in both California and New York, doctors saw an increase in a rare lung infection, *Pneumocystis* pneumonia (at the time known as *Pneumocystis carinii* pneumonia). At first, the disease was thought to be limited to gay men; then cases were reported in users of injection drugs, then Haitians. In 1982, cases were also appearing in Europe. Eventually, it became clear that blood transfusions also put people at risk. This was a real problem for people with hemophilia because the blood concentrate they needed exposed them to up to 5,000 individual blood donors.

The diagnosing of children with AIDS led to the incorrect belief that casual contact could lead to infection. In the United States and in many other countries around the world, there was an "epidemic of fear and prejudice."[95] By the end of 1986, there were cases in Africa, the Americas, Asia, Europe, and Oceania (i.e., Australia and surrounding regions).[96] In October 1987, AIDS became the first disease debated on the floor of the United Nations General Assembly.[97] The American Medical Association urged its members to break the confidentiality of their patients and warn the sexual partners of people they were treating.[98]

Ryan White became a poster child for HIV/AIDS after his middle school barred him from attending because he had AIDS, which he contracted through his treatments for hemophilia. He became a national spokesperson on the importance of AIDS education and died a month before graduating high school. In August 1990, Congress passed the Ryan White Comprehensive AIDS Resources Emergency (CARE) Act (often referred to as the Ryan White CARE Act) in his honor. It has been reauthorized four times, most recently in 2009.[99]

According to the World Health Organization, there are approximately 36.7 million people around the world living with HIV/AIDS.[100] The vast majority of people living with HIV are in low- and middle-income countries, not the United States. Many of these countries have other public health challenges. If a person is HIV positive and has access to the current sophisticated medicines, HIV/AIDS can be a chronic disease. See the list below of Famous People Do Get HIV/AIDS for some famous people who are or were HIV positive. Early in the epidemic particularly, there was stigma associated with being HIV positive. Thus, the list of famous people who have been open about their HIV diagnosis is a short one. Many of the celebrities now known to have been HIV positive did not reveal their HIV status until just before they died, or the news came out after their death. Others used, or are still using (as in the case of Magic Johnson), their influence to increase HIV awareness.

- Rock Hudson: One of the most beloved movie stars of the 1950s and 60s, Rock Hudson died in late 1985 of AIDS-related complications. Hudson's revelation of his infection with the disease was viewed as an event that could transform the public's perception of AIDS.
- Earvin "Magic" Johnson: One of basketball's all-time greats, Magic Johnson's HIV diagnosis led to groundbreaking dialogue in the sports community regarding whether a person infected with HIV should be allowed to play competitive sports. He has been open about the sexually promiscuous lifestyle he led prior to his infection. He is still alive.
- Freddy Mercury: Lead singer of Queen, a top-selling rock band. He tested positive in 1987 and died of AIDS-related pneumonia 4 years later. He died 1 day after publicly acknowledging that he had AIDS.
- Keith Haring: Known for street murals and cartoon figures. He was diagnosed with AIDS in 1988 and died 2 years later.
- Eric "Eazy-E" Wright: Eazy-E was a rap legend and known as the "Godfather of Gangsta Rap." He died at 31, one month after acknowledging he had AIDS.
- Elizabeth Glaser: Not really famous until after she was diagnosed, she became famous through her efforts to fight AIDS. She contracted the disease through a blood transfusion and passed it on to both of her children. She founded the Elizabeth Glaser Pediatric AIDS Foundation.
- Isaac Asimov: A prolific writer of science fiction novels, he died of AIDS-related complications in 1992, but his cause of death was not revealed until 10 years *after* his death.
- Arthur Ashe: The first African American man to win a Grand Slam tennis title, he is well known for his humanitarian and civil rights efforts. Ashe was diagnosed 4 years before going public. He died a year later from AIDS-related pneumonia.
- Anthony Perkins: A famous actor, he was well known as Norman Bates in Alfred Hitchcock's 1960 film *Psycho*. He chose to ignore that he was ill until a tabloid newspaper speculated that he had AIDS. He died 2 years later.
- Andy Bell: Lead singer of the English synth-pop duo Erasure. In 2004 he announced he was HIV-positive and expressed concern about the complacency of gay men about HIV.
- Greg Louganis: A diver who won four gold medals in the 1984 and 1988 Olympics. Louganis announced his HIV status in his autobiography, Breaking the Surface. He is still alive.
- Alvin Ailey: A renowned modern dance choreographer, in 1958 he formed the Alvin Ailey American Dance Theater in New York City. Ailey died of AIDS in 1989. Ailey asked his doctor to hide his diagnosis to protect his family from the stigma.
- Robert Mapplethorpe: Artist and photographer Robert Mapplethorpe was known for his choice of controversial subject matter. He died in 1989 of

AIDS complications. He was 42 years old. Since his death, his Robert Mapplethorpe Foundation has raised millions of dollars for medical research in the fight against AIDS and HIV.

- Rudolf Nureyev: A Soviet-born dancer known to celebrate both classical ballet and modern dance in the same performance, he was afraid to acknowledge the condition because of concern that the United States would refuse him entry. He died in 1993.
- Michael Jeter: An American actor of film, stage, and television. Six years before his 2003 death, the actor went public and became a speaker about living with an HIV diagnosis.
- Chuck Panozzo: Panozzo, of the band Styx, announced in 2001 that he is gay and living with HIV. He has acted as both an advocate for gay rights and HIV awareness.
- Charlie Sheen: Sheen announced in November 2015 that he is HIV positive. The actor revealed he had been diagnosed about 4 years earlier. "It's a hard three letters to absorb. It's a turning point in one's life," Sheen said.

Mad Cow Disease

As you read about earlier, the scientific name for mad cow disease is bovine spongiform encephalopathy (BSE), and it is a prion disease. Cows are herbivores, which mean they eat plants—namely, grass. But in the modern world of agriculture, cows are fed commercial feed. In the 1980s bone meal was used as an ingredient in cattle feed. Bone meal is a mixture of finely and coarsely ground animal bones and slaughterhouse waste products. What was later discovered was that the cooking procedures did not destroy infectious BSE prion material. The infectious agent remains viable at over 1,100°F. In the United States, meal made from the solid soybean residue by-product, created after extracting soybean oil, is a main source of protein in cattle feed. In Europe, soybeans do not grow well. Before the mad cow disease epidemic of the 1980s, in Europe, bone meal was an inexpensive alternative for feeding cattle. It is likely that cattle contracted BSE from consuming bone meal made from sheep that had scrapie. (Scrapie is a transmissible spongiform encephalopathy disease. Sheep in the United Kingdom had been known to have scrapie for 200 years.)[101]

BSE is a fatal neurodegenerative disease (a disease resulting in deterioration of the central nervous system, especially the neurons in the brain) in cattle that causes a spongy degeneration in the brain and spinal cord. The disease has an incubation period of 4 to 5 years and for cattle is fatal within weeks to months of onset.[101]

BSE was initially recognized in cattle in the United Kingdom in 1986; by 1993, there were more than 1,000 cases per week. While protein supplements containing sheep and cattle offal were banned in the United Kingdom in 1988, it was not until 1991–1992 that the ban was strictly enforced. Why did this matter to humans? As noted, BSE remains viable even after being heated to very high temperatures—much higher than the temperatures at which we cook food. In March 1996, it was announced that 10 people had Creutzfeldt-Jakob disease (CJD), a rare, degenerative, invariably fatal brain disorder. (We now know they had a variant, vCJD.) The cause was linked to eating meat from cattle infected with mad cow disease. According to the World Health Organization, there were more than 220 cases of vCJD worldwide, with 177 cases occurring in the United Kingdom and 27 cases in France. Only four cases were reported in the United States, and the evidence suggests that all of the cases were acquired while outside the United States.[101,102] Although many drugs have been tested, none have proven effective at treating CJD.

Ebola

Ebola is one of the world's most deadly diseases. It can kill between 30% and 90% of people who become infected. Ebola has an incubation period of 2 to 21 days, and during that time, the virus cannot be detected. It is not until symptoms develop that Ebola can be detected.

In 2014, an epidemic of Ebola started in Guinea, West Africa. Precisely how it started is unknown. In an under resourced country, health officials have many competing priorities. The area where the epidemic started also has a high incidence of Lassa fever, making it harder to pinpoint the origin. Lassa fever is also a hemorrhagic disease, but far less deadly than Ebola.

Three and a half months after the beginning of the epidemic, 30 people had died and no one had correctly identified the virus. A man with Ebola arrived in Conakry, the capital. Within a week, 5 more people were sick, and within a month, 47 people were sick.[103]

The clue that helped correctly identify the disease as Ebola was that for some unknown reason, victims would get the hiccups. In March, a Doctors Without Borders physician in Brussels read the report of the outbreak in Guinea. He immediately suspected that it was Ebola. Because it was the most expeditious method, blood samples from Guinea were sent to Paris, France, for testing. Not only did the samples contain Ebola, but they were the deadliest species of Ebola. By the end of March 2014, experts from Doctors Without Borders, the World Health Organization, the CDC, and the Red Cross had poured into Guinea.[103]

While there was an international effort to help stem the epidemic, many people did not understand what was happening. Foreigners in what looked like spacesuits entered their villages and isolated people who were sick before the villagers understood why this tactic was important (**FIGURE 8-13**). What the villagers observed was their relatives going to see the foreigners and never returning. The measures intended to bring about the natural decline of the epidemic were, in fact, alienating people from seeking help. Nonetheless, like all epidemics that follow a period of increasing numbers of cases and then decreasing number of cases, this epidemic also waned, but not before killing more than 10,000 people.

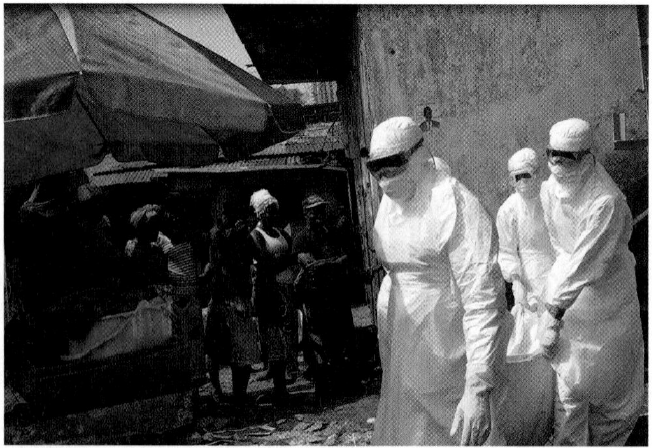

FIGURE 8-13 Red Cross workers, wearing protective suits, carry the body of a person who died.

In Summary

Pathogens that cause illness in humans are bacteria, viruses, fungi, and parasites. Fortunately, your body helps protect you from becoming ill. Your skin, eyes, ears, nose, and mucous membranes help ward off infection. Your saliva and stomach acid also help protect you from illness, as does your immune system.

The following vaccines are recommended if you did not receive them when you were younger: human papillomavirus (HPV); measles, mumps, rubella (MMR); varicella; and hepatitis B. Other important vaccines are tetanus, diphtheria, and acellular pertussis (TdaP); *Haemophilus influenza* type b; pneumococcal polysaccharide; hepatitis A; and meningococcal. Also, every year you should get a flu shot. Vaccines help protect you from diseases that can make you very sick, some of which have devastating sequelae. They also help protect people who cannot get vaccinated themselves.

While you are in college you may be exposed to a large number of diseases. They include bacterial vaginosis, bronchitis/chest cold, common cold, foodborne illness, influenza, meningococcal meningitis, mononucleosis, bacterial STDs (including chlamydia, gonorrhea, syphilis, and trichomoniasis), viral STDs (including genital herpes, hepatitis A and B, HIV, and HPV), strep throat, and urinary tract infection. These diseases range from mild, mostly causing discomfort (e.g., the common cold), to extremely serious (e.g., HIV).

The best defense against infectious diseases is to take a holistic approach to your health—eating well, sleeping enough, washing your hands, washing produce before you eat it, getting vaccinated, and using protection when you have sex. If you do get an infection, prevent sharing it with your friends by covering your sneezes and coughing into your elbow, not your hand. Be conscientious about throwing away your used tissues. If you have a bacterial infection, you should take all the medicine you are prescribed in the way it is prescribed. The host (you), the pathogen (the disease), and environmental factors are all important keys to understanding an infectious disease.

Key Terms

antibiotics
bacteria
contact transmission
direct transmission
endemic
epidemic
etiology
fungi
herd immunity
host
immunity
noncontact transmission
pandemic
parasite
pathology
prions
prognosis
subclinical infection
virus

Student Discussion Questions and Activities

1. Discuss the similarities and differences between historic and current pandemics.
2. With the exception of people who have medical reasons not to, should everyone be required to get vaccinations?

3. Explain the difference between bacteria and viruses.
4. Explain the differences between airborne, vehicle-borne, and vector-borne transmission and between infectious and contagious diseases.
5. What makes it possible to eradicate an infectious disease?
6. Complete your own vaccination schedule (see the following chart). Are you up to date on your vaccinations?

Vaccine	Date	Doctor/Health Clinic's Name and Address
Tetanus, diphtheria, and pertussis		
Haemophilus influenza type b (Hib)		
Pneumococcal		
Influenza		
Measles, mumps, rubella		
Varicella		
Hepatitis A		
Hepatitis B		
Human papillomavirus		
Meningococcal		

7. How can infectious diseases be prevented?
8. The CDC recommends an annual flu vaccination. Why does it not always work? If you do get the flu even after getting a vaccination, does the vaccination help?
9. If you have a bacterial infection, why should you take all the medicine you are prescribed?

References

1. National Health Service. (2015.) How long do bacteria and viruses live outside the body? Retrieved from http://www.nhs.uk/chq/Pages/how-long-do-bacteria-and-viruses-live-outside-the-body.aspx.
2. Fenner, F., Henderson, D. A., Arita, I., Jezek, Z., & Ladnyi, I. D. (1988). *Smallpox and its eradication (history of international public health, no. 6)*. Geneva, Switzerland: World Health Organization; 1460.
3. Robbins, F. C., & Daniel, T. M. (1999). *Polio*. Rochester, NY: University of Rochester Press.
4. Dobell, C. (2015). *Antony van Leeuwenhoek and his "Little Animals": Being Some Account of the Father of Protozoology & Bacteriology and His Multifarious Discoveries in These Disciplines*. Wolcott, New York: Scholar's Choice.
5. Ryan, K. J. (2015). *Sherris medical microbiology* (6th ed.). New York: McGraw-Hill; 2014.
6. National Meningitis Association. (n.d.). Serogroup B meningococcal disease outbreaks on U.S. college campuses. Retrieved from http://www.nmaus.org/disease-prevention-information /serogroup-b-meningococcal-disease/outbreaks/
7. Food and Drug Administration. (2012). Pathogenic *Escherichia coli* group. In: *Bad bug book, foodborne pathogenic microorganisms and natural toxins* (2nd ed.). Washington, DC: US Department of Health and Human Services; 68–81.
8. Centers for Disease Control and Prevention (CDC). (2018). Lyme disease. Retrieved from http://www.cdc.gov/lyme/index.html
9. Centers for Disease Control and Prevention (CDC). (2017). Fact sheet: Syphilis. Retrieved from http://www.cdc.gov/std/syphilis/STDFact-Syphilis.htm
10. Watson, J. T., Gayer, M., & Connolly, M. A. (2007). Epidemics after natural disasters. *Emerging Infectious Diseases, 13*(1), 1–5. doi: 10.3201/eid1301.060779
11. Noji, E. K. (1997). *The public health consequences of disasters*. New York: Oxford University Press.
12. Surmieda, M. R., Lopez, J. M., Abad-Viola, G., Miranda, M. E., Abellanosa, I. P., Sadang, R. A, . . . White, F. M. (1992). Surveillance in evacuation camps after the eruption of Mt. Pinatubo, Philippines. *MMWR. CDC Surveillance Summaries, 41*(4), 9–12.

13. World Health Organization. (2005). Epidemic-prone disease surveillance and response after the tsunami in Aceh Province, Indonesia. *Weekly Bulletin; Epidemiological Information Received*, *80*(18), 160–164.
14. World Health Organization (WHO) & Ministry of Health of Pakistan. (2006, April 22–28). Pakistan earthquake. *Weekly Morbidity and Mortality Report (WMMR)*. Retrieved from http://www.who.int/hac/crises/international/pakistan_earthquake/sitrep/Pakistan_WMMR_VOL23_03052006.pdf
15. Yan, H., Almasy, S., & Santiago, C. (2017, September 21). Puerto Rico governor: Power could be out for months. CNN World. Retrieved from http://www.cnn.com/2017/09/20/americas/hurricane-maria-caribbean-islands/index.html
16. Centers for Disease Control and Prevention (CDC). (2016). Water, sanitation, & hygiene (WASH)-related emergencies & outbreaks: Emergency water supply preparation. Retrieved from https://www.cdc.gov/healthywater/emergency/drinking/emergency-water-supply-preparation.html
17. Semmelweis, I. (1983). *The etiology, concept, and prophylaxis of childbed fever.* Madison, Wisconsin: University of Wisconsin Press.
18. World Health Organization. (2017). Cholera. Retrieved from http://www.who.int/mediacentre/factsheets/fs107/en
19. Snow, J. (1965). *Snow on cholera.* New York, NY: Hafner.
20. Davis, C. J., & Krueger, J. M. (2012). Sleep and cytokines. *Sleep Medicine Clinics*, 7(3), 517–527.
21. Nielsen, H. G. (2013). Exercise and immunity. In: M. Hamlin, N. Draper, & Y. Kathiravel, (Eds.), *Current issues in sports and exercise medicine.* Rijeka, Croatia: InTech; 126.
22. Ahmed, U., & Tanwir, F. (2015). Association of periodontal pathogenesis and cardiovascular diseases: A literature review. *Oral Health and Preventive Dentistry,13*, 21-27.
23. Leite, R. S., Marlow, N. M., & Fernandes, J. K. (2013). Oral health and type 2 diabetes. *American Journal of the Medical Sciences, 345*(4), 271–273.
24. Lafon, A., Pereira, B., Dufour, T., Rigouby V, Giroud M, Béjot Y, Tubert-Jeannin S. (2014). Periodontal disease and stroke: A meta-analysis of cohort studies. *European Journal of Neurology, 21*, 1155–1161.
25. Martinez de Tejada, B., Gayet-Ageron, A., Combescure, C., Irion, O., & Baehni, P. (2012). Association between early preterm birth and periodontitis according to USA and European consensus definitions. *Journal of Maternal-Fetal and Neonatal Medicine*, *25*(11), 2160–2166.
26. Touger-Decker, R., & van Lovern, C. (2003). Sugars and dental caries. *The American Journal of Clinical Nutrition*, 78(4), 881S–892S.
27. Al-Tarakemah, Y., & Darvell, B. W. (2016) On the permanence of tooth bleaching. *Dent Mater, 32*(10):1281–1288. doi: 10.1016/j.dental.2016.07.008
28. Yaacob, M., Worthington, H. V., Deacon, S. A., Deery, C., Walmsley, A. D., Robinson, P. G., & Glenny, A-. M. (2014). Powered versus manual toothbrushing for oral health. *Cochrane Database of Systematic Reviews.* doi: 10.1002/14651858.CD002281.pub3
29. Dyer, D., Addy, M., & Newcombe, R. G. (2000). Studies in vitro of abrasion by different manual toothbrush heads and a standard toothpaste. *Journal of Clinical Periodontology*, *27*(2), 99–103.
30. Sambunjak, D., Nickerson, J. W., Poklepovic, T., Johnson, T. M., Imai, P., Tugwell, P., & Worthington, H. V. (2011). Flossing for the management of periodontal diseases and dental caries in adults. Cochrane Oral Health Group. The Cochrane Library. doi: 10.1002/14651858.CD008829.pub2
31. Eke, P. I., Dye, B. A., Wei, L., Thornton-Evans, G. O., & Genco, R. J. (2012). Prevalence of periodontitis in adults in the United States: 2009 and 2010. *Journal of Dental Research, 91*(10, 914-920. doi: 10.1177/0022034512457373
32. Ozturk, A. B., Damadoglu, E., Karakaya, G., & Kalyoncu, A .F. (2011). Does nasal hair (vibrissae) density affect the risk of developing asthma in patients with seasonal rhinitis? *International Archives of Allergy and Immunology*, *156*(1), 75–80.
33. Informed Health Online [Internet]. (2016, September 21). How does the immune system work? Retrieved from https://www.ncbi.nlm.nih.gov/pubmedhealth/PMH0072548/
34. U.S. Department of Health and Human Services, National Institutes of Health, National Institute of Allergy and Infectious Diseases, National Cancer Institute. Understanding the immune system: How it works. NIH Publication No. 03-5423. Retrieved from http://www.imgt.org/IMGTeducation/Tutorials/ImmuneSystem/UK/the_immune_system.pdf
35. Fleming-Dutra, K. E., Mangione-Smith, R., & Hicks, L. A. How to prescribe fewer unnecessary antibiotics: Talking points that work with patients and their families. Retrieved from http://www.aafp.org/afp/2016/0801/p200.html
36. Centers for Disease Control and Prevention (CDC). (2015). Improving antibiotic use. Retrieved from http://www.cdc.gov/features/antibioticuse/index.html
37. Holmes A. H., Moore L. S., Sundsfjord A., Steinbakk M., Regmi S., Karkey A., Guerin P. J., Piddock L. J., (2016) Understanding the mechanisms and drivers of antimicrobial resistance. Lancet. 387 (10014): 176-87.
38. Centers for Disease Control and Prevention (CDC). (2015). About antimicrobial resistance. Retrieved from https://www.cdc.gov/drugresistance/about.html
39. Centers for Disease Control and Prevention (CDC). (2015). Antibiotics aren't always the answer. Retrieved from http://www.cdc.gov/Features/GetSmart
40. Jepson, R. G., Williams, G., & Craig, J. C. (2012). Cranberries for preventing urinary tract infections. Cochrane Database of Systematic Reviews. doi: 10.1002/14651858.CD001321.pub5.
41. Jepson, R. G., Mihalijevic, L., & Craig, J. C. (1998). Cranberries for preventing urinary tract infections. Cochrane Database of Systematic Reviews. doi: 10.1002/14651858.CD00132.
42. WebMD. (n.d.). 10 ways to prevent yeast infections. Retrieved from http://www.webmd.com/women/guide/10-ways-to-prevent-yeast-infections
43. Centers for Disease Control and Prevention (CDC). (2013). STD curriculum for clinical educators: Vaginitis module. Retrieved from www2a.cdc.gov/stdtraining/ready-to-use/Manuals/Vaginitis/vaginitis-notes-2013.docx
44. de Bary, W.T. (1972) The Buddhist Tradition: In India, China and Japan. New York, NY: Vintage
45. Hume, E.H. (2012). The Chinese Way in Medicine. Whitefish, MT: Literary Licensing, LLC
46. Parry, J. (2008) No vaccine for the scaremongers. *Bulletin of the World Health Organization, 86*(6), 425–426.
47. United Nations. (2015). Millenium development Goal 4: Reduce child mortality. Retrieved from http://www.un.org/millenniumgoals/childhealth.shtml
48. Plotkin, S. A., Orenstein, W. & Offit, P. (2008) *Vaccines: Expert consult, 5e (Expert Consult Title: Online + Print)*. Philadelphia, PA: Saunders
49. NIAID. (n.d.). Vaccine types. Retrieved from http://www.niaid.nih.gov/topics/vaccines/understanding/pages/typesvaccines.aspx

50. Centers for Disease Control and Prevention (CDC). (2015). Immunization schedules for children in easy-to-read formats. Retrieved from http://www.cdc.gov/vaccines/schedules/easy-to-read/child.html
51. Centers for Disease Control and Prevention (CDC). (2015). Immunization schedules for preteens and teens in easy-to-read formats. Retrieved from http://www.cdc.gov/vaccines/schedules/easy-to-read/preteen-teen.html
52. Centers for Disease Control and Prevention (CDC). (2015). Immunization schedules for adults in easy-to-read formats. Retrieved from http://www.cdc.gov/vaccines/schedules/easy-to-read/adult.html
53. Centers for Disease Control and Prevention (CDC). (2015). Immunization for travelers. Retrieved from http://www.cdc.gov/vaccines/pubs/downloads/f_imz_travelers.pdf
54. Atkinson, W., Wolfe, C., Hamborsky, J. (2011) *Epidemiology and Prevention of Vaccine-Preventable Diseases, 12th Edition (The Pink Book)*. Washington, DC: Public Health Foundation Publications.
55. Centers for Disease Control and Prevention (CDC). (2015). Measles: it isn't just a little rash parent infographic. Retrieved from http://www.cdc.gov/measles/parent-infographic.html
56. Centers for Disease Control and Prevention (CDC). (2018). Shingles (herpes zoster). Retrieved from http://www.cdc.gov/shingles/hcp/clinical-overview.html
57. Wakefield, A. J., Murch, S. H., Anthony, A., Linnell, J., Casson, D. M., Malik, M., Berelowitz, M., Dhillon, A. P., Harvey, P., Davies, S. E., Walker-Smith, J. A. (1998). Ileal-lymphoid-nodular hyperplasia, non-specific colitis, and pervasive developmental disorder in children. *Lancet*, *351*(9103), 637–641.
58. Tate, N. (2015, February 18). Disneyland measles outbreak likely originated in Philippines. Newsmax Health. Retrieved from http://www.newsmax.com/Health/Health-News/measles-disney-land-vaccine/2015/02/18/id/625552
59. Zipprich, J., Winter, K., Hacker, J., Xia D., Watt J., Harriman K. (2015). Measles outbreak—California, December 2014–February 2015. *Morbidity and Mortality Weekly Report*. 64(6), 153–154.
60. Alexander, A. (2015). NO, it's not my job to vaccinate my kid just to keep *Yours* safe. YourTango. Retrieved from http://www.yourtango.com/no-its-not-my-job-to-vaccinate-my-kid-just-to-keep-yours-safe
61. Erwin, P. C., & Bialek, R. (2015). A matter of perspective: Seeing Cuban and United States health systems through a cultural lens. *American Journal of Public Health*. 105, 1509–1511.
62. Centers for Disease Control and Prevention (CDC). (2015). Vaccines: About. Retrieved from http://www.cdc.gov/vaccines/about/terms/glossary.htm#commimmunity. Accessed 5 /25 /2015,
63. Smart Global Health. (2015). Infectious diseases: The CSIS global health policy center. Retrieved from http://www.smartglobalhealth.org/issues/entry/infectious-diseases/
64. Centers for Disease Control and Prevention (CDC). (2018). Malaria. Retrieved from http://www.cdc.gov/malaria/
65. Porter, R. (1997). The Greatest Benefit to Mankind: A Medical History of Humanity. New York, NY: W.W. Norton & Company, Inc.
66. Centers for Disease Control and Prevention (CDC). (2015). Basic TB facts. Retrieved from http://www.cdc.gov/tb/topic/basics/default.htm
67. Centers for Disease Control and Prevention (CDC). (2015). About Zika virus disease. Retrieved from http://www.cdc.gov/zika/about/index.html
68. Centers for Disease Control and Prevention (CDC). (2015). Zika virus: Symptoms, diagnosis, & treatment. Retrieved from http://www.cdc.gov/zika/symptoms/index.html
69. Centers for Disease Control and Prevention (CDC). (2015). Zika virus: Prevention. Retrieved from http://www.cdc.gov/zika/prevention/index.html
70. Centers for Disease Control and Prevention (CDC). (2015). Zika virus: Transmission. Retrieved from http://www.cdc.gov/zika/transmission/index.html
71. Centers for Disease Control and Prevention (CDC). (2018). World map of areas with risk of Zika. Retrieved from https://wwwnc.cdc.gov/travel/page/world-map-areas-with-zika
72. Centers for Disease Control and Prevention (CDC). (2016). West Nile virus. Retrieved from https://www.cdc.gov/westnile/index.html
73. Centers for Disease Control and Prevention (CDC). (2016). West Nile virus: Prevention and control. Retrieved from https://www.cdc.gov/westnile/prevention/index.html.
74. Centers for Disease Control and Prevention (CDC). (2016). West Nile virus & dead birds. Retrieved from https://www.cdc.gov/westnile/faq/deadbirds.html
75. Centers for Disease Control and Prevention (CDC). (2016). Lyme disease. Retrieved from https://www.cdc.gov/lyme/index.html
76. Centers for Disease Control and Prevention (CDC). (2016). Signs and symptoms of untreated Lyme disease. Retrieved from https://www.cdc.gov/lyme/signs_symptoms/index.html
77. Centers for Disease Control and Prevention (CDC). (2016). Lyme disease: Data and statistics. Retrieved from https://www.cdc.gov/lyme/stats/index.html
78. Centers for Disease Control and Prevention (CDC). (2016). Cold versus flu. Retrieved from https://www.cdc.gov/flu/about/qa/coldflu.htm
79. Mayo Clinic. (2017). Overview: common cold. Retrieved from http://www.mayoclinic.org/diseases-conditions/common-cold/home/ovc-20199807
80. WebMD. (2017). Flu or cold? Know the differences. Retrieved from http://www.webmd.com/cold-and-flu/cold-guide/flu-cold-symptoms#2
81. Centers for Disease Control and Prevention (CDC). (2004.) CDC Smallpox fact sheet. Retrieved from http://emergency.cdc.gov/agent/smallpox/overview/disease-facts.asp
82. World Health Organization. (2015). Smallpox. Retrieved from http://www.who.int/csr/disease/smallpox/en
83. Jenner, E. (1798.) *An Inquiry Into The Causes And Effects Of The Variolae Vaccinae A Disease Discovered in Some of the Western Counties of England, Particularly Gloucestershire, and Known by the Name of the Cow Pox.* London, England: Sampson Low.
84. Centers for Disease Control and Prevention (CDC). (2014). Fact sheet: Chlamydia. Retrieved from http://www.cdc.gov/std/Chlamydia/STDFact-Chlamydia.htm
85. Centers for Disease Control and Prevention (CDC). (2014). Fact sheet: Genital herpes. Retrieved from http://www.cdc.gov/std/Herpes/STDFact-Herpes.htm
86. Centers for Disease Control and Prevention (CDC). (2014). Fact sheet: Gonorrhea Retrieved from http://www.cdc.gov/std/Gonorrhea/STDFact-gonorrhea.htm

87. Centers for Disease Control and Prevention (CDC). (2012.) Prion diseases. Retrieved from http://www.cdc.gov/ncidod/dvrd/prions/.
88. National Institute of Neurological Disorders and Stroke (NINDS). (2015). Kuru information page. http://www.ninds.nih.gov/disorders/kuru/kuru.htm
89. Lindenbaum, S. (2013). *Kuru sorcery: Disease and danger in the new guinea highlands* (2nd ed.). Mountain View, CA: Paradigm Publishers.
90. DeWitte, S. N. (2014). Mortality risk and survival in the aftermath of the medieval black death. *PLoS One*, 9(5), e96513.
91. Centers for Disease Control and Prevention (CDC). (2015). Plague. Retrieved from http://www.cdc.gov/plague
92. Ziegler, P. (2009). *The black death.* New York: Harper Perennial Modern Classics; 16.
93. Trilla, A., Trilla, G., & Daer, C. (2008). The 1918 "Spanish flu" in Spain. *Clinical Infectious Diseases*. 47(5), 668–673.
94. Barry, J. M. (2005). *The Great Influenza: The Story of the Deadliest Pandemic in History*. New York, NY: Penguin Books.
95. Boffey, P. M. (1985, September 20) U.S. counters public fears of AIDS. *The New York Times*. U.S. counters public fears of AIDS. *The New York Times*. Retrieved from https://archive.nytimes.com/www.nytimes.com/library/national/science/aids/092085sci-aids.html
96. Anonymous. (1986). AIDS newsletter. *Great Britain Bureau of Tropical Hygiene*, *2*(1).
97. Mann, J. & Tarantola, D. J. M. (Eds.) (1996). AIDS in the World II (vol 2): New York, N.Y.: Oxford University Press.
98. Wilkerson, I. (1988, July 1). A.M.A. urges breach of privacy to warn potential AIDS victims. *The New York Times*. Retrieved from http://partners.nytimes.com/library/national/science/aids/070188sci-aids.html
99. Health Resources and Services Administration. (2016.) Ryan White HIV/AIDS Program Legislation. Retrieved from http://hab.hrsa.gov/abouthab/legislation.html
100. WHO | HIV/AIDS. Retrieved from http://www.who.int/gho/hiv/en
101. WHO | bovine spongiform encephalopathy (BSE). Retrieved from http://www.who.int/zoonoses/diseases/bse/en
102. World Health Organization. (2016). Variant Creutzfeldt-Jakob disease. Retrieved from http://www.who.int/mediacentre/factsheets/fs180/en
103. Stern, J. E. (2014, October). Hell in the hot zone: Why a massive international effort has failed to contain the Ebola epidemic. *Vanity Fair*. Retrieved from http://www.vanityfair.com/news/2014/10/ebola-virus-epidemic-containment

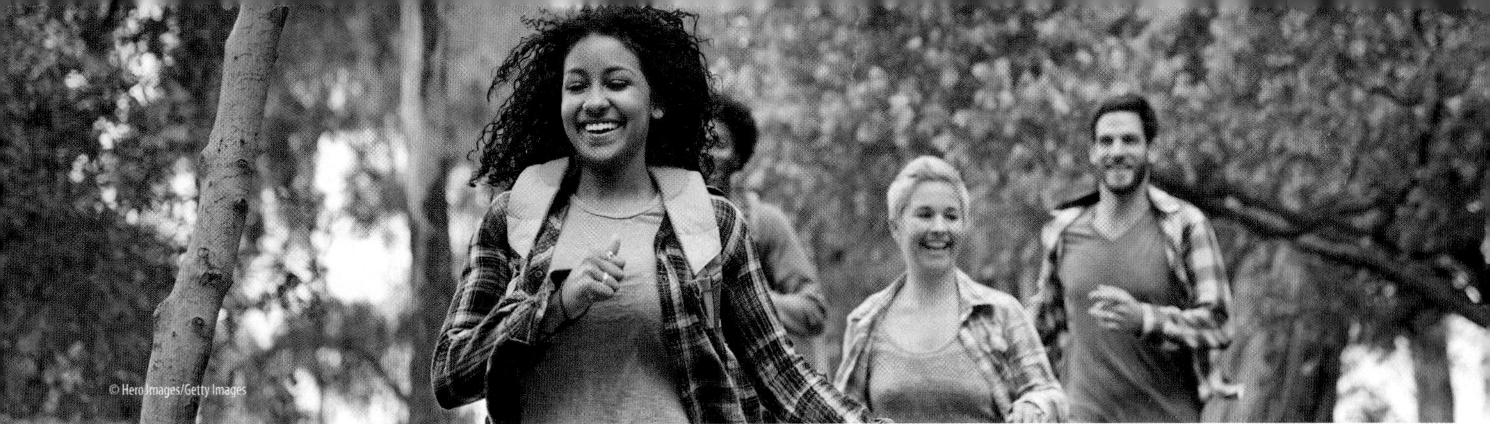
© Hero Images/Getty Images

CHAPTER 9

The Bandage Brigade: Injuries and Accidents

CHAPTER OBJECTIVES

- Define and understand the common causes of injuries.
- Recognize behaviors that increase the risk of injuries.
- Help develop skills for the prevention of injuries.
- Identify ways that students and communities can work to reduce injuries in their environment.

You likely got your first injury when you were just learning to walk. That unsteady balance of toddlers means they fall and sustain scrapes and bruises. You also got scrapes and bruises on the playground as you grew up. If you are lucky, you never experienced anything more serious. But by this point in your life, there's a good chance you have had more severe injuries. Maybe you sustained a concussion while playing football, broke a bone (or worse) in a car crash, ingested something poisonous, burned yourself while cooking in the kitchen—the list goes on. There are behaviors you can choose that in some instances will minimize the likelihood that you will be seriously injured. In this chapter, we'll talk about unintentional injuries. For information about intentional self-injury, see Chapter 6.

Sports Injuries

Sports injuries have been a part of human history for a long time. A 2006 study examined the skulls of Roman gladiators to review the types of injuries these sport contestants sustained.[1] While contestants in modern sports don't necessarily die from their participation, that does not mean they are entirely safe.

The Centers for Disease Control and Prevention (CDC), the population health community, and your primary care provider all send the message to be

athlete exposures A unit of susceptibility to injury equal to one athlete participating in one game or practice in which the athlete is exposed to the possibility of athletic injury. For college-aged individuals, this measure does not include injuries among those participating in recreational team or individual sports activities.

physically active. (See Chapter 3.) For most people, being physically active means taking part in sports and in physically active recreational activities. As part of that participation, injuries can, and do, occur. Each year emergency departments treat more than 2.6 million children age 19 years and younger for sports- and recreation-related injuries. Among college athletes, for all sports combined, the injury rates for games were 13.8 per 1,000 **athlete exposures** (AEs) and for practices were 4.0 per 1,000 AEs.[2]

Of the many sports in which you can participate, the types and likelihood of injury depend on the sport. Among collegiate athletes, football has the highest injury rates for both practices (9.6 injuries per 1,000 AEs) and games (35.9 injuries per 1,000 AEs) (see Tales of Public Health box). **TABLE 9-1** presents the most

TABLE 9-1 Types and Rates of Injury by Sport

Sport	Injury	Injury Rate
Archery	Lacerations, puncture wounds, rotator cuff tear or irritation, rotator cuff impingement, muscle strains, dislocated shoulder (repetitive stress injury)	4.4/10,000[4]
Badminton	Shoulder injuries caused by overuse, wrist injuries, knee and ankle injuries	5.04/1,000 player hours[5]
Basketball	Wrist, ankle, finger, medial knee ligament, and hamstring sprains; Achilles and patellar tendonitis; shin splints; shoulder injuries; contusions from thrown projectiles	9.9/1,000 AEs for games and 4.3/1,000 AEs for practices[6]
Baseball	Rotator cuff injury, thrower's elbow, tennis elbow, medial (elbow) ligament injury, shoulder instability	5.8/1,000 AEs for games and 1.9/1,000 AEs for practices[7]
Bobsled	Hamstring pulls, fatal head and spinal cord injuries, wrist fractures, shoulder injuries, ligament tears	No data available
Boxing	Cuts and bruises, sprains, strains, concussions, fractures, shoulder dislocation	An average of 8,716 injuries annually, with an increase in the annual number of injuries during the 19-year study period; rate of injury was 12.7/1,000 participants[8]
Cheerleading	Not as frequent as other sports, but tend to be catastrophic: wrists, shoulders, ankles, head, neck	Lower extremity (30–37% of all cheerleading injuries), upper extremities (21–26%), head/neck (16–19%), and trunk (7–17%). Concussion rates in cheerleading 0.06/1,000 AEs. Catastrophic injuries 2.0/100,000 college participants and 0.4/100,000 high school participants[9]
Curling	Knee muscle strains, shoulder tendonitis, pulled hip flexors, back strain	2/1,000 AEs[10]

Cycling	Achilles tendonitis, patellar tendonitis, collarbone and the carpal bone on the thumb side of the hand fractures, saddle sores, lower back and neck pain	26.5/100 participants[11]
Diving	Smacking the water, scrapes and contusions from hitting the board (usually minor), wrist, shoulder, back repetitive motion injuries, spinal cord injuries (95% of which are from diving into water that is not deep enough)	1.71/1,000 AEs (men: 1.94/1,000; women: 2.49/1,000)[12]
Equestrian	Head injury from a fall, crushing injuries by horse or horse kick, bruises, cuts, facial abrasions, arm fractures, joint sprains	About 20% over participants' lifetime of riding[13]
Fencing	Fencer's elbow, patellar (knee) tendonitis, patellofemoral syndrome	2.5/100 Olympic participants[14]
Field hockey	Hand, forearm, face, ankle, foot, knee injuries in form of sprains, strains, fractures, contusions, concussions	0.94/1,000 AEs[15,16]
Figure skating	Overuse: foot or spine stress fractures, shin splints, muscle strains, tendonitis, jumper's knee, ankle bursitis. Traumatic: ankle sprains and fractures, shoulder or knee dislocation, head injuries, muscle tears, lacerations	1/1,000 Olympic participants[17]
Football (American)	Concussions, overuse injuries (back and knee), heat injuries, traumatic injuries (knee, ankle, shoulder)	Concussion: 0.39/1,000 AEs[18]
Golf	Low back pain, shoulder pain (impingement syndrome and rotator cuff problems), golfer's or thrower's elbow and tennis elbow, overuse injuries of the wrist flexor and extensor tendons	35.2/100 golfers over the past year[19]
Gymnastics	Labral (SLAP) tears, Achilles tendinitis, wrist injuries, ACL injuries, foot and ankle injuries, muscle strain	Men: 8.78/1,000 AEs Women: 9.37/1,000 AEs[20]
Handball	Ankle and finger sprains, contusions	11.1 to 23.5/1,000 match hours[21]
Ice hockey	Lacerations (cuts) to the head, scalp, and face; neck and spinal injuries; knee sprains and shoulder separation and dislocation	14.2/1,000 player games[22]
Inline skating	Wrist fractures and sprains; head injuries; abrasions; knee, foot, ankle, and shoulder injuries	3.9/1,000 participants[23]
Lacrosse	Sprains and strains; concussions; head, face, lower leg, ankle, foot, and knee injuries	1.96/1,000 AEs (men: 2.26/1,000; women: 1.54/1,000)[24]
Luge	Contusions of extremities, neck strains, concussions, fractures mostly due to crashes	7.1/1,000 track runs[25]
Martial arts	Sprains; strains; pain; ruptures and injuries to ankle, feet, hips, knees, and/or shoulder; bulging and degenerative disc disease; stress fracture; temporomandibular joint dysfunction	228.07/1,000 AEs[26]

(continues)

TABLE 9-1 Types and Rates of Injury by Sport *(continued)*

Sport	Injury	Injury Rate
Racquetball	Tennis elbow, rotator cuff injuries, ankle sprains	No data available
Rowing	Primarily overuse: knee, lumbar spine, and ribs	No data available
Rugby	Dislocated shoulder, thumb sprains, acromioclavicular (AC) joint injury, hamstring and rotator cuff strains, contusions	9.2/1,000 player hours[27]
Running	Groin strain, iliotibial band syndrome (runner's knee), Achilles tendonitis, hamstring injury, shin splints, calf strain, ankle strain, plantar fasciitis (heel pain)	10/1,000 hours of running exposure[28]
Sailing	Minor cuts, contusions, avulsions, mild burns	Injuries: 4.6/1,000 days of sailing Severe injuries: 0.57/1,000 days of sailing[29]
Skateboarding	Sprained or fractured wrist, fingers, arms, legs, and feet; head injuries; abrasions and contusions	8.9/1,000 participants[23]
Skiing	Medial knee ligament injury, fractured collarbone, shoulder separation joint injury, medial meniscus injury, thumb sprain	4 to 9.1/1,000 skier days[30]
		26.4/100 athletes[31]
Snowboarding	Wrist sprain and fracture, elbow contusions and dislocations, rotator cuff injuries, broken collarbones, concussions, other head and neck injuries	15/1,000 snowboarder days[30]
Soccer	Ankle sprain; torn ligament or tendon or muscle strain; knee ligament tears; groin muscle injury; calf, shin, and hamstring injuries	Women: 0.7/1,000 hours of exposure Men: 0.6/1,000 hours of exposure[32]
Squash	Ankle, knee, leg, arm, and lower back strains and sprains; eye and head injuries; dehydration	44.5/100 players[33]
Swimming	Swimmers shoulder (overuse injury)	1.54/1,000 AEs (men: 1.48/1,000; women: 1.63/1,000)[12]
Table tennis	Muscle strain; lower back injuries; knee, wrist, shoulder, and ankle joint injuries	No data available
Tennis	Tennis elbow; bursitis of the elbow, shoulder, and wrist; tendonitis; impingement syndrome; frozen shoulder; Achilles tendinitis and rupture; iliotibial band syndrome; osteoarthritis of the knee; torn rotator cuff; shoulder separation; wrist and ankle sprains; hamstring pulls or tears; muscle sprains and strains; knee ligament injuries; torn knee cartilage; blisters; plantar fasciitis; stress fractures	0.04 to 3.0/1,000 playing hours[34]
		6.1/1,000 playing hours[35]

Trampoline	Fractures, injury to ligaments, contusions, lacerations, dislocations	More than 1 million hospital visits over 9-yr period. Twenty-nine percent had fractures, including upper and lower extremity and axial skeleton.[36]
Triathlon	Injuries occurred during running (50%), cycling (43%), and swimming (7%). Contusions and abrasions, ligament and capsular injuries, muscle and tendon injuries, fractures	Data were collected both retrospectively and prospectively. Incidence of an injury/1,000 training hours was 0.69 (retrospective) and 1.39 (prospective) during training and 9.24 (retrospective) and 18.45 (prospective) during competition.[37]
Volleyball	Achilles tendonitis; ankle or AC joint sprain; finger fracture; calf, hamstring, or quadriceps strain; jumper's knee; rotator cuff tear	Women: 4.1 to 4.6/1,000 AEs[38]
		2.6/1,000 hours[39]
		Beach: 3.1/1,000 competition hours[40]
Wrestling	Bruises and contusions, sprains (particularly ankle and wrist), strains, overtraining, dehydration. More serious injuries: rotator cuff injuries, shoulder separation and dislocation, anterior cruciate and posterior cruciate ligament injuries, elbow dislocation, neck strain, whiplash, cervical fractures	7.25/1,000 AEs[41]

AEs, athlete exposures.

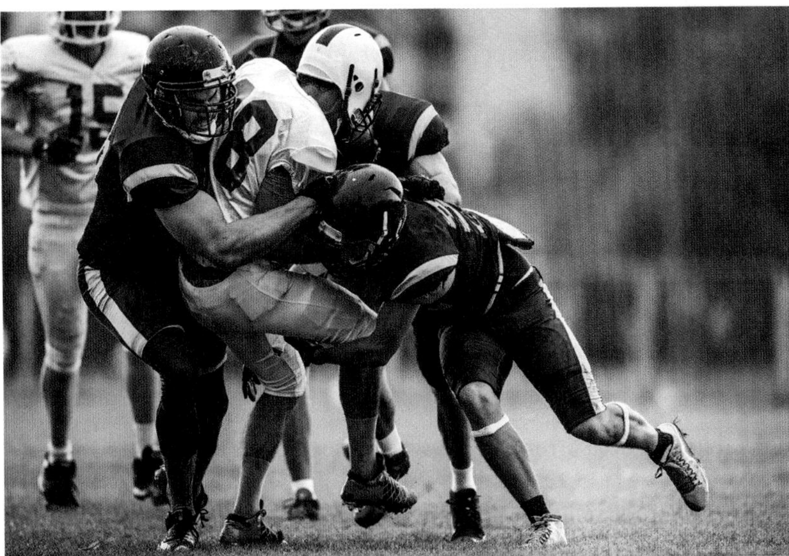

common types of injury and the injury rates associated with different sports. The stated injury rates are reported in many ways: player hours, AEs, and player days. Because most of the injury data are from medical literature specific to a sport, they are constrained by how the study author reports the data.

TALES OF PUBLIC HEALTH

Chronic Traumatic Encephalopathy and Football

Chronic traumatic encephalopathy (CTE) is a progressive, degenerative disease of the brain found in athletes (and others) with a history of repetitive brain trauma, including symptomatic concussions as well as hits to the head. More recently, there have been confirmed cases of CTE in retired professional football players and other athletes who have a history of repetitive brain trauma. This trauma triggers progressive degeneration of the brain tissue.[3]

These changes in the brain can start months, years, or even decades after the brain trauma occurred. The symptoms of CTE include memory loss, confusion, impaired judgment, impulse control problems, aggression, depression, anxiety, suicidality, parkinsonism, and, eventually, progressive dementia.[3]

The number of hits to the head needed to trigger CTE is unknown. Not everyone with a history of repeated brain trauma develops this disease. Just because you have some or many of the symptoms of CTE does not necessarily mean you have the disease itself.[3]

Some football players only receive a diagnosis of CTE after their deaths. A few of these players, including Jovan Belcher, Shane Dronett, Dave Duerson, Aaron Hernandez, and Tiaina Baul "Junior" Seau, Jr., committed suicide likely because of their CTE. In 2015, the Pro Football Hall of Fame inducted Junior Seau without addressing the circumstances of his death. In 2013, the NFL and retired players and players' families reached a settlement in a class-action lawsuit.

chronic traumatic encephalopathy A progressive degenerative disease of the brain found in athletes (and others) with a history of repetitive brain trauma, including symptomatic concussions and hits to the head.

When you are going to participate in either team or individual sports, make sure you have the right protective equipment, that the equipment fits properly, and that you wear it every time you are participating in the sport. The partial list includes helmets, wrist guards, knee or elbow pads, safety goggles, mouth protectors, and safety gloves. Be sure to drink plenty of water. Being well hydrated is particularly important in hot or humid environments. Before you start exercising, make sure you do a proper warm up. Warming up increases blood flow to your muscles, warms the connective tissues, and lubricates your joints. The 5 to 10 minutes you spend warming up is important. Preventing an injury is better than treating one.

RICE/PRICE

What should you do if you experience an injury such as a sprain, strain, contusion, muscle pull, or tear? You can use RICE or PRICE. Both terms are related. RICE stands for Rest, Ice, Compression, and Elevation, and PRICE adds Protection to the recommendation. Traditionally, with a soft muscle injury, these therapies have been the treatment of choice. As noted by researchers,[42,43] however, there is not much scientific basis for these forms of therapy; the practices occur largely as a practical, easy to implement, and time-honored treatment.

- **Protection**: The goal of protection is to prevent further injury. Depending on what body part you have injured, you may need a sling, splint, crutches, or a cane.
- **Rest**: After an injury, you want to rest to allow your body to heal. You may need to take a break from the activity you were doing that caused the injury or pain.[44]
- **Ice**: Cold reduces pain and swelling. One researcher recommended melting ice water as the most effective method of applying cold to the injury.[45] If you are using ice, do not place it directly on your skin. Put a towel between the ice pack and your skin. Use the ice or cold pack for 10 to 20 minutes, and then take a break. (A bag of frozen vegetables also works well for this.) Do this for at least three times per day, but doing it more often is better. If after 2 to 3 days, there is no more swelling, you may apply heat to the area if it still hurts. Just as with ice, if you are using a heat pack, do not place it directly on your skin.[44]

- **Compression**: Compression, or wrapping the injured area with an elastic bandage, both helps to decrease swelling and provides additional support to the injured area. Be sure not to wrap the elastic bandage too tightly or you may cause swelling below the injury. If you have wrapped the bandage too tightly, you may feel numbness, tingling, or swelling below the bandage. Call your primary care health provider if you need to wrap the injury for more than 48 to 72 hours.[44] The researchers who systematically reviewed the literature[43] concluded that there is no consistent information about the duration of compression that helps best.
- **Elevation**: Any time you are sitting or lying down, elevate the injured area to help decrease swelling. Ideally, the injured extremity should be higher than your heart. In practice, that means if your ankle or knee is injured, you should be lying down. If your wrist is injured, try using a piece of cloth or a scarf as a sling to help keep your arm up and close to your body.[44]

Traumatic Brain Injury

Traumatic brain injury (TBI) is a complex injury with a full spectrum of symptoms and disabilities. It is often the result of an acute event. After you break a leg or an arm, you are the same person you were before the injury. Following a TBI, your life has changed in dramatic ways. TBI is an acquired brain injury that happens when a sudden trauma causes damage to the brain. It can result when a person's head suddenly and violently hits an object or when an object pierces the skull and enters the brain.[46]

A TBI can range from mild to severe. A mild TBI can cause headaches, confusion, lightheadedness, dizziness, blurred vision, ringing in the ears, fatigue, a change in sleep patterns, behavioral or mood changes, and trouble with memory, concentration, attention, or thinking. A person with a moderate or severe TBI may show the same symptoms as a person with a mild

traumatic brain injury
Damage to the brain caused by an external physical force that may produce a diminished or altered state of consciousness and causes diminution of cognitive abilities or physical functioning. A person who has experienced this type of injury may have trouble with cognitive, emotional, and behavior functioning and may have permanent physical or psychosocial impairments.

YOU'VE HURT YOURSELF. SHOULD YOU TOUGH IT OUT OR SEE A HEALTH CARE PROVIDER?

While you may want to be a hero and not see a healthcare provider, there are times when it is the right thing to do. You should see a healthcare provider if any of the following are true:

1. **You can identify the exact moment you got hurt.** If you know the moment you hurt yourself, it is likely that the injury may be serious. Maybe you were in the weight room and heard a pop or you were on a trampoline and rolled your ankle. These are instances when you have likely injured yourself severely enough to see a healthcare provider.
2. **You can't walk.** If you hurt your foot or ankle such that you cannot bear weight on it, that is a sign you have likely broken a bone. Even if you have not broken anything, seeing a healthcare provider is a good idea because it may help prevent further injury.
3. **Your joint is unstable.** Even if it does not hurt, if your joint locks up, is unstable, or does not work the way it should, get it checked out by a healthcare provider.
4. **You have pulled your muscle and there is a bruise or a divot.** If you have pulled a muscle and it looks deformed where it hurts or there is a large bruise, the muscle strain is serious and you should seek medical care.
5. **Any symptom after a head injury should be seen by a healthcare provider.** If your head injury caused you to see double; lose consciousness; be dizzy, confused or nauseous, seek medical care.
6. **Your injury gets worse over time.** If your injury does not get better, or the situation where it used to hurt when you exercised but now it hurts afterwards as well, it is time to seek medical care.
7. **You have numbness or radiating pain down your arm or leg.** Back or neck pain is especially tricky. The neck and back have many important and vulnerable structures. Treatment will depend on what is injured.

As a general rule—if you are in enough pain that it disrupts your ability to function or sleep, see a healthcare provider.

TBI. This person may also have prolonged and more serious symptoms. These symptoms include a headache that gets worse or does not go away, repeated vomiting or nausea, convulsions or seizures, an inability to awaken from sleep, dilation of one or both pupils, slurred speech, weakness or numbness in the extremities, loss of coordination, and increased confusion, restlessness, or agitation.[46] A TBI can affect a person for the rest of his or her life, including personality changes.[47]

Causes of TBI

FIGURE 9-1 shows the leading causes of TBI. More than half of TBIs occur in children (0 to 14 years). Of TBIs that occur in people over age 65 years, 81% are due to falls. Examples of falls that may cause TBIs include falling out of bed, slipping in the bath, and falling down steps or from a ladder. Motor vehicle crashes, which can also involve motorcycles, bicycles, and pedestrians, are the third-leading cause of TBI.[47] Other common causes are violence, such as domestic violence or child abuse, including shaken baby syndrome, which is caused by violent shaking of an infant. (See Chapter 10.) There is increasing evidence that sports injuries, particularly American football, are an important cause of TBI. High-impact or extreme sports (e.g., boxing, lacrosse, skateboarding, hockey) also put the participant at risk of a TBI. Explosive blasts and other events during combat often result in TBI. TBI also occurs when shrapnel or other combat debris penetrate the head.[48]

Treatment of TBI

Although TBIs are classified as mild, moderate, and severe, even a mild brain injury is serious. It is important to seek prompt attention even for a "mild" injury.[48] Little can be done to reverse the initial brain damage caused by trauma. Medical personnel focus on preventing further injury by ensuring proper oxygen supply, maintaining adequate blood flow, and controlling blood pressure. Doctors perform imaging tests to help determine the diagnosis and prognosis.

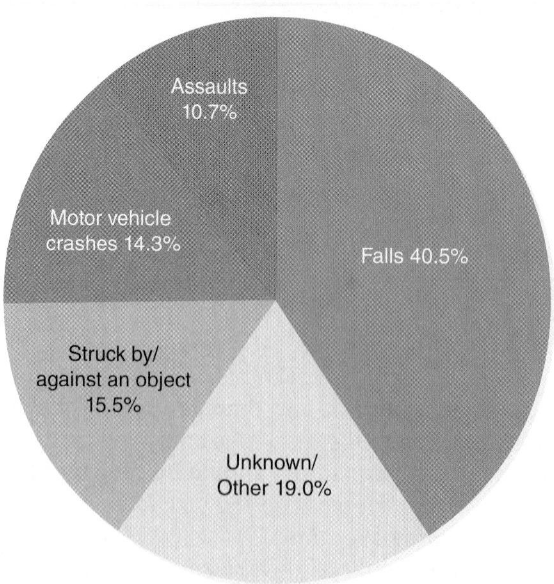

FIGURE 9-1 Leading causes of TBI.

Centers for Disease Control and Prevention, National Center for Injury Prevention and Control. (2017). Traumatic brain injury & concussion. TBI: Get the facts. Retrieved from https://www.cdc.gov/traumaticbraininjury/get_the_facts.html

TALES OF PUBLIC HEALTH

Don't Try This at Home

As evidenced by **FIGURE 9-2**, some people are incredibly lucky. The people whose injuries are shown in the figure sustained injuries that could have been life threatening. Both of them survived their experience. One did not even realize what had happened to him.

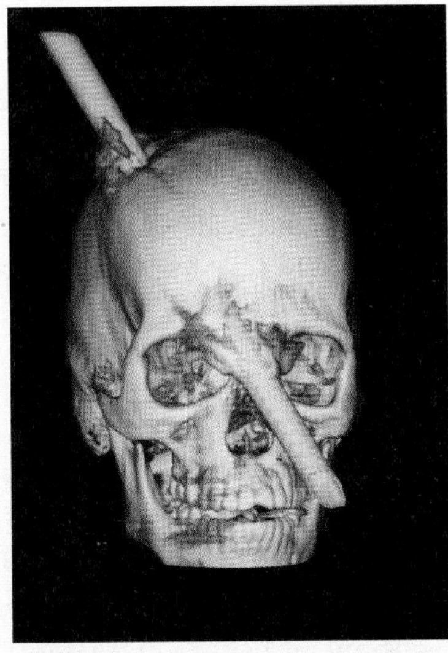

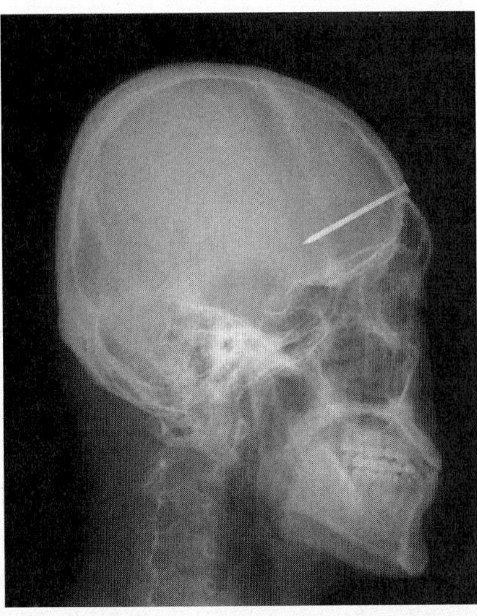

FIGURE 9-2 Don't try this at home: X-rays and computed tomography (CT) scan of men with traumatic brain injuries.

Patients with mild to moderate injuries may have X-rays while moderate to severe cases will have a computed tomography (CT) scan.[46]

A patient with moderate to severe injuries will likely have individually tailored rehabilitation. Such rehabilitation may include one or more of the following: physical therapy, occupational therapy, speech/language therapy, physiatry (physical medicine), psychology/psychiatry, and social support.[46]

Approximately half of severely head-injured patients will need surgery to remove or repair ruptured blood vessels or bruised brain tissue. Disabilities stemming from a TBI depend on the severity of the injury, the location of the injury, and the age and general health of the individual.

Serious head injuries may result in the following:

- *Stupor*—the person is unresponsive, but can be aroused briefly.
- *Coma*—the person is totally unconscious, unresponsive, unaware, and unarousable.
- *Vegetative state*—the person is unconscious and unaware of surroundings but continues to have a sleep–wake cycle and periods of alertness.
- *Persistent vegetative state*—the person loses cognition and can perform only certain involuntary actions on his or her own. Because the lower brain stem is still healthy and functioning, the patient can blink, open and move the eyes, breathe, laugh or cry (although not as an emotional response), move the arms or legs (as a reflex rather than intentionally), and smile.

Injuries in the Streets: Car Crashes and Pedestrian, Bicycle, and Motorcycle Injuries

You have probably heard it said that you are more likely to die in a car crash than in a plane crash, right? Well, it's true. In fact, one of the most dangerous things people do—seemingly without considering the danger—is get in a car. Unintentional injuries are the leading cause of death for people 1 to 44 years of age.[49] Of those injuries, in 2016, there were more than 38,000 deaths due to automobile crashes. Among people age 15 to 24 years, there were more than 7,000 deaths, or 16.2/100,000 people 15 to 24 years of age. Of deaths due to automobile crashes, 71% were among males, and 29% were among females.

Regardless of any other advice you receive regarding cars and driving, the most important one is: Always, always, always to wear your seat belt! According to the CDC, adult seat belts are the most effective way to save lives and reduce injuries if there is a crash.[50] In you are in a serious crash, wearing your seat belt reduces serious injuries and deaths by about half.[51]

Air bags are not a replacement for seat belts. The two *together* provide the best protection for adults.[52] Air bags are designed to supplement seat belts and help distribute the force exerted on the person during a crash to minimize the likelihood of injury. Air bags must work quickly: The time between the initial impact of a car hitting an object and when the person hits the steering wheel or instrument panel is 8 to 40 milliseconds.[53] The combination of air bags and seat belts reduces fatalities by 50%. Seat belts without air bags reduce fatalities by 45%, and air bags alone reduce fatalities by 13%.[52] As seen in **TABLE 9-2**, depending on the body region, air bags plus seat belts significantly reduce injuries.

Drivers and adult front seat passengers must wear seat belts in the District of Columbia and all states except New Hampshire. Thirty-four states have primary enforcement of seat belt laws, and 15 states have secondary enforcement. The District of Columbia and 28 states have laws requiring seat belt use for all rear-seat passengers. Regardless of what your state requires regarding seat belt use, the

ROAD TRAFFIC CRASHES

The World Health Organization estimates that every year there are 1.25 million deaths attributable to road traffic crashes.[54]

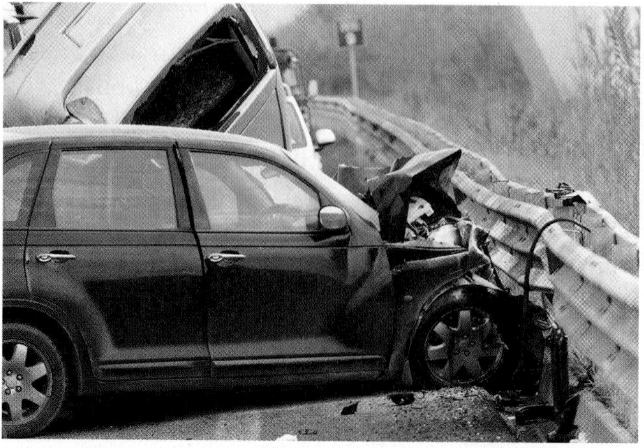

TABLE 9-2 Estimated Effectiveness of Occupant Protection Systems in Reducing the Likelihood of Moderate and Serious Injury[52]

System Used	Major Body Region			
	Head	Chest	Upper Extremity	Lower Extremity
Moderate Injury				
Air bag plus lap–shoulder belt	***85%***	***62%***	***58%***	***59%***
Air bag alone	***57%***	10%	41%	–5%
Manual lap–shoulder belt	***70%***	48%	***51%***	52%
Serious Injury				
Air bag plus lap–shoulder belt	***85%***	35%	46%	***72%***
Air bag alone	43%	–26%	61%	39%
Manual lap–shoulder belt	***60%***	***58%***	57%	***83%***
*Note: **Bold italics*** indicates statistically significant difference from the risk of unrestrained drivers.				

U.S. Department of Transportation. National Highway Traffic Safety Administration. (2001). Fifth/sixth report to Congress—effectiveness of occupant protection systems and their use.

safest choice is always to wear a seat belt. Go to www.cdc.gov/motorvehiclesafety/seatbelts/states.html to see the restraint use fact sheet for your state.

Enforcement of the law can be primary or secondary. Primary enforcement allows police to stop the driver solely for the stated infraction (not wearing a seat belt, talking on a handheld device, texting, etc.). Secondary enforcement allows police to ticket the driver for the infraction only when stopped for other reasons, such as speeding.

Motor vehicle crashes are caused by a variety of factors, including driver distraction, fatigue, drunk driving, speeding, aggressive driving, and weather conditions. In addition to talking on your cell phone (even hands-free) or texting, there are many other distractions, including rubbernecking (slowing down to look at an accident), eating, changing a CD or radio station, and interacting with other passengers in the car. According to the American Automobile Association (AAA) Foundation for Traffic Safety, drivers spend more than half their time focused on things other than driving.[55]

Driver fatigue, which is particularly prevalent in the hours when people usually sleep (between 11:00 p.m. and 8:00 a.m.), is the time of highest risk. Signs of driver fatigue include feeling like the eyelids are heavy, frequent yawning, drifting over road lines, and varying vehicle speed for no reason. The best way to avoid driver fatigue is to make sure you are well rested before you start your drive. Other ways include taking a break from driving at least every 2 hours, sharing the driving duties whenever possible, and abstaining from drinking alcohol or taking medicine that causes drowsiness before driving. If you feel drowsy or not alert, pull your car over and take a nap. Getting to your destination a little later is better than not getting there at all.

Almost 30 people in the United States die every day in automobile crashes involving alcohol.[56] This means a person dies every 51 minutes due to an alcohol-impaired driver. Almost one-third of traffic-related deaths (10,076)

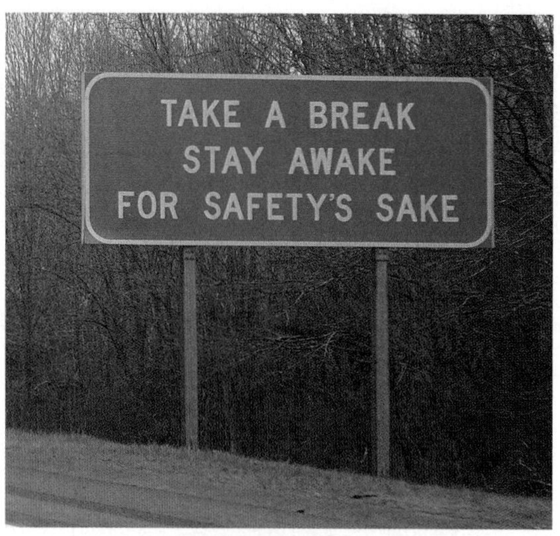

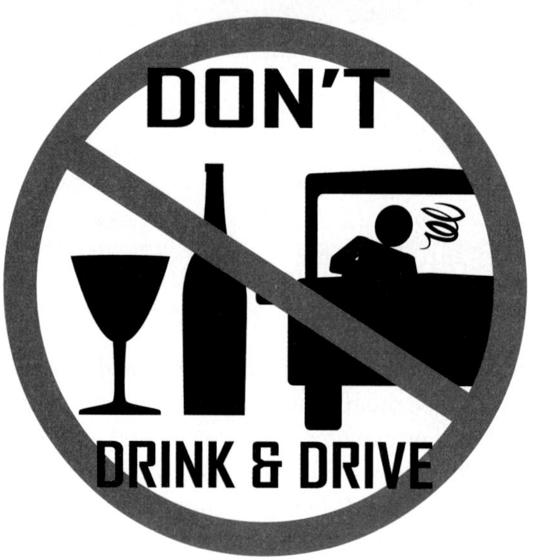

in 2013 were due to alcohol.[56] The only way to prevent this type of car crash is not to drink and drive. If you and your friends are going to drink and need to drive afterward, choose a designated driver in advance. The designated driver should not drink at all. Admittedly, being the one sober person in a group of friends who are drunk may not be as much fun as drinking, but arriving home safely is well worth the sacrifice. Drinking and driving can have consequences from which you will never recover. Go to YouTube and search for "Drunk Driving Kills" to view a public service announcement that will really make you think.

Speeding in an automobile creates multiple potential problems. It increases the risk of crashes, reduces the amount of time the driver has to avoid the problem, and makes the crash more severe if it does happen. According to the Advocates for Highway and Auto Safety, increasing driving speed from 40 mph to 60 mph doubles the energy released in a crash.[57] Every year approximately 10,000 people die in speeding-related crashes, accounting for almost one-third of all traffic fatalities.[57] Speeding is not limited to highways. A 3-mile stretch of road driven at 50 mph saves 104 seconds compared to driving the same stretch of road at 35 mph. Choosing to drive at or below the posted speed limits will make the roads safer for everyone.

FACT VS. FICTION

Camera Enforcement of Speed Limits

Myth: Speed cameras are just a way for cities to make money and don't make people slow down.

Fact: Speeding is a factor in most collisions, especially ones where there are injuries and fatalities. Encouraging people to slow down helps to reduce or eliminate injuries and fatalities. Like many cities resorting to cameras to monitor speeding, in 2007, police in Rockville, Maryland, installed two cameras to detect speeders in front of a local high school. It was one of the city's worst speeding locations. About 2,800 vehicles pass the cameras every day. When the cameras were first installed, there were approximately 75 citations issued per day; 2 years later, it is only 16 per day. The cameras in front of the high school were placed there after someone speeding through the school zone killed a student who was crossing the street.

Most people know aggressive driving when they see it. Aggressive driving behaviors include aggressive tailgating, flashing lights at other drivers, directing rude gestures or verbal abuse at other drivers, deliberately preventing other drivers from moving their vehicle, and failing to yield the right of way. If you encounter an aggressive driver when you are on the road, the best advice is to not engage them. Remain calm and do your best to keep your distance from them. If the situation is dangerous, call 9-1-1 to report them.

Inclement weather is a factor in driving that people simply cannot control. Heavy rain, hail, snowstorms, ice, fog, and high winds all make driving more difficult. If you can, avoid driving during periods of inclement weather; this is the safest option. Otherwise, because all of these conditions affect the ability to see, you need to slow down, anticipating that it will take more time to stop if you need to do so. If you need to stop, pull off the road, out of traffic, and wait until driving conditions improve.

Cell Phones and Driving

The most common distraction for drivers these days is their cell phone. Driving and cell phones are dangerous together. A substantial portion of the population believes that drivers using cell phones are a serious traffic safety problem. Yet the AAA reported that over half of U.S. drivers acknowledged using a cell phone while driving in the past 30 days, and one in seven persons admitted to sending a text message while driving.[58] Although the evidence suggests otherwise, many people believe that talking on a hands-free cell phone is safer than using a handheld device. But talking (even hands-free) and driving can distract drivers from the road. Distracted driving is a deadly behavior. Federal estimates suggest that distraction contributes to 16% of all fatal crashes, leading to around 5,000 deaths every year. The ultimate goal is for people to pay attention and not use cell phones at all while driving.[55] Many states have enacted laws regarding use of handheld devices, hands-free devices, and texting. Depending on the state where you live, laws can range from a total ban to no laws at all.

Bicycles

According to the Sightline Institute, bicycles are "a sustainable wonder."[59] Riding a bicycle is the most energy-efficient mode of travel, and it is good for you and the environment. Worldwide, bicycles outnumber automobiles almost two to one, and their production outpaces that of cars by three to one. A human walking spends three times as much energy per pound than the same person riding a bicycle.[59] Cycling is good for your heart, your muscles, your waistline, your coordination, and your mental health.

The 2009 data on mode of transportation (the most recent data available) for all trips taken in the United States estimate that 1.0% are by bicycle, and 10.4% are by foot. In large cities, these numbers are slightly higher, with 1.1% by bicycle and 12.7% by foot. Among major U.S. cities, those with extensive bicycle lanes have a higher rate of commuting by bicycle compared to other cities. Concern about safety is one of the most commonly stated reasons for not bicycling and walking.[60] Using questionnaire data from seven Seattle-area hospitals over a 3-year period, researchers found that cyclists wore helmets 51% of the time. The risk of a serious injury was increased by colliding with a motor vehicle, traveling at more than 15 mph, and being either under age 6 years or over 39 years of age (compared to age 20 to 39 years). Risk for serious injury was not influenced by helmet use.[61]

BY THE NUMBERS

Cyclists

As seen in **TABLE 9-3**, the number of cyclists ($n = 818$) killed in 2015 was 12.2% higher than the number killed the previous year. The percentage of fatalities among cyclists has been increasing since 2004.[63] Not everyone is at equal risk. The cyclist fatality rate per capita was almost six times greater for males than for females. Alcohol involvement—either for the motor vehicle operator or the cyclist—was reported in more than 37% of fatal cyclist crashes. Of the cyclists who died in 2015, 26% of them had blood alcohol concentrations of 0.01 g/dL or greater.[62, 63]

TABLE 9-3 Cyclist Fatalities in Traffic Crashes, 2004–2015

Year	Number of Cyclist Fatalities	Percentage of Total Fatalities
2004	727	1.7%
2005	786	1.8%
2006	772	1.8%
2007	701	1.7%
2008	718	1.9%
2009	628	1.9%
2010	623	1.9%
2011	682	2.1%
2012	734	2.2%
2013	749	2.3%
2014	729	2.2%
2015	818	2.3%

Fatality Analysis Reporting System (FARS), 2004-2012. Final File, 2013 Annual Report File (ARF) and 2006-2014 final File, 2015 Annual Report.

PROTECT YOURSELF WHEN RIDING A BIKE

- Don't drink and ride.
- Wear a bicycle helmet.
- Make sure you are visible when you ride—wear fluorescent or reflective clothing.
- Use bike lights.

Motorcycles

Older riders, female riders, and more of them! Motorcycle ownership is at an all-time high. According to the CDC, the average age of people riding motorcycles is increasing, and more women than ever before are riding.[64] There are

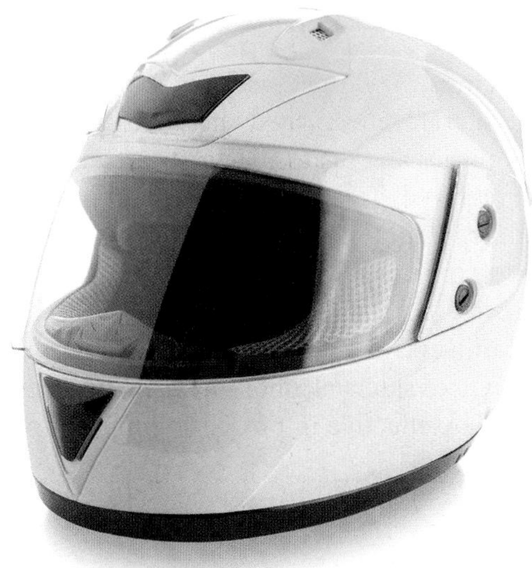

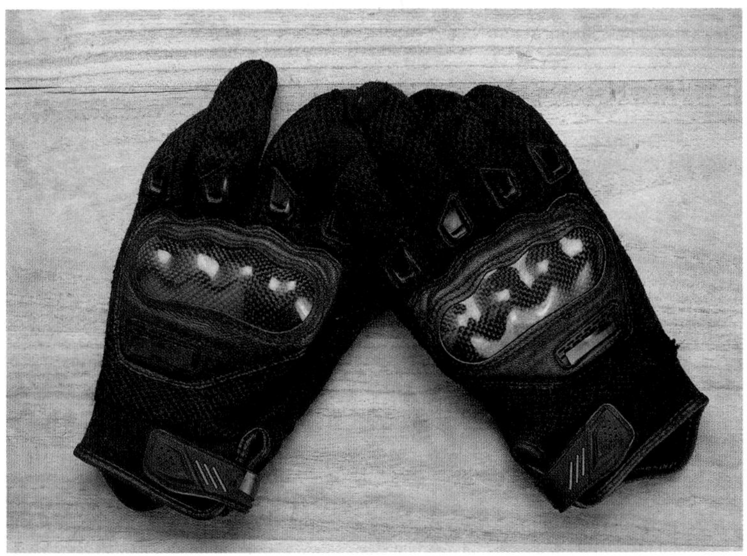

Wear protective clothing you want to crash in, not what you want to ride in. (A) A full-face helmet protects your head. Even with a lot of experience, crashes happen. Wearing a full-face helmet will help protect your face. (Imagine a crash where your face is dragged along the pavement for 20 feet!) It also protects you from bugs. Make sure to buy one that passes safety standards. (B) Gloves with ability to feel the levers and offer flexibility are the right choice. Gloves are important because in a crash, people instinctively extend their hands to protect themselves.

benefits to riding a motorcycle, such as costing less than a car to buy, insure, and operate. Distractions common in a car are typically absent when riding a motorcycle: no phones, no messing with music, no eating, and often no passengers. It's easier to find a space to park a motorcycle than a car, and motorcycles are more maneuverable. It's also easy to go incredibly fast with little or no effort, which is definitely part of the appeal for some people.

If you ride a motorcycle, always wear the most and best protective gear you can. Wear gear that will protect you from wind chill, flying bugs and debris, and road rash if you should slide out. Most people who ride motorcycles will crash at some point. It's a good idea to take a Motorcycle Safety Foundation course.[65] The book, *Proficient Motorcycling,* has a lot of advice that is worth considering. There are some crucial differences between cars and motorcycles. Understanding those differences can help protect you from getting seriously hurt or killed.

Riding a motorcycle is risky, but the approach taken by the person driving the motorcycle can go a long way to reducing that risk. In 2015, motorcycle crashes killed almost 5,000 people,[66] an increase of 70% since 2000. A recent review of the literature evaluated the effectiveness of interventions to prevent motorcycle injuries and deaths. Helmets are effective, especially where they are universally required. Training was found to have a positive effect, but not when it was totally voluntary. In terms of clothing, motorcyclists wearing protective gear were significantly less likely to be admitted to a hospital if they were wearing motorcycle jackets, pants, and gloves. A systematic review of helmet laws found that universal helmet laws increased use and reduced injuries and deaths.[67] The CDC considers alcohol impairment detection, enforcement, and sanctions likely to be effective in preventing injuries and deaths based on

RIDE SOBER!
IN 2015, 27% OF THE
MOTORCYCLE RIDERS WHO DIED
IN MOTOR VEHICLE CRASHES
WERE DRUNK.
SOURCE: NHTSA.GOV

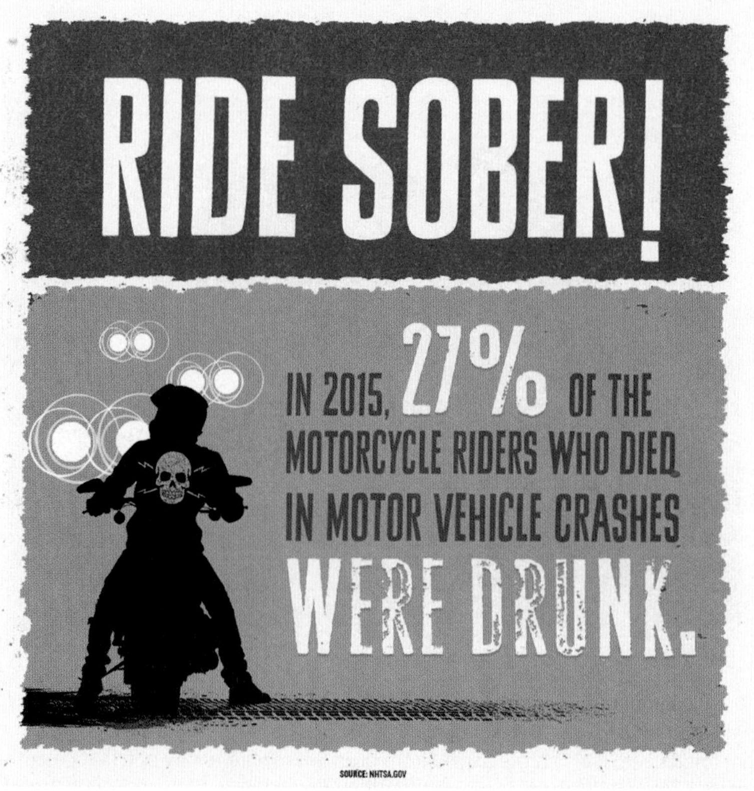

Ride sober.

Courtesy of U.S. Department of transportation. "Ride Sober" poster. Accessed at https://www.trafficsafetymarketing.gov/get-materials/motorcycle-safety/stop-impaired-riding

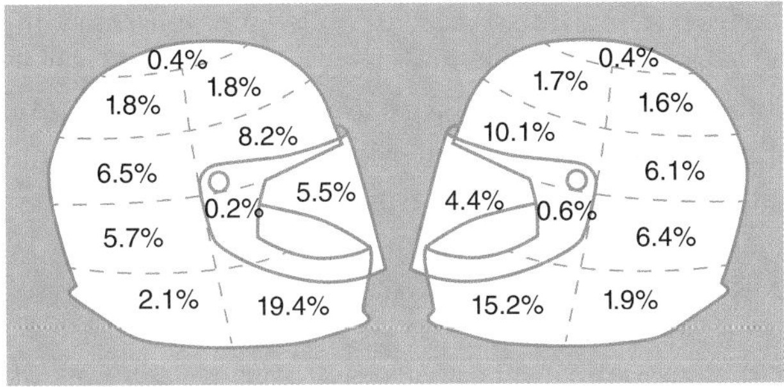

FIGURE 9-3 Why full-face helmets are a good idea. Distribution of impact locations on motorcycle helmets.

Center for Disease Control and Prevention. Motorcycle Safety: How To Save Lives And Save Money. Accessed at https://www.cdc.gov/motorvehiclesafety/pdf/mc2012/motorcyclesafetybook.pdf

the balance of evidence from high-quality evaluations. Only state motorcycle helmet laws are demonstrated to be effective in preventing fatalities in several scientific evaluations with consistent results.[64] The National Highway Traffic Safety Administration (NHTSA) agrees that wearing a helmet when riding a motorcycle is the single most effective means of reducing the number of people who are injured or die as a result of a motorcycle crash.[68]

As with driving a car, driving a motorcycle while intoxicated is dangerous. In a study performed by NHTSA, the effects of alcohol on motorcycle riding skills were examined. The study notes that alcohol intoxication is a serious risk factor for a fatal crash, particularly on a motorcycle. The study used professional drivers on a test track. The results showed there were observable changes in motorcycle control and rider behavior indicating impairment. It took the intoxicated drivers longer to respond. The riders prioritized bike stability over other tasks they were expected to perform. One way to protect the bike's stability was to go faster. However, going faster increases other risks.[69]

A full-face helmet is the correct choice for riding a motorcycle because it offers the most protection. It protects the eyes and face with a face shield and protects the chin as well. For motorcyclists, the protective effect of a helmet is to lower the collision impact for the head.[70] **FIGURE 9-3** demonstrates how motorcycle helmets absorb impact.[71]

Everyone who uses the road, be it in cars or on motorcycles or bicycles, needs to respect each other and foster a safer transportation environment for everyone.

Pedestrian Safety and Injuries: Walk With Care

Walking is good for you. Whether you are walking your dog, walking to visit a friend, or walking to class or work, taking precautions to arrive at your destination safely is worthwhile. The lessons parents and teachers taught you about how to walk safely still apply. It is always best to walk on sidewalks and cross at intersections in a crosswalk, paying attention to traffic signals. If there are no sidewalks, walk as far to the left as possible, and walk facing traffic. Put your cell phone or other electronic device in your pocket so you are paying attention to what is going on around you, particularly when crossing the street. If you are wearing headphones, pull them off or turn off the volume when crossing the street. Even when you have a walk signal, it is always wise to look both ways before crossing. Be a good citizen and be aware of others who are distracted; speak up if you see someone in danger.[72]

When people are walking while talking or texting on their mobile phone, they exhibit reduced situational awareness, distracted attention, and unsafe behavior. Using data on injuries in hospital emergency departments from 2004 through 2010, researchers found that mobile phone–related injuries among pedestrians increased compared to total pedestrian injuries, and in 2010 they exceeded mobile phone–related injuries for drivers. Pedestrian injuries associated with mobile phone use were higher for males and people under 31 years of age. The researchers concluded that using a mobile phone while walking puts pedestrians at risk of accident, injury, or death.[73]

If you are walking at night, carry a flashlight and wear retroreflective clothing (i.e., clothing that reflects light toward its source) so that drivers see you.[74] Be aware of cars that are turning or backing up. Driveways and alleys may pose extra danger.

Motor Vehicle Traffic–Related Pedestrian Deaths

Of all motor vehicle deaths in 2016, 16% were pedestrians, which translates to almost 6,000 pedestrian deaths. A pedestrian is killed every 1.5 hours and the rate was highest among those 50 to 54 years of age. From 2001 to 2010, the rate was highest among American Indians/Alaska Natives. Males are more than twice as likely as females to die as a pedestrian. Rates are highest in large central metro areas.[75]

Drowning

Every day, about ten people die from unintentional drowning. From 2005 to 2014, there were an average of more than 3,500 accidental drownings.[76] Of those who died, 80% were males. At all ages, African Americans die of drowning at significantly higher rates than do Caucasians.

Why do African Americans have higher rates of drowning? The reasons include lower access to swimming pools and swimming lessons. Published rates of drowning are based on the population as a whole, not participation in swimming-related activities. Researchers hypothesize that if the rates were based on actual participation, there would be a much larger disparity between Caucasian and African American drowning rates.[77]

Research shows that formal swimming lessons can reduce the risk of drowning.[78] A study on the constraints of swimming among minority youth found that even when the researchers accounted for income, African American students had significantly lower swimming ability than Caucasian or Hispanic youth. Fear of injury and drowning was a strong predictor of no or low swimming ability. Fear of the water, whether by a parent or child, trumps concerns about finances as a reason for not learning to swim. Concern about getting their hair wet was also an issue for African American girls.[79]

Other factors influence drowning risk for the entire population. A four-sided isolation fence (separating the pool area from the house and yard) reduces a child's risk of drowning 83% compared to three-sided property-line fencing, separating the pool from the street, but not from the house.[80] While young children are more likely to drown in home swimming pools, the percentage of drownings in lakes, rivers, and oceans increases with age. The CDC reports that 57% of fatal and 57% of nonfatal drownings among individuals 15 years and older occurred in natural settings.[81]

Alcohol use is involved in 70% of drowning deaths among adolescents and adults associated with water recreation. Drinking alcohol significantly increased the likelihood of drowning. Sun exposure and heat intensify the

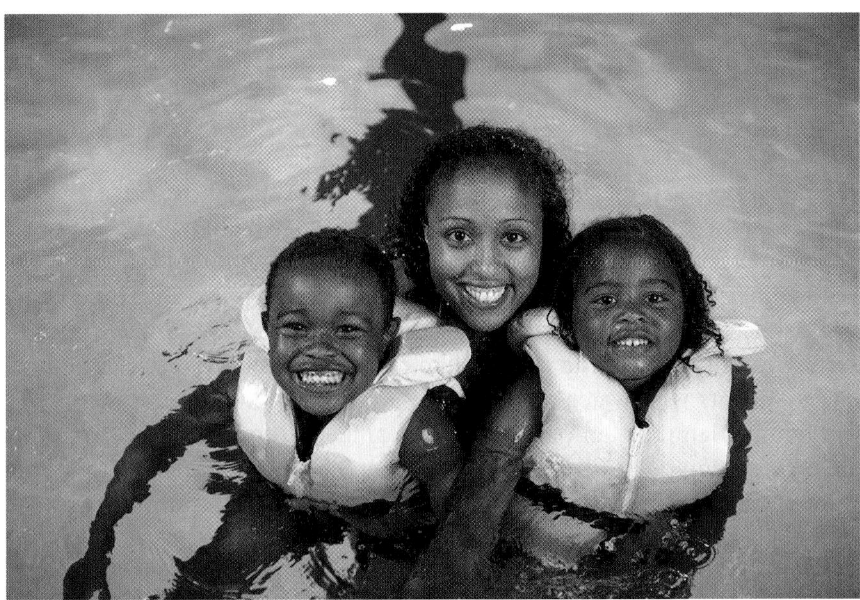

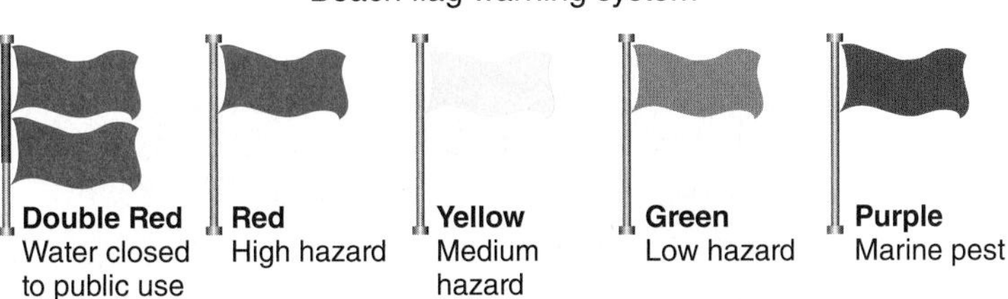

FIGURE 9-4 Beach warning flags.

effects of alcohol. On boats, men tend to drink more and behave in riskier ways than women do.[82]

Tips to being safe in the water include the following[83]:

- *Use the buddy system.* Don't swim alone.
- *Learn cardiopulmonary resuscitation (CPR).* Seconds do count. CPR performed by bystanders has saved lives and improved outcomes for drowning victims.
- *Learn to swim.* It is never too late.
- *Use U.S. Coast Guard–approved life jackets.* Float toys, such as noodles or inner tubes are just that—toys—and are not intended to keep a swimmer safe.
- *Don't mix alcohol and swimming.*

An additional tip if you are in a natural water setting is to know and obey warnings represented by colored beach flags (**FIGURE 9-4**). Watch for dangerous waves and signs of a rip current. If you do get caught in a rip current, swim parallel to shore until you are free of the current. Then swim diagonally toward the shore.[83]

Burns

A burn is harm to the body's tissue caused by heat, chemicals, electricity, sunlight, or radiation. Burns are extremely common, with 486,000 burns receiving medical treatment in hospitals in 2011, 3,240 deaths occurring in 2013 due to fire/smoke inhalation, and 40,000 burn-related hospitalizations in 2010. Many minor burns may be treated at clinics, in a doctor's office, or at home.[84]

Tanning

The media often projects images that imply being tan is attractive and desirable—it's sexy! But no matter how you do it—whether you get a tan on a beach or a tanning bed—it is undeniably harmful. Indoor tanning is widespread among young adults in the United States, despite scientific evidence that it is a risk factor for skin cancer. College students' belief that tanning improves their appearance makes them more likely to tan.[85] Other research shows that college students who watch reality television beauty shows are more likely to use a tanning lamp or tan outdoors.[86] Researchers from Tennessee found that appearance trumped health among college students in deciding whether or not to tan. The researchers used an appearance-focused intervention that included exercise, choosing fashions that do not require a complementary tan, and the use of sunless tanning products to reduce tanning behaviors.[87]

You want to and need to preserve your skin (**FIGURE 9-5**)[88]. The sun affects the cells that renew your skin, contributing to wrinkles and lots of brown spots. Tanning ages your skin and increases the risk of skin cancer. In the past

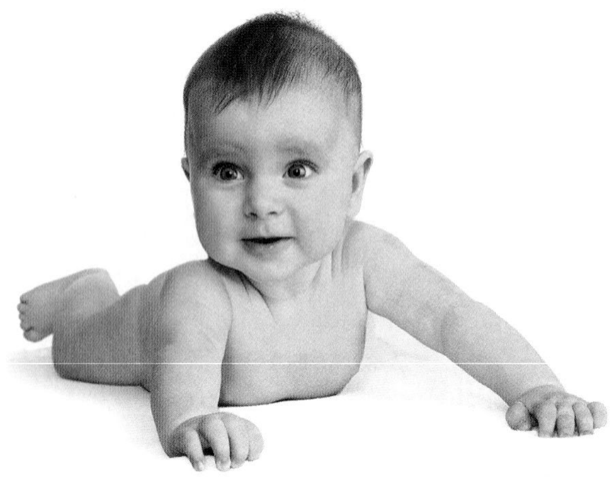

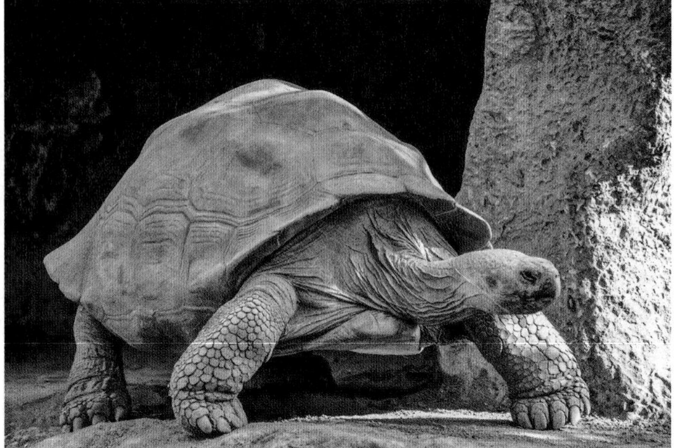

FIGURE 9-5 What kind of skin do you want?

FACT VS. FICTION

Tanning

Myth 1: A base tan is "nature's sunscreen."

Fact: Sun damages your cells regardless of your skin color. A tan means that you have already damaged your skin.

Myth 2: Sunscreen is toxic.

Fact: There has been concern about sunscreen containing oxybenzone. However, a recent study found it to be nontoxic.[91] If you are still concerned, you can choose sunscreen made with titanium. Make sure you use enough sunscreen: Apply about 1 ounce or a shot-glass amount of SPF 30 or higher. Apply at least 20 minutes before going outside. Reapply sunscreen at least every 2 hours, or more frequently if you are swimming or sweating.

Additional options include choosing sun-protective clothing and a wide-brimmed hat, and sitting in the shade.[92]

Myth 3: Sun doesn't cause wrinkles.

Fact: Exposing your skin to the sun causes changes such as wrinkles and sagging. It also causes internal changes to the structure and function of the skin.[93]

Myth 4: Using a tanning bed gives a person a "healthy glow."

Fact: Whether you lie in the sun or a tanning bed, you are exposing yourself to harmful UV rays that damage your skin. You increase your risk for melanoma with every tan.[94]

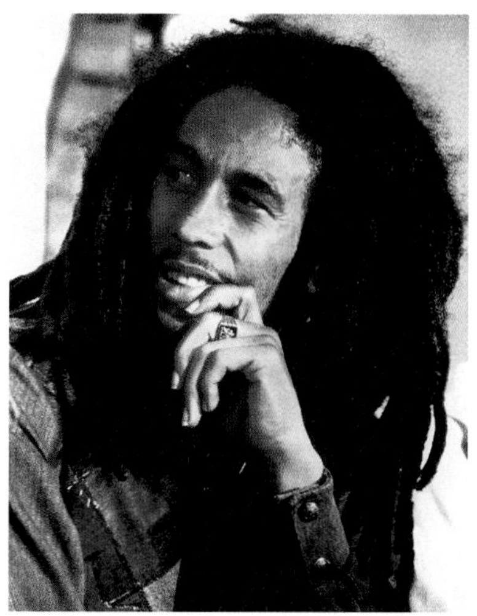

Jamaican singer and musician, Bob Marley, died of acral lentiginous melanoma when he was 36 years old.

40 years, the risk of melanoma has increased among 18- to 39-year-olds by 800% in women and 400% in men.[89] The incidence of nonmelanoma skin cancer also has increased,[90] and exposure to tanning increases the risk.

Even if you have dark skin tone, you should use sunscreen. Anyone can get skin cancer. It is true that the darker your skin, the more melatonin you have, and this does help protect you. However, people of color can get sunburned and have the same poor outcomes as people who are light skinned.[95] Despite the fact that Caucasians have higher rates of melanoma, overall survival is better for them than (in order) Hispanics, Asian American/Native American/Pacific Islanders, and Blacks.[96]

Some celebrities have shunned tanning: They are taking the glamour and prestige out of being tanned. Among the celebrities who do not tan are Amanda Seyfried, Amy Adams, Anna Kendrick, Anne Hathaway, Cate Blanchett, Emma Stone, Emma Watson, Evan Rachel Wood, Gwen Stefani, Keira Knightley, Kirsten Dunst, Michelle Williams, Naomi Watts, Nicole Kidman, Scarlett Johansson, Taylor Swift, and Zooey Deschanel.

Be Safe in Your Home: House Fires

The majority of deaths due to fires are in homes without a working smoke alarm. Manufacturers of smoke alarms specify where they should be placed (wall or ceiling). Newly built housing should have smoke alarms powered by the building's electrical system. Otherwise, battery-powered smoke alarms are acceptable. Every floor of your home should have a smoke alarm. The alarm should be clearly audible in all bedrooms over background noise levels with intervening doors closed.[97] Federal law requires dormitories to have smoke detectors in good working order. Group housing should have smoke detectors in sleeping areas, in every room in the path leading to the sleeping area, and on each story, including the basement.[98] State regulations regarding smoke alarms can be found at www.ajfire.org/uploads/smoke_alarm_requirements.pdf. If your smoke alarm is battery powered, change the batteries annually.

Keep emergency phone numbers and other pertinent information posted close to your telephone.

BY THE NUMBERS

Fires

- Between 2011 and 2015, there were an average of 4,100 fires per year in dormitories, fraternities, sororities, and related buildings.
- Most fires occur in the evening between 5:00 p.m. and 11:00 p.m.
- September and October are the most common months for dormitory fires.
- Cooking equipment was involved in 87% of dormitory-type fires.

Have an escape plan to leave your house or apartment if there is a fire. If you live in a dormitory, practice all fire drills as if they were a real fire. Know the dorm's evacuation plan. Depending on the age and construction of your home, fire can spread rapidly. Walk through your home and inspect all possible exit and escape routes. Think about your floor plan and find two exits from each room. Windows can serve as emergency exits. Practice evacuating your home twice a year. Designate a meeting place with other occupants of your home a safe distance away from the house. Never go back into a burning building to look for missing people or pets. That is the responsibility of the fire department. Treat every alarm as if it were a real fire. Wait until you are out of the building to call the fire department.[99]

If you find yourself trapped in a burning building, you will need to employ important survival tactics. Smoke rises, so drop to the ground and crawl to an

TALES OF PUBLIC HEALTH

The Station Nightclub Fire

On February 20, 2003, the band Great White was headlining at The Station, a rock-and-roll club in West Warwick, Rhode Island. At the beginning of the show, the tour manager set off pyrotechnics, which are designed to produce a controlled spray of sparks. The sparks from the pyrotechnics ignited the acoustic foam on both sides of the drummer's alcove.[100]

Patrons thought the flames were part of the show. Only when the fire reached the ceiling and smoke began to pour down did people realize they were in danger. Almost instantly, the entire stage was engulfed in flames, with the band members bolting for the exit door. In a little over 5 minutes, flames filled the club.

As the flames spread, most patrons headed for the front doors. Someone had chained two of the four exits shut. A bouncer initially forbade patrons from using the stage door, creating a bottleneck at the front door. More than one patron reported the bouncer stating that that door was "for the band only."

The club's official licensed capacity was 404 people. There were 462 people in attendance; of them, 100 people died and 230 were injured. After the fire, the National Fire Protection Association enacted strict new code provisions for fire sprinklers and crowd management in nightclub-type venues.

To see a video about a survivor of The Station fire and his experience, search for NFPA and the station fire.

exit if you are trapped in a burning building. If it is safe to leave, exit the building as quickly as possible. Because smoke inhalation is a problem, cover your nose and mouth with a cloth, preferably one that is moist. Test doorknobs and the space around the door with the back of your hand to feel the temperature. If it is warm, try another escape route. If it is cool, open the door slowly. Close it quickly if smoke enters the room. Never use an elevator during a fire.[97] To understand how quickly a situation can become deadly, see the Tales of Public Health box.

If you are trapped inside, call the fire department for assistance. If you can't get to a phone, yell out a window for help. Wave or hang something out the window to attract attention. Open the windows only slightly at the top and bottom. If smoke enters through the window, close it quickly.[97]

First Aid

TABLE 9-4 describes the different types of burns and lists the signs and treatment for each type of burn.

The treatment a burn victim receives in the first few minutes after the burn can make a huge difference in the severity of the injury. The priority is to smother the flames. If a person's clothing is on fire, direct the person to "stop, drop, and roll." Remove all of the person's burned clothing. If clothing adheres to the skin, cut or tear around the burned area. It is imperative to remove all jewelry, belts, and tight clothing from the burned areas and from around the burn victim's neck, because burned areas swell immediately.[97]

TABLE 9-4 Types of Burns, Signs, and Treatment[97]

Description	Signs	Treatment
First-degree burns: involve the top layer of skin (Sunburn is a first-degree burn.)	▪ Red ▪ Painful to touch ▪ Skin shows mild swelling	▪ Apply cool, wet compresses, or immerse in cool, fresh water. Continue until pain subsides. ▪ Cover the burn with a sterile, nonadhesive bandage or clean cloth. ▪ Do *not* apply ointments or butter to burn. ▪ Over-the-counter pain medications may be used to help relieve pain and reduce inflammation. ▪ First-degree burns usually heal without further treatment. However, if a first-degree burn covers a large area of the body, or the victim is an infant or elderly, seek emergency medical attention.
Second-degree burns: involve the first two layers of skin	▪ Deep reddening of the skin ▪ Pain ▪ Blisters ▪ Glossy appearance from leaking fluid ▪ Possible loss of some skin	▪ Immerse in fresh, cool water, or apply cool compresses. Continue for 10 to 15 minutes. ▪ Dry with clean cloth and cover with sterile gauze. ▪ Do *not* break blisters. ▪ Do *not* apply ointments or butter to burns. ▪ Elevate burned arms or legs. ▪ Take steps to prevent shock: lay the victim flat; elevate the feet about 12 inches. Cover the victim with a coat or blanket. Do *not* place the victim in the shock position if a head, neck, back, or leg injury is suspected, or if it makes the victim uncomfortable. ▪ Further medical treatment is required. Do *not* attempt to treat serious burns unless you are a trained health professional.

(continues)

TABLE 9-4 Types of Burns, Signs, and Treatment[97] *(continued)*

Description	Signs	Treatment
Third-degree burns: penetrate the entire thickness of the skin and permanently destroy tissue	▪ Loss of skin layers ▪ Often painless (Pain may be caused by patches of first- and second-degree burns that surround third-degree burns.) ▪ Skin is dry and leathery. ▪ Skin may appear charred or have patches that appear white, brown, or black.	▪ Cover burn lightly with sterile gauze or clean cloth. (Don't use material that can leave lint on the burn.) ▪ Do *not* apply ointments or butter to burns; these may cause infection. ▪ Take steps to prevent shock: lay the victim flat; elevate the feet about 12 inches. ▪ Have person sit up if face is burned. Watch closely for possible breathing problems. ▪ Elevate burned area higher than the victim's head when possible. Keep person warm and comfortable, and watch for signs of shock. ▪ Do *not* place a pillow under the victim's head if the person is lying down and there is an airway burn. This can close the airway. ▪ *Immediate* medical attention is required. Do *not* attempt to treat serious burns unless you are a trained health professional.

Centers for Disease Control and Prevention (CDC). Burns.

Thunder and Lightning

Around the world, lightning strikes the earth more than 100 times each second or 8 million times per day.[101] In the United States, lightning strikes about 25 million times a year. For an average person in the United States, the lifetime risk of being struck by lightning is estimated at 3.3 in 10,000, and the risk of being killed by lightning is 28.6 in 1,000,000.[101] Although the odds of being struck by lightning are not high, it is important to take precautions seriously.

FACT VS. FICTION

Lightning

Myth: Lightning never strikes the same place twice.

Fact: Lightning often strikes the same place repeatedly, especially if it is a tall, pointy, isolated object. The Empire State Building is struck nearly 23 times per year.[102]

If you hear thunder, lightning is close enough for you to be in danger. Even when there is a blue sky above you, if you hear thunder, it is important to seek shelter. Lightning can travel up to 10 miles horizontally before touching the ground. If there is a thunderstorm, the safest place to be is inside in a significant, closed shelter. Buildings like rain shelters or sheds do not provide protection because they lack a grounding mechanism. According to the CDC, when you are inside during a thunderstorm, you should avoid water and electrical equipment, including corded phones. Stay away from open windows.[103] Wait for at least 30 minutes after the last time you hear thunder before you go outside.

If there are no buildings around, the next best choice is a hardtop automobile, which will also provide protection. If you are outside with no option of going inside, take the precautions described in the box below.

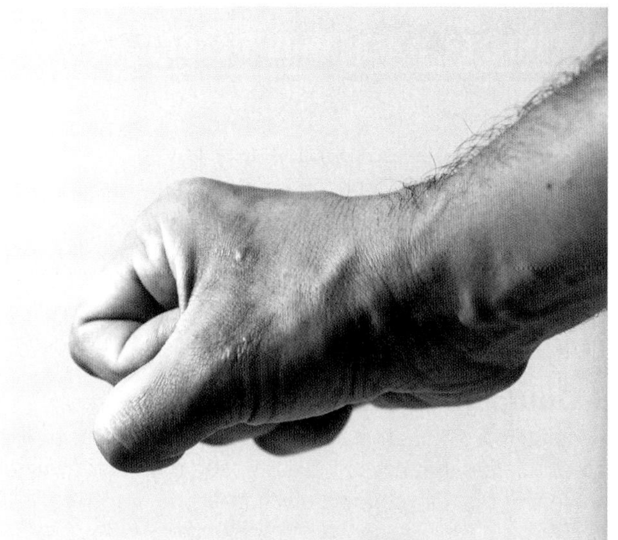

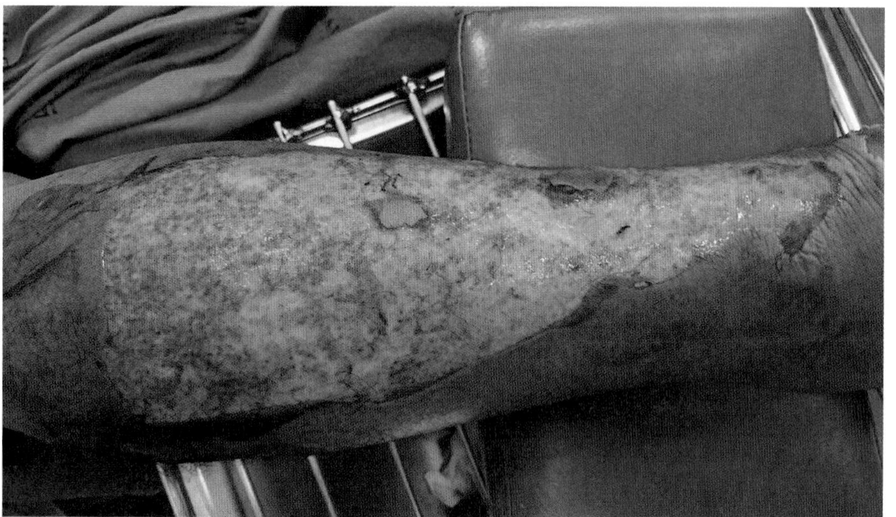

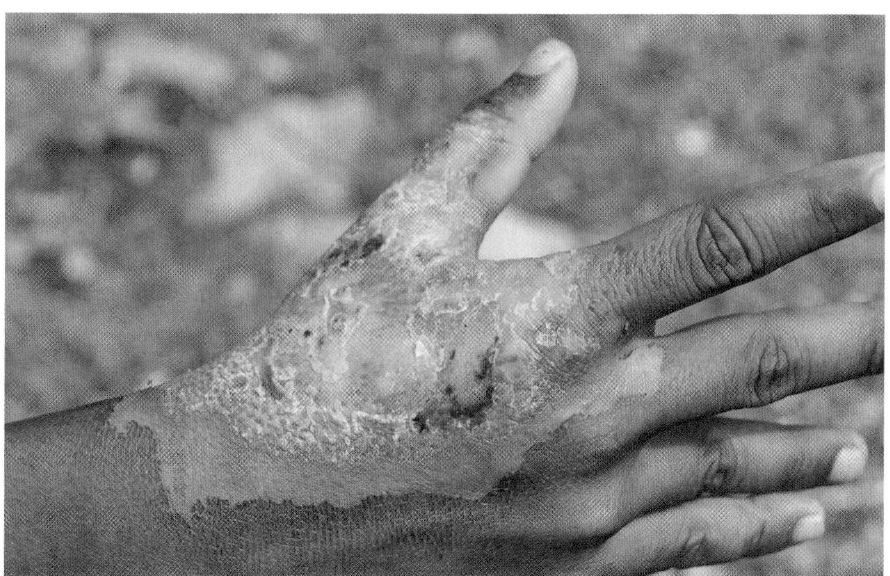

(A) First-degree burn. (B) Second-degree burn. (C) Third-degree burn.

IF THERE'S NO SHELTER, WHERE SHOULD I GO?[104]

In a Forest

Retreat to a group of small trees surrounded by taller trees, or find a dry, low area like a depression or ravine. Avoid lone trees and other tall objects as well as rocky outcrops and ledges.

In an Open Area

Look for a dry, low-lying area such as a valley and become the smallest target possible. Minimize your contact with the ground, and do not lie down flat.

Anywhere Outdoors

You can take shelter in a car or other safe shelter, but not a tent. In all cases, avoid bodies of water and areas that have high flash-flood potential. Avoid objects such as barbed wire fences that can conduct electricity.

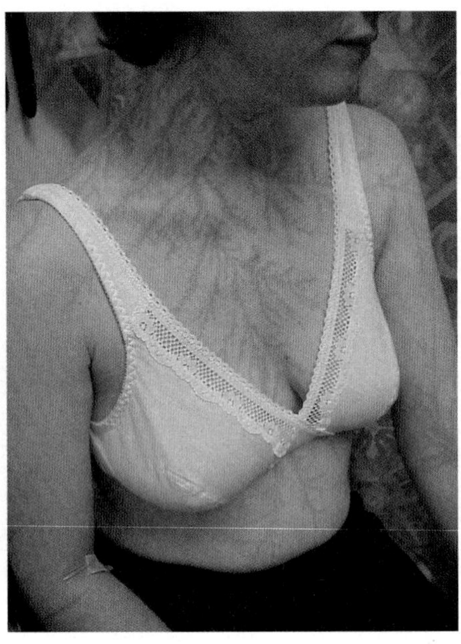

FIGURE 9-6 Lichtenberg figure from lightning.

Reproduced from Mahajan, A. L., Rajan, R., & Regan, P. J. (2008). Lichtenberg figures: cutaneous manifestation of phone electrocution from lightning. Journal of Plastic, Reconstructive & Aesthetic Surgery, 61(1), 111-113.

When someone is struck by lightning, get emergency help as soon as possible. If more than one person is struck by lightning, treat the unconscious person first. Although the person may appear to be dead, with no pulse or breath, he or she may respond to CPR. Treat conscious persons next. Common injuries include burns, wounds, and fractures. Lightning fatalities are usually caused by a heart attack.[105]

The electrical discharge from lightning can leave a tattoo-like scar with fractal properties, called a Lichtenberg figure (**FIGURE 9-6**).[106]

Poisonings

Poisonings happen more often than you think. In 2016, more than 2.8 million calls were made to poison control centers because someone had been exposed to **poison**. Another 54,000 calls were made for animals exposed to poisons. While 60% of exposures are to children (defined by the American Association of Poison Control Centers as younger than age 20 years), 94.8% of deaths due to poisoning are to people 20 years and over.[107]

poison A substance that can cause illness or death of a living organism when introduced or absorbed.

COMMON POISONOUS SUBSTANCES

The following is a list of the most common poisonous substances to which adults are exposed (in order of frequency):

- Analgesics
- Sedative/hypnotics and antipsychotics
- Antidepressants
- Cardiovascular drugs
- Cleaning substances (household)
- Alcohols
- Pesticides
- Bites and envenomations (being bitten or stung by a venomous animal/insect)
- Anticonvulsants
- Antihistamines
- Cosmetics/personal care products
- Hormones and hormone antagonists
- Stimulants and street drugs
- Fumes/gases/vapors
- Chemicals
- Antimicrobials
- Cold and cough preparations
- Muscle relaxants
- Hydrocarbons
- Topical preparations
- Gastrointestinal preparations
- Foreign bodies, toys, and miscellaneous objects
- Miscellaneous drugs

Poison is any substance that can harm you. Substances that may be safe when used correctly can also be poisonous. If a substance can harm you when used incorrectly, by the wrong person, or in the wrong amount, it is a poison.[108] Some substances are poison when swallowed or inhaled, others when they get on the skin or in the eyes. Poisons can be ingested, inhaled, injected, or absorbed.

If you live with young children, most of the adult exposures are also on the list for children. Household cleaning substances are of particular concern. In addition to adult exposures, children also commonly ingest vitamins, plants, dietary supplements (including herbal and homeopathic), deodorizers, and arts/crafts/office supplies.[107]

Every poisoning is distinct and unique. Treatment advice will depend on the type and the amount of poison. If a person is unconscious or has trouble breathing, call 9-1-1. Then call 1-800-222-1222, which will connect you to your local poison control center. Do *not* wait for signs of poisoning.

When accidents happen, get help. If a person inhaled poison, get him or her to fresh air right away. If a person has poison on his or her skin, remove any clothing that may have poison on it. Rinse the skin for 15 to 20 minutes. If the person got poison in his or her eye, rinse the eyes with running water for 15 to 20 minutes. If a person takes the wrong medicine or too much medicine, do *not* try to administer first aid. Call 1-800-222-1222.[109]

Preventing Poisoning due to Medicines

Never take expired medication, and never take medicine in the dark. If you are prescribed multiple medications, it is easy to be confused about what you have and have not taken. Pill organizers are inexpensive and easy to use. Read the warning labels on your prescription medications and follow the directions. Some medications cannot be taken with other medicines or with alcohol.[110]

Today, over-the-counter medicine comes in packaging designed to prevent tampering. If you think there is a problem, don't take the medicine. Return the medicine to the store manager where you bought it. Prescription medicines are available in childproof bottles. While childproof containers have helped reduce the number of poisonings, a determined child can manage to open them.[111]

Carbon Monoxide Poisoning

Carbon monoxide is an odorless, colorless gas that is poisonous. Cars, appliances, grills, gas ranges, furnaces, and gas clothes dryers can give off carbon monoxide. The signs of carbon monoxide poisoning are similar to those of the flu, including a headache, dizziness, weakness, upset stomach, vomiting, chest pain, and confusion. If you think you have been exposed to carbon monoxide, immediately go outside and call poison control (1-800-222-1222). If you feel better when you go outside but the symptoms return when you reenter your house or apartment, suspect carbon monoxide exposure. Call 9-1-1 and have the fire department check for carbon monoxide. If carbon monoxide is present, you cannot return home until the source has been repaired.

Make sure gas appliances have a seal of a national testing agency, such as the Underwriters Laboratories. Make sure gas appliances are properly vented. Never use a gas range or oven for heating your house. Never use gas camp stoves or grills inside the house. Generators should be at least 20 feet away from any window, door, or vent. Never run your car inside an attached garage, even if the garage door is open.[112]

Drug Poisoning, Intoxication, and Overdose

On February 2, 2014, the actor, director, and producer of film and theater, Philip Seymour Hoffman, died of an overdose, caused by an "acute mixed drug intoxication including heroin, cocaine, benzodiazepines, and amphetamine."[113] While this story received a lot of attention when it happened because it involved

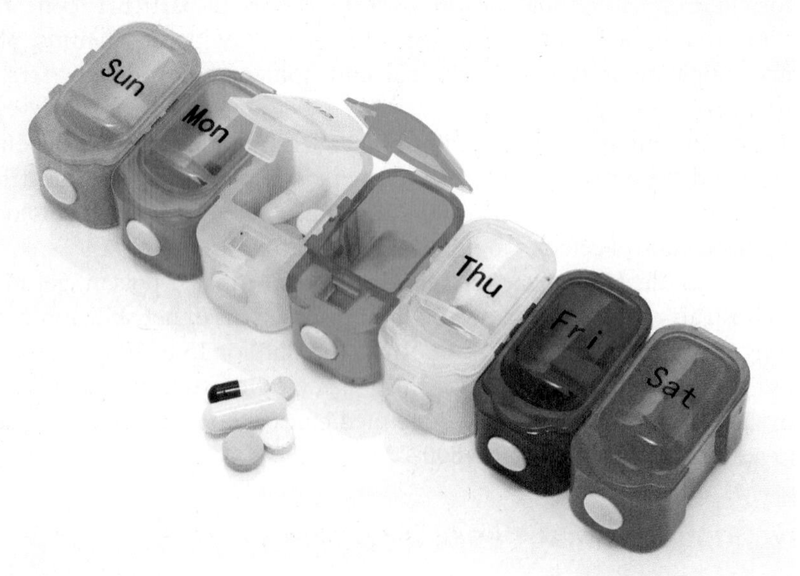

Pill organizer.

KEEPING YOUR PET SAFE

Foods that are perfectly safe for you may be dangerous to your pet. To learn more about foods to avoid feeding your pets, visit the American Society for the Prevention of Cruelty to Animals (ASPCA) web page and search for people foods to avoid feeding your pets.

Although this list is not exhaustive, foods you should not feed your pets include the following: alcoholic beverages, apple seeds, apricot pits, avocados, candy (particularly chocolate—which is toxic to dogs, cats, and ferrets—and any candy containing the toxic sweetener xylitol), cherry pits, coffee (grounds, beans, and chocolate-covered espresso beans), eggs (raw), fat trimmings, garlic and garlic powder, grapes and raisins, gum (can cause blockages, and sugar-free gums may contain the toxic sweetener xylitol), hops (used in home beer brewing), macadamia nuts, milk and dairy products, onions and onion powder, peach pits, plum pits, persimmon seeds, potato leaves and stems (green parts), raw meat and fish, rhubarb leaves, salt, sugary foods and drinks, tea and other items containing caffeine, tomato leaves and stems (green parts), walnuts, xylitol (artificial sweetener that is toxic to pets), and yeast dough. If you are concerned, call the ASPCA at 1-888-426-4435. They specialize in the treatment of animal poisoning.

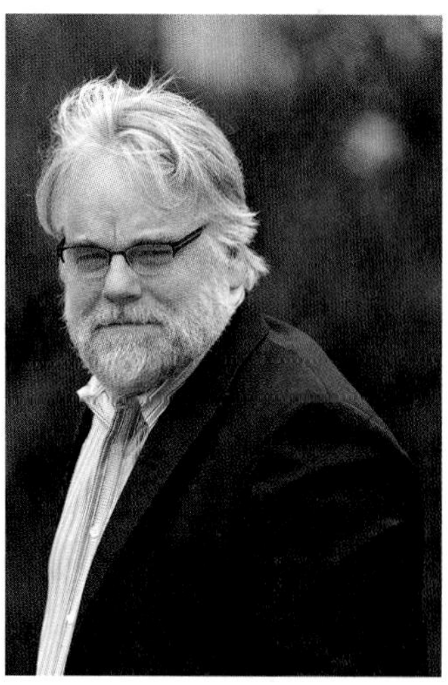

Phillip Seymour Hoffman.

a celebrity, what most people don't know is that approximately 100 people die every day from **drug overdose**. In addition, the stereotypes that many people hold about the types of people who die of drug overdoses do not mirror reality. Most people who have drug problems have regular lives: school or jobs, friends, families. Drug use and overdose are an epidemic that affects a broad swath of American society. What many adolescents and young adults consume is a polypharmacy of whatever they can get: alcohol, legal pharmaceuticals, and illegal street drugs.[114]

drug overdose Taking too much of a substance, whether it is a prescription drug, over-the-counter medication, or a supplement. It may be legal or illegal. It can be intentional or unintentional. If you have taken enough of the substance to have a harmful effect, you have overdosed. The severity of the overdose is dependent upon the individual (physical and medical history), the drug, and the amount of the drug consumed. It can cause serious medical complications, the most severe being death.

Drug overdoses can be accidental or intentional and can result from taking prescription or illegal drugs. Earlier in this section, we focused on medication overdose, here we will be talking primarily about illegal drugs.

An overdose happens when a person's metabolism cannot detoxify the drug fast enough to avoid inadvertent consequences. A person's body weight and personal sensitivity to the drug and the ingredients used to cut or dilute the drug all affect how toxic it is for an individual. An amount that is safe for one person may be too much for another person's body to handle. The concept of "safety" is used here in a relative way; it does not imply that taking illegal drugs is in any way a good idea or safe. An overdose may result in dangerous symptoms or death.

Alcohol Poisoning

College is a time when many people drink alcohol, and they often drink heavily. If you are going to drink, it is helpful to understand what alcohol does to your body. Alcohol is a depressant, in that it depresses the nerves controlling involuntary functions, like breathing and your gag reflex (which prevents choking). Too much alcohol will eventually cause you to stop breathing and inhibit your gag reflex. Because it is common for someone who has drunk too much to vomit, there is a danger of choking on the vomit and dying by asphyxiation if the person is unconscious.[115]

It is possible for blood alcohol concentration (the amount of alcohol in the bloodstream) to rise even if a person has passed out. The alcohol a person has already consumed and is in their stomach will continue to be digested and enter their bloodstream. It is not safe to assume that a person who drank too much will be okay if they go to sleep.[115]

The signs that a person may have an alcohol overdose include breathing slower than eight breaths per minute; or irregular breathing, vomiting, mental confusion; or you cannot wake the person, seizure, and a low body temperature. If a person has these symptoms, call 9-1-1 for help. Even if you or the person is too young to be legally drinking alcohol, it is a better choice to get help.[115]

Many people believe that there are easy ways to get sober, such as drinking coffee, taking a cold shower, eating something, sleeping it off, or walking it off. However, what you really need is time. Time is the only thing that reduces your blood alcohol level.

Heroin

Heroin comes from morphine, which is extracted from the seedpods of Asian (opium) poppy plants. It is highly addictive. Symptoms of a heroin overdose are shallow, slow, and labored breathing or absence of breathing. Overdose also causes a person's mouth to become dry and the pupils to become very small, or "pinpoint." The person's blood pressure may be low, and because the person is not getting enough oxygen, his or her nails and lips may look bluish. The person may be delirious and disoriented. These symptoms indicate a life-threatening condition, so seek medical care immediately.[116]

Cocaine

Cocaine is an illegal stimulant drug that affects the central nervous system. It is derived from the *Erythroxylum coca* plant. It is a white powder that can be snorted, injected, or made into crack and smoked. Symptoms of cocaine overdose may include anxiety and nervousness or distress, chest pain, enlarged pupils, euphoria, and increased heart rate and blood pressure. At higher doses, these symptoms may be exaggerated and include hyperthermia (seriously elevated body temperature), seizures, and stroke. Seek treatment if someone who has used cocaine experiences any of these symptoms. Medications will be given to counteract the symptoms, to lower the heart rate and blood pressure, and to treat the anxiety or agitation.[117]

Methamphetamine

Methamphetamine is a common illegal street drug. Taking a large amount of methamphetamine can cause agitation, increased heart rate and blood pressure, paranoia, seizures, severe stomach pain, and stroke. In extreme cases, a person's heart can stop, or the person can go into a coma. Long-term use of methamphetamine can cause both psychological problems (insomnia, paranoia, and delusional behavior) and physical problems (severe weight loss, missing and rotted teeth [called "meth mouth"], and skin sores).[118] Meth mouth is caused by the lack of saliva, extended periods of poor oral hygiene, high sugar intake, and bruxism (teeth grinding).

Synthetic Cannabinoids

Synthetic cannabinoids—commonly referred to as K2, Spice, and synthetic marijuana—are becoming a large public health problem due to their increasing popularity and their unpredictable toxicity. Synthetic cannabinoids, although chemically similar to THC—the active ingredient in marijuana—have higher rates of toxicity than natural marijuana.[119] The year 2015 brought an increase in

BY THE NUMBERS

Recreational Drug Use

One recent study of an emergency department in Switzerland noted that almost 70% of visits for recreational drug use were among men. Of the patients, 19% were 16 to 20 years old and 37% were 21 to 30 years old. The most commonly used recreational drug was cocaine, but the list also included cannabis, benzodiazepines ("downers"), opioids, and amphetamines. Forty-four percent of the patients had used more than one drug. The authors concluded that most visits to the emergency department were for medical problems related to illicit drugs, psychiatric disorders, or both.[121]

the number of hospitalizations and calls to poison control centers due to consumption of synthetic cannabinoid. Users can experience anxiety and agitation, nausea, high blood pressure, seizures, hallucinations, and paranoia.[120]

Drug Overdose Overview

It isn't just the drugs that are bad for you. Sometimes the drugs include by-products that come from the manufacturing process. They may also be cut or diluted at any point along the distribution chain to improve the dealers' profit margin. In choosing a cutting agent, a drug manufacturer or dealer wants to find a chemical that is inexpensive, easy to obtain, relatively nontoxic, and similar in physical attributes to the drug to be adulterated. Given some of the agents that have been used to dilute drugs, relative toxicity is likely the least important of these characteristics. Agents used to cut drugs include flour, sugar, salt, rat poison, and ground plasterboard.

Overuse and Repetitive Motion Injuries

There is a fine line between **overuse injury** and **repetitive motion injuries**. Overuse injuries are the most common type of injury sustained by people participating in physical activities. These injuries are usually the result of poor training techniques, poor body mechanics, or both. An overuse injury results from stressing the joints, muscles, or other tissues without allowing them enough time between events to recover. Examples of overuse injuries include runner's knee, swimmer's shoulder, **tennis elbow** (inflammation of the tendons of the elbow), shin splints, and iliotibial band syndrome (pain along the outside of the thigh and knee).

Repetitive motion injuries describe injuries associated with repetitive tasks, forceful exertions, or sustained/awkward positions. These are injuries to the tendons, ligaments, muscles, or nerves, caused by performing the same motion over and over again during normal daily activities.[122] Among the common overuse and repetitive motion injuries are Achilles tendinopathy, tendinosis, bursitis, patellofemoral pain syndrome, plantar fasciitis, rotator cuff disorders, and tennis elbow.

overuse injury Muscle or joint injury caused by repetitive trauma.

repetitive motion injuries Temporary or permanent injuries to muscles, nerves, ligaments, and tendons caused by doing the same motion over and over again; also called repetitive stress injuries.

tennis elbow Soreness or pain on the outer part of the elbow that occurs when a person damages the tendons that connect the muscles in the forearm to the elbow.

Achilles Tendinopathy

If you have had a problem with your Achilles tendon (the tendon that begins in the middle of your calf and connects to your heel bone), your perception may be that it was a sudden event. Usually, however, these problems are the result of many tiny tears in the tendon that have happened over time. When you play

TENDINOSIS VS. TENDINITIS VS. TENDINOPATHY[125]

The suffix *itis* means inflammation; thus, the term *tendinitis* refers to a tendon injury that involves an acute injury with inflammation.

The suffix *osis* indicates a pathology of chronic degeneration without inflammation. The term *tendinosis* refers to an accumulation over time of microscopic tendon injuries that do not heal properly. Although there may be inflammation in the initial stages of the injury, it is the inability of the tendon to heal that causes the pain and disability.

Tendinopathy is a more general term that does not suggest the pathology of the injury.

sports that involve a lot of stop-and-go motions or pushing off, you raise the risk of Achilles tendon microtears.[123]

The main symptoms of Achilles tendinopathy include swelling in the ankle area and pain, which can be either mild or severe, and may develop and progress slowly. Causes of overuse injuries include muscle imbalance, poor core stability, lack of good muscle strength, biomechanical issues like flat feet, training improperly, focusing on how much weight you are lifting rather than proper technique, and lack of flexibility.[124]

Treatment depends on the length and seriousness of the symptoms. Rest and time off from sports are important, particularly for high-impact sports.

Tendinosis

Tendinosis is an accumulation over time of small-scale injuries that do not heal properly. Although you cannot see a tendinosis injury on the outside of your body, it can occur in your wrist, forearm, elbow, shoulder, knee, or heel.

When your muscles do more work than they can handle, they sustain some damage. When the demand is gradual, your muscle and tendon tissues heal and become stronger. However, if you continue to perform the activity before the tendon has a chance to heal, gradually you develop more of these microinjuries until you feel pain. As with Achilles tendinopathy, tendon injuries require patience. It is helpful to remember that tendons heal more slowly than muscles do.[125]

Bursitis

Bursae (singular: *bursa*) are small fluid-filled sacs situated in places where friction would otherwise occur; they cushion and lubricate where tendons, ligaments, skin, muscles, or bones rub against each other. Bursitis is the painful inflammation of the bursae.[126] Overuse or repeated motions can cause bursitis. People who repeat the same movement over and over, whether in their jobs, sports, or daily activities, have a greater chance of developing bursitis. Typing on a keyboard, gardening, and cooking can all cause bursitis. Putting continual pressure on the same area day after day can also cause bursitis.

Patellofemoral Pain Syndrome

Patellofemoral pain syndrome is pain in the front of the knee. It often occurs in teenagers, manual laborers, and athletes. Overuse, injury, excess weight, and sometimes wearing down or softening of the cartilage under the knee can cause patellofemoral pain syndrome.[127] The primary symptom of patellofemoral pain syndrome is knee pain, especially when sitting with bent knees, squatting, jumping, or using the stairs (especially going down stairs).

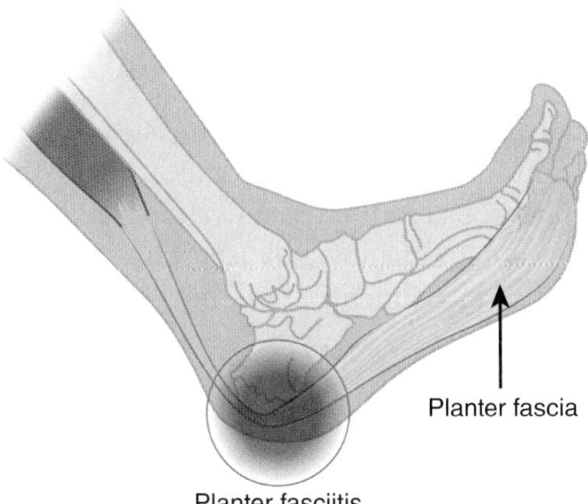

Plantar fasciitis.

Plantar Fasciitis

Plantar fasciitis is the most common cause of heel pain. Straining the ligament that supports the arch causes plantar fasciitis. While it is common in people who are middle-aged, it also occurs in younger people who are on their feet a lot, such as athletes or soldiers.[128]

plantar fasciitis An inflammation of the tissue that runs across the bottom of the foot and connects the heel bone to the toes (plantar fascia).

Conditions that increase the likelihood of getting plantar fasciitis include having high arches or flat feet; overpronating (a tendency of the feet to roll too far inward when walking or running); wearing shoes that are worn out or don't fit properly; walking, standing, or running for long periods, especially on hard surfaces; and being overweight.[128]

Rotator Cuff Disorders

Rotator cuff disorders happen when the tissues in the shoulder are irritated or injured. This disorder can be an inflammation of the tendons or a bursa; impingement, where the tendon is squeezed and rubs against the bone; or a partial or complete tear of the tendons in the rotator cuff.

Rotator cuff injuries are relatively common. Every time you raise your arm, you are using your rotator cuff. Over time, wear and tear occurs. This, in turn, leads to thinning and fraying of the rotator cuff tendons and reduced blood supply. Sports or other activities that require you to raise your arms frequently, such as tennis, swimming, or house painting, can lead to rotator cuff injuries.

Tennis Elbow (Lateral Epicondylitis)

Tennis elbow is soreness or pain on the outer part of the elbow and occurs when a person damages the tendons that connect the muscles in the forearm to the elbow. Not surprisingly, playing tennis or other racquet sports can cause this injury. Other sports or work activities that require repetitive and vigorous use of the forearm raise a person's risk of tennis elbow. While most people who get tennis elbow are older than 30 years of age, anyone can get it. Usually, there is no acute event that leads to tennis elbow. The symptoms develop gradually and get worse over time.[129]

Final Thoughts on Overuse and Repetitive Motion Injuries

If you consider some of the causes of overuse injuries, it is easy to see why they happen as frequently as they do. Doing too much too soon, doing exercises too intensely, not varying one's activity or exercise routine, not doing proper conditioning before playing sports, not using the proper equipment or form, or simply doing too much of the activity are all considered causes of these types of injuries.[130]

Overuse and repetitive motion injuries cause substantial morbidity. These injuries range from an occasional annoyance to significant loss of function. For many people whose jobs require repetitive motions, even a minor loss of function can be devastating. Imagine a dancer who can't dance or a musician who can't play his or her instrument. These injuries have a huge direct economic impact in the workplace.

Falls

Although falls are not just something that happen to toddlers and the elderly, they are primarily a problem for older adults and the most common reason older adults lose their independence. Even though younger adults are at much lower risk than the elderly, falls can still be a problem. In a population-based study in Canada, falls were the leading cause of nonfatal injuries among 12- to 24-year-olds.[131]

The factors that cause falls among the elderly can also cause falls among younger individuals. There are three main categories of risk: biological risk factors, environmental risk factors, and behavioral risk factors.

Biological Risk Factors

One biological risk factor is having a balance disorder, a condition that makes the person feel unsteady or dizzy. People describe feeling as though they are moving, spinning, or floating. Balance disorders can be caused by health conditions, medications, ear infections, a head injury, or anything else that affects the inner ear or brain. Unfortunately, balance disorders can start suddenly and with no obvious cause.[132] The most common balance disorders include the following:

- *Positional vertigo*—a brief episode of vertigo (unsteadiness) triggered by a change in head position.
- *Labyrinthitis*—an infection or inflammation of the inner ear that causes dizziness and a loss of balance.
- *Ménière disease*—episodes of vertigo, hearing loss, ringing or buzzing in the ear, and a feeling of fullness in the ear.
- *Vestibular neuronitis*—an inflammation of the vestibular nerve (one of the nerves that help with hearing and balance) that can be caused by a virus, primarily causing vertigo.
- *Mal de Debarquement syndrome*—a feeling of continuously rocking or bobbing, typically after being on an ocean cruise or in a boat. Usually, the symptoms recede within a few hours or days after returning to land. Severe cases, however, can last months or even years, and the cause remains unknown.

Diseases that cause gait (a person's manner of walking) disorders raise a person's risk for falls. Huntington disease, ataxia, cerebral palsy, a brain tumor, multiple sclerosis, spinal cord trauma, muscular dystrophy, and congenital hip dysplasia are just a few of the diseases that cause problems with a person's gait. If the cause is treatable, a person's gait will improve with treatment. Physical therapy can also help with gait disorders.[133]

Numbness in the feet and legs can also be a problem. This numbness isn't simply the sensation of having your foot "fall asleep." Diabetes, a herniated disc, vitamin B_{12} deficiency, multiple sclerosis, and fibromyalgia can all cause numbness, which raises the risk for falls.[134]

Many of the biological risks for falls increase with age. Some causes are genetic, with variable age of onset, and others occur young in life. If you are experiencing these symptoms with no obvious minor cause, you should see a health professional.

Medications can also raise the risk of falling. Almost any drug that acts on your brain or your circulation can cause falls. Drugs that sedate you or make you sleepy, drugs that lower your blood pressure, and drugs that alter your heart rate, either giving you slow or rapid heart rate, can cause falls. See **TABLE 9-5** for a partial list of drugs that raise the risk of falling.

Environmental Risk Factors

Most homes (apartments or houses) contain potential hazards for falls, although the hazards alone don't cause the falls. Poor lighting, clutter, and tripping hazards, such as the floor being slippery or uneven and frayed or loose rugs, all increase the risk of falls. These hazards can also exist in office settings. Stairs are inherently hazardous and stairway accidents can cause severe injury and even death. Careful stairway design can substantially reduce the potential for injury

TABLE 9-5 Drugs That Increase the Risk of Falls

Type of Drugs	Examples by Brand Names
Sedatives (benzodiazepines)	Xanax Onfi Klonopin Tranxene Librium Valium Prosom Ativan Serax Restoril Halcion
Drugs for schizophrenia or bipolar disorder	Thorazine Haldol Prolixin Risperdal Seroquel Zyprexa
Opioid analgesics	All opioid and related analgesics Codeine (only available as a generic) Avinza Kadian Ultram OxyContin
Antidepressants	Effexor Cymbalta

by providing the means to retrieve your balance. Holding on to the stair railing when going up or down stairs is an important part of fall prevention.

During icy and snowy conditions, falls increase. If you live in an area that has serious winter weather, short of moving to a different location, this hazard is a fact of life. When you are walking, pay attention to the path ahead of you. Be aware of changes in the walking surface from safe to slippery. Take your time and proceed at a safe pace. Where possible, avoid slippery surfaces, such as icy areas and snow banks. Wear appropriate footwear, such as boots with treaded soles. Better to change shoes once you get to your destination than to suffer an injury trying to make do with the wrong footwear! Use handrails when they are available. If you are holding on to the handrail, you can prevent a slip from becoming a fall. Make sure you get the ice and snow off your shoes so that you don't create indoor hazards.

Behavioral Risk Factors

Many people think that a job where most of the workers sit in a chair in an office would not be a dangerous setting. But falls are the most common source of injury in an office. The National Safety Council says employees are 2.5 times more likely to suffer a disabling fall in an office setting than anywhere else. Standing on chairs, particularly rolling office chairs, is an invitation for falling. It is much better to use a step stool or stepladder.[135]

The behavioral risk factor for falls that most applies to college-aged individuals is drinking. In a study of Canadian adolescents and young adults, drinking alcohol was positively associated with a serious injury in the previous year.[136] Binge drinking is endemic among college students. Binge drinkers are usually more impulsive than are people who do not binge drink, and this impulsivity is likely exacerbated by drinking alcohol. Falls are among the injuries that occur when binge drinking. Alcohol use is an important risk factor for falls among young adults.[136]

Occupational Falls

According to the Bureau of Labor Statistics, in the United States there were 5,190 fatal work injuries in 2016, for a rate of 3.6 per 100,000 full-time workers. The causes of death for 11% of women and 17% of men were falls, slips, or trips. Falls, slips, and trips were the leading cause of death for construction laborers, roofers, and carpenters. More than 82% of the deaths due to falls, slips, or trips were falls to a lower level, with a quarter being a fall of 10 feet or less.[137,]

Occupations in the construction industry have the highest frequency of fall-related deaths. Health services, wholesale, and retail industries have the most nonfatal fall injuries. Healthcare support, building cleaning and maintenance, transportation and material moving, and construction and extraction occupations are particularly at risk of fall injuries.

Fall injuries create a considerable financial burden, including workers' compensation and medical costs. In the United States, the estimated annual cost due to falls is approximately $70 billion. Many other countries have similar challenges regarding falls. The international public health community has a keen interest in developing strategies to reduce the toll of fall injuries with the goal of improving the culture of safety. The ability of the country to decrease the number of injuries and deaths due to falls requires the joint effort of a broad group of organizations, including regulators, industry leaders, professional associations, labor unions, employers, safety professionals, and researchers.[138]

Hearing Loss and Music

Most college students today listen to music through earbuds or headphones via their phone or other device. Have you ever wondered whether listening to music this way could damage your ears or hearing? Unfortunately, it can. People frequently wear headphones and earbuds for an extended period, and if not used correctly, hearing loss can occur.

There was a time when excessive noise exposure in the workplace was a leading cause of hearing loss. Today many young people are losing their hearing due to excessive noise exposure from portable stereo earphones. Noise-induced hearing loss is a result of loudness and duration of exposure, especially when using headphones or earphones at a high volume for extended periods.[139] Noise-induced hearing loss is not limited to using headphones or earbuds; listening to the car radio with the music at a high volume or frequently attending music concerts or clubs can also be a problem. The latter is particularly an issue when you are close to the speakers.

The inner part of the ear contains tiny hair cells (nerve endings). You hear because the hair cells change the sound into electric signals, which the brain recognizes as sound. These tiny hair cells are easily damaged.[140]

The lowest sound that humans can hear is 20 decibels (dB) or lower, and normal talking is usually between 40 and 60 dB. Headphones usually have a maximum volume of 105 to 120 dB. When you go to a music concert, the sound is between 110 and 120 dB; however, right in front of the speakers, the sound can be as high as 140 dB. Being a musician, sound crew member, recording engineer, or employee at a club increases the risk of hearing loss because of extended exposure to noise at high volumes.[140]

How to Protect Your Hearing

If you are using earbuds, resist the temptation to turn up the volume to block outside sounds. The general concept is if the person standing or sitting next to you can hear your music, the volume is too high. You can also protect yourself by decreasing the amount of time you wear headphones or earbuds.[140]

When you go to a concert, if you can afford custom-fit musician earplugs, they are the best choice. Otherwise, foam or silicone earplugs will help reduce the noise level. Using tissues to block the noise will not protect your hearing. Position yourself at least 10 feet or more from the speakers. Move around the venue; the quieter the spot, the better it is for your hearing. Don't let your friends yell in your ear just to be heard. Give your ears a rest for at least 24 hours after exposure to loud music.[140]

How Much Time Can You Safely Be Exposed to Noise Without Harm?

It is unclear how long you can be exposed to noise without it harming you. The National Institute for Occupational Safety and Health (NIOSH)[141] and the Occupational Safety and Health Administration (OSHA)[142] are two federal agencies responsible for protecting worker safety. The two agencies recommend very different maximum noise exposure levels and durations. What the discrepancy between the agencies' recommendations demonstrates is that we do not yet know the maximum time you can listen to loud noises without causing harm. What we do know is the louder the noise, the shorter amount of time you can listen to it before damage to your hearing occurs. **TABLE 9-6** provides examples of common noises, how loud they are, and NIOSH's recommendation for level of noise exposure duration.

TABLE 9-6 Examples of Noise Levels and Recommended Maximum Duration[143–148]

Sound Level	Examples	NIOSH Recommended Maximum Duration[141]
10 dB	Leaves rustling, calm breathing	
40 dB	Average home noise	
40-60 dB	Normal talking	
70 dB	Inside a car at 60 mph	
75 dB	Vacuum cleaner	
80 dB	Alarm clock	
80-89 dB	Heavy traffic, noisy restaurant, blender or food processor	
90 dB		2 hrs 31 min
92 dB	Jazz concert	1 hr 35 min
90-95 dB	Shouted conversation, yelling	
95 dB	Inside a subway car	47 min 37 sec
97 dB		30 min
96-100 dB	Motorcycle	
100 dB		15 min
102 dB		9 min 27 sec
105 dB	Helicopter close by	4 min 43 sec
110 dB		1 min 29 sec
16-115 dB	Snowmobile, leaf blower, busy video arcade	
115 dB		28 seconds
120 dB	Thunderclap	
120-129 dB	Sports crowd, rock concert, loud symphony	
128 dB	Loudest human scream	
130 dB	Typical professional DJ system, stock car races	
140-149 dB	Gun shot, siren at 100 ft.	

National Institute for Occupational Safety and Health. NIOSH publication no. 98-126, Criteria for a recommended standard, occupational noise exposure, revised criteria 1998 - 98-126.pdf. 1998;98-126(7/19/2015)

When to Call the Doctor

If you have ringing in your ears or your hearing is muffled for more than 24 hours after exposure to loud music, call your healthcare professional. They may recommend having your hearing checked by an audiologist. Other signs that you need to see a doctor about your hearing include the following: Some sounds are louder than they should be, you can understand men's voices more easily than women's, you are having trouble distinguishing high-pitched sounds, you find yourself continually turning up the volume on the television or radio, your ears feel full, or you have ringing in your ears.[140]

Fashionable Feet at Any Price?

If you are a woman who loves to wear high heels, you may imagine someday having your own pair of Manolo Blahniks. Some women love to wear high heels, though most women do not realize exactly how harmful wearing high heels can be on their body. High heels, which are shoes with a heel that is 2-inches or higher, can cause various foot, knee, hip, and back/pelvis injuries and other problems. Wearing high heels is bad for your posture, your gait, and your balance.

Wearing high heels puts your foot in a plantar-flexed positioned (toes pointing downward) (**FIGURE 9-7**). This position shifts your legs and pelvis forward and puts most of your body weight on the balls of your toes. To offset this shift, you balance yourself by having your upper body lean backward. This posture puts unhealthy pressure on your lower back and sacroiliac joint (near the bottom of your spine).

The postural change caused by high heels also affects your walking pattern. Due to the position of your feet, your calf muscles cannot generate the force needed to push off the ground. To compensate, your hip and knee muscles work harder. Your knees tend to stay bent during the entire walking movement because of the increased weight shifted forward.

Walking in high heels requires a significant amount of balance and lower leg strength. The higher the heel, the more your body weight is pushed forward, and the more unstable you are. Wearing high heels also exacerbates low back pain. High heels cause your pelvis to tip forward. This change in posture alters

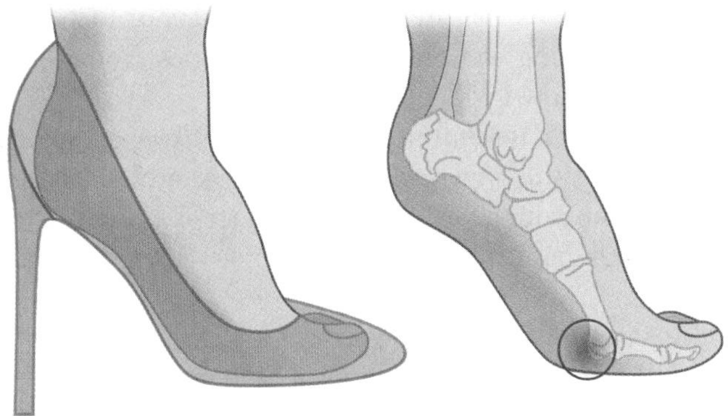

FIGURE 9-7 Foot in a plantar-flexed position.

MORTON'S NEUROMA

Morton's neuroma is a thickening of the tissue around one of the nerves leading to the toes. It can cause a sharp, burning pain in the ball of the foot. The toes also may sting, burn, or feel numb.[149]

the alignment of the spine and makes it difficult for your body to maintain its natural center of gravity.

Your hips, knees, and ankles are also affected by wearing high heels. When you overwork your thigh muscles, you put extra strain on the knee joint and the patellar tendon. This strain makes you more susceptible to a knee injury. High heels increase the pressure on the inside of the knee by as much as 30% and can shorten your hamstring muscles. Wearing high heels can also cause specific foot injuries, such as hammertoes, blisters, bunions, and neuromas. Wearing high heels causes the foot to become turned more to the outside. This position changes your foot posture and the biomechanics of the foot and ankle joints during walking.

Although all high heels have the potential to cause problems, the ultra-narrow heels of stilettos are particularly risky. A chunky heel has more surface area and distributes the body weight more evenly, making the feet much more stable when compared to stilettos or spindle heels.[150]

According to the American Academy of Orthopaedic Surgeons, 43.1 million Americans have foot problems. Eight out of every 10 women say their shoes are painful, and women are nine times more likely to develop foot problems because of poorly fitted shoes than are men.[151]

Do You Have to Give Up Your Heels?

Many women may not want to give up high heels, even if that is the healthiest choice. Luckily, there are ways to minimize the damage wearing high heels can do.[152]

1. *Choose sensible heels.* Select shoes with low heels—an inch and a half or less—and a wide heel base. Narrow, stiletto-type heels provide little support, and 3-inch or higher heels may shorten the Achilles tendon. The broader the heel, the more evenly it will spread your weight.[152]
2. *Wear soft insoles to reduce the impact on your knees.*[152]
3. *Make sure your shoes are the right size,* so your foot doesn't slide forward, increasing the pressure on your toes. Your toes should have ample room to wiggle inside the shoe.[152]
4. *Wear heels on days that require limited walking or standing.*[152]
5. *Don't wear your high heels all day.* Wear athletic shoes on the way to and from your work. The best choice is to wear shoes that allow you to walk naturally. Another alternative is not to wear heels every day.[152]
6. *Make sure you stretch every day.* Stretch your calf muscles and feet. The following are a couple of useful stretches:
   - Holding onto a handrail, stand on the edge of a step with your shoes off. Putting your weight on the balls of your feet and your heels off the edge, drop your heels down to stretch.
   - Put a pencil on the floor and pick it up with your toes.[152]

Work Can Be Dangerous to Your Health: Sweatshops

What Is a Sweatshop?

In these types of manufacturing facilities, sometimes called **sweatshops**, workers endure poor working conditions, long hours, low wages, exposure to toxic substances, and other labor law violations. Sweatshops are especially

sweatshops According to the U.S. Department of Labor definition, a factory that violates two or more labor laws.

TALES OF PUBLIC HEALTH

The Triangle Shirtwaist Factory Fire of 1911[155]

In the early 1900s in the United States, most workers had few, if any, rights. Unions were rare, and working conditions were dreadful, with grueling hours and minimal wages. On Saturday afternoon, March 25, 1911, at the Triangle Shirtwaist Factory in New York City, there was a horrific fire. The fire broke out at 4:45 in the afternoon. Within minutes, the top three floors were engulfed in flames. Many of the staff, mostly recently immigrated women, some as young as 14 years old, were trapped in a building that claimed to be fireproof. In less than 20 minutes, 146 people were dead either from burning to death or leaping to their deaths from 100 feet up.

Although many garment workers in New York City had better wages and working conditions, the owners of the Triangle Shirtwaist Factory refused to recognize unions or to institute safety measures. Although it was unsafe, the building had only two staircases, instead of three. An iron fire escape that stopped at the second floor was considered the third staircase. Exit doors opened inward rather than outward, making it nearly impossible to open the doors amid the crush of panic-stricken workers. Additionally, the managers often locked the exits to prevent workers from sneaking out for a break and to prevent theft. Those locked doors prevented workers from escaping the fire. Boxes of scrap fabric blocked other exits. Workers tried to use the fire escape. The weight of the people and the heat of the fire caused the fire escape to collapse. Workers six stories up fell to their deaths. Elevator operators could fit only 10 people at a time into the elevator. Some people flung themselves down the elevator shaft to escape the fire.

This fire motivated America to protect its workers.

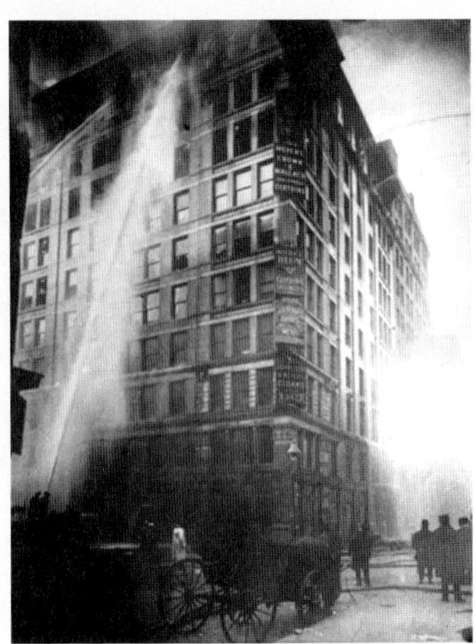

Triangle Shirtwaist Fire.

Department of Labor. (n.d.). The Triangle Shirtwaist Factory fire of 1911: About the fire. Retrieved from https://www.dol.gov/shirtwaist/about.htm.

common in developing countries, where labor law enforcement is weak or nonexistent.[153]

As an example, on April 24, 2013, a nine-story building housing five garment factories in Savar, Bangladesh, collapsed. More than 1,100 people died. The day before it collapsed, the owner dismissed safety concerns, saying, "This building will stand a hundred years."[154]

The International Labor Organization (ILO) estimates that there are 215 million children involved in child labor worldwide, more than half of them doing hazardous work. It also estimates that 6 million children and 15 million adults are in forced labor.[156]

Sadly, most of your clothes are probably made in a sweatshop. Most Americans know very little about the working conditions where their clothes were manufactured. People are forced by their life situations to work in conditions that most reasonable people would find unacceptable. These conditions involve child labor, physical abuse of workers, cheating workers of their already low wages, and sexual pressure on young women by male supervisors.[157]

There have been news stories about the garment industry and its involvement in sweatshops. But these companies are not alone. Goods we all use every day—tires, auto parts, shoes, toys, computer parts, electronics, nearly every kind of manufactured product you can think of—are made in sweatshops.

College Students Are Powerful

One of the greatest accomplishments of the anti-sweatshop movement is in the college apparel market. Universities contract with garment companies to produce their branded apparel. Students refusing to buy sweatshop-produced clothing have had an enormous impact on this multibillion-dollar market. In this instance, students have leverage unavailable to most consumers. Student groups like the United Students Against Sweatshops have been able to pressure universities and colleges to force their suppliers to accept independent inspections and make the necessary improvements (or else lose a highly lucrative dedicated market).[158]

▸ Why Are Injuries a Public Health Issue?

Unintentional injuries are one of the leading causes of death for every age group, from infants to seniors. Among people 1 to 44 years of age, they are the leading cause of death. Working to reduce unintentional injuries is important for individuals, families, communities, and the country. When a teenager drinks alcohol and drives, then crashes, injuring and possibly killing themselves, passengers, and perhaps others on the road, it is preventable. When a new parent is exhausted, his or her baby won't stop crying, and the parent shakes the infant out of frustration, it causes a preventable injury. When an older person falls and injures himself or herself, it is avoidable. We know how to prevent many of these injuries from happening.

Taking a public health approach to prevention of injuries is important. Traditional public health approaches involve monitoring risk factors, designing and testing interventions that address the problems, creating interventions for the community, and finally evaluating the impact of these interventions. Prevention of injuries improves the overall health of the population.

Race/Ethnicity and Injuries

Looking at the data from the CDC's injury data system, for nonfatal injuries by all causes, there are not significant differences by race or ethnicity (**TABLE 9-7**). This finding makes sense because, for many causes of injuries, there is no inherent reason why one group should necessarily have higher rates. (Note that here we use the terminology used by the CDC in categorizing race and ethnicity.) Whites have higher rates than Blacks or Hispanics for injuries due to falls, foreign bodies, poisoning, bicycle injuries, motorcycle injuries, and injuries due to machinery. Blacks have higher injury rates as motor vehicle occupants and from fire-related injuries.

There are, however, race-based discrepancies in how individuals are treated once they arrive at a hospital.[159] Using data from the National Hospital Ambulatory Medical Care Survey to study disparities in treatment of mild TBI, researchers found that compared to Caucasians, African Americans are more likely to be treated by a medical resident (a physician who is still in training) than by a staff physician, emergency medical technician, or another care provider. In this study, there were no other differences in care by race or ethnicity.[159]

Another study used 9 years of data from the National Automotive Sampling System Crashworthiness Data System to compare three components of crash survival by race and ethnicity for drivers with serious injuries. Race/ethnicity was not associated with overall survival or with survival requiring treatment at a hospital. Once at the hospital, compared to Whites, Blacks were 50% less likely to survive for 30 days. Although there was no way to test either explanation within their dataset, among the possible explanations considered were that the Blacks were in poorer health before the crash and that the hospitals to which they were taken were not as good as the hospitals to which the Whites were taken.[159]

Many publications outline the socioeconomic and racial/ethnic disparities in the quality of health care. The causes of those disparities appear to be multifactorial. These factors may be socioeconomic, or may include physician biases, race, and differential access to quality care. With the creation of the Patient Protection and Affordable Care Act of 2010, lack of insurance should be less important than in the past.

TABLE 9-7 Injuries by Race/Ethnicity

Ethnicity	Injuries	Population	Injuries/1,000 Population
All races	28,649,449	316,128,839	90.63
White non-Hispanic	17,263,328	200,918,513	85.92
Black	3,281,197	43,696,271	75.09
Hispanic	2,778,291	51,177,185	54.29
Other non-Hispanic	674,681	20,336,870	33.18
Not stated	4,651,952	—	—

CDC's WISQARS™ (Web-based Injury Statistics Query and Reporting System).

In Summary

This chapter has described many of the ways injuries can and do happen. In addition, it has offered keys to prevent many of these injuries.

Following the rules of the road when driving, including wearing your seat belt, driving within the speed limit, keeping your cell phone put away, and not drinking alcohol when driving will all help prevent injuries to you and others.

Warming up before participating in sports, wearing the proper equipment, and resting if you are injured are all important. Allow injuries to heal fully. Knowing how to swim and practicing good safety behaviors when around water are essential to avoid drowning.

Be mindful of all the different types of burn hazards. Consider the immediate and long-term benefits of not tanning. Know what to do in case of a fire in your home or other building. If you are outside during a thunder and lightning storm, go inside if possible.

Know how to keep yourself safe from poisoning. Keep the phone number for poison control (1-800-222-1222) posted near your phone. Take only medicines prescribed for you, and take them as prescribed. Make the choice not to use street drugs, even if they are technically legal.

Finally, be mindful of the lifestyle choices you make and how they can affect your health. Limit the volume and time you spend listening to music with earbuds or earphones. If you choose to wear high heels, minimize the time you wear them and follow the advice given in this chapter.

Remember the saying, "An ounce of prevention is worth a pound of cure."

Key Terms

athlete exposures
chronic traumatic encephalopathy
drug overdose
overuse injury
plantar fasciitis
poison
repetitive motion injuries
sweatshops
tennis elbow
traumatic brain injury

Student Discussion Questions and Activities

1. Think about your behavior in the streets, whether you are driving a car or motorcycle, riding a bicycle, or walking. Have you done things that raise your risk of injuries? Do you think you will change your behavior based on what you have learned? Why or why not?
2. Do you think driving restrictions should be stricter or more lenient? Why?
3. Why do you think there are variations in injury rates by gender?
4. Do you and your classmates know how to swim? Do you think being able to pass a swimming test should be required for college graduation?
5. Have you taken a CPR course? Do you think everyone should know how to administer CPR?
6. What do you think about the fact that college students are more motivated to not tan based on appearance rather than health? Do you think movie stars refusing to tan will help motivate students to not

tan? When responding, consider the downsides of tanning discussed in this article: http://www.elephantjournal.com/2015/05/tawny-willoughby-changing-the-face-of-skin-cancer-graphic-images/.

7. Does your home have working smoke alarms? Do you have an escape plan at home? Have you ever had a home fire drill so that you would know what to do in the event of a fire? Do you think it would be useful?

References

1. Kanz, F., & Grossschmidt, K. (2006). Head injuries of Roman gladiators. *Forensic Science International, 160*(2-3), 207–216.
2. Hootman, J. M., Dick, R., & Agel, J. (2007). Epidemiology of collegiate injuries for 15 sports: Summary and recommendations for injury prevention initiatives. *Journal of Athletic Training, 42*(2), 311–319.
3. Boston University Research CTE Center. About the center. Retrieved from http://www.bu.edu/cte/about/
4. Palsbo, S. E. (2012). Epidemiology of recreational archery injuries: Implications for archery ranges and injury prevention. *Journal of Sports Medicine and Physical Fitness 52*(3), 293–299.
5. Yung, P. S., Chan, R. H., Wong, F. C., Cheuk, P. W., & Fong, D. T. (2007). Epidemiology of injuries in Hong Kong elite badminton athletes. *Research in Sports Medicine, 15*(2), 133–146.
6. Randall, D., Hertel, J., Agei, J., Grossman, J., & Marshall, S. W. (2007). Descriptive epidemiology of collegiate men's basketball injuries: National collegiate athletic association injury surveillance system, 1988–1989 through 2003–2004. *Journal of Athletic Training, 42*(2), 194-201.
7. Dick, R., Sauers, E. L., Agel, J., Keuter, G., Marshall, S.W., McCarty, K., McFarland, E. (2007). Descriptive epidemiology of collegiate men's baseball injuries: National collegiate athletic association injury surveillance system, 1988-1989 through 2003-2004. *Journal of Athletic Training, 42*(2), 183–193.
8. Potter, M. R., Snyder, A. J., & Smith, G. A. (2011). Boxing injuries presenting to U.S. emergency departments, 1990-2008. *American Journal of Preventive Medicine, 40*(4), 462–467.
9. LaBella, C. R., Mjaanes, J., & Council on Sports Medicine and Fitness. (2012). Cheerleading injuries: Epidemiology and recommendations for prevention. *Pediatrics, 130*(5), 966–971.
10. Reeser, J. C., & Berg, R. L. (2004). Self reported injury patterns among competitive curlers in the United States: A preliminary investigation into the epidemiology of curling injuries. *British Journal of Sports Medicine, 38*(5), E29.
11. Heesch, K. C., Garrard, J., & Sahlqvist, S. (2011). Incidence, severity and correlates of bicycling injuries in a sample of cyclists in Queensland, Australia. *Accident Analysis and Prevention, 43*(6), 2085–2092.
12. Kerr, Z. Y., Baugh, C. M., Hibberd, E. E., Snook, E. M., Hayden, R., & Dompier, T. P. (2015). Epidemiology of national collegiate athletic association men's and women's swimming and diving injuries from 2009/2010 to 2013/2014. *British Journal of Sports Medicine, 49*(7), 465–471.
13. Havlik, H. S. (2010). Equestrian sport-related injuries: A review of current literature. *Current Sports Medicine Reports*, 9(5), 299–302.
14. Junge, A., Engebretsen, L., & Mountjoy, M. L., Alonso, J. M., Renström, P. A., Aubry, M. J., Dvorak, J. (2009). Sports injuries during the summer Olympic games 2008. *American Journal of Sports Medicine, 37*(11), 2165–2172.
15. Gardner, E. C. (2015). Head, face, and eye injuries in collegiate women's field hockey. *American Journal of Sports Medicine*, 43(8):2027-2034.
16. National Collegiate Athletic Association (NCAA). (2015). NCAA: Field Hockey Injuries. Retrieved from https://www.ncaa.org/sites/default/files/NCAA_FieldHockey_Injuries_HiRes.pdf
17. Ruedl, G., Schobersberger, W., Pocecco, E., Blank, C., Engebretsen, L., Soligard, T., Steffen, K., Kopp, M., Burtscher, M. (2012). Sport injuries and illnesses during the first winter Youth Olympic Games 2012 in Innsbruck, Austria. *British Journal of Sports Medicine, 46*(15), 1030–1037.
18. Kerr, Z. Y., Hayden, R., Dompier, T. P., & Cohen, R. (2015). Association of equipment worn and concussion injury rates in national collegiate athletic association football practices: 2004-2005 to 2008-2009 academic years. *American Journal of Sports Medicine, 43*(5), 1134–1141.
19. Fradkin, A. J., Cameron, P. A., & Gabbe, B. J. (2005). Golf injuries—common and potentially avoidable. *Journal of Science and Medicine in Sport, 8*(2), 163–170.
20. Westermann, R. W., Giblin, M., Vaske, A., Grosso, K., & Wolf, B. R. (2015). Evaluation of men's and women's gymnastics injuries: A 10-year observational study. *Sports Health, 7*(2), 161–165.
21. Moller, M., Attermann, J., Myklebust, G., & Wedderkopp, N. (2012). Injury risk in Danish youth and senior elite handball using a new SMS text messages approach. *British Journal of Sports Medicine, 46*(7), 531–537.
22. Tuominen, M., Stuart, M. J., Aubry, M., Kannus, P., & Parkkari, J. (2015). Injuries in men's international ice hockey: A 7-year study of the international ice hockey federation adult world championship tournaments and Olympic winter games. *British Journal of Sports Medicine, 49*(1), 30–36.
23. Kyle, S. B., Nance, M. L., Rutherford, G. W., Jr., & Winston, F. K. (2002). Skateboard-associated injuries: Participation-based estimates and injury characteristics. *Journal of Trauma, 53*(4), 686–690.
24. Xiang, J., Collins, C. L., Liu, D., McKenzie, L. B., & Comstock, R. D. (2014). Lacrosse injuries among high school boys and girls in the United States: Academic years 2008–2009 through 2011–2012. *American Journal of Sports Medicine, 42*(9), 2082–2088.
25. Cummings, R. S., Jr., Shurland, A. T., Prodoehl, J. A., Moody, K., & Sherk, H. H. (1997). Injuries in the sport of luge. Epidemiology and analysis. *American Journal of Sports Medicine, 25*(4), 508–513.
26. Yiemsiri, P., & Wanawan, A. (2014). Prevalence of injuries in wushu competition during the 1st Asian martial arts games 2009. *Journal of the Medical Association of Thailand, 97*(Suppl 2), S9–S13.
27. Schwellnus, M. P., Thomson, A., Derman, W., Jordaan, E., Readhead, C., Collins, R., Morris, I., Strauss, O., Van der

Linde, E., Williams, A. (2014). More than 50% of players sustained a time-loss injury (>1 day of lost training or playing time) during the 2012 super rugby union tournament: A prospective cohort study of 17,340 player-hours. *British Journal of Sports Medicine, 48*(17), 1306–1315.

28. Hespanhol Junior, L. C., Pena Costa, L. O., & Lopes, A. D. (2013). Previous injuries and some training characteristics predict running-related injuries in recreational runners: A prospective cohort study. *Journal of Physiotherapy, 59*(4), 263–269.
29. Nathanson, A.T., Baird, J., & Mello, M. (2010). Sailing injury and illness: Results of an online survey. *Wilderness and Environmental Medicine, 21*(4), 291–297.
30. Hagel, B. (2005). Skiing and snowboarding injuries. *Med Sport Sci, 48*, 74–119.
31. Johansen, M. W., Steenstrup, S. E., Bere, T., Bahr, R., & Nordsletten, L. (2015). Injuries in world cup telemark skiing: A 5-year cohort study. *British Journal of Sports Medicine, 49*(7), 453–457.
32. Esquivel, A. O., Bruder, A., Ratkowiak, K., & Lemos, S. E. (2015). Soccer-related injuries in children and adults aged 5 to 49 years in US emergency departments from 2000 to 2012. *Sports Health, 7*(4), 366–370.
33. Berson, B. L., Rolnick, A. M., Ramos, C. G., & Thornton, J. (1981). An epidemiologic study of squash injuries. *American Journal of Sports Medicine, 9*(2), 103–106.
34. Pluim, B. M., Staal, J. B., Windler, G. E., & Jayanthi, N. (2006). Tennis injuries: Occurrence, aetiology, and prevention. *British Journal of Sports Medicine, 40*(5), 415–423.
35. Maquirriain, J., & Baglione, R. (2015). Epidemiology of tennis injuries: An eight-year review of Davis Cup retirements. *European Journal of Sport Science, 12*, 1–5.
36. Loder, R. T., Schultz, W., & Sabatino, M. (2014). Fractures from trampolines: Results from a national database, 2002 to 2011. *Journal of Pediatric Orthopaedics, 34*(7), 683–690.
37. Zwingenberger, S., Valladares, R. D., Walther, A., Beck, H., Stiehler, M., Kirschner, S., Engelhardt, M. Kasten, P. (2014). An epidemiological investigation of training and injury patterns in triathletes. *Journal of Sports Science*, 2014:32(6), 583–590.
38. Agel, J., Palmieri-Smith, R. M., Dick, R., Wojtys, E. M., & Marshall, S. W. (2007). Descriptive epidemiology of collegiate women's volleyball injuries: National collegiate athletic association injury surveillance system, 1988–1989 through 2003–2004. *Journal of Athletic Training, 42*(2), 295–302.
39. Verhagen, E. A., Van der Beek, A. J., Bouter, L. M., Bahr, R. M., & Van Mechelen, W. (2004). A one season prospective cohort study of volleyball injuries. *British Journal of Sports Medicine, 38*(4), 477–481.
40. Bahr, R., Reeser, J. C., & Federation Internationale de Volleyball. (2003). Injuries among world-class professional beach volleyball players. The federation internationale de volleyball beach volleyball injury study. *American Journal of Sports Medicine, 31*(1), 119–125.
41. Yard, E. E., Collins, C. L., Dick, R. W., & Comstock, R. D. (2008). An epidemiologic comparison of high school and college wrestling injuries. *American Journal of Sports Medicine, 36*(1), 57–64.
42. Ueblacker, P., Haensel, L., & Mueller-Wohlfahrt, H. W. (2016). Treatment of muscle injuries in football. *Journal of Sports Science, 34*(24), 2329–2337.
43. van den Bekerom, M. P., Struijs, P. A., Blankevoort, L., Welling, L., van Dijk, C. N., & Kerkhoffs, G. M. (2012). What is the evidence for rest, ice, compression, and elevation therapy in the treatment of ankle sprains in adults? *Journal of Athletic Training, 47*(4), 435–443.
44. WebMD. (2017). Rest, ice, compression, and elevation (RICE) - topic overview. Retrieved from http://www.webmd.com/first-aid/tc/rest-ice-compression-and-elevation-rice-topic-overview
45. Mac Auley, D. C. (2001). Ice therapy: How good is the evidence? *International Journal of Sports Medicine, 22*(5), 379–384.
46. National Institute of Neurological Disorders and Stroke. (2015). Traumatic brain injury information page. Retrieved from http://www.ninds.nih.gov/disorders/tbi/tbi.htm
47. Centers for Disease Control and Prevention (CDC). (2015). Get the facts: Traumatic brain injury: Injury center. Retrieved from http://www.cdc.gov/traumaticbraininjury/get_the_facts.html
48. Mayo Clinic. (2015). Traumatic brain injury. Retrieved from http://www.mayoclinic.org/diseases-conditions/traumatic-brain-injury/basics/definition/con-20029302
49. Centers for Disease Control and Prevention (CDC). (2015). Leading causes of death by age group—2015. Retrieved from https://www.cdc.gov/injury/wisqars/pdf/leading_causes_of_death_by_age_group_2015-a.pdf
50. Centers for Disease Control and Prevention (CDC). (2015). Seat belts: Get the facts. Retrieved from http://www.cdc.gov/Motorvehiclesafety/seatbelts/facts.html
51. National Highway Traffic Safety Administration. (2015). Final regulatory impact analysis amendment to federal motor vehicle safety standard 208: Passenger car front seat occupant protection. (1984). DOT-HS-806-572. (7/19/2015).
52. National Highway Traffic Safety Administration. (2015). Fifth /sixth report to Congress: Effectiveness of occupant protection systems and their use. 2001. (7/19/2015).
53. Car and Driver. (2015). The physics of: Airbags. Retrieved from http://www.caranddriver.com/features/the-physics-of-airbags-feature
54. National Highway Traffic Safety Administration. (2015). Third report to Congress: Effectiveness of occupant protection systems and their use. 1996(7/19/2015).
55. World Health Organization. (2018). Road traffic injuries. Retrieved from http://www.who.int/mediacentre/factsheets/fs358/en/
56. AAA Foundation for Traffic Safety. (2015). Distracted driving. Retrieved from https://www.aaafoundation.org/distracted-driving
57. National Highway Traffic Safety Administration. (2015). 2013 data: Alcohol-impaired driving - 812102.pdf. Retrieved from http://www-nrd.nhtsa.dot.gov/Pubs/812102.pdf
58. Advocates for Highway and Auto Safety. (2018). Speeding. Retrieved from http://saferoads.org/wp-content/uploads/2018/01/2018-Roadmap-Report-FINAL2.pdf
59. AAA Foundation for Traffic Safety. (2015). Report: Cell phones and driving research update. Retrieved from https://www.aaafoundation.org/sites/default/files/CellPhonesandDrivingReport.pdf
60. Sightline Institute. (2006). Why bikes are a sustainable wonder. Retrieved from http://www.sightline.org/research/bicycle/
61. Jacobsen, P., & Rutter, H. (2012). Cycling safety. In Pucher, J., Buehler, R., eds. *City cycling: Urban and industrial environments* (pp. 141–156). Cambridge, MA: MIT Press.
62. Rivara, F. P., Thompson, D. C., & Thompson, R. S. (2015). Epidemiology of bicycle injuries and risk factors for serious injury—1997. *Injury Prevention, 21*(1), 47–51.

63. National Highway Traffic Safety Administration. (2017). 2015 data: Pedal cyclists. Retrieved from https://crashstats.nhtsa.dot.gov/Api/Public/Publication/812382/
64. Centers for Disease Control and Prevention (CDC). (2012). People who ride: Motorcycle safety. Retrieved from http://www.cdc.gov/motorvehiclesafety/mc/guide/ride.html
65. Consumer Reports. (2013). 10 motorcycle safety tips for new riders. Retrieved from http://www.consumerreports.org/cro/2013/04/10-motorcycle-safety-tips-for-new-riders/index.htm
66. National Highway Traffic Safety Administration. (2017). Traffic Safety Facts: Motorcycles. Retrieved from https://crashstats.nhtsa.dot.gov/Api/Public/ViewPublication/812353.pdf
67. Peng, Y., Vaidya, N., Finnie, R., Reynolds, J., Dumitru, C., Njie, G., . . . Compton, R. P. (2017). Universal motorcycle helmet laws to reduce injuries: A community guide systematic review. *American Journal of Preventive Medicine, 52*(6), 820-832.
68. Goodwin, A., Kirley, B., Sandt, L., Hall, W., Thomas, L., O'Brien, N., & Summerlin, D. (2013). *Countermeasures that work: A highway safety countermeasures guide for state highway safety offices* (7th ed.). Washington, DC: National Highway Traffic Safety Administration.
69. Creaser, J. I., Ward, N. J., Rakauskas, M. E., Boer, E., Shankwitz, C., & Nardi, F. (2007). Effects of alcohol on motorcycle riding skills. DOT HS 810 877. Washington, DC: Department of Transportation.
70. Richter, M., Otte, D., Lehmann, U., Chinn, B., Schuller, E., Doyle, D., . . . Krettek, C. (2001). Head injury mechanisms in helmet-protected motorcyclists: Prospective multicenter study. *The Journal of Trauma: Injury, Infection, and Critical Care, 51*(5), 949–958.
71. Hough, D. L. (2008). *Proficient motorcycling.* Irvine, CA: Bow Tie Press.
72. Safe Kids. (n.d.). Pedestrian safety tips. Retrieved from http://www.safekids.org/sites/default/files/documents/pedestrian_safety_tips_1.pdf
73. Nasar, J. L., & Troyer, D. (2013). Pedestrian injuries due to mobile phone use in public places. *Accident Analysis and Prevention, 57*, 91–95.
74. National Highway Traffic Safety Administration. (2014). 2012 data: Pedestrians. Retrieved from https://crashstats.nhtsa.dot.gov/Api/Public/Publication/812493
75. Naumann, R. B., & Beck, L.F. (2013). Motor vehicle traffic-related pedestrian deaths — United States, 2001–2010. *Morbidity and Mortality Weekly Report, 62*(15), 277–282.
76. Centers for Disease Control and Prevention (CDC). (2016). Unintentional drowning: Get the facts. Retrieved from https://www.cdc.gov/homeandrecreationalsafety/water-safety/waterinjuries-factsheet.html
77. Branche, C. M., Dellinger, A. M., Sleet, D. A., Gilchrist, J., & Olson, S. J. (2004). Unintentional injuries: The burden, risks and preventive strategies to address diversity. In I. L. Livingston (Ed). *Praeger handbook of Black American health: Policies and issues behind disparities in health.* 2nd ed. (pp. 317–327). Westport, CT: Praeger Publishers.
78. Brenner, R. A., Taneja, G. S., Haynie, D. L., Trumble, A. C., Qian, C., Klinger, R. M., & Klebanoff, M. A. (2009). Association between swimming lessons and drowning in childhood. *Archives of Pediatrics & Adolescent Medicine, 163*(3), 203.
79. Irwin, C., Irwin, R., Martin, N., & Ross, S. (2010). Constraints impacting minority swimming participation PHASE II. Retrieved from http://www.usaswimming.org/_Rainbow/Documents/121d4497-c4be-44a6-8b28-12bf64f36036/2010%20Swim%20Report-USA%20Swimming-5-26-10.pdf
80. Thompson, D. C., & Rivara, F. P. (2000). Pool fencing for preventing drowning in children. *Cochrane Database of Systematic Reviews,* CD001047.
81. Laosee, O. C., Gilchrist, J., & Rudd, R. (2012). Drowning 2005–2009. *Morbidity and Mortality Weekly Report, 61*(19), 344–347.
82. Driscoll, T. R., Harrison, J. A., & Steenkamp, M. (2004). Review of the role of alcohol in drowning associated with recreational aquatic activity. *Injury Prevention, 10*, 107–113.
83. Centers for Disease Control and Prevention (CDC). (2014). Unintentional drowning: Get the facts. Retrieved from http://www.cdc.gov/HomeandRecreationalSafety/Water-Safety/waterinjuries-factsheet.html
84. American Burn Association. (2015). Burn incidence and treatment in the United States: 2015. Retrieved from http://www.ameriburn.org/resources_factsheet.php
85. Yoo, J. J., & Hur, W. M. (2014). Body-tanning attitudes among female college students. *Psychological Rep, 114*, 585–596.
86. Fogel, J., & Krausz, F. (2013). Watching reality television beauty shows is associated with tanning lamp use and outdoor tanning among college students. *Journal of the American Academy of Dermatology, 68*(5), 784–789.
87. Hillhouse, J., Turrisi, R., Stapleton, J., & Robinson, J. (2008). A randomized controlled trial of an appearance-focused intervention to prevent skin cancer. *Cancer*, 113(11), 3257–3266.
88. Skin Cancer Foundation. (2015). Appearance trumps health as an anti-tanning argument. Retrieved from http://www.skincancer.org/prevention/tanning/appearance-trumps-health
89. Reed, K. B., Brewer, J. D., Lohse, C. M., Bringe, K. E., Pruitt, C. N., & Gibson, L. E. (2012). Increasing incidence of melanoma among young adults: An epidemiological study in Olmsted County, Minnesota. *Mayo Clinic Proceedings, 87*(4), 328–334.
90. Christenson, L. J., Borrowman, T. A., & Vachon, C. M. (2005). Incidence of basal cell and squamous cell carcinomas in a population younger than 40 years. *Journal of the American Medical Association, 294*(6), 681–690.
91. Bora, N. S., Pathak, M. P., Mandal, S., Mazumder, B., Policegoudra, R., Raju, P. S., & Chattopadhyay, P. (2017). Safety assessment and toxicological profiling of a novel combinational sunprotective dermal formulation containing melatonin and pumpkin seed oil. *Regulatory Toxicology and Pharmacology, 89*, 1–12.
92. Watson, S. (2012). 12 ways to wreck your skin. Retrieved from http://www.webmd.com/beauty/skin/how-to-wreck-your-skin
93. Amano, S. (2016). Characterization and mechanisms of photoageing-related changes in skin. Damages of basement membrane and dermal structures. *Experimental Dermatology, 25*, 14–19.
94. Centers for Disease Control and Prevention (CDC). (n.d.). Tanned skin is not healthy skin. Retrieved from https://www.cdc.gov/cancer/skin/pdf/tanned_skin_not_healthy_skin_hi.pdf
95. Skin Cancer Foundation. (2016). Dark skin tones and skin cancer: What you need to know. Retrieved from http://www.skincancer.org/prevention/skin-cancer-and-skin-of-color
96. Dawes, S. M., Tsai, S., Gittleman, H., Barnholtz-Sloan, J. S., & Bordeaux, J. S. (2016). Racial disparities in melanoma survival. *Journal of the American Academy of Dermatology, 75*(5), 983–991.
97. Centers for Disease Control and Prevention (CDC). (n.d.). Burns. Retrieved from https://www.cdc.gov/masstrauma/factsheets/public/burns.pdf

98. United States Fire Administration. (n.d.). State-by-state residential smoke alarm requirements. Retrieved from http://www.thewfsf.org/sap_usa_files/FEMA_StateSmokeAlarmRequirementsMay2010.pdf
99. National Fire Protection Association. (2015). Escape planning. Retrieved from http://www.nfpa.org/safety-information/for-consumers/escape-planning
100. National Fire Protection Association. (2015). NFPA: The Station nightclub fire. Retrieved from http://www.nfpa.org/safety-information/for-consumers/occupancies/nightclubs-assembly-occupancies/the-station-nightclub-fire
101. Ritenour, A. E., Morton, M. J., McManus, J. G., Barillo, D. J., & Cancio, L. C. (2008). Lightning injury: A review. *Burns, 34*(5), 585–594.
102. National Oceanic and Atmospheric Administration, National Weather Service. (n.d.). Lightning myths and facts. Retrieved from http://www.lightningsafety.noaa.gov/myths.shtml
103. Centers for Disease Control and Prevention (CDC). (2015). Stay safe during lightning. Retrieved from http://www.cdc.gov/features/lightning-safety/index.html
104. Wild Backpacker. (2015). Surviving a lightning storm. Retrieved from http://www.wildbackpacker.com/wilderness-survival/articles/surviving-a-lightning-storm/
105. Lightning safety tips. (2015). Retrieved from https://www.health.ny.gov/publications/3109.pdf
106. Twisted Sifter. (2015). Lichtenberg figures: The fractal patterns of lightning strike scars. Retrieved from http://twistedsifter.com/2012/03/lichtenberg-figures-lightning-strike-scars/
107. Gummin, D. D., Mowry, J. B., Spyker, D. A., Brooks, D. E., Fraser, M. O. & Banner, W. (2017). 2016 Annual Report of the American Association of Poison Control Centers' National Poison Data System (NPDS): 34th Annual Report. *Clinical Toxicology (Phila), 55*(10), 1072–1254. DOI: 10.1080/15563650.2017.1388087
108. Health Resources and Services Administration. (2015). General questions on poisons: Poison help. Retrieved from http://www.poisonhelp.hrsa.gov/faqs/general-questions-on-poisons/index.html
109. Health Resources and Services Administration. (2015). First steps in a poisoning emergency: Poison help. Retrieved from http://www.poisonhelp.hrsa.gov/faqs/basic-first-aid-tips/index.html
110. Centers for Disease Control and Prevention (CDC). (2013). Tips to prevent poisonings: Home and recreational safety. Retrieved from http://www.cdc.gov/HomeandRecreationalSafety/Poisoning/preventiontips.htm
111. Baird, J. S. (1990). Child-proof containers. *Pediatric Emergency Care, 6*(3), 254.
112. Centers for Disease Control and Prevention (CDC). (2015). Carbon monoxide poisoning - frequently asked questions. Retrieved from http://www.cdc.gov/co/faqs.htm
113. Schwirtz, M. (2014, February 28). Hoffman killed by toxic mix of drugs, official concludes. *New York Times*. Retrieved from http://www.nytimes.com/2014/03/01/nyregion/hoffman-killed-by-toxic-mix-of-drugs-official-concludes.html?ref=arts&_r=1
114. Pollack, H. (2014, February 7). 100 Americans die of drug overdoses each day. How do we stop that? *Washington Post*. Retrieved from http://www.washingtonpost.com/news/wonkblog/wp/2014/02/07/100-americans-die-of-drug-overdoses-each-day-how-do-we-stop-that/
115. National Institute on Alcohol Abuse and Alcoholism (NIAAA). (2015). Facts about alcohol overdose (or alcohol poisoning). Retrieved from https://www.collegedrinkingprevention.gov/parentsandstudents/students/factsheets/factsaboutalcoholpoisoning.aspx
116. U.S. National Library of Medicine. (2013). Heroin overdose. Retrieved from https://www.nlm.nih.gov/medlineplus/ency/article/002861.htm
117. U.S. National Library of Medicine. (2013). Cocaine intoxication. Retrieved from https://www.nlm.nih.gov/medlineplus/ency/article/000946.htm
118. U.S. National Library of Medicine. (2013). Methamphetamine overdose. Retrieved from https://www.nlm.nih.gov/medlineplus/ency/article/007480.htm
119. Mills, B., Yepes, A., & Nugunt, K. (2015). Synthetic cannabinoids. *American Journal of the Medical Sciences, 350*(1), 59–62.
120. National Institute on Drug Abuse. (2015). Emerging trends. Retrieved from http://www.drugabuse.gov/drugs-abuse/emerging-trends#spice
121. Liakoni, E., Dolder, P. C., Rentsch, K., & Liechti, M. E. (2015). Acute health problems due to recreational drug use in patients presenting to an urban emergency department in Switzerland. *Swiss Medical Weekly, 28*(9), 145.
122. Johns Hopkins Medicine. (n.d.). Health library: Repetitive motion injury. Retrieved from http://www.hopkinsmedicine.org/healthlibrary/conditions/physical_medicine_and_rehabilitation /repetitive_motion_injury_85,P01176
123. WebMD. (2015). Achilles tendon problems - topic overview. Retrieved from http://www.webmd.com/a-to-z-guides/achilles-tendon-problems-topic-overview
124. Physioworks. (2017). Overuse injuries. Retrieved from http://physioworks.com.au/injuries-conditions-1/overuse-injuries
125. Tendinosis.org. (2015). What is tendinosis? Retrieved from http://www.tendinosis.org/index.shtml
126. WebMD. (2015). Bursitis symptoms, treatment (shoulder, hip, elbow, and more). Retrieved from http://www.webmd.com/pain-management/arthritis-bursitis
127. WebMD. (2015). Patellofemoral pain syndrome - topic overview. Retrieved from http://www.webmd.com/pain-management/knee-pain/tc/patellofemoral-pain-syndrome-topic-overview
128. WebMD. (2014). Plantar fasciitis - symptoms, treatments, causes of plantar fasciitis. Retrieved from http://www.webmd.com/a-to-z-guides/plantar-fasciitis-topic-overview?page=2
129. American Academy of Orthopaedic Surgeons. (2015). Tennis elbow (lateral epicondylitis). Retrieved from http://orthoinfo.aaos.org/topic.cfm?topic=a00068
130. WebMD. (2014). Overuse injuries - topic overview. Retrieved from http://www.webmd.com/a-to-z-guides/overuse-injuries-topic-overview
131. Mo, F., Turner, M. C., Krewski, D., & Merrick, J. (2006). Adolescent injuries in Canada: Findings from the Canadian Community Health Survey, 2000–2001. *International Journal of Injury Control and Safety Promotion, 13*(4), 235–244.
132. National Institute on Deafness and Other Communication Disorders. (2014). Balance disorders. Retrieved from http://www.nidcd.nih.gov/health/balance/pages/balance_disorders .aspx
133. U.S. National Library of Medicine. (2013). Walking abnormalities. Retrieved from https://www.nlm.nih.gov/medlineplus/ency/article/003199.htm
134. Healthline. (2015). Is it fibromyalgia? Common causes of numbness in the legs and feet. Retrieved from http://www.healthline.com /health/fibromyalgia/numbness-in-legs-and-feet#Numbness1
135. National Safety Council. (2013). Recognizing hidden dangers: 25 steps to a safer office. Retrieved from http://www

.safetyandhealthmagazine.com/articles/recognizing-hidden-dangers-25-steps-to-a-safer-office-2. Accessed 9/7/2015, 2015.

136. Kool, B., Ameratunga, S., & Jackson, R. (2009). The role of alcohol in unintentional falls among young and middle-aged adults: A systematic review of epidemiological studies. *Injury Prevention, 15*(5):341–347.

137. U.S. Bureau of Labor Statistics. (2014). Census of fatal occupational injuries, 2018. Retrieved from https://www.bls.gov/iif/oshwc/cfoi/cfch0015.pdf

138. Centers for Disease Control and Prevention (CDC). (2014). Fall injuries prevention in the workplace - NIOSH workplace safety and health topic. Retrieved from http://www.cdc.gov/niosh/topics/falls/

139. Stony Brook University School of Medicine Department of Surgery. (2012). Headphones & earphones can cause permanent hearing loss. Retrieved from http://medicine.stonybrookmedicine.edu/surgery/blog/headphones-and-earphones-can-cause-permanent-hearing-loss-what-you-need-to-know

140. National Library of Medicine. Hearing loss and music. Retrieved from http://www.nlm.nih.gov/medlineplus/ency/patientinstructions/000495.htm. Accessed 7/19/2015, 2015.

141. National Institute for Occupational Safety and Health. (1998). Criteria for a recommended standard, occupational noise exposure, revised criteria. 1998 NIOSH publication no. 98-126. 98–126.

142. U.S. Department of Labor. (2008). Occupational noise exposure. Retrieved from https://www.osha.gov/SLTC/noisehearingconservation/

143. Center for Hearing and Communication. (n.d.). Common environmental noise levels. Retrieved from http://chchearing.org/noise/common-environmental-noise-levels/

144. American Academy of Otolaryngology - Head and Neck Surgery. (2018). Noise and hearing protection: Patient health information. Retrieved from http://www.entnet.org/content/noise-and-hearing-protection

145. Decibelcar. (n.d.). Decibel equivalent table (what's how loud). Retrieved from http://www.decibelcar.com/menugeneric/87.html

146. IAC Acoustics. (2018). Comparative examples of noise levels. Retrieved from http://www.industrialnoisecontrol.com/comparative-noise-examples.htm

147. Noisehelp. (2018). Noise level chart. Retrieved from http://www.noisehelp.com/noise-level-chart.html

148. Alpine Hearing Protection. (n.d.). 5 sound levels in decibels. Retrieved from https://www.alpinehearingprotection.com/5-sound-levels-in-decibels/

149. Mayo Clinic. (2015). Morton's neuroma. Retrieved from http://www.mayoclinic.org/diseases-conditions/mortons-neuroma/basics/definition/CON-20026482

150. WebMD. (2015). Pictures of worst shoes: Foot pain, high heels, flip flops, and more. Retrieved from http://www.webmd.com/pain-management/ss/slideshow-worst-shoes-for-your-feet

151. Pappas, S. (2012). Fashion's high price: How heels damage the body. Retrieved from http://www.livescience.com/18690-high-heels-foot-damage.html

152. American Osteopathic Association. (2015). The real harm in high heels. Retrieved from http://www.osteopathic.org/osteopathic-health/about-your-health/health-conditions-library/womens-health/Pages/high-heels.aspx

153. Oxfam Australia. (n.d.). Are your clothes made in sweatshops? Retrieved from https://www.oxfam.org.au/what-we-do/ethical-trading-and-business/workers-rights/are-your-clothes-made-in-sweatshops/

154. Ahmed, S., & Lakhani, L. (2013). Bangladesh building collapse recovery efforts end, toll at 1,127 dead - CNN.com. Retrieved from http://www.cnn.com/2013/05/14/world/asia/bangladesh-building-collapse-aftermath/

155. U.S. Department of Labor. (2015). The Triangle Shirtwaist Factory fire of 1911. Retrieved from http://www.dol.gov/shirtwaist/introduction.htm

156. U.S. Department of Labor. (2015). ILAB - Office of child labor, forced labor, and human trafficking (OCFT). Retrieved from http://www.dol.gov/ilab/child-forced-labor/

157. Blumgart, J. (2013). Sweatshops still make your clothes. Salon.com. Retrieved from http://www.salon.com/2013/03/21/sweatshops_still_make_your_clothes/

158. Bazarian, J. J., Pope, C., McClung, J., Cheng, Y. T., & Flesher, W. (2003). Ethnic and racial disparities in emergency department care for mild traumatic brain injury. *Academic Emergency Medicine, 10*(11), 1209–1217.

159. Haskins, A. E., Clark, D. E., & Travis, L. L. (2013). Racial disparities in survival among injured drivers. *American Journal of Epidemiology, 177*(5), 380–387.

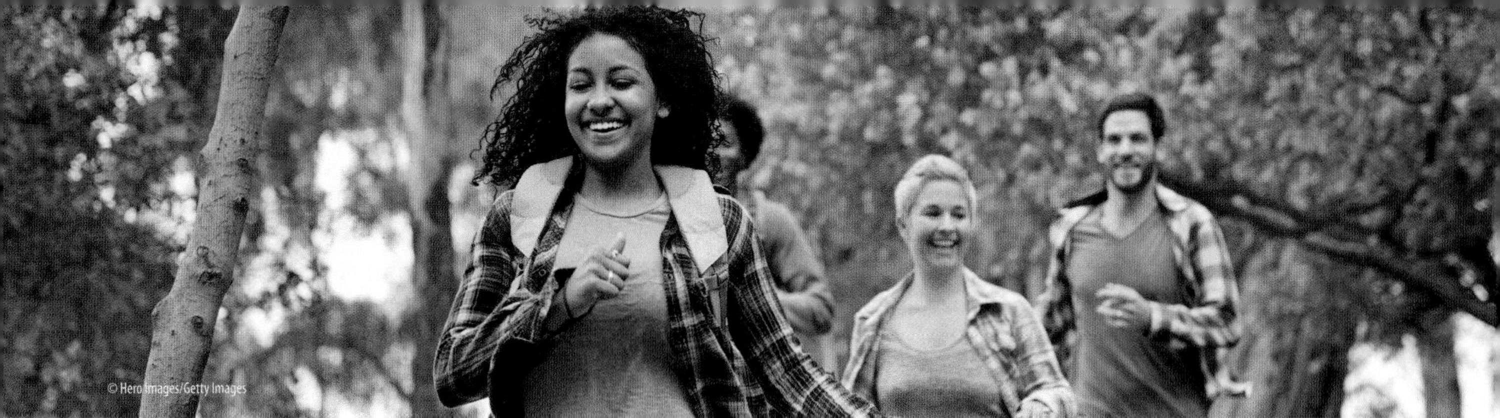
© Hero Images/Getty Images

CHAPTER 10

Be On the Right Side: Prevent Violence

CHAPTER OBJECTIVES

- Explain the social-ecological model of violence.
- Discuss the types of violence that occur at home and within communities.
- Recognize the difference between healthy and unhealthy relationships.
- Illustrate ways to reduce sexual violence on college campuses.
- Explore the prevalence of guns in our society.

"Many who live with violence day in and day out assume it is an intrinsic part of the human condition. But this is not so. Violence can be prevented. Violent cultures can be turned around . . ."
—**Nelson Mandela**, *South African Anti-Apartheid Revolutionary, Politician, and Philanthropist*

At times it seems like violence is all around us. Almost daily, the news includes reports of shootings, stabbings, rapes, and other violent crimes. You wouldn't think that we would need to define violence, but the World Health Organization (WHO) offers this definition: "the intentional use of physical force or power, threatened or actual, against oneself, another person, or against a group or community, which either results in or has a high likelihood of resulting in injury, death, psychological harm, maldevelopment, or deprivation."[1]

Violence is an extreme form of aggression, and it has many causes. These causes include learned behavior from violence in the home or neighborhood, exposure to violence in the media, frustration and external stressors such as poverty, and a tendency to see other people's actions as hostile even when they are not. Additional factors increase the risk of aggression, such as drinking, insults, and environmental factors like heat and overcrowding.

Violence is complicated. Many factors influence the likelihood of the use of violence against oneself or others. The goal of studying violence and trying to understand it is to prevent violence before it happens. The **social-ecological model of violence** prevention considers how individuals relate to one another and their external environment.

social-ecological model of violence A framework for understanding the multifaceted and interactive effects among individual, relationship, community, and societal factors to recognize the reasons that put people at risk for violence or protect them from experiencing or perpetrating violence.

Social-Ecological Model of Violence

In 1998, the journal, *Violence Against Women,* published an article by Lori Heise that proposed a social-ecological model to understand the origins of gender-based violence.[2] This model has been widely used not only for understanding gender-based violence but also for violence in general. The approach theorized that violence has multiple causes that arise from a combination of personal, situational, and societal factors.

FIGURE 10-1 demonstrates the levels of influence within violence. It also helps public health officials determine prevention strategies at the various levels.

Individual Level

The individual level identifies biological and personal history factors that increase the likelihood that a person will be either a victim or a perpetrator of violence. These factors include age, low educational achievement, being unemployed or having insufficient income, a history of alcohol or illicit substance abuse, being a victim of **abuse** as either a child or an adult, a history of violent behavior, having few or no friends, or having a psychological or personality disorder.

abuse The cruel and violent treatment of a person or animal.

The Centers for Disease Control and Prevention (CDC)[3] proposes several strategies that address the individual level within the social-ecological model:

- *In-home programs* that help parents to understand age-appropriate infant and toddler behavior and that teach skills for age-appropriate infant and toddler care
- *School-based programs* that help students at various developmental stages acquire the necessary social, emotional, and behavioral skills to build positive relationships
- *After-school tutoring programs* to increase academic performance
- *Classroom-based health curriculums* that teach students in developmentally appropriate ways to cope with loss and disappointment, and to learn the warning signs for depression
- *Group sessions* that increase knowledge and understanding of healthy dating relationships

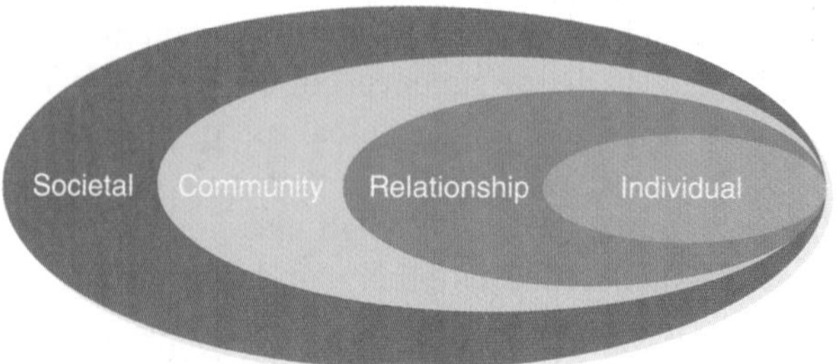

FIGURE 10-1 Social-ecological model of violence prevention.

Centers for Disease Control and Prevention. (2018). The Social-Ecological Model: A Framework for Prevention. Retrieved from https://www.cdc.gov/violenceprevention/overview/social-ecologicalmodel.html

The goal is for individuals to learn healthy behaviors and the appropriate responses when they witness unhealthy or problematic behaviors. Because people feel unsure about the right thing to do, many programs give people an opportunity to practice what to do or say to a friend or family member who demonstrates unacceptable behaviors.

Relationship/Interpersonal Level

This level focuses on families, friends, classmates—basically anyone contributing to our social network. Because our social network influences how people respond to stressors, family and friends can affect how you behave.

When you live with others, even people you love, there are disagreements, tensions, or struggles. How your parents or family members dealt with issues influences how you will deal with them. If your parents disciplined you using violence, you might think that is the right way to behave, or you may think about how much you disliked being hit and choose not to do that to others. Factors that raise the risk for violence include poor communication between parents, marital instability, divorce or separation, poor parental supervision of children, association with aggressive or delinquent peers, or an emotionally unsupportive family.[3]

The CDC's recommendations to improve healthy relationships include the following[2]:

- A peer-to-peer program that teaches youth how they can promote positive dating models within their circle of friends
- Relationship workshops for couples to work on respectful communication strategies
- Within child-parent centers, offer education and family support to promote positive child development
- Pair elders from a senior center with preschool children to increase the emotional support young children receive
- A mentoring program that pairs youth with caring adults

Community Level

This level focuses on settings or institutions in which social relationships take place. How much or how little violence occurs is partly dependent on how the organizational system, such as schools, workplaces, and neighborhoods, function.

Community-level factors that affect the level of violence include the social connectedness of the residents, how quickly residents move in and out of neighborhoods, the lack of neighborhood organization, the income level of the neighborhood, the economic and recreational opportunities presented by the neighborhood, and the physical layout of a neighborhood. If the neighborhood lacks support from the police and judicial system and if there is a general tolerance for violence within the neighborhood, with weak community sanctions for perpetrators, there is likely to be more violence.[3]

The following examples are among the CDC's strategies to address issues at the community level[3]:

- Neighborhood residents organize and make physical improvements to their environment.
- Community associations work with the mayor's office to develop a series of after-school programs for youth.
- A school district, from elementary to high schools, creates, implements, monitors, and evaluates a policy to prevent **bullying**.

bullying The abuse and mistreatment of someone vulnerable by someone else who is stronger or more powerful.

- A city develops safe recreational areas for residents.
- A city focuses on improving the business district to increase employment opportunities.

Societal Level

At a societal level, factors that either create a level of acceptance or intolerance for violence come into play. The more we see ourselves in others, the less violence there will be in society.

Factors that affect violence at a societal level include a social norm that violence is an acceptable way to resolve conflict and that the consequences for those who perpetrate violence are minimal, as well as health, economic, and educational policies. Violence occurs more where there are inequalities due to gender, religion, culture, sexual orientation, or race. It is problematic when society grants one group control over another, for example, men over women or one religious group over another.

Examples of societal-level strategies to reduce violence include the following[2]:

- A national media campaign to create awareness and change societal norms about the way people think concerning violence
- Legislation to encourage employers to offer family-leave options and both paternity and maternity leave
- A media campaign designed to reduce the stigma associated with self-directed violence being considered as just a mental health problem
- Legislation that provides tax incentives to businesses that partner with school districts to provide learning-based technology and other academic resources to disadvantaged communities

Nobody wants to be a victim of violence, whether the violence is at the hands of another individual or at the societal level. To help prevent violence, it is important to treat others with respect. It is essential at all levels within the social-ecological model to implement programs and policies that can reduce risk factors and increase protective factors.

PROTECT YOURSELF FROM VIOLENCE

If you are a woman, you have probably experienced the feeling when you are walking alone at night that you are being followed. Your adrenaline starts pumping, and your heart rate speeds up.

If it is an option, prevention is the best choice to protect yourself from violence. Choose well-lit streets and be aware of what is going on around you. Keep your keys in your hand as you approach your door or car. If you walk alone at night frequently, vary your route and times of travel. If a confrontation is unavoidable, try to talk your way out of trouble. Giving up your money, wallet, or purse is a better choice than giving up your life.[4]

In situations where violence is unavoidable, be prepared to defend yourself. Remember these following tips:

- Be *loud* and push back against the attacker. These actions indicate you won't be an easy victim.
- Know the most vulnerable body parts (see figure). The most easily damaged body parts are the eyes, nose, ears, neck, groin, and knees. If the attacker is wearing sneakers or other soft shoes, the instep is also vulnerable.
- Remember, if you are attacked, it is not the time to be gentle.

Your college or town likely has self-defense classes. Take one. Take another. The more prepared you are, the easier it will be to react if you need to do so.

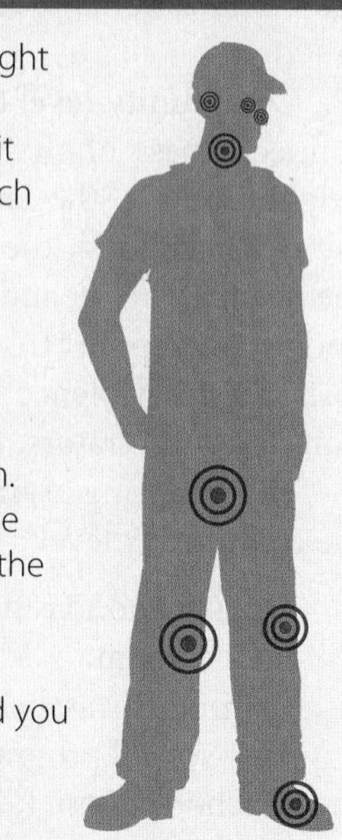

Violence Across the Lifespan: Child Abuse, Intimate Partner Violence, and Elder Abuse

Living in a home where there is violence is upsetting and frightening. Violence at home is always wrong. If you are a victim of violence, it is important to remember that it is not your fault. Abusive behaviors may include a wide range of actions, including excessive yelling, unreasonable demands, excessive criticism, belittling, ignoring, humiliating, demeaning punishment, withholding praise or affection, and exposure to or witnessing violence perpetrated on others. Abuse may be any one or a mixture of **neglect**, emotional, physical or **sexual abuse**.

- Neglect, whether intentional or not, occurs when a parent or caregiver fails to provide a child or elderly person with the basic needs such as love, food, shelter, adequate supervision, and/or medical care.
- **Emotional abuse** is when a person is deprived of love, affection, and attention or when the perpetrator continually speaks in a negative or hurtful way and makes the victim feel worthless.
- Physical violence includes hurting the victim by hitting, slapping, shoving, pushing, biting, kicking, or burning. This also includes throwing things and hurting animals.
- Sexual violence is when, without consent, the perpetrator touches the victim's body in a sexual way or forces the victim to have sex.

neglect Not meeting the basic needs of a person who requires care: physical, medical, educational, and emotional.

sexual abuse Unwanted sexual activity, with perpetrators using force, making threats, or taking advantage of victims not able to give consent.

emotional abuse Any act, including confinement, isolation, verbal assault, humiliation, intimidation, or any other treatment that may diminish the sense of identity, dignity, and self-worth of the victim.

Child Maltreatment

Young children understand their world through their connections with parents, extended family members, and other caregivers. The relationships between the adults in a child's world have a huge impact on the child. When the relationships are healthy and supportive, it improves the child's health and well-being. Safe, stable, nurturing relationships and environments are fundamental to healthy brain development. These relationships also shape the child's physical, emotional, social, behavioral, and intellectual capabilities.

Safe Haven Laws

Safe haven laws provide the option for parents in crisis to leave unharmed infants without criminal penalties so that the child becomes a ward of the state. The intent of these laws is to protect the infant, but they also protect the parents by making them immune to prosecution. **TABLE 10-1** provides the length of time states allow to relinquish an infant under safe haven laws. This information was current through December, 2016. If you are considering relinquishing your infant under a safe haven law, be sure to check with your state, as they frequently amend laws.[5]

safe haven laws Laws that allow any person statutorily defined by law, usually a parent, to abandon an unharmed newborn baby at a designated location. These laws were enacted in response to an increased number of infant abandonments and infanticides.

Most states allow either parent to relinquish his or her infant to a designated safe haven. Georgia, Maryland, Minnesota, Puerto Rico, and Tennessee allow only the mother to surrender the infant, but Maryland and Minnesota allow the mother to approve another person to deliver the relinquished infant on her behalf. Idaho specifies that the parent who relinquishes the infant be the custodial parent. The District of Columbia requires that the custodial parent be a resident of the District to be eligible to relinquish the infant. Some states allow the parent to approve another person to surrender the baby, while in others, the relinquishing person must have legal custody of the child. Still other states do not specify who may relinquish a child.[4] Clearly, there is no nationwide

TABLE 10-1 Length of Time to Relinquish an Infant Under Safe Haven Laws

States	Length of Time to Relinquish
Alabama, Arizona, California, Colorado, Hawaii, Michigan, Mississippi, Puerto Rico, Tennessee, Utah, Washington, Wisconsin	72 hours
Florida, Georgia, Massachusetts, Minnesota, New Hampshire, North Carolina, Oklahoma	7 days
Maryland	10 days
Delaware, District of Columbia, Iowa, Virginia, Wyoming	14 days
Alaska	21 days
Arkansas, Connecticut, Idaho, Illinois, Indiana, Kentucky, Louisiana, Maine, Montana, Nebraska, Nevada, New Jersey, New York, Ohio, Oregon, Pennsylvania (28 days), Rhode Island, Vermont, West Virginia	30 days/1 month
Kansas, Missouri	45 days
South Carolina, South Dakota, Texas	60 days
New Mexico	90 days
North Dakota	1 year

Child Welfare Information Gateway, ed. (2017). Infant safe haven laws. Washington, DC: U.S. Department of Health and Human Services, Children's Bureau.

consensus on this issue, other than the recognition that this option is necessary to protect infants.

States vary in what they consider a safe haven. Some states allow only hospitals, emergency medical service providers, or healthcare facilities. Other states also include fire stations or police stations, emergency medical personnel responding to 9-1-1 calls, or churches, provided there is a person present when the infant is relinquished.[5]

The remaining rules regarding relinquishment vary by state, including issues regarding medical care, notification of the local child welfare department, the gathering of family medical history, legal repercussions, and information about referrals. Thirteen states and the District of Columbia guarantee parental anonymity. Safe haven laws in 27 states and Puerto Rico protect against compelling the parent to provide information. Most states protect against criminal liability for the parents who safely relinquish their infants. If there is evidence of child abuse or neglect, the parent forfeits anonymity and immunity from prosecution.[5]

Shaken Baby Syndrome (Abusive Head Trauma)

What was previously called shaken baby syndrome is now referred to as abusive head trauma in the medical community. This violent occurrence is the leading cause of child abuse deaths in the United States. The trauma and ensuing

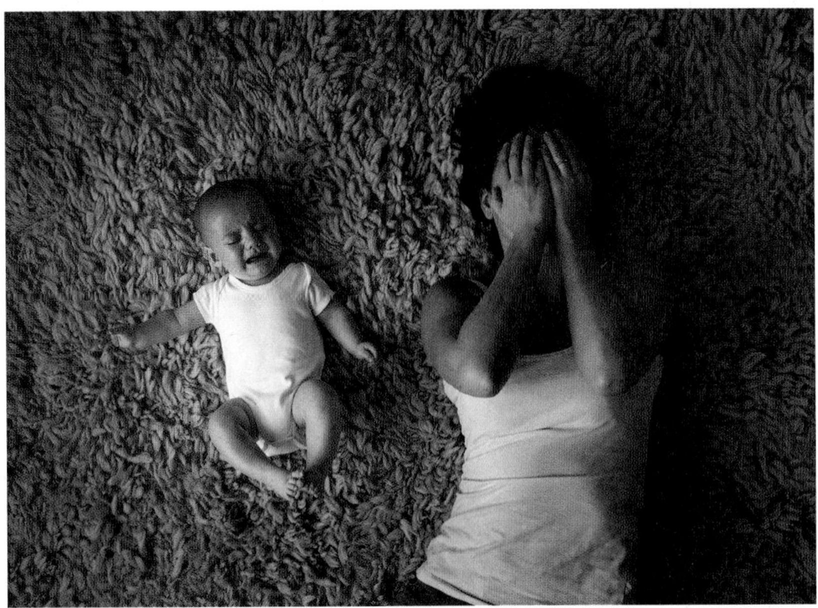

© SolStock/E+/Gettyimages.

traumatic brain injury result from either violently shaking an infant (hence the previous name) or from blunt trauma to the head, often in response to the infant's crying.[6] Infants' crying, including long spells of crying inconsolably, is normal developmental behavior. For a caregiver, inconsolable crying can be extremely frustrating, but shaking, throwing, hitting, or hurting a baby is never an appropriate response.[6] It is important that when you become a parent, you have realistic expectations about child development.

Abusive head trauma causes serious health consequences for nearly all victims. At least one of every four babies who are violently shaken dies from this form of child maltreatment. Shaking a baby can cause bleeding in the brain. A baby who has been severely shaken may vomit, have seizures, and be irritable. In more severe cases, babies may lose consciousness, breath irregularly, or not have a pulse. While the most serious consequence is death, a severely shaken baby can lose his or her hearing, or become blind or mentally retarded as a result.[7]

Child Abuse

Child maltreatment includes all types of abuse and neglect of a child under the age of 18.[8] In the United States, in 2015, there were 683,000 victims of abuse and **child neglect** reported to **Child Protective Services**. This is likely an underestimate of the actual rate of abuse and neglect because many cases are not reported. In 2015, about1,670 children died because of abuse and neglect.[8]

child neglect A form of child abuse that occurs when a person who is responsible for the child fails to care for the minor's emotional or physical needs.

Child Protective Services A state governmental agency that responds to reports of child abuse or neglect. Different states use different names, such as Department of Children and Family Services or Department of Social Services.

Many factors increase the risk for abuse or neglect, such as the child's age. Children under 4 years of age are at greatest risk for severe injury and death from abuse. According to the relationship/interpersonal-level of the socio-ecological model, in situations where there is a lot of stress, abuse and neglect are more likely to occur. The stress can be from a family history of violence, drug or alcohol abuse, poverty, and chronic health problems. Isolated families, in that the adults do not have nearby friends, relatives, or a social support network, are also at risk. At the community level, neighborhoods that are poor, that experience ongoing violence, and where neighbors are not well connected, are more likely to have problems with child abuse and neglect.[9]

TABLE 10-2 lists indicators of child abuse, whether physical, sexual, or neglect. It is hard to imagine how devastating child abuse can be.

TABLE 10-2 Indicators of Child Abuse[10,11]

Physical Indicators	Sexual Indicators	Neglect Indicators
Injuries to the eyes or both sides of the head or body	Difficulty and/or pain when sitting or walking	Obvious malnourishment, listlessness, or fatigue
Frequently appearing injuries, such as bruises, cuts, and/or burns, especially if the child is unable to provide an adequate explanation of the cause. These may appear in distinctive patterns, such as grab marks, human bite marks, cigarette burns, or impressions of other instruments.	Injury to genital area	Untreated need for glasses, dental care, or other medical attention
Rope marks or burns	Injury to genital area	Stealing or begging for food
Fractures/broken bones	Sexual victimization of other children	Lack of personal care: poor personal hygiene, torn and/or dirty clothes
Destructive, aggressive, or disruptive behavior	Sexually suggestive, inappropriate, or promiscuous behavior or verbalization	Child inappropriately left unattended or without supervision
Passive, withdrawn, or emotionless behavior	Pregnancy at less than 12 years	Inadequate clothing for weather
Fear of going home or fear of parent(s)	Expressing age-inappropriate knowledge of sexual relations	Frequent absence from or tardiness to school

Data from New York Office of Children & Family Services. Signs of Child Abuse or Maltreatment. Retrieved from: http://ocfs.ny.gov/main/prevention/signs.asp

physical abuse The intentional use of force against a child that has a high likelihood of harm for the child's health, survival, development, or dignity. This includes hitting, beating, kicking, shaking, biting, strangling, scalding, burning, poisoning, and suffocating. Much physical violence against children in the home is inflicted with the object of punishment. This type of abuse often does not occur in isolation, but as part of a constellation of behaviors, including authoritarian control, anxiety-provoking behavior, and a lack of parental warmth.

BY THE NUMBERS

How Much Does Child Abuse Cost?[12]

While it may appear insensitive to estimate the cost of child abuse, it is important to understand how much of a societal burden child maltreatment creates. CDC estimated the average lifetime cost per victim of nonfatal child maltreatment includes:

- $35,787 in childhood healthcare costs
- $11,593 in adult medical costs
- $158,938 in productivity losses
- $8,508 in child welfare costs
- $7,428 in criminal justice costs
- $8,807 in special education costs

The estimated average lifetime cost per death includes:

- $15,524 in medical costs
- $1,385,916 in productivity losses

The total lifetime estimated financial costs associated with just 1 year of confirmed cases of child maltreatment (**physical abuse**, sexual abuse, psychological abuse, and neglect) are approximately $183 billion.

(NOTE: All costs recalculated based on inflation to March, 2018)

TALES OF PUBLIC HEALTH

A True Story From the *Dallas Morning News*[13]

(Warning: This story is very upsetting, and the *Dallas Morning News* series is even more graphic than this description.)

This is the story of Lauren, *the girl in the closet*. Lauren was adopted at birth, but her adoptive parents' lawyer did not terminate the biological mother's parental rights. When the biological mother wanted Lauren back, the switch from her adoptive parents' home to living with her biological mother was gradual. During the process, the adoptive parents maintained that Lauren's biologic mother abused her, but the judge awarded full custody to the biologic mother. When her adoptive parents gave Lauren, then 20 months old, back to the biologic mother, she was a dimpled, smiley toddler.

Some time around Lauren's second birthday, her biologic mother began locking her in the bathroom. Over the next 6 years, the confinement and starvation got progressively worse. Twice when Child Protective Services came to check on her, Lauren was seated at the table with food in front of her, but her parents told her not to eat. Another complaint was filed, but by the time Child Protective Services came, the family had moved. Another time the biological mother and stepfather lied about their identity.

When the police finally came looking for 8-year-old Lauren, they found a child that looked like a 3-year-old. She weighed 25.6 pounds, only 2 pounds more than when she was 2 years old. Her hair was matted, and her eyes were sunken. For the year before her rescue, she was locked in a 4-by-9-foot closet. She slept there and went to the bathroom there.

She had difficulty sitting up, and could not stand up. She was extremely thin and emaciated. Her hair was broken and sparse. She had sunken eyes, hollowed cheeks, and several teeth missing in the front. She had more than two dozen cigarette burns and puncture wounds across her back and face. Her hair was lice-infested, almost translucent, and her esophagus was clogged with feces, carpet fibers, and plastic. She was also sexually abused.

The psychologist at the hospital stated, "We had seen abuse cases, but nothing to the extent . . . as her story unfolded." Even in a hospital full of sick and injured children, the damage was shocking. It was so horrific that the hospital staff needed the services of a psychologist.

At age 8, Lauren was not potty-trained, did not know how to use silverware, and would not wear shoes because they hurt her feet. She did not recognize the sun and had never seen a television. Her parents had sold her to pedophiles. As the police said, they treated their dogs better than they treated Lauren.

Her mother told the police: "I never loved Lauren. I never wanted her," "When my other kids hurt, I hurt. When Lauren hurt, I felt nothing." Lauren's mother and stepfather were convicted of felony injury to a child. Both received a sentence of life in prison. They will be eligible for parole in 2031 when Lauren is 38.

Lauren was reunited with the adoptive parents who raised her.

In the words of a child psychologist: "Neglect is probably the most pervasive and devastating form of abuse that any child can endure. It will last longest and affect more areas of functioning in a child's life than had the child simply been abused or molested."[13]

Child Maltreatment Around the World

Child maltreatment is a problem in the United States and around the world. In addition to abuse and neglect, issues include child labor, trafficking, sexual exploitation, female genital mutilation, and child marriage.[14] Some of these practices occur primarily in the developing world while others occur around the world, including in the United States.

Child Labor

In the United States, we live with the understanding that all children will go to school. U.S. child labor laws, enacted in 1938, ensure that when young people work, conditions are safe, and it does not jeopardize their health, well-being, or educational opportunities.[15] For many children, particularly in the world's poorest countries, this is not their reality. UNICEF estimates that 150 million children around the world engage in child labor. Working is child labor when those working are too young or doing work that is hazardous in that it may compromise their physical, mental, social, or educational development. In developing countries, approximately 13% of children aged 5 to 14 years are required to work.

West and Central Africa 25
Sub-saharan Africa 25
Eastern and Southern Africa 25
Least developed countries 22
World* 13
South Asia 12
Latin America and Caribbean 11
Middle East and North Africa 9
East Asia and Pacific* 8
Central and Eastern Europe and the Commonwealth of Independent States 5
0 10 20 30
Percentage of children

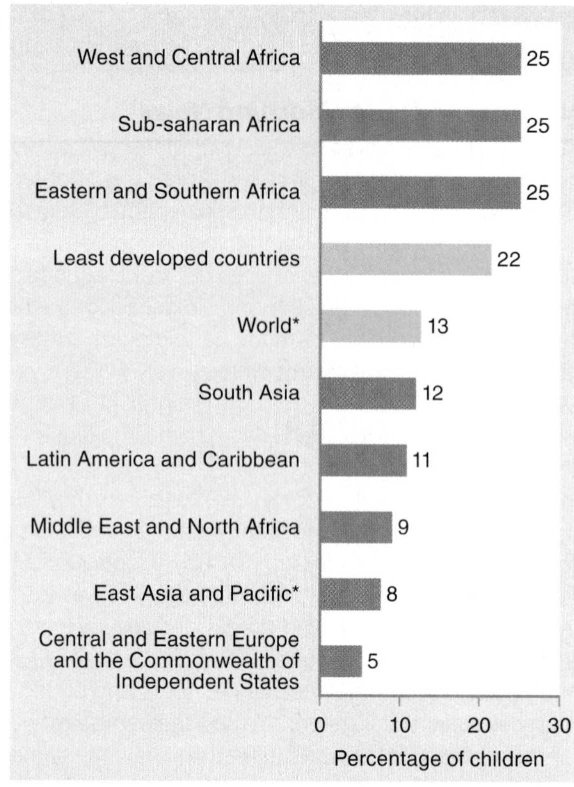

* Excludes China.
Notes: Estimates based on a subset of 90 countries covering 71 per-cent of the global population of children aged 5 to 14 (excluding China, for which comparable data are not available in UNICEF global databases). Regional estimates represent data from countries covering at least 50 per-cent of the regional population.

FIGURE 10-2 Percentage of children aged 5 to 14 years engaged in child labor.

Data from UNICEF. (2018). In the world's poorest countries, around 1 in 4 children are engaged in child labour. Retrieved from http://data.unicef.org/topic/child-protection/child-labour/#sthash.MmRMVsDg.dpuf

In sub-Saharan Africa, 25% of children are working. In South Asia, 12% of children aged 5 to 14 years are doing potentially harmful work. **FIGURE 10-2** shows the percentage of children aged 5 to 14 years engaged in child labor by region.[16]

Trafficking

Trafficking of children is defined as the "recruitment, transportation, transfer, harboring, and/or receipt" of a child for the purpose of exploitation. In 2010, the International Labour Organization estimates that 115 million children were engaged in hazardous work.[17] The types of labor children are forced into include bonded labor (a form of slavery which exchanges labor as a means of repayment of a loan), camel jockeying, child domestic labor, commercial sexual exploitation and prostitution, drug couriering, and child soldiering. Between 1.8 and 2 million children are sexually trafficked. In at least 17 countries around the world, "tens of thousands" of children are forced into armed conflicts, as fighters, but also in supportive roles as cooks, porters, messengers, spies, and sexual partners.[18,19]

Around the world, children are trafficked into the drug trade. Children "are often paid in drugs" to increase the likelihood that they will become drug addicts themselves, entrapping them even further. If they become dependent on drugs from the supplier, they are less likely to run away. Because the drugs they are carrying or dealing are illegal, children who are apprehended are often treated as criminals.[18,20]

Trafficked children may also work as beggars. Forced begging is considered child trafficking, even when done by family members. Children who are forced to beg are commonly beaten, either by the individuals who force them to work or by the people from whom they beg money. Children who beg are required to work long hours, are intimidated and punished by police, and required to give up most of the money they get. In some cases, teachers construe the Koranic teachings of charity and humility to coerce young children to beg.[18,21]

The United States is both a source of trafficking as well as a transit country. This country is one of the top destination points for victims of child trafficking and exploitation. According to UNICEF: "Cases of human trafficking have been reported in all 50 U.S. states; anyone can be trafficked regardless of race, class, education, gender, age, or citizenship when forcefully coerced or enticed by false promises."[18]

Sexual Exploitation

Sexual exploitation includes child prostitution (regardless of where it occurs), trafficking children and adolescents for sex trade, child sex tourism, production and distribution of child pornography, and the use of children in public or private sex shows. Sexual exploitation often occurs with other forms of violence. Around the world, approximately 120 million girls under the age of 20 have been forced to have sexual intercourse or perform other sexual acts. Although boys are also at risk, there are no numerical estimates, but experts believe it occurs to a lesser extent than among girls.[22]

FIGURE 10-3 shows the percentage of girls, aged 15 to 19 years old, who experienced forced sexual acts in the last year. This figure shows some countries as having no victims of forced sexual intercourse; this does not mean there were no victims. After rounding, the estimates came to zero.[22]

Female Genital Mutilation and Cutting

According to the WHO, the practice of Female genital mutilation and cutting (FGM/C) refers to "all procedures involving partial or total removal of the female external genitalia or other injury to the female genital organs for non-medical reasons."[23]

This practice has continued because it is a tradition and aligned with social norms and ethnicity. FGM/C is more common among middle-aged women than among adolescents. In many places where FGM/C occurs, it is widely supported, without question by both men and women. People who believe otherwise may face condemnation, harassment, and ostracism.[22]

STOP
FEMALE CIRCUMCISION
IT IS
DANGEROUS
TO
WOMEN'S HEALTH
FAMILY PLANNING ASSOCIATION OF UGANDA

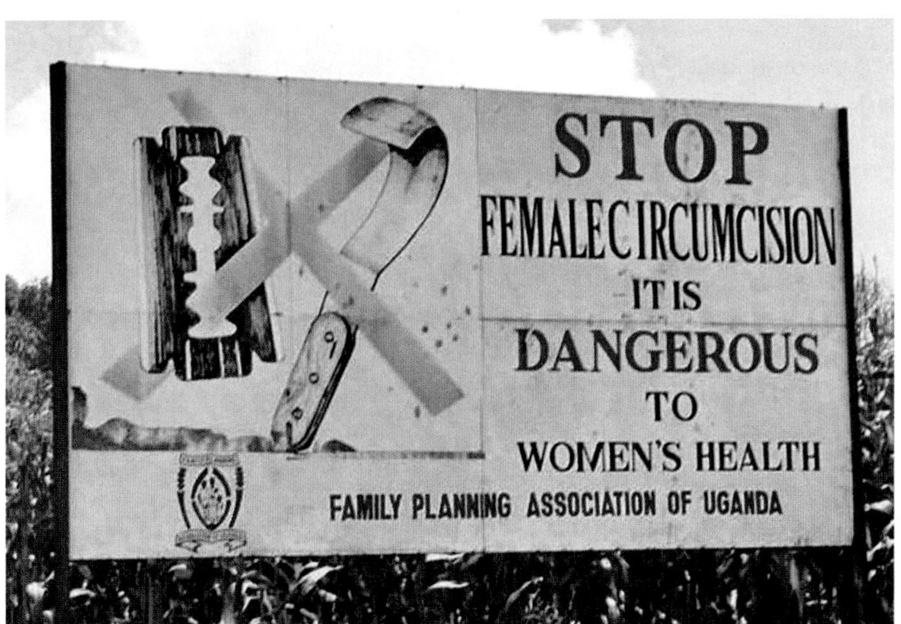

Image used with permission from Reproductive Health Uganda.

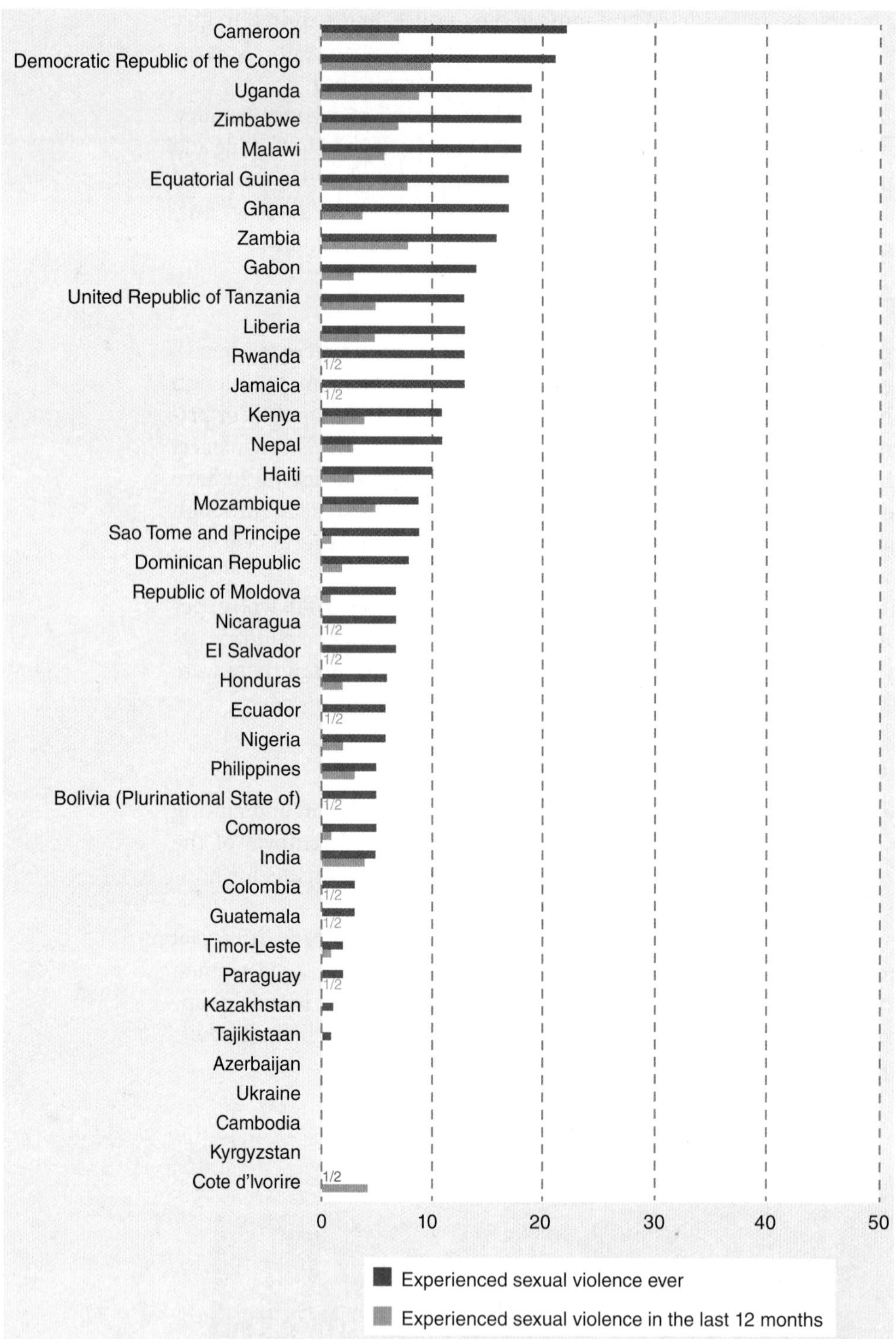

FIGURE 10-3 Percentage of girls aged 15 to 19 years who experienced forced sexual intercourse or other forced sex acts, ever and in the last 12 months.

Data from UNICEF. (2017). Worldwide, around 15 million adolescent girls aged 15 to 19 have experienced forced sex in their lifetime. Boys are also at risk, although a global estimate is unavailable. Retrieved from http://data.unicef.org/child-protection/sexual-violence.html#sthash.xA18bbba.dpuf

Attitudes about FGM/C vary widely across countries. Where the practice occurs in African and Middle Eastern countries, most girls and women think it should end.[24] In Djibouti, Egypt, Eritrea, Guinea, Mali, Sierra Leone, Somalia, and Sudan more than 80% of girls and women, aged 15 to 49 years, have had their genitalia mutilated or cut. In the other countries where FGM/C occurs, the percentage is smaller.[23,24] (There was a 2017 documentary about this called *The Cut*.)

Child Marriage

In the United States, most people grow up with the belief that when they are adults, they get to marry the person of their choice. Yet worldwide, among women 20 to 24 years of age, approximately one-quarter were child brides, meaning families pressured the girls into arranged marriages before the age of 18. Some child brides are as young as 8 or 9 years old. There are many reasons why this happens, including poverty, the idea that marriage will provide "protection" for the girl, family honor, social norms, customary or religious laws that tolerate the practice, an inadequate legislative framework, and the state of a country's civil registration system. In reality, being married early often isolates the girl, puts her at risk of early pregnancy, ends her schooling and opportunities for a career or vocational training, and increases her risk of being a victim of **intimate partner violence**.[25]

intimate partner violence A pattern of assaultive and coercive behaviors that includes the threat or infliction of physical, sexual, or psychological abuse that is used by a current or former intimate partner for the purpose of intimidation and control over the victim.

In countries where the primary expectation for girls is to become wives and mothers, they have limited opportunities for other options. Rigid gender and cultural beliefs also help promote child marriage. Growing up in a rural environment and in poverty increase the risk for a girl's parents to have her get married early. Latin America and the Caribbean are the only regions where child marriage is not declining: the prevalence there has remained the same for the last 30 years.[26]

BY THE NUMBERS

Child Marriage

South Asia has the highest rates of child marriage with almost half of all girls marrying before the age of 18 and about 17% before the age of 15.[25] Bangladesh has the highest rate of child marriage at 65%, followed by India (47%), Nepal (41%), and Afghanistan (40%). Although there are less data for boys, in Comoros, Nepal, the Marshall Islands, Nauru, Honduras, Lao People's Democratic Republic, and Madagascar, between 11% and 13% of boys were married before the age of 18 years.[25]

Intimate Partner Violence

What used to be called domestic abuse is now referred to as intimate partner violence. While the definition of intimate partner violence (IPV) varies from study to study, it is a pattern of assaultive and coercive behaviors that includes the threat or infliction of physical, sexual, or psychological abuse. Perpetrators use these behaviors for the purpose of intimidation and control over the victim.[27] Although not equally distributed, the victim can be a woman or a man and IPV can occur in homosexual as well as heterosexual couples. Verbal abuse, imprisonment, humiliation, **stalking**, and denial of access to financial resources, shelter, or services are all behaviors classified as IPV.[28] Research shows having a secondary education, having more income, and a formal marriage offers protection, but not a guarantee, from IPV. Alcohol abuse, cohabitation, young age, holding the belief that abuse is acceptable, having outside sexual partners, experiencing childhood abuse, growing up with domestic violence, and experiencing or perpetrating other forms of violence in adulthood increase the risk of IPV.[29]

stalking Repeated visual or physical proximity, nonconsensual communication, and/or verbal, written, or implied threats directed at a person to arouse fear. It is unusual in that the individual behaviors may be legal, such as sending flowers, writing love notes, or waiting outside a person's place of work.

Individual factors that put a person at risk for IPV victimization also put a person at risk of being a perpetrator (the one who commits the act of violence). Risk factors include low self-esteem, lower educational attainment, low income, being young, aggressive or delinquent behavior as a young person, heavy alcohol and drug use, depression, anger, hostility, antisocial or borderline personality disorder, a prior history of being physically or psychologically abusive, having few friends or generally being isolated, unemployment, emotional dependence and insecurity, belief in strict gender roles, such as male dominance and the

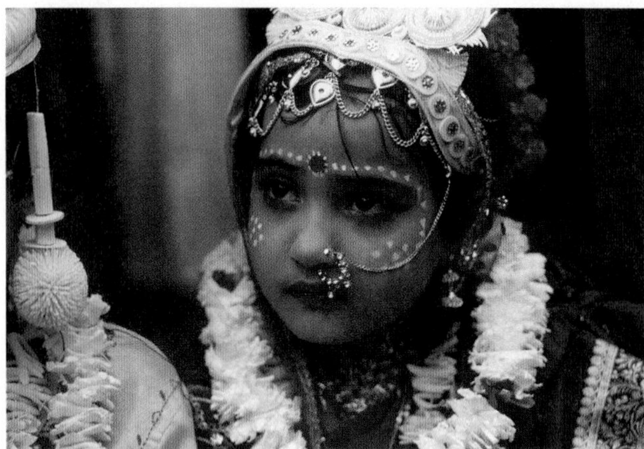

Child brides are a global problem. India is a country with one of the worst records of forcing children into early marriage.

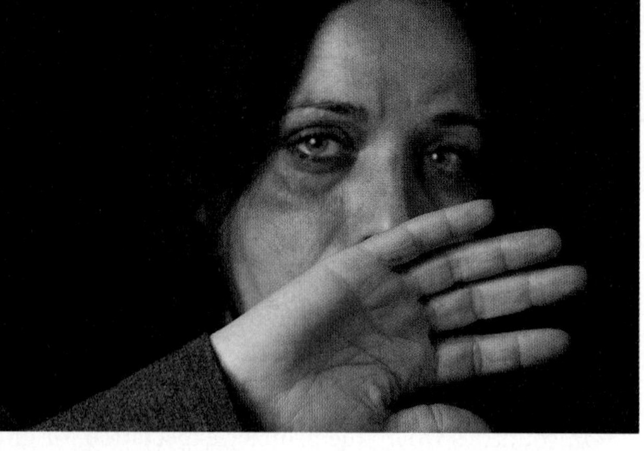

Domestic violence.

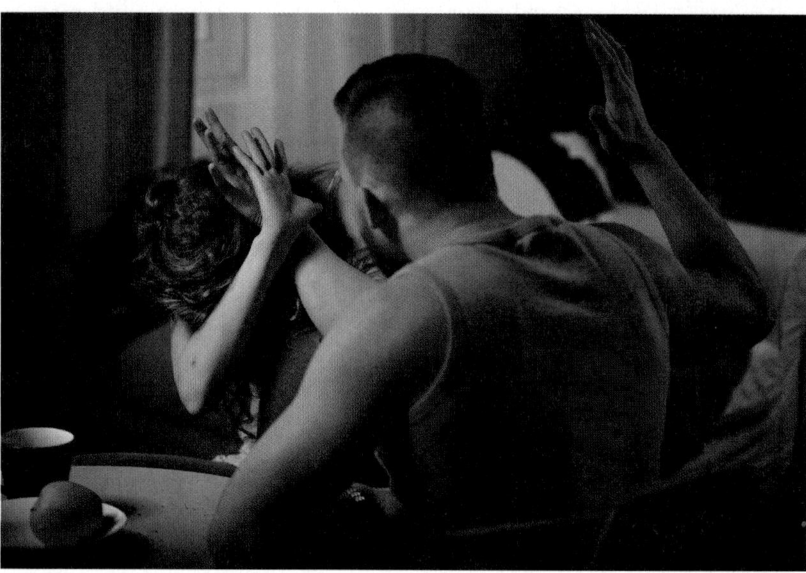

Intimate partner violence is unacceptable.

belief that aggression in relationships is acceptable, desire for power and control in relationships, and a history of physical discipline as a child.[29]

Relationship factors that increase the risk of IPV include marital conflicts and instability, including fights, tensions, separations, and divorce. If one partner is dominant and exerts control of the relationship, rather than it being a partnership, there is an increased risk. Economic stresses and unhealthy family relationships and interactions also affect the likelihood of IPV.[29]

Community factors also come into play, where weak community sanctions, such as others in the neighborhood being unwilling to intervene if they witness violence, increase the risk of IPV. Neighborhoods that are poor and overcrowded experience more IPV. Societal norms that support traditional gender roles make the likelihood of IPV more likely. These include the beliefs that women should stay at home and not be in the paid workforce, that women should be subservient to men, and that it is the husband/father's right to make decisions.

Consequences of IPV

IPV has lifelong consequences that include mental, physical, and reproductive health. **FIGURE 10-4** itemizes some consequences.[32]

BY THE NUMBERS

The Financial Cost of Intimate Partner Violence

In 2003, the CDC estimated the financial costs of intimate partner violence against women.[30] The costs are staggering. Updating the CDC data to 2017 dollars, IPV costs were between $9.3 billion to $10.3 billion. This estimate includes $6.8 billion for medical and mental health services, $1.44 billion in lost productivity from paid and nonpaid work for nonfatal victims and another $1.44 billion lost in lifetime earnings of IPV homicide victims. Breaking down the IPV costs further, included $613 million for rape, $8.2 billion for physical assault, $614 million for stalking, and $1.65 billion in the value of lost lives. Although this is a huge amount of money, these costs are considered an underestimate because they do not include things like social services and criminal justice costs.[30]

THE POWER OF SOCIAL MEDIA CAMPAIGNS

Facebook—Instagram—Pinterest—Twitter—YouTube—Snapchat—Tumblr—and the list goes on. The power of social media and the ability to spread a message is clear. The Pew Research Center found that 79% of Americans use Facebook, 24% use Twitter, 31% use Pinterest, and 32% use Instagram.[31] The wisdom is that facts tell, but stories sell.

The following are just some of the social media campaigns focused on bringing attention to violence against women:

- #metoo
- https://nomore.org/ (listed as a resource, but also running a social media campaign)
- #nevermore
- #stopviolenceagainstwomen
- Strength of a Survivor photo project
- https://blogs.oxfam.org/en/blogs/17-05-31-can-social-media-help-end-violence-against-women-and-girls
- https://www.polishedman.com/

Physical

- Bladder and kidney infections
- Circulatory conditions
- Cardiovascular disease
- Fibromyalgia
- Irritable bowel syndrome
- Chronic pain syndromes
- Central nervous system disorders
- Gastrointestinal disorders
- Joint disease
- Migraines and headaches

Reproductive

- Pelvic inflammatory disease
- Sexual dysfunction
- Sexually transmitted infections, including HIV/AIDS
- Delayed prenatal care
- Preterm delivery
- Pregnancy complications, such as inadequate weight gain, infections, and bleeding
- Adverse pregnancy outcomes, such as low birth weight, preterm delivery, and perinatal deaths
- Unintended pregnancy
- Vaginal bleeding

Psychological

- Anxiety
- Depression
- Symptoms of post-traumatic stress disorder (PTSD)
- Antisocial behavior
- Suicidal behavior
- Low self-esteem
- Inability to trust others, especially in intimate relationships
- Fear of intimacy
- Emotional detachment
- Sleep disturbances

FIGURE 10-4 Consequences of intimate partner violence.

Regardless of the type of abuse, IPV can lead to mental health consequences for the victims. A 2002 study examined outcomes by type of abuse (physical or psychological, with psychological further divided by power/control and verbal abuse). Among the mental health outcomes that were significantly increased included depressive symptoms, heavy alcohol use, and drug use (tranquilizer, painkiller, recreational drugs). Not surprisingly, the more severe the abuse, the worse the outcomes. The most common mental health response is depression. In a study of abused women, 63% had major depression compared to 9.3% in the general population.[33]

Mental health consequences include depression, anxiety, posttraumatic stress disorder, antisocial behavior, suicidal behavior, low self-esteem, and sleep disturbance. In addition, it causes people to distrust others, particularly in intimate relationships.[32]

The physical health consequences of IPV may be the direct result of violence, such as bruises, knife wounds, broken bones, headaches, as well as pain and injury at the point of physical contact. There is also a strong and consistent relationship between abuse and other physical conditions, including cardiovascular, gastrointestinal, endocrine, and immune problems. Victims of abuse have worse health-related quality of life, more healthcare utilization, and more pain.[32,34] Women physically abused by a spouse or live-in partner were significantly more likely than other women to define their health as fair or poor.[35]

There are a large number of health conditions associated with IPV, including pain conditions (migraines and headaches, fibromyalgia, and other chronic pain syndromes), asthma, bladder and kidney infections, circulatory conditions, cardiovascular disease, irritable bowel syndrome, central nervous system disorders, gastrointestinal disorders, and joint disease.[32] Research shows women with a history of IPV were more likely to smoke, binge drink, and be obese.[36]

There is a strong relationship between being in an abusive relationship and poor reproductive outcomes. Women who suffer from IPV are more likely to have sexually transmitted diseases, vaginal bleeding or infection, and urinary tract infections.[37] Victims are more likely to become pregnant unintendedly.[38] Once pregnant, women are more likely to have pregnancy complications (e.g., inadequate weight gain, infections, and bleeding), as well as more adverse pregnancy outcomes (low birth weight, preterm delivery, and neonatal death).[39-41]

Victimization in the LGBTQ Community

Individuals who identify as LGBTQ have equal or higher rates of IPV compared to people who identify as heterosexual. This is true for both women and men. According to the CDC, 44% of lesbians, 61% of bisexual women, and 35% of heterosexual women experienced rape, physical violence, or stalking by an intimate partner. Among men, 26% of gay men, 37% of bisexual men, and 29% of heterosexual men experience rape, physical violence, or stalking by an intimate partner. The data show that women experience these events at younger ages. Among bisexual women who were victims of rape, almost half of them experienced their first completed rape between the ages of 11 and 17 years.[42] Among those within the LGBTQ community, individuals who are transgender are at the greatest risk of assault.

People who are LGBTQ may feel an additional sense of isolation or vulnerability. Not only have their bodies experienced a violation, but their identity as well. LGBTQ individuals are less likely to report a sexual assault. They may fear not being taken seriously. They may fear the authorities will revictimize them because of their sexual orientation. If they are not "out," they may fear the information becoming public, and explaining the situation may require more of them than it would a heterosexual person.

Violence in Immigrant Communities

Using data from the Sexual Assault Among Latinas study, researchers reported on a national sample of adult Latino women living in the United States. The participants were predominantly from Mexico or of Mexican descent or from Cuba. The study asked women about stalking, physical assaults, weapon

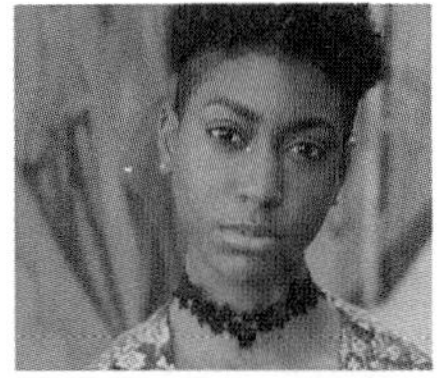
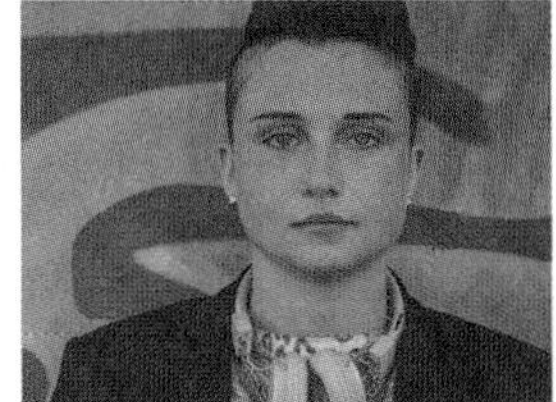
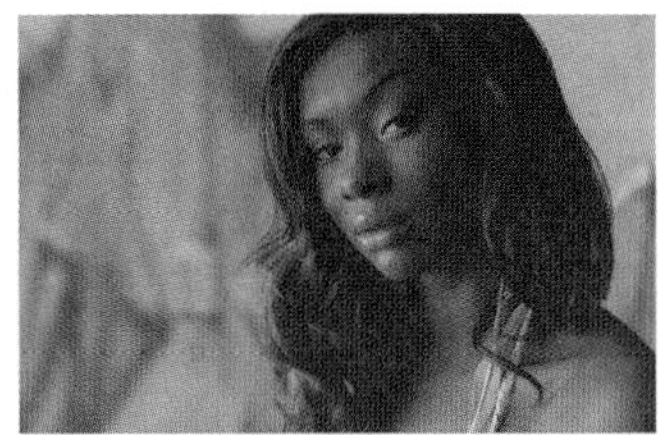

WE BELIEVE YOU.

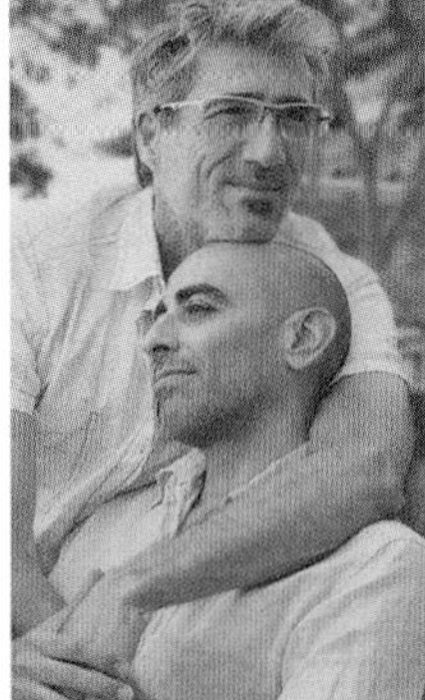
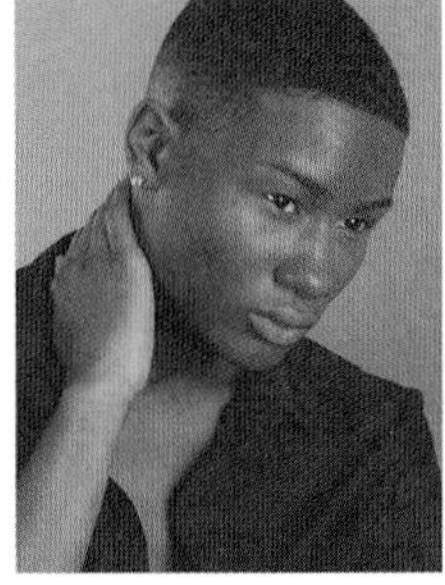
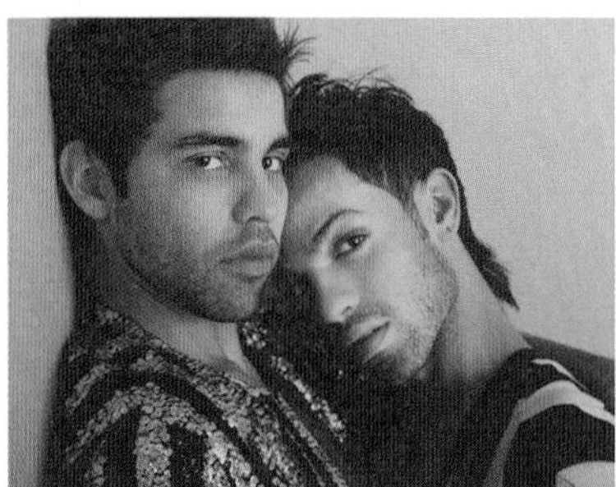
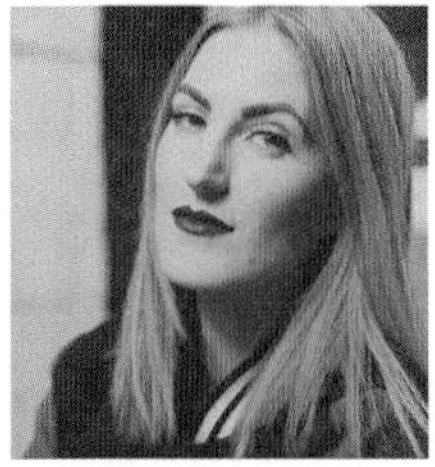

SEXUAL VIOLENCE **HAPPENS IN ALL COMMUNITIES.**
You have the right to live free from sexual violence. You have the right to receive help regardless of your sexual orientation, gender identity or expression, age, immigration status, race, ethnicity, nationality, or your religious or spiritual beliefs.

Sexual assault crisis programs provide free and confidential **services in English and Spanish. These services include:**
· certified sexual assault victim advocates
· short-term counseling and support groups
· information and referrals to other social and legal services
· accompaniment and support in the hospital, police department and court

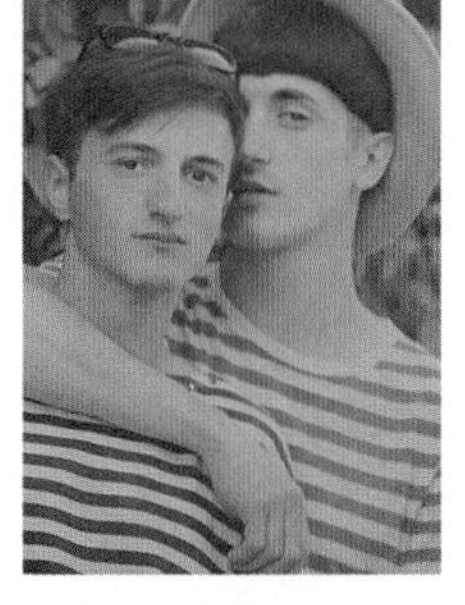

Call the 24-hour, free and confidential hotline:
1-888-999-5545 (English)
1-888-568-8332 (Español)

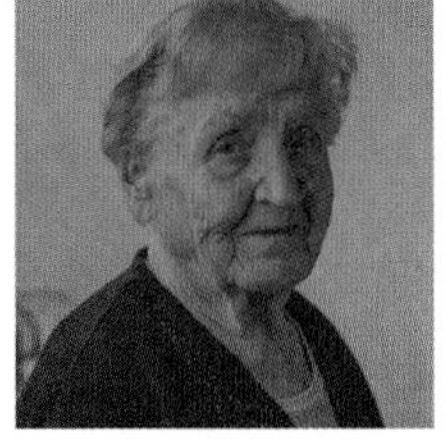

CONNECTICUT ALLIANCE
TO END SEXUAL VIOLENCE
Support. Advocate. Prevent.
EndSexualViolenceCT.org formerly CONNSACS

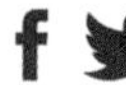

Follow us on social media:

This project was supported by Grant No. 2012-WF-AX-0015 awarded by the Office on Violence Against Women, U.S. Department of Justice. The opinions, findings, conclusions and recommendations expressed in this material do not necessarily reflect the views of the Department of Justice, Office on Violence Against Women.

Same sex abuse.

Reproduced with permission Connecticut Alliance to End Sexual Violence.

assaults, physical assaults in childhood, threats, threats with weapons, sexual assault, attempted sexual assault, sexual fondling, and witnessed victimization. More than half reported at least one lifetime victimization incident, and 66% experienced more than one victimization incident.[43] Starting where this study left off, other researchers studied the relationship of documentation status as it related to violence and help-seeking behaviors among those women. Factors that influence the risk of violence among women who are immigrants include isolation from social support networks, language fluency, cultural norms, economic needs, and documentation status. When abusive husbands sponsor their wives, it creates a situation in which the husband may use their spouse's documentation status to control her.[44]

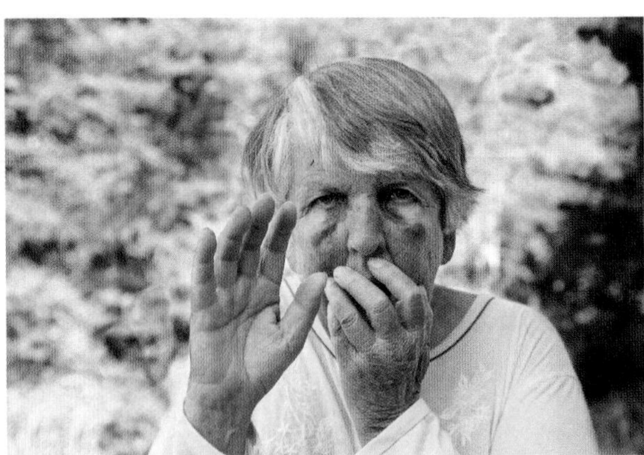

Elder abuse.

Additionally, individuals within immigrant communities may be more vulnerable because the victim's alternatives to living with the abusive spouse are more limited than people who have family around. Thus, they have fewer options to escape the violence, and those options they have are more difficult than for people with a broader network.[45]

While there may be no significant differences between legal status and reported victimization rates or types of perpetrators, undocumented women were less likely to seek formal help than those with permanent status.[41]

Elder Abuse

The definition of elder abuse is very much like that of child abuse. Elder abuse is any knowing, intentional, or negligent act by a caregiver or any other person that causes harm or a serious risk of harm to a vulnerable adult. All states have laws relating to prevention of elder abuse.[46]

As discussed previously, neglect, and physical, emotional, and sexual abuse can all apply to the elderly. In addition, there are specific types that mainly occur among the elderly.[46] These include the following:

- *Exploitation*: illegally taking, misusing, or concealment of funds, property, or assets of a senior for someone else's benefit
- *Abandonment*: desertion of a vulnerable elder by a person who has assumed responsibility for care or custody of that person
- *Self-neglect*: when a person fails to perform essential, self-care tasks, and, as such, threatens his or her health or safety

How Much of a Problem Is Elder Abuse?

systematic review A focused literature review that identifies, appraises, selects, and synthesizes all of the high-quality research relevant to a particular question.

Elder abuse is not only a global public health problem, but it is a human rights problem as well. A recent **systematic review** concluded that elder abuse is "common, fatal and costly."[47] In North America, while abuse occurs in approximately 10% of cognitively intact older adults,[48] the rate among individuals with dementia is almost five times higher.[49] Minorities suffer higher rates of elder abuse. In African American populations, Beach and colleagues found that financial exploitation was three times as high and psychological abuse was four times as high compared to non–African–Americans.[50] In a study from Los Angeles, 40% of Latino adults age 66 years and older had suffered some form of abuse or neglect within the previous year. Nearly 25% reported psychological abuse, 11% reported physical assault, 9% reported sexual abuse, 17% reported financial exploitation, and 12% reported caregiver neglect.[51]

Unhealthy Relationships: Dating Violence and Date Rape

Unhealthy Relationships

The definition of an unhealthy relationship is one in which physical, sexual, psychological, or emotional violence takes place. While even healthy relationships have stressful times, these harmful behaviors characterize unhealthy relationships.[52]

These harmful behaviors include, but are not limited to, the following:

- Pressure to change who you are for your partner
- Being worried when you disagree with your partner
- Feeling pressure to not see your friends or family
- Having to justify where you are when you aren't at home
- Your partner attempting to control or manipulate you
- Feeling pressure to not participate in things you enjoy
- Feeling obligated to have sex, even against your will
- Lack of fairness and equity in the relationship
- You and your partner have no common friends
- A partner attempting to control how you dress and behave
- You have a lack of privacy
- Your partner monitors your social networking sites and/or your phone
- There is an unequal control or resources

If your partner ever tries to hurt you physically or forces you to have sex against your will, these are clear signs that the relationship is not healthy. The choice is to either get help or end the relationship. Your goal is to be in a relationship that allows for individuality, brings out the best in both partners, and encourages personal growth. Speaking with a mental health counselor may help. You may choose to see a counselor on your own or with your partner. Remember that you can only change yourself, and it is your partner's responsibility to change his or her behavior. Having a counselor can help you work out challenges in the relationship.[52]

Everybody deserves to be in a safe and healthy relationship.[53] Loveisrespect.org's description is "the ultimate resource to engage, educate and empower youth to prevent and end abusive relationships." Their website has a quiz on if your relationship is healthy. It is a quick evaluation. They also have related quizzes on topics including whether you are a good partner, whether abusers can change, and how would you help.[54]

It is sometimes hard to understand other people's motivations. An abusive partner may believe it is his or her right to control the person he or she is dating. An abusive partner may believe they know best. An abusive partner may believe it is his or her job to be in charge. Whatever the reason, it is a learned behavior

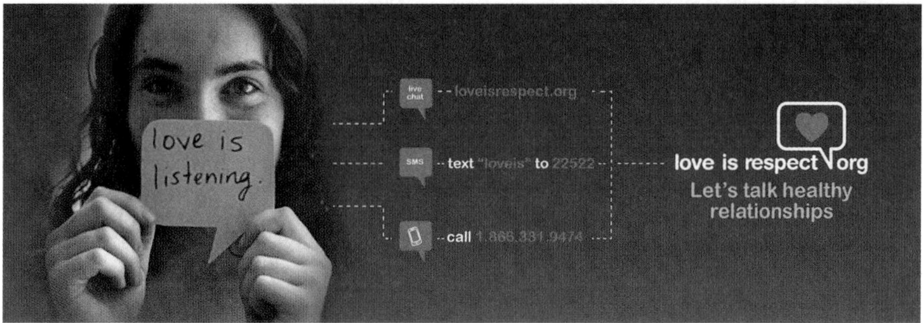

Love is respect.

and it is a choice. Everyone has the chance to make the correct choice, and if needed, to learn to make the correct choice.[53]

Anyone can be abusive, and anyone can be the victim. Abusers and victims can be of any age, race, sexual orientation, or gender, regardless of economic background.

Abusive LGBTQ Relationships

Lesbian, gay, bisexual, transgender, and queer couples experience abusive relationships at the same rate and in the same ways as heterosexual couples do. Depending on your circumstances, where you live, whether your family is supportive, and your school or work environment may all affect your feelings about acknowledging abuse. Remember that regardless of your sexual orientation, you deserve to be in a safe and healthy relationship.[55] Consent within a relationship does not depend on sexual orientation. It is just as important within an LGBTQ relationship as it is within a heterosexual relationship.

Some obstacles you might face in asking for help include the following:

- *Embarrassment*: If you are not out or are still questioning your sexual orientation or gender identity, an abusive partner may use this against you. The abusive partner may intimidate you or focus on your insecurities.[55]
- *Fear of not being taken seriously*: You may worry that in reporting abuse, others won't believe you, that lesbians don't do this to one another, or that the abuse is mutual. An abusive partner may tell you that no one will believe that LGBTQ relationships are abusive or that others will take you seriously.[55]
- *Fear of retaliation, harassment, or bullying*: If you are out, an abusive partner may threaten to expose you to others who don't know: your family, your straight friends, or your workplace. Threatening to do things that will make your life more difficult is not being respectful or supportive.[55]
- *Good intentions*: You may feel uncomfortable with the idea of exposing bad things about the LGBTQ community. Do not believe that one person doing harmful things will reflect poorly on others. In these instances, your safety and well-being are more important.[55]
- *Concerns about legal protection*: You may have all the legal protections that heterosexual people do. Each state has its laws about what you need to obtain a restraining order. Go to www.loveisrespect.org/resources/teen-dating-violence-laws/ to see your state's laws.[56]
- *Loss of community*: If you are part of a religious community or a family that disapproves of LGBTQ people, you may worry that being outed to them will strain that relationship and the acknowledgement of abuse will make it worse. It is important to build a support system around you so that when you need help you can get it.[55]

How to Leave an Abusive Relationship

Have you decided to leave an abusive relationship? Understand that for many, the most dangerous time in an abusive relationship is when it is ending. Because abusive relationships are about power, when you make the decision to leave, your abusive partner is losing control over you. You should have a plan.[53]

Remember, you don't owe your abusive ex-partner anything. This person did you harm, emotionally, physically, or sexually. It truly does not matter why they did it, but you do not owe them an explanation, or a returned phone call. You owe yourself peace of mind. Be clear that you do not want to talk with them or text with them. Block them on Facebook and consider changing your phone number and your email address. You want to make it extremely difficult for them to contact you.

HOW TO HELP A FRIEND IN AN ABUSIVE RELATIONSHIP[57]

1. Be there to talk with your friend. Do it in private.
2. Tell your friend you are worried about his or her safety.
3. Be supportive.
4. Offer specific help. Do what you can to help your friend, depending on what the person needs. The person may just need someone with whom to talk, transportation, or help with childcare.
5. Don't blame the person.
6. Help your friend make a safety plan.
7. Encourage your friend to get organized help (domestic abuse agency, the police, or the court system).
8. Whether your friend decides to leave or stay in the relationship, remain supportive.
9. Encourage your friend to see family and friends outside the relationship.
10. Remember you can't rescue your friend, but you can be there to support them.

U.S. Department of Health and Human Services, Office on Women's Health in the Office. (2017). How to help a friend who is being abused. Retrieved from https://www.womenshealth.gov/violence-against-women/get-help-for-violence/how-to-help-a-friend-who-is-being-abused.html#pubs

If you decide to meet your ex-partner, do it in public and bring a trusted friend with you. Make sure you are not alone. You may find it helpful to keep a written list of why you wanted out of the relationship. In addition, keep a list of what you want to say to your ex. Don't get involved in his/her manipulation. Be sure you are giving them a clear message that the relationship is over. If you see them at school, and the abuse continues, go to the school authorities (faculty, guidance counselor, healthcare facility). Have a friend meet you between classes, and make sure you are not alone with the person.

Make sure you employ technology safety as well. Change your online passwords, particularly if your ex-partner knows them. Block his or her phone number and remove it from your phone. "Love is respect" also suggests changing his or her name in your contact list with a reminder of why you left them. Make sure to update the privacy settings for social media. Turn off location or check-ins so your ex cannot follow you. Set your profile settings to need approval for friends to tag you in a picture or ask your friends not to tag pictures of you. Make sure your ex did not install spyware on your phone and computer. (See http://nnedv.org/downloads/SafetyNet/NNEDV_SpywareAndSafety_2013.pdf for advice about spyware.[58])

Revenge Porn

Revenge porn is the distribution of sexually explicit images or photos without the consent of the individuals shown. It is used to continue a relationship or blackmail the individuals shown. As of March, 2018, 38 states and the District of Columbia have revenge porn laws. Offenses range from misdemeanors to felonies.

Rape

The FBI's current definition of rape is "penetration, no matter how slight, of the vagina or anus with any body part or object, or oral penetration by a sex organ of another person, without the consent of the victim." The FBI expanded their definition because the previous definition excluded many sex offenses, including oral or anal penetration, penetration with objects, and the rape of males.[59] Many women are raped when they are young, with more than half of rape victims being younger than 18. These same women were twice as likely to report being raped as an adult. In these instances, a current or former husband, cohabiting partner,

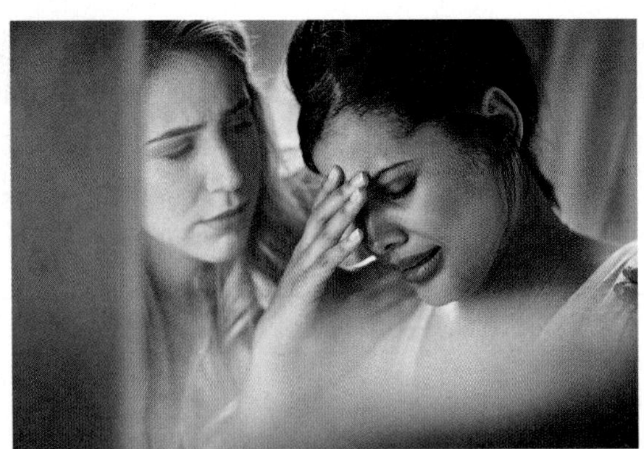

Comforting a friend.

date rape Forcible sexual intercourse by a male acquaintance of a woman, during a date or other voluntary social engagement. The fact that the parties knew each other or that the woman willingly accompanied the man are not legal defenses to a charge of rape. In instances of date rape, the woman did not intend to submit to the sexual advances and resisted verbally and/or physically.

boyfriend, or date primarily perpetrates this violence against women. A woman's risk of injury increases when the assailant is a current or former intimate partner.[59]

Using data from the National Violence against Women Survey conducted by the National Institute of Justice, the U.S. Department of Justice, and the CDC, researchers found that in the United States, 1 in 6 women and 1 in 33 men have been victims of a completed or attempted rape in their life. This translates to more than 876,000 rapes committed against women and more than 11,000 rapes committed against men in the year before the survey.[28] These are probably underestimates because they do not include rapes perpetrated against children or adolescents, the homeless, individuals living in group facilities, or people who do not have telephones.[28]

Rape is real, and rape is painful. There are many kinds of rape: **date rape**, spousal rape, incest, rape by a known assailant, and rape by an unknown assailant.

TALES OF PUBLIC HEALTH

From Rape Culture in the Alaskan Wilderness[60–62]

This is a true story about Jane (not her real name).

Jane lives in the tiny village of Tanana, Alaska, population 254. The town is about 130 miles northwest of Fairbanks. It was a trading settlement for the Koyukon and Tanana Athabascans long before European contact. To reach Tanana, which is near the intersection of the Tanana and Yukon Rivers, you can fly or arrive by boat. In the summer of 2014, the state began work on a road connecting the bush community to the Alaska road system. This is a single-lane gravel road that puts you 6 miles upstream and a 20-minute boat ride from Tanana. When Jane was 13, she was sleeping in the room she shared with her sisters. A man, whom she had known all her life and who was drunk and aggressive, stumbled into her room and climbed on top of her. "He tried to get into my clothes. He tried putting his hands under my shorts and inside my shirt." She felt dirty. She cried. But she didn't tell her parents. The following summer at her family's fish camp, she awoke to another man pulling at her clothes and reaching between her legs. After that, she locked her bedroom door and stayed awake until all the guests visiting her parents had passed out or gone home. She has been repeatedly molested. Now she avoids being alone with men and boys.

When Jane spoke to her sisters, she learned she was not the only one. She was also told to "leave it alone." No one talks about it, but everyone knows it happens. A village elder raped his daughters and granddaughters. Only when he did it to a girl in another family was he arrested. After his stint in jail and some time down river, he is back on the village tribal council. Jane's great aunt was molested and raped by her uncle for years. He did the same thing to the aunt's daughter. Most of the time nothing is reported and nothing is done. Hence, nothing changes.

In 2013, Jane joined the new 4-H club in Tanana. Cynthia Erickson, owner of the town's general store, runs the 4-H club. The club quickly became a place where kids shared their stories of sexual and domestic violence and alcohol and drug abuse. When the 4-H club was asked to speak at a conference in Fairbanks, Jane spoke about her abuse and what she saw happening all around her:

> *A local woman who was gang raped until she could barely walk. A young boy who was sexually assaulted by an older man and later killed himself. Tribal elders who commanded respect, but whose behavior didn't . . . It's happening in his house, in her house, even in your own bed.*

Immediately after the presentation, things seemed to change. A few months later, Cynthia Erickson asked the 4-H kids if they thought their presentations had made a difference. The answer was clearly no.

Alaska is the rape capital of the U.S. At 80 rapes per 100,000 people, it is three times the national average. Of Alaskan women, 59% have been victims of sexual assault, intimate partner violence, or both. As high as those numbers are, they are likely an underestimate. Why? Many of the industries are male dominated. Unlike most of the United States, there are more males than females. The vast wilderness, with few police, and no roads, means getting help is difficult. The culture exacerbates the situation, where silence is the norm and people keep private things private.

In small communities where everyone knows everyone else and is likely related to them by blood or marriage, accusing people is a problem. If you report a crime, you are the one blamed. Cynthia Erickson tells of a woman from her hometown. After enduring beatings by her husband for decades, she moved with her children to Fairbanks. People viewed her as having broken up the family, as if she were supposed to endure the abuse.

Date Rape

Date rape (sometimes called acquaintance rape) usually refers to a rape in which there has been some sort of romantic or potentially sexual relationship between the two parties. Even if there was consensual sex in the past, it is still illegal to force sex upon another person. Date rape is nonconsensual, but force isn't necessarily part of it. If the victim is unable to give consent because they are asleep, or have passed out from drugs or alcohol, it is rape. When people think about rape, they often think of a stranger breaking into their home or jumping out of a shadowy place and attacking. But many people know their rapist.

What is not consent? If one person is saying "no" and the other is ignoring them, that isn't consent. It is incorrect to assume that clothing choice, flirting, or kissing another person is an invitation for sex. Pressuring another person into having sex is not consent. Nor is assuming that because you have had sex in the past, that it is okay now without communication about sexual engagement.

Consent vs. Coercion and Lack of Consent

We don't talk enough about what consent is and what constitutes consent or lack of consent. It is important in a healthy relationship that people feel comfortable talking about what they want to do or don't want to do. In this context, we mean that consent is a voluntary agreement from both partners to engage in sexual activity and that both people say yes, on their terms.

Consent means agreement on each step and making no assumptions about what the other person is comfortable doing; that there is voluntary agreement to engage in sexual activity. Consent means that when a person says no, that is what they mean. There is a need to respect everybody's boundaries.

The definition of coercion is the practice of persuading someone to do something by using force or threats. Using guilt or reacting with anger, resentment, or sadness at being told no is coercion. If your partner does not respect your need to consent, that is a problem. Other red flags are when they pressure you to do something you don't want to do or don't accept that you are not consenting.

In a healthy relationship, partners discuss and respect boundaries. Consent once doesn't mean consent always. Consent must be clear, verbal, sober, and affirmative.

Date Rape Drugs

Date rape drugs are used to assist a sexual assault, and they are also known as "club drugs." These drugs are powerful and dangerous. They often have no color, smell, or taste, so you can't tell if you are being drugged. They can be slipped into your drink when you are not looking. These drugs make you weak and confused so that you are unable to refuse sex or defend yourself. If you are drugged, you might not remember what happened while you were drugged. Date rape

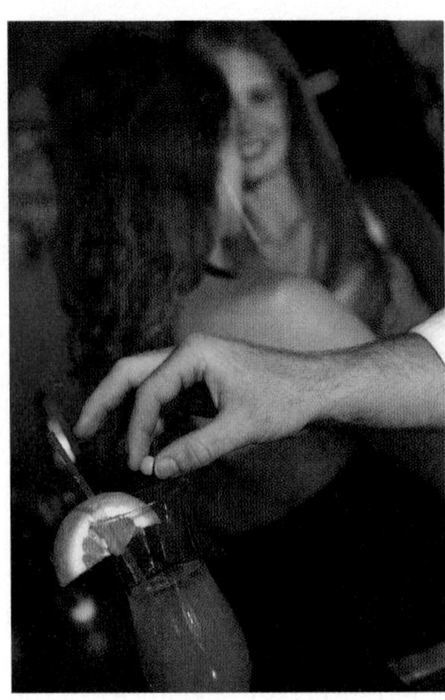

Date rape drugs.

TALES OF PUBLIC HEALTH

One Man's Terrifying Experience With Date Rape[64]

This is a story of one man's experience of being a victim of date rape. The author, Richard Morgan, is a writer.

Richard had arrived in New York after a long bus ride, to visit a man he had met a few weeks earlier. The man was "handsome: 30, well-built, tall with long black hair, and a surfer's laugh." After a shower, his host made him a celebratory drink: it was Gatorade laced with GHB.

Over the course of the weekend, Richard was drugged repeatedly, and he was semiconscious the entire time. As he described it: "I had received anal sex twice in my life before that night. By weekend's end, it was 17 times, according to my fog-of-war count. Eyes squeezed shut, the tally was the only thing I focused on at times—like a ticking clock in a solitary confinement cell."

Although Richard said no and wanted to stop, his rapist ignored his pleas. Accompanying the multiple rapes was Lady Gaga's "I Like It Rough." Richard could see the front door to the apartment, but there was no way to get there. And even if he physically could have gotten away, it would have meant running through the streets of New York naked.

Some people have a hard time imagining that men get raped. But they do. Not all rapes are a man dragging an innocent woman into a dark alley or woods. The reality of rapes is complicated. Rape covers a broad spectrum: war-crime rape, date rape, rape as a ritual for pledging a fraternity, spousal rape, incest, rape with known assailants, rape with unknown assailants. When people discuss male victims of rape, the first thought is pedophilia. Truly, anyone can be raped.

After his rape, Richard wanted nothing to do with sex. "I realized there was a whole extra circle of Hell, hidden horrors done to my unconscious body with no way of ever knowing fully what happened."

Richard's response to his rape has been to dedicate himself to kindness, hope, and intimacy, with the hope that telling his story can serve a purpose.

drugs are used on both females and males.[63] If you are drinking alcohol at a party, try not to put your cup down.

The three most common date rape drugs are:

- *Rohypnol* (generic name flunitrazepam). In some parts of the United States, other drugs have replaced Rohypnol. These are Klonopin (generic name clonazepam) and Xanax (generic name alprazolam).[59] Other names for Rohypnol are Rophies, Roofies, Roach, Rope, Ruffies, the "date rape" drug, Mexican valium, Costa Rican Quaaludes, Forget pill, and Forget me pill.[61]
- *GHB*, which is short for gamma hydroxybutyric acid, is a central nervous system depressant.[63] Other names for GHB are Grievous Bodily Harm

(GBH), Liquid X, Liquid E, Liquid Ecstasy, Easy Lay, G, Vita-G, G-Juice, Georgia Home Boy, Great Hormones, Somatomax, Bedtime Scoop, Soap, Gook, Gamma 10, and Energy Drink.[63]

- *Ketamine* is a dissociative anesthetic, which means that it distorts a person's perception of sight and sound and produces feelings of detachment from the environment and self.[63] Other names for Ketamine are Cat Valium, Cat Tranquilizer, K, Special K, Super K, Vitamin K, Kit Kat, Purple, and Jet.[63]

Rapes on Campus

Think about the following statistics: Up to 90% of college campus rapes occur as date rapes. The U.S. Department of Education is investigating colleges and universities for **Title IX** sexual violence issues.[65] Only 40% U.S. colleges or universities offer any sort of sexual assault training to their staff and rarely is this training offered to the general student population. Even fewer colleges train campus security officers on how to respond to a report of date rape. Approximately two-thirds of schools are out of compliance with the Clery Act, which requires all colleges and universities to keep and disclose information about crimes on and near their campuses. Only 25% of college women who have been raped describe the encounter as rape. Of college men, 43% admit that they have used coercive behavior to have sex, including ignoring when a woman said no. Up to 80% of the date rapes by men against women occur when the woman is intoxicated. Forty percent of men assume that alcohol consumption by a woman indicates she is a willing sexual partner. One in twelve college-age men admit having fulfilled the definition of rape or attempted rape, yet virtually none identify themselves as rapists. Date rape is the least reported of all violent crimes.[66]

Title IX A comprehensive federal law that prohibits discrimination on the basis of sex in any federally funded education program or activity.

Part of the problem with date rape is that even when men describe their own behavior as coercive, they don't think of themselves as rapists; and women don't see themselves as being raped even when they have been. What this means in practical terms is that the behavior continues because nothing is done to stop the practice. When a school does nothing, it legitimizes the behaviors.

Mattress Performance (Carry That Weight)

Emma Sulkowicz was a sophomore at Columbia University when she alleged a male student who was supposedly her friend raped her. The university cleared her attacker of wrongdoing. In protest, Sulkowicz carried a mattress to protest campus sexual assault (**FIGURE 10-5**). She even carried it to Columbia's graduation ceremony.[67]

REAL CONSENT

No one who uses lies or alcohol to persuade someone sexually has real consent.

It is hard to ignore a woman carrying a mattress everywhere she goes when she is on campus. Her position was, that as long as her rapist was at the same school, she would carry her mattress.

According to Sulkowicz, what began as consensual sex devolved into rape. She says that the young man "pushed her legs against her chest, choked her, slapped her, and anally raped her" in her dorm room, as she struggled. When two friends acknowledged that he had been abusive toward them as well, she pressed charges with the university administration. According to Title IX, universities must adjudicate sexual-assault claims (see the box on Title IX).[68]

Sulkowicz claims that Columbia University administrators made errors during the hearing process. The young man denied the charges. Columbia did

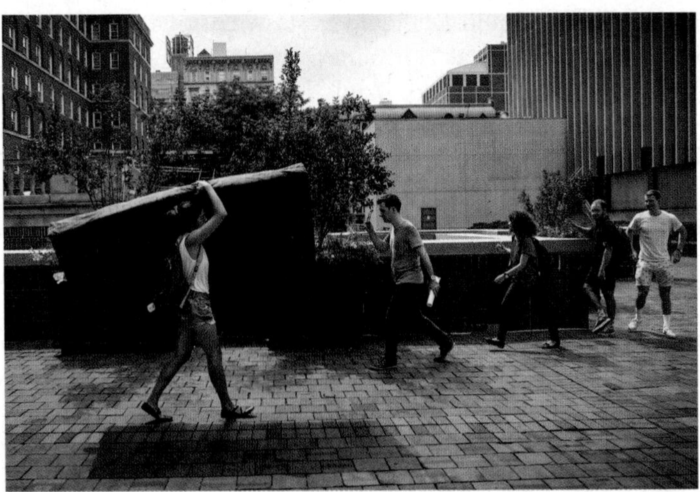

FIGURE 10-5 Emma Sulkowicz carried a mattress in protest of the university's lack of action after she reported being raped during her sophomore year.

REGARDING TITLE IX: YOUR SCHOOL MUST RESPOND PROMPTLY AND EFFECTIVELY TO SEXUAL VIOLENCE[69]

- Students have the right to report the incident to the school; the school must investigate what happened, and your complaint should be resolved promptly and equitably.
- Students can report sexual violence to campus or local law enforcement. Even if there is a criminal complaint, the school still has requirements under Title IX.
- The school must adopt and publish procedures for resolving complaints of sexual violence. The resolution must be prompt and equitable.
- The school must ensure you are aware of Title IX rights and available resources.
- All students are protected by Title IX.

not hear her charges for 6 months and then found in his favor. When Sulkowicz appealed the decision, a dean refused to overturn the verdict.[68]

In response, Sulkowicz used the mattress as the centerpiece of her senior art thesis. To her, the mattress symbolized the university's flawed handling of her complaint. The young man graduated the same day. He has steadfastly maintained he did not rape Emma Sulkowicz. He has sued the university[68] and administration officials for what he calls a "harassment campaign" after the university cleared him.[67] He requested in his lawsuit that the university prohibit Sulkowicz from carrying the mattress during graduation. He also claimed the university supported her in committing gender-based harassment against him.[70]

Shortly after Sulkowicz began her protest, a group of Columbia students, calling themselves "Carry That Weight Together," began to help her carry her mattress around campus. The movement went beyond Columbia to more than 130 college and university campuses, documenting their standing in solidarity with survivors of sexual assault and domestic violence with #carrythatweight. Both Sulkowicz's and other supporters' goal was to shift the way rape survivors are treated by university administrators. By carrying mattresses, the action made the problem more public. It is a powerful visual symbol. By bringing sexual assault into the public sphere, it helps survivors realize they aren't alone.[71] As the website https://www.knowyourix.org/ says, "Everyone needs Title IX because the cost of school should NOT include sexual violence."[72]

TALES OF PUBLIC HEALTH

The Hunting Ground[73]

There is much more to this CNN documentary about sexual assault on American college campuses than is presented here. However, what is presented here makes it clear that universities are not on the side of the sexual assault victim.

There is a long history of sexual assault on American college campuses. However, just because it has been happening for a long time does not make the colleges' and universities' response to it acceptable.

In general, many students (women and men) find when they go to an administrator to report being sexually assaulted, there is a lot of victim blaming.

- "What were you wearing?"
- "What were you drinking?"
- "How much did you drink?"
- "You shouldn't go out in short skirts."
- "Drop out of school until it blows over."
- "How did you say no?"
- "You don't know what he is going through and neither do I. He could be having a really hard time."
- "Despite the fact that I had a written admission from him, I did not have enough evidence. The facts that I presented to them only proved that he loved me."

Is it surprising then that 88% of sexual assaults on campus do not get reported?

From administrators to the filmmakers:

- "The first job of an administrator is to protect the institution from harm, not the student from harm."
- "You make it difficult for the student to report. So you don't have 200 or 1,000 reported assaults. So, you artificially keep the numbers low."
- "They discourage students from going to the police because it creates a public record."
- "It is in the interest of the college to actually suppress all knowledge that a rape has happened."

In 2012, 45% of colleges reported no sexual assaults on their campuses.

After a sexual assault, a Harvard law student went to her dean of students. What she was told was, "I just want to make sure, above all else, that you don't talk to anyone about this. It could be bad for everyone if people start rallying around having him removed from campus."

University	Years	Reported Sexual Assaults	Suspension/Expulsions
Harvard University	2009–2013	135	10 suspensions
University of California at Berkeley	2008–2013	78	3 suspensions
Dartmouth College	2002–2013	155	3 expulsions
Stanford University	1996–2013	259	1 expulsion
University of North Carolina	2001–2013	136	0 expulsions
University of Virginia	1998–2013	205	0 expulsions*

*Over the same time period, University of Virginia had 183 expulsions for cheating and other honor code violations.

One interpretation might be that women are lying. It is rare that women make false allegations of rape. Between 95% and 98% of women are telling the truth when they report being sexually assaulted.

Universities protect perpetrators across the board because they have a financial incentive to do so. Perpetrators who are found responsible for rape are much more likely to sue institutions than survivors are.

Below is a table of *actual* sanctions men received for being found responsible for a sexual assault.

University	Actual Sanction for Sexual Assault
Columbia University	Suspended for 1 semester
Indiana University	Suspended over summer vacation
Yale University	Suspended for 1 day
University of Colorado, Boulder	$75 fine
University of Toledo	$25 fine
Brandeis University	Given a warning
University of Colorado	Assigned a paper to "reflect on your experience"
Occidental College	Required to construct a poster board listing 10 ways to approach a girl you like
Occidental College	50 hours of community service at a rape crisis center
James Madison University	Expelled upon graduation

NInety-five percent of college presidents say their institutions handle sexual assault reports "appropriately." Yet more than 100 colleges and universities are currently under federal investigation for their handling of sexual assault complaints.

Stalking

Depending on the definitions used, researchers estimate that between 1 million and 5.3 million persons are stalked in the United States each year.[74] Stalking is a criminal activity, consisting of the repeated following and harassing of another person. Stalking is unusual as a criminal behavior because the individual actions that constitute stalking are not illegal. Sending flowers, writing love notes, waiting for a person outside his or her place of work, are not illegal and are desirable actions, if wanted. However, when they are intended to instill fear, they become illegal. Although most antistalking laws are gender-neutral, most perpetrators are men and most victims are women.[74]

Stalking is about one person trying to control another.[75] The ability of the stalker to control the victim is the reward. The normal responses to being stalked are all rewards to the stalker: screaming, threatening, and arguing are evidence to a stalker that they are in control.

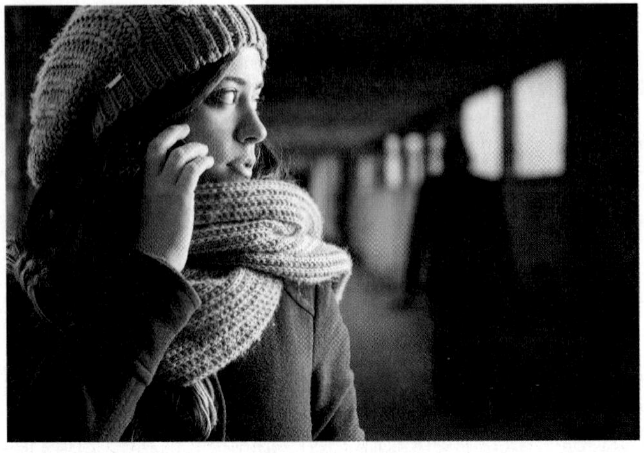

Stalking.

How to Stop a Stalker

Do not take being a victim of stalking lightly. File a complaint against the stalker, and ask the police about seeking a protective order against the person who is stalking you. The punishment for violating a protective order varies by state, from a misdemeanor to a felony. To find your state's laws on stalking go to the Stalking Resource Center website. (See the resource list at the end of the chapter).[76] Because laws change, the American Bar Association recommends verifying the information.

Cooperate with prosecutors. Sometimes victims fear that involving the law will provoke more and worse behavior from the perpetrator. Victims should be as proactive as possible using the legal system.[77]

Protect yourself. Stalkers have a mental health problem that is not the victim's responsibility. If you are the victim of stalking, you need to protect yourself and those around you. Inform neighbors, coworkers, and security guards about the stalker. If the stalker uses the telephone to call you, ask the police to tap the phone line.[77]

Collect evidence. If you are the victim of stalking, collect and preserve evidence. Keep a diary of stalking and other crimes the perpetrator commits. If the perpetrator destroys property, take a photograph of that as well as any injuries the perpetrator inflicts. If the stalker writes you letters or notes or leaves you phone messages, do not destroy or erase them.[77]

TALES OF PUBLIC HEALTH

Passage of America's First Anti-Stalking Laws[78]

Rebecca Schaeffer (November 6, 1967–July 18, 1989) was an American model and television and film actress.

She began working as a model in high school. At 17, Rebecca moved to New York City. After being on the cover of *Seventeen* magazine, she was cast in the television show, *My Sister Sam*. Robert John Bardo murdered Schaeffer after stalking her over a period of 2 to 3 years.

In 1987, Bardo traveled to Los Angeles. He went to the Warner Brothers studio, hoping to meet with Schaeffer. The security guards turned him away. A month later, he returned with a knife, but again, the security guards prevented him from gaining access to Schaeffer.

Bardo returned to Tucson and paid a private detective to find Schaeffer's home address through the California Department of Motor Vehicles. Because he was under age, his brother helped him buy a handgun. Returning to Los Angeles, he rang Schaeffer's doorbell. She answered the door, and after a short conversation asked him to leave. He returned later that evening. When Schaeffer answered the door, he shot her at point-blank range. She died in the hospital.

Bardo was convicted of capital murder and sentenced to life imprisonment without parole for her murder. Schaeffer's death helped prompt the 1990 passage of America's first antistalking laws.

Bullying: The Power Imbalance

Bullying can take many forms. It can be face-to-face, by mail, by email, by phone or text, or over social media. Bullying can be emotional or physical. The target can be nonspecific, or it can be that the target is different from the bully religiously, physically, racially, or because of gender identity. The definition of bullying is as follows:

> *Bullying is unwanted, aggressive behavior among school-aged children that involves a real or perceived power imbalance. The behavior is repeated, or has the potential to be repeated, over time.*[79]

The behaviors can include physical fighting, stealing, making threats, name calling, teasing, giving "dirty" looks, purposefully excluding someone from a group, and spreading rumors.[79,80]

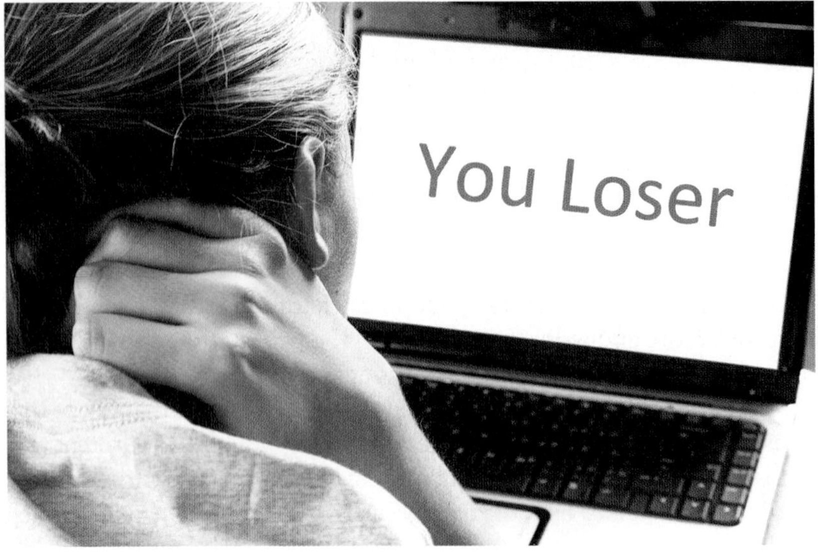

© chrisboy2004/E+/Gettyimages.

The National Center for Education Statistics surveyed over 25 million students aged 12–18 years. More than 20% reported they were bullied at school during the 2012–2013 school year. Almost 7% reported having been cyberbullied (bullied online through email or social media[81]). There is noticeably more bullying in sixth and seventh grade than during other grades. All of the behaviors that constitute bullying: being made fun of, called names, or insulted; had rumors spread, threatened with harm; pushed, shoved, tripped, or spit on; forced to do things they didn't want to do; or intentionally excluded from activities occurred at higher rates among sixth and seventh graders than at later grades.

cyberbullying A form of bullying that takes place over digital devices like cell phones, computers, and tablets. It can occur through SMS, text, and apps, or online in social media, forums, or gaming where people can view, participate in, or share content. It includes sending, posting, or sharing negative, harmful, false, or mean content about someone else. It can include sharing personal or private information about someone else that is intended to cause embarrassment or humiliation.

Cyberbullying peaked among tenth graders.[82] Cyberbullying includes mean text messages or emails, rumors sent by email or on a social media site, and embarrassing pictures, videos, websites, or fake profiles.[83]

It is true that kids who are cyberbullied are often bullied in person as well. Because of the reach of technology, kids who are cyberbullied never get a reprieve. Additionally, messages can be posted anonymously and spread quickly. Once it is out, it is difficult to take back and sometimes impossible to trace.[83]

Children Involved in Bullying

Children's involvement in bullying is complicated. Often kids play multiple roles in the group: the one who bullies, the one who is bullied, the witnesses, and the ones who assist. There are reasons why kids who bully do so. They may be aggressive or easily frustrated, they may be having issues at home, they may have learned that violence is a way to handle anger or frustration, or they may have friends who bully others. The child who is doing the bullying may not be bigger or stronger than the one being bullied. Although the power on the part of the child who does the bullying may be due to size and physical strength, it can also be due to popularity or other characteristics. Children who participate in bullying behavior need to understand that it is wrong to bully others and that their behavior is unacceptable.[79]

Children perceived as vulnerable and unable to defend themselves are more likely to be bullied. They may be less popular or seen as different from their peers. This difference may have to do with weight, clothing worn, being new to a school, or simply "uncool" by whatever definition is current.[78]

There are roles other than bully that kids play in bullying situations. Kids may assist in the bullying and encourage others to participate in this behavior.

There are kids who reinforce the bullying by providing an audience. While they are not actively engaging in bullying, they likely encourage the one who does the bullying. There are outsiders, who remain separate from the situation, neither participating nor defending the bullied. There are also kids who defend the bullied child.[79]

There are things you can do if you witness a situation where a child or children are bullying one another. It is important to send a message that bullying behavior is unacceptable. Intervene immediately and get others to help if needed. Stay calm and separate those involved. Make sure everyone is safe. If there are any immediate needs for medical or mental health attention, address that as well. Remember to model respectful behavior.[79]

Young Adults

The behaviors that are considered bullying among school-aged kids may still occur among college-aged individuals. Bullying-like behaviors, either in person or via technology among college-aged people include hazing, harassment, and stalking. Many of these behaviors are, under state and federal law, crimes when committed by individuals over the age of 18. They may have serious consequences for the person.

BY THE NUMBERS

Bullying

A study at a northeastern public university explored bullying by students and teachers. The researchers sampled 1,025 undergraduates. Almost a quarter of students reported that they had seen students bully other students occasionally, and 2.8% very frequently. Five percent reported that other students bullied them occasionally, and 1.1% very frequently. Students reported 12.8% had seen teachers bullied by others occasionally, and 1.9% very frequently. Teachers also bullied students in the sample, 4.2% occasionally and 0.5% very frequently. Of the students, 3.2% acknowledged they had bullied others occasionally, and 1.9% very frequently. Male students bullied significantly more than females.[84]

How You Can Help or Get Help

If you or a friend is the target of these behaviors, don't keep it to yourself. Talk to someone you trust. If the behavior violates campus policies or laws, report it to your campus or community law enforcement. If the behavior is sexual harassment, the college's Title IX coordinator is likely the right person to approach. Many colleges have an ombudsperson whose job it is to handle concerns and complaints. This person should be able to direct you to the appropriate resource to resolve the issue.

Hazing

hazing Any action or situation, with or without the consent of the participants, which recklessly, intentionally, or unintentionally endangers the mental, physical, or academic health or safety of a student.

Hazing has been around as a behavior for a long time. For a long time, it was part of the college experience for many people. Hazing is a form of interpersonal violence that can jeopardize the health and safety of students.[85] Hazing as an activity dates back to the ancient and medieval eras.

It includes many actions that are unacceptable. Hazing includes physical injury, assault or battery, kidnapping or imprisonment, intentionally placing a person at risk of mental or emotional harm, degradation, humiliation, forced consumption of any liquid or solid, placing an individual in physical danger, which includes abandonment, and impairment of physical liberties, or other interference with academic endeavors.

Hazing among U.S. college students is widespread, including among fraternities and sororities, student organizations, and athletic teams. Included among hazing practices are alcohol consumption, humiliation, isolation, sleep-deprivation, and sex acts. Students do not always consider these types of experiences as hazing, even though they are.[86]

A study of almost 12,000 students at 53 college and universities found that hazing practices were common across student groups. Researchers also found a gap between the number of students who experienced hazing and the number that identified their experience as such.[86]

Hazing is now illegal in most states and on most college campuses. Most colleges have hazing prevention policies and response procedures for hazing incidents, based on their educational mission. Search for hazing prevention and state laws to see what your state's laws are regarding hazing.[87]

It is important to understand how serious the consequences of hazing can be. A 2008 study[88] reported on a survey of death events linked to bullying or hazing. This study covered more than 50 years of reports. At least 250 deaths were the result of "bullying, hazing, or ragging." Of all the reports, 76% contained a history of bullying, and 22% contained a history of hazing or ragging.

Gun Violence: Too Many Guns?

How Prevalent Is Gun Violence in America?

According to CNN, in the United States, the rate of gun ownership is the highest in the world at 88.8 firearms for every 100 people.[89] The second highest is Yemen, a country listed by the U.S. Department of State as a high-security threat due to terrorist activities and civil unrest.[90] In Yemen, there are 54.8 firearms for every 100 people. That means that in Yemen, a country the State Department deems as dangerous, there are 40% fewer guns per person than in the United States.[89]

Research shows there is a relationship between firearms and violence, such that the more guns in a household the more likely there is to be a

BY THE NUMBERS

Guns in the United States

Sixty-two percent of people who own guns in the United States own more than one gun. Of those owning guns, 74% own a rifle or shotgun, 68% handguns, 17% semiautomatic weapons, and 8% other weapons. Why do people own guns? Sixty-seven percent say for protection against crime, 66% for target shooting, and 58% for hunting.[89]

In 2011, the homicide (murder) rate in the United States was 4.7 per 100,000 residents, the lowest level since 1963. Even as the murder rate dropped, there was little change in the percentage of murders committed with guns. Firearms were used in 68% of murders. But this rate does not reflect everybody's experience. From 2002 to 2011, the average homicide rate for males was 3.6 times higher than the rate for females. Young adults, ages 18 to 24 years, had the highest homicide rates. The average homicide rate for African Americans was 6.3 times higher than the rate for Caucasians.[91] The United States has the highest homicide rate of the world's developed nations.

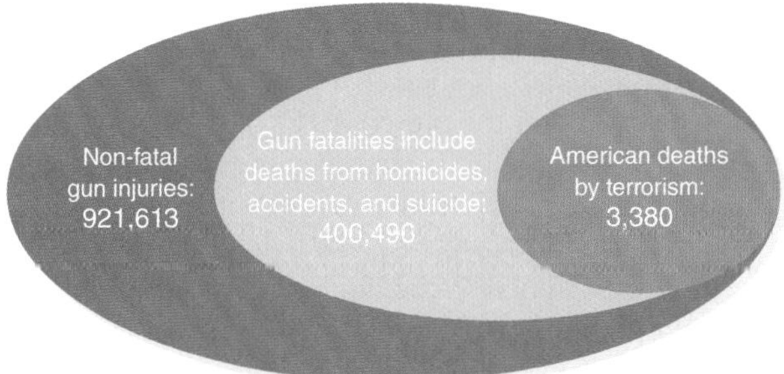

FIGURE 10-6 Compared to terrorism deaths, there are 120 times as many fatalities due to homicides, accidents, and suicide, and almost 273 times as many nonfatal injuries due to guns.

Data from CNN. Retrieved from http://www.cnn.com/2015/12/04/us/gun-violence-graphics/

gun-related homicide. The relationship was true even when the researchers considered other factors associated with violence, including poverty, urbanization, unemployment, alcohol consumption, and nonlethal violent crime.[92] States that have a higher rate of gun ownership have significantly higher homicide victimization rates. Household guns are used to kill men, women, and children.[93] A study of Arizona motorists reviewed self-reports of drivers. Having a gun in the car was an indicator for aggressive and illegal behavior while driving.[94]

After the October 2015 shooting at a community college in Oregon, President Barak Obama asked the news organizations to compare the number of persons killed by guns within the United States with the number of U.S. citizens killed by terrorists (**FIGURE 10-6**). To compute the number of persons who died by firearms from 2001 to 2013, CNN used data from the CDC. Between 2001 and 2013, 406,496 people died by firearms on U.S. soil, including homicides, accidents, and suicides. Data on U.S. citizens killed by terrorists overseas came from the U.S. State Department. From 2001 to 2013, overseas 350 U.S. citizens were killed. Inside the United States, another 3,380 people were killed in domestic acts of terrorism. More than 120 times as many people died from firearms compared to terrorism over this 12-year period.[95]

In addition to the number of deaths due to guns, there are even more nonfatal gun injuries. In the period between 2001 and 2013, there were more than 900,000 nonfatal injuries due to guns. As many deaths as there are due to guns, a person is more than twice as likely to be injured as killed due to guns.[95]

Who Owns Guns?

Every time there is a mass shooting in the United States, there is another discussion about gun control. There are pros and cons to restrictions on gun ownership (**TABLE 10-3**); however, the rigidity of the two sides' positions makes it difficult to have a calm and meaningful conversation about the issue. However, it is important to think about who and why people want guns. There is no simple answer.

The primary reason people cite as their reason for wanting guns is for protection.[98] It is also a common reason provided by incarcerated youth who are in jail or prison for gun-related crimes. If guns used in crimes were initially obtained for protection, there is little reason to believe youth will willingly give them up.[99]

GUN VIOLENCE RESEARCH: HOW THE DICKEY AMENDMENT FROZE FEDERAL FUNDING

In 1993, a group of researchers published an article in the *New England Journal of Medicine*. They concluded that the presence of a gun in the house made it 2.7 times more likely for there to be a homicide in the home. Rather than make you safer, guns increased the risk of death to a family member or acquaintance.[96]

The National Rifle Association responded by trying to eliminate the center that funded the study, the National Center for Injury Prevention at the CDC. While Congress did not abolish the center, they added the Dickey Amendment to the Omnibus Consolidated Appropriations Bill for fiscal year 1997. The language said, "none of the funds made available for injury prevention and control at the CDC may be used to advocate or promote gun control." It was unclear exactly what research was or was not permitted. As a result, support for firearm injury prevention research quickly dried up. In the 2012 funding, Congress approved a similar prohibition for the National Institutes of Health.

Since 1997, there has essentially been a ban on federal funding for gun violence research.

TABLE 10-3 Pros and Cons of Gun Restrictions

Pro-Gun Ownership: Gun Restrictions Are Not the Answer	Anti-Gun Ownership: We Should Have More Gun Restrictions
■ Symbol of freedom ■ Feeling of security ■ If guns are banned, outlaws will find a way to have guns. ■ Most gun owners are responsible. ■ Causes of mass shootings are all different and we don't know why. ■ Gun registries can be used by governments to control the people. ■ Current gun laws are poorly executed.	■ Guns are not safe. There are many accidents involving inexperienced or careless individuals. ■ Many criminals can legally buy guns. ■ Current gun registration laws are inadequately enforced, and there are significant loopholes in the current gun laws. ■ Kids love showing off or playing with adult things. ■ Semiautomatic weapons should be for military use only. ■ There are many scenarios in which gun availability puts people at increased risk of death, such as an abusive spouse killing a partner and a depressed person successfully committing suicide.

The Pew Research Center found that gun owners view themselves differently than other adults. They are more likely to self-identify as an "outdoor person" (68% vs. 51%), or as "a typical American" (72% vs. 62%), and to acknowledge "honor and duty" as core values (59% vs. 48%). Those who own guns also are twice as likely as those who don't own guns to identify as a "hunter, fisher, or sportsman" (37% vs. 16%).[97]

In 2004, Kyle Cassidy wondered why people bought guns. He took three cross-country trips to photograph gun owners at home and ask them why. The people he met were a cross-section of the people who live in the United States. You can see their answers at Slate.com if you search for "Kyle Cassidy."

Regardless of your position on gun ownership, there is no doubt that when there are children in the house, owners should store firearms to make them inaccessible to children. They need to be unloaded, locked in a gun safe, and

BY THE NUMBERS

Who Owns Guns?

Who owns guns? Based on data from the Pew Research Center, gun ownership varies by region of the country.[97]

- By region:
  - Southerners: 38%
  - Midwesterners: 35%
  - Westerners: 34%
  - Northeasterners: 27%

The only statistical difference between those percentages is for those in the northeastern United States, who are significantly less likely than the rest of the country to have a gun.

- By race/ethnicity:
  - Blacks: 19%
  - Whites: 41%
  - Hispanics: 20%

Blacks may be less likely than Whites to keep guns; however, they are significantly more likely to be a shooting victim.

- By age:
  - 18- to 29-year-olds: 26%
  - 30- to 49- year-olds: 32%
  - Over 50 years old: 40%
- By place of residence:
  - City dwellers: 25%
  - Suburbanites: 36%
  - Rural residents: 51%
- By political party:
  - Republicans: 49%
  - Democrats: 22%
  - Independents: 37%
- By ideology:
  - Conservatives: 41%
  - Moderates: 36%
  - Liberals: 23%

stored separately from ammunition. The ammunition should be kept in a locked storage box.

Alcohol and Guns

The association between alcohol and interpersonal violence is clear. Studies show that the effects of alcohol, including lack of self-discipline, increased mood swings, and reduced cognitive functioning, result in higher rates of violence.[100] When a violent individual with a gun has been drinking, the opportunity to do a great deal of harm is readily available.[101]

A study from Chicago used city, state, and national data to look at the relationship between gunshot wounds and proximity to establishments with liquor licenses, both package stores and taverns. While there was no association when looking at the city as a whole, in certain areas, it was highly statistically significant, meaning that the association was not by chance. In five of the city's regions, the likelihood of a gunshot wound was more than 500 times as high near a liquor store and 21 times as high near a tavern.[102] Where are the liquor stores near you? Are these areas safe?

Does Conceal and Carry Actually Work?

Many people believe that the ability to carry a concealed handgun both makes them safer and reduces crime. A recent study evaluated the connection between crime rates and concealed gun permits in four states: Florida, Michigan, Pennsylvania, and Texas.[103] The researchers looked at 12 years of data, from 1998 to 2010. They compared handgun licenses for each county and arrest data from the FBI's Uniform Crime Rates, which includes arrests for homicide, rape, robbery, aggravated assault, burglary, theft, and arson.[103]

The researchers found no connection between allowing concealed weapons and crime rates.[103] The study was in response to the Texas legislators' decision to allow concealed handguns on campuses. An earlier study from California found an association between the right to carry a gun with increases in violent crime.[104]

Many people believe that allowing people to carry guns will make them safer. A 2010 study conducted by ABC News and the Bethlehem Police Department at Pennsylvania's Muhlenberg College confronted the subject of putting guns in classrooms. The videos listed here, from ABC News, showed people's reaction when faced with an active shooter. Police are trained and retrained as to how to respond correctly in such a difficult situation. The experiment was done with a police department to test the ability of average people without crisis training to react and protect themselves, with a gun, under stress. This experiment was in response to a real situation in which a former student with a gun killed five and injured 22 people. Officers trained six students with different levels of firearm experience during a gun-safety class, and then gave them a handgun with fake bullets that they would wear

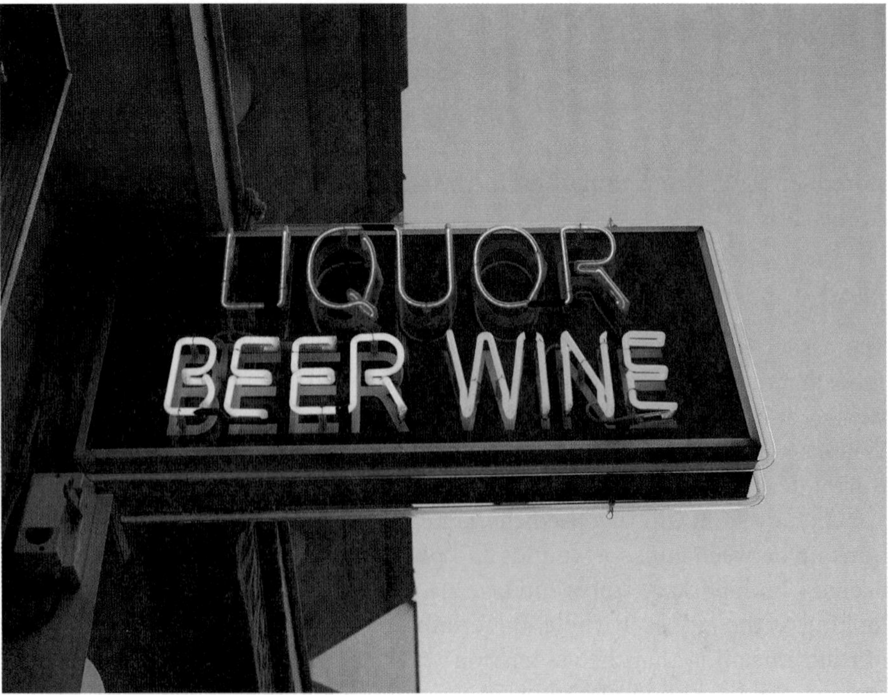

during class. At random times, an armed intruder would burst into the classroom and open fire. The question of interest was, if someone in the lecture hall had a gun, would this have protected him or her or other students? While the students expected to defend themselves, *none* was successful. Not even the self-described gun enthusiast. The titles of these videos suggest the experimenter's answer: "Proof that concealed carry holder's live in a dream world." Search YouTube for "Proof that Concealed Carry permit holders live in a dream world, Part One" and "Proof that Concealed Carry permit holders live in a dream world, Part Two" to view the videos.

The worst mass shooting in Australian history occurred in 1996. A 28-year-old man walked into a café, ate lunch, pulled a semiautomatic weapon out of his bag and proceeded to kill 35 people and injure 23. In response, Australian lawmakers enacted gun control legislation, banning certain types of guns, including automatic and semiautomatic rifles and shotguns. The Australian government also instituted a gun buyback program that netted 650,000 banned firearms. All new gun purchases now require a permit. As a result, Australia's homicide rate by firearms dropped by about 42% in the 7 years after the law passed, and its firearm suicide rate fell by 57%.[105]

Shootings on School Property

There are a surprising number of school shootings. Many shootings on school property have a particular target. In these instances, the shooter and the victim know each other. The causes are varied but include marital discord and students unhappy with a faculty member. There are also shootings that result from disagreements.

When people think of school shootings, they usually think of mass shootings. While mass shootings make national news, the other types are reported locally. Mass school shootings make national news and become synonymous with the idea of mass shootings: Columbine, Sandy Hook, Parkland. There is no agreement on the definition of a mass shooting. A Congressional Research Service report developed a definition for their report.[106] Mass shootings occur in relatively public places and involve four or more deaths, not including the

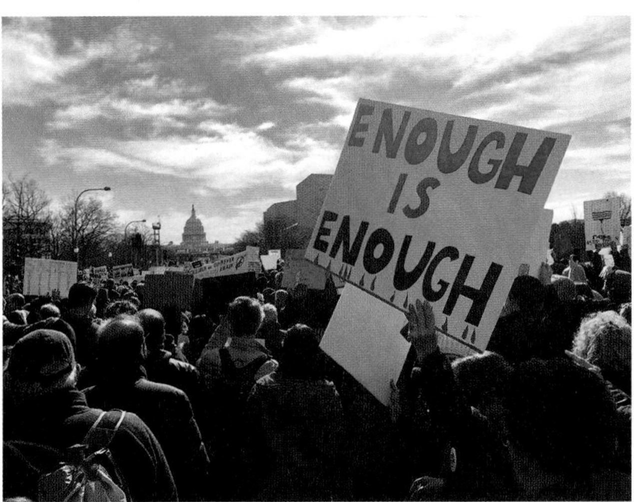

Photo showing Parkland students protesting gun violence at the Capital.

shooter. The choice of victims are somewhat indiscriminate, and the violence is not a means to an end, so it neither includes killings in the name of an ideology nor does the shooter gain anything by the violence.

TABLE 10-4 lists the shootings on school property from the 1950s through March of 2018. The factors used to create this table were that a shooting involved a gun being intentionally fired. The shooting occurred on school ground or a school bus and included all causes for the violence. Accidental discharge of firearms was not included, even if it involved an injury. There are increasing numbers of incidents, as well as deaths due to gun violence over time. There were more gun incidents on school properties in 2014 and 2015 than in all of the 1950s, 1960s, and 1970s. For the first time in 2014, there were shootings in preschools. From this table, we see that the average number of deaths per year on school property has steadily increased over the years.

In February of 2018, a heavily armed perpetrator killed 17 students and injured another 17 people. With their acts of witness and advocacy, the

TABLE 10-4 Shootings on School Property

Year(s)	Number of Incidents	Number of Deaths	Average Number of Deaths per Year	Number of Injuries	Number of School Shootings by Type of School*				
					College	High School	Junior High/ Middle School	Elementary School	Preschool
1950s	17	13	1.3	8	3	11	3	–	–
1960s	18	44	4.4	64	4	9	3	2	–
1970s	27	30	3.0	75	4	12	6	5	–
1980s	38	48	4.8	164	5	18	8	7	–
1990s	61	86	8.6	145	8	37	14	2	–
2000s	61	106	10.6	137	15	34	10	3	–
2010–2012	22	54	18	39	7	14	4	2	–
2013	38	28	28	36	13	17	5	3	–
2014	61	27	27	49	26	25	1	7	2
2015	61	35	35	56	27	17	5	9	2
2016	38	17	17	42	13	21	2	1	–
2017	49	22	22	37	19	20	–	8	–
2018 (January–March)	26	28	112	41	9	14	2	–	–

*School level not included when shooting was either into/on a school bus or in a K—12 school.

survivors of the Marjory Stoneman Douglas High School have changed gun politics in the United States in a way that politicians have been unable to do. A month after the shooting, tens of thousands of students across the United States left their schools as a demand for action on gun violence. As one student put it, "We are tired of thoughts and prayers, and we're ready to finally do something."[107]

While college campuses are safe, every instance of gun violence increases the volume of the arguments, both for and against guns on campuses. The issue remains highly divisive.

All states allow citizens who meet the requirements to carry concealed weapons. Ten states allow carrying concealed weapons on public college campuses, including Arkansas, Colorado, Georgia, Idaho, Kansas, Mississippi, Oregon, Texas, Utah and Wisconsin. Nineteen others ban concealed weapons on campuses, including California, Florida, and New York; and 23 others, including Alabama and Arizona, leave the decision to the colleges or state board of regents.[109]

TALES OF PUBLIC HEALTH

Concealed Carry

From an opinion piece in the New York Times: "I'm a Responsible Gun Owner? Seriously?[110]

Zachary Stone is a 22-year-old student at the University of Texas at Austin. The first time he shot a gun, Zachary missed a 4-foot tall, 2-foot wide target from only 9 feet away. Ten minutes later, an instructor certified his concealed handgun license application. In Texas, it takes more training to become a manicurist than it does to carry a handgun.

After almost no training and a 10-minute test, the State of Texas considers Zachary responsible enough to carry a gun. According to the Texas Department of Public Safety, 99.7% of the 2014 applicants got a license. Zachary is a founder of the University of Texas Students Against Guns on Campus. Hosting a university debate on the topic, Zachary asked, "Given that the system allows me—lacking firearm experience—to get a license, would you be comfortable if we sat with each other in class, upon learning I'm secretly carrying a gun?"

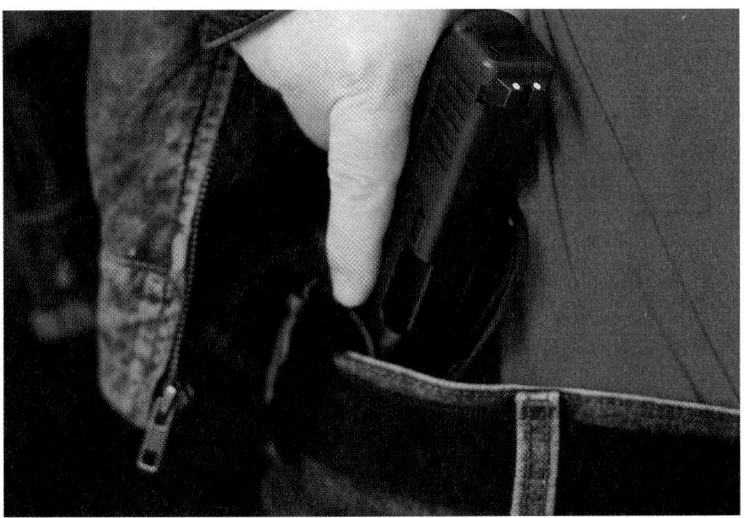

A student showed his 9-millimeter Glock handgun on the University of Utah campus.

GUNS ON COLLEGE CAMPUSES

"No thinking, responsible person who knows anything about the teenage or young adult brain would openly advocate that students at any university be allowed to openly carry firearms on campus."[108] Lewis Diuguid, Journalist

Lewis Diuguid, Journalist.

Gun Violence as a Public Health Issue

According to the American Academy of Pediatrics, a gun in the home is 43 times more likely to be used to kill a friend or family member than a burglar or other criminal. In his book, *Private Guns, Public Health*, David Hemenway argues that a significant portion of serious, intentional violence would be less deadly if guns were not so readily available.[111] The answer to how to reduce the violence isn't simply that there are too many guns. It has to do with who owns

UP FOR DEBATE

Are Guns a Public Health Issue?

Things to consider:

- After every major shooting, the polls show strong support for tougher gun regulations. Yet regulations never seem to pass.
- The Second Amendment to the United States Constitution reads: "A well regulated Militia, being necessary to the security of a free State, the right of the people to keep and bear Arms, shall not be infringed." Does this affect the conversation?
- A Florida law banned pediatricians from talking to parents about gun *safety*. In 2017, the United States Circuit Court of Appeals for the 11th Circuit concluded the law was unconstitutional.
- The number of people who die and the number of injuries from firearms annually
- Maybe instead of banning guns, there should be more education
- Criminals won't obey gun laws

guns, what kinds of guns people own, how people store their guns, and why people own them.[111]

Police Use of Force

Police are authorized to use deadly force only when they fear for their lives or the lives of others. Currently, reporting by police departments to the FBI is voluntary. According to FBI statistics, there are only about 400 shootings by police annually. But since 2011, less than 3% of state and local police agencies reported shootings to the FBI.[112] It is widely acknowledged that the FBI counts of police shootings are underreported. In October 2015, at a crime summit, the FBI director said,

> "It is unacceptable that the *Washington Post* and the *Guardian* newspaper from the UK are becoming the lead source of information about violent encounters between [U.S.] police and civilians. That is not good for anybody,"[113]

To understand how pervasive police shootings are in the United States, consider the following. In the United States (population 316.1 million) in the first 24 days of January 2015, there were 59 shootings. In England and Wales (population 56.9 million), there were 55 shootings in the last 24 years.[114] This means, according to the World Bank, the United States has a per capita intentional homicide rate five times that of the UK. The police in Iceland had one fatal shooting in 71 years. Stockton, California, with a smaller population than Iceland, had three fatal shootings between January and May of 2015. In the United States, the police shot more people in March of 2015 than in 19 years in Australia (1992–2011). In 2013, Finnish police fired just six bullets.[114]

Even though the numbers are high, they do not tell the whole story. In 2015, 1,136 people were killed by the police. The rate of people killed by race per million population was 2.92 Whites/million population, 7.15 Blacks/million population, 3.48 Hispanics/Latinos/million population, 3.4 Native Americans/million population, and 1.34 Asian/Pacific Islanders/million population. The police kill a disproportionate number of Black Americans, at twice the rate of Whites or Hispanic/Latinos. In 2015, 32% of Blacks killed by police were unarmed, as were 25% of Hispanic and Latino people. Only 15% of White people killed were unarmed. Twenty-seven percent of individuals killed by police in 2015 had mental health issues.[115]

The Counted[115] is an interactive database monitoring police killings in the United States. You can explore the database at www.theguardian.com by searching for "The Counted" to learn more about people's stories.

There are many stories in the news about police abuse of authority and excess force. In 2000, the National Institute of Justice published a report on police attitudes toward abuse of authority.[116] The authors surveyed a representative national sample. (A sample that accurately reflects the members of the population. Here the sample represents all police in the United States.) When police use excess force, it raises questions regarding their authority, especially when the victim is a minority. Below are some results from the survey. The percentages are officers agreeing or agreeing strongly with the statement.

- Always following the rules is not compatible with getting the job done (43%).
- It is sometimes acceptable to use more force than is legally allowable to control someone who physically assaults an officer (25%).
- Police are not permitted to use as much force as is often necessary in making arrests (31%).

- Officers used more force than necessary to make an arrest (78%).

One of the issues that arises is whether officers should and do report misconduct of other officers.

- It is not unusual for a police officer to ignore improper conduct of other officers (52%).
- Police officers do not always report serious abuse by fellow officers (61%).
- Reporting on fellow officers will result in being deliberately ignored by others (67%).

The National Institute of Justice reports race as a troublesome issue for American police. Black and nonblack officers viewed issues about citizen's race and social class differently and about how those characteristics affected the likelihood of police abuse. Approximately 17% of the sample reported police treat Whites better than they treat Blacks and other minorities. However, 51% of Black officers acknowledged that Whites receive better treatment. Fifty-seven percent of Black officers said that police officers use more physical force against Blacks and other minorities compared to White citizens. Of Black officers, 14% believed that police use more physical force against people who are poor than those who are middle-class.[116]

Many police departments do not use excessive force. Results of the survey show that most police officers in the United States disapprove of the use of excessive force.[116]

There are international laws and standards on lethal use of force. None of the state or Washington, DC, laws comply with international laws and standards. Nine states and Washington, DC, currently have no laws regarding use of lethal force by law enforcement officers.[117]

Because of the number of firearms among the general population, police officers have to be prepared for the worst when confronting a suspect. They must make split-second decisions about how to react. This means that any unexpected movement can be mistaken as someone reaching for a firearm, even if the suspect turns out to be unarmed.[117]

There are many cases where officers rush into volatile situations and save people's lives. These instances are less likely to be reported in the press than the use of excess force.

When Police Use Fatal Force

No federal agency in the United States tracks the number of shots fired by police departments. Starting in 2015, the *Washington Post* newspaper began cataloging every fatal shooting by police officers in the line of duty. Their database is compiled from news reports, public records, social media, and other sources. Nearly a quarter of the incidents involved individuals with mental illness. Most police agencies had not provided officers with appropriate training to de-escalate encounters with people in a mental or emotional crisis. One-quarter of the shootings occurred when suspects fled. Although many police departments discourage officers from pursuing suspects, unless the person presents an immediate threat, police expect people to obey their commands. When people don't listen to them, the encounter can quickly escalate. One-tenth of people shot by the police were unarmed. According to their findings, unarmed Black men were seven times as likely to be fatally shot as unarmed White men. **TABLE 10-5** tracks the use of fatal force by police, by the race of the victim. Although more White individuals were shot by police

TABLE 10-5 Police Use of Fatal Force by Race of Victim

Year	Race					
	White	Black	Hispanic	Other	Unknown	Total
2015[119]	497	259	172	38	29	995
2016[120]	466	233	160	42	62	963
2017[121]	406	197	160	32	67	862*

*2017 numbers are as of mid-November 2017.
The Washington Post. (2017). Fatal force. Retrieved from https://www.washingtonpost.com/graphics/national/police-shootings-2017/

than Black individuals, when you consider that non-Hispanic Whites make up approximately three-quarters of the population and Blacks or African Americans make up approximately 13%, it becomes clear that the rate at which Blacks are killed is much higher than for Whites.[118]

On a more egalitarian note, in 2015, the indictments of police officers tripled compared with previous years. Six percent of the 2015 shootings were filmed by body cameras. In three-quarters of the fatal shootings, either the police or someone else was under attack. In these instances, police may have only a fraction of a second to make a life-or-death decision.

Murder and Capital Punishment

In 2016, there were more than 17,000 murders and nonnegligent manslaughters in the United States, an 8.6% increase from 2015. It was the third year in a row in which the homicide rate increased.[120] The majority of homicides (68%) used firearms, including handguns, rifles, shotguns, and other or unstated firearms. Other homicide methods included 13% used knives, 6% personal weapons (hands, fists, or feet), 4% blunt objects like clubs or hammers, 1% each used fire, narcotics, strangulation, and asphyxiation, less than 1% each used poison, explosives, and drowning. There was another 7% where the weapon was not stated or listed as other.[123]

For Uniformed Crime Reporting purposes, the definition of murder or nonnegligent manslaughter is the willful killing of one person by another. This definition includes any death caused by injuries received in a fight, argument, assault, or commission of a crime. Not included in this category are suicides, fetal deaths, traffic fatalities (including those involving driving under the influence of alcohol), attempted murders, or accidental deaths.[122,123,124] Eighty-one percent of the time the victim and offender know each other (**FIGURE 10-7**).

The majority of murders occur between 7:00 p.m. and 3:00 a.m. About half of murders (54%) occur in a person's home. Twenty-three percent occur on highways, roads, alleys, or sidewalks, 6% in parking lots, 3% in fields or woods, 2% in bars, and 12% in other places.[124] Causes given by defendants as to why they committed murder are presented in **TABLE 10-6**.

As shown in Figure 10-7, both the victim and the offender are most often between the ages of 20 and 29 years.[124]

MURDER and NONNEGLIGENT MANSLAUGHTER by WEAPON/FORCE USED[1] *Percent Distribution, 2013*

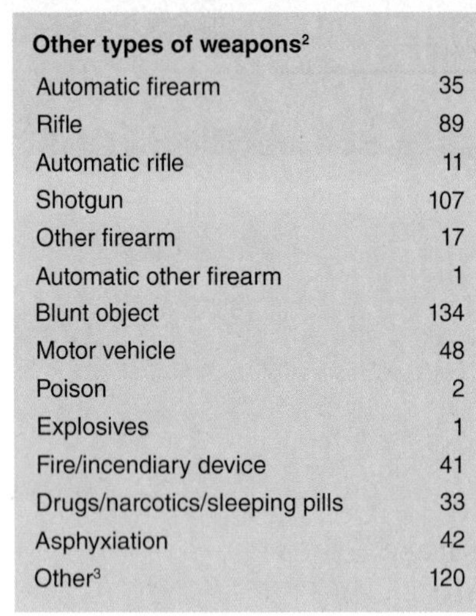

Other types of weapons[2]	
Automatic firearm	35
Rifle	89
Automatic rifle	11
Shotgun	107
Other firearm	17
Automatic other firearm	1
Blunt object	134
Motor vehicle	48
Poison	2
Explosives	1
Fire/incendiary device	41
Drugs/narcotics/sleeping pills	33
Asphyxiation	42
Other[3]	120

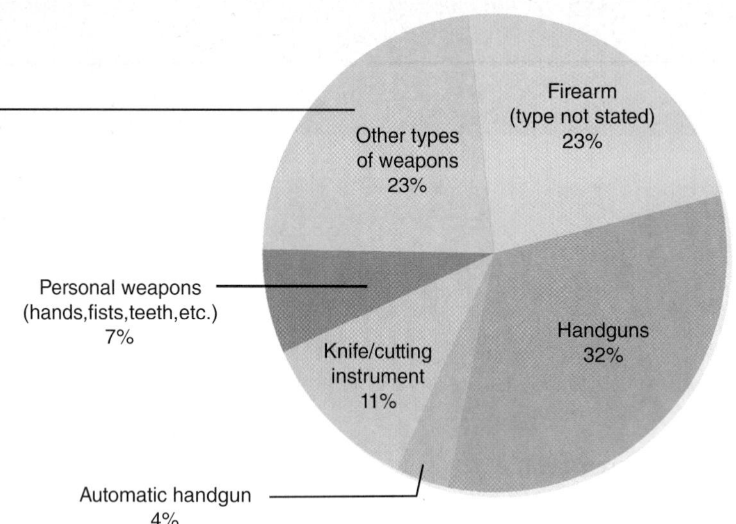

RELATIONSHIP of the VICTIM to the OFFENDER

	Percent with known victim/offender relationship	
Total	**100%**	
Stranger	**19%**	
Known to victim	**81%**	
Acquaintance		33%
Spouse		7%
Boyfriend/girlfriend		7%
Friend		5%
Child		5%
Otherwise known		11%
All other relationships		13%

[1]*LEAs may report multiple weapons per offense type.*
[2]*Due to rounding, the percentages do not add to 23 percent.*
[3]*Other includes drowning, strangulation, suffocation, gas, etc.*

AGE of VICTIM and OFFENDER[1]

40%
35%
30%
25%
20%
15%
10%
5%
0%

< 10 years, 10-19 years, 20-29 years, 30-39 years, 40-49 years, 50-59 years, 60-69 years, 70-79 years, 80-89 years, 90 and over, Unknown age

Victim — Offender

[1]*The victim of Murder and Nonnegligent Manslaughter was most often 20-29 years old (1,062) and the offender was most often 20-29 years old (1,509).*

FIGURE 10-7 FBI Information about murder.

Criminal Justice Information Services Division, Federal Bureau of Investigation, U.S. Department of Justice. Data from the National Incident-Based Reporting System.

TABLE 10-6 Why People Kill Each Other[124]

Cause	Percentage of Murders
Argument	22%
Drug dealing	3%
Lover's quarrel	3%
Other (including assault on a law enforcement officer, juvenile gangs, and mercy killing)	20%
Gangland	1%
Other felony	3%
Unknown	48%

Federal Bureau of Investigation. (2014). Murder and nonnegligent manslaughter. Retrieved from https://www.fbi.gov/about-us/cjis/ucr/nibrs/2013/the-advantage-of-nibrs-data/murder-and-nonnegligent-manslaughter

Homicides by Race and Ethnicity

The number of homicides was decreasing over time, but started rising again in 2015.[121] Between 1993 and 2012, the violent crime rate in the United States, including homicide, robbery, rape, and aggravated assault, dropped by 48%.[125] There is wide agreement that we do not yet fully know why the crime rate dropped.[126] There are competing theories, but it is likely a combination of various social, economic, and environmental factors, such as growth in income and an aging population.

Even as the homicide rate has fallen over time (even given the recent rise), the decrease is not spread evenly across gender, racial, or ethnic lines. Regardless of race or ethnicity, being male increases the likelihood of being a murder victim. Compared to being White, Black or African American males are 6.5 times as likely to be a murder victim. Hispanics also have higher homicide rates than non-Hispanic Whites. But Hispanics are not a homogenous group. Depending on the country of origin, the likelihood of being a murder victim varies. Using 5 years of data, a researcher found that Puerto Ricans had a rate of 6.5/100,000 population, Mexicans had a rate of 5.2/100,000 population, and Cubans had a rate of 4.3/100,000 population. There were no data for other countries of origin.[127]

Those Left Behind

For every murdered person, family members, friends, neighbors, and others are left behind to cope with the loss. Nothing in life prepares you for having a loved one murdered. Most people live with the hope that the people they love will live into old age. The death of someone you love is always a shock, but when the cause of death is murder, it is a much more intense experience, with the sorrow and loss compounded by a sense of injustice and helplessness. Those left behind face an extended period of emotional struggle to rebuild their devastated life.[128]

Survivors have many reactions to the initial crisis. These include, but are not limited to, preoccupation with personal loss, horror at the thought of the victim's suffering, a need to know minute details about the death, panic attacks, restlessness and insomnia, inability to concentrate, rage at the assailant, fear for one's own life or that of loved ones, self-blame that the survivor did or did not do something to prevent the murder, anger that others cannot bring the victim back, and hopelessness and helplessness.

For a much more complete discussion of issues for the family members of homicide victims, see http://www.pomc.org/survivors.html, the website for Parents of Murdered Children, Inc.

Capital Punishment

capital punishment The lawful infliction of death as a punishment; the death penalty.

The first use of **capital punishment** in America was in 1608 in Jamestown Colony. At the end of the Revolutionary War, 11 colonies wrote new constitutions, and all allowed capital punishment. In 1790, the First Congress passed legislation that authorized the death penalty for robbery, rape, murder, and forgery of public securities. In the eighteenth century, there were 162 executions and in the nineteenth century, there were 1,391.[129]

In 1967, there was a moratorium (temporary suspension of activity) on capital punishment while the U.S. Supreme Court considered the question of whether it was constitutional.[129] In 1972, the Supreme Court ruled that there must be a degree of consistency in the application of the death penalty.[130] In 1976, Florida, Georgia, and Texas enacted death penalty laws, which the Supreme Court upheld.[129]

Currently, 31 states, as well as the U.S. military and U.S. federal government, have the death penalty. Nineteen states and the District of Columbia have abolished the death penalty. **FIGURE 10-8** shows a map of states with the death penalty and how each state executes.

There are many arguments for and against the death penalty. Among these are morality, constitutionality, whether the death penalty acts as a deterrent, retribution (society seeking revenge for a wrong committed), irrevocable mistakes, the cost of executing a person versus life in prison, how race and income affect the likelihood of receiving the death penalty, and the quality of the defendant's attorney.

As shown in **TABLE 10-7**, the murder rate in states without capital punishment is consistently lower than in states with capital punishment. This trend was also true for each year in the decade preceding the years shown.[131]

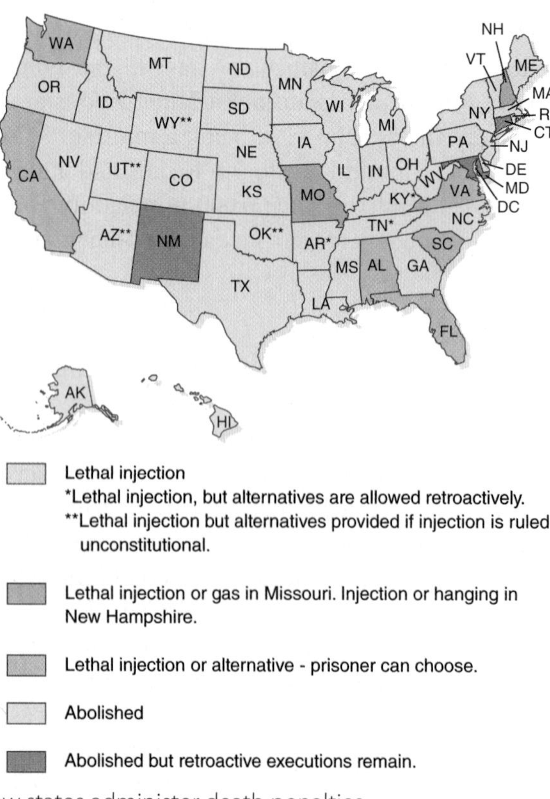

FIGURE 10-8 How states administer death penalties.

Reproduced with permission from Death Penalty Information Center.

TABLE 10-7 Does the Death Penalty Act as Deterrence?

Year	Murder Rate per 100,000 population in Death Penalty States	Murder Rate per 100,000 population in Non–Death Penalty States	Percent Difference
2000	5.70	4.25	35%
2001	5.82	4.25	37%
2002	5.82	4.27	36%
2003	5.91	4.10	44%
2004	5.71	4.02	42%
2005	5.87	4.03	46%
2006	5.90	4.22	40%
2007	5.83	4.10	42%
2008	5.72	4.05	41%
2009	5.26	3.90	35%
2010	5.00	4.01	25%
2011	4.89	4.13	18%
2012	4.95	4.09	21%
2013	4.72	3.88	22%
2014	4.75	3.70	28%
2015	5.17	4.26	21%
2016	5.63	4.49	25%

Deterrence: States Without the Death Penalty Have Had Consistently Lower Murder Rates | Death Penalty Information Center. (2018). Deathpenaltyinfo.org. Retrieved from https://deathpenaltyinfo.org/deterrence-states-without-death-penalty-have-had-consistently-lower-murder-rates

Serial Killers

While serial killers (people who murder three or more people) are rare, they attract the attention of the media. Much of what the public *knows* about serial killers is the result of television shows and movies, rather than fact. This description of serial killers comes primarily from an FBI report, "Serial Murder: Multi-Disciplinary Perspectives for Investigators."

The most famous historical serial killer is Jack the Ripper, who was responsible for killing female prostitutes in the Whitechapel district of London in 1888. Between August 31 and November 9, 1888, five prostitutes were killed, all with their necks slashed and abdomens mutilated. As time passed, the mutilations became increasingly severe. Although the London Metropolitan Police interviewed more than 2,000 people, the murders went unsolved.

The FBI report reviewed the usual *misconceptions* about serial killers as follows:[132]

- *Serial killers are dysfunctional loners.* Serial killers often have families, homes, jobs, and appear as normal members of their community. They may not be suspects because they fit in so well. Robert Yates killed 17 prostitutes

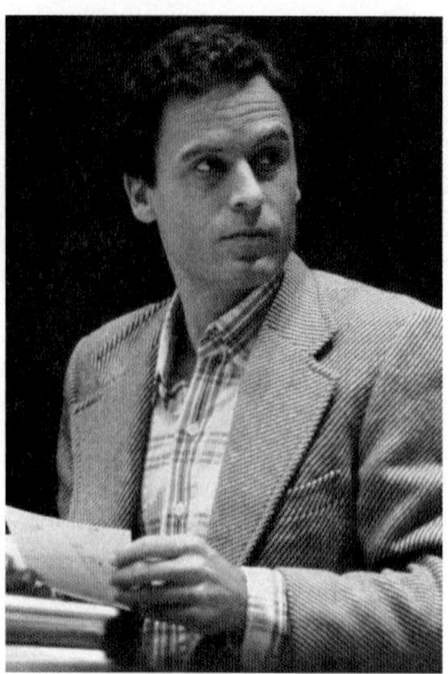

Ted Bundy was an American serial killer, kidnapper, rapist, and necrophile. He confessed to killing 30 women and indulged in sexual acts with the corpses. Bundy decapitated at least 12 victims and kept their heads as trophies in his apartment. Bundy was executed in the electric chair in 1989.

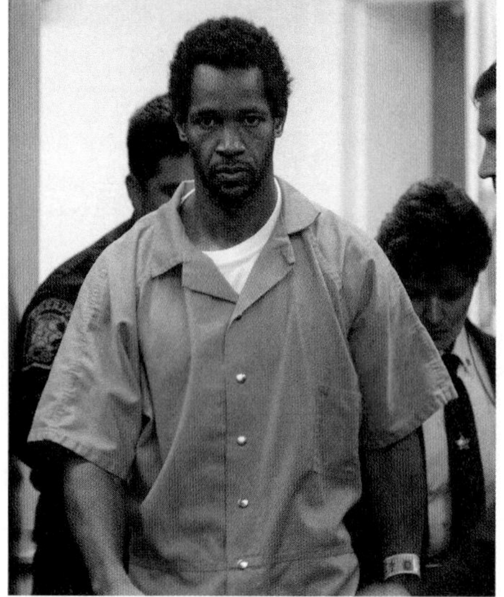

John Allen Muhammad was an American serial killer. He killed 17 people. He killed people around Washington, DC, allegedly as part of a plot to kill his wife and regain custody of his children. Muhammad was executed by lethal injection in 2009.

in Spokane, Washington, in the 1990s. He was married, a father of five, lived in a middle-class neighborhood, and was a decorated U.S. Army National Guard helicopter pilot.

- *Serial killers are all White males.* The racial spectrum of serial killers is similar to the racial spectrum of the United States. In addition to Caucasians, there have been Asian, Hispanic, and African American serial killers.
- *Sex motivates serial killers.* Sometimes sex drives serial killers, but other motivations include anger, thrill seeking, financial gain, and attention.[132] Over a 3-week period in October of 2002, John Allen Muhammad and Lee Boyd Malvo killed 10 people in the Washington, DC, metro area. Their motivations were anger and thrill seeking.
- *Serial killers travel and operate interstate.* Usually, serial killers have a very defined geographic area where they are comfortable.

- *Serial killers cannot stop killing.* Some serial killers stop murdering before being caught. Dennis Rader, also known as the BTK (Bind, Torture, and Kill) Killer, murdered 10 victims between 1974 and 1991 in and near Wichita, Kansas. His arrest was in 2005.
- *All serial killers are insane or are evil geniuses.* Most serial killers suffer from a variety of personality disorders, including psychopathy (mental illness) and antisocial personality (a type of mental condition where the person is manipulative, exploitative, and violates the rights of others). Under legal definitions, most are not insane.
- *Serial killers want to get caught.* Most serial killers plan their offenses with great care. As they proceed, they may feel empowered. With time and experience, they may take chances because they believe they *can't* be caught.

Violence in the Name of Hate

Hate Crimes

There are public health consequences of **hate crimes**. Bigotry and discrimination because of hatred affect the health of populations. A study from Boston found lesbian, gay, bisexual, and transgender youths as the targets of discrimination were more likely to report suicidal ideation.[133] People who personally perceived any major lifetime discrimination were more likely to have major depression.[134] Arab Americans who lived in the United States after 9/11/2001 were the targets of discrimination. As a result, they were more likely to experience increased psychological distress, reduced levels of happiness, and worse health status.[135] As eloquently noted, by Dr. Sandro Galea, "... that hatred and intolerance pervade our daily lives, with real and substantial impacts on the health of populations."[136]

hate crimes A violent crime motivated because of the victim's perceived membership in a specific group.

Hate crimes are violent crimes motivated because of the victim's perceived membership in a specific group. This membership may include ethnicity, gender

"Hate, it has caused a lot of problems in this world, but it has not solved one yet."
—**Maya Angelou,** *Poet and Author*

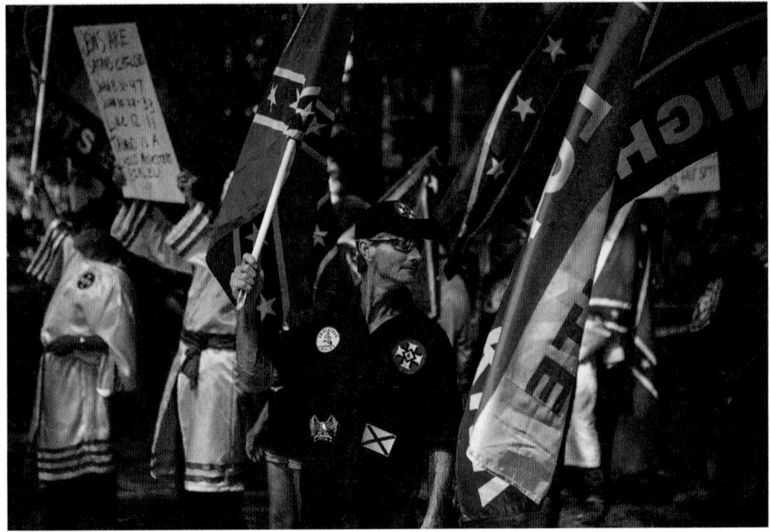

Hate Crimes

identity, language, nationality, religion, sexual orientation, disability, or physical appearance. These crimes may involve physical assault, damage to property, bullying, harassment, verbal abuse, cybercrimes, or hate mail. They can occur almost anywhere, including college campuses. Hate crime laws are typical "penalty enhancement" statutes that increase the penalty if the choice of the victim or target is because of his or her personal characteristics. Vandalism usually carries a light sentence for the criminal if caught. Painting a swastika on a synagogue will result in a heavier sentence. Bias-incidents are noncriminal actions motivated by hate.

Unfortunately, hate crimes are disturbingly common. According to the FBI, the number of hate crimes reported to the police in the United States decreased from 5,922 in 2013 to 5,462 in 2014.[137] According to the Bureau of Justice, nearly two-thirds of all hate crimes go unreported to the police.[138] Thus the FBI's numbers are much lower than reality. The FBI's number is limited to single-bias incidents, which means there is only one reason the people or institutions are the targets. (An example of multiple biases would be a person targeted because they were a specific race and disabled.) Beginning in January 2015, the FBI expanded the list of biases to include more religions and anti-Arab under the race/ethnicity/ancestry category. Although the constitution guarantees free speech, recently there is an increase in harsh, hateful rhetoric against immigrants.

Victims of hate crimes may be reluctant to go to the police. If a victim perceives the police as being discriminatory, they will be less likely to report a crime. Some immigrants may feel there is a language barrier that prevents them from reporting. Others believe it is unacceptable to report crimes to the police. Other reasons may be police nonparticipation and miscategorization of hate crimes. The actual number of hate crimes is probably closer to 200,000 to 300,000 per year.

A 2015 Gallup poll found that 43% of Americans harbor some degree of prejudice toward Muslims. After September 11, anti-Muslim hate crimes multiplied and are about five times as frequent as they were before 2001. Americans dislike Muslims more than any other religious group. Yet Muslim Americans are the most likely of all religious groups to disavow individual attacks against civilians.[139]

TALES OF PUBLIC HEALTH

Three Stories of Hate Crimes

1. Seven teens in Suffolk County, New York, admitted to being part of a gang that targeted Hispanics for violence. Three of the teens, all aged 19 years, pleaded guilty to gang assault, conspiracy, and attempted assault as a hate crime. The teens were walking near a train station in November of 2008, looking for targets. The group spotted 37-year-old Marcelo Lucero, and one boy punched him in the face. Attempting to defend themselves, Lucero and his friend swung their belts at the boys. During the confrontation, a belt hit one boy in the head. The teen took his knife and stabbed Lucero in the chest.[140]
2. Initially, it looked like the death of James C. Anderson was a hit-and-run accident. Anderson was an African American who worked at an automobile plant in Jackson, Mississippi. Two carloads of White teenagers had been partying all night and drove to Jackson looking to "mess with" some African Americans. The teens beat Anderson while yelling, "white power" and racial slurs. One group left, but Ray Dedmon drove a Ford pickup truck over Anderson, killing him. According to witnesses, he used his cell phone reporting that "I ran that nigger over."[141]
3. Deah Barakat was a 23-year-old dentistry student at the University of North Carolina. Yusor Abu-Salha, Barkarat's 21-year-old wife, was an incoming dental student at the University of North Carolina. Razan Abu-Salha, Yusor's 19-year-old sister, was an undergraduate at North Carolina State.

   They were much like other Americans their age. Barakat was a fan of SportsCenter, liked country music and playing basketball. Razan was a gaming enthusiast, who liked Call of Duty and listened to Nicki Minaj. They believed in service to their community. Both volunteered to help feed the homeless and organized health fairs.

   On February 10, 2015, Craig Hicks, who faces the death penalty, shot and killed all three. Yusor had told her father, "Daddy, I think he hates us for who we are and how we look."[142]

While the FBI reports hate crimes from police reports, the U.S. Department of Justice reports numbers based on the victim's accounts of the crime and what they perceive as the motivation for being a victim. Among hate crime victims, approximately 58% reported more than one reason. Over time, the motivations for hate crimes have changed, with the largest increase being in crimes based on ethnicity. The definition of ethnicity is a victim's "ancestral, cultural, social, or national affiliation." As seen in **TABLE 10-8**, in 2004, 22% of hate crimes were because of ethnicity. By 2012, more than half of hate crimes were motivated by bias against the victim's ethnicity.[143]

Lesbian, gay, bisexual, and transsexual people have often been the target of violence because of who they love. A partial history of anti-LGBT violence in the United States:[144]

- In 1973, an arsonist set fire at the UpStairs Lounge, a New Orleans gay bar. A fire was set at the bottom of the stairs and swept up. The lounge had barred windows and no emergency exit, resulting in 32 deaths.
- In 1978, Harvey Milk, a pioneering gay activist and politician in San Francisco, was shot to death by a former colleague. Also murdered was the mayor, who, although straight, was a strong ally to the LGBT community. (There was a 2008 movie about this called *Milk*.)
- In 1992, a U.S. Navy Seaman, Allen Schindler, was nearing time for completion of his military service. A shipmate beat Schindler to death. The day after the murder he said he hated homosexuals and was disgusted by them. He said he would do it again.
- Brandon Teena was a young female-to-male transgender from Nebraska. Two supposed friends, enraged when they learned that he was transgender, raped and murdered him in 1993. (There was a 1999 movie about this called *Boys Don't Cry*.)
- Matthew Shepard was killed in 1998 because he was gay. Two men that he met in a Laramie, Wyoming, bar beat him to death.

TABLE 10-8 Victims' Perceptions Of Offender Bias In Hate Crimes, 2004, 2011 to 2015

Offender Bias	2004	2011–2015
Ethnicity	22%	35.4%
Race	58%	48.1%
Association§	23%	22.5%
Religion	10%	16.7%
Gender	12%	29.3%
Sexual orientation	22%	22.1%
Disability	11%	15.6%
Perceived characteristics*	19%	6.6%

§Motivated by victim's association with persons having certain characteristics.
*Motivated by offender's perception of victim's characteristics.
Bureau of Justice Statistics, National Crime Victimization Survey, 2003-2012.

- Pfc. Barry Winchell was beaten to death with a baseball bat in 1999 while he was sleeping. The perpetrator was a fellow service member. Although Winchell didn't identify as gay, he was dating a transgender woman.
- In 2000, Ronald Gay went on a shooting rampage at a gay bar in Roanoke, Virginia. He didn't like that people made jokes about his name.
- In 2002, a California teen, Gwen Araujo, was beaten by a group of men when they discovered she was transgender.
- In 2008, Larry King, a gay, gender-nonconforming 15-year-old was shot in the head by a classmate at their junior high school. The murderer was enraged that King had a crush on him.
- In 2013, James Dixon was flirting with Islan Nettles on a street in New York City. When Dixon realized she was transgender, he struck her, causing her to fall and hit her head. But he kept on hitting her.

TALES OF PUBLIC HEALTH

After a Shooting at a Gay Nightclub

On June 12, 2016, there was a shooting at Pulse, an LGBTQ nightclub in Orlando, Florida. At least 50 people died with dozens more injured.

From Alex Darke, a gay man living in Texas, in response to this shooting:

Earlier today, a friend remarked: "I don't understand. The way you are reacting, it's almost like you knew someone in the club."

Here's the thing you need to understand about every LGBT person in your family, your work, and your circle of friends: We've spent most of our lives being aware that we are at risk.

When you hear interviewers talking to LGBT folks and they say "It could have been here. It could have been me," they aren't exaggerating. I don't care how long you've been out, how far down your road to self-acceptance and love you've traveled, we are always aware that we are at some level of risk.

... and when I reach to hold Matt's hand in the car? I still do the mental calculation of "ok, that car is just slightly behind us so they can't see, but that truck to my left can see right inside the car." If I kiss Matt in public, like he leaned in for on the bike trail the other day, I'm never fully in the moment. I'm always parsing who is around us and paying attention to us. There's a tension that comes with that ... a literal tensing of the muscles as you brace for potential danger. For a lot of us, it's become such an automatic reaction that we don't even think about it directly any more. We just do it.

Every LGBT person you know knows what I'm talking about. Those tiny little mental calculations we do over the course of our life add up ... and we just got hit with a stark reminder that those simmering concerns, those fears ... they probably won't ever go away. We'll never be free of them. Additionally, now we just got a lesson that expressing our love could result in the deaths of "others" completely unrelated to us. It's easy to take risks when it's just you and you've made that choice. Now there's this subtext that you could set off someone who kills other people who weren't even involved. And that's just a lot.

I live in Texas and was not personally affected by this tragedy. Don't get me wrong: nothing will change. I will still hold my husband's hand in public. I will still kiss him in public. We'll still go out and attend functions and hold our heads high.

But we will be doing those mental calculations for the rest of our lives. Those little public displays of affection you take for granted with your spouse. They come with huge baggage for us. Every single one is an act of defiance, with all that entails.

So do me a favor. Reach out to that LGBT person in your life. Friend, coworker, or family. Just let them know you are thinking of them and you love them. That will mean the world to them right now. I promise you.

Courtesy of Alex Darke.

Diversity Builds Acceptance

Stotzer and Hossellman studied whether or not increasing the number of Black and Latino college students (often considered "historically disadvantaged") and Asian college students (described as the "model minority"), as well as the percentage of minority faculty, affected the incidence of hate crimes. Using data

LBGT flag.

HATRED

Hatred for others begins with dehumanizing them. Hating a person for what makes them different from you. Effectively you are taking the position that the other person is "less than human." As noted at the website, Empathy as a Cure for Hatred:

> *"Hatred fills the heart and leads the hater to concentrate fully on the object of hate, thus preventing that time and energy to be spent growing and nurturing things."*[146]

from more than 400 colleges and universities, the researchers found a "promising relationship" between more diversity among students and fewer hate crimes on campus. The authors concluded that having a diverse student body, where there are many perspectives, significantly contributes to students' educational experience.[144]

Genocide: Mass Violence Because of Hate

World history has many examples of hate-filled violence. Mass violence in the name of hate is hate crimes taken to an extraordinary level. Sadly, there is no shortage of examples, including genocide of Native Americans, the genocide of Armenians, killing of Cambodians by the Khmer Rouge, Serbs targeting the Croatians, and the government of Sudan against the Darfuri civilians. We discuss briefly three instances of mass violence in the name of hate.

Slavery (Violence Because of Race)

The history of slavery spans nearly every culture, nationality, and religion from ancient times, even before the time of Christ.[147] The slave trade from Africa to the Americas lasted more than 300 years and enslaved more than 12.5 million Africans. Most slave merchants sold people in the Caribbean and Brazil; less than 4% of the Africans came to North America.

The cotton industry in the Deep South depended on slavery as an integral part of the economy. As cotton growth expanded West, slaves were forced to migrate, and owners often split up families.[148] Violence was used to control the slaves and masters or overseers beat their slaves for reasons real or imagined.

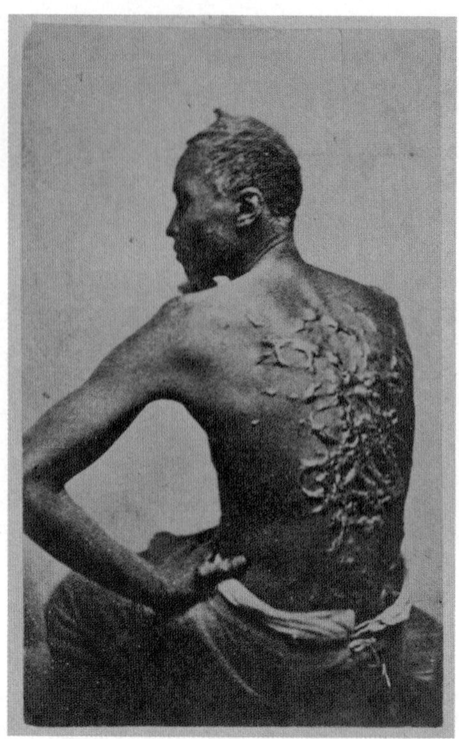

Whipped slave. Photo taken at Baton Rouge, LA, 1863. The guilty overseer was fired.

Image courtesy Library of Congress Prints and Photographs Division Washington, D.C. 20540 USA http://hdl.loc.gov/loc.pnp/pp.print

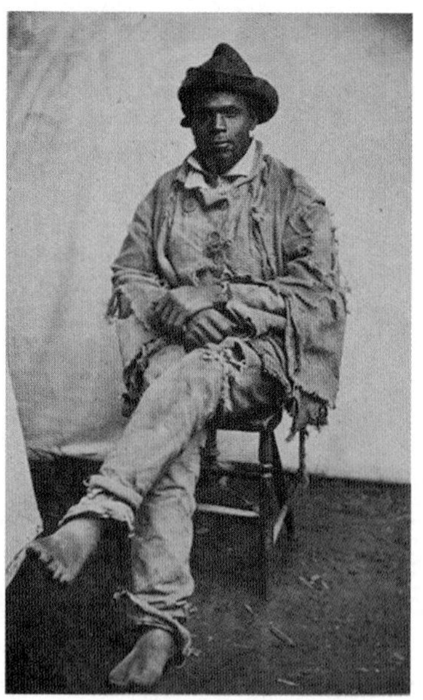

A slave who escaped and served as Union soldier. This picture was taken just after he reached a Union Army camp.

Courtesy of Photographers William D. McPherson and his partner Mr. Oliver, New Orleans.

Anti-Semitism (Violence Because of Religion)

Anti-Semitism is prejudice against, hatred of, or discrimination against Jews. The Holocaust was the mass murder of some 6 million European Jews (as well as members of some other persecuted groups, such as Romani (gypsies) and homosexuals, by the German Nazi regime during the Second World War. Adolf Hitler, the anti-Semitic Nazi leader, viewed Jews as inferior and a threat to German racial purity. His final solution was the building of concentration camps to exterminate the Jews.

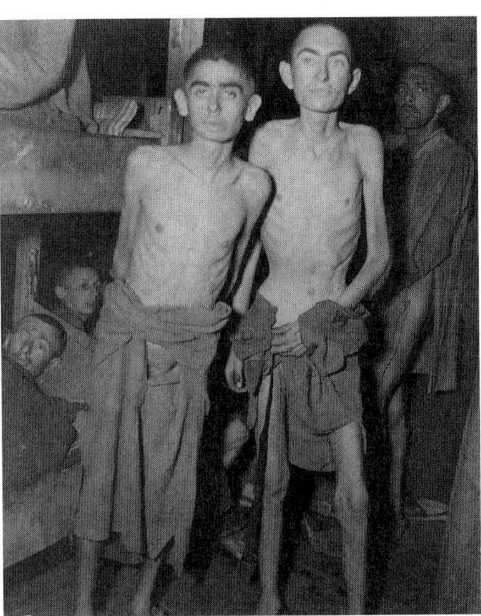

Survivors of the Dachau concentration camp soon after liberation by U.S. troops. Ampfing, Germany, May 4, 1945.

Reproduced from National Archives and Records Administration, College Park, MD.

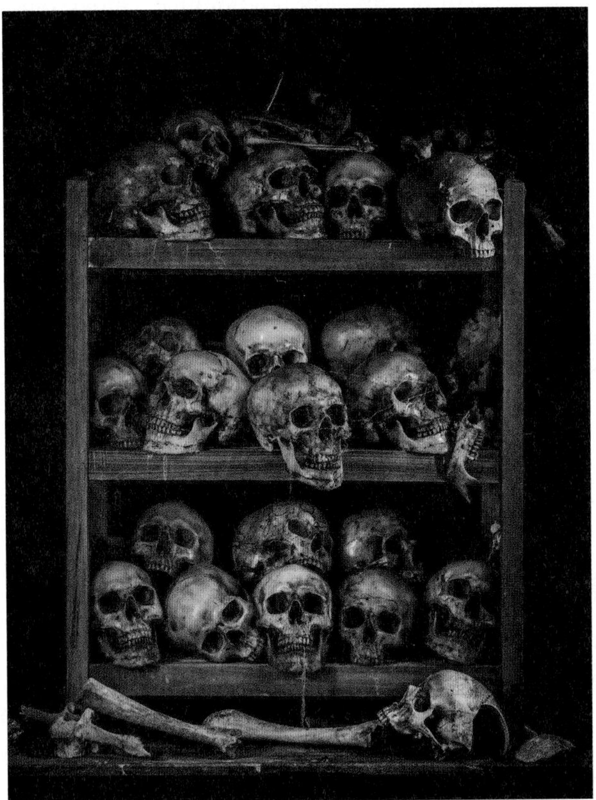

Well over 500,000 people died in Rwanda. Most of them clubbed, hacked, stabbed, or shot to death. Their unburied bones are gathered and displayed at memorial centers all across the country.

Ethnic Cleansing (Violence Because of Ethnicity)

Social identities reflect the way people and groups of people establish divisions within their society. These groups may be attributable to gender, class, or ethnic identity. When one group within a society controls another, problems may arise. Seeing people as "other" than yourself helps to divide society.

In Central Africa, for much of the 20th century, there was a longstanding conflict between the Hutu and Tutsi peoples. A large number of people died because of this conflict. In 1972, the Tutsi army slaughtered between 80,000 and 200,000 Hutus. In the 1994 Rwandan genocide, the Hutu militias targeted the Tutsis, killing between 800,000 and 1 million people. All of this violence is because the Hutu and Tutsi people view the other as ethnically different.

It may be human nature to fear what we do not understand. To the extent that we see others as different from ourselves, it is easier to justify committing violence against them.

In Summary

Violence is complicated. Many things influence whether a person will perpetrate violence and where the perpetrator will direct their violence. There are many points along the lifespan where a person may be a victim: as a baby, as a child, in a romantic relationship, and as an older person. No one deserves abuse. If you are in an abusive relationship, seek help. Hate crimes are common and occur because of prejudice and ignorance. Understanding about differences among people and their traditions helps to promote tolerance and decrease violence.

Key Terms

abuse
bullying
capital punishment
child neglect
Child Protective Services
cyberbullying
date rape
emotional abuse
hate crimes
hazing
intimate partner violence
neglect
physical abuse
safe haven laws
sexual abuse
social-ecological model of violence
stalking
systematic review
Title IX

Student Discussion Questions and Activities

1. Is there ever a time when violence is justified?
2. What should students do to reduce sexual violence on campus?
3. Does your state and/or school allow guns on campus? Do you think it makes you safer? Has reading this chapter changed your position on this?
4. Do you think there is too much violence on TV and in video games? Do you think it affects violence in real life?
5. Do you think more intensive licensing of guns, much like we do with driving a car, would help prevent gun violence? Would limiting the type of guns (like banning personal ownership of assault rifles) help?
6. How and why do people learn to be violent?
7. How does your college handle sexual assaults?
8. Mahatma Gandhi, the leader of the Indian independence movement in British-ruled India, once said, "Victory attained by violence is tantamount to a defeat, for it is momentary." Do you agree?

Resources

Violence is terrifying and traumatic, whether it is emotional, sexual, physical, or more than one. Knowing what to do is a struggle. It is important to understand you are not alone. Resources are listed here, but there are others out there. Help yourself or your friends to connect to one or more of these resources.

Black Women's Blueprint	http://www.blackwomensblueprint.org/
Breakthrough	http://us.breakthrough.tv/
Culture of Respect	http://cultureofrespect.naspa.org/
End Rape on Campus	http://endrapeonecampus.org
Family Violence Prevention & Services Resource Centers	http://www.acf.hhs.gov/programs/fysb/fv-centers
Futures Without Violence	http://www.futureswithoutviolence.org/
Generation Progress: It's On US	http://www.genprogress.org
Green Dot	https://www.livethegreendot.com/
Know Your IX	http://knowyourix.org/
Live your dream	http://www.liveyourdream.org/get-help/domestic-violence-resources.html
Love is Not Abuse	https://www.breakthecycle.org/sites/default/files/pdf/lina-curriculum-college.pdf
Love is Respect	http://www.loveisrespect.org/ 1-866-331-9474 Text Loveis to 22522
Man Up	http://manupcampaign.org/
National Alliance Ending Sexual Violence	http://endsexualviolence.org/
National Coalition Against Domestic Violence	http://www.ncadv.org/
National Domestic Violence Hotline	http://www.thehotline.org/ 1-800-799-SAFE (7233) 1-800-787-3224 (TDD)
National Sexual Violence Resource Center	http://www.nsvrc.org/
National Teen Dating Abuse Helpline	866-331-9474
NO MORE Campaign	http://nomore.org/
One in Four, Inc.	http://www.oneinfourusa.org/themensprogram.php
PreventConnect	http://www.preventconnect.org/
Rape, Abuse & Incest National Network	www.rainn.org 1.800.656.HOPE
Stalking Resource Center	http://victimsofcrime.org/our-programs/stalking-resource-center
Stop Sexual Assault in School	http://stopsexualassaultinschools.org/
Teens on Line	https://teenlineonline.org/ Call 310-855-4673 Text Teen to 839863
Victim & Survivor Resources	http://youth.gov/youth-topics/teen-dating-violence/resources

References

1. World Health Organization. (2016). Definition and typology of violence. Retrieved from http://www.who.int/violenceprevention/approach/definition/en/
2. Heise, L. L. (1998). Violence against women: An integrated, ecological framework. *Violence Against Women, 4*(3), 262–290
3. Centers for Disease Control and Prevention. (2011). The social-ecological model: A framework for violence prevention. Retrieved from http://www.cdc.gov/ViolencePrevention/pdf/SEM_Framewrk-a.pdf
4. Pinola, M. (2011). Basic self-defense moves anyone can do (and everyone should know). Retrieved from https://lifehacker.com/5825528/basic-self-defense-moves-anyone-can-do-and-everyone-should-know
5. Child Welfare Information Gateway, ed. (2017). Infant safe haven laws. Washington, DC: U.S. Department of Health and Human Services, Children's Bureau. Retrieved from https://www.childwelfare.gov/pubPDFs/safehaven.pdf
6. Carbaugh, S. F. (2004). Understanding shaken baby syndrome. *Advances in Neonatal Care, 4*(2), 105–114; quiz 15–17.
7. Centers for Disease Control and Prevention. (2012). Head's up: Prevent shaken baby syndrome. Retrieved from http://www.cdc.gov/concussion/HeadsUp/sbs.html
8. Centers for Disease Control and Prevention. (2015). Child maltreatment prevention. Retrieved from http://www.cdc.gov/ViolencePrevention/childmaltreatment/index.html
9. Centers for Disease Control and Prevention. (2014). Understanding child maltreatment. Retrieved from http://www.cdc.gov/violenceprevention/pdf/understanding-cm-factsheet.pdf
10. University System of Maryland. (2016). Reporting abuse and neglect in the university system of Maryland. Retrieved from https://www.umuc.edu/faculty/upload/child-abuse-and-neglect-faq.pdf
11. New York State Office of Children & Family Services. (n.d.). Signs of child abuse or maltreatment. Retrieved from http://ocfs.ny.gov/main/prevention/signs.asp
12. Centers for Disease Control and Prevention. (2012). CDC online newsroom press release. Child abuse and neglect cost the United States $124 billion. Retrieved from http://www.cdc.gov/media/releases/2012/p0201_child_abuse.html
13. Farwell, S. (2013, October). Interactives: The girl in the closet. *Dallas Morning News*. Retrieved from http://res.dallasnews.com/interactives/2013_October/lauren/#.Vjzcu2CFO74%29
14. UNICEF. (2012). Global statistics on children's protection from violence, exploitation, and abuse. Retrieved from http://www.unicef.org/protection/files/1412886011_Global_Statistics_on_CP_Brochure_HR_.pdf
15. U.S. Department of Labor. (2016). Child labor—wage and hour division. Retrieved from http://www.dol.gov/whd/childlabor.htm
16. UNICEF. (2013). UNICEF Statistics: An estimated 150 million children are engaged in child labour. Retrieved from http://data.unicef.org/child-protection/child-labour.html
17. International Labour Organization. (2010). Facts on child labour 2010. Retrieved from http://www.ilo.org/wcmsp5/groups/public/@dgreports/@dcomm/documents/publication/wcms_126685.pdf
18. UNICEF. (n.d.). Child trafficking. Retrieved from http://www.unicefusa.org/mission/protect/trafficking
19. International Labour Organization: International Programme on Elimination of Child Labour. (2015). Child labour and armed conflict. Retrieved from http://www.ilo.org/ipec/areas/Armedconflict/lang--en/index.htm
20. International Labour Organization. (2009). Training manual to fight trafficking in children for labour, sexual and other forms of exploitation. Retrieved from http://www.unicef.org/protection/Textbook_1.pdf
21. Delap, E. (2009). Begging for change: Research findings and recommendations on forced child begging in Albania/Greece, India and Senegal. London: Anti-Slavery International. Retrieved from https://digitalcommons.ilr.cornell.edu/cgi/viewcontent.cgi?article=3914&context=globaldocs
22. UNICEF. (2014). UNICEF Statistics: Sexual violence. Retrieved from http://data.unicef.org/child-protection/sexual-violence.html
23. World Health Organization. (2015). Eliminating female genital mutilation: An interagency statement. Retrieved from http://apps.who.int/iris/bitstream/10665/43839/1/9789241596442_eng.pdf
24. UNICEF. (2015). UNICEF Statistics: Female genital mutilation and cutting. Retrieved from http://data.unicef.org/child-protection/fgmc.html
25. UNICEF. (2015). Child marriage. Retrieved from http://data.unicef.org/child-protection/child-marriage.html
26. Girls Not Brides. (2015). About child marriage. Retrieved from http://www.girlsnotbrides.org/
27. Kiely, M., El-Mohandes, A. A., El-Khorazaty, M. N., Blake, S. M., & Gantz, M. G. (2010). An integrated intervention to reduce intimate partner violence in pregnancy: A randomized controlled trial. *Obstetrics and Gynecology, 115*(2 Pt 1), 273–283.
28. Tjaden, P., & Thoennes, N. (2000). Extent, nature, and consequences of intimate partner violence: Findings From the National Violence Against Women Survey. Retrieved from https://www.ncjrs.gov/pdffiles1/nij/181867.pdf
29. Abramsky, T., Watts, C. H., Garcia-Moreno, C., Devries, K., Kiss, L., Ellsberg, M., Jansen, H.A., Heise, L. (2011). What factors are associated with recent intimate partner violence? Findings from the WHO multi-country study on women's health and domestic violence. *BMC Public Health*, 11, 109-2458-11-109.
30. Centers for Disease Control and Prevention. (2015). Intimate partner violence. Retrieved from http://www.cdc.gov/violenceprevention/intimatepartnerviolence/
31. Greenwood, S., Perrin, A., & Duggan, M. (2016, November 11). Social Media Update 2016: Facebook usage and engagement is on the rise, while adoption of other platforms holds steady. Retrieved from http://www.pewinternet.org/2016/11/11/social-media-update-2016/
32. Centers for Disease Control and Prevention. (2015). Intimate partner violence: Consequences. Retrieved from http://www.cdc.gov/violenceprevention/intimatepartnerviolence/consequences.html
33. Campbell, J. C., & Lewandowski, L. A. (1997). Mental and physical health effects of intimate partner violence on women and children. *Psychiatric Clinics of North America, 20*(2), 353–374.
34. Leserman, J., & Drossman, D. A. (2007). Relationship of abuse history to functional gastrointestinal disorders and symptoms: Some possible mediating mechanisms. *Trauma Violence & Abuse, 8*(3), 331–343.
35. Plichta, S. B. (1996). Violence, health and use of health services. In M. M. Falik, & K. S. Collins, eds. *Women's health and care seeking behavior: The commonwealth fund survey* (pp. 237–270). Baltimore, MD: Johns Hopkins University Press.

36. Bosch, J., Weaver, T. L., Arnold, L. D., & Clark, E. M. (2015). The impact of intimate partner violence on women's physical health: Findings from the Missouri behavioral risk factor surveillance system. *Journal of Interpersonal Violence*, Aug. doi: 10.1177/0886260515599162
37. Campbell, J., Jones, A. S., Dienemann, J., Kub, J., Schollenberger, J., O'Campo, P., Gielen, A.C., Wynee, C.. (2002). Intimate partner violence and physical health consequences. *Archives of Internal Medicine*, *162*(10), 1157–1163.
38. Spivak, H. R., Jenkins, L., VanAudenhove, K., Lee, D., Kelly, M., Iskander, J., Centers for Disease Control and Prevention (CDC). (2014). CDC grand rounds: A public health approach to prevention of intimate partner violence. *Morbidity and Mortality Weekly Report, 63*(2), 38–41.
39. Janssen, P. A., Holt, V. L., Sugg, N. K., Emanuel, I., Critchlow, C. M., & Henderson, A. D. (2003). Intimate partner violence and adverse pregnancy outcomes: A population-based study. *American Journal of Obstetrics and Gynecology*, *188*(5), 1341–1347.
40. Moraes, C. L., Amorim, A. R., & Reichenheim, M. E. (2006). Gestational weight gain differentials in the presence of intimate partner violence. *International Journal of Gynecology and Obstetetrics, 95*(3), 254–260.
41. Yost, N. P., Bloom, S. L., McIntire, D. D., & Leveno, K. J. (2005). A prospective observational study of domestic violence during pregnancy. *Obstetrics and Gynecology*, *106*(1), 61–65.
42. Centers for Disease Control and Prevention. (2010). NISVS: An Overview of 2010 Findings on Victimization by Sexual Orientation. Retrieved from https://www.cdc.gov/violenceprevention/pdf/cdc_nisvs_victimization_final-a.pdf
43. Cuevas, C. A., Sabina, C., & Milloshi, R. (2012). Interpersonal victimization among a national sample of Latino women. *Violence Against Women*, *18*(4), 377–403.
44. Zadnik, E., Sabina, C., & Cuevas, C. A. (2014). Violence against Latinas: The effects of undocumented status on rates of victimization and help-seeking. *Journal of Interpersonal Violence*, *31*(6), 1141–1153.
45. Hass, G. E., Dutton, M. A., & Orloff, L. E. (2000). Lifetime prevalence of violence against Latin immigrants: Legal and policy implications. *International Review of Victimology*. *7*, 93–113.
46. Administration for Community Living. (2014). What is elder abuse? Retrieved from http://www.aoa.gov/AoA_programs/elder_rights/EA_prevention/whatisEA.aspx
47. Dong, X. Q. (2015). Elder abuse: Systematic review and implications for practice. *Journal of the American Geriatrics Society, 63*(6), 1214–1238.
48. Acierno, R., Hernandez, M.A., & Amstadter, A.B., Resnick, H.S., Steve, K., Muzzy, W, Kilpatrick, D.G.. (2010). Prevalence and correlates of emotional, physical, sexual, and financial abuse and potential neglect in the United States: The national elder mistreatment study. *American Journal of Public Health, 100*(2), 292–297.
49. Wiglesworth, A., Mosqueda, L., Mulnard, R., Liao, S, Gibbs, L., & Fitzgerald, W. (2010). Screening for abuse and neglect of people with dementia. *Journal of the American Geriatrics Society*, *58*(3), 493–500.
50. Beach, S. R., Schulz, R., Castle, N. G., & Rosen, J. (2010). Financial exploitation and psychological mistreatment among older adults: Differences between African Americans and non-African Americans in a population-based survey. *Gerontologist*, *50*(6), 744–757.
51. DeLiema, M., Gassoumis, Z. D., Homeier, D. C., & Wilber, K. H. (2012). Determining prevalence and correlates of elder abuse using promotores: Low-income immigrant Latinos report high rates of abuse and neglect. *Journal of the American Geriatrics Society*, *60*(7), 1333–1339.
52. University of Washington Tacoma Student Health Services. (2015). Healthy vs. unhealthy relationships. Retrieved from http://www.tacoma.washington.edu/studentaffairs/SHW/documents/Health topics/Healthy vs Unhealthy Relationships.pdf
53. Love is Respect. (2015). Why people abuse. Retrieved from http://www.loveisrespect.org/is-this-abuse/why-people-abuse/
54. Love is Respect. (2015). Empowering youth to end dating abuse. Retrieved from http://www.loveisrespect.org/#quizhome
55. Love is Respect. (2015). Healthy LGBTQ relationships. Retrieved from http://www.loveisrespect.org/healthy-relationships/healthy-lgbtq-relationships/
56. Love is Respect. (2015). National survey of teen dating violence laws. Retrieved from http://www.loveisrespect.org/resources/teen-dating-violence-laws/
57. U.S. Department of Health and Human Services, Office on Women's Health in the Office. (2017). How to help a friend who is being abused. Retrieved from https://www.womenshealth.gov/violence-against-women/get-help-for-violence/how-to-help-a-friend-who-is-being-abused.html#pubs
58. National Network to End Domestic Violence. (2013). NNEDV: Spyware and safety. Retrieved from http://nnedv.org/downloads/SafetyNet/NNEDV_SpywareAndSafety_2013.pdf
59. Federal Bureau of Investigation. (2014). New rape definition in frequently asked questions. Retrieved from https://www.fbi.gov/about-us/cjis/ucr/recent-program-updates/new-rape-definition-frequently-asked-questions.
60. Bernard, S. (2014, September 11). Rape culture in the Alaskan wilderness. *The Atlantic*. Retrieved from https://www.theatlantic.com/health/archive/2014/09/rape-culture-in-the-alaskan-wilderness/379976/
61. Shedlock, J. (2014, May 3). Tanana resident, 20, arraigned for allegedly killing 2 Alaska state troopers. *Alaska Dispatch News*. Retrieved from http://www.adn.com/article/20140503/tanana-resident-20-arraigned-killing-2-alaska-state-troopers
62. Friedman, S. (2014, July 21). Alaska starts work on road to Tanana. *Newsminer.com: The voice of interior Alaska*. Retrieved from http://www.newsminer.com/news/local_news/alaska-starts-work-on-road-to-tanana/article_60f1730a-1139-11e4-a6ed-001a4bcf6878.html
63. MedicineNet.Com. (2015). Date rape drug: Learn the street names of these drugs. Retrieved from http://www.medicinenet.com/date_rape_drugs/article.htm
64. Morgan, R. (2014, July 1). My own rape shows how much we get wrong about these attacks. *Washington Post*. Retrieved from https://www.washingtonpost.com/posteverything/wp/2014/07/01/my-own-rape-shows-how-badly-we-stereotype-perps-and-victims/
65. U.S. Department of Education. (2014). U.S. Department of Education releases list of higher education institutions with open Title IX sexual violence investigations. Retrieved from http://www.ed.gov/news/press-releases/us-department-education-releases-list-higher-education-institutions-open-title-ix-sexual-violence-investigations.

66. Health Research Funding. (2014). 39 date rape statistics on college campuses. Retrieved from http://healthresearchfunding.org/39-date-rape-statistics-college-campuses/
67. Izadi, E. (2015, May 20). Columbia student protesting campus rape carries mattress during graduation. *Washington Post*. Retrieved from https://www.washingtonpost.com/news/grade-point/wp/2015/05/19/columbia-student-protesting-campus-rape-carries-mattress-during -commencement/
68. Grigoriadis, V. (2014, December 29). Meet the college women who are starting a revolution against campus sexual assault. *New York Magazine*.
69. U.S. Department of Education. (2014). Know your rights: Title IX requires your school to address sexual violence. Retrieved from https://www2.ed.gov/about/offices/list/ocr/docs/know-rights-201404-title-ix.pdf
70. Vilensky M. (2015, May 19). Columbia student graduates while carrying mattress. *Wall Street Journal*. Retrieved from http://www.wsj.com/articles/columbia-student-graduates-while-carrying-mattress-1432052902
71. Nathanson, R. (2014, December 1). Conversation on campus sexual assault: Columbia student Emma Sulkowicz's protest inspires nationwide actions. *Rolling Stone*. Retrieved from http://www.rollingstone.com/politics/news/how-carry-that-weight-is-changing-the-conversation-on-campus-sexual-assault-20141201
72. Know Your IX. (n.d.). Get updates on the Title IX rulemaking process. Retrieved from https://www.knowyourix.org/
73. Dick, K. (2016). The hunting ground. [Movie].
74. Owens, J. G. (2015). Why definitions matter: Stalking victimization in the United States. *Journal of Interpersonal Violence*, *31*(12), 2196–2226. doi: 10.1177/0886260515573577
75. Brewster, M.P. (2003). Power and control dynamics in prestalking and stalking. *Journal of Family Violence*, *18*(4), 207–217.
76. National Center for Victims of Crime. (2012). Stalking Resource Center. Retrieved from http://victimsofcrime.org/our-programs/stalking-resource-center
77. Thefreedictionary.com. (2015). How to stop a stalker: Legal definition of how to stop a stalker. Retrieved from http://legal-dictionary.thefreedictionary.com/How+to+Stop+a+Stalker
78. Wikipedia.org. (2018). Rebecca Schaeffer. Retrieved from https://en.wikipedia.org/wiki/Rebecca_Schaeffer
79. U.S. Department of Health and Human Services. (2015). What is bullying? Retrieved from http://www.stopbullying.gov/what-is-bullying/
80. Tarshis, T. P., & Huffman, L. C. (2007). Psychometric properties of the peer interactions in primary school (PIPS) questionnaire. *Journal of Developmental and Behavioral Pediatrics*, *28*(2), 125–132.
81. Stopbullying.gov. (2018). What is cyberbullying? Retrieved from https://www.stopbullying.gov/cyberbullying/what-is-it/index.html
82. National Center for Education Statistics. (2013). Student reports of bullying and cyber-bullying: Results from the 2011 school crime supplement to the national crime victimization survey. Retrieved from https://nces.ed.gov/pubs2013/2013329.pdf
83. U.S. Department of Health and Human Services. (2015). What is cyberbullying? Retrieved from http://www.stopbullying.gov/cyberbullying/what-is-it/
84. Chapell, M., Casey, D., De la Cruz, C., Ferrell, J., Forman, J., Lipkin, R., Newsham, M., Sterling, M., Whittaker, S. (2004). Bullying in college by students and teachers. *Adolescence*, *39*(153), 53–64.
85. Office of the Dean of Students. (n.d.). What is hazing? Retrieved from https://deanofstudents.umich.edu/article/what-hazing
86. Allan, E. J., & Madden, M. (2012). The nature and extent of college student hazing. *International Journal of Adolescent Medicine and Health*, *24*(1), 83–90.
87. Hazingprevention.org. (2015). State laws: Hazing prevention. Retrieved from http://hazingprevention.org/home/hazing/statelaws/
88. Srabstein J. (2008). Deaths linked to bullying and hazing. *International Journal of Adolescent Medicine and Health*, *20*(2), 235–239.
89. Huffington Post. (2012). Armed to the teeth: Gun ownership in America. Retrieved from http://big.assets.huffingtonpost.com/transparency.jpeg
90. U.S. Department of State. (2015). Yemen travel warning. Retrieved from http://travel.state.gov/content/passports/en/alertswarnings/yemen-travel-warning.html
91. Cooper, A., & Smith, E. L. (2013). Homicide in the U.S. known to law enforcement, 2011. Retrieved from http://www.bjs.gov/index.cfm?ty=pbdetail&iid=4863
92. Miller, M., Azrael, D., & Hemenway, D. (2002). Rates of household firearm ownership and homicide across US regions and states, 1988–1997. *American Journal of Public Health*, *92*(12), 1988–1993.
93. Miller, M., Hemenway, D., & Azrael, D. (2007). State-level homicide victimization rates in the US in relation to survey measures of household firearm ownership, 2001–2003. *Social Science and Medicine*, *64*(3), 656–664.
94. Miller, M., Azrael, D., Hemenway, D., & Solop, F. I. (2002). 'Road rage' in Arizona: Armed and dangerous. *Accident Analysis and Prevention*, *34*(6), 807–814.
95. CNN. (2015). American deaths in terrorism vs. gun violence. Retrieved from http://www.cnn.com/2015/10/02/us/oregon-shooting-terrorism-gun-violence/index.html
96. Kellermann, A. L., Rivara, F. P., Rushforth, N. B., et al. (1993). Gun ownership as a risk factor for homicide in the home. *New England Journal of Medicine*, *329*(15), 1084–1091
97. Pew Research Center. (2014). The demographics and politics of gun-owning households. Retrieved from http://www.pewresearch.org/fact-tank/2014/07/15/the-demographics-and-politics-of-gun-owning-households/
98. Gallup. (2005). Gun ownership and use in America. Retrieved from http://www.gallup.com/poll/20098/gun-ownership-use-america.aspx
99. Sheley, J. F., & Wright, J. D. (1993). Motivations for gun possession and carrying among serious juvenile offenders. *Behavioral Science & the Law*, *11*(4), 375–388.
100. Darke, S. (2010). The toxicology of homicide offenders and victims: A review. *Drug and Alcohol Review*, *29*(2), 202–215.
101. Chermack, S. T., & Taylor, S. P. (1995). Alcohol and human physical aggression: Pharmacological versus expectancy effects. *Journal of Studies on Alcohol*, *56*(4), 449–456.
102. Crandall, M., Kucybala, K., Behrens, J., Schwulst, S., & Esposito, T. (2015). Geographic association of liquor licenses and gunshot wounds in Chicago. *The American Journal of Surgery*, *210*(1), 99–105.
103. Phillips, C. D., Nwaiwu, O., Lin, S., Edwards, R, Imanpour, S-. H., & Ohsfeldt, R. (2015). Concealed handgun

licensing and crime in four states. *Journal of Criminology*, 2015. doi: 10.1155/2015/803742.

104. Aneja, A., Donohue III, J. J., & Zhang, A. (2011). The Impact of right-to-carry laws and the NRC Report: Lessons for the empirical evaluation of law and policy. Retrieved from https://crimeresearch.org/wp-content/uploads/2015/03/Aneja-Donohue-and-Zhang-ALER.pdf
105. Grimson, M. (2015). Port Arthur massacre: The shooting spree that changed Australia's gun laws. NBC news. Retrieved from http://www.nbcnews.com/news/world/port-arthur-massacre-shooting-spree-changed-australia-gun-laws-n396476
106. Bjelopera, J. P., Bagalman, E., Caldwell, S. W., Finklea, K. M., & McCallion, G. (2013, March 18). Public mass shootings in the United States: Selected implications for federal public health and safety policy. Congressional Research Service. Retrieved from https://fas.org/sgp/crs/misc/R43004.pdf
107. Rosenblatt, K., Chuck, E., & Sperling, J. (2018, March 14). Students demand action on gun violence with nationwide walkout. *NBC News*. Retrieved from https://www.nbcnews.com/news/us-news/national-school-walkout-marks-month-parkland-mass-shooting-n856386)
108. Diuguid, L. (2015, December 7). Guns on college campus in hands of students wrong solution to prevent mass shootings. *The Kansas City Star*. Retrieved from http://www.kansascity.com/opinion/opn-columns-blogs/lewis-diuguid/article48445285.html
109. National Conference on State Legislatures. (2017). Guns on campus: Overview. Retrieved from http://www.ncsl.org/research/education/guns-on-campus-overview.aspx
110. Stone, Z. (2015, December 13). I'm a responsible gun owner? Seriously? *The New York Times*. Retrieved from http://www.nytimes.com/2015/12/13/opinion/is-this-really-how-you-get-your-gun.html?_r=0
111. Hemenway, D. (2006). *Private guns, public health*. Ann Arbor, MI: University of Michigan Press.
112. Kindy, K., Tate, J., Jenkins, J., Rich, S., Alexander, K., & Lowery, W. (2015, May 30). Fatal shootings in 2015 approaching 400 nationwide. *Washington Post*. Retrieved from https://www.washingtonpost.com/national/fatal-police-shootings-in-2015-approaching-400-nationwide/2015/05/30/d322256a-058e-11e5-a428-c984eb077d4e_story.html
113. Tran, M. (2015, October 8). FBI chief: 'Unacceptable' that Guardian has better data on police violence. *The Guardian*. Retrieved from http://www.theguardian.com/us-news/2015/oct/08/fbi-chief-says-ridiculous-guardian-washington-post-better-information-police-shootings
114. *The Guardian*. (2015, June 9). By the numbers: US police kill more in days than other countries do in years. Retrieved from http://www.theguardian.com/us-news/2015/jun/09/the-counted-police-killings-us-vs-other-countries
115. *The Guardian*. (2015, June 1). The Counted: People killed by police in the United States in 2015— interactive. Retrieved from http://www.theguardian.com/us-news/ng-interactive/2015/jun/01/the-counted-police-killings-us-database#
116. Weisburd, D., Greenspan, R., Hamilton, E. E., Williams, H, & Bryan, K. A. (2000). Police attitudes toward abuse of authority: Findings from a national study. Retrieved from https://www.ncjrs.gov/pdffiles1/nij/181312.pdf
117. Amnesty International USA. (2015). Deadly force: Police use of lethal force in the United States. Retrieved from http://www.amnestyusa.org/research/reports/deadly-force-police-use-of-lethal-force-in-the-united-states?page=2
118. *The Washington Post*. (2015, December 26). 2015 Police shootings investigation. Retrieved from https://www.washingtonpost.com/graphics/national/police-shootings-year-end/
119. *The Washington Post*. (2015, December). Fatal force. Retrieved from https://www.washingtonpost.com/graphics/national/police-shootings/
120. *The Washington Post*. (2016). Fatal force. Retrieved from https://www.washingtonpost.com/graphics/national/police-shootings-2016/
121. *The Washington Post*. (2017). Fatal force. Retrieved from https://www.washingtonpost.com/graphics/national/police-shootings-2017/
122. Federal Bureau of Investigation. (2016). Uniform crime reports: 2016 crime in the United States. Retrieved from https://ucr.fbi.gov/crime-in-the-u.s/2016/crime-in-the-u.s.-2016/topic-pages/tables/table-1
123. Federal Bureau of Investigation. (2014). Uniform crime reports: 2014 crime in the United States. Retrieved from https://www.fbi.gov/about-us/cjis/ucr/crime-in-the-u.s/2014/crime-in-the-u.s.-2014
124. Federal Bureau of Investigation. (2013). Murder and nonnegligent manslaughter. Retrieved from https://www.fbi.gov /about-us/cjis/ucr/nibrs/2013/the-advantage-of-nibrs-data/murder-and-nonnegligent-manslaughter
125. Weisser, M. (2014, April 12). It's clear violent crime is decreasing, but less clear why. *The Huffington Post*. Retrieved from http://www.huffingtonpost.com/mike-weisser/violent-crime-cities_b_4760996.html
126. Chettiar, I. M. (2015, February). Locking more people up is counterproductive. *The Atlantic*. Retrieved from http://www.theatlantic.com/politics/archive/2015/02/the-many-causes-of-americas-decline-in-crime/385364/
127. Centers for Disease Control and Prevention. (2014). Vital signs: Leading causes of death, prevalence of diseases and risk factors, and use of health services among Hispanics in the United States—2009–2013. Retrieved from http://www.cdc.gov/mmwr/preview/mmwrhtml/mm6417a5.htm
128. National Organization of Parents of Murdered Children. (n.d.). Survivors of homicide victims. Retrieved from http://www.pomc.org/survivors.html
129. Thefreedictionary.com. (n.d.). Capital punishment—legal definition of capital punishment. Retrieved from http://legal-dictionary.thefreedictionary.com/capital+punishment
130. *Furman v. Georgia*, 408 US 238 (Supreme Court 1972). Retrieved from https://scholar.google.com/scholar_case?case=3510234117314043073&hl=en&as_sdt=2&as_vis=1&oi=scholarr
131. Death Penalty Information Center. (2015). Deterrence: States without the death penalty have had consistently lower murder rates. Retrieved from http://www.deathpenaltyinfo.org/deterrence-states-without-death-penalty-have-had-consistently-lower-murder-rates#stateswithvwithout
132. Morton, R. J. (2008). Serial murder: Multi-disciplinary perspectives for investigators. NCJ 223848. https://www.ncjrs.gov/App/Publications/abstract.aspx?ID=245787
133. Duncan, D. T., & Hatzenbuehler, M. L. (2014). Lesbian, gay, bisexual, and transgender hate crimes and suicidality among a population-based sample of sexual-minority

adolescents in Boston. *American Journal of Public Health, 104*(2), 272–278.

134. Kessler, R. C., Mickelson, K. D., & Williams, D. R. (1999). The prevalence, distribution, and mental health correlates of perceived discrimination in the United States. *Journal of Health and Social Behavior, 40*(3), 208–230.
135. Padela, A. I., & Heisler, M. (2010). The association of perceived abuse and discrimination after September 11, 2001, with psychological distress, level of happiness, and health status among Arab Americans. *American Journal of Public Health, 100*(2), 284–291.
136. Boston University. (2015). The public health consequences of hate. Retrieved from http://www.bu.edu/sph/2015/01/18/the-public-health-consequences-of-hate/
137. Federal Bureau of Investigation. (2014). Latest *Hate crime statistics* report released. Retrieved from https://www.fbi.gov/news/stories/2014/december/latest-hate-crime-statistics-report-released
138. Langton, L., Planty, M., & Sandholtz, N. (2013). Bureau of Justice Statistics (BJS): Hate crime victimization, 2003–2011. Retrieved from http://www.bjs.gov/index.cfm?ty=pbdetail&iid=4926
139. Younis M. (2015). Perceptions of Muslims in the United States: A review. Retrieved from http://www.gallup.com/opinion/gallup/187664/perceptions-muslims-united-states-review.aspx?g_source=religious identity&g_medium=search&g_campaign=tiles
140. Jabali-Nash N. (2010). Four New York teens sentenced in 2008 hate crime. *CBS News.* Retrieved from http://www.cbsnews.com /news/four-new-york-teens-sentenced-in-2008-hate -crime/
141. Severson K. (2011, August 8). Video intensifies interest in a Mississippi killing. *The New York Times.* Retrieved from http://www.nytimes.com/2011/08/09/us/09hate.html
142. Talbot M. (2015, June 22). The story of a hate crime. *The New Yorker.* Retrieved from https://www.newyorker.com/magazine/2015/06/22/the-story-of-a-hate-crime
143. Langton L., & Masucci, M. (2017). Hate crime victimization, 2004-2015: Statistical tables. Retrieved from https://www.bjs.gov/index.cfm?ty=pbdetail&iid=5967
144. Advocate.com. (2016, June 15). A brief history of anti-LGBT violence. Retrieved from http://www.advocate.com/politics/2016/6/15/brief-history-anti-lgbt-violence
145. Stotzer, R. L., & Hossellman, E. (2012). Hate crimes on campus: Racial/ethnic diversity and campus safety. *Journal of Interpersonal Violence, 27*(4), 644–661.
146. Kindness Above Malice. (2011). Empathy as a cure for hatred. Retrieved from http://www.kindnessabovemalice.org/empathy-as-a-cure-for-hatred/
147. Code of Hammurabi. Retrieved from https://web.archive.org/web/20110514033802/http://www.wsu.edu/~dee/MESO/CODE.HTM
148. History.com. (n.d.). Congress abolishes the African slave trade: March 2, 1807. Retrieved from http://www.history.com/this-day-in-history/congress-abolishes-the-african-slave-trade

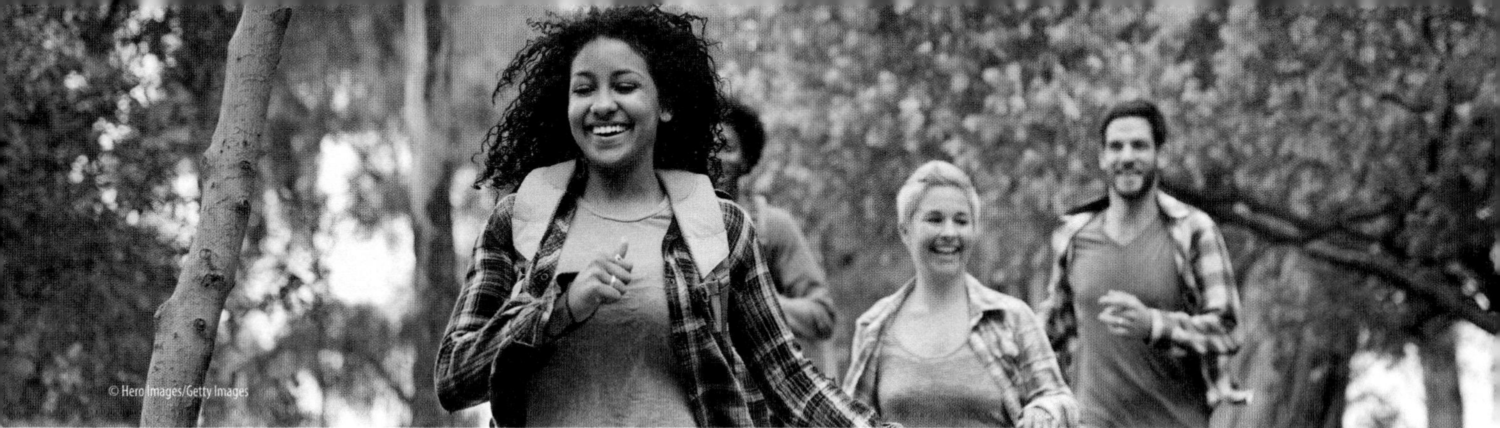
© Hero Images/Getty Images

CHAPTER 11

Environmental Health: Nurture Nature

CHAPTER OBJECTIVES

- Identify the various sources of energy we use as well as the pros and cons of each type.
- Understand how food must be kept safe, from the grower until it reaches your table.
- Understand what pesticides are and how their use affects the environment.
- Describe why individuals choose bottled versus tap water, and explain the differences between the two choices and how these differences impact the environment.
- Recognize how pervasive plastic is in our environment and the consequences of its use.
- Explain the implications of global warming and climate change and what individuals can do to help.
- Explain how to protect yourself from air pollution.
- Understand the extent of our everyday exposures to toxicants.
- Identify natural disasters, and know how to protect yourself.
- Recognize the role of environmental justice.

Environmental health is a broad and increasingly important field. Reading this chapter will help you appreciate the importance of the choices we make, because many of the choices we make on a daily basis have effects on the environment. Using public transportation or walking versus driving, recycling items versus throwing them away, drinking from the tap versus buying bottled water—even the small choices we make can have long-term environmental effects. If everyone makes better choices, our world will be a healthier and more enjoyable place in which to live.

Sources of Energy

Most of the energy we use in the United States comes from nonrenewable sources, especially fossil fuels. Nonrenewable energy sources include coal, petroleum, natural gas, and uranium. We use the energy these sources produce

TABLE 11-1 Major Sources of Energy and Usage in the United States[1]

Source	Percentage of U.S. Electricity Generation in 2017
Coal	30.1%
Natural gas	31.7%
Nuclear	20%
Hydropower	7.5%
Other renewables	9.6%
Biomass	1.6%
Geothermal	0.4%
Solar	1.3%
Wind	6.3%
Petroleum	0.5%
Other gases	<1%

to make electricity; to heat and cool our homes, office buildings, and stadiums; and to fuel our cars. Although the use of renewable sources like wind and sun is growing, they provide a small proportion of the energy we consume. **TABLE 11-1** presents the major sources of energy and usage in the United States.

fossil fuels Natural fuels formed in the geological past from remains of ancient plants and animals and used as fuel.

greenhouse gases A group of gases, including carbon dioxide, methane, nitrous oxide, ozone, and fluorocarbons, that allow sunlight to pass through the atmosphere and reach the earth's surface. These gases trap the sun's heat like a blanket, warming the earth. They need to be present in specific amounts; however, when too much is present, the earth warms more than is needed.

solar power Power obtained by harnessing the energy of the sun's rays.

Fossil Fuels

Fossil fuels—that is, coal, petroleum, and natural gas—come from the decomposition of dead plant and animal life that existed on the earth millions of years ago. More than 60% of the energy we use in the United States is from fossil fuels.[2] The infrastructure required to use fossil fuels as a source of energy is already built. Fossil fuels can be easily transported from the source to a power-generating plant.

However, there are many disadvantages of fossil fuels, most importantly that they harm the environment and human health. Use of fossil fuels creates **greenhouse gases** and acid rain. Liquid run-off from coal and oil production pollutes the local water supplies. You will read much more about the consequences of our reliance on fossil fuels in this chapter.

Solar Power

One solution to reduce pollution that is gaining in popularity is the use of **solar power**. Solar power is the conversion of sunlight into electricity. One of the best things about solar energy is that it is a renewable and sustainable source of energy. The National Aeronautics and Space Administration (NASA) estimates that our sun will be around for another 6.5 billion years.[4] Also, the amount of

HYDRAULIC FRACTURING OR FRACKING

Fracking is the process of drilling down into the earth followed by injection of fracking fluid (primarily water, with sand or other proppants) under high pressure. This process creates cracks in the deep rocks to allow natural gas to flow out. (A proppant is a solid material, typically sand, treated sand, or human-made ceramic materials, designed to keep the hydraulic fracture open.)

Fracking is highly controversial. Proponents advocate its use because it produces gas for energy and improves energy independence (reduces U.S. dependence on foreign imports of petroleum and other foreign energy sources). If done correctly, supporters believe it can reduce air pollution and water use compared to other fossil fuels. Opponents argue that there are environmental problems associated with fracking, including ground and surface water contamination, air and noise pollution, and the potential to trigger earthquakes. A less direct problem is that it will slow the adoption of renewable energy sources.[3]

sunlight the earth receives is significantly more than is needed to supply the entire world with energy.[5] Although manufacturing, transporting, and installing solar power systems all cause pollution, harnessing solar energy does not. The amount of solar power generation has increased dramatically since 2009. The amount of pollution produced in the creation of solar power systems is minimal compared to that produced by conventional energy sources. Without subsidies, solar panels can be expensive. But many utility companies offer incentives, which reduce or may even eliminate the cost. Solar power systems require little maintenance, and the technology is improving.

Wind Power

wind power Power obtained by harnessing the energy of the wind.

Wind power is created by harnessing the energy of the wind to generate electricity. Wind farms consist of many individual wind turbines connected to an electric power transmission network. The amount of wind energy almost doubled between 2009 and 2013.[6] Like solar power, wind energy is clean and renewable (**FIGURE 11-1**). Because turbines come in a variety of sizes, they can

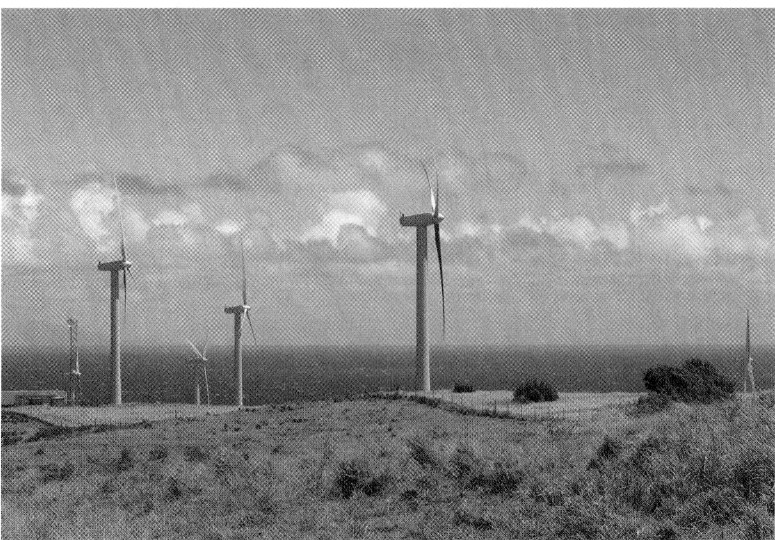

FIGURE 11-1 Use of renewable energy is an effective way to reduce greenhouse gas emissions.

Image Courtesy of U.S. Environmental Protection Agency.

be adapted for use in many settings, but they need to be placed where the wind speed is high. In rural areas, wind turbines can be used as a source of earnings from electricity generation. One of the biggest concerns about wind turbines is that they are unsafe for birds. Some people find wind turbines ugly, and the turbines make noise, between 50 and 60 decibels. People's self-reports of health effects include migraine headaches, dizziness, and poorer sleep.[7,8] Wind turbines are expensive to set up. Because they are mostly located in rural areas, there is a concomitant need for transmission lines.[9]

methane A colorless, odorless flammable gas that is the main constituent of natural gas. It traps heat in the atmosphere and, as such, contributes to the warming of the earth.

carbon dioxide A colorless, odorless gas produced by burning carbon and organic compounds and by respiration. It is naturally present in air (about 0.03%) and is absorbed by plants in photosynthesis. It traps heat in the atmosphere and, as such, contributes to the warming of the earth.

Nuclear Energy

Two different processes produce nuclear energy: nuclear fission and nuclear fusion, although power plants only use nuclear fission. Nuclear-fueled power plants produce energy by harnessing the power of atoms. Nuclear fission is the division of one atom into two. Nuclear fusion is the combination of two lighter atoms into a larger one.

Pros of Nuclear Energy: The Good

Nuclear power produces less pollution than other sources of power. It does not produce **methane**, **carbon dioxide**, and nitrous oxide, the primary greenhouse gases that come from burning fossil fuels. In 2017, approximately 20% of the energy used in the United States came from nuclear power plants.[1]

FIGURE 11-2 provides a map of nuclear power plant locations in the United States. Let's look at the benefits of using nuclear power.

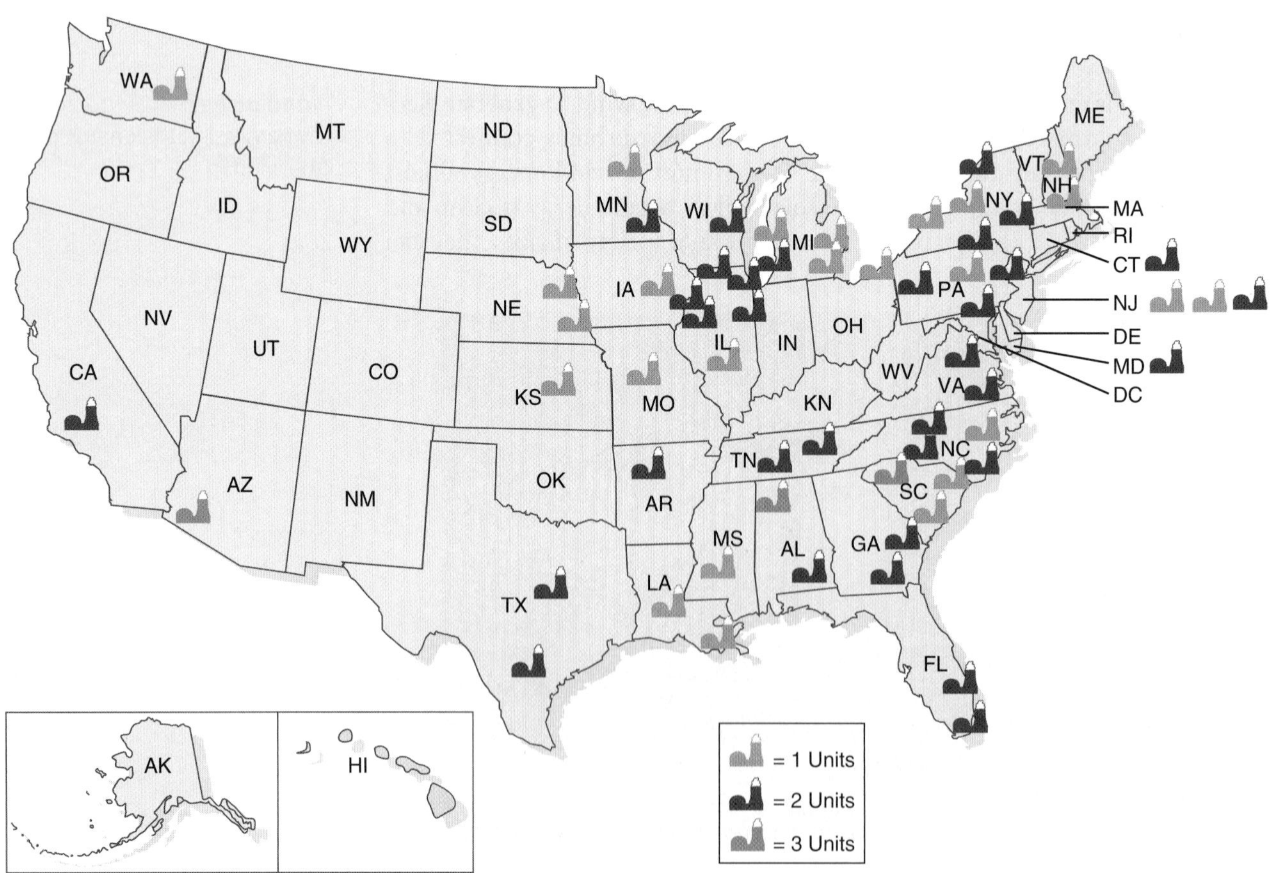

FIGURE 11-2 Location of nuclear power plants in the United States.

U.S. Nuclear Regulatory Commission. (2017). Map of power reactor sites. Retrieved from https://www.nrc.gov/reactors/operating/map-power-reactors.html

1. Low Pollution. Overall, nuclear power production produces a fraction of the greenhouse emissions produced by fossil fuels. Comparing the entire spectrum of the energy chains for electricity generation for nuclear power and energy created by fossil fuels, nuclear power emits 40 to 100 timesless CO_2 than do fossil-fuel chains.[10] **Nuclear energy** has the least effect on the earth's atmosphere because it does not discharge carbon dioxide, which is the primary greenhouse gas. Except during transportation, there is little impact on air pollution because of nuclear power use.[11]

nuclear energy Energy released during nuclear fission, especially when used to generate electricity

2. Low Operating Costs. Electricity produced by nuclear power is inexpensive. The cost of the uranium, the fuel used in this process, is low. Also, even though the expense of setting up nuclear power plants is moderately high, the expense of running them is quite low. The usual life of a nuclear reactor is anywhere from 40 to 60 years, depending on how often and in what capacity it is used. Together, these variables make the expense of delivering power low. Even if the cost of uranium increases, the impact on the cost of power is still low.[11]

3. Reliability. With the current consumption rate of uranium, we have enough to last for another 70 to 80 years. In fact, experts believe that the supply of uranium is going to last much longer than that of fossil fuels.[11] When producing energy, a nuclear power plant can run uninterrupted for as long as a year. While solar energy and wind energy are dependent on weather conditions, there are no weather constraints on a nuclear power plant, and it can run without disruption in any climatic condition.

4. Superiority to Fossil Fuels. Some nuclear energy innovations have made it a much more feasible choice than fossil fuels. Compared to fossil fuels, nuclear power has high energy density. Nuclear power plants require relatively less fuel than power plants that utilize fossil fuels. Nuclear fission produces approximately 10 million times more energy than is produced by a fossil fuel atom.

The greatest benefit from nuclear energy is that it does not depend on fossil fuels. Fluctuating oil and gas prices do not impact nuclear power costs. Coal and natural gas power plants discharge carbon dioxide into the air, creating environmental issues. With nuclear power plants, carbon emissions are insignificant.[11]

5. Renewable? Nuclear energy is not a renewable resource. The supply of uranium, nuclear energy's fuel, is limited. However, by using breeder and fusion reactors, we can create other fissionable element(s). One such element is plutonium, produced by the by-products of chain reaction. Also, once scientists understand how to control atomic fusion, the same reactions that fuel the sun, we could have almost unlimited energy.[11]

Cons of Nuclear Energy: The Bad

1. Environmental Impact. One of the main issues about nuclear energy is the environmental impact. The uranium used by nuclear reactors presents environmental hazards all along the production chain, from mining to refining to transportation to disposal after its use. Because it is radioactive and dangerous, dumping it in a landfill is not an option. Each nuclear power plant creates approximately 20 metric tons of spent nuclear fuel every year. According to the Nuclear Regulatory Commission, as of 2017, there were 99 nuclear reactors in the United States, which means we produce almost 2,000 metric tons of spent nuclear fuel every year.[12] The waste emits radiation and high temperatures, suggesting that eventually it will destroy the container that holds it. The radioactivity can damage all living things.[11]

2. Radioactive Waste Disposal. In addition to spent fuel, nuclear power plants create low-level radioactive waste by contaminating items with radioactive material. Low-level radiation waste comes from medical sources, industry, as well as nuclear power plants. These contaminated items include, but are not limited to, contaminated protective shoe covers and clothing, rags, mops, filters, reactor water treatment residues, equipment, tools, medical tubes, swabs, needles, syringes, and laboratory animal carcasses and tissues.[13] Even low-level radioactive waste takes a long time to achieve adequate safety levels.

3. Uranium Is Finite. Like other sources of fuel, uranium that fuels nuclear power is finite. It is expensive to mine, refine, and transport. Uranium production creates considerable waste during all stages, from mining to transport. These steps require proper handling or may result in environmental contamination.

4. As a Target. Nuclear power plants are potentially a prime target for terrorist activities. If a power plant was successfully targeted, immense havoc and destruction could result.[11]

Nuclear Accidents: The Ugly

Nuclear accidents, when they happen, create serious health issues for people living near the power plant. Although there have been other accidents, the three most well-known ones are Three Mile Island (1979), Chernobyl (1986), and Fukushima Daiichi (2011).

The Three Mile Island accident was a partial nuclear meltdown in reactor number 2 of the Three Mile Island Nuclear Generating Station in Pennsylvania. Significant amounts of nuclear reactor coolant leaked, releasing unknown amounts of radioactive gases. There was no convincing evidence that the radiation released during the Three Mile Island accident increased cancer risk[14]; however, the accident resulted in new nuclear industry regulations.[15]

In 1986, there was a disastrous accident at the Chernobyl Nuclear Power Plant in the Ukraine. It was the worst nuclear accident in history. An explosion and fire released large quantities of radioactivity into the atmosphere, which spread over much of the western Soviet Union and Europe. The Chernobyl accident released 200 times as much radioactivity as the atomic bombs dropped on Hiroshima and Nagasaki during World War II.[16] The Chernobyl accident contaminated more than 38,600 square miles of land. It forced the evacuation of more than 350,000 people. A recent publication reported 4,000 cases of solid cancers from 1992 to 2009 among emergency workers.[17] Twenty years after Chernobyl, there were still food restrictions in place as a result of the accident.[16] Ukrainian scientists believe that as a result of the accident, Chernobyl will not be habitable by humans for at least 20,000 years.[18]

An earthquake followed by a tsunami in Japan in 2011 caused the Fukushima Daiichi nuclear disaster. The incident involved equipment failures, with three nuclear meltdowns and release of radioactive materials. The original evacuation zone was 1.25 miles around the plant and progressively increased so that by 27 hours after the earthquake, it was enlarged to almost 12.5 miles, and 2 weeks later to 18.5 miles. Six weeks after the earthquake, the government extended the evacuation zone to specific areas up to 31 miles. A month after the catastrophe, the Japanese government increased its official safe radiation exposure level from 1 mSv to 20 mSv. A millisievert (mSv) is the average amount of radiation present in the general environment to which an individual is exposed in a year's time, exclusive of **radon** gas. Physicians for Social Responsibility believe that increasing the allowable radiation exposure level allowed the Japanese government to downplay the dangers produced by the accident.[19]

radon A colorless, gaseous radioactive element produced by the decay of radium.

The exclusion zone now contains radioactive cesium (**FIGURE 11-3** and **FIGURE 11-4**). Cesium-137 has a half-life of 30 years.[20] It takes approximately 10 half-lives for any radionuclide to disappear; thus, it will be more than 300 years before the exclusion zone is habitable by humans. Once radioactive cesium enters an ecosystem, it contaminates water, soil, plants, and animals. Cesium-137 is present in a large range of foods, including freshwater fish 200 miles from Fukushima.[19] Radioactive cesium bioaccumulates, bioconcentrates, and biomagnifies as it moves up the food chain (see the box on radiation exposure).

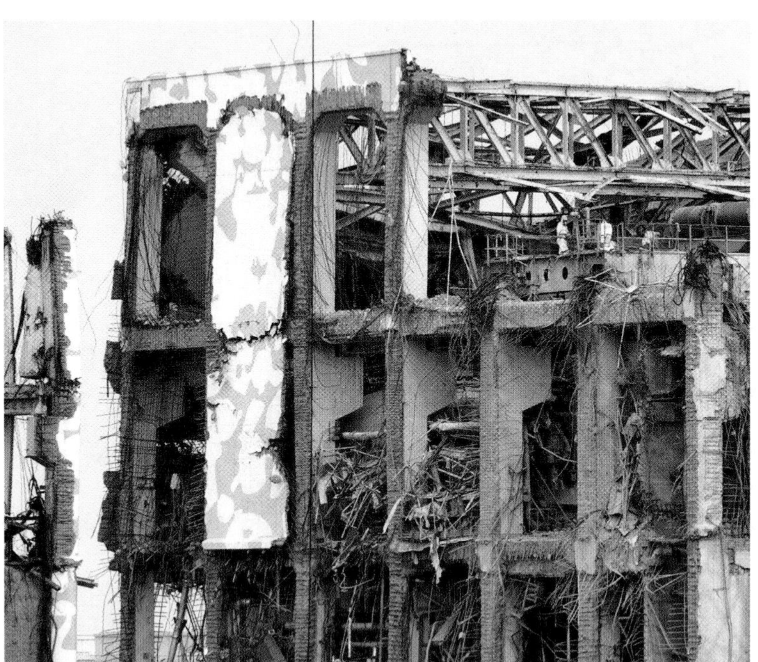

FIGURE 11-3 The fourth reactor at Fukushima on February 20, 2012, almost a year after the accident.

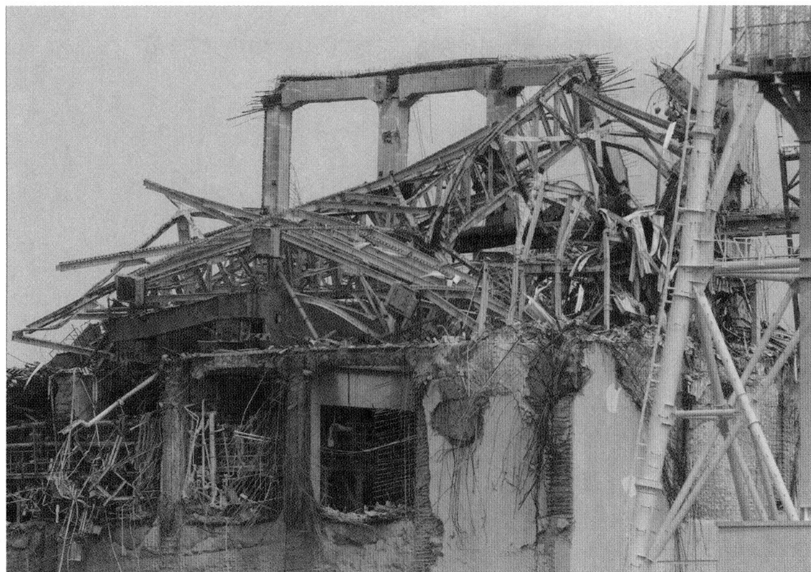

FIGURE 11-4 Destroyed top of reactor Number 3, one year after disaster.

RADIATION EXPOSURE TERMS

Bioaccumulation—accumulation of chemicals in the tissue of organisms through any route, including respiration, ingestion, or direct contact.

Bioconcentration—accumulation of a chemical in the tissues of an organism as a result of direct exposure to the surrounding medium. It does not include dietary intake.

Biomagnification—the process whereby the tissue concentration of a contaminant increases as it passes up the food chain.

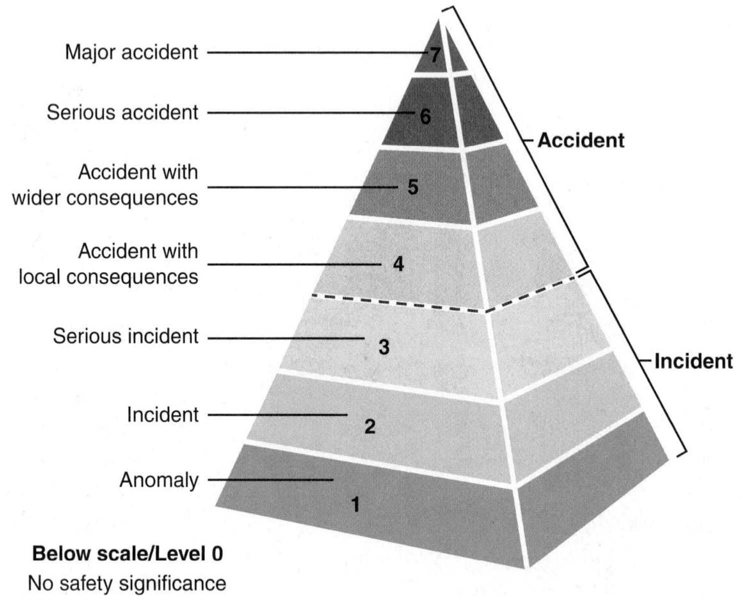

FIGURE 11-5 The International Atomic Energy Agency introduced the International Nuclear and Radiological Event Scale in 1990.

U.S. Nuclear Regulatory Commission. (2017). International Nuclear and Radiological Event Scale (about emergency preparedness). Retrieved from https://www.nrc.gov/about-nrc/emerg-preparedness/about-emerg-preparedness/emerg-classification/event-scale.html

Both Chernobyl and Fukushima Daiichi disasters rated seven on the International Nuclear and Radiological Event Scale. A rating of seven is the most serious accident possible. These two events are the only ones rated as a seven. See **FIGURE 11-5**.

Food Safety: What Can Go Wrong from the Farm to the Table

Whether your food comes from a backyard garden or you purchase it at a farmer's market or a grocery store, food must be handled correctly all along the supply chain to avoid contamination.

Irrigation and Wash Water

pesticides Substances used for destroying insects or other organisms harmful to cultivated plants or animals.

Using water safely is critical to fruit and vegetable production. Water can spread harmful microorganisms across a large area. Before harvesting, water is used to irrigate plants (**FIGURE 11-6**), to cool crops, to protect crops from frost, and to convey fertilizers and **pesticides**. It is used to wash tools as well as workers' hands and for drinking. After harvest, it is used to wash and transport, cool, and apply

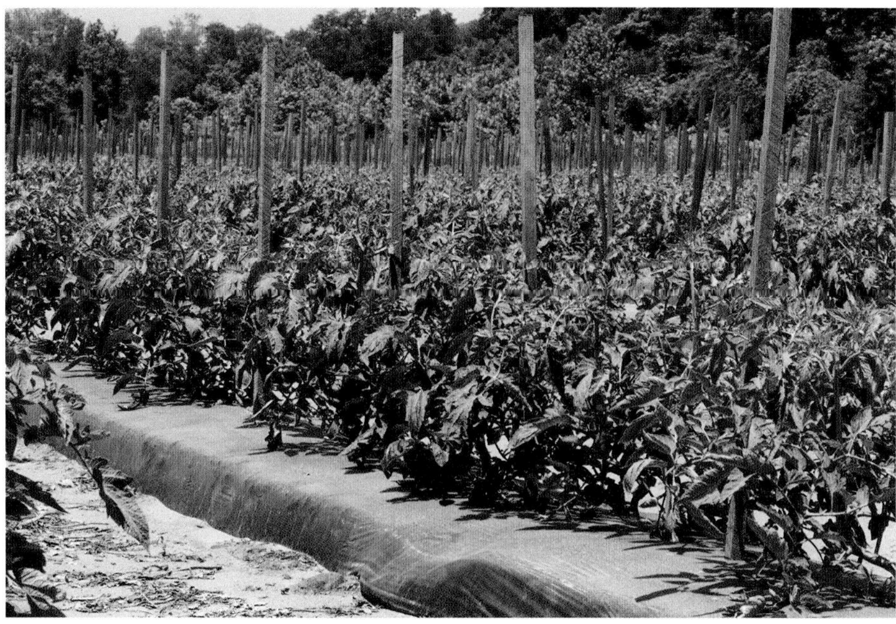

FIGURE 11-6 Peppers and tomatoes being grown with drip irrigation, which eliminates most of the potential for irrigation water to contact the fruit.

protective coatings to produce, and it is also used for hand washing and drinking. Water used after harvesting must meet standards set for drinking water.[21]

Water for agriculture comes from three sources: surface water, well water, and municipal water supplies. Surface water includes ponds, lakes, rivers, and streams. Because the water is openly available, there is no control over potential contamination. There may be many sources of contamination upstream, such as wild and domestic animal contamination, runoff from manure, sewage, and drainage from animal operations. Surface water presents the highest risk for contamination.[21]

Well water presents an intermediate risk. If a well is correctly sited, constructed, and maintained, it is a reliable source of safe water. However, if the well is too close to an area prone to flooding, septic tanks, cesspools, manure storage areas, or other sources of contamination, it may be contaminated by harmful microorganisms. The risks increase if the well were not constructed correctly or maintained properly.[21]

The safest water for agriculture comes from a municipal water supply.[21] Because it is intended for drinking, federal laws mandate high standards regarding chemicals and microorganisms. Municipalities test their water regularly to ensure it is safe to drink.[21]

Risks From Animals: Manure, Feathers, Fur, and Skin

Animal waste often contains high concentrations of human pathogens—that is, viruses, bacteria, and parasites. Farms that raise livestock, such as cattle, swine, and poultry, produce large amounts of animal waste. Giant livestock farms have thousands to tens of thousands of animals crowded into small areas. The way these farms store and use animal manure has a profound effect on public health and the environment. Fish farms also produce large quantities of waste by-products.[22]

Pathogens from animal manures and other waste can potentially contaminate water, land, and air. Some of these pathogens can live in the environment for days, weeks, or months. Farmers use animal waste as fertilizer. But if the farmer uses too much or applies it incorrectly, the runoff can pollute water sources.[23]

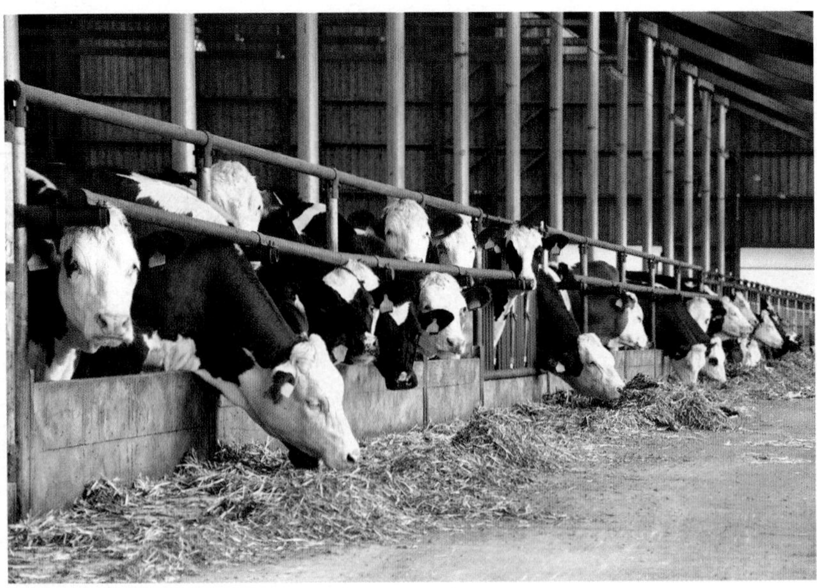

Livestock farm.

TABLE 11-2 Common Gases From Livestock[26]

Gas	Source	Effects and Characteristics	Solution
Carbon dioxide	Animal respiration	Respiratory distress Headaches Death (with prolonged high exposure)	Maintain proper ventilation at all times.
Carbon monoxide	Combustion equipment in a confined area		
Ammonia	By-product of manure decomposition	20–25 ppm: eye irritant 1,500 ppm: coughing and froth at the mouth 5,000 ppm: death	Maintain sufficient ventilation to prevent ammonia levels from rising above 25 ppm. Rinse equipment frequently and leave at least 0.5 inch of water in pits or on floor.
Methane	Animal waste decomposition	Highly combustible at 50,000 ppm Colorless, odorless, tasteless	All manure storage areas should be well ventilated. Prohibit open sparks or flames near storage facilities.
Hydrogen sulfide "manure gas"	Bacteria in manure	At < 1 ppm, smells like rotten eggs At higher levels, gas paralyzes the sense of smell 1,000 ppm: can cause death	Provide extra ventilation during manure agitation. Use precautions when entering a manure pit. If you suspect high hydrogen sulfide levels, leave the building immediately.

ppm, parts per million.

Animal manure pits are one way farmers store animal waste. These pits must be properly maintained and ventilated because as the manure decays and ferments, it can produce deadly gases: ammonia, carbon dioxide, hydrogen sulfide, and methane (**TABLE 11-2**). These gases are hazardous and highly toxic. They can cause human illnesses, oxygen depletion, and explosions.[23,24]

Researchers analyzed reports of major accidents related to manure exposure. Of the 61 accidents, 72% were due to inhalation of manure gas, 18% involved falls into manure containers, and 10% were methane explosions. There were 49 deaths, with 24% of deaths occurring during attempts to rescue the primary victims. Almost one-third of these accidents were falls into manure pits or manure gas explosions.[25]

Harvester and Handler Health and Hygiene

The Centers for Disease Control and Prevention (CDC) estimates that each year in the United States approximately 48 million people get a laboratory-confirmed foodborne illness. That is about 15% of the population. Fresh produce causes more cases of illness than any other type of food. Personal health practices play a major role in helping to prevent contamination risks.[27] Periodically, the CDC publishes a progress report on food safety. The 2014 report is shown in **FIGURE 11-7**.

Keeping Healthy and Clean

It is important for people who work with food to be healthy. You would not want someone who is unhealthy to touch the food you are about to eat. It is essential for workers who are sick not to have direct or indirect contact with fresh produce. A person with a cut on the hand should wash and bandage the wound, then wear plastic gloves to prevent disease transmission. Workers should turn away from the food when coughing or sneezing. Overall, good hygiene is essential: bathing or showering, wearing clean clothes, and keeping fingernails short. Washing hands frequently is also an effective way to keep fresh produce safe.[28]

The Occupational Safety and Health Administration (OSHA) has standards regarding locating, supplying, and maintaining sanitary facilities. There must be at least one toilet and hand washing station for every 20 workers. The toilets can be portable or permanent but must be either within a quarter mile walk from the field or workers provided with vehicle access.[29]

Traceability and Recall Programs

The U.S. Food and Drug Administration (FDA) is responsible for protecting the public's health by ensuring the safety of the U.S. food supply. When a foodborne

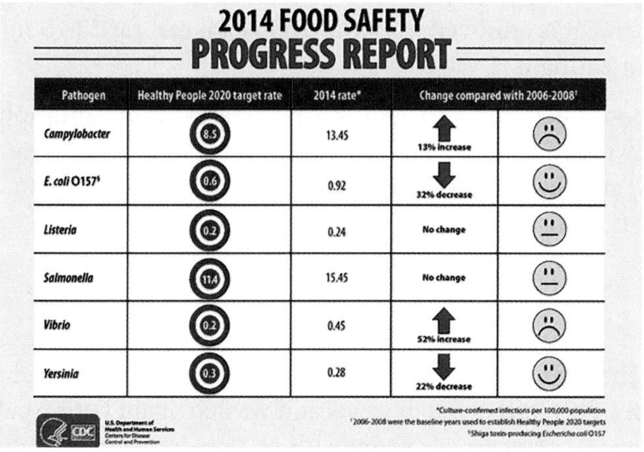

2014 FOOD SAFETY PROGRESS REPORT

Pathogen	Healthy People 2020 target rate	2014 rate*	Change compared with 2006-2008†	
Campylobacter	8.5	13.45	13% increase	☹
E. coli O157§	0.6	0.92	32% decrease	☺
Listeria	0.2	0.24	No change	😐
Salmonella	11.4	15.45	No change	😐
Vibrio	0.2	0.45	52% increase	☹
Yersinia	0.3	0.28	22% decrease	☺

*Culture-confirmed infections per 100,000 population
†2006-2008 were the baseline years used to establish Healthy People 2020 targets
§Shiga toxin-producing *Escherichia coli* O157

U.S. Department of Health and Human Services, Centers for Disease Control and Prevention

FIGURE 11-7 America's 2014 report card for food safety.

Centers for Disease Control and Prevention. (2018). Foodborne Diseases Active Surveillance Network (FoodNet). Retrieved from https://www.cdc.gov/foodnet/index.html

© Bro Studio/Shutterstock.

HOW PRODUCE TRACEABILITY WORKS

Each produce item has a Global Trace Item Number that identifies the brand owner and information about the particular produce, including what it is and how it is packaged. The numbers are used to follow the produce from the grower to the packer and distributor to the store. There are specific rules to follow if the produce gets repackaged. The Global Trace Item Number is part of the bar code on the boxes of produce. Also, both the seller and the store receiving the product have an extensive list of items they must keep track of, including the buyer/seller, product description, quantity purchased/sold, shipment identification number, transporter of produce, locations shipped from and to, and receipt dates. Sellers must keep their data for 2 years.[30]

disease outbreak occurs and the evidence is definitive, there is a recall. In response to concerns about foodborne disease outbreaks, the fresh produce industry has created a Produce Traceability Initiative.[30] This initiative makes it possible to track produce from the grower to the seller to the consumer. Produce traceability allows health agencies to identify quickly and accurately the source of produce believed to be the cause of a foodborne disease outbreak.

Once You Get Food Home: Preventing Foodborne Illness

Meat

The simple messages for meat safety at home are clean, separate, cook, and chill.[31]

Always wash your hands with warm water and soap, scrubbing for 20 seconds, before handling food and after touching raw meat.[32] Use clean plates, serving dishes, and utensils to serve food. Always keep surfaces clean.

Make sure raw meat, poultry, and fish do not come into contact with other food. Once you have cooked the food, put it on a clean plate. Do not put it back on the plate that held raw ingredients.[31]

The safest way to know if meat and poultry are sufficiently cooked is to use a food thermometer. Place the thermometer in the thickest part of the food. Follow the manufacturer's directions about how long the thermometer should be in place before reading it. The following temperatures can be considered general guidelines:

- Cook raw poultry (whole, parts, or ground) to 165°F.
- Cook raw ground meat (beef, pork, lamb, and veal) to 160°F.
- Cook raw beef, pork, lamb, and veal steaks, chops, and roasts to 145°F. Once the meat is removed from the oven, let it rest for 3 to 5 minutes before cutting or eating it.

When food is between 40°F and 140°F, bacteria rapidly multiply. To prevent bacterial growth, you should promptly refrigerate food. Do not leave it out for more than 2 hours. If perishable food is left out for longer than 2 hours, the safest choice is to discard it.[31]

Produce

When you bring produce home, do not wash fruits and vegetables until you are ready to use them. If you feel like you need to wash your produce before storing it, dry it thoroughly with a paper towel and wash it again before eating.[33]

When you are ready to use your produce, you do need to wash it to remove dirt and, if it isn't organic, pesticides. But fancy produce wash isn't necessary. A study from the University of Maine[34] found that tap water worked as well, if not better than, produce wash. Do not use soaps, washes, or detergents. You can use a vegetable brush to help wash away microorganisms. If you are concerned about your tap water, you can use distilled water. While organic or homegrown produce may not have pesticide residue on it, it should still be washed. Dust, dirt, and microbes can contaminate even organic produce, and you don't want to eat any of those. Soak produce like broccoli and lettuce for 1 to 2 minutes in cold water. If you are going to peel your vegetables, wash them first or you will transfer the bacteria from the skin to the inside of the vegetable.[33]

Mold can spread inside of moist, soft produce such as tomatoes. If the fruit or vegetable is completely moldy, just throw it away. If there is mold on a hard fruit or vegetable, such as an apple, you can safely cut away the mold, wash it thoroughly, and eat it.[33]

Food Waste

Americans lead the world in food waste—throwing away large quantities of food every year. This includes both uneaten leftovers and food that is spoiled. According to *The Guardian*,[35] about 60 million tons of produce, worth approximately $160 billion, is wasted every year.

Most wasted food ends up in landfills. In part because of the U.S. obsession with blemish-free fruits and vegetables, produce is discarded at every stop along the chain: the fields where it is grown, warehouses and packaging plants, during distribution, in supermarkets and restaurants, and in our refrigerators.

Reducing the amount of food we waste is important for individuals and for your community. On a personal level, when you buy food and throw it away you are wasting money. You spend time shopping and (maybe) cooking. But if you end up throwing food away, you have wasted your time. When food goes into a landfill, it produces methane, which is not good for the environment. Sometimes food goes directly from the field to the landfill.

If you cook for yourself, here are some tips to help reduce food waste[36]:

- Plan your shopping based on how many meals you will cook and eat at home.
- "Shop" in your refrigerator first. Cook or eat what is there before you buy more.
- Plan your meals to use up ingredients in your refrigerator.
- Produce that may be past its prime can still be used in casseroles, stir-fries, soups, omelets, or made into stock.

Organic vs. Natural vs. Conventional Produce. When you shop at the grocery store, you see foods labeled as organic or natural. Organic produce is labeled as such, and some stores identify some produce as being grown conventionally. In general, food categories are defined as follows:

- *Organic:* The U.S. Department of Agriculture (USDA) defines organic food as being produced using sustainable agricultural production practices. It does not allow conventional pesticides; fertilizers made with synthetic ingredients or sewage sludge; bioengineered products; or ionizing radiation. Organic meat, poultry, eggs, and dairy products come from animals that are not given antibiotics or growth hormones.[37]
- *Natural:* The FDA has no definition for the term *natural*, however, the agency allows its use to describe food that does not contain added color, artificial flavors, or synthetic substances.[38] The FDA's policy does not address food production methods, such as pesticides; nor does it address processing or manufacturing methods, such as thermal technologies, pasteurization, or irradiation.

A SIMPLE WAY TO TELL IF PRODUCE IS ORGANIC

Most fruits and vegetables have a product label. Some labels claim that the product is organic. Look at the code number on the label. This code is what the cashiers use to determine the price of a product. If the label has four numbers, it is conventional produce. If the produce has five numbers and the first is a 9, the produce is organic.

conventional farming Farming techniques that make use of synthetic chemical fertilizers, pesticides, herbicides and may include genetically modified organisms.

- *Conventional:* **Conventional farming** varies from farm to farm as well as country to country. Conventional farms usually are large-scale enterprises, with single crops grown continuously over many seasons, extensive use of synthetic pesticides and fertilizers, and dependence on agribusiness.[39]

What do these food categories, and the associated farming techniques, have to do with the environment? How people farm affects the environment. Conventional farming uses chemicals to manage weeds and pests. Pesticides used to increase produce production end up in the groundwater. Nutrient runoff creates dead zones in rivers, lakes, and oceans. A **dead zone** means there are such low oxygen levels in the water that animals either leave the area or die, creating biological deserts.[40]

dead zone A low-oxygen area within the world's oceans or lakes. Because most organisms need oxygen to live, in these areas organisms cannot survive.

The USDA has identified over 400 insects and pests and more than 70 fungi that are now resistant to one or more pesticides. Pollinator species, like bees, are crucial to agriculture because they pollinate billions of dollars' worth of crops. Pesticides and fungicides contaminate pollen that bees collect to feed their hives.[41]

The rising demand for food and other agricultural products means that native vegetation is cleared off of land. As one example, to create farmland, lowland rainforests in Indonesia and Amazon rainforests were destroyed. Habitat loss threatens entire ecosystems and many species. Deforestation, in turn, helps elevate levels of carbon dioxide and other greenhouse gases. There is a loss of wetland and wildlife habitat and reduced genetic diversity in crops and livestock. The long-term negative effects on the environment are not yet fully appreciated.

The choice between organic and conventional produce involves a balance. While **organic farming** practices reduce the environmental impact of agriculture, they harvest less produce per acre of farmland. While organic farming uses less energy than conventional farming, it requires more land use to produce the same amount of food.[42] As the population of the world increases, the need for food grows with it. As noted in the *Washington Post*, the environmental benefits of organic farming will not matter if we have to sacrifice more land, including old-growth forests, to create more organic farms.[43]

organic farming A type of farming that takes a holistic approach that is both sustainable and harmonious with the environment. It includes, but is not limited to, not using pesticides, fertilizers, genetically modified organisms, antibiotics, or growth hormones.

Pesticides: Agricultural Hazards (What Are Workers Exposed To? What Are We Eating?)

You've heard of pesticides and know they aren't good if found on your food. But what are they and what is the risk? Pesticides are biocidal agents (a chemical agent used to destroy or deter living organisms) used to control a wide variety of organisms that pose a threat to health or compete for food or other materials. They are released intentionally into our environment. The term pesticide includes herbicides (to kill weeds), insecticides (to kill insects), fungicides (to kill fungus), rodenticides (to kill rodents), and others. Pesticide use is common around the world. They are used in agriculture and in homes, parks, schools, and buildings.

Some pesticides are useful and help to prevent disease. Pesticides are used to kill mosquitos that transmit diseases, such as malaria, yellow fever, and West Nile virus. Malaria was once the world's most serious endemic disease. In 2016, according to the CDC, there were an estimated 216 million cases of malaria around the world and 445,000 people, mostly children, died from the disease, mostly in Africa.[44] Pesticides are also used to protect domestic animals from fleas. Pesticides prevent termites from eating the structure of your home. Farmers use pesticides to prevent insects from destroying their crops.

Pesticide use can be costly, especially to health and the environment. Acute poisoning from pesticides causes respiratory, gastrointestinal, nervous system, skin, eye, and cardiovascular illnesses.[45] The most common health effect is skin irritation.[46] The long-term effects of pesticides include cognitive and psychomotor dysfunction and neurodegenerative disorders. One of the difficulties in studying the long-term effects of pesticide exposure is that those exposed usually have a long history of exposure that includes cumulative exposure to many different pesticides as well as current exposures at home and work. A systematic review of exposure to pesticides found many serious sequelae. In addition to neurotoxicity, there was evidence of neurodegenerative disease, poor reproductive outcomes, and genotoxicity (genetic damage to cells).[46]

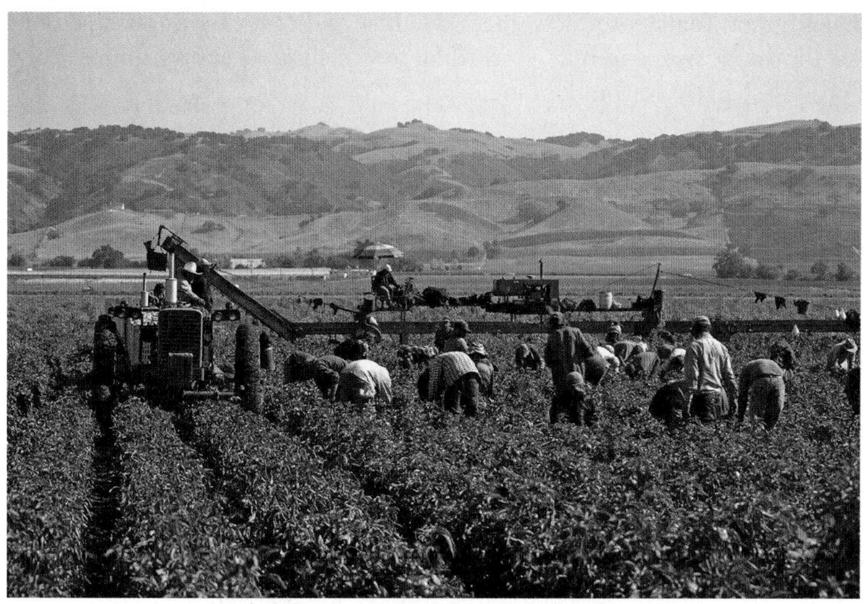

Many studies examining the role of pesticides on development of cancer were conducted among workers with occupational exposure, including farmers, pesticide applicators, workers in pesticide factories, landscapers, lumberjacks, and golf course workers. Among these individuals, pesticide exposure raised the risk of non-Hodgkin lymphoma and leukemia. There were increased risks for brain cancer, breast cancer, kidney cancer, pancreatic cancer, prostate cancer, and stomach cancer. Research on kidney cancer also found increased risk for the children of exposed workers.[47]

Children are the most vulnerable to pesticide exposure. Although you might suspect higher rates in rural areas, children who live in poor, urban areas—specifically, in crowded, substandard housing—are at high risk from chemical pesticides. They are exposed at home, at school, and at day care centers, where these pesticides are applied to control cockroaches, rats, and other vermin. Children often play on the ground, and young children have hand-to-mouth behaviors. The result is that children absorb more pesticides from the environment than do adults. Pesticides persist on indoor surfaces such as rugs and furniture. In addition, children have less ability to detoxify and rid the body of pesticides.[48]

When deciding how much pesticide exposure is safe, regulators consider one pesticide at a time. This approach is flawed because often pesticides are used as mixtures. Mixtures increase the toxic effect on the insects, but at the same time, they increase the toxic effect on humans, raising the risk of cancer and other serious health problems.

Because there are few restrictions on using multiple pesticides, growers often apply different pesticides to adjoining fields or different pesticides one after another. The result is that the people who live, work, or go to school nearby are exposed to the pesticide mixture. This exposure to multiple pesticides poses even greater risk than exposure to a single pesticide.

How Risky Is It to Eat Pesticides?

There has been a decline in pesticide residues since Congress passed the Food Quality Protection Act. The USDA[49] monitors pesticide residues on agricultural products, with an emphasis on food consumed by infants and children. Their Pesticide Data Program regularly evaluates fresh and processed fruit and vegetables, grains, dairy products, meat, poultry, and other foods such as honey, infant formula, fish, and nuts. According to Consumer Reports, almost a third of produce had two or more pesticides.[50]

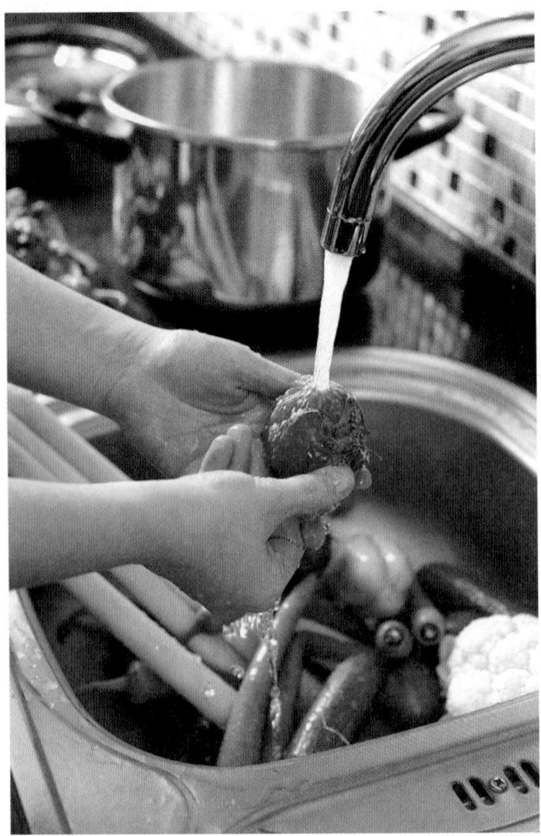

Most synthetic pesticides, including the toxic ones, are banned from organic farming. But because there are pesticides in the air and water, pesticides may end up on organic produce. Before you eat it, wash produce under running water whether it is organic or conventional. As noted earlier in this chapter, washing only with water is equally effective as using soap or produce wash. If you are washing a hard fruit or vegetable, you can use a vegetable brush to help remove dirt, germs, and pesticide residues. Rub soft produce to remove these contaminants.

While organic is the safest choice, it is not always available, and it is not always affordable. For your health, it is better to eat conventional fruits and vegetables than to skip them because you cannot afford organic ones. **TABLE 11-3** shows the Environmental Working Group's recommendations for produce to always buy organic as well as those which are least likely to retain pesticides.[51] The lists are updated annually.

TABLE 11-3 Environmental Working Group Recommendations

Dirty Dozen	Clean Fifteen
Produce the EWG recommends to always buy organic	**Fruits and vegetables that are the least likely to retain pesticide residues**
Strawberries	Avocados
Spinach	Sweet corn
Nectarines	Pineapples
Apples	Cabbage
Grapes	Onions
Peaches	Frozen sweet peas
Cherries	Papayas
Pears	Asparagus
Tomatoes	Mangoes
Celery	Eggplant
Potatoes	Honeydew melon
Sweet bell peppers	Kiwis
	Cantaloupe
	Cauliflower
	Broccoli

Data from Environmental Working Group. (2016). The EWG's 2016 shopper's guide to pesticides in produce.

Water Quality and Quantity

Bottled vs. Tap: Think About What You Drink

Bottled water is everywhere. People buy bottled water by the caseload because they like its taste, believe it is safe, and find it convenient. There were approximately 10 billion gallons of bottled water sold in the United States at a cost of around $12.3 billion in 2013.[52] On average, every person in the United States uses 173 bottles of water a year.[53] It is calorie-free and convenient to carry around and is certainly healthier than drinking soda. The International Bottled Water Association writes about "bottled water's allure." This allure includes associations with healthfulness, convenience, safety, and value.[52]

Marketing for bottled water implies that bottled water is the best and the purest beverage you can drink. Some bottled water actually does come from springs and other pristine sources, but between 25%[54] and 49%[55] of bottled water comes from a municipal water supply. After companies treat and purify the water, they sell it to consumers at an extraordinary price markup. One website estimated that if your monthly water bill cost the same as the least expensive bottled water, you would spend $9,000 a month. Because bottlers are not required to list the source of their water on the label, most people are surprised to learn that they are paying a lot of money for tap water. As Eric Goldstein, codirector of the urban program at the Natural Resources Defense Council,[54] says, "No one should think that bottled water is better regulated, better protected, or safer than tap."

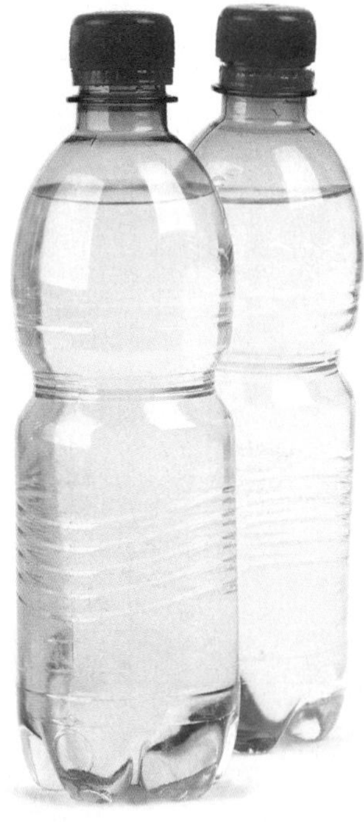

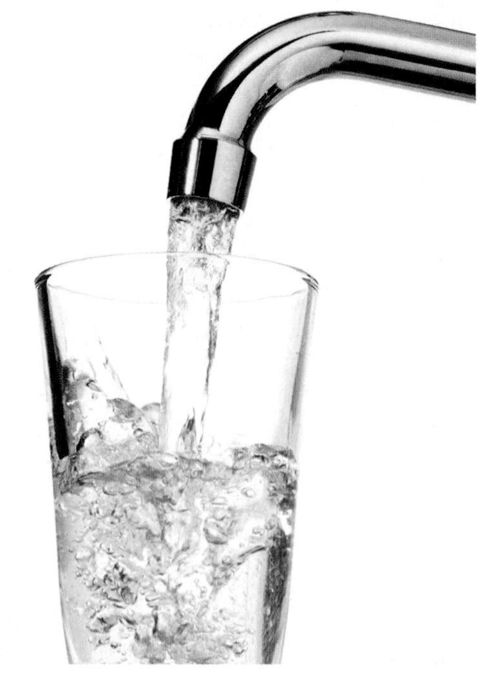

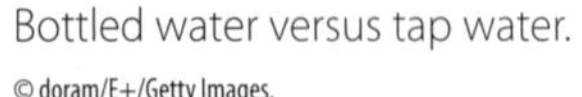

Bottled water versus tap water.

© doram/E+/Getty Images. © Brian Hagiwara/Stockbyte/Getty Images.

Is Bottled Water Safer Than Tap Water?

According to the Mayo Clinic, bottled and tap water are equally safe. While the FDA oversees bottled water and the Environmental Protection Agency (EPA) oversees tap water, both agencies use similar safety standards. Among the FDA's requirements, manufacturers must use sanitary conditions when they

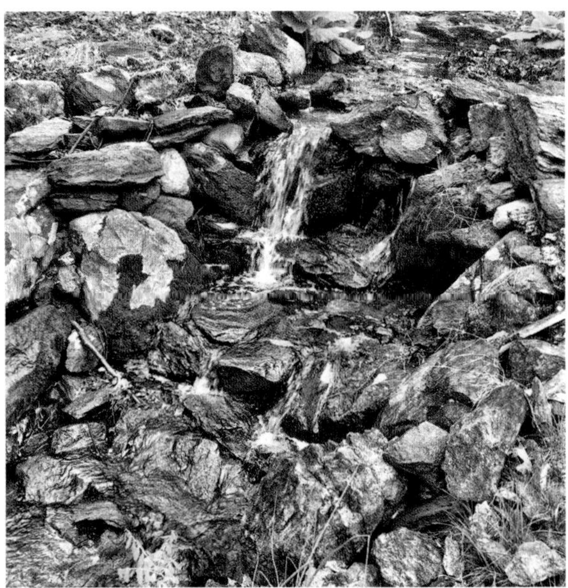

What companies want you to think is the source of their bottled water.

process, bottle, and transport water. The manufacturer must protect the water from contaminants by sampling and testing the source of the water and the bottled water. The EPA requires municipal water suppliers to report annually to customers about the source of the water, the contaminant levels, and potential health effects. The EPA does not monitor private wells, which should be tested at least annually for contaminants.[56] Nationally, 95% of the population uses a community water system.[57]

Do Tap Water and Bottled Water Taste Different?

Many people think that bottled water tastes better than tap water. A French research team conducted a taste test of six French bottled waters and six French municipal tap waters. The authors identified three main tastes that coincide with the amount of minerals in the water. The report concluded that most people could not distinguish between bottled water and tap water when the tap water was chlorine-free.[58] An earlier study from Belfast, Ireland, found that people could not differentiate between the tastes of bottled and tap water. The author concluded that the demand for bottled water went beyond taste or smell.[59]

Deciding Between Tap Water and Bottled Water

It is true that the taste of tap water varies by water source. As such, taste may be a perfectly reasonable basis for deciding which type of water to drink. Other common considerations include what is in the water (e.g., tap water often has fluoride added, which helps keep teeth healthy), whether the convenience of bottled water offsets its cost, and whether a person's living situation demands one option versus the other (e.g., a person may live in a rural area where safe tap water is not available).

If you choose tap water but feel you must filter it, filtration options, from least to most expensive, are pitcher filters, filters that attach to the water faucet, reverse osmosis filters, and under-the-counter water filters. All choices can filter your water, and there is no one "right" answer. In deciding whether to filter water, think about your budget, how much water you use, maintenance, and what types of

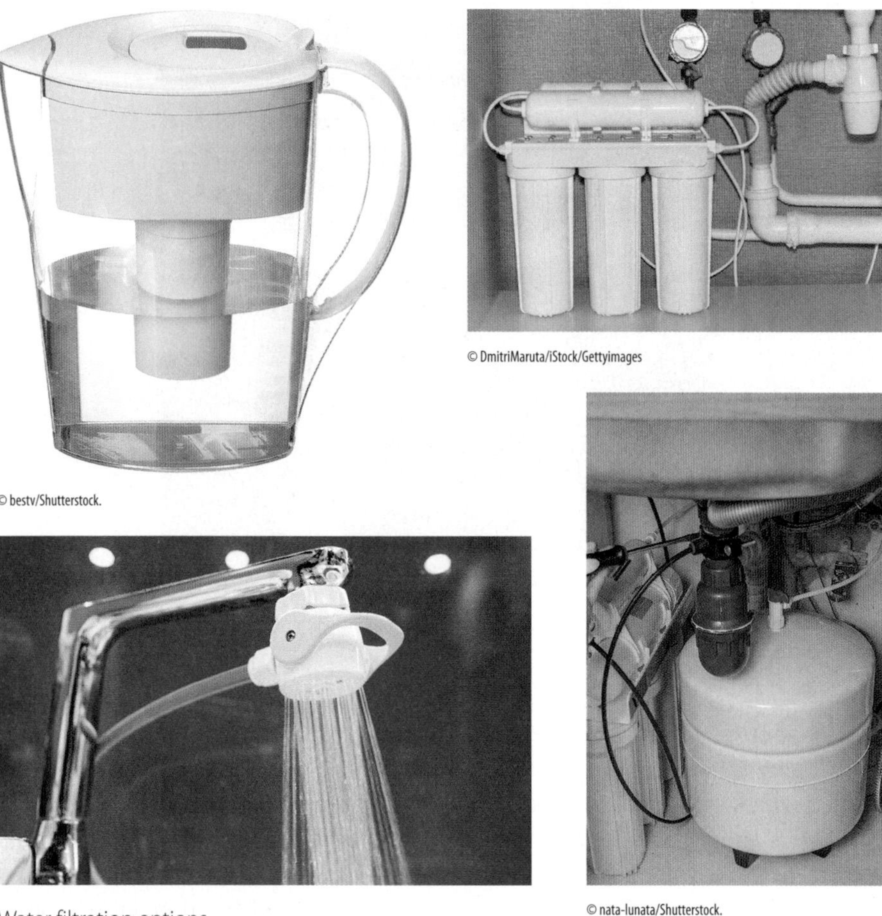

© bestv/Shutterstock.

© DmitriMaruta/iStock/Gettyimages

© nata-lunata/Shutterstock.

Water filtration options.

© quangmooo/Shutterstock.

contaminants are in your water. All the choices have good and bad points, so pick a filter that fits your budget, has NSF (formerly National Sanitation Foundation) certification, and reduces the particular contaminants in your water system.[60]

If you want to read more about drinking water, consult the EPA report, *Water on Tap*.[61] Visit the EPA website to find reports on your local water supply.[62]

Clean water is essential for our survival. With global climate change, protecting our water sources and promoting efficient water use are crucial.

Water Quality

Usually, water is safe if it comes from a public water system in the United States that is run and maintained by the municipal government. The EPA sets health standards regarding contaminants in drinking water.[63]

Water can contain microorganisms, such as bacteria and parasites, or chemicals from industrial waste or spraying crops. Minerals can enter the water system, either from natural deposits in the ground or from pipes. It is the responsibility of the EPA to make sure the water is safe to drink.[63] The frequency of testing depends on the location and size of the public water system. Consumers should receive an annual report on compliance testing for contaminants.

The EPA maintains a Safe Drinking Water Hotline at 800-426-4791. The hotline is open 10:00 a.m. to 4:00 p.m. Eastern time, Monday to Friday. The hotline provides information on many topics related to drinking water, including local drinking water quality, drinking water standards, public drinking water systems, and source water protection. Recorded messages are also available 24 hours a day, 7 days a week, in both English and Spanish.[64]

TALES OF PUBLIC HEALTH

The Flint, Michigan, Water Crisis

In 2014, the corrosive Flint River water caused lead in aging pipes to leach lead into the municipal water supply. As a result, between 6,000 and 12,000 children in Flint, Michigan, were exposed to drinking water with high levels of lead. These children may experience a range of serious health problems.

To understand how this crisis came to pass, some background details are necessary. By 2011, Flint was in a state-declared financial emergency. To address the emergency, in December 2011, the governor appointed an emergency manager to manage the city's affairs (referred to as a state of "receivership"). By the time Flint's financial emergency ended in April 2015, Flint had had three emergency managers, with one serving twice. This bureaucratic organization was connected to the incident because the governor gave the emergency manager expanded powers to run local government. The emergency manager was allowed to strip local elected leaders of their power, had unilateral authority to cut pay, outsource city services, merge departments, and change employee contracts. Moreover, the emergency managers were accountable only to the governor.[65] Thus, key decisions that would affect tens of thousands of people were being made by a succession of individuals rather than by committees of knowledgeable people invested in the long-term welfare of the city's inhabitants.

Another relevant bit of background: Well before this crisis started, a study of the Flint River concluded that using the water would be an ongoing problem and more expensive than treating lake water.[66]

In 2013, the Flint City Council voted to join the Karegnondi Water Authority (KWA). When Detroit announced it would no longer supply Flint with water, Flint needed a new source because the KWA water system would not be ready until 2016. Michigan's Department of Environmental Quality, Genesee County, and Flint's water department decided to use the Flint River water until KWA was ready.[67]

In April 2014, the city switched its source of water to the Flint River. Within a month, residents started to complain about the water's color, taste, and smell. Residents reported rashes and eye irritations. In the fall of 2014, the General Motors engine plant in Flint announced it would stop using Flint River water because it was corroding their engine parts.[68]

In January 2015, in the time span of 1 week, Flint was found to be in violation of the Safe Drinking Water Act. An official contradicted the finding, saying that the Flint River water was safe to drink.[69] Then the University of Michigan–Flint found some campus water samples were high in lead.

The EPA questioned the water treatment process, but the state said they were doing it correctly. A group of citizens filed a lawsuit to force the authorities to reconnect Flint to Detroit's water, but a judge rejected the injunction. In July of 2015, a spokesperson for the state of Michigan told people that "anyone who is concerned about lead in the drinking water in Flint can relax. It does not look like there is any broad problem with the water supply freeing up lead as it goes to homes." After a pediatrician realized that many children had lead poisoning, the county declared a public health emergency. Water filters were given to residents, and finally in October of 2015, Flint was reconnected to Detroit's water supply.[68]

How and why did this crisis happen? There is no simple answer to this question.

This story is one of political failure and environmental injustice. As will be discussed later, race and economic status were unfortunate but unmistakable players in the story. The population of Flint is 65% non-White, and 42% of people live below the poverty level.[70] Furthermore, the structure of overlapping and mismatched government authorities guaranteed that when there were problems, it was easy for officials to blame someone else.[71]

None of the people or agencies who should have done the right thing by treating the Flint River water did so. The residents started complaining about the water immediately (**FIGURE 11-8**). Six months after the residents started complaining, city officials said that Flint River water was safe to drink. It took the Michigan Department of Environmental Quality almost a year to document the problem, but they did not immediately fix the problem. It took a year and a half before Detroit again became Flint's water source. However, because of the corrosive nature of the Flint River water, the damaged pipes continued to leach lead.

Because Flint was economically depressed, the state took over. Those in charge made decisions based only on finances, without considering potential consequences. There were many agencies and no one responsible for the decisions. Rather than address the issues, officials blamed others. The Michigan Department of Environmental Quality should not have allowed the switch to Flint River water. Once it was allowed, corrosion-controlling additives should have been added initially.

Would this situation have happened if Flint had been wealthy, with a predominantly White population? Likely not. Burton, Michigan, is 7 minutes and 4.5 miles from Flint, but a world away. Burton is 88% White, the median household income is 1.8 times higher than in Flint, and the median value of homes is also 1.8 times higher than in Flint. Burton has clean, inexpensive water, and Flint does not. In 2014, the water in Flint was almost 2.5 times as expensive as the water in Burton.[72]

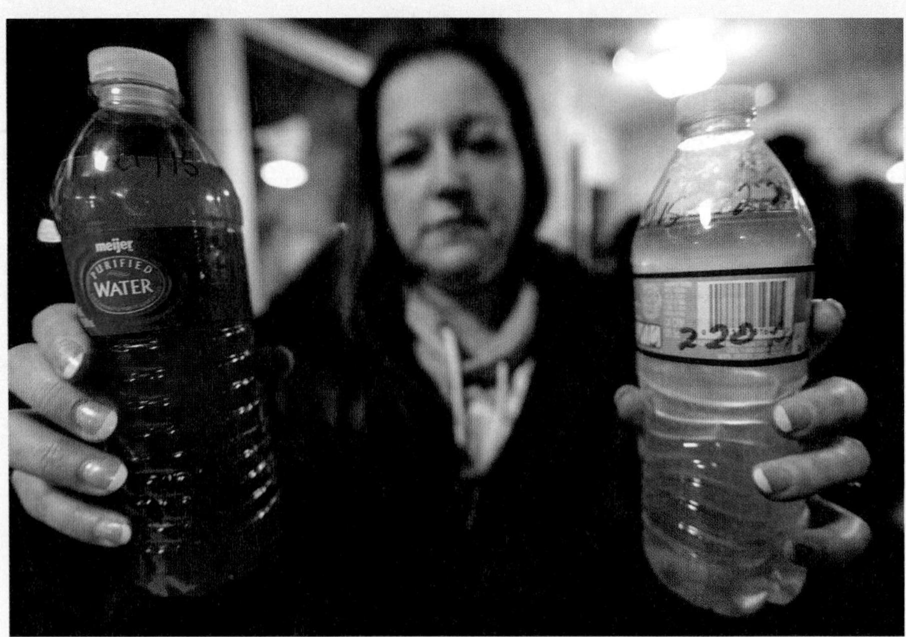

FIGURE 11-8 Flint, Michigan, resident shows what tap water looks like when it comes from the Flint River.

There is a hero in this story: Dr. Mona Hanna-Attisha, a pediatrician at a public hospital in Flint. A friend told her that the city of Flint wasn't doing anything to prevent lead from pipes from leaching into the water, which meant the children were being exposed to lead. There is no safe blood level of lead for children. Lead exposure can affect nearly every system in the body, including the brain. Because lead exposure often occurs with no obvious symptoms, it frequently goes unrecognized.[73] Among the problems elevated lead levels cause are slowed growth and development, behavior and attention problems, hearing problems, and lowered IQ scores.[74]

Dr. Hanna-Attisha started a crusade. She compared lead levels in blood samples before and after the switch to Flint River water. The percentage of children with lead poisoning doubled and in some neighborhoods tripled. Where water lead levels were the highest, the number of kids with lead poisoning was highest. She announced her findings at a press conference and drew lots of criticism. But as the doctor pointed out, her job is to take care of the kids, and once her story got out, the world began to listen.[75]

Follow-up: There are multiple lawsuits pending. In one case, the U.S. District Court ruled that Flint, Michigan, residents could bring a lawsuit requiring the state and city to replace water lines with lead-free piping at no cost to consumers. A class action lawsuit against the state of Michigan and the governor was dismissed by a federal judge, but a similar lawsuit was allowed to proceed. The Michigan attorney general filed criminal charges against public officials responsible for the water crisis.[76–78]

As of January 2017, lead levels in Flint's water were determined to no longer exceed federal limits. Nonetheless, residents were advised to continue using filtered water for cooking and drinking.[79]

Environmental Impact of Plastic

The issue with bottled water is not simply that there are cheaper ways to get water. Plastic bottles and plastics in general have a huge environmental impact. While most of this discussion revolves around plastic bottles, there are many other sources of plastic that pollute the environment.

Too Many Plastic Bottles

The world does not need more plastic bottles. That bottle of water you bought today takes nearly 1,000 years to degrade.[80] Approximately 70% of the plastic bottles people buy are thrown away rather than recycled. The United States alone uses more than 50 billion bottles of water every year. Given our current rate of recycling, this year's 35 billion bottles will be with us for the next 1,000 years. In 1 year, enough bottles are thrown away to wrap around the earth more than 50 times.[81]

It isn't only the sheer number of bottles that pose an environmental concern; it's also the resources it takes to produce them. Creating the bottles for water and transporting those filled bottles consume a lot of natural resources and create pollution.[82] Imagine a plastic bottle filled one-quarter of the way with oil. That is the amount of fossil fuels it takes to make a single bottle. In addition to using natural resources to make the bottles, manufacturing plastic bottles produces millions of tons of carbon dioxide, a greenhouse gas. It takes more water to produce a bottle than the bottle will hold. To help understand how much energy plastic bottles consume, the total carbon footprint of one 500-mL (17-ounce) bottle of water in North America is 82.8 grams of carbon dioxide.[83] This estimate includes manufacturing the bottle, the distribution and transportation to the store, and retail energy use. In comparison, driving a compact car produces 254 grams of carbon dioxide per mile. Thus, if you drank one bottle of water every day, necessitating the production of seven bottles of water in a week, it is the equivalent of the emissions generated by driving 2.3 miles.[84] It may not sound like much, but when you consider how many bottles of water are sold every year, it quickly adds up to a very large number.

Another place your plastics end up is in the ocean. There is an area of the Pacific Ocean called the North Pacific Subtropical Gyre. (It is one of five major oceanic gyres.) The North Pacific Subtropical Gyre is the biggest ecosystem on earth and comprises 20 million square kilometers (more than 7.7 million square miles).[85] This **gyre** is formed by the North Pacific Current, the California Current, the North Equatorial Current, and the Kuroshio Current. In the center of the North Pacific Subtropical Gyre is an area called the **Great Pacific Garbage Patch.**[86] The area in the center of a gyre is calm and stable. The circular motion of the currents draws debris into the center, where it becomes trapped. See **FIGURE 11-9** to get a sense of how much plastic is in the water. Even more compelling is what all this plastic does to wildlife. **FIGURE 11-10** shows an albatross that died from ingesting plastic.

gyre A large system of rotating ocean currents. They rotate clockwise in the Northern Hemisphere and counterclockwise in the Southern Hemisphere.

Great Pacific Garbage Patch A concentration of marine debris in the North Pacific Ocean. It has exceptionally high concentrations of plastics, chemical sludge, and other debris. Most of the debris is suspended beneath the surface of the ocean.

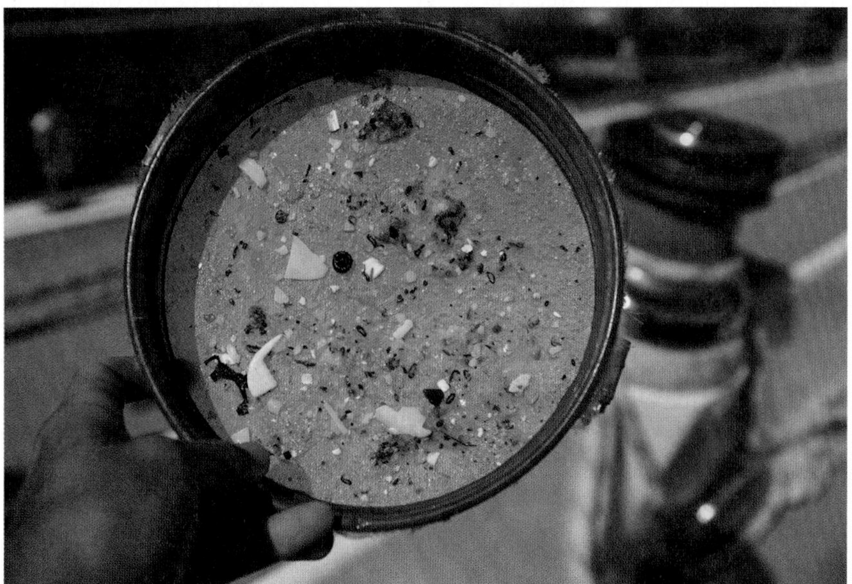

FIGURE 11-9 A trawl sample of microplastics from the North Pacific Subtropical Gyre.

Reproduced with permission from Plastic Free Seas.

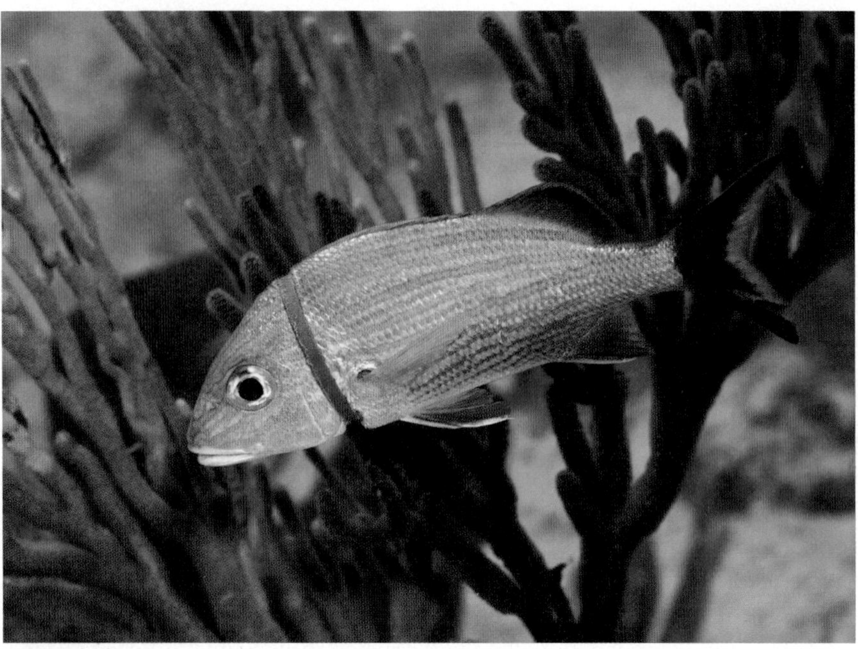

FIGURE 11-10 A discarded plastic band in the Caribbean Sea threatens the life of a blue striped grunt fish.

When people hear the term "garbage patch," they likely think of large pieces of trash floating on the ocean. But the Great Pacific Garbage Patch is made up of tiny pieces of plastic that are not biodegradable. They break up into smaller and smaller pieces of plastic.

If you were to look at the garbage patch, you wouldn't see it. All of the tiny pieces of plastic make the water look cloudy. Oceanographers and ecologists believe that the seafloor beneath the Great Pacific Garbage Patch may look more like that trash heap because about 70% of debris settles on the bottom of the ocean.[86]

There are many different types of debris, but most of it is plastics. Because plastics do not biodegrade, they simply turn into smaller and smaller pieces. Most of the debris in the Great Pacific Garbage Patch comes from plastic water bottles, plastic bags, bottle caps, and Styrofoam cups. Scientists estimate that there are about 1.9 million pieces of plastic per square mile.

Bioplastics and Biodegradable Plastics[87]

We live in a world filled with plastic—it isn't just water bottles. Think back to the beginning of your day and you will realize how many things you use are made from plastic; from bottles and grocery bags to pens and food wrap. Discarded plastics are a significant cause of pollution in our communities and around the globe.

We make plastics from petroleum. Mostly we think of plastics as low-cost, disposable items such as produce bags at the grocery store. However, there is nothing disposable about most plastics. On average, we use plastic bags for 12 minutes before discarding them, yet they take years to break down in the environment. Getting rid of plastics is extremely challenging. There are many different kinds of plastics, and there are specific ways to recycle each type of plastic. You may have noticed a number inside the triangular recycling symbol on plastic items (**FIGURE 11-11**). This number indicates the chemical used to make the plastic. **TABLE 11-4** explains what the plastics are made of, their uses, and what they become when recycled.[88]

FIGURE 11-11 Recycling symbols.

We use plastics in mind-boggling amounts. According to the Earth Policy Institute, over 1 trillion plastic bags are used every year worldwide. In the United

TABLE 11-4 What Recycling Numbers Mean and Uses[88]

Number	Composition	Common Uses	Recycled Into
1	Polyethylene terephthalate	Soda bottles, water bottles, salad dressing containers, mouthwash bottles, peanut butter containers	Tote bags, furniture, carpet, paneling, polar fleece
2	High-density polyethylene	Milk jugs, household cleaner containers, juice bottles, shampoo bottles, cereal box liners, detergent bottles, motor oil bottles, yogurt tubs, butter tubs, toiletry bottles	Pens, recycling containers, picnic tables, lumber, benches, fencing, detergent bottles
3	Polyvinyl chloride	Food wrap, plumbing pipes, detergent bottles	Paneling, flooring, speed bumps, decks, roadway gutters
4	Low-density polyethylene	Squeezable bottles, shopping bags, clothing, carpet, frozen food, bread bags, some food wraps	Compost bins, paneling, trash can liners and cans, floor tiles, shipping envelopes
5	Polypropylene	Yogurt containers, ketchup bottles, syrup bottles, medicine bottles	Brooms, auto battery cases, bins, pallets, signal lights, ice scrapers, bicycle racks
6	Polystyrene (Styrofoam)	Compact disc cases, egg cartons, meat trays, disposable plates and cups	Egg cartons, vents, foam packing, insulation
7	Miscellaneous (everything that doesn't fit into other categories)	Sunglasses, iPod cases, computer cases, nylon, 3- and 5-gallon water bottles, bullet-proof materials	Plastic lumber and other custom-made products

Barrett, M. (2013). The numbers on plastic bottles: What do plastic recycling symbols mean? Natural Society. Retrieved from http://naturalsociety.com/recycling-symbols-numbers-plastic-bottles-meaning/

States alone, we use and throw away 100 billion plastic bags every year. Those 100 billion plastic bags require 12 million barrels of oil per year to manufacture.[89]

Making Better Plastics

Making plastics that break down more quickly is better for the environment. With increasing interest in protecting the environment, there has been an emphasis on creating these more environmentally friendly plastics. To date, the primary solutions include **bioplastics**, plastics made from recycled plastic, and biodegradable plastics.

bioplastics A type of biodegradable plastic derived from biological substances rather than from petroleum.

Bioplastics are made from natural materials, like cornstarch. Bioplastics made from cornstarch take less energy to produce than regular plastics. Because they are plant based, bioplastics produce fewer greenhouse gases as they degrade. Corn-based plastics are significantly better for the environment than oil-based plastics. Unfortunately, the 100% compostable claims are true only in commercial, high-heat facilities. Corn-based plastic bottles will last as long as petroleum-based plastic bottles in a regular landfill site.

One solution is to recycle plastic materials into new items, like park benches, instead of making these items from raw materials. What is unclear

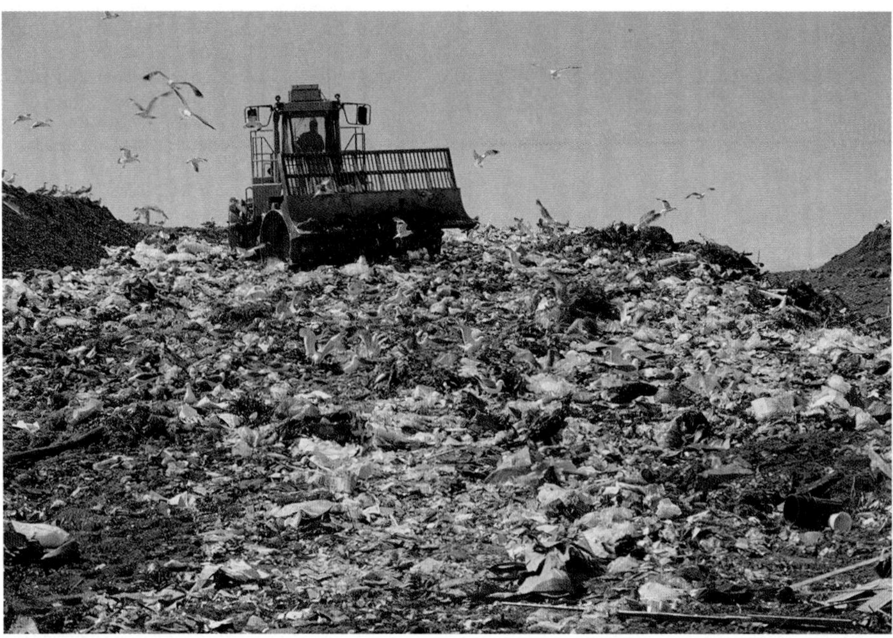

is if this process results in a net saving of energy and water and a reduction in greenhouse gas emissions.

Biodegradable plastics are modified during production to decompose more quickly. They contain additives, causing them to decay more rapidly in the presence of light and oxygen. Biodegradable plastics are made from normal plastics (think petrochemical), and as they decompose, they may leave a toxic residue. For the most part, you cannot compost them.

These "environmentally friendly" plastics are not the magic bullet their manufacturers portray them to be. Some biodegradable plastics produce methane, a greenhouse gas that increases global warming. Some biodegradable plastics require high temperatures to decompose and may take years to break down. Growing corn to make plastics uses land that could be used to grow food.

How to Cut Down on Plastics

The best solution is to reduce our dependence on plastics. Some cities, counties, and states are working on strategies to reduce the number of single-use plastic bags.[90]

At a community level, increasingly common strategies are outright bans on plastic bags, per-bag charges, and per-bag rebates for recyclable bags. As the environmentally conscious say, "Reduce, repair, reuse, recycle."

Global Warming/Climate Change: We Are the Problem

Many people use global warming and climate change interchangeably, but they mean different, though related, things. Global warming is an increase in the earth's average temperature due to rising levels of greenhouse gases. Climate change is a long-term shift in the earth's climate. Thus, global warming is one aspect of climate change. There are side effects of global warming, including melting glaciers, heavier rainstorms, more frequent droughts, and more severe storms and other weather events.

The scientific consensus on climate change and global warming is that the earth has been getting warmer over the last century. According to the

TRY IT!

Reducing Use of Plastic

There are many things you can do to reduce your use of plastic. Even if you cannot avoid plastic all the time, every time you do, it helps the environment. The following is a list of relatively easy ways to reduce your use of plastic[91]:

- Use reusable shopping bags.
- Don't use plastic straws, even in restaurants.
- Give up chewing gum; it is made from synthetic rubber (plastic).
- When you have the option, such as when buying orange juice or milk, choose products sold in cardboard rather than plastic containers.
- Buy bulk food and store it in a reusable container.
- Try not to use plastic knives, forks, and spoons. If you are buying food to go and don't need these utensils, ask the restaurant to not put them in the bag.
- Pack your lunch in reusable containers.
- Don't use disposable razors. Instead choose a razor with replaceable blades.

STOP
PLASTIC
POLLUTION
RE
DUCE
USE
CYCLE
BYOB
BRING YOUR
OWN BAG
Ban plastic bags
Shop with
reusable bags
and help protect
the environment
SAVE EARTH
LOVE EARTH

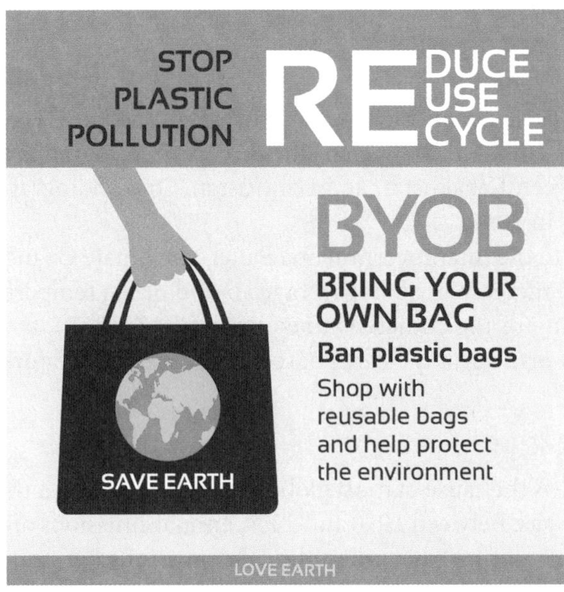

Intergovernmental Panel on Climate Change, the average temperature has risen approximately 1.33°F over the past 100 years, and more than half of that increase has occurred since 1979, especially over the Northern Hemisphere.[92] The 2013 update of the report shows a slightly higher increase.[93] The primary sources of global warming include the increases in carbon dioxide and other greenhouse gases from the burning of fossil fuels, land clearing, agriculture, and other human activities. Before the Industrial Revolution (approximately 1760 to 1840), the levels of carbon dioxide were about 280 parts per million by volume. The current levels are greater than 380 parts per million by volume, a 35% increase. Evidence of warming includes rising sea levels and decreases in snow and ice. Sea levels rising and seawater moving inland can cause erosion, flooding, and contamination of water systems and agricultural land. This will result in a loss of habitats for fish, birds, plants, and humans. Low-lying islands could end up completely submerged. As an example, **FIGURE 11-12** shows Venice, Italy, a coastal city, during the 2008 floods.[94] Satellite data from 1978 onward show that the average area of Arctic sea ice has shrunk by 2.7% per decade.[92] In the Northern Hemisphere, 1983–2012 was likely the warmest 30-year period

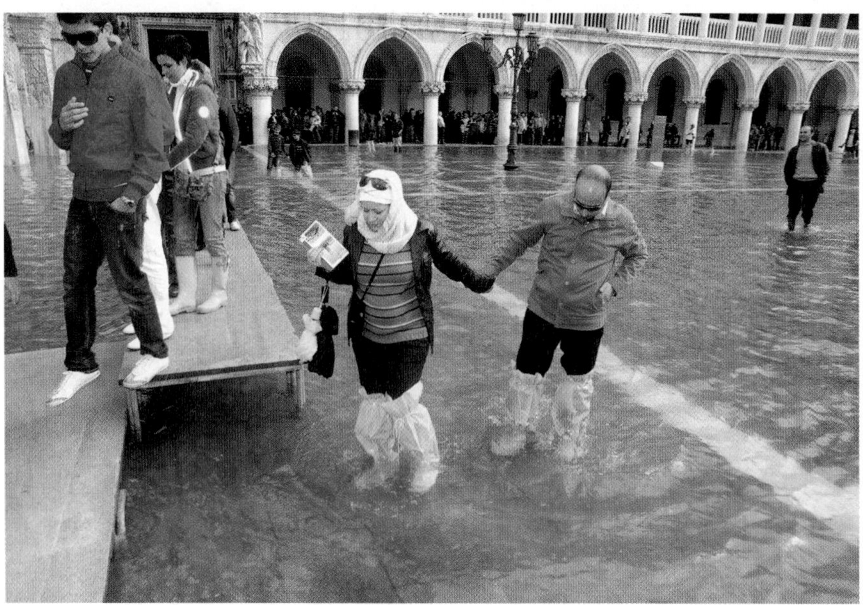

FIGURE 11-12 Venice, Italy, during the historic flood of 2008.
© Roman Stetsyk/Shutterstock.

of the last 1,400 years. Almost the entire surface of the globe is warming.[93,95] As an example, see **FIGURE 11-13**, which shows NASA photographs of the Aral Sea, which lies between Kazakhstan and Uzbekistan. One photograph was taken in 2000 and other in 2014.

According to the Intergovernmental Panel on Climate Change, the evidence of the observed increase in global average air and ocean temperatures indicates that the warming of the climate is unequivocal.[92] **FIGURE 11-14** shows the projected surface warming of the earth based on recent temperature changes.

Causes of Change

Carbon dioxide is the cause of most global warming, making it the most important greenhouse gas. Between 1970 and 2004, annual emissions of carbon dioxide grew by 80%. Up until 2000, carbon dioxide emissions per unit of energy supplied were declining, but this has reversed since then and continues to increase. These increases are mainly due to fossil fuel use. The atmospheric concentrations of methane and nitrous oxide are increasing as well, also attributable primarily to fossil fuel use, and agriculture.[92] According to the Intergovernmental Panel on Climate Change, humans cause climate change. Humans contributed to rising sea levels (very likely), changes in wind pattern (likely), increased temperatures of extreme hot nights, cold nights, and cold days (likely), and more likely than not are responsible for the increased risk of heat waves, droughts, and the frequency of heavy precipitation. The idea that the degree of the changing climate is natural variation is, in their estimation, *very unlikely*.[92]

Polar Vortex

The polar vortex is a zone of frigid upper-level winds that circles the Arctic. In North America, we feel the effects of the polar vortex during the winter. When the polar vortex is strong, the cold air mass stays in the polar regions. As a result, the winter weather is milder in North America, Europe, and Asia. When the polar vortex weakens, it becomes unstable and may break apart, causing bitterly cold weather in the mid-latitudes. (Mid-latitudes are 30 to 60 degrees north or south of the equator—roughly from the northern half of the United

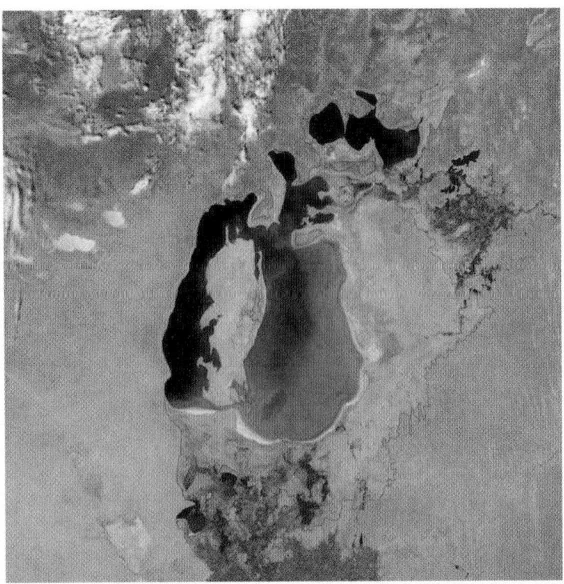

August 25, 2000

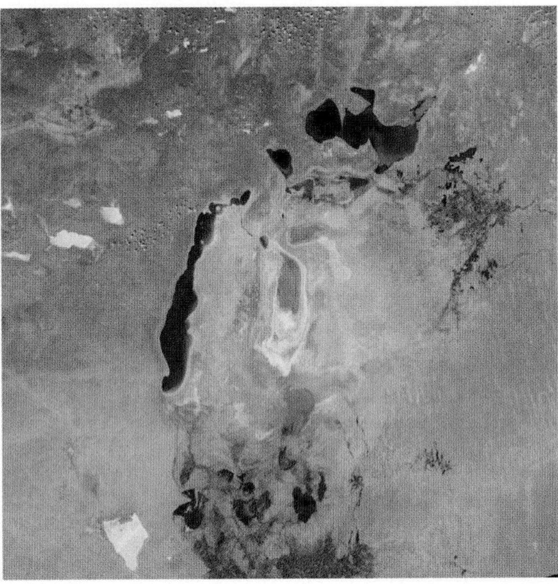

August 19, 2014

FIGURE 11-13 The Aral Sea shrinking over a 14-year period.

National Geographic. (2015, December 29). See before-and-after photos of the changing environment. Retrieved from https://news.nationalgeographic.com/2015/12/151229-before-after-earth-features/

States to southern Canada.) **FIGURE 11-15** provides a picture of what it looks like when the polar vortex weakens and areas of the United States experience the extremely cold air moving southward from the North Polar region.[96]

Many climate scientists believe that because there are natural variations in the weather, these natural variations partially explain why recently there have been extremes of cold weather. Just because there is climate change does not mean we do not have weather. Weather patterns are driven by the jet streams and other global atmospheric phenomena. These atmospheric phenomena can even cause opposite effects in different parts of the globe.[97]

Projected Climate Change

Greenhouse gas emissions will continue to increase because the burning of fossil fuels remains our primary source of energy. Continued and increasing

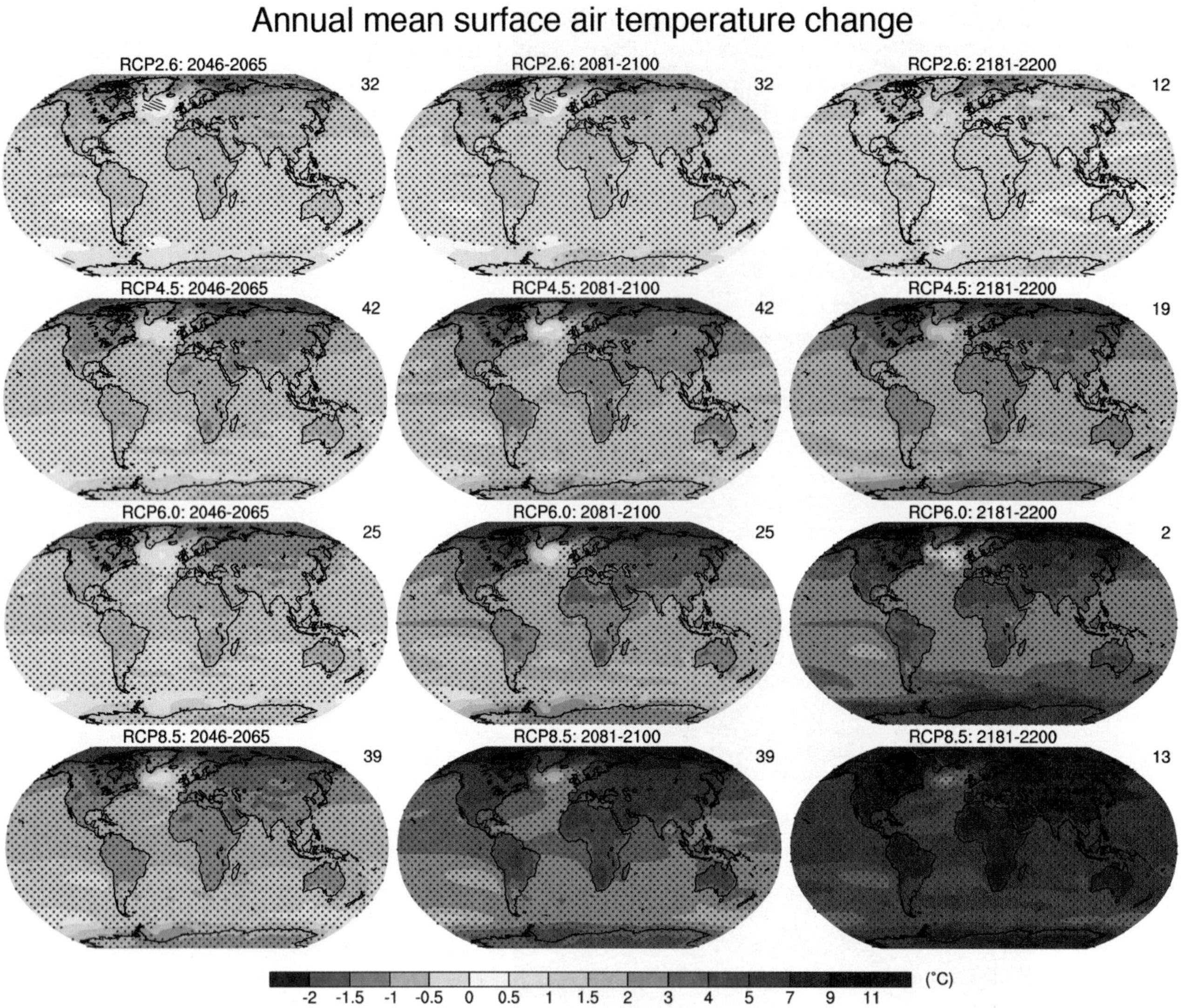

Annual mean surface air temperature change

RCP2.6: 2046-2065 32
RCP2.6: 2081-2100 32
RCP2.6: 2181-2200 12
RCP4.5: 2046-2065 42
RCP4.5: 2081-2100 42
RCP4.5: 2181-2200 19
RCP6.0: 2046-2065 25
RCP6.0: 2081-2100 25
RCP6.0: 2181-2200 2
RCP8.5: 2046-2065 39
RCP8.5: 2081-2100 39
RCP8.5: 2181-2200 13

-2 -1.5 -1 -0.5 0 0.5 1 1.5 2 3 4 5 7 9 11 (°C)

FIGURE 11-14 Projected surface temperature changes for the late 21st century.

Environmental Protection Agency. (n.d.). Future of climate change. Retrieved from https://www.epa.gov/climate-change-science/future-climate-change

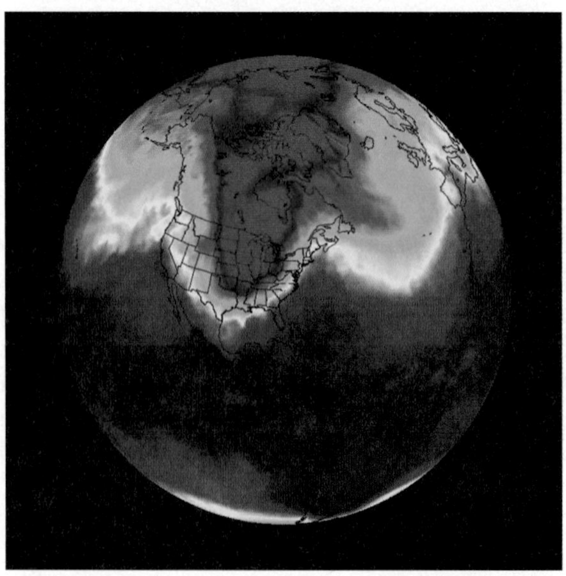

FIGURE 11-15 Visualization of polar vortex invasion in January of 2014.

NASA's Goddard Space Flight Center Video and images courtesy of NASA/JPL.

greenhouse gas emissions mean that the global climate change that is currently seen will get worse. Even if greenhouse gases were held constant at the year 2000 levels, the earth's temperature would continue to rise.

These changes are important and significant. By the mid-2000s, annual river runoff and water availability will increase in some areas, such as high latitudes and tropical wet areas. At the same time, it will decrease in other regions, such as the mid-latitudes and tropics. Semi-arid areas like the western United States will have reduced water due to climate change.

These changes have a devastating effect on particular ecosystems: tundra, boreal forest and mountain regions (sensitivity to warming), Mediterranean ecosystems (reduced rainfall), tropical rainforests, mangrove and salt marshes, coral reefs, and sea ice biomes. Oceans are becoming more acidic. The expectation is that they will continue to acidify, which will have an adverse impact on marine shell-forming organisms like coral and the species that depend on them.

Scientists predict drastic changes around the globe. **TABLE 11-5** presents just some of the projected changes due to climate change.

As stated in the Intergovernmental Panel on Climate Change's 2013 report, "Continued emissions of greenhouse gases will cause further warming and changes in all components of the climate system. Limiting climate change will require substantial and sustained reductions of greenhouse gas emissions."[93] Currently, there is no single answer to this problem. Changes, particularly on a global scale, come slowly. Governments need to integrate climate policies into their overall policies.[92]

On December 12, 2015, climate history was made at the 2015 United Nations Climate Change Conference. On that day, representatives from 195 nations reached an agreement to commit nearly every country to reduce greenhouse gas emissions and thereby slow climate change. Traditionally, agreements have exempted developing nations such as China and India, even though they are two of the top four countries with the highest carbon dioxide emissions in the world. The agreement requires every country to address climate change. Ban Ki-moon, the Secretary-General of the United Nations, declared, "For the first time, we have a truly universal agreement on climate change, one of the most crucial problems on earth."[98]

The conference participants committed to limiting global temperature increase to less than 2°C (or 3.6°F). All countries must report regularly on their progress and set new goals every 5 years. Developed countries will support the

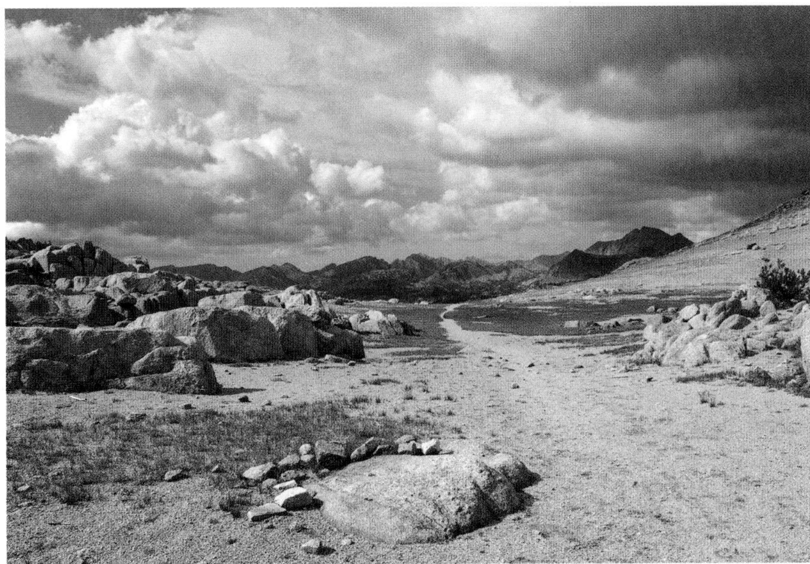

Ecosystems.

TABLE 11-5 Projected Climate Impact by Continent[92]

Africa	■ By 2020, increased water stress for between 75 and 250 million people ■ Severe compromise in agriculture, affecting food security and making malnutrition more severe ■ By the end of the 2000s, rise in sea level, affecting low-lying coastal communities
Asia	■ By the 2050s, decrease in fresh water from rivers in Central, South, East, and Southeast Asia ■ Flooding of coastal areas ■ Expected increase in illness and death from diarrheal disease associated with floods and droughts
Australia and New Zealand	■ By 2020, a significant loss of biodiversity in areas like the Great Barrier Reef ■ Intensification of water security problems in southern and eastern Australia and New Zealand ■ By 2030, a decline in agriculture and forestry in southern and eastern Australia and eastern New Zealand ■ By 2050, rising sea levels and increases in the severity and frequency of storms and coastal flooding
Europe	■ Increase in inland flash floods, more frequent coastal flooding, and increased erosion ■ Glacier retreat, reduced snow cover, and species loss ■ In southern Europe, increasing high temperatures and drought, heat waves, and increased frequency of wildfires
Latin America	■ By midcentury, change in vegetation from semi-arid to arid ■ Loss of biodiversity ■ Decrease in crop and livestock productivity ■ Changes in precipitation, affecting water availability
North America	■ Decrease in water in western mountains ■ Over the century, increase in intensity and duration of heat waves
Polar Regions	■ Reduction in the thickness and extent of glaciers, ice sheets, and sea ice, in turn affecting migratory birds and mammals ■ Detrimental impact on indigenous infrastructure
Small Islands	■ Sea level rise and deterioration of coastal communities ■ By midcentury, water reduction, possibly resulting in inability to meet needs ■ Increased invasion of non-native species

Data from Intergovernmental Panel on Climate Change. Climate change 2007: Synthesis report; summary for policy makers.

efforts of developing countries. Countries will mobilize $100 billion per year through 2025, with a new target to be set after that.[99] On Earth Day (April 22) 2016, 177 countries signed the agreement. When the United States pulled out of the Paris Accords, we became the only other country besides Syria to not participate. Although the Trump administration stated that "the United States will cease all implementation" of the climate agreement, polls show that most U.S. citizens support climate change measures. In response, California, New York, and Washington governors, mayors across the country, and many Fortune 500 companies committed to reducing greenhouse gas emissions.

The adverse effects of climate change will not be distributed evenly across populations. Currently, there is unequal access to resources. People who are poor, who experience food insecurity, and who live in places with conflict

BY THE NUMBERS

According to the June 2017 Associated Press-NORC Center for Public Affairs Research poll, few Americans support withdrawal from the Paris Agreement to reduce greenhouse gas emissions.[100]

Overall

29% strongly or somewhat support withdrawal.
23% neither support nor oppose.
46% somewhat or strongly oppose withdrawal.

By Political Party

51% of Republicans support withdrawal.
69% of Democrats oppose withdrawal.

By Belief in Climate Change

Not believing in climate change makes you three times as likely as those who believe that climate change is happening to support withdrawal.

Other Numbers

44% believe withdrawal will hurt the country's reputation.
43% are concerned that withdrawal will harm the global efforts to fight climate change.
50% believe withdrawal will harm the U.S. economy.

TRY IT!

Reducing Greenhouse Gas

Here are a few easy things you can do to reduce greenhouse gas emissions and help the environment:

- *Use water efficiently*. It is a precious resource. Simple things like not running the water while you shave or brush your teeth help reduce water waste. Repair all toilet and faucet leaks immediately. If you have a dishwasher, run it only when it is full. This both reduces carbon dioxide and saves you money.[101]
- *Driving efficiently helps the environment*. Go easy when using both the gas pedal and brakes, avoiding hard accelerations and hard braking. Don't idle your car for more than 30 seconds. Unload unnecessary items from the trunk of your vehicle, and if you have a removable roof rack, remove it when it isn't needed. If you have a four-wheel drive vehicle, use the two-wheel drive option when it is safe to do so.[101]
- When possible, leave your car at home. Using public transportation, walking or biking, or carpooling helps the environment. As the EPA notes, not driving your car just 2 days per week can reduce your greenhouse gas emissions by an average of 2 tons per year.[101]
- When you buy a car, consider choosing a fuel-efficient vehicle. The labels on cars have been redesigned to provide fuel economy and environmental ratings.[103] See the labels at www.fueleconomy.gov/feg/Find.do?action=bt1.

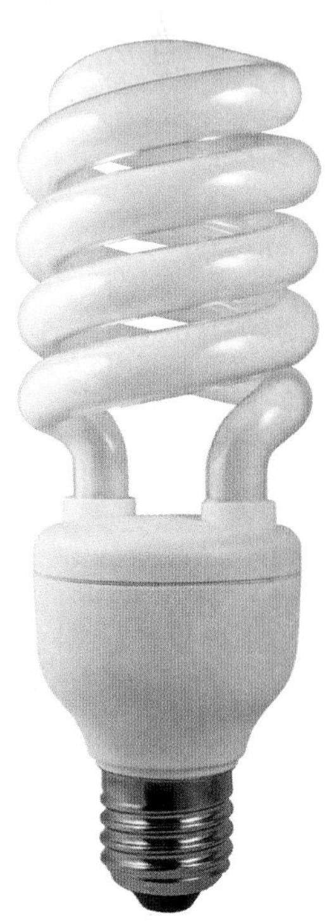

A lightbulb certified by the ENERGY STAR program.

and high rates of disease will fare worse than those with more resources. As resources such as water and food decrease, the discrepancies will be magnified.

Each of us plays a role in greenhouse gas emissions. You can help reduce greenhouse gases by buying locally grown in-season produce, eating more produce (and thus less meat), driving your car less, using energy-saving light bulbs, powering down electronics when not in use, not wasting water, and recycling as many items

TRY IT!

Your Household's Carbon Footprint

The EPA offers an online app that allows you to calculate your household's carbon footprint. It can be found by searching "Carbon Footprint Calculator" on the EPA site.

as possible. Small actions each individual takes will help the environment.[101] When you buy light bulbs, choose ones certified by the ENERGY STAR program. They use 70% to 90% less energy than traditional bulbs and last 10 to 25 times longer. They also save you money on your electricity bill.[102] Recycling at home helps conserve energy, reduces pollution, and reduces greenhouse gas emissions. Composting your food and yard waste reduces both the amount of garbage in landfills and greenhouse gases. Many communities recycle some or all of the following: newspaper, cardboard and other paper, glass bottles and jars, and a variety of plastics.

There are more involved actions you can take to help the environment. There are many environmental groups that you can join that already have active agendas. Visit the START organization's "Environmental Organizations" page (www.startguide.org/orgs/orgs08.html) to find links to broadly focused environmental groups (e.g., Sierra Club, Greenpeace USA), environmental groups focused on climate change, environmental groups focused on energy and mining, forest protection groups, conservation groups, environmental research and public policy groups, and other specific-focus environmental groups.

Engage in the political process by voting. There are many opportunities to do more, from working for candidates whom you support, to community organizing, to helping at the polls. Eventually, you may want to run for a political office yourself!

Think about policies that make a difference for the environment. Maybe you think we should eliminate coal-fired power plants, or raise gas taxes, or encourage subsidies for workers who use public transit. The important thing is to engage actively to help improve the world.

Health Effects of Climate Change

In all likelihood, as climate change continues, there will be an enormous impact on human health. Not everyone is equally at risk. Low- and middle-income

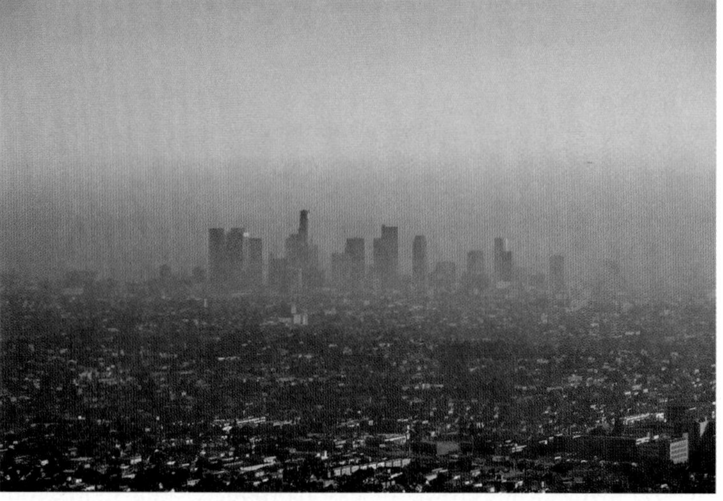

Los Angeles smog.

countries and the most disadvantaged populations will likely feel the effects more profoundly. Within high-income countries, medically vulnerable populations will be the most affected.

Weather-related outcomes due to climate change that impact human health include extreme weather events, rising temperatures, rising sea levels, and increasing **air pollution**. These outcomes, in turn, affect the social and environmental determinants of health, including clean air, safe drinking water, sufficient food, and safe housing.

air pollution A condition in which toxic chemicals or compounds are in the air, at levels that pose a health risk.

Extreme heat is one of the deadliest weather-related hazards. Heat waves directly contribute to cardiovascular- and respiratory-related deaths. In 2003, Europe experienced a heat wave that produced the hottest summer on record since 1540.[104] It is also important to consider that much of Europe does not use air conditioners.[105] During that heat wave, there were an additional 70,000 deaths in Europe over the expected number.[106]

The combination of extreme heat with a lack of rain results in drought situations. Drought conditions have a direct impact on crop production, which leads to a rise in food prices. In the period from 2001 to 2015, there were 12 years in which there were droughts that the National Oceanic and Atmospheric Administration (NOAA) registered as billion-dollar disaster events.[107] As warned by

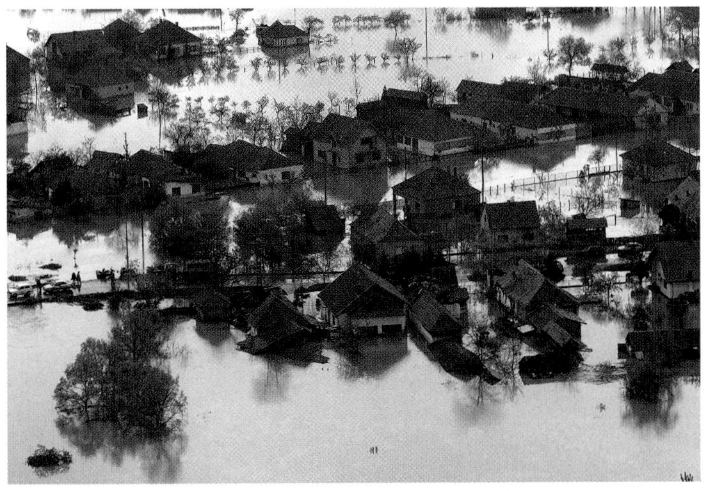

Flood.

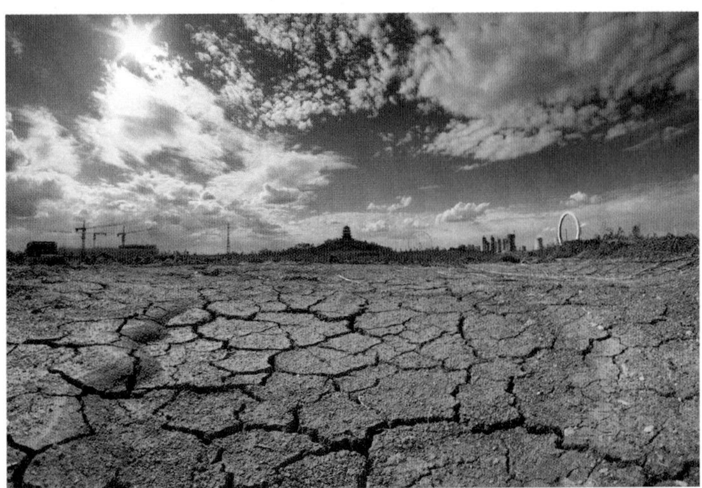

Drought.

the World Health Organization (WHO), climate change is likely to increase the number and severity of droughts on a global scale.[108]

At the other end of the drought spectrum is flooding. Flooding is expected to increase in frequency and severity over the next century.[109] When flooding occurs, it may contaminate fresh water, increase the risk of water-borne diseases, and create opportunities for breeding for disease-carrying insects like mosquitos.[108] Drownings and physical injuries also result. After a storm is over, other water-related issues arise, such as mold-related illnesses.[110]

Rising sea levels present another problem, because more than half the world's population lives less than 40 miles from the ocean. As was seen with Hurricane Katrina (2005) and Superstorm Sandy (2012), these megastorms are highly destructive. The aftermath of Hurricane Katrina left 90% of New Orleans covered in flood water, with many structures destroyed or uninhabitable. People had no place to live and limited drinking water, food spoiled and became scarce, and the risk of mosquito-borne diseases escalated.[111] In the aftermath of Katrina, there were gastrointestinal tract infections, respiratory infections, dehydration, and open wounds.[112] Residents of New Orleans experienced general psychological distress and posttraumatic stress as a result of the hurricane.[113] Following Superstorm Sandy, New York City and surrounding areas experienced severe flooding and loss of power. Three weeks after the storm, four New York City hospitals were still closed for patients, the result being that other hospitals were filled to capacity, with operating rooms booked into the evenings and on weekends.[114] Three years after the storm, people were still experiencing heightened anxiety and posttraumatic stress disorder.[115]

Climate changes affect water-borne diseases and those transmitted by insects. As the climate changes, the geographic range of insect vectors will expand and increase the risk of vector-borne diseases, such as those carried by fleas, ticks, and mosquitoes. **TABLE 11-6** presents vector-borne diseases, their incidence, and the likelihood that climate change will alter the distribution of the disease.

TABLE 11-6 Climate Change and Vector-Borne Diseases

Disease	Vector	Number of New Cases per Year	Present Distribution	Likelihood of Climate Change Altering the Distribution
Malaria	Mosquito	214 million[116]	Tropics and subtropics	Very likely
Schistosomiasis	Water snail	238 million[117]	Tropics and subtropics	Very likely
Lymphatic filariasis	Mosquito	120 million[118]	Tropics and subtropics	Likely
Sleeping sickness (African trypanosomiasis)	Tsetse fly	4,000	Tropical Africa	Likely
Leishmaniasis	Phlebotomine sand fly	900,000–1.3 million[119]	Asia, southern Europe, Africa, Americas	Likely
River blindness (onchocerciasis)	Black fly	750,000[120] (prevalence)	Africa, Latin America	Very likely
Chagas disease (American trypanosomiasis)	Triatomine bug	28,000 in the Americas[121]	Central and South America	Likely

Dengue fever	Mosquito	2.4 million[122]	All tropical countries	Very likely
Yellow fever	Mosquito	84,000–170,000 severe cases and 29,000–60,000 deaths[123]	Tropical South America, Africa	Likely
West Nile virus	Mosquito	2,060 cases in United States[124]	Africa, Europe, Middle East, North America, West Asia	Very likely
Lyme disease	Tick	329,000 cases in United States[125,126]	Everywhere except Antarctica	Very likely

World Health Organization. (2015). 10 facts on malaria. Retrieved from http://www.who.int/features/factfiles/malaria/en/; Vos, T., Flaxman, A. D., Naghavi, M., Lozano, R., Michaud, C., Ezzat, M., . . . Memish, Z. A. (2012). Years lived with disability (YLDs) for 1160 sequelae of 289 diseases and injuries 1990–2010: A systematic analysis for the Global Burden of Disease Study 2010. Lancet, 380(9859), 2163–2196.; World Health Organization. (2016). Lymphatic filariasis. Retrieved from http://www.who.int/mediacentre/factsheets/fs102/en/; World Health Organization. (2016). Leishmaniasis. Retrieved from http://www.who.int/mediacentre/factsheets/fs375/en/; Nettleman, M. D. (2015, November 5). Onchocerciasis: Background. Retrieved from http://webcache.googleusercontent.com/search?q=cache:T6Ge0Cc0JM4J:emedicine.medscape.com/article/224309-overview+&cd=1&hl=en&ct=clnk&gl=us; Pan American Health Organization & World Health Organization. (2016). Chagas disease. Retrieved from http://www.paho.org/hq/index.php?option=com_topics&view=article&id=10&Itemid=40743; Brady, O. J., Gething, P. W., Bhatt, S., Messina, J. P., Brownstein, J. S., Hoen, A. G., . . . Hay, S. I. (2012). Refining the global spatial limits of dengue virus transmission by evidence-based consensus. PLoS Neglected Tropical Disease, 6(8), e1760.; World Health Organization. (2016). Yellow fever. Retrieved from http://www.who.int/mediacentre/factsheets/fs100/en/; Centers for Disease Control and Prevention. (2016). Preliminary maps and data for 2015. West Nile Virus. Retrieved from http://www.cdc.gov/westnile/statsmaps/preliminarymapsdata/index.html; Nelson, C., Saha, S., Kugeler, K. J., Delorey, M. J., Shankar, M. B., Hinckley, A. P., & Mead, P. S. (2015). Incidence of clinician-diagnosed Lyme disease, United States, 2005–2010. Emerging Infectious Diseases, 21(9), 1625–1631.; U.S. Environmental Protection Agency. (2015). Climate change indicators in the United States. Retrieved from https://www3.epa.gov/climatechange/science/indicators/health-society/lyme.html; GRID Arendal. (2016). Vital climate graphics: Spread of major tropical vector-borne diseases. United Nations Environment Programme. Retrieved from http://www.grida.no/publications/vg/climate/page/3093.aspx.

Measuring the health effects of climate change is an imprecise science. We have addressed only a subset of the possible health outcomes of climate change. The WHO estimates that between the years 2030 and 2050, there will be an additional 250,000 deaths per year due to heat exposure, 48,000 due to diarrhea, 60,000 due to malaria, and 95,000 due to childhood undernutrition.[128]

FIGURE 11-16 presents a visual summary of the health effects of climate change.

Air Quality: Indoors and Outdoors

Indoor Air Pollution

Indoor air quality is the quality of the air in and around buildings, especially as it relates to health. Common sources of indoor air pollution include tobacco smoke, mold and pollen, pesticides, some household products, radon, carbon monoxide, and building materials such as asbestos, paints, varnishes, lead, and formaldehyde.[129]

There are several types of devices designed to clean air and remove some pollutants. High-efficiency particulate air (HEPA) filters remove particles, as do electronic air cleaners. There are also residential gas-phase air filters, but none removes all of the gas pollutants usually present in a house. For example, residential gas-phase filters will not remove carbon dioxide. The critical question is whether cleaning the air will reduce adverse health effects. According to the EPA,[130] the ability of a cleaning device to remove particles from the air does not indicate that it will also reduce adverse health effects from indoor pollutants, particularly in sensitive populations such as children, people with asthma and allergies, and the elderly. There are no studies evaluating whether gas-phase filtration or other types of air cleaners, such as ultraviolet germicidal irradiation cleaners and photocatalytic oxidation cleaners, reduce health symptoms. There is not much evidence that air-cleaning devices reduce asthma symptoms from small particles, such as animal dander and dust mites. Larger particles often

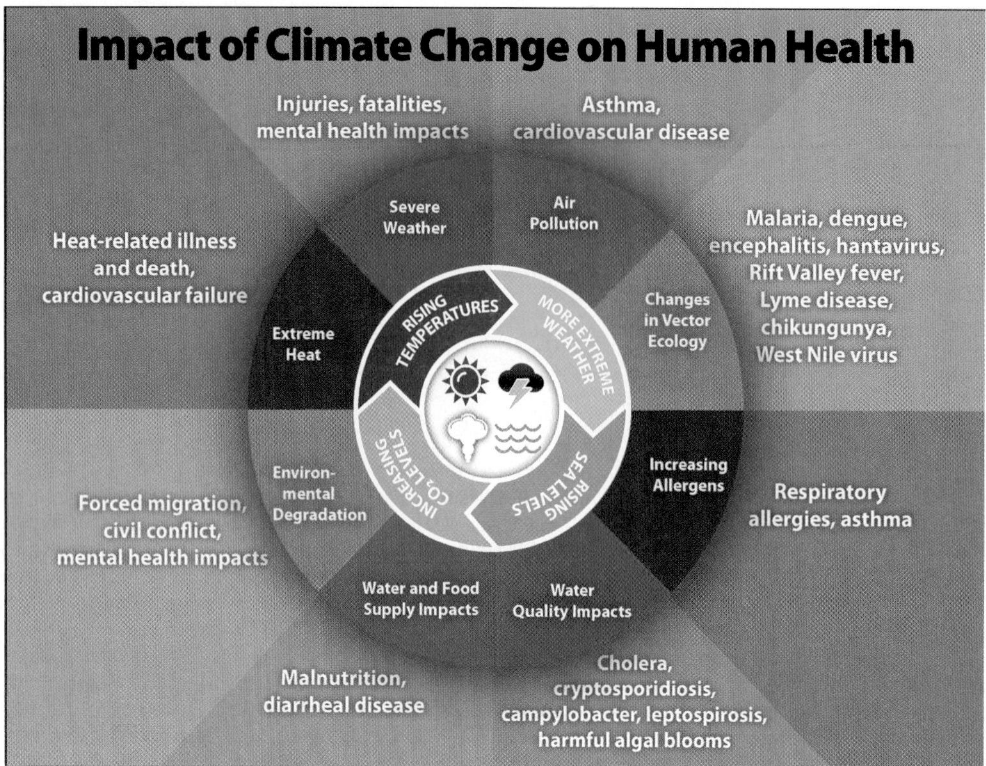

FIGURE 11-16 Health effects of climate change.

Centers for Disease Control and Prevention. (2016). Climate and health: Climate effects on health. Retrieved from http://www.cdc.gov/climateandhealth/effects/default.htm

settle before the filtration system can remove them, so washing sheets at least weekly, dusting hard surfaces, and frequent vacuuming of carpets and upholstery are also necessary.

Should you invest in one of these devices? Researchers conducted a study to test methods of reducing indoor air pollution and increasing symptom-free days in children with asthma who live with a smoker. Although the use of air cleaners did result in a significant reduction in indoor particulate matter concentrations and a substantial increase in symptom-free days, it was not enough to prevent exposure to secondhand smoke.[130,131]

Radon

Radon is a serious indoor air pollutant. Radon is a radioactive, colorless, odorless, tasteless gas that occurs naturally as the decay product of radium and is a health hazard. The only way to know if you have radon in your home is to test for it. While there are many regions in the country with radon, radon mitigation systems do lower the level of radon. For a map showing radon zones in the United States, go to www.epa.gov and search for "Radon Map."

Environmental Tobacco Smoke Exposure

environmental tobacco smoke exposure Exposure to tobacco smoke from being exposed to someone else's cigarette, cigar, or pipe smoke. It can also be described as the material in indoor air that originates from tobacco smoke.

Secondhand smoke, or **environmental tobacco smoke exposure**, refers to exposure to tobacco smoke from someone else's cigarette, cigar, or pipe smoke. Breathing in secondhand smoke is also called passive or involuntary smoking. Secondhand smoke has been proven to be harmful. The only way to be fully protected is to eliminate tobacco use in homes, offices, and public places.[132–134] Some states have introduced laws to make it illegal to smoke in cars with children.

Tobacco smoke is made up of solid particles and gases. There are more than 7,000 different chemicals in tobacco smoke. Between 30 and 60 of these chemicals

are **carcinogens**, meaning they cause cancer in animals, humans, or both. The solid particles comprise about 10% of tobacco smoke and include "tar" and nicotine, and the gases or vapors make up about 90% of tobacco smoke. While the primary gas is carbon monoxide, tobacco smoke also contains formaldehyde, acrolein, ammonia, nitrogen oxides, pyridine, hydrogen cyanide, vinyl chloride, N-nitrosodimethylamine, and acrylonitrile. Vinyl chloride is a known carcinogen,[135] and formaldehyde is a probable carcinogen.[136] Research has shown N-nitrosodimethylamine[137] and acrylonitrile[138] to cause cancer in animals.

carcinogen A substance capable of causing cancer in living tissue.

Mainstream Smoke and Sidestream Smoke. Mainstream smoke is inhaled and then exhaled by the smoker. Sidestream smoke enters the air directly from the burning end of a cigarette, cigar, or pipe. Concentrated sidestream smoke contains higher concentrations of several chemicals than the mainstream smoke inhaled by the smoker, including 2-naphthylamine,[139] N-nitrosodimethylamine,[137] 4-aminobiphenyl,[140] and carbon monoxide. The U.S. Department of Health and Human Services, the International Agency for Research on Cancer, and the EPA have not classified carbon monoxide for human carcinogenicity.

In a room with people smoking, both smokers and nonsmokers will have similar exposure to environmental tobacco smoke because 85% comes from sidestream smoke. Mainstream smoke exposure is limited to the time it takes to smoke the cigarette, but sidestream smoke remains in the room.

Environmental tobacco smoke exposure raises the risk of illness in children, especially respiratory illnesses like bronchitis and pneumonia. It also increases the risk of sudden infant death syndrome in young infants. Among adults who have never smoked, secondhand smoke can cause heart disease, lung cancer, and strokes.[132–134]

Between 1981 and 1989, the Philip Morris Tobacco Company studied the effects of secondhand smoke using mice. They found that sidestream smoke is nearly four times more toxic than mainstream smoke, and it is more likely to cause tumors.[141]

Race, Ethnicity, and Income. Exposure to secondhand smoke is not evenly distributed across the population. Although cotinine (a marker of smoke exposure that can be measured in blood, saliva, and urine) levels have declined in all racial and ethnic groups, data from the CDC's National Health and Nutrition Examination Survey show that levels are higher among non-Hispanic Black Americans than non-Hispanic White Americans and Mexican Americans. Secondhand smoke exposure is more than twice as high among people whose incomes are below the poverty line.[142] **FIGURE 11-17** presents these findings graphically.

Occupation. There are differences in environmental tobacco smoke exposure, depending on what your job is. While these differences have decreased over time, they are still significant. As more states and communities adopt clean indoor air laws, exposure to secondhand smoke decreases. When measured using the National Health and Nutrition Examination Survey III data, Black male workers, construction/manufacturing sector workers, and blue-collar and service workers had the highest serum cotinine levels.[143]

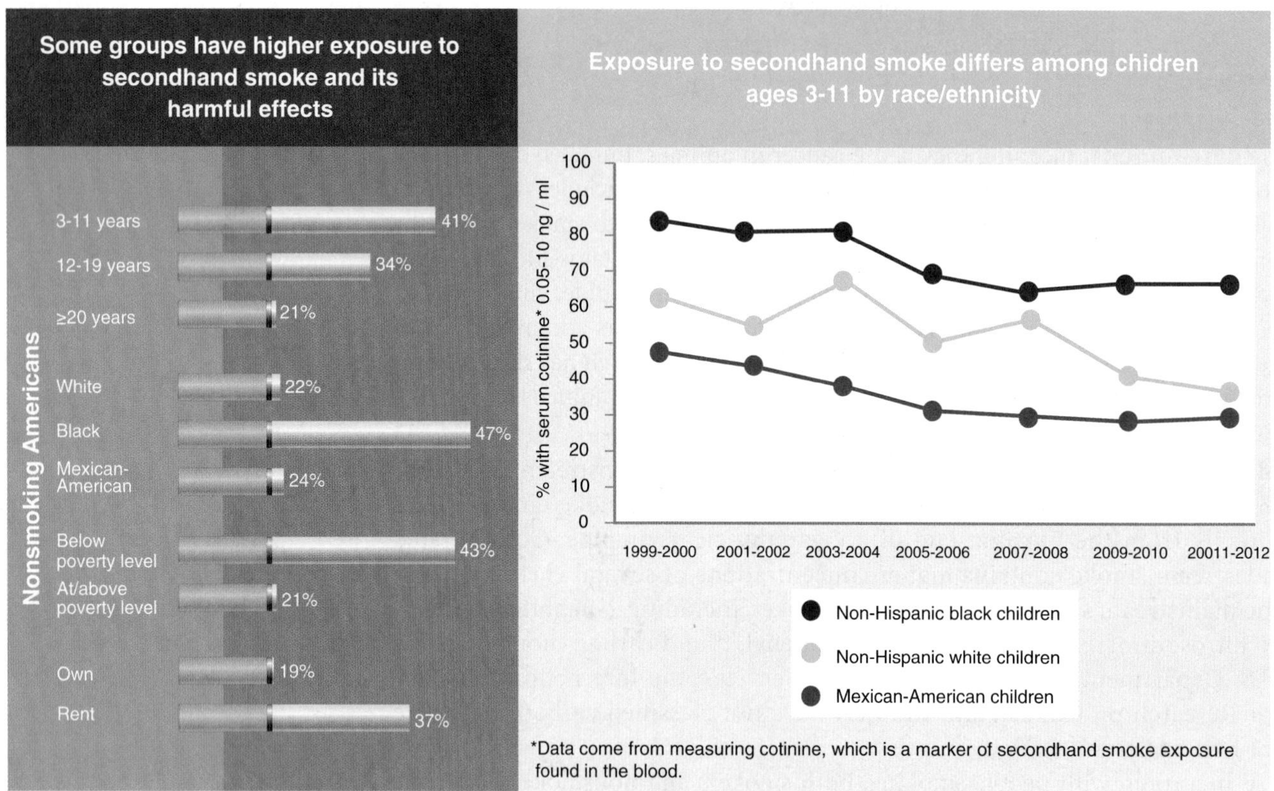

FIGURE 11-17 Your exposure to secondhand smoke depends on who you are.

Centers for Disease Control and Prevention. (2015). Vital signs: Secondhand smoke infographics. Retrieved from http://www.cdc.gov/vitalsigns/tobacco/infographic.html

TRY IT!

How to Protect Yourself From Indoor Air Pollutants

The simplest way to protect yourself from indoor air pollutants is to avoid using toxic chemicals. However, if you do choose to use chemicals, follow these tips to help keep you safe and healthy in your indoor environment[144]:

- Make sure household cleaners list all of the chemicals.
- Limit the use of disinfecting products in your home. While disinfectants do deter microorganisms, overuse can lead to superbugs (bacteria that are resistant to several types of antibiotics.)[145]
- Limit the use of pesticides on lawns. Children and pets track lawn pesticides into the house. Using organic lawn care methods is a better choice. Note that the EPA considers disinfectants a type of pesticide.
- Choose non-PVC flooring and wall covering to minimize exposure to chemical additives such as phthalate plasticizers. (PVC is polyvinyl chloride. It is a carcinogen and is a common element in flooring.)
- If you are doing construction or renovations, select solid woods and formaldehyde-free insulation.
- Choose fragrance-free personal care items. Make sure to open a window when using nail polish and acetone nail polish remover.
- Choose a dry cleaner that offers safer alternatives such as liquid carbon dioxide or wet cleaning. Dry cleaners usually use perchloroethylene (also called tetrachloroethylene). The International Agency for Research on Cancer classifies this chemical as a probable carcinogen.[146]

ARE "GREEN" CLEANERS REALLY BETTER?

Some people may want to use cleaners from "green" companies that exclude chemicals with known or suspected toxicities. On the upside, green cleaners are more environmentally friendly. On the downside, they are more expensive and require more effort for the same level of visual cleanliness. The bottom line is you don't need chemicals to get your house clean. With some effort on your part, you can clean your house with baking soda and vinegar. Chemicals don't make your house cleaner, but they do make cleaning easier.

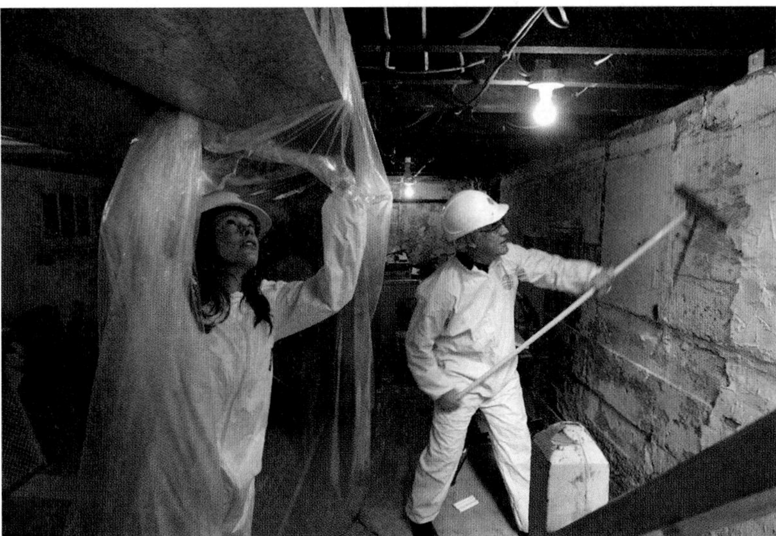

Sick Building Repair.

Buildings With Medical Problems

Buildings can also have problems that affect our health. A building that has a problem may have either a building-related disease or **sick building syndrome**. A building-related disease is a distinct illness that can be traced to a specific cause, such as allergies or asthma caused by dust or mold in the ventilation system.[147]

sick building syndrome A situation in which the occupants of a building experience acute health- or comfort-related effects that seem to be linked directly to the time spent in the building. No specific illness or cause can be identified. The complainants may be localized in a particular room or zone or may be widespread throughout the building.

One of the most famous building-related disease occurrence was in 1976, when there was an outbreak of pneumonia among people attending a convention of the American Legion in Philadelphia. The cooling tower of the convention hotel's air conditioning system contained bacteria[147] that spread through the building,[149] causing more than 200 cases of the disease. The bacterium was subsequently named *Legionella* after the Legionnaires.

Sick building syndrome occurs when the inhabitants of a building experience acute health effects or discomforts that are related to the time they spend in the building. The issue may be localized in a single room, a few rooms, or the entire building. Often the occupants have a variety of nonspecific symptoms without identification of a specific illness or cause.[150]

Sick building syndrome is controversial because there are no specific causes, there are no tests available to diagnose a building, people experience nonspecific symptoms, and there is no treatment. Sick building syndrome is amorphous, making it difficult to prevent. Although a medical care provider cannot diagnose a specific disease, the symptoms, such as nausea or headaches, can be treated and provide individuals with symptomatic relief.

Depending on the ventilation system in the building, spending time in a problematic building may expose you to something of a low-level chemical stew. The location of the free-air intake vents may affect what the building occupants breathe. Potential problems include the following:

- If there is a parking garage in the building or a loading dock, carbon monoxide may enter the ventilation system.
- If smokers gather outside near the air intake vents, the building occupants may be exposed to secondhand smoke.
- If exterminators spray pesticides, these chemicals can be added to the mix of other air contaminants, as can cleaning solutions.

When possible, opening a window can help relieve these conditions by drawing in fresh air.

Many new office buildings have the problem of simply not getting enough fresh air. The American Society of Heating, Refrigerating, and Air Conditioning Engineers recommends appropriate distances from potentially noxious fumes to make sure the air coming into the ventilation systems is fresh.[151]

Outdoor Air Pollution

Air pollution occurs when there are gases, dust, or fumes in the air, which are harmful or even poisonous. Before there were large cities and big industries, nature kept the air clean. Wind and rain kept the air clean by dispersing gases and washing dust away. Plants absorbed carbon dioxide and replaced it with oxygen. The increase in urbanization and industrialization overloaded the system so that plants cannot keep the air clean.

One of the jobs of the EPA is to control hazardous air pollutants. Under the Clean Air Act, there are 187 pollutants for which the EPA is responsible.[152] Most of the toxic air pollutants come from human-made sources, including cars, trucks, buses, factories, refineries, power plants, building materials, and cleaning compounds.

Air Quality Index

The air quality index (AQI) is a guide that the EPA uses to report daily air quality. It tells you how clean or polluted the air you are breathing is. It also tells you what associated health effects might be of concern. The EPA calculates the AQI for five major air pollutants regulated by the Clean Air Act: ground-level ozone, particle pollution (also known as particulate matter), carbon monoxide, sulfur dioxide, and nitrogen dioxide. For each of these pollutants, there are national air quality standards to protect public health.

The AQI is a scale that goes from 0 to 500. The higher the AQI value, the greater the level of air pollution and the greater the health concern. **TABLE 11-7** provides the index value and air quality conditions.

TALES OF PUBLIC HEALTH

September 11, 2001

On September 11, 2001, terrorists flew planes into the World Trade Center in New York City. Less than 2 hours after the attack, both towers collapsed, causing damage to numerous other buildings nearby. Hundreds of thousands of tons of toxic dust spread across lower Manhattan, releasing a variety of airborne toxicants. Those exposed to dust related to the incident were more likely to develop respiratory symptoms. Individuals who were at risk for respiratory health outcomes were those caught in the dust and debris cloud and people, such as rescue, recovery, and cleanup workers, who arrived at the World Trade Center site early and/or worked longer hours there. Delayed mask and respirator use was also related to developing respiratory problems. People who worked and lived in lower Manhattan continued to have lower respiratory symptoms related to the 2001 attacks for years afterward.[152,153]

TABLE 11-7 Air Quality Index

SAQI Value	Air Quality Conditions	Condition Symbolized by the Color
0 to 50	Good	
51 to 100	Moderate	
101 to 150	Unhealthy for sensitive groups	
151 to 200	Unhealthy	
201 to 300	Very unhealthy	
301 to 500	Hazardous	

Natural Air Pollution

Most, but not all, air pollution is human-made; however, there are other sources of air pollution that nature produces. Forest fires, erupting volcanoes, and radioactive decay of rocks are all natural sources of air pollution. Lightning is the leading cause of naturally occurring forest fires. Annually in the United States, there is an average of more than 10,500 fires caused by lightning, with more than 3.8 million acres burned each year.[154] These fires produce huge swathes of smoke.

Volcanoes are created when the molten rock (magma) erupts onto the surface of the earth. Rock fragments, gases, and ashes are ejected from inside the earth. Giant volcanic eruptions can spew so much ash and dust into the atmosphere that they block out significant amounts of sunlight and disrupt air travel. To illustrate the environmental impact that major eruptions can have, the following list describes the most significant eruptions in the last two centuries[155]:

- The eruption of Mt. Tambora (1815) in what is now Indonesia cast a veil of ash around the world and lowered global temperatures by more than 5°F.[155]
- A series of eruptions of Mt. Krakatoa (1883) created a tsunami (a series of ocean waves generated by sudden displacements in the sea floor, landslides, or volcanic activity) 150 feet high in Indonesia. The volcanic ash circled the earth in 2 weeks and lingered for years.[155]
- Mt. Novarupta in Alaska erupted in 1912. Ash from the volcano fell for 3 days, accumulating 1 foot deep. The eruption also caused the top of Mt. Katmai, 6 miles from Mt. Novarupta, to collapse.[155]
- Mt. Pinatubo in the Philippines erupted in 1991. It had not shown any significant activity for 500 years. The average worldwide temperature decreased by 1°F for several years. Sulfur dioxide, mixed with water and oxygen in the atmosphere, creating sulfuric acid and contributing to the destruction of the ozone layer.[155]

Effects of Pollution from Vehicle Exhaust

Air pollution exacerbates many illnesses, including asthma, chronic obstructive pulmonary disease, cardiovascular disease, lung cancer, and diabetes. Children and the elderly are at increased risk from the harmful effects of vehicle exhaust. Nearly half of Americans live in areas that do not meet federal air quality standards.[156]

In 2013, in the United States there were more than 6.6 million children (9.0%) younger than 18 years old with a diagnosis of asthma.[157] It isn't surprising, given the relationship between vehicle exhaust and asthma, that the prevalence of asthma is highest among urban children.[158] Vehicle exhaust adversely affects lung function among asthmatics because it contains particulate matter that causes respiratory problems. Even if a child doesn't have asthma, exposure to traffic-related air pollution in infancy negatively impacts lung function in adolescence.[159]

Southern California is highly urbanized and has some of the worst air quality in the United States.[160] The 2015 report of the Multiple Air Toxics Exposure Study is round 4 of a study to examine cancer risks due to air toxins. The 2005 report found that 90% of the cancer risk in Southern California was due to motor vehicles and other mobile sources.[161] The implementation of emission control programs means that toxic emissions have been declining. The most recent report shows an almost 57% decrease in cancer risk compared to the

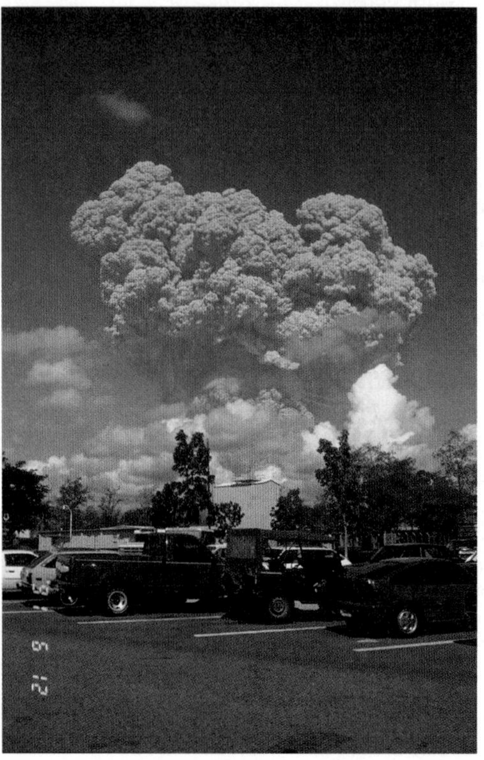

In 1991, Mount Pinatubo erupted in the Philippines. This eruption sent ash plumes 12 miles high.
Courtesy of United States Geological Survey.

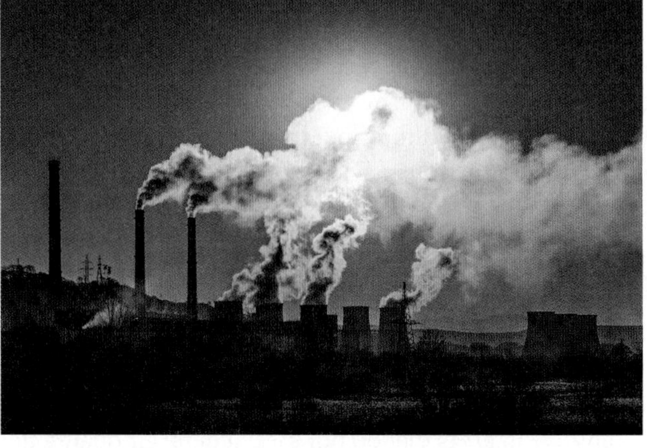

Greenhouse gas emissions.

previous period. The report's authors noted that reducing toxic air contaminants may not be as effective in reducing risks in lower-income communities.[160]

Gases Contribute to Air Pollution

Any gas would qualify as pollution if it reached a high enough concentration to do harm. Theoretically, that means there are dozens of different pollution gases. In practice, about 10 different substances cause the greatest concern:

1. *Sulfur dioxide:* Burning fossil fuels and smelting mineral ores release sulfur dioxide (chemical symbol, SO_2). Exposures as short as 5 minutes can produce adverse respiratory effects, including bronchoconstriction (tightening of the airways causing cough, wheezing, and shortness of breath) and increased asthma symptoms.[162] Sulfur dioxide dissolves easily to form sulfuric acid, an important component of acid rain. Coal-fired power plants are the world's biggest source of sulfur dioxide air pollution.
2. *Carbon monoxide:* Carbon monoxide (chemical symbol, CO) is an odorless, colorless gas, formed from the incomplete burning of fuels, such as gasoline, kerosene, natural gas, oil, coal, or wood. Carbon monoxide is also a component of cigarette smoke and vehicle exhaust. Carbon monoxide reduces the availability of oxygen to the body's organs (like the heart and brain) and tissues. At high levels, this gas can cause death.[162]
3. *Carbon dioxide:* Carbon dioxide (chemical symbol, CO_2) is a colorless gas that contributes to global warming. In solid form, it is dry ice. When people breathe, they exhale carbon dioxide. Burning fossil fuels, such as coal, oil, gasoline, natural gas, and diesel fuel, also produces carbon dioxide. Exposure to carbon dioxide can cause hyperventilation, vision damage, lung congestion, central nervous system injury, abrupt muscle contractions, elevated blood pressure, and shortness of breath. At concentrations above 10%, it can cause convulsions, unconsciousness, or death.[164]
4. *Nitrogen oxides:* Nitrogen oxides are a group of gases composed of nitrogen and oxygen and include nitrogen dioxide (NO_2), nitric oxide (NO), and nitrous oxide (N_2O). When combined with volatile organic compounds, nitrogen oxides form smog. Nitrous oxide is a greenhouse gas that contributes to climate change. Exposure to low levels of nitrogen oxides in smog can irritate the eyes, nose, throat, and lungs. It can cause coughing, shortness of breath, fatigue, and nausea. Longer exposure can trigger severe respiratory problems.[165]
5. *Volatile organic compounds (VOCs):* These chemicals, which are both naturally occurring and human-made, evaporate easily at room temperatures and pressures, so they readily become gases. They are used as solvents in many paints, waxes, and varnishes. When VOCs combine with nitrogen oxides, they form smog. The health effects of VOCs depend on the compound, ranging from no health effect to being highly toxic.[166]
6. *Particulates:* **Particulates** are tiny particles in the air and include dust, dirt, soot, and smoke.[167] Soot and smoke are large and dark enough to be seen. Other particulates are so small that one needs a microscope to see them. Particulate matter is formed from burning fuels, grilling food over charcoal or gas, and burning leaves, brush, and wood. In cities, most particulates come from traffic fumes. High concentrations of particulates present a serious health hazard.[168] This form of pollution causes premature death in people with heart or lung disease. It also causes heart and increased respiratory problems, including aggravating asthma, decreased lung function, and difficulty breathing.[162]

particulates Tiny particles in the air, including dust, dirt, soot, and smoke. Once a person inhales these particles, they can cause serious health effects.

ACID RAIN

Acid rain is defined as any precipitation with high levels of nitric and sulfuric acids. It can also be snow or fog. The most important cause of acid rain is the burning of fossil fuels by coal-burning power plants, factories, and automobiles. Acid rain makes lakes, streams, wetlands, and other aquatic environments toxic to crayfish, clams, fish, and other aquatic animals as well as harming other animals in the food chain. Acid rain also damages forests.[163]

ozone A gas composed of three atoms of oxygen. It is harmful to breathe. The layer in the atmosphere composed of this gas prevents most harmful short-wave ultraviolet B sun rays from reaching the ground.

7. *Ozone:* **Ozone** (chemical symbol, O_3) is a pale blue gas with a distinct smell. In the upper atmosphere, a band of ozone called the ozone layer protects us by screening out harmful ultraviolet radiation from the sun. Even at low concentrations, ozone is a toxic pollutant that can damage health.[169] Breathing ozone can trigger chest pain, coughing, throat irritation, and airway inflammation. It also can reduce lung function and harm lung tissue. Ozone can worsen bronchitis, emphysema, and asthma.[162] It is a key ingredient of smog.
8. *Chlorofluorocarbons (CFCs):* CFCs were used as refrigerants, in aerosol cans as propellants, and as solvents. These compounds are being phased out of use because they contribute to ozone depletion. Direct exposure to CFCs can cause a broad range of health effects, from confusion, drowsiness, coughing, sore throat, difficulty breathing, and eye redness and pain to unconsciousness, shortness of breath, and irregular heartbeat.[170]
9. *Unburned hydrocarbons:* Petroleum and other fuels are composed of organic compounds based on chains of carbon and hydrogen atoms. When hydrocarbons burn incompletely, they can release carbon monoxide, contributing to smog.
10. *Heavy metals, including but not limited to lead, cadmium, and mercury:* Lead occurs naturally in rocks and soil and also comes from burning fossil fuels. Lead is primarily used in the manufacture of batteries. Homes built before 1978 often have lead-based paints, and homes built before 1986 have water pipes joined with lead solder.[171] Depending on the level of exposure, lead can adversely affect the nervous system, kidney function, the immune system, the reproductive and developmental systems, and the cardiovascular system.[162] Cadmium is primarily used as an ingredient in batteries.[172] Mercury is a naturally occurring metal. Methylmercury is the most common mercury compound and builds up in the tissue of fish.[173] It is important to pay attention to what kinds of fish you eat and whether they are high in mercury. If you frequently eat fish high in methylmercury, it can accumulate in your bloodstream over time. Avoiding fish high in mercury is of particular importance if you are pregnant or feeding a young child because it is toxic to the central and peripheral nervous systems.[174] **TABLE 11-8** presents the level of mercury in commonly consumed fish.[175]

Toxic Exposures and Sequelae

Exposure to toxic pollutants may increase your chances of health problems. Pollutants also impact the environment. According to the WHO, in 2012, an estimated 12.6 million people died around the world as a result of living or working in an unhealthy environment. The causes included pollution, chemical exposures, climate change, and radiation.[176]

TABLE 11-8 Mercury in Fish

Lowest Mercury			
Anchovies	Flounder	Oysters	Shad (American)
Arctic char	Haddock (Atlantic)	Perch (ocean)	Shrimp
Butterfish	Hake	Plaice	Sole (Pacific)
Catfish	Herring	Pollock	Squid
Clams	Mackerel (North Atlantic, chub)	Salmon (canned)	Tilapia
Crab (domestic)		Salmon (fresh)	Trout (freshwater)
Crawfish	Mullet	Sardines	Whitefish
Croaker (Atlantic)	Mussels	Scallops	Whiting
Moderate Mercury: Limit to 6 Servings or Less per Month			
Bass (striped, black)	Halibut (Atlantic)	Mahi-mahi	Snapper
Carp	Halibut (Pacific)	Monkfish	Tuna (canned chunk light)
Cod (Alaskan)	Jacksmelt (silverside)	Perch (freshwater)	
Croaker (White Pacific)		Sablefish	Tuna (skipjack)
	Lobster	Skate	Weakfish
High Mercury: Limit to 3 Servings or Less per Month			
Bluefish	Mackerel (Spanish, gulf)	Sea bass (Chilean)	Tuna (yellowfin)
Grouper		Tuna (canned albacore)	
Highest Mercury: Avoid Eating			
Mackerel (king)	Orange roughy	Swordfish	Tuna (bigeye, ahi)
Marlin	Shark	Tilefish	

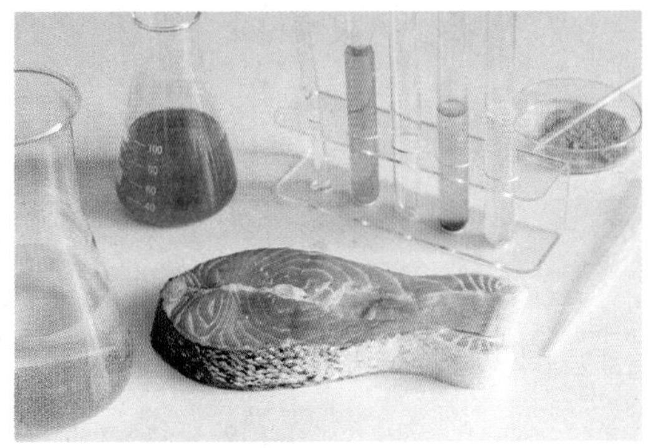

Test Salmon in Laboratory.

Around the world, 23% of deaths and 26% of deaths among children under age 5 years are due to environmental risks that can be improved. Some of the causal environmental factors are well known, including unsafe drinking water and sanitation, air pollution, indoor solid fuel stoves, and, to a lesser extent, climate change and the built environment (housing, workplaces, land use, and roads).[176]

Among the important environmental factors include air pollution, chemical or biological agents in soil and water, ultraviolet and ionizing radiation, noise, electromagnetic fields, occupational risks (physical, chemical, biological, and psychosocial risks and working conditions), the built environment, agricultural methods, human-made climate change, and behavior related to environmental factors, such as the availability of safe water for hand washing.[176] **TABLE 11-9** lists some of the important diseases and the main intervention areas for each illness.

TABLE 11-9 Diseases With Environmental Causes and Main Areas for Intervention[176]

Disease	Main Areas for Intervention
Infectious and Parasitic Diseases	
Respiratory infections	Household and ambient air pollution, secondhand tobacco smoke, housing improvements
Diarrheal diseases	Water, sanitation, hygiene, agricultural practices, climate change
Intestinal roundworm infections	Water, sanitation, hygiene, wastewater management
Malaria	Environmental modification and manipulation to reduce vector breeding sites and reduce contact with disease-carrying mosquitos; mosquito-proof drinking water storage
Trachoma	Access to domestic water supplies, latrines, fly control, personal hygiene
Schistosomiasis	Feces management, safe water supply, safe agricultural practices
Lymphatic filariasis	Modification of drainage and wastewater ponds, freshwater collection, and irrigation schemes
Leishmaniasis	Housing, cleanliness of area around the home, worker protections
Dengue fever	Management of bodies of water around the house, removal of standing water
Hepatitis B and C	Occupational transmission in sex and migrant workers (hepatitis B), accidental needlestick injuries in healthcare workers (hepatitis B and C)
Tuberculosis	Exposure of miners and other occupational groups to airborne particles such as silica or coal dust, exposure in settings such as prisons, hospitals, and overcrowded housing
Noncommunicable Diseases	
Cancers	Household and ambient air pollution, secondhand tobacco smoke, ionizing radiation, ultraviolet radiation, chemicals, worker protection
Mental, behavioral, and neurologic disorders	Occupational stress, disasters, forced resettlements, entertainment and alcohol industry occupations, head trauma, chemicals, noise, bright lights, poor air quality and odors

Cataracts	Ultraviolet radiation, household air pollution
Hearing loss	Occupational exposure to high noise levels
Cardiovascular diseases	Household and ambient air pollution, secondhand tobacco smoke, exposure to lead, stressful working conditions, shift work
Chronic obstructive pulmonary disease	Household and ambient air pollution, exposure to workplace dust
Asthma	Air pollution, secondhand smoke, indoor mold and moisture exposure, occupational exposure to allergens
Musculoskeletal diseases	Occupational stressors, prolonged sitting at work and poor work posture, need to carry large quantities of water (or other heavy burdens) over significant distances

Data from Prüss-Üstün, A., & Corvalán, C. (2006). Preventing disease through healthy environments. Towards an estimate of the environmental burden of disease. Geneva: World Health Organization.

As agencies and researchers get better at identifying occupational diseases, we can work toward methods that protect the worker. Some of the well-known occupational diseases include the following:

- *Asbestosis:* Exposure to high levels of asbestos over an extended period allows the fibers to become lodged in the person's lungs, irritating and scarring the lung tissue. As the disease progresses, the lung tissue becomes scarred, making it harder to breathe.[180] People who worked in mining, milling, manufacturing, and installation and removal of asbestos before the late 1970s are at risk, including asbestos miners, aircraft and auto mechanics, construction workers, electricians, shipyard workers, boiler operators, and railroad workers.[181]
- *Silicosis:* Breathing in tiny bits of silica, a mineral that is part of sand, rock, and mineral ores, causes silicosis. It is common for workers in mining, glass manufacturing, and foundry work to be exposed to silica. Like asbestos, exposure to silica causes scarring in the lungs. Those exposed to silica can develop silicosis in a few weeks, or it may take decades. Silicosis can cause significant lung damage.[182]
- *Lead poisoning:* Although many uses of lead are banned, it is still an ingredient in thousands of products, including lead-based paints, solder, electrical fittings, and plumbing fixtures. Construction or demolition projects of older buildings may expose a worker to lead. The range of exposures varies from minimal to extensive. OSHA requires employers to use engineering controls and work practices, where possible, to reduce worker exposure to lead. Depending on the job, an employer may be required to provide workers with protective clothing and respiratory protection.[183]
- *Noise-induced hearing loss:* Chronic exposure to loud noises contributes significantly to hearing loss. Many workplaces have loud noises, including airports, police firing ranges, and anywhere that has noisy machines.

Occupational Exposure

The Occupational Safety and Health Administration is the federal agency responsible for assuring that every working person in the United States has safe and healthful working conditions. OSHA assesses toxic exposures in the workplace, namely risk factors leading to cancers, respiratory diseases, and circulatory disease, among others.

For many workers, the environments in which they live and work are the same. Thus, the toxic hazards affect not only the worker but their families and communities as well. One typical example is agricultural pesticide use. Workers may be exposed to the pesticides during and after spraying. They may absorb the chemicals through their skin. They may ingest the chemicals if they do not wash sufficiently to remove the chemicals from their hands. Additionally, the chemicals may remain in the air, contaminate the water, and remain on their clothes as residue. Family and community members all experience the same exposures. Finally, the chemicals leach into the soil and groundwater.[177]

The health and safety of workers have improved over time. The Tales of Public Health box describes the first known account of an occupational cancer.

TALES OF PUBLIC HEALTH

Percivall Pott and Chimney Sweeps[178]

In 1775, English surgeon Percivall Pott described a link between environmental toxins to which chimney sweeps were exposed and the development of cancer. At the time, being a chimney sweep was a common profession in England.

Pott had found a large number of cases of scrotal cancer among his male patients. The common factor was that all of them worked as "climbing boys" when they were young. Traditionally, master sweepers would hire climbing boys—small boys who were orphans or from indigent families—to climb inside the flues and brush them clean. The climbing boys also used metal scrapers to remove the tar deposited by wood smoke. The boys could be as young as 7 years old. Some grew up to be assistants to the master sweeper. Because this was the 1700s, the boys had no safety clothing and there were no safety regulations to protect them. Many of the boys died of suffocation due to breathing in dust and soot. Others died when they got stuck in narrow flues and suffered catastrophic injuries.

Pott studied a large number of climbing boys and concluded that the cancer was due to prolonged exposure to soot. Other doctors reported similar findings, and 100 years later, the United Kingdom outlawed the use of climbing boys.[179]

Percivall Pott's description of cancer among chimney workers was the first description of an occupational cancer.

Occupational Cancers

Many toxins are carcinogenic in animals and may be carcinogenic in humans. Millions of U.S. workers are exposed to these toxins. The International Agency for Research on Cancer has tested fewer than 2% of the chemicals or physical agents manufactured or processed in the United States.[184] The National Institute for Occupational Safety and Health (NIOSH) estimates that workplace exposure causes between 45,000 and 92,000 cases of cancer in 1 year.[185] This assessment is likely an underestimate of the actual number of cases. As researchers gather more information about toxic exposures that cause cancer, that number will be revised upwards. It is important to understand that exposure to occupational carcinogens, can, to a large extent, be avoided.[186,187] NIOSH provides an extensive list on its website of potential occupational carcinogens.[188]

Little Things Matter

These are not just theoretical issues that affect other people. We are all exposed to dozens, if not hundreds, of chemicals. Even mild exposures to common toxins are bad for you and worse for young children. Chemical companies spread the idea that there are few consequences of toxins on brain development. Even low amounts of lead, polychlorinated biphenyl, organophosphate pesticides, or polybrominated diphenyl ethers (flame retardants found in furniture and clothing) have been shown in U.S. studies to increase the likelihood of developing mental disorders. Except for carcinogens, toxins are regulated as if there were a safe level, below which exposure would not harm a person. Go to YouTube and search for "Little Things Matter: The Impact of Toxins on the Developing Brain" to hear Dr. Bruce Lanphear of Simon Fraser University discuss the impact of toxins on the developing brain and explain why it matters.

Natural Disasters and Emergency Preparedness

There is an extensive list of natural disasters that can create havoc: avalanches, tornadoes, earthquakes, floods, hurricanes, lightning strikes, tsunamis, wildfires, and volcanoes. Although many of these disasters can occur anywhere, some areas are more prone to experience a particular type of natural disaster. It is important to know whether you are living in an area that experiences natural disasters. Do you live in Tornado Alley (discussed in the tornadoes section)? Have there been mudslides where you are living? Is there a volcano close by that has shown recent activity? Once you know the answer to such questions, you can plan accordingly. The important thing to remember is, planning ahead and keeping calm in a disaster will help a lot.

Being safe in a natural disaster is often dependent on planning. It is always useful to have emergency kits ready. The following information box lists the items that the CDC recommends including in a first aid kit. If you have special medical needs, you should add the necessary items to your own first aid kit.

FIRST AID KIT[189]

Drugs and Medications

- Soap and clean water to disinfect wounds
- Antibiotic ointment
- Individually wrapped alcohol swabs
- Aspirin and non-aspirin tablets
- Prescriptions and any long-term medications (keep these current)
- Diarrhea medicine
- Eye drops

NOTE: Important medical information and most prescriptions can be stored in the refrigerator, which provides protection from fires.

Dressings

- Bandages
- Clean sheets torn into strips
- Elastic bandages
- Rolled gauze
- Cotton-tipped swabs
- Adhesive tape roll

Other First Aid Supplies

- First aid book
- Writing materials

Food and Medicine

- Clean containers for water
- A 3- to 5-day supply of water at 5 gallons per day per person
- A 3- to 5-day supply of food that doesn't go bad and doesn't need refrigeration
- If you have a baby, formula and/or baby food

Safety Items

- Fire extinguisher
- Battery-powered radio
- Flashlights and extra batteries
- Sleeping bags or blankets
- Iodine tablets or chlorine bleach to purify water for drinking

Personal Care Products

- Hand sanitizer
- Cleaning cloths (like baby wipes) in case you don't have clean water
- Soap
- Toothpaste
- Tampons or pads
- If you have a baby, diapers

(continues)

- Scissors
- Tweezers
- Thermometer
- Bar soap
- Tissues
- Sunscreen
- Paper cups
- Plastic bags
- Safety pins
- Needle and thread
- Instant cold packs for sprains
- Pocket knife
- Splinting material

Emergency Car Kit

Always keep an emergency kit in your car.

- Food that doesn't go bad and doesn't need refrigeration
- Flares
- Jumper cables
- Maps (because service to your cell phone may be disrupted!)
- A first aid kit and instructions
- A fire extinguisher
- Sleeping bags
- Flashlight and extra batteries

If service is available, having a global positioning system (GPS) can help during an emergency, too.

Make sure you gather emergency supplies, including enough food and water for 3 to 5 days and supplies for performing first aid. Have important information written down (see the following discussion of tornadoes). Have an evacuation plan, including, if possible, more than one exit from each room. If possible, turn off the utilities to your home.

Establish your priorities, including what important items you can hand-carry with you and the order of importance. If you have a vehicle and time permits, make sure your emergency car kit is in order, decide what additional items you would take, and plan other actions to complete before evacuating, such as locking doors and windows. Before actually evacuating in the vehicle, make sure the gas tank is full. If you don't have a vehicle, arrange with friends or family for transportation. Make sure to gather your important documents and put them in a waterproof container. If you have a pet, find a local emergency pet shelter.

If you are ordered to evacuate, take only essential items with you. Disconnect appliances before you leave. Follow the designated evacuation routes, but expect heavy traffic. Do not, under any circumstances, walk or drive across flooded roads.

Remember, in an emergency, your priority should be safety above all else.

Landslides and Mudslides[190]

The definition of a landslide is a mass of rock, earth, or other debris moving down a hill or mountain slope. Mudslides or debris flows are fast-moving landslides that tend to flow in channels. Landslides occur when there is a disturbance in the natural stability of a slope. Instability may be due to heavy rainfall, earthquakes, or a volcanic eruption. Mudslides often occur on steep slopes. Lack of vegetation, either due to fires or people removing the vegetation, make slopes particularly vulnerable to landslides and mudslides. Other areas at higher risk of landslides or mudslides include areas with steep slopes or canyons, areas where landslides have previously occurred, hillsides that have been altered for construction, and channels along a river.

Landslides and mudslides pose both direct and indirect health hazards. The debris and water from slides can cause massive damage to humans and buildings. They can also break electric, water, gas, and sewage lines. Roadways covered in mud and water both endanger motorists and disrupt access to health care.

It is important to know whether you live in an area prone to landslides or mudslides. If you have recently moved, you can find out by contacting local authorities. Also, ask the authorities about emergency evacuation plans. If you live in such an area, consider evacuating if the prediction is for intense storms and rainfall. Develop emergency and evacuation plans for your family, including a communication plan in case of separation, and become familiar with the recommendations provided in this section on natural disasters for before, during, and after the event.

During an intense storm, listen to the radio or television for information and emergency instructions from local officials. Be aware of nature's warning signs: a sudden increase or decrease in the water level; tilted trees, telephone poles, fences, or walls; and rumbling sounds from an approaching landslide. If danger is imminent, move as quickly as possible away from the path of the slide to high ground. After a landslide or debris flow, listen for emergency instructions from local authorities. Do not enter the path of the landslide! Always report broken utility lines to authorities.

Tornadoes

A tornado is a violently rotating column of air that extends from the base of a thunderstorm to the ground.[191] Tornadoes may be a variety of shapes. They are often dark due to the soil and debris they pick up as they move. Tornadoes move at an average of 35 miles per hour. Usually, tornadoes travel about 5 miles before they dissipate. The diameter of a tornado can vary from 300 feet to 1 mile. A tornado over a body of water is called a waterspout.

Knowing what to do when you see a tornado, or when you hear a tornado warning, can help you to keep yourself and your family safe. During a tornado, there are extremely high winds. Flying and falling objects are a hazard. The wreckage after a tornado also poses additional injury risks. Although you cannot prevent tornadoes, being prepared and exercising good judgment will minimize the risks.

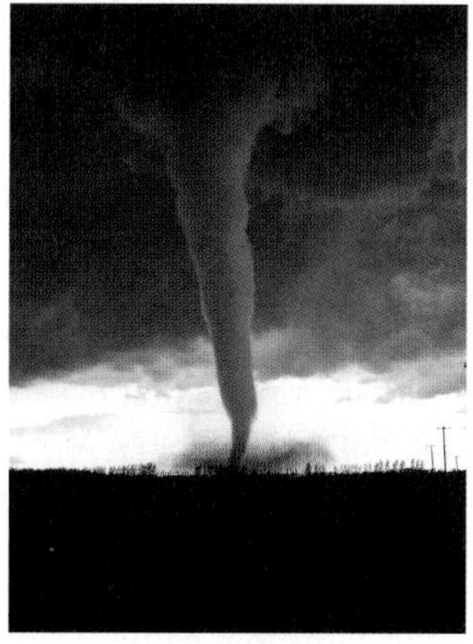

Funnel cloud touching the ground near Elie, Manitoba.

WHERE IS TORNADO ALLEY?

Tornadoes can and do occur everywhere in the United States as well as Australia, Europe, Africa, Asia, and South America. Tornado Alley is the name given to the area in the United States that tends to experience the strongest and most violent tornadoes. This area includes South Dakota, Nebraska, Kansas, Oklahoma, northern Texas, and eastern Colorado.[191]

Write Down Important Information[189]

Long before weather conditions turn ominous, you can begin to prepare for a tornado. It is useful to have a list of important information, including phone numbers of the police and fire station, medical centers, the utility companies, and your landlord or property manager. Know your neighbors' names and telephone numbers. Write down a brief medical history of important information such as medication allergies or medications you take regularly. Know your account numbers for your bank. Also, write down the year, model, and vehicle identification number (VIN) of your car.

Keep critical documents in a fireproof and waterproof safe. These documents include birth certificates, social security cards, car titles, and a list and photograph of anything that is of high monetary value. If anything you own has a serial number, write this information down as well. (If you don't have a safe, copying these items and giving the copies to a trusted relative or friend is another option.)

Before and During a Tornado

When you live in an area that is prone to tornadoes, if there are thunderstorms, turn on the radio or television to get emergency information from local authorities. Currently, the average lead time authorities have for tornado warnings is 13 minutes.[191] Most areas prone to tornadoes have a siren system to alert people to tornado watches and tornado warnings. You can also get information from a NOAA weather radio.[192] There are unofficial NOAA weather apps for both iPhones and Android phones. If conditions worsen, be prepared to take shelter, and if there is a tornado warning, seek shelter immediately.

Because tornadoes can form rapidly, there isn't always time for a warning. If it is raining or there are clouds, you may not see the funnel. Dark or green-colored sky, dark, low-lying clouds, large hail and a loud noise that sounds like a freight train are all signs that a tornado may occur. If you notice any of these weather conditions, take cover immediately, and keep tuned to local radio and television stations or a NOAA weather radio.

If you see a funnel cloud nearby, take shelter immediately. If you see a funnel cloud that is far away, and you have time without endangering yourself, alert the newsroom of a local radio or television station.

The key to surviving a tornado and reducing the risk of injury lies in planning, preparing, and practicing. Know where your first-aid kit and fire extinguishers are. If you reside in a place that has utility cutoffs, know where they are and how to turn them off if necessary. Most deaths and injuries from tornadoes are from flying debris. An important thing to remember is to avoid windows. The goal is to stay on the lowest floor available. The safest place is the interior part of a basement. If there is no basement, go to the first floor and choose a center hallway, a bathroom without windows, or a closet. Protect your head with anything available: a heavy table, a sleeping bag, a mattress,

TORNADO WATCH VS. TORNADO WARNING

A *tornado watch* means the weather conditions favor the formation of tornadoes, for example, during a severe thunderstorm.

A *tornado warning* means a tornado funnel is sighted or indicated by weather radar.

or, if nothing else is available, your hands. Avoid areas where there are very heavy objects on the floor above where you are.[189] The least safe place to be during a tornado is in a motor vehicle. If there is no obvious shelter, lie on the ground at the lowest point available, such as a ditch, away from trees, and protect your head. Long-span buildings, like shopping malls, are particularly dangerous during tornadoes because the roof is usually supported only by the external walls. Their construction makes them prone to collapsing. In public buildings, use the same guidelines as in a house: the lowest floor possible and away from windows.

If you have special needs, such as mobility issues, you should make a list of your specific capabilities, medications, needs, and limitations. Keep that list near you. Prepare someone who lives nearby to assist you in an emergency. This person should have a copy of your list as well as a spare key to your house. To the extent possible, follow the general instructions regarding where to go in the event of a tornado. If no assistance is available and you cannot get out of bed or a chair, protect yourself from falling objects by covering yourself with pillows.

Mold

You may not think of mold as a natural disaster along the lines of hurricanes and tornadoes, but it often is a result of these events and therefore must be considered in the discussion of health risks resulting from natural disasters. After natural disasters involving water (e.g., hurricanes, floods, tornadoes), the excess moisture and standing water increase the likelihood that there will be mold. People with asthma and allergies and those who are immune suppressed will be more sensitive or susceptible to mold. Individuals who are sensitive to mold may suffer from a stuffy nose, irritated eyes, wheezing, or skin irritation. Those who are allergic to mold will likely experience respiratory problems. People with suppressed immune systems may develop mold infections in their lungs. Mold may cause similar problems in otherwise healthy people.[193]

If your house or apartment building has mold, you may smell it, or you may see it if the walls are discolored from the mold. The goal is to dry out your house as quickly as possible to prevent mold from growing. Open doors and windows and use large fans and dehumidifiers to dry out the building. Items like carpet, carpet padding, some clothing, paper, and wood that cannot be thoroughly cleaned and dried should be removed to prevent mold growth. The EPA offers advice about cleaning up mold.[194] If you are cleaning up mold yourself, use an N95 mask to filter out airborne particles. The CDC offers a list of approved manufacturers of these masks.[195]

Earthquakes

Like other natural disasters, survival and minimizing the health effects is dependent on preparation and planning. Although recently California has had the most severe earthquakes, there are other fault zones in the United States. Other states that have had earthquakes since 2000 include Alabama, Alaska, Colorado, Florida, Hawaii, Illinois, Indiana, Oklahoma, Virginia, and Washington. Even if an earthquake is not severe, it can cause substantial injuries.[196]

Magnitude measures how strong an earthquake is. The magnitude of an earthquake is related to the area of the fault (a break or fracture in the ground that happens when the earth's tectonic plates move or shift) on which it occurs; the larger the fault area, the larger the earthquake.[196]

Floods[197]

Even small floods can be disastrous. Know the location of your community's emergency shelters. Much of the disaster planning for other disasters applies here as well. Know how to turn off electrical power, gas, and water lines before you evacuate your home. Buy a fire extinguisher and make sure everyone living there knows how to use it. Install or have your landlord install a sump pump. (Sump pumps remove accumulated water, usually in the basement.) If you live in a flood zone, the electric components (switches, sockets, circuit breakers, and wiring) should be at least 12 inches above the projected flood elevation.

Hurricanes[198]

Hurricanes cause high winds, flooding, heavy rain, and storm surges (high tidal waves).

Food and Water Safety After a Hurricane

Throw out spoiled food. This may seem obvious, but in stressful situations, people don't always make good choices. If the food has a strange smell, color, or texture, throw it away. If canned food has been punctured, is damaged, or is bulging, throw it away. If foods that need to be kept cold (meat, eggs, fish, poultry, and leftovers) have been out of a refrigerator for more than 2 hours, throw them away.

If canned food came in contact with floodwater, but is otherwise intact, once you clean off the can, it is safe to use. Remove the label and dip the cans in a mixture of water and household bleach; the mixture should be 80 parts water to 1 part bleach (i.e., 5 cups [40 oz.] water and 1 tablespoon [0.5 oz.] bleach). Make sure to label the cans with a permanent marker, so you know what is in them.

After a hurricane, local officials will announce when the tap water is safe for drinking or washing. Until you are sure it is safe, use bottled water. If bottled water is not available, you can use water purification tablets or water that has been boiled at a rolling or full boil for 1 to 5 minutes. Boiling water will kill microorganisms, but it will not remove solids, metals, or minerals. If there are solids in the water, they will settle to the bottom of the pot as the water cools.

Remaining Safe After a Hurricane

Never use an electrical appliance if it got wet. Do not unplug anything without first turning off the power to the outlet. When the power is out, flashlights are much safer than candles. If candles are your only choice, always stay near them when lit. Because hurricanes can damage a building, if you hear shifting or unusual noises, vacate the house right away.

Do not use gas- or coal-burning equipment intended for outside use, inside your house. These items have not been designed for inside use and can emit carbon monoxide, which is very dangerous. Do not use a gas oven to heat your home.

Fallen or damaged power lines are dangerous. Call the utility company to report them. Dust from damaged buildings may be toxic. Be sure to use a breathing mask and wash the dust off your body. Flooding often brings mosquitoes that carry disease. Wear long pants, long-sleeved shirts, and socks. Use insect repellant that contains either DEET (diethyltoluamide) or picaridin.

Lightning[199]

It is important to avoid lightning whenever possible. Be aware of the weather. If you hear thunder, lightning is close enough to strike you. If you are outside, find a safe, enclosed shelter, including a house, office, shopping center, or hardtop vehicle. If you are in an open area, away from any shelters, crouch down with your head tucked to your chin and your hands over your ears. Do not lie down; you want to be as low and as small as possible, but minimize your contact with the ground. If you are with a group of people, do not stay bunched together. The group should separate to reduce the number of injuries if the lightning strikes the ground. According to the CDC, when you are inside during a thunderstorm, avoid water and electrical equipment, including corded phones. Stay away from open windows. (See Chapter 9 for more information on lightning.)

Do not leave your pet outside during a lightning storm. Bring pets inside the house.

If someone else is struck by lightning, call 9-1-1.

Tsunamis

Tsunamis are a series of long high waves created by an earthquake, landslide, volcanic eruption, meteorite, or other disturbance. A tsunami can occur anywhere along most of the U.S. coastline.[200] Tsunamis occur most frequently in the Pacific Ocean because there is a large number of active submarine earthquake zones.[201]

Natural tsunami signs include earthquake shaking, water rapidly receding from the beach, and loud rumbles, like a train, coming from the ocean. Tsunamis are dangerous because they cause the water level and currents to rise rapidly. In a tsunami, there can be multiple dangerous waves.[201]

As with most natural disasters, the primary public health concerns after a tsunami are clean drinking water, food, shelter, and medical care.

Wildfires[202]

As the population expands, more and more people live in areas prone to wildfires. If you see a wildfire, report it by calling 9-1-1. If you receive evacuation orders, follow them promptly. Know where you will go, either to a friend whose home is not in danger or to an emergency shelter. Weather apps on your phone often report that conditions are favorable for wildfires. If you live where wildfires are common, you should keep your car's fuel tank full and your car in good working order. Keep emergency supplies and a change of clothes in the car.

Do not return to your house or building after a fire until authorities say it is safe. Use caution, even after the fire is out, as there can still be hot spots. Wear a mask and use water to wet debris, minimizing dust. Discard any food exposed to heat, smoke, or soot.

The U.S. Forest Service and other agencies responsible for public lands deal with tens of thousands of wildfires each year.[203] Each year, there is an average of more than 73,000 wildfires in the United States. They burn about 7.3 million acres of land and more than 2,600 structures. Wildfires are almost impossible to prevent and difficult to control. The Forest Service manages fires by thinning grass, brush, and trees, to reduce the risk of bigger and more severe fires.

In public areas, you may see signs such as the one shown in **FIGURE 11-18**. These signs describe the danger level of a fire. Managers may impose restrictions or close public lands.[204]

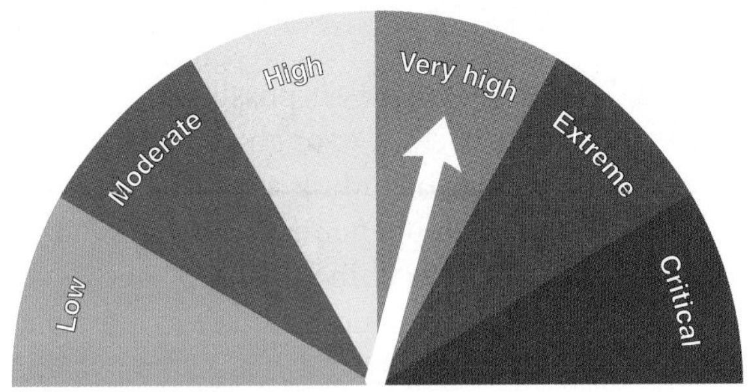

FIGURE 11-18 National Fire Danger Rating System.

National Park Service. (n.d.). Understanding fire danger. Retrieved from https://www.nps.gov/articles/understanding-fire-danger.htm

Climate Change and Wildfire Risks

Global warming is a major contributor to the frequency of wildfires, particularly in the western United States, which has had an increased frequency of droughts. The fire season is lasting longer, and the drier conditions increase the probability of fires. Thunderstorms are becoming more severe, with more lightning and, in turn, more fires.[205]

Climate exerts a powerful effect on the number and distribution of insects. Warmer temperatures lead to more rapid development and survival as well as shifts in the range of insect species. Not only will they reproduce and grow more quickly, but also they are likely to survive longer.[205] As insect infestation increases, they consume more foliage, killing trees and thus producing more fuel for fires.[205]

Volcanoes[206]

See earlier in this chapter under natural air pollution a description of volcanoes. If you live in an area with an active volcano, local authorities will provide you with information about how to prepare. Disaster planning is much like planning for other natural disasters. The CDC adds sturdy shoes and a manual can opener to the emergency supply kit for volcanoes. Evacuation recommendations are similar to those for other disasters.

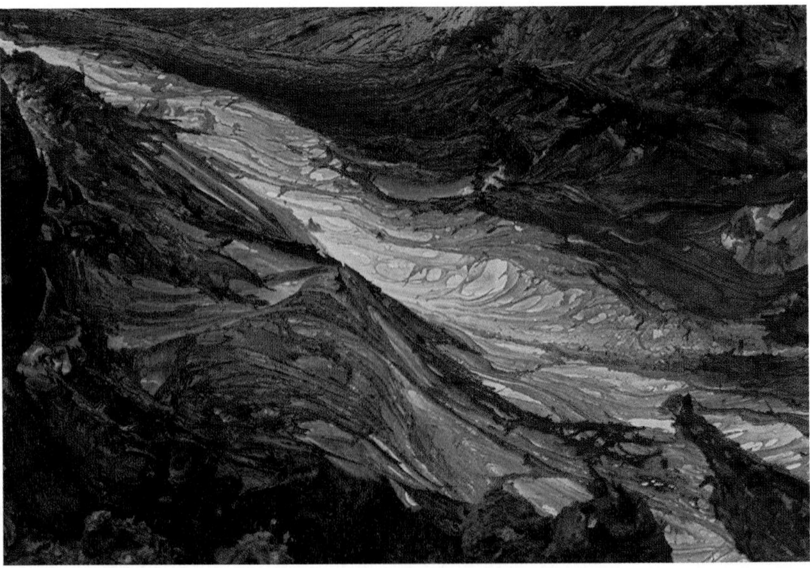

Lava flow from an active volcano.

If you are told to shelter in place, close and lock all windows and outside doors. Turn off all heating or air conditioning systems and fans. Shut the fireplace damper. Make sure you have a working radio. Your safest place is above ground level in an interior room without windows. If you have a pet, bring it with you and be sure to have food and water for it.

Environmental Justice

According to the EPA, the definition of environmental justice is "the fair treatment and meaningful involvement of all people regardless of race, color, national origin, or income with respect to the development, implementation, and enforcement of environmental laws, regulations, and policies."[208] What this means is that there should be an equitable distribution of environmental risks and benefits. Historically, the locations of environmentally hazardous facilities are in predominantly minority neighborhoods. Such facilities include waste disposal plants, manufacturing facilities, landfills, incinerators, and other potentially toxic facilities.

TALES OF PUBLIC HEALTH

Warren County, North Carolina[209]

Warren County, North Carolina, is poor, rural, and overwhelmingly Black.

In 1981, Governor James B. Hunt Jr. convinced the state general assembly to pass a law allowing governors the right to choose hazardous waste facility sites prior to and essentially without a public hearing. The state government decided that Warren County would be an excellent place to dump 6,000 truckloads of soil laced with toxic polychlorinated biphenyl. In September 1982, the trucks arrived with the goal of leaving the soil in a newly constructed hazardous waste site. The Warren County citizens expressed concern that the chemicals would leach into their drinking water. To stop the trucks, people lay down in the roads leading to the landfill. There were 6 weeks of marches and nonviolent street protests. More than 500 people were arrested.

While the people lost their battle, they did spark a national movement. It was the beginning of the national movement for environmental justice.

Is there a relationship between the racial composition of neighborhoods, household income levels, and the environmental hazards in those areas? A study from 2008 used national census tract-level data and the EPA's industrial air pollutant concentration data to examine the answer to this question. In the United States, non-Hispanic Blacks are more likely to live in neighborhoods with environmental hazards than are any of the other racial/ethnic groups studied. Non-Hispanic Whites also live in environmentally hazardous neighborhoods but not as frequently as non-Hispanic Blacks. Hispanics and non-Hispanic Pacific Islanders more often live in environmentally hazardous neighborhoods compared to non-Hispanic Native Americans and non-Hispanic Asian Americans, but less frequently than non-Hispanic Blacks and non-Hispanic Whites. For individual income levels, the researchers compared the environmental quality of the neighborhood by race. At each annual income level from under $10,000 up to $200,000, non-Hispanic Blacks had the highest neighborhood toxic concentrations, followed by non-Hispanic Whites and Hispanics. These results show that Blacks, Whites, and Hispanics with similar incomes live in neighborhoods of dissimilar environmental quality.[210]

A more recent study from California found somewhat similar results. The differences are likely due to the population distribution by ethnicity.

The likelihood of living in a highly polluted community compared to non-Hispanic Whites was highest for Hispanics, and in decreasing order, African Americans, Native Americans, Asian/Pacific Islanders, and other or multiracial groups. The authors concluded that burden of environmental health hazards disproportionately affects communities of color.[211]

A Federal Response to Issues of Environmental Health Disparities

The EPA, National Institute of Environmental Health Sciences, and National Institute on Minority Health and Health Disparities are jointly supporting a collaborative research effort to address environmental disparities. The centers funded by these agencies support research efforts, mentoring, capacity building, research translation, and information dissemination to help eliminate environmental health disparities. There are currently five centers funded.[212] See **TABLE 11-10**.

A Health Activist Fights Back

Majora Carter is from the South Bronx neighborhood in New York City. As an American urban revitalization strategist and public radio host, she works on issues of environmental justice.

Go to Ted.com and search for "Majora Carter: Greening the Ghetto" to watch her talk about fighting for environmental justice in the South Bronx.

TABLE 11-10 Research Efforts to Help Eliminate Environmental Health Disparities

Center	Focus
University of Arizona	■ Build sustainable tribal environmental health disparities research capacity. ■ Effectively partner with tribes to address their environmental health concerns. ■ Support sustainable tribal environmental approaches for improving community health.
University of Southern California	■ Examine whether environmental exposures, coupled with exposures to psychosocial and built environment stressors, lead to excessive gestational weight gain and postpartum weight retention in local Hispanic women and increased childhood obesity risk.
Johns Hopkins University	■ Examine the role of indoor air pollution exposures on chronic obstructive pulmonary disease in low-income U.S. communities. Understand the role of obesity and poor diets as factors that are common in low-income communities and that may increase susceptibility to indoor pollution exposure.
Harvard University	■ Focus on multiple health outcomes across the life course with evidence for environmental health disparities (birth outcomes, childhood growth rates, and cardiovascular mortality). ■ Study the influence of housing and the neighborhood environment on multiple exposures and health outcomes.
University of New Mexico	■ Address the environmental health disparities experienced by the Native American population. ■ Examine and compare mechanisms of toxicity in mining waste metal mixtures of different composition across Navajo, Sioux, and Crow populations. ■ Study the distribution of contaminants, cultural practices, and genetic origins of the three tribes to sort out the health effects of metal mixtures in tribal communities.

In Summary

Everyone should be concerned about the environment in which we live. The choices we make can have consequences for a very, very long time. But for some of the issues raised, there isn't one "right" answer. For example, one might consider organic farming better because it doesn't use pesticides. On the other hand, conventional farming produces more food per acre, which is important when you consider how many people there are in the world and that they all need to eat. It is important to understand the balance between the benefits of pesticides (that they help prevent serious diseases) and the risks of pesticides (that exposure can harm people).

Selecting the source of our energy requires that we, as a society, make some hard choices. While burning fossil fuels in the short term may be the least expensive option, in the long run it is not the wisest choice. Aside from the fact that we are using up a nonrenewable source, we are destroying the planet and making the quality of the air we breathe less healthy.

Using water safely is critical to fruit and vegetable production. Farmers who raise animals, particularly on a large scale, must deal with animal waste products to avoid endangering public health. Farm workers need to maintain their own health to prevent transmitting illness to the public.

You have read about how to prepare for natural disasters. If you live in an area prone to disasters, being prepared may make a huge difference in the future.

Every day we make choices about whether we recycle. The more we recycle, the better it is for the environment. Plastic bottles and other plastic items are particularly important to recycle so they don't end up polluting the oceans. Choosing to drink tap water is clearly better for the environment, but sometimes it is not an option. If you buy bottled water, make sure you recycle your bottles.

As the environmentally conscious say, "Reduce, repair, reuse, recycle."

Key Terms

air pollution
bioplastics
carbon dioxide
carcinogens
conventional farming
dead zone
environmental tobacco smoke exposure
fossil fuels
Great Pacific Garbage Patch
greenhouse gases
gyre
methane
nuclear energy
organic farming
ozone
particulates
pesticides
radon
sick building syndrome
solar power
wind power

Student Discussion Questions and Activities

1. In thinking about the benefits and trade-offs of conventional versus organic farming, which type of farming do you think is the right choice? Why?
2. Think about how much plastic you use in a day. How much do you recycle, and how much do you throw away? What ideas do you have to minimize the amount of plastic you use?

3. This chapter discusses various sources of energy, including fossil fuels, nuclear power, solar power, and wind power. Which do you think is the right choice? (Note, there is no one right choice.) Do you think the United States will move away from burning fossil fuels?
4. What actions do you take to minimize your personal contribution to global warming? Are there any new actions suggested in this chapter that you can adopt? What can you do to minimize global warming?
5. Do you drink bottled water regularly? Does it taste better than tap water? Does the likelihood that you are paying an inflated price for tap water when you buy bottled water change your mind about buying bottled water?
6. Do you live in an area prone to any natural disasters, such as Tornado Alley or coastal areas prone to earthquakes? Even if you don't, emergencies can happen. Do you have an emergency plan? Create one for yourself.

References

1. U.S. Energy Information Administration. (2018). What is U.S. electricity generation by energy source? Retrieved from https://www.eia.gov/tools/faqs/faq.cfm?id=427&t=3
2. U.S. Energy Information Administration. (2017). Energy in brief: What are the major sources and users of energy in the United States? Retrieved from http://www.eia.gov/energy_in_brief/article/major_energy_sources_and_users.cfm
3. Jackson, R. B., Vengosh, A., Carey, J. W., Davies, R., Darrah, T. H., O'Sullivan, S., & Petron, G. (2014). The environmental costs and benefits of fracking. *Annual Review of Environment and Resources, 39*(1), 327–362.
4. National Aeronautics and Space Administration. (2016). What is the sun's lifetime going to be? Retrieved from http://image.gsfc.nasa.gov/poetry/ask/a10395.html
5. U.S. Department of Energy. (2005). Basic research needs for solar energy utilization. Retrieved from http://science.energy.gov/~/media/bes/pdf/reports/files/Basic_Research_Needs_for_Solar_Energy_Utilization_rpt.pdf
6. Bullis, K. (2014). Smart wind and solar power. *MIT Technology Review.* Retrieved from https://www.technologyreview.com/s/526541/smart-wind-and-solar-power/
7. Jalali, L., Nezhad-Ahmadi, M. R., Gohari, M., Bigelow, P., & McColl, S. (2016). The impact of psychological factors on self-reported sleep disturbance among people living in the vicinity of wind turbines. *Environmental Research, 148*, 401–410.
8. Michaud, D. S., Feder, K., Keith, S. E., Voicescu, S. A., Marro, L., Than, J., . . . van den Berg, F. (2016). Exposure to wind turbine noise: Perceptual responses and reported health effects. *Journal of the Acoustical Society of America, 139*(3), 1443.
9. Conserve Energy Future. (2016). Wind energy: Pros and cons of wind energy. Retrieved from http://www.conserve-energy-future.com/pros-and-cons-of-wind-energy.php
10. Reference: Jiang, Z. (2011). Nuclear Power Development for Greenhouse Gas Emission Reduction in China. Advances in Climate Change Research. 2(2):75–78
11. Conserve Energy Future. (2016). Nuclear energy pros and cons. Retrieved from http://www.conserve-energy-future.com/pros-and-cons-of-nuclear-energy.php
12. U.S. Nuclear Regulation Commission. (2015). Operating nuclear power reactors (by location or name). Retrieved from http://www.nrc.gov/info-finder/reactors/
13. U.S. Nuclear Regulation Commission. (2015). Low-level waste. Retrieved from http://www.nrc.gov/waste/low-level-waste.html
14. Hatch, M. C., Beyea, J., Nieves, J. W., & Susser, M. (1990). Cancer near the Three Mile Island nuclear plant: Radiation emissions. *American Journal of Epidemiology, 132*(3), 397–412; discussion 413–417.
15. U.S. Nuclear Regulatory Commission. (2013). Backgrounder on the Three Mile Island accident. Retrieved from http://www.nrc.gov/reading-rm/doc-collections/fact-sheets/3mile-isle.html.
16. Fairlie, I., & Sumner, D. (2006). The other report on Chernobyl (TORCH). Retrieved from http://www.chernobylreport.org/?p=summary
17. Kashcheev, V. V., Chekin, S. Y., Maksioutov, M. A., Tumanov, K. A., Kochergina, E. V., Kashcheeva, P. V., . . . Ivanov, V. K. (2015). Incidence and mortality of solid cancer among emergency workers of the Chernobyl accident: Assessment of radiation risks for the follow-up period of 1992–2009. *Radiation and Environmental Biophysics, 54*(1), 13–23.
18. Lallanilla, M. (2013, September 25). Chernobyl: Facts about the nuclear disaster. Retrieved from http://www.livescience.com/39961-chernobyl.html
19. Starr, S. (2012). Costs and consequences of the Fukushima Daiichi disaster—physicians for social responsibility. Physicians for Social Responsibility. Retrieved from http://www.psr.org/environment-and-health/environmental-health-policy-institute/responses/costs-and-consequences-of-fukushima.html
20. University of Washington, Environmental Health and Safety. (n.d.). Radioactive decay calculator. Retrieved from https://www.ehs.washington.edu/rso/calculator/activity_calc.shtm
21. Penn State Extension Farm Food Safety Team, Penn State Extension and Penn State Department of Food Science. (2015). Safe uses of agricultural water. Retrieved from http://extension.psu.edu/food/safety/farm/gaps/safe-uses-of-agricultural-water
22. Sobsey, M. D., Khatib, L. A., Hill, V. R., Alocilja, E., & Pillai, S. (2006). Pathogens in animal wastes and the impacts of waste management practices on their survival, transport and fate. Retrieved from http://fyi.uwex.edu/manureirrigation/files/2014/03/ASABE_2006_Pathogens-in-Animal-Wastes-and-Impacts-of-Waste-Management-Practices.pdf
23. National Institutes of Health. (2016). Tox Town: Animal waste. Retrieved from https://toxtown.nlm.nih.gov/text_version/locations.php?id=4

24. State Compensation Insurance Fund. (2016). Manure pits. Retrieved from http://content.statefundca.com//safety/safetymeeting/SafetyMeetingArticle.aspx?ArticleID=431
25. Knoblauch, A., & Steiner, B. (1999). Major accidents related to manure: A case series from Switzerland. *International Journal of Occupational and Environmental Health, 5*(3), 177–186.
26. Schwab, C. V., Lorimor, J., & Miller, L. (1993). Manure storage poses invisible risks. National Ag Safety Database. Retrieved from http://nasdonline.dev.conceptualarts.com:8080/1265/d001069/manure-storage-poses-invisible-risks.html
27. Penn State Extension. (2015). Food safety: Worker health and hygiene. Retrieved from http://extension.psu.edu/food/safety/farm/gaps/worker-health-and-hygiene
28. Lucey, J. (2015). Personal hygiene and food safety tips. Food Quality and Safety. Retrieved from http://www.foodqualityandsafety.com/article/personal-hygiene-and-food-safety/
29. Occupational Safety and Health Administration. (2016). Agricultural operations: Hazards and controls. Retrieved from https://www.osha.gov/dsg/topics/agriculturaloperations/hazards_controls.html
30. The Produce Traceability Initiative. (2016). The PTI vision: Supply chain-wide adoption of electronic traceability. Retrieved from http://www.producetraceability.org/
31. FoodSafety.gov. (2016). 50 years of Super Bowl and food safety changes. Retrieved from http://www.foodsafety.gov/blog/2016/01/50-years.html
32. Centers for Disease Control and Prevention. (2015). Show me the science—how to wash your hands. Retrieved from http://www.cdc.gov/handwashing/show-me-the-science-handwashing.html
33. Larson, L. (2015, January 19). Seven myths about washing your produce. Modern Farmer. Retrieved from http://modernfarmer.com/2015/01/7-myths-washing-produce/
34. Center for Food Safety. (2016). The truth about produce wash. Retrieved from http://www.centerforfoodsafety.org/healthy-home/3274/cfs-healthy-home/tips-for-a-healthy-home/3474/the-truth-about-produce-wash#
35. Goldenberg, S. (2016, July 13). Half of all US food produce is thrown away, new research suggests. *The Guardian*. Retrieved from https://www.theguardian.com/environment/2016/jul/13/us-food-waste-ugly-fruit-vegetables-perfect?CMP=share_btn_tw
36. U.S. Environmental Protection Agency. (n.d.). Reducing wasted food at home. Retrieved from https://www.epa.gov/recycle/reducing-wasted-food-home
37. U.S. Department of Agriculture. (2004). Organic certification: How does USDA define the term organic? Retrieved from http://www.usda.gov/wps/portal/usda/usdahome?parentnav=FAQS_BYTOPIC&FAQ_NAVIGATION_ID=ORGANIC_FQ&FAQ_NAVIGATION_TYPE=FAQS_BYTOPIC&contentid=faqdetail-3.xml&edeployment_action=retrievecontent
38. U.S. Food and Drug Administration. (2016). About FDA: What is the meaning of "natural" on the label of food? Retrieved from http://www.fda.gov/aboutfda/transparency/basics/ucm214868.htm
39. U.S. Department of Agriculture. (2007). Sustainable agriculture: Definitions and terms. Alternative Farming Systems Information Center. Retrieved from http://afsic.nal.usda.gov/sustainable-agriculture-definitions-and-terms-1
40. National Oceanic and Atmospheric Administration. (2014). What is a dead zone? Retrieved from http://oceanservice.noaa.gov/facts/deadzone.html
41. Pettis, J. S., Lichtenberg, E. M., Andree, M., Stitzinger, J., Rose, R., & vanEngelsdorp, D. (2013). Crop pollination exposes honey bees to pesticides which alters their susceptibility to the gut pathogen *Nosema ceranae*. *PloS One, 8*(7), e70182.
42. Tuomisto, H. L., Hodge, I. D., Riordan, P., & Macdonald, D. W. (2012). Does organic farming reduce environmental impacts? A meta-analysis of European research. *Journal of Environmental Management, 112*, 309–320.
43. Palmer, B. (2012, November 12). Organic vs. conventional farming: Which uses less energy? *Washington Post*.
44. Centers for Disease Control and Prevention. (2018). Malaria. Retrieved from http://www.cdc.gov/malaria/index.html
45. Alarcon, W. A., Calvert, G. M., Blondell, J. M., Mehler, L. N., Sievert, J., Propeck, M., . . . Stanbury, M. (2005). Acute illnesses associated with pesticide exposure at schools. *JAMA, 294*(4), 455.
46. Sanborn, M., Kerr, K. J., Sanin, L. H., Cole, D. C., Bassil, K. L., & Vakil, C. (2007). Non-cancer health effects of pesticides. *Canadian Family Physician, 53*, 1712–1720.
47. Bassil, K. L., Vakil, C., Sanborn, M., Cole, D. C., Kaur, J. S., & Kerr, K. J. (2007). Cancer health effects of pesticides. *Canadian Family Physician, 53*, 1704–1711.
48. Landrigan, P. J., Claudio, L., Markowitz, S. B., Berkowitz, G. S., Benner, B. L., Romero, H., . . . Wolff, M. S. (1999). Pesticides and inner-city children: Exposures, risks, and prevention. *Environmental Health Perspectives, 107*(Suppl 3), 431–437.
49. U.S. Department of Agriculture. (2016). Pesticide Data Program. Retrieved from https://www.ams.usda.gov/datasets/pdp.
50. Consumer Reports. (2015). Pesticides in produce. Retrieved from http://www.consumerreports.org/cro/health/natural-health/pesticides/index.htm?loginMethod=auto©rightYear=2016
51. Environmental Working Group. (2016). The EWG's 2016 shopper's guide to pesticides in produce. Retrieved from https://www.ewg.org/foodnews/summary.php
52. Rodwan, J. G. (2014). Bottled water 2013: Sustaining vitality. *Bottled Water Reporter*, 12–22.
53. Statistic Brain. (2015). Bottled water industry statistics. Retrieved from http://www.statisticbrain.com/bottled-water-statistics/
54. Postman, A. (2016, January 5). The truth about tap. Natural Resources Defense Council. Retrieved from https://www.nrdc.org/stories/truth-about-tap
55. Consumer Reports. (2011). Bottled water doesn't mean better. Retrieved from http://www.consumerreports.org/cro/magazine-archive/2011/september/food/bottled-water/overview/index.htm
56. Zeratsky, K. (2015). Is tap water as safe as bottled water? Mayo Clinic. Retrieved from http://www.mayoclinic.org/healthy-lifestyle/nutrition-and-healthy-eating/expert-answers/tap-vs-bottled-water/faq-20058017
57. U.S. Environmental Protection Agency. (2014). Population served by community water systems with no reported violations of health-based standards. Retrieved from https://cfpub.epa.gov/roe/indicator.cfm?i=45
58. Teillet, E., Urbano, C., Cordelle, S., & Schlich, P. (2010). Consumer perception and preference of bottled and tap water. *Journal of Sensory Studies, 25*(3), 463–480.
59. Wells, D. L. (2005). The identification and perception of bottled water. *Perception, 34*(10), 1291–1292.
60. Consumer Reports. (2016). Water filter buying guide. Retrieved from http://www.consumerreports.org/cro/water-filters/buying-guide.htm.

61. U.S. Environmental Protection Agency. (2009, December). Office of Water. Water on tap: What you need to know. Retrieved from http://www.bottledwater.org/files/EPA%20Water%20on%20Tap%20(2009).pdf
62. U.S. Environmental Protection Agency. (2016). Ground water and drinking water. Retrieved from http://www.epa.gov/your-drinking-water
63. WebMD. (2016). Safe drinking water: Tap water, bottled water, and water filters. Retrieved from http://www.webmd.com/women/home-health-and-safety-9/safe-drinking-water#2
64. U.S. Environmental Protection Agency. (2016). Safe drinking water hotline. Retrieved from https://www.epa.gov/ground-water-and-drinking-water/safe-drinking-water-hotline
65. Longley, K. (2011). Emergency manager Michael Brown appointed to lead Flint through second state takeover. *Michigan Live*. Retrieved from http://www.mlive.com/news/flint/index.ssf/2011/11/emergency_manager_michael_brow.html
66. Cavanaugh, P. (2011). Analysis of the Flint River as a permanent water supply for the city of Flint. Retrieved from https://www.scribd.com/doc/64381765/Analysis-of-the-Flint-River-as-a-Permanent-Water-Supply-for-the-City-of-Flint-July-2011
67. Smith, L. (2015, December 17). Reporter's notebook: Some state officials still in denial or misinformed over Flint River decision. Michigan Radio. Retrieved from http://michiganradio.org/post/reporter-s-notebook-some-state-officials-still-denial-or-misinformed-over-flint-river-decision#stream/0
68. Brush, M., Williams, R., Smith, L., & Scullen, L. (2015, December 21). Timeline: Here's how the Flint water crisis unfolded. Michigan Radio. Retrieved from http://michiganradio.org/post/timeline-heres-how-flint-water-crisis-unfolded#stream/0
69. City of Flint, Michigan. (2014). City of Flint 2014: Annual water quality report. Retrieved from https://www.cityofflint.com/wp-content/uploads/CCR-2014.pdf
70. U.S. Census Bureau. (2016). QuickFacts: Flint City, Michigan. Retrieved from http://www.census.gov/quickfacts/table/PST045215/2629000
71. Trounstine, J. (2016, February 8). How racial segregation and political mismanagement led to Flint's shocking water crisis. *Washington Post*.
72. Lin, J. C. F., Rutter, J., & Park, H. (2016, January 21). Events that led to Flint's water crisis. *New York Times*. Retrieved from https://www.nytimes.com/interactive/2016/01/21/us/flint-lead-water-timeline.html
73. Centers for Disease Control and Prevention. (2016). Lead. Retrieved from http://www.cdc.gov/nceh/lead/
74. MedLine Plus. (2016). Lead poisoning. U.S. National Library of Medicine. Retrieved from https://www.nlm.nih.gov/medlineplus/ency/article/002473.htm
75. Gupta, S., Tinker, B., & Hume, T. (2016, January 22). Flint doctor's fight to expose lead poisoning. CNN.com. Retrieved from http://www.cnn.com/2016/01/21/health/flint-water-mona-hanna-attish/
76. Michigan Radio Newsroom & Shaffer, C. (2016, July 8). Federal court allows Flint lead lawsuit to proceed. Michigan Radio. Retrieved from http://michiganradio.org/post/federal-court-allows-flint-lead-lawsuit-proceed
77. Dennis, B. (2016, December 20). Four more officials charged with felonies in Flint water crisis. *The Washington Post*. Retrieved from https://www.washingtonpost.com/news/energy-environment/wp/2016/12/20/four-more-officials-charged-with-felonies-in-flint-water-crisis/?utm_term=.43068baf9dc3
78. Lo, T. (2017, February 3). Flint class action lawsuit thrown out by federal judge. *JDJournal*. Retrieved from http://www.jdjournal.com/2017/02/03/flint-class-action-lawsuit-thrown-out-by-federal-judge/
79. Berman, M., & Dennis, B. (2017, January 24). Flint water falls below federal lead limits, but residents are still asked to use filtered water. *The Washington Post*. Retrieved from https://www.washingtonpost.com/news/post-nation/wp/2017/01/24/flint-water-falls-below-federal-lead-limits-but-residents-still-asked-to-use-filtered-water/?utm_term=.870d32b23627
80. O'Connor, K. (2011, October 31). The impact of plastic water bottles. Postconsumers.com. Retrieved from http://www.postconsumers.com/education/how-long-does-it-take-a-plastic-bottle-to-biodegrade/
81. Ban the Bottle. (n.d.). Bottled water facts. Retrieved from https://www.banthebottle.net/bottled-water-facts/
82. Gleick, P. H., & Cooley, H. S. (2009). Energy implications of bottled water. *Environmental Research Letters, 4*(1).
83. Elua.com. (2013). Bottled water and our environment. Retrieved from http://elua.com/wp-content/uploads/2013/08/Elua-Bottled-Water-and-Our-Environment.pdf.
84. U.S. Department of Energy. (2016). Reduce climate change. Retrieved from http://www.fueleconomy.gov/feg/climate.shtml
85. Karl, D. M. (1999). A sea of change: Biogeochemical variability in the North Pacific Subtropical Gyre. *Ecosystems, 2*, 181–214.
86. National Geographic Society. (2016). Great Pacific Garbage Patch. Retrieved from http://nationalgeographic.org/encyclopedia/great-pacific-garbage-patch/
87. Woodford, C. (2016, June 8). Bioplastics and biodegradable plastics. Explain That Stuff. Retrieved from http://www.explainthatstuff.com/bioplastics.html
88. Barrett, M. (2013, February 6). Your guide to plastic recycling symbols: The numbers on plastic. Natural Society. Retrieved from http://naturalsociety.com/recycling-symbols-numbers-plastic-bottles-meaning/
89. Reuseit. (2015, May 27). Facts about the plastic bag pandemic. Retrieved from http://www.reuseit.com/blog/Facts-About-the-Plastic-Bag-Pandemic/
90. National Conference of State Legislators. (2016). State plastic and paper bag legislation. Retrieved from http://www.ncsl.org/research/environment-and-natural-resources/plastic-bag-legislation.aspx
91. Green Education Foundation. (2016). Tips to use less plastic. Retrieved from http://www.greeneducationfoundation.org/nationalgreenweeksub/waste-reduction-tips/tips-to-use-less-plastic.html
92. Intergovernmental Panel on Climate Change. (2007). Climate change 2007: Synthesis report; Summary for policy makers. Retrieved from http://www.ipcc.ch/pdf/assessment-report/ar4/syr/ar4_syr_spm.pdf
93. Intergovernmental Panel on Climate Change. (2013). Climate change 2013: The physical science basis; Summary for policymakers. Retrieved from https://www.ipcc.ch/pdf/assessment-report/ar5/wg1/WGIAR5_SPM_brochure_en.pdf
94. *National Geographic*. (2016). Sea level rise. Retrieved from http://ocean.nationalgeographic.com/ocean/critical-issues-sea-level-rise/
95. Down to Earth Climate Change. (2016). Global climate change: Evidence and causes. Retrieved from http://globalclimate.ucr.edu/resources.html

96. Samenow, J. (2016, November 2). Polar vortex shifting due to climate change, extending winter, study finds. *The Washington Post*. Retrieved from https://www.washingtonpost.com/news/capital-weather-gang/wp/2016/10/31/polar-vortex-shifting-due-to-climate-change-extending-winter-study-finds/?utm_term=.41836bb8bf89
97. Cornell University. (2017). What is a polar vortex? Cornell Climate Change. Retrieved from http://climatechange.cornell.edu/what-is-a-polar-vortex/
98. Davenport, C. (2015, December 13). Nations approve landmark climate accord in Paris. *New York Times*. Retrieved from https://www.nytimes.com/2015/12/13/world/europe/climate-change-accord-paris.html?_r=0
99. Center for Climate and Energy Solutions. (2016). Outcomes of the U.N. climate change conference in Paris. Retrieved from http://www.c2es.org/international/negotiations/cop21-paris/summary
100. The Associated Press-NORC Center for Public Affairs Research. (2017, June). Views on the Paris Climate Agreement. Retrieved from http://www.apnorc.org/projects/Pages/Views-on-Paris-Agreement.aspx
101. U.S. Environmental Protection Agency. (2016). Retrieved from https://www3.epa.gov/climatechange/wycd/
102. U.S. Environmental Protection Agency. (n.d.). Light bulbs. Retrieved from https://www.energystar.gov/products/lighting_fans/light_bulbs
103. U.S. Environmental Protection Agency. (2016). Fuel economy. Retrieved from https://www.epa.gov/fuel-economy
104. World Meteorological Organization. (2010). WMO: Unprecedented sequence of extreme weather events. PreventionWeb.net. Retrieved from http://www.preventionweb.net/news/view/14970
105. Noack, R. (2015, July 22). Europe to America: Your love of air-conditioning is stupid. *The Washington Post*.
106. Robine, J. M., Cheung, S. L., Le Roy, S., Van Oyen, H., Griffiths, C., Michel, J. P., & Herrmann, H. R. (2008). Death toll exceeded 70,000 in Europe during the summer of 2003. *Comptes Rendus Biologies, 331*(2), 171–178.
107. National Centers for Environmental Information. (2016). U.S. billion-dollar weather and climate disasters. Retrieved from http://www.ncdc.noaa.gov/billions/events
108. World Health Organization. (2016). Climate change and health. Retrieved from http://www.who.int/mediacentre/factsheets/fs266/en/
109. Edenhofer, O., Pichs-Madruga, R., Sokona, Y., Farahani, E., Kadner, S., Seyboth, K., . . . Minx, J. C. (2014). Climate change 2014: Mitigation of climate change. Contribution of Working Group III to the Fifth Assessment Report of the Intergovernmental Panel on Climate Change. Retrieved from https://www.ipcc.ch/pdf/assessment-report/ar5/wg3/ipcc_wg3_ar5_full.pdf
110. American Public Health Association. (n.d.). Extreme rainfall and drought. Retrieved from http://www.cdc.gov/climateandhealth/pubs/precip-final_508.pdf
111. On the Cutting Edge. (2012). The health effects of Hurricane Katrina. Retrieved from https://serc.carleton.edu/NAGTWorkshops/health/case_studies/hurricane_Katrina.html
112. McMichael, A. J. (2015). Extreme weather events and infectious disease outbreaks. *Virulence, 6*(6), 543–547.
113. Chan, C. S., & Rhodes, J. E. (2014). Measuring exposure in Hurricane Katrina: A meta-analysis and an integrative data analysis. *PLoS One, 9*(4), e92899.
114. Mogul, F. (2012, November 19). 4 NYC hospitals still closed by Hurricane Sandy. Medpage Today. Retrieved from http://www.medpagetoday.com/publichealthpolicy/generalprofessionalissues/36013
115. Burling, S., & Urgo, J. L. (2015, July 30). Report: Health effects of Hurricane Sandy still linger. *Philadelphia Inquirer*. Retrieved from http://www.emergencymgmt.com/disaster/Report-Health-effects-of-Hurricane-Sandy-still-linger.html
116. World Health Organization. (2015). 10 facts on malaria. Retrieved from http://www.who.int/features/factfiles/malaria/en/
117. Vos, T., Flaxman, A. D., Naghavi, M., Lozano, R., Michaud, C., Ezzat, M., . . . Memish, Z. A. (2012). Years lived with disability (YLDs) for 1160 sequelae of 289 diseases and injuries 1990–2010: A systematic analysis for the Global Burden of Disease Study 2010. *Lancet*, (9859), 2163–2196
118. World Health Organization. (2016). Lymphatic filariasis. Retrieved from http://www.who.int/mediacentre/factsheets/fs102/en/
119. World Health Organization. (2016). Leishmaniasis. Retrieved from http://www.who.int/mediacentre/factsheets/fs375/en/
120. Nettleman, M. D. (2015, November 5). Onchocerciasis: Background. Retrieved from http://webcache.googleusercontent.com/search?q=cache:T6Ge0CcOJM4J:emedicine.medscape.com/article/224309-overview+&cd=1&hl=en&ct=clnk&gl=us
121. Pan American Health Organization & World Health Organization. (2016). Chagas disease. Retrieved from http://www.paho.org/hq/index.php?option=com_topics&view=article&id=10&Itemid=40743
122. Brady, O. J., Gething, P. W., Bhatt, S., Messina, J. P., Brownstein, J. S., Hoen, A. G., . . . Hay, S. I. (2012). Refining the global spatial limits of dengue virus transmission by evidence-based consensus. *PLoS Neglected Tropical Disease, 6*(8), e1760.
123. World Health Organization. (2016). Yellow fever. Retrieved from http://www.who.int/mediacentre/factsheets/fs100/en/
124. Centers for Disease Control and Prevention. (2016). Preliminary maps and data for 2015. West Nile Virus. Retrieved from http://www.cdc.gov/westnile/statsmaps/preliminarymapsdata/index.html
125. Nelson, C., Saha, S., Kugeler, K. J., Delorey, M. J., Shankar, M. B., Hinckley, A. P., & Mead, P. S. (2015). Incidence of clinician-diagnosed Lyme disease, United States, 2005–2010. *Emerging Infectious Diseases, 21*(9), 1625–1631.
126. U.S. Environmental Protection Agency. (2015). Climate change indicators in the United States. Retrieved from https://www3.epa.gov/climatechange/science/indicators/health-society/lyme.html
127. GRID Arendal. (2016). Vital climate graphics: Spread of major tropical vector-borne diseases. United Nations Environment Programme. Retrieved from http://www.grida.no/publications/vg/climate/page/3093.aspx
128. Hales, S., Kovats, S., Lloyd, S., & Campbell-Lendrum, D. (2014). Quantitative risk assessment of the effects of climate change on selected causes of death, 2030s and 2050s. World Health Organization. Retrieved from http://apps.who.int/iris/bitstream/10665/134014/1/9789241507691_eng.pdf?ua
129. MedlinePlus. (2016). Indoor air pollution. U.S. National Library of Medicine. Retrieved from https://www.nlm.nih.gov/medlineplus/indoorairpollution.html
130. U.S. Environmental Protection Agency. (2015). Guide to air cleaners in the home. Retrieved from https://www.epa.gov/indoor-air-quality-iaq/guide-air-cleaners-home#indoor-air
131. Butz, A. M., Matsui, E. C., Breysse, P., Curtin-Brosnan, J., Eggleston, P., Diette, G., . . . Rand, C. (2011). A randomized trial of air cleaners and a health coach to improve indoor air quality for inner-city children with asthma and secondhand

smoke exposure. *Archives of Pediatrics and Adolescent Medicine, 165*(8), 741–748.

132. U.S. Department of Health and Human Services. (2006). *The health consequences of involuntary exposure to tobacco smoke: A report of the Surgeon General.* Atlanta, GA: Centers for Disease Control and Prevention, National Center for Chronic Disease Prevention and Health Promotion, Office on Smoking and Health.
133. Centers for Disease Control and Prevention. (2010). A report of the Surgeon General: How tobacco smoke causes disease: What it means to you. Retrieved from https://www.cdc.gov/tobacco/data_statistics/sgr/2010/consumer_booklet/pdfs/consumer.pdf
134. U.S. Department of Health and Human Services. (2014). The health consequences of Smoking—50 years of progress: A report of the Surgeon General. Retrieved from http://www.surgeongeneral.gov/library/reports/50-years-of-progress/
135. Agency for Toxic Substances and Disease Registry. (2014). ToxFAQs for vinyl chloride. Retrieved from http://www.atsdr.cdc.gov/toxfaqs/tf.asp?id=281&tid=51
136. National Cancer Institute. (2011). Formaldehyde and cancer risk. Retrieved from http://www.cancer.gov/about-cancer/causes-prevention/risk/substances/formaldehyde/formaldehyde-fact-sheet
137. Agency for Toxic Substances and Disease Registry. (2015). ToxFAQs for N-nitrosodimethylamine. National Institutes of Health. Retrieved from http://www.atsdr.cdc.gov/toxfaqs/tf.asp?id=883&tid=173
138. Agency for Toxic Substances and Disease Registry. (2011). ToxFAQs for acrylonitrile. Retrieved from http://www.atsdr.cdc.gov/toxfaqs/TF.asp?id=446&tid=78
139. National Toxicology Program, Department of Health and Human Services. (2014). 2-naphthylamine. Retrieved from https://ntp.niehs.nih.gov/ntp/roc/content/profiles/naphthylamine.pdf
140. Feng, Z., Hu, W., Rom, W. N., Beland, F. A., & Tang, M. S. (2002). 4-aminobiphenyl is a major etiological agent of human bladder cancer: Evidence from its DNA binding spectrum in human p53 gene. *Carcinogenesis, 23*(10), 1721–1727.
141. Schick, S., & Glantz, S. (2005). Philip Morris toxicological experiments with fresh sidestream smoke: More toxic than mainstream smoke. *Tobacco Control, 14*, 396–404.
142. Centers for Disease Control and Prevention. (2015). Vital signs: Secondhand smoke infographics. Retrieved from http://www.cdc.gov/vitalsigns/tobacco/infographic.html
143. Arheart, K. L., Lee, D. J., Dietz, N. A., Wilkinson, J. D., Clark, J. D., III, LeBlanc, W. G., . . . Fleming, L. E. (2008). Declining trends in serum cotinine levels in U.S. worker groups: The power of policy. *Journal of Occupational and Environmental Medicine, 50*(1), 57–63.
144. Toxics Use Reduction Institute. (2011). Ten tips to improve indoor air quality. Retrieved from http://www.turi.org/TURI_Publications/Tip_Sheet_Series/Ten_Tips_to_Improve_Indoor_Air_Quality
145. NIH News in Health. (2014). Stop the spread of superbugs. National Institutes of Health. Retrieved from https://newsinhealth.nih.gov/issue/feb2014/feature1
146. Agency for Toxic Substances and Disease Registry. (2013). Tetrachloroethylene toxicity. Retrieved from http://www.atsdr.cdc.gov/csem/csem.asp?csem=14&po=10
147. U.S. Environmental Protection Agency. (1991). Indoor Air Facts No. 4 (revised): Sick building syndrome. Retrieved from https://www.epa.gov/sites/production/files/2014-08/documents/sick_building_factsheet.pdf
148. Legionnaire's disease may be spread by water. (1978, October 3). *Wilmington Star News.*
149. Kotulak, R. (1986, August 31). Legionnaires disease less mysterious, still deadly. *Chicago Tribune.*
150. Joshi, S. M. (2008). The sick building syndrome. *Indian Journal of Occupational and Environmental Medicine, 12*(2), 61–64.
151. American Society of Heating, Refrigeration, and Air-Conditioning Engineers, Inc. (2010). Ventilation for acceptable indoor air quality (ASHRAE 62.1-2010). Retrieved from https://www.techstreet.com/ashrae/standards/ashrae-62-1-2010?gateway_code=ashrae&product_id=1720986
152. U.S. Environmental Protection Agency. (2015). Initial list of hazardous air pollutants with modifications. Retrieved from https://www.epa.gov/haps/initial-list-hazardous-air-pollutants-modifications
153. Ekenga, C. C., & Friedman-Jimenez, G. (2011). Epidemiology of respiratory health outcomes among World Trade Center disaster workers: Review of the literature 10 years after the September 11, 2001 terrorist attacks. *Disaster Medicine and Public Health Preparedness,* 5(Suppl 2), S189–S196.
154. NYC 9/11 Health. (2016). A Message from the Commissioner of the New York City Department of Health and Mental Hygiene. Retrieved from http://home.nyc.gov/html/doh/wtc/html/know/know.shtml
155. National Interagency Fire Center. (2014). 2013 national report on state and agency fires and acres burned. Retrieved from http://www.nifc.gov/fireInfo/fireInfo_stats_YTD2013.html
156. Sappenfield, M. (2010, April 18). Five biggest volcano eruptions in recent history. CSMonitor.com. Retrieved from http://www.csmonitor.com/Science/2010/0418/Five-biggest-volcano-eruptions-in-recent-history
157. Goldenberg, S. (2014, April 29). Almost half of Americans live with unhealthy levels of air pollution. *The Guardian.* Retrieved from https://www.theguardian.com/environment/2014/apr/30/americans-unhealthy-levels-air-pollution
158. Centers for Disease Control and Prevention. (2016). FastStats: Asthma. Retrieved from http://www.cdc.gov/nchs/fastats/asthma.htm
159. Aligne, C. A., Auinger, P., Byrd, R. S., & Weitzman, M. (2000). Risk factors for pediatric asthma. Contributions of poverty, race, and urban residence. *American Journal of Respiratory and Critical Care Medicine, 162*(3 Pt 1), 873–877
160. Schultz, E. S., Hallberg, J., Bellander, T., Bergstrom, A., Bottai, M., Chiesa, F., . . . Melen, E. (2016). Early-life exposure to traffic-related air pollution and lung function in adolescence. *American Journal of Respiratory and Critical Care Medicine, 193*(2), 171–177.
161. Barbosa, S., Bermudez, R., Cassmassi, J., Cheung, K., Eden, R., Lee, S.-M., . . . Zhang, X. (2015). Multiple Air Toxics Exposure Study in the South Coast air basin. Retrieved from http://www.aqmd.gov/docs/default-source/air-quality/air-toxic-studies/mates-iv/mates-iv-final-draft-report-4-1-15.pdf?sfvrsn=7
162. Wargo, J. (2006). *The harmful effects of vehicle exhaust: A case for policy change.* North Haven, CT: Environment and Human Health. U.S. Environmental Protection Agency. (2016). Criteria air pollutants. Retrieved from https://www.epa.gov/criteria-air-pollutants
163. *National Geographic.* (2016). Acid rain facts, acid rain information, acid rain pictures, acid rain effects. Retrieved from

http://environment.nationalgeographic.com/environment/global-warming/acid-rain-overview/

164. National Institutes of Health. (2016). Tox Town: Carbon dioxide. Retrieved from https://toxtown.nlm.nih.gov/text_version/chemicals.php?id=6
165. National Institutes of Health. (2016). Tox Town: Nitrogen oxides. Retrieved from https://toxtown.nlm.nih.gov/text_version/chemicals.php?id=19
166. National Institutes of Health. (2015). Tox Town: Volatile organic compounds (VOCs). Retrieved from https://toxtown.nlm.nih.gov/text_version/chemicals.php?id=31
167. U.S. Environmental Protection Agency. (n.d.). Particulate matter (PM) pollution. Retrieved from https://www.epa.gov/pm-pollution
168. National Institutes of Health. (2016). Tox Town: Particulate matter. Retrieved from https://toxtown.nlm.nih.gov/text_version/chemicals.php?id=21
169. U.S. Environmental Protection Agency. (n.d.). Ozone pollution. Retrieved from https://www.epa.gov/ozone-pollution
170. National Institutes of Health. (2016). Tox Town: Chlorofluorocarbons (CFCs). Retrieved from https://toxtown.nlm.nih.gov/text_version/chemicals.php?id=9
171. National Institutes of Health. (2016). Tox Town: Lead. Retrieved from https://toxtown.nlm.nih.gov/text_version/chemicals.php?id=16
172. National Institutes of Health. (2016). Tox Town: Cadmium. Retrieved from https://toxtown.nlm.nih.gov/text_version/chemicals.php?id=63
173. National Institutes of Health. (2016). Tox Town: Mercury. Retrieved from https://toxtown.nlm.nih.gov/text_version/chemicals.php?id=17
174. World Health Organization. (2016). Mercury and health. Retrieved from http://www.who.int/mediacentre/factsheets/fs361/en/
175. National Resources Defense Council. (2015). The smart seafood buying guide. Retrieved from https://www.nrdc.org/stories/smart-seafood-buying-guide?gclid=CjwKEAjwqpK8BRD7ua-U0orrgkESJADlN3YBgHJT3Y_SOVCTD2Bzs5BxrJsWPRrZfszhmpDdK0_PQxoCQ0vw_wcB
176. Prüss-Ustün, A., Wolf, J., Corvalán, C., Bos, R., & Neira, M. (2016). Preventing disease through healthy environments. World Health Organization. Retrieved from http://www.who.int/quantifying_ehimpacts/publications/preventingdisease.pdf
177. International Labour Organization. (n.d.). Introduction to occupational health and safety. Retrieved from http://training.itcilo.it/actrav_cdrom2/en/osh/intro/inmain.htm
178. Brown, J. R., & Thornton, J. L. (1957). Percivall Pott (1714–1788) and chimney sweepers' cancer of the scrotum. *British Journal of Independent Medicine, 14*(1), 68–70.
179. Bleeker, J. (2012). Occupational diseases. National Chimney Sweep Guild. Retrieved from http://www.ncsg.org/chimney_sweeps/occupational_diseases.aspx
180. Mayo Clinic Staff. (2014). Asbestosis: Causes. Mayo Clinic. Retrieved from http://www.mayoclinic.org/diseases-conditions/asbestosis/basics/causes/con-20019671
181. Mayo Clinic Staff. (2014). Asbestosis: Risk factors. Mayo Clinic. Retrieved from http://www.mayoclinic.org/diseases-conditions/asbestosis/basics/risk-factors/con-20019671
182. American Lung Association. (2016). Learn about silicosis. Retrieved from http://www.lung.org/lung-health-and-diseases/lung-disease-lookup/silicosis/learn-about-silicosis.html
183. Occupational and Health Safety Administration. (2005). Lead hazards. Retrieved from https://www.osha.gov/OshDoc/data_Hurricane_Facts/LeadHazards.pdf
184. Straif, K. (2008). The burden of occupational cancer. *Occupational and Environmental Medicine, 65*(12), 787–788.
185. U.S. Cancer Statistics Working Group. (2015). *1999–2012 incidence and mortality web-based report*. Retrieved from https://nccd.cdc.gov/uscs/
186. Boffetta, P. (2004). Epidemiology of environmental and occupational cancer. *Oncogene, 23*(38), 6392–6403.
187. Centers for Disease Control and Prevention. (2015). Cancer policy. NIOSH workplace safety and health topic. Retrieved from http://www.cdc.gov/niosh/topics/cancer/
188. Centers for Disease Control and Prevention. (2012). Occupational cancer. Carcinogen list. NIOSH safety and health topic. Retrieved from http://www.cdc.gov/niosh/topics/cancer/npotocca.html
189. Centers for Disease Control and Prevention. (2014). Tornadoes. Retrieved from http://emergency.cdc.gov/disasters/tornadoes/
190. Centers for Disease Control and Prevention. (2014). Landslides and mudslides. Retrieved from http://emergency.cdc.gov/disasters/landslides.asp
191. National Oceanic and Atmospheric Administration. (2011). Tornadoes 101. Retrieved from http://www.noaa.gov/stories/tornadoes-101
192. National Oceanic and Atmospheric Administration. (2016). NOAA weather radio all hazards. Retrieved from http://www.nws.noaa.gov/nwr/
193. Centers for Disease Control and Prevention. (2015). Natural disasters and severe weather: Mold after a disaster. Retrieved from http://emergency.cdc.gov/disasters/mold/index.asp
194. U.S. Environmental Protection Agency. (2016). Mold. Retrieved from https://www.epa.gov/mold
195. Centers for Disease Control and Prevention. (2014). NIOSH-approved N95 particulate filtering facepiece respirators. Retrieved from http://www.cdc.gov/niosh/npptl/topics/respirators/disp_part/n95list1.html
196. Centers for Disease Control and Prevention. (2014). Earthquakes. Retrieved from http://emergency.cdc.gov/disasters/earthquakes/index.asp
197. Centers for Disease Control and Prevention. (2013). Floods. Retrieved from http://emergency.cdc.gov/disasters/floods/
198. Centers for Disease Control and Prevention. (2015). Hurricanes and other tropical storms. Retrieved from http://emergency.cdc.gov/disasters/hurricanes/index.asp
199. Centers for Disease Control and Prevention. (2014). Lightning. Retrieved from http://emergency.cdc.gov/disasters/lightning/
200. Centers for Disease Control and Prevention. (2013). Tsunamis. Retrieved from http://emergency.cdc.gov/disasters/tsunamis/index.asp
201. NOAA Center for Tsunami Research (2005). FAQ results. Retrieved from http://nctr.pmel.noaa.gov/faq_display.php?kw=15
202. Centers for Disease Control and Prevention. (2015). Wildfires. Retrieved from http://emergency.cdc.gov/disasters/wildfires/index.asp
203. U.S. Forest Service. (n.d.). Fire. Retrieved from http://www.fs.fed.us/managing-land/fire

204. National Park Service. (n.d.). Understanding fire danger. Retrieved from https://www.nps.gov/fire/wildland-fire/learning-center/fire-in-depth/understanding-fire-danger.cfm
205. National Park Service. (n.d.). Global warming and wildfires. Retrieved from https://www.nwf.org/Wildlife/Threats-to-Wildlife/Global-Warming/Global-Warming-is-Causing-Extreme-Weather/Wildfires.aspx
206. Stange, E. E., & Ayres, M. P. (2010). Climate change impacts: Insects. *eLS*. Retrieved from http://www.els.net/WileyCDA/ElsArticle/refId-a0022555.html
207. Centers for Disease Control and Prevention. (2012). Volcanoes. Retrieved from http://emergency.cdc.gov/disasters/volcanoes/index.asp
208. U.S. Environmental Protection Agency. (2016). Environmental justice. Retrieved from https://www.epa.gov/environmentaljustice
209. National Resources Defense Council. (2016). The environmental justice movement. Retrieved from https://www.nrdc.org/stories/environmental-justice-movement
210. Downey, L., & Hawkins, B. (2008). Race, income, and environmental inequality in the United States. *Sociological Perspectives, 51*(4), 759–781.
211. Cushing, L., Faust, J., August, L. M., Cendak, R., Wieland, W., & Alexeeff, G. (2015). Racial/ethnic disparities in cumulative environmental health impacts in California: Evidence from a statewide environmental justice screening tool (CalEnviroScreen 1.1). *American Journal of Public Health, 105*(11), 2341–2348.
212. U.S. Environmental Protection Agency. (2016). Centers of excellence on environmental health disparities research. Retrieved from https://www.epa.gov/research-grants/centers-excellence-environmental-health-disparities-research

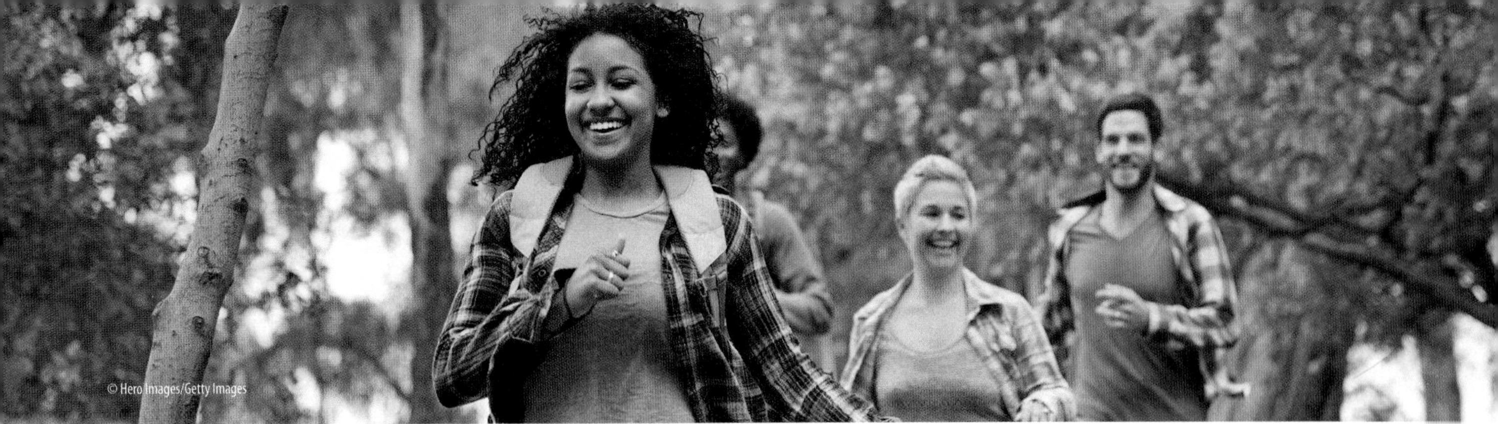
© Hero Images/Getty Images

CHAPTER 12

Aging, Dying, and Death

CHAPTER OBJECTIVES

- Review common physical and mental health problems that occur as we age, including dementia and depression.
- Describe what you can do to promote healthy aging.
- Recognize the importance of having all your information well organized.
- Explain the choices to be made in a living will.
- Describe palliative care and hospice care and the role each may play in the dying process.
- Discuss Medicare and insurance coverage issues regarding hospice care.
- Define grief, and describe the various ways people grieve.

TALKING ABOUT HOW WE DIE

"The sooner we start talking about how we die, the better."[1]
—**Jessica Nutik Zitter**, M.D., *New York Times*

Death occurs when all of the vital body functions stop, including the heartbeat, brain activity (including activity in the brain stem), and breathing. Death can come in many ways, whether at the end of a terminal illness or as the result of an unexpected accident. When someone has a terminal illness, the person, the person's family and friends, and the person's primary care providers generally have time to prepare for the impending death. When death comes from an unexpected accident or medical condition, the family and friends may not have the opportunity to say goodbye.

In 2016, there were 2,744,248 deaths in the United States, or 849.0 deaths per 100,000 members of the population. **Life expectancy** for the U.S. population was 78.6 years.[2] However, the main causes of death vary by age. As you can see in **TABLE 12-1**, for people between 1 and 44 years of age, the leading

life expectancy The number of years that an average person will live.

10 Leading causes of death by age group, United States - 2016

	Age Groups										
Rank	<1	1-4	5-9	10-14	15-24	25-34	35-44	45-54	55-64	65+	Total
1	Congenital anomalies 4,816	Unintentional injury 1,261	Unintentional injury 787	Unintentional injury 847	Unintentional injury 13,895	Unintentional injury 23,984	Unintentional injury 20,975	Malignant neoplasms 41,291	Malignant neoplasms 116,364	Heart disease 507,118	Heart disease 635,260
2	Short gestation 3,927	Congenital anomalies 433	Malignant neoplasms 449	Suicide 436	Suicide 5,723	Suicide 7,366	Malignant neoplasms 10,903	Heart disease 34,027	Heart disease 78,610	Malignant neoplasms 422,927	Malignant neoplasms 598,038
3	SIDS 1,500	Malignant neoplasms 377	Congenital anomalies 203	Malignant neoplasms 431	Homicide 5,172	Homicide 5,376	Heart disease 10,477	Unintentional injury 23,377	Unintentional injury 21,860	Chronic low. respiratory disease 131,002	Unintentional injury 161,374
4	Maternal pregnancy comp. 1,402	Homicide 339	Homicide 139	Homicide 147	Malignant neoplasms 1,431	Malignant neoplasms 3,791	Suicide 7,030	Suicide 8,437	Chronic low. respiratory disease 17,810	Cerebro-vascular 121,630	Chronic low. respiratory disease 154,596
5	Unintentional injury 1,219	Heart disease 118	Heart disease 77	Congenital anomalies 146	Heart disease 949	Heart disease 3,445	Homicide 3,369	Liver disease 8,364	Diabetes mellitus 14,251	Alzheimer's disease 114,883	Cerebro-vascular 142,142
6	Placenta cord. membranes 841	Influenza & pneumonia 103	Chronic low. respiratory disease 68	Heart disease 111	Congenital anomalies 388	Liver disease 925	Liver disease 2,851	Diabetes mellitus 6,267	Liver disease 13,448	Diabetes mellitus 56,452	Alzheimer's disease 116,103
7	Bacterial sepsis 583	Septicemia 70	Influenza & pneumonia 48	Chronic low. respiratory disease 75	Diabetes mellitus 221	Diabetes mellitus 792	Diabetes mellitus 2,049	Cerebro-vascular 5,353	Cerebro-vascular 12,310	Unintentional injury 53,141	Diabetes mellitus 80,058
8	Respiratory distress 488	Perinatal period 60	Septicemia 40	Cerebro-vascular 50	Chronic low. respiratory disease 206	Cerebro-vascular 575	Cerebro-vascular 1,851	Chronic low. respiratory disease 4,307	Suicide 7,759	Influenza & pneumonia 42,479	Influenza & pneumonia 51,537
9	Circulatory system disease 460	Cerebro-vascular 55	Cerebro-vascular 38	Influenza & pneumonia 39	Influenza & pneumonia 189	HIV 546	HIV 971	Septicemia 2,472	Septicemia 5,941	Nephritis 41,095	Nephritis 50,046
10	Neonatal hemorrhage 398	Chronic low. respiratory disease 51	Benign neoplasms 31	Septicemia 31	Complicated pregnancy 184	Complicated pregnancy 472	Septicemia 897	Homicide 2,152	Nephritis 5,650	Septicemia 30,405	Suicide 44,965

National Vital Statistics System, National Center for the Health Statistics, CDC.

cause of death is unintentional injuries. The exact cause of the injury differs by age. For children aged 1 to 4 years, it is drowning; for individuals aged 5 to 24 years, it is motor vehicle crashes; and for individuals aged 25 to 64 years, the primary cause of injury death is unintentional poisoning. For individuals aged 10 to 34 years, the second leading cause of death is suicide. For people 45 to 64 years of age, malignant neoplasms (cancer) are the leading cause of death. For those 65 years of age and over, heart disease is the leading cause. Looking at the population as a whole, the leading causes of death, in order, are heart disease, cancer, unintentional injuries, and chronic lower respiratory disease.[3]

Aging

What happens to our bodies as we age? Your body is a reflection of both your genetic makeup and the physical and social environment in which you live. In combination, these factors, along with personal behavior, affect our health as we age. (See Chapters 6 and 11 to learn more specifics about how stress and the environment can affect health.)

Gerontologists study aging to learn about what makes people vulnerable to diseases and disabilities as they age. From their research, we have learned that, over time, the accumulation of damage to and loss of our cells affect

TALES OF PUBLIC HEALTH

Centenarians

A centenarian is someone who lives to be 100 or more years old. According to the United Nations, in 2000, there were approximately 180,000 centenarians around the world and by 2050 there will likely be 2.2 million people over age 100.[6] Super-centenarians are people who live to or past their 110th birthday.

Why do some people live so long? Scientists do not know how much of longevity is due to genes that help you live a long time or how much is due to a noticeably better lifestyle.

Here are some people who lived to be over age 100:

1. Jeanne Calment lived to be 122 years old. According to the Guinness Book of World Records,[7] Jeanne Calment was born in 1875 and died in 1997. She took up fencing at age 85, rode her bicycle until 100, and lived independently until 110 years of age.
2. Strom Thurmond lived to be 100 years old. He represented South Carolina in the U.S. Senate from 1954 until 2003. He left the Senate at age 100, making him the oldest serving senator in U.S. history. He died 6 months after leaving office.
3. Irving Berlin was an American composer and lyricist. He composed over 3,000 songs, including "God Bless America" and "White Christmas." He died of a heart attack at age 101.
4. Albert Hoffman was a Swiss scientist. He was the first person to synthesize, ingest, and learn of the psychedelic effects of lysergic acid diethylamide (LSD). He lived to be 102 years old.
5. Queen Elizabeth the Queen Mother was the wife of King George VI and mother of Queen Elizabeth II (currently the Queen of England) and Princess Margaret. She was the matriarch of the British Royal Family and died at 101 years.

major organs, including the heart, kidneys, brain, and lungs. Gradually, this process results in a decrease in physical and mental capacity. For example, blood vessels and arteries in the heart may become stiff, which leads to high blood pressure and other cardiovascular problems. The size and density of your bones and muscle mass may decrease with age, increasing your risk of fractures and impairing balance.[4] Impaired balance can lead to falls, which are dangerous in old age because they cause injury and may lead to a decline in functional abilities.[5]

Even though all of us get older, not everyone will experience the same effects of aging. You may know someone who is 85 years old and requires little to no help to live independently and someone else the same age or even younger who needs full-time care.

Our Health as We Age

Common health problems among the elderly include hearing loss, osteoarthritis (a painful inflammation of the joints), chronic obstructive pulmonary disease (a disease that affects the lungs and makes it hard to breathe), diabetes, depression, dementia, cancer, influenza, pneumonia, and heart disease. (See Chapters 2 and 3 for more specifics on diabetes.) It is common for older adults to have more than one health problem at the same time. Management of these coexisting conditions becomes particularly complicated if multiple medications, treatments, or specialists are required. There is also a group of distinct health issues common in old age that fall under the heading of "geriatric syndromes." These problems include pressure ulcers (bed sores), falls, incontinence (lack of voluntary control over urination or defecation), and delirium. Although not major diseases, these syndromes can negatively impact one's ability to function.[8,9]

As we age, everyday activities can become difficult. Seemingly simple tasks that we may take for granted when we are younger, such as dressing or bathing ourselves, eating, or using the toilet, can become challenging when we are older. These activities, which allow us to meet our own basic health and social needs, are referred to as **activities of daily living**. Other activities that allow someone to live independently, such as driving, managing money, cleaning, and shopping, are referred to as "instrumental activities of daily living." Reduced ability to do these activities may be the result of a chronic illness or health-related disability. For example, osteoarthritis may prevent someone from being able to engage in activities that require hand movement, such as dressing or eating. Limited eyesight could affect one's ability to read the label of a prescription bottle. A chronic pulmonary disease can hinder one's ability to be mobile and climb the stairs to a bedroom. These are just a few examples of how age-related health issues can affect daily life.[10]

activities of daily living Routine activities that people usually do every day without needing assistance, such as eating and bathing.

dementia A chronic or persistent disorder of the mental processes caused by brain disease or injury and marked by memory disorders, personality changes, and impaired reasoning.

Having difficulty with these activities usually progresses slowly over time. If the limits to activities of daily living start to affect one's ability to live independently, often family members will arrange for someone to come into the person's home to help, or they may move the person into an assisted-living facility, nursing home, or with a family member. Because most people tend to feel more comfortable in their own home than in other settings, home health aides are often used first before relocating someone to an assisted-living facility.

Alzheimer's disease A progressive type of dementia in which people suffer damage to brain cells that causes loss of memory and other important mental functions.

Dementia

Dementia is an example of a health problem that prevents someone from living independently. As we age, we may have more and more trouble remembering things like where we placed the house keys or whether we locked the car door. In many cases, this type of memory loss is normal. Dementia, however, refers to a decline in mental ability to the degree that it adversely affects daily living. Dementia consists of a range of symptoms associated with declining cognitive function, including memory loss, and it is caused by damage to brain cells.

There are many different types of dementia. **Alzheimer's disease** is one of the most common. People with Alzheimer's disease first suffer damage to brain cells in the hippocampus region of the brain (the area associated with learning and memory). This damage may begin over a decade before any symptoms, such as memory loss, appear. It is related to the accumulation of certain proteins in the brain that make it difficult for brain cells to communicate with one another. This damage spreads to other regions of the brain and causes brain tissue to shrink (**FIGURE 12-1**).[11]

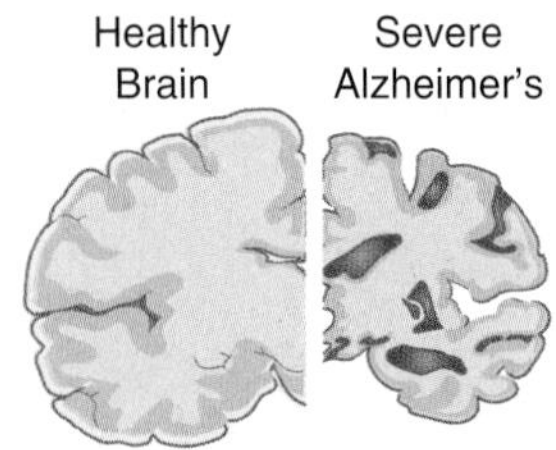

FIGURE 12-1 Cross section of a brain. The right side shows brain tissue that has shrunk due to Alzheimer's disease.

U.S. Department of Health and Human Services, National Institute on Aging. (n.d.). Alzheimer's disease fact sheet. Retrieved from https://www.nia.nih.gov/health/alzheimers-disease-fact-sheet#participating

Over 5.7 million people in the United States have Alzheimer's disease, and the vast majority of them are over the age of 65 years. Researchers estimate that by 2050, almost 14 million Americans will have Alzheimer's disease[12] (**FIGURE 12-2**). This disease can be devastating not only for those who are affected but also for their loved ones. It can be upsetting to witness someone losing their ability to recognize a loved one or recall simple things. Beyond the emotional effects of Alzheimer's disease, this disease can be very costly to families and the healthcare system. Alzheimer's disease costs the United States over $230 billion per year in long-term and hospice care. In addition, lost wages for caretakers or the unpaid care of a loved one who has Alzheimer's disease total over $450 billion.[13]

Alzheimer's disease is progressive, meaning it gets worse over time and cannot be reversed. It starts off mild and progresses to moderate and then severe. It is not clear what causes Alzheimer's disease. Research suggests it is a complex combination of genetics, environmental factors, and lifestyle factors. Scientists continue to seek out the causes of the complex brain changes that occur in Alzheimer's disease.[11,14-19]

RECOGNIZING ALZHEIMER'S DISEASE

The following 10 warning signs and symptoms are suggestive of Alzheimer's disease:

1. Memory loss that disrupts daily life
2. Challenges in planning or solving problems
3. Difficulty completing familiar tasks at home, work, or leisure
4. Confusion with time or place
5. Difficulty understanding visual images and spatial relationships
6. New problems with words in speaking or writing
7. Tendency to misplace things and inability to retrace steps
8. Decreased or poor judgment
9. Withdrawal from work or social activities
10. Changes in mood or personality

If someone you know displays any of these symptoms, seek medical help.

Alzheimer's Association. (2018). 10 early signs and symptoms of Alzheimer's. Retrieved from https://www.alz.org/alzheimers_disease_10_signs_of_alzheimers.asp

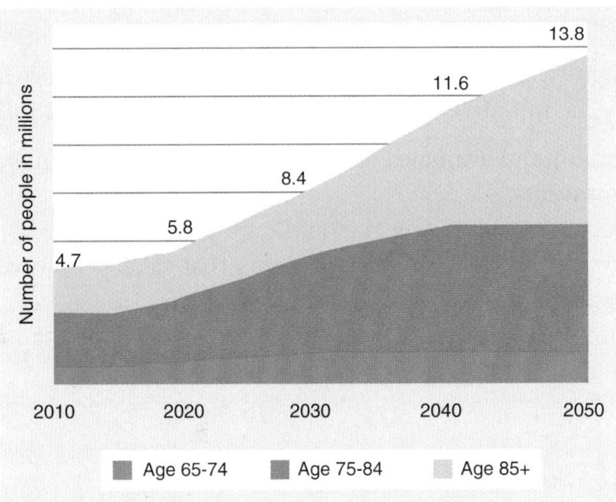

FIGURE 12-2 Graph of Alzheimer's disease projections.

Centers for Disease Control and Prevention. (2017). Alzheimer's disease: Promoting health and independence for an aging population at a glance 2017. Retrieved from https://www.cdc.gov/chronicdisease/resources/publications/aag/alzheimers.htm

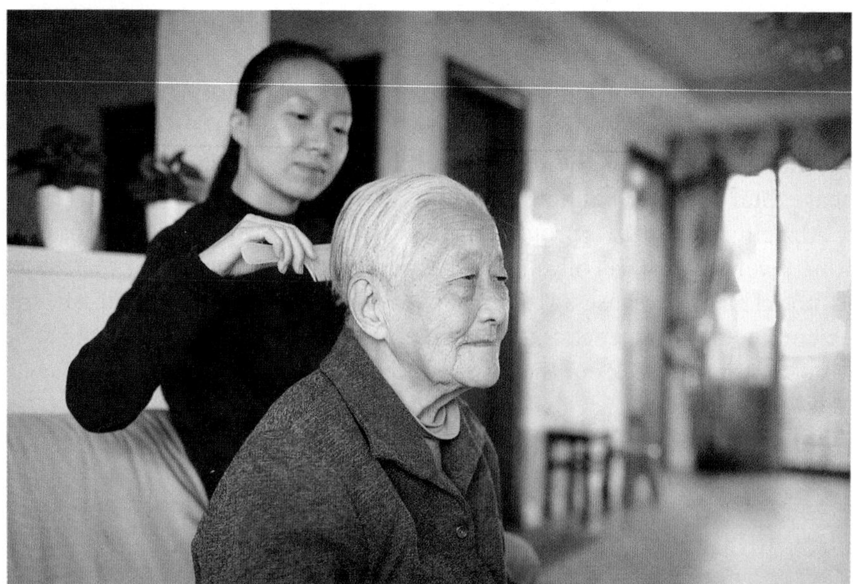

Although aging cannot be slowed down, there are some steps individuals can take (both when they are old and throughout their life) toward reducing the risk of dementia, including the following:

- Avoid tobacco.
- Maintain a healthy weight.
- Exercise regularly.
- Eat a healthy diet that focuses on whole grains, fruits, vegetables, fish, and nuts.
- Stay socially engaged.

You can help yourself and those around you by implementing these suggestions in your life.

Public health agencies at the local and state levels can help in the fight against dementia. The Centers for Disease Control and Prevention's Healthy Aging program, along with the Alzheimer's Association, developed the Healthy Brain Initiative. This road map provides public health agencies with an outline as to how they can foster cognitive function in all adults, address issues for those with cognitive impairment, and provide aid and support for caretakers (**FIGURE 12-3**). The initiative suggests that these agencies do the following:

1. Monitor and evaluate cognitive functioning among members of their community.
2. Educate and empower the public about dementia.
3. Develop policies and partnerships that take people with cognitive impairment into consideration.
4. Maintain a competent workforce that has an understanding of cognitive health and impairment.[17]

Depression

In addition to increasing physical health issues, mental health problems are also prevalent with aging. Why is that? Depression is more common among people with chronic illnesses, and older adults are more likely to have one or more chronic illnesses. With nearly 7 million adults aged 65 years and older who have depression, it is the most common mental health issue among the elderly.

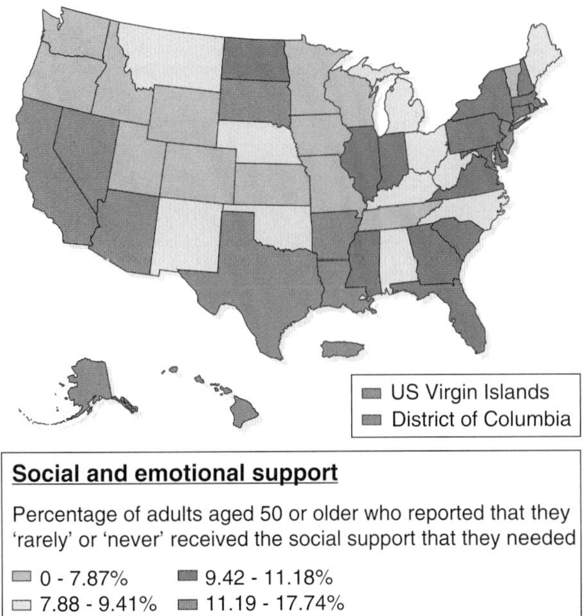

FIGURE 12-3 Map of social and emotional support.

Centers for Disease Control and Prevention and National Association of Chronic Disease Directors. (2008). The State of Mental Health and Aging in America: Issue Brief #1: What do the data tell us? Retrieved from https://www.cdc.gov/aging/pdf/mental_health.pdf

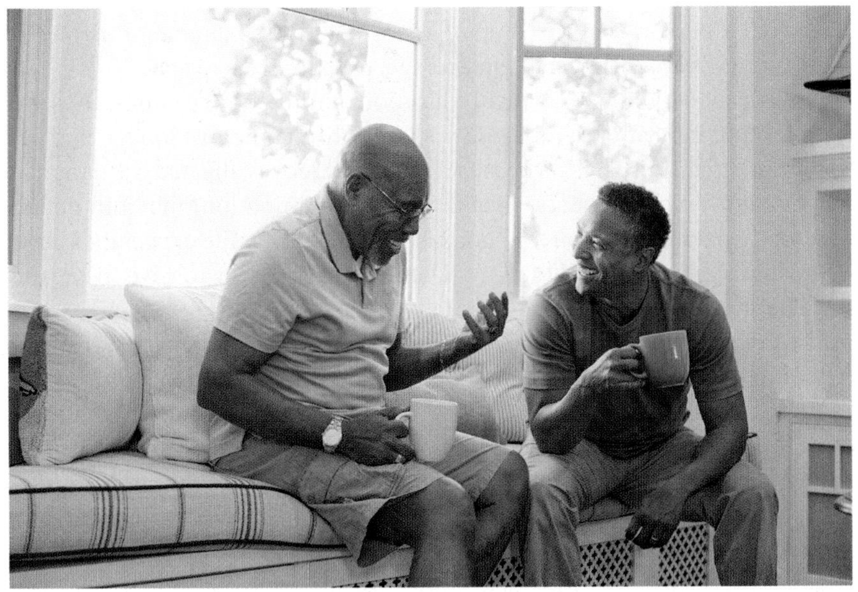

Many of the signs and symptoms of depression among older adults are the same for people of any age, including sleep disturbances, weight loss, and feelings of despair. Medication and counseling are indicated to treat depression in this population.

Despite being a treatable condition, depression often goes undiagnosed in older adults. While it may be common, it should not be ignored or considered a natural part of aging. Older adults can experience life changes that cause stress or feelings of sadness, such as the death of a loved one, retirement, or new physical limitations. Many adults adjust to these changes in time, but if feelings of sadness or signs of depression persist, they need to seek help. Receiving adequate social support is critical in managing depression among the elderly.[18] (See Chapter 6 for more specific information about depression.)

TALES OF PUBLIC HEALTH

Chicago Heat Wave

In the book *Heat Wave: A Social Autopsy of Disaster in Chicago*, Eric Klinenberg revisits the devastating 1995 weeklong heat wave in Chicago, Illinois.[19] During this week, the heat index rose to as high as 126°F. More than 700 people died that week from heat-related causes—more than from any other meteorological event in the city's history. Why did so many perish?

Klinenberg's analysis of the underlying social issues that may have contributed to these deaths revealed that many of the people who died were elderly and living alone. Also, more males died than did females; Klinenberg argued that this disparity was due to men being less likely to have social ties or to reach out for help. Klinenberg attributed the deaths to an increase in social withdrawal, degradation of public spaces, and citizens not being entitled to social protection. As a result of this crisis, after the heat wave, Chicago invested in support services, established hotlines and phone banks to check in with senior residents, made taxis available to transport the elderly, and established cooling centers in the event of future heat waves.

Healthy Aging

What people consider "old" has changed drastically over the last few centuries, as life expectancy has increased. Life expectancy is the number of years that an average person will live. In the United States, infants born in 1900, on average, were expected to live to age 47 years. Today, thanks in part to public health interventions such as immunizations and control over infectious diseases,[20] the life expectancy of an infant is almost 79 years.[21] Life expectancy changes depending on how old a person is at the time of assessment. For example, someone who lives to age 65 years is expected, on average, to then live to age 84.

Life expectancy differs by race, education, and income; Whites, those with a high level of education, and those with a high income live longer than their counterparts. This disparity is because life expectancy is affected by many social determinants: access to quality health care, discrimination, the built environment, food systems, and more.[22] For a fascinating look at life expectancy around the world, listen to the TED talk by Dan Buettner, "How to Live to be 100+" (available at www.ted.com). In this talk, Buettner explores four areas of the world where the life expectancy is much longer than in other areas, exploring what it is about these communities that may contribute to a longer life.

What can we do to promote healthy aging? Many of the things we talk about in this textbook! Eating well, exercising regularly, avoiding tobacco and other harmful substances, being social, and managing stress throughout your life are all ways to maintain physical and mental health. Much of the time we do not determine our environment, but we can control some of the individual factors mentioned here. Maintaining a social network and feeling a connection to your

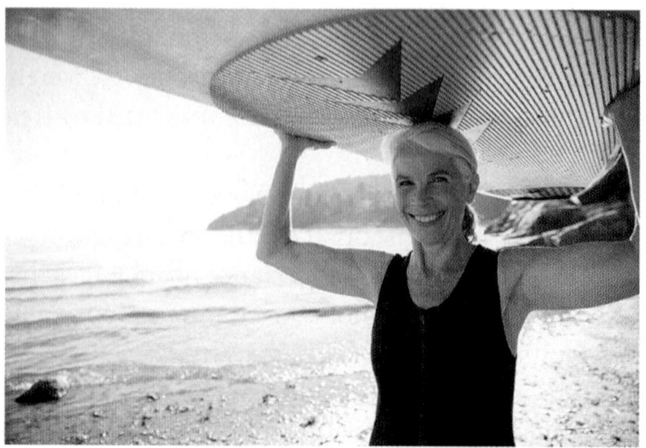

community adds to your mental well-being. Creating a safe and supportive neighborhood is crucial to maintaining good health.[8]

TALES OF PUBLIC HEALTH

A Different Sort of Hobby in New Zealand[23]

Apparently, there is a different sort of hobby among retirees in New Zealand. They form clubs to build coffins, either for personal use or to donate for charity.

Different clubs use different materials. The Rotorua Club buys wood and cuts it into shape. They devise the best way to secure handles. Other clubs use kits made from particleboard. The coffins must meet national standards. In New Zealand this means the coffin must be waterproof and strong enough to hold a body.

Members paint and decorate coffins to best represent their individual personalities. Not surprisingly, these coffins cost much less than what funeral homes charge for a casket. But the real goal is to participate in a social club and to have an individualized coffin. People choose their own color to paint the coffin and often use them to tell a story that means something. People have decorated them with pictures of Elvis, racing cars, soccer team colors, trees, and abstract patterns.

The Kiwi Coffin Club's motto is "fine and affordable underground furniture." However, people use the coffins creatively until their final use. Among the uses people have devised include coffee tables, liquor cabinets, and a garage storage cupboard.

As one reporter said, in describing a coffin-building club, "I won't say that people were dying to join. After all, this is a grave matter."

Innis, M. (2017, February 25). 'Affordable underground furniture': D.I.Y. coffin clubs catch on in New Zealand. *New York Times*. Retrieved from https://www.nytimes.com/2017/02/25/world/australia/new-zealand-diy-coffins.html

Being Organized for the Future

Following the recommendations to promote healthy aging and living can help increase the length and quality of one's life. Ultimately, however, everyone alive will someday die. Ideally, your loved one's dying and death should be peaceful. Although most of us will die in ways that are out of our control, there are healthy ways to approach death. Everybody thinks about death in a different way, and how they feel will affect how they approach their own death or the death of a loved one. Respecting others' feelings and differences can help them have a peaceful death. The more prepared the dying person is, the easier it will be for family members.[24]

Getting Things in Order

Sometimes in life, no matter how careful you are, something disastrous happens. If something terrible happened and you became incapacitated, would your family know what to do and where to find your important papers? Here is a guide to organizing relevant information.

Your goal should be to have a master folder or electronic document that contains all your essential information. Whether you are creating it for yourself or helping a family member do it, it is an important step to take. This document should be both convenient and safely accessible if needed.

Before you start, gather your records to make the process easier. The safest place to keep important documents is in a fireproof safe or a safe deposit box. These documents include your birth certificate, your Social Security card, your passport, any official documents or records that may be hard to replace, and (if you are from another country) any immigration papers. It is also a good idea to photograph or scan the documents, so you have a digital copy of them. Be sure these digital files are as safe as your paper documents.

The list presented in **TABLE 12-2** includes many of the important pieces of information you will need to consolidate, but remember that everyone's life is different, so you probably want to personalize the list. Programs are available

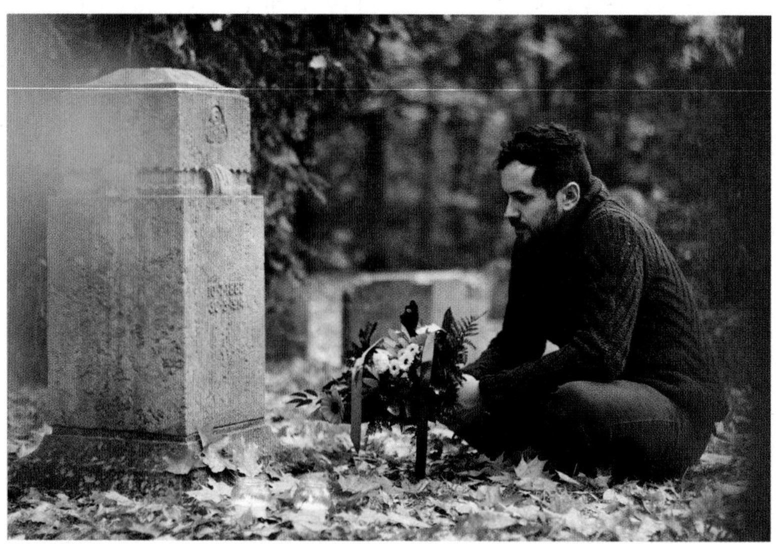

TABLE 12-2 Getting Things in Order

Category	Information to Include
Personal information	Current address, email address, all phone numbers that apply (home, work, cell), date and place of birth, employment details (name and address of where you work, your supervisor's name), person to contact in an emergency
Important contacts	Parents, children, nearest relatives, physician(s), lawyer(s), will executor, medical power of attorney, accountant, financial advisor, neighbor(s), pharmacy, home repair people (general maintenance person, contractor, plumber, electrician), babysitter, veterinarian, work personnel manager/human resources, auto repair. Include name, address, and phone numbers for each.
Important bills to be paid	Rent/mortgage, utility services (electricity, gas, water, garbage collection), insurance company, loans, credit card(s)
Health information	Allergies, dietary restrictions, medication list, immunization records, previous surgeries and treatments (include the dates and diagnosis)
Emergency planning	Emergency contacts and phone numbers (designate more than one person); location of fire extinguisher, smoke alarms, and gas and water shutoffs; emergency meet-up location(s)
Insurance information	Homeowners, auto, medical, life, disability, and other insurance. Include contact information for agents/brokers and policy numbers.
Financial accounts	All accounts, including bank(s), investment firm(s), credit card(s), and loan information. Include individual contact, if applicable, institution name, phone numbers, and account numbers.
Will and medical directives	Name of executor and person who has medical power of attorney, location of will/living trust and any medical directives
Important property location	Car/truck information (registration and insurance information), home purchase papers/deeds, other home inventory items (jewelry, furniture, etc.)
Pet information	Name and description of each pet, veterinary contact information, important medical information

on the Internet to help you get organized, and books are also available. Use the approach that works best for you. The information you need, if for yourself, should include information on your spouse and children, if applicable. If you are doing this for one or both parents, include their current spouse (if not your parent), all of your siblings, half-siblings, and nieces and nephews, as needed.

Today, everybody has many usernames and passwords to remember for online accounts. It is important to keep them safe and secure. In the event of an emergency, however, it is important that someone else be able to access the online accounts. Sharing a password hint that would not make sense to a stranger is a safe strategy.

Remember that once created, this information needs to be updated regularly. This update should be done at least once per year, although more frequently is better. The initial creation will be time-consuming. After that, the updates should be relatively quick.

TALES OF PUBLIC HEALTH

This Can Happen to Anyone[25]

As reported in a *New York Times* article, in July 2009, Chanel Reynold's life turned upside down. Her husband, 43-year-old José Hernando, was riding his bicycle near Lake Washington in Seattle, Washington, when a van turned into the path of his bicycle, killing him.

Chanel and José owned a house they had bought in 2008. They had a 5-year-old son. They had drafted wills but had not signed them. Chanel did not know how much money was in their checking account. They had little in emergency savings, and the passwords to an unknown number of accounts had been stored only in José's head. The thought that kept running through Chanel's mind was that she didn't know if she could sustain her family by herself. This is not where you want to be.

It took Chanel months of sleuthing to sort out her financial accounts. The experience prompted her to create a website that anyone can use to help maintain all important information in one place. You can find it online at www.gyst.com.

As noted in the *New York Times* article, in 2011 only 43% of adults in the United States had a will. Of those who were 45 to 64 years old, only 56% had wills.

You might be thinking, "This type of story can't happen to me. I'm young and in college. I have plenty of time to take care of this stuff." Hopefully it won't happen to you, but the idea that it can't just because you are young is wrong. In her first 2 years of college, one of the authors of this book had three friends die. One was murdered, one died of an infectious disease (for which he should have been vaccinated), and one died in a car crash. Hopefully such a tragedy will not happen to you. But in case it does, do your family and friends a favor, and be prepared.

Data from Lieber R. A shocking death, a financial lesson and help for others. *New York Times*. January 12, 2013. Business: B1. Accessed 2/2/2017.

Parental Wishes

It is hard to accept that one day your parents will die, and talking about it is difficult. If you are lucky, they will stay in good health and live for a very long time. While this is what we all hope for, how life works out is sometimes different. Many people die without sharing their wishes with their family. As hard as this conversation, or rather series of conversations, may be, it is one of the best things you can do for one another. It is much better for both you and your parents to be prepared and to discuss all the relevant details beforehand. By doing so, you can carry out their wishes and know that you are doing the right thing. Among the things that need to be sorted out are their finances, their estate plans, and their memorial wishes. Completing this process will also help you plan for yourself.

If your parents or guardians are still living, you should ask them the following important questions,[26] many of which are described in greater detail elsewhere in this chapter:

1. What are the names, addresses, and phone numbers of people who are critical to the process? This information includes financial and legal professionals, accountant and financial planners, and physicians.

will A legal declaration of a person's wishes regarding the disposal of his or her property, or estate, after death.

2. Do they have a **will**? If they don't, they need one. If they do, you need to know how old the will is, where it is, and who is the executor. If it is more than 5 years old, they should review it.
3. Do they have a living will and power of attorney? Ask to see these documents, so you know what their wishes are and who is empowered to make decisions for them.
4. Are the beneficiaries (people who will inherit their belongings) listed on relevant documents up to date? Beneficiaries listed on insurance policies, pensions, and investments often supersede what is in a will. Make sure the policies are up to date.
5. What financial accounts do they have, and what are the details? You need a list of all bank accounts, brokerage accounts, and mutual fund accounts and the associated account numbers, usernames, and passwords. They may not want to share this information now. If that is the case, have them store the information where you can find it after they have passed away.
6. What insurance do they have and where are the policies? Insurance policies they may have include health, life, automobile, homeowners or renters, disability, and long-term care. Understand what their coverage includes and phone numbers to claim or cancel services.
7. Where is the financial paperwork? You need to know where they keep the titles to any properties they own, as well as any loan documents. Additionally, you need to know where they keep their previous tax returns.
8. Do they want to stay in the family home or would they consider moving? If so, what are their wishes about where to move? At some point, the family home may become a burden; for example, they may become unable to climb the stairs or take care of the house. Do they prefer in-home care? An assisted-living facility? Would they rather live with a family member, and if so, with whom? If they want to stay at home, as many people do, can the house be modified to accommodate their needs?
9. Are they signed up to be an organ donor? Ask them their wishes so that you can do what they want. If they want to be an organ donor, know where they keep their cards. In many states, this wish is stated on the driver's license.
10. How do they envision their memorial service? What kind of funeral do they want? Do they want to be cremated? Do they already own a burial plot or plots? If yes, where are they, and where is the documentation?
11. Where are the safe-deposit box and its key? The executor of the estate may be able to get into the safe-deposit box without a key, but it will likely be expensive. It is better to know where the key is.

Estate Planning

Doing estate planning helps to protect your family and your property when you die or if you become incapacitated. Estate planning for you or a family member includes the following:

- Determining who will get your possessions when you die
- Naming an executor to carry out your wishes and take care of your affairs
- Naming the guardian(s) for minor children
- Avoiding probate (a court process by which a will is proved valid or invalid)
- Preparing for a time when you cannot make financial or medical decisions

Although most people do not need all of these, among the documents that are part of an estate plan include a living will, a will, a power of attorney, and a living trust.[27]

Living Will

When people think of wills, they think of the document that determines who is going to get what after a person's death. A **living will**, also called an **advance directive** or a healthcare directive, does not address monetary or property matters; it provides individuals with an opportunity to express their end-of-life wishes before reaching that point. Without such a document, family members have to guess what their loved one would want. If various family members have differing ideas about what a person wants, disputes may arise.

living will A written statement, such as an advance directive, detailing a person's desires regarding medical treatment should the person lose his or her ability to express informed consent.

advance directive A legal document that outlines a patient's end-of-life care preferences.

A painful example of the need for a living will is the case of Terri Schiavo. At the age of 26 years, she had a cardiac arrest. Before being resuscitated, Terri sustained massive brain damage. Approximately 1 year after the cardiac arrest, her doctors certified her to be in a persistent vegetative state (a condition in which a medical patient is completely unresponsive to psychological and physical stimuli and displays no sign of higher brain function, being kept alive only by medical intervention). Her husband wanted to have her feeding tube removed, but her parents disagreed. A highly public and acrimonious battle between her family members followed. For 7 years Terri's husband and parents battled in the courts. The governor of Florida, the president of the United States, and Congress all were involved in the decision-making process. Had Terri had a living will, none of this would have happened.

There are many considerations in end-of-life decision making. If you have questions about what any of the following terms mean, ask your physician or primary care provider for an explanation. Their answers should help you decide if you want any or all of these measures. For interventions that help maintain life (such as ventilation, feeding tube, dialysis), you will need to decide not only whether you want them, but also for how long you would want them.[28] Terms related to life-sustaining measures include the following:

resuscitation The action or process of reviving someone from unconsciousness or apparent death.

- **Resuscitation**: The act of bringing someone back to life—for example, cardiopulmonary resuscitation (CPR) if the person's heart stops beating.

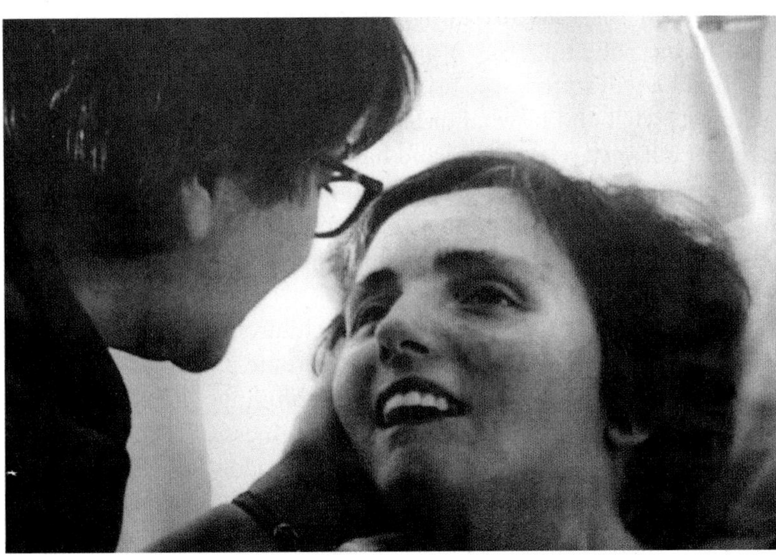

Terri Schiavo.

CPR helps maintain partial blood flow to the brain and the body. Defibrillation (electric shock to the heart) is often needed to get the heart beating again.

- *Mechanical ventilation*: A mechanical means used to help a person breathe. Think about how long you would want to be on a ventilator (the machine that supports breathing).
- *Tube feeding*: The process of using a medical device to provide nutrition to a person who cannot feed himself or herself. Think about how long you would want to have a feeding tube.
- *Dialysis*: Use of a specialized machine to clean waste and excess water from a person's body when the person's kidneys do not function. Many patients have dialysis for years to treat chronic conditions.[29] In this instance, however, we are speaking about end-of-life treatments. Think about how long you would want to have dialysis.
- *Antibiotics or antiviral medications*: Drugs used to combat bacterial or viral infection. If you were at the end of your life, would you want doctors to treat an infection aggressively?
- *Palliative care*: Care that provides patients with symptomatic relief from pain while at the same time honoring other wishes, such as avoiding invasive treatments.
- *Organ donation*: Use of a recently deceased person's viable organs to treat an ill or injured person. You can specify your willingness to donate organs in the living will. See the detailed section later in this chapter about organ donation.

The requirements for a living will vary by state. Many people choose to hire a lawyer to prepare their living will. Others buy software packages to lead them through the process. If you choose the do-it-yourself approach, make sure to choose a program that is reputable.

As part of the living will, you should specify a medical power of attorney, as discussed later in this section.[30]

Will

A basic will allows you to designate who gets your property. If, for example, you want to leave a favorite piece of jewelry to your best friend, this document is the place to say so. Wills also designate the executor to carry out the wishes expressed in the will and name a guardian(s) for any children and property. Dying without a will (referred to as intestate) means the state's laws will determine who gets what and in what order. Depending on your state's laws, if you are in a nontraditional relationship and have no will, your significant other may inherit nothing. Wills are also useful if you want to give a gift conditionally, such as leaving an adult child money, but on the condition that the child goes through rehabilitation for a drug abuse problem or is willing to take over the family business.

Many states protect spouses and minor children from being left nothing in a will. If you decide to go the do-it-yourself route, make sure you follow the laws of your state so that your will is legal and binding. There is a requirement for two witnesses in most states. The reason for witnesses is because, by the time the will is in force, the person making the will is no longer available to state his or her preferences. Witnesses must be over the age of 18 years and cannot be a will beneficiary. Not all states require witnesses.[31]

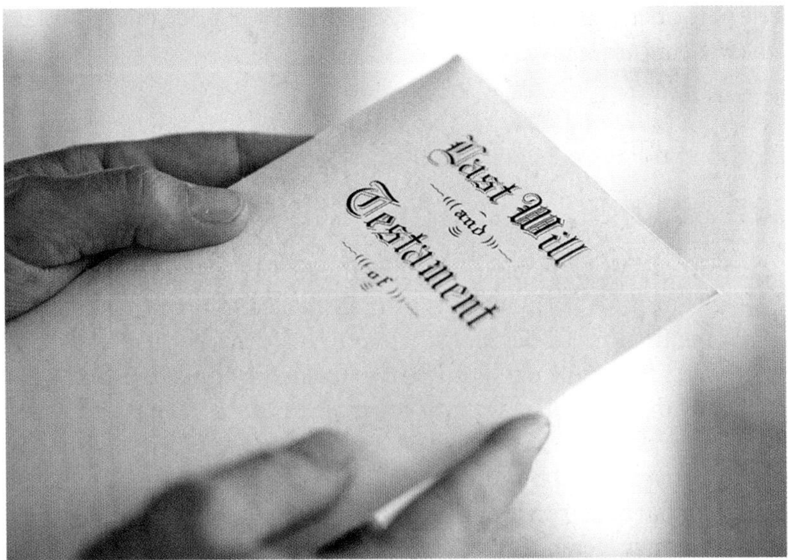

© Tetra Images/Getty Images

Financial Power of Attorney

As the name suggests, a financial power of attorney authorizes someone to take care of your finances when you are not able to do so. If your power of attorney is "durable," it continues if you are incapacitated. You can stipulate exactly what powers you want the person to have regarding your finances. As you might guess, it is critical to pick someone whom you totally trust.

Living Trust

The purpose of a living trust is to pass on ownership of property and to help avoid probate, that is, when the validity of the terms of a will is determined by a court. A living trust transfers ownership of property into a trust and names the person as the trustee; it also names the successor trustee(s) who are the beneficiaries for the property. When the person (trustee) dies, ownership of the trust automatically transfers the property to the successor trustee(s) (beneficiaries). Do you need one? You do not need a living trust if you do not have much property and everything is being left to your spouse, children, or will be assumed by creditors because you have debt. Having a lawyer create a living trust usually costs more than drawing up a simple will.[27]

Memorial Societies

Memorial societies were set up to help with a variety of funeral planning needs and to give members the benefit of "group discounts." The cost to join ranges from $30 to $50, and for most memorial societies, it is a one-time cost. Being a member ensures that funeral costs are kept low at the time of death. The memorial society should be a member of the Funeral Consumers Alliance (FCA), a nonprofit group. Their mission is to protect consumers' rights to a meaningful and dignified funeral that they can afford.[32]

Many societies have negotiated reduced rates for **cremation** or burial with cooperating funeral homes. All of the FCA sites advise against prepaying for

cremation To reduce a body to ashes by fire, especially as a funeral rite.

a funeral. Membership in a society is reciprocal, so if a person dies in another state, the benefits are transferrable.[32]

The Path to Acceptance: Palliative Care and Hospice

terminally ill A patient with a disease that cannot be cured and will likely cause death within approximately 6 months of diagnosis.

Many **terminally ill** patients and their families face a point in their journey where they transition from seeking to prevent death to managing the dying process. Sometimes these decisions, while never easy, are relatively clear-cut. Other times, it may not be obvious when to make this transition. Some patients or their family members may want to continue to try more invasive, expensive, and "heroic" measures to cure an illness, or just to try to buy more time. Unfortunately, disagreements about this process within a family can lead to challenging and uncomfortable situations. This is one reason it is so important to try to establish these preferences as early as possible—even before the prospect of death enters the picture so clearly. Through early planning, families can avoid these difficult decisions as much as possible while the process of death and dying is underway. Establishing legal documents, such as living wills, trusts, and advance directives (discussed earlier), is one way to avoid these discrepancies; however, even with these documents in place, the death and dying process is seldom free from stress and conflict. It is hard to let a loved one go.

palliative care Specialized medical care for people with serious illness. This type of care is focused on providing relief from the symptoms and stress of a serious illness.

hospice A program or facility designed to provide palliative care and emotional support to the terminally ill patient in a home or homelike setting so that quality of life is maintained and family members may be active participants in care.

Essentially, the overall goals of **palliative care** and **hospice** programs are to increase the quality of life and decrease pain and symptoms. If everyone accepts these goals, the specifics of the decisions should be easier. Understanding the different types of care and available treatment options can help everyone affected come to a common understanding, have a more informed conversation, and reach more satisfying decisions.

Palliative and hospice care represent a positive change in health care that has occurred over the past few decades. While the U.S. healthcare system has always sought to do everything possible to prevent death, in recent decades, it has focused more on the science and practice of improving the many steps and emotions associated with the act of dying.[33,34]

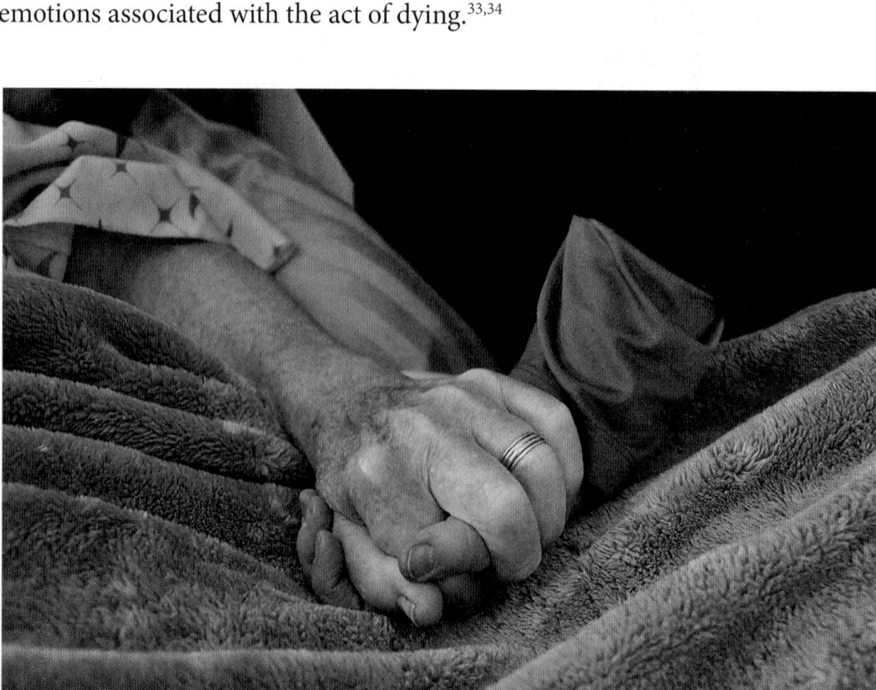

Palliative Care

Palliative and *hospice care* are terms used to describe the kind of care given to people to ease the pain and suffering that often accompany the dying process. Palliative care focuses on improving patients' quality of life by addressing their physical, emotional, and spiritual needs, and supporting their families as they struggle with dying, death, and loss.[35] Rather than giving medicine to cure a disease, one goal of palliative medicine is to help patients manage pain and other unwanted symptoms that often accompany the dying process. Palliative care is usually, but not always, provided when there is no hope for treatment. Sometimes, the patient and family may decide that the chances of curing the disease and making a full recovery are so small that it is not worth the pain or anguish, or even the expense, of pursuing **heroic treatments**. In fact, illness or disease does not have to be categorized as terminal for someone to qualify for palliative care benefits under many insurance companies and Medicare. Sometimes palliative care is provided to ease the pain of another treatment where the goal is to cure the disease. One example of palliative care is alleviating the effects of nausea associated with chemotherapy. It is often an important part of treatment as well as when dying.

heroic treatments Health care or therapy that is likely to be ineffective or, worse, that may cause increased pain or further damage to a patient's health. Heroic procedures are usually undertaken as a last resort, recognizing that lesser treatment will result in death.

Provision of palliative care is often part of a comprehensive care program for the following conditions:

- Alzheimer's disease
- Cancer
- Chronic obstructive pulmonary disease
- Congestive heart failure
- HIV/AIDS
- Parkinson's disease
- Stroke

A variety of approaches are taken to provide palliative care and may include various types of treatments, including the following:

- Pain medications
- Physical therapy
- Massage
- Counseling
- Acupuncture
- Medical marijuana

Hospice Care

Hospice care is often thought of as being interchangeable with palliative care because both play important roles in the process of dying. But while palliative care can be used to relieve the side effects of treating illnesses where there may still be hope for successful treatment, hospice care is specifically concerned with easing the dying process and is usually delivered through a comprehensive hospice program.

Hospice care occurs when a patient and/or the family has conceded that death is inevitable and imminent. It seeks to allow terminally ill patients to live as comfortably as possible in the last weeks of life and provides a holistic approach to the end-of-life care. This approach includes medical services, emotional support, and spiritual resources for people who are in the last stages of a serious illness. Hospice services also help family members manage the day-to-day details and emotional issues that come with the approach of a loved one's death. Their goal is to keep the patient comfortable, to improve the quality of

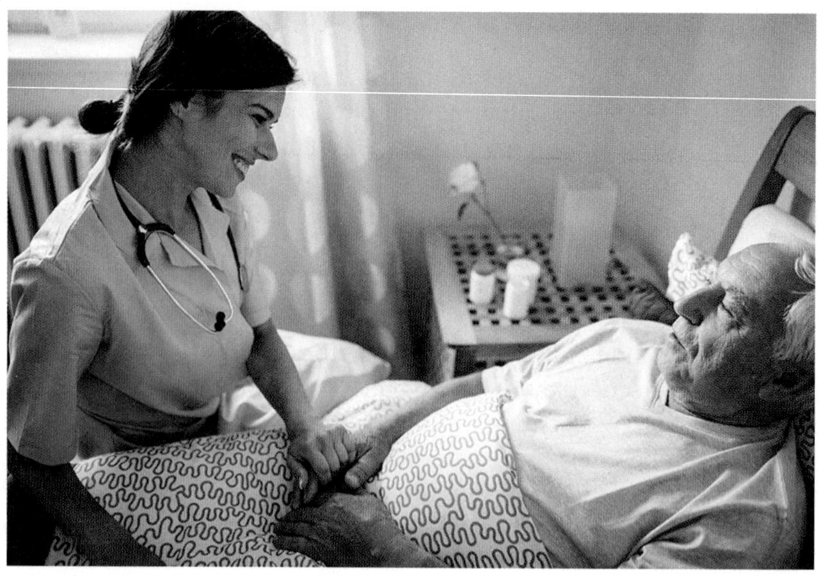

© wavebreakmedia/Shutterstock

life for the whole family, and to allow people to die with dignity. Hospice programs may provide services in the home or at a hospice center.[36]

Hospice team members are available as needed, depending on where the family is in the process. Sometimes they come in to see the dying person weekly or daily, but they are available 24 hours a day, 7 days a week if needed. The medical care focuses on the control of pain and the management of side effects and symptoms. The assistance that hospice provides to the family includes counseling and support and helping to guide the family through end-of-life issues and closure. **Bereavement**, the process of dealing with death through grieving, challenging the process, accepting the outcome, and/or letting go of someone who has died, can be extremely difficult for everyone affected by the dying process—patients and family members alike. The hospice team may also help with everyday chores like preparing meals and running errands.[36]

bereavement The process of dealing with death through grieving, challenging, accepting, and/or letting go of someone who has died.

It is important to recognize that seeking hospice is not about "giving up" or speeding up the dying process. It is about making the absolute best of the dying process. This usually means ensuring as much comfort as possible for the dying person and his or her loved ones.

Typically, to be eligible for hospice care, the person must have a condition from which he or she will not recover. Also, the person's life expectancy must be 6 months or less. Sometimes people who receive hospice care live longer than the expected 6 months. Even if the person lives longer than 6 months, he or she can continue to receive care from the hospice team.

Medicare and Insurance and Hospice

It is also important that insurance and cost issues don't entangle what is already a challenging process, so it is helpful to understand these matters to the extent that you can.

Because the Medicare insurance program covers all Americans older than 65 years of age, it may not surprise you that around 80% of people receiving hospice care are Medicare enrollees. The good news is that virtually all insurance programs, including Medicare, Medicaid (insurance coverage for those of low income or with certain chronic illnesses), and commercial insurance plans, cover the cost of hospice services.[36] For people who have no insurance coverage at all, such as undocumented residents, many community-based hospice programs will seek to provide services regardless of ability to pay.[37] (See Chapter 14 for more specifics about insurance coverage.)

For people insured through Medicare, hospice programs are paid for as part of the Medicare Part A benefit, which covers hospital services. In fact, nearly all hospice centers in the United States (around 9 out of 10) are certified by Medicare and are reimbursed by the Medicare hospice benefit.[38] The hospice benefits provided by Medicare, Medicaid, and commercial plans tend to be comprehensive and provide a broad range of care and services for patients and families in need. These benefits usually include hospice services provided to the family of the patient, such as counseling and bereavement programs.

For Medicare or a private health plan (commercial insurance) to pay hospice benefits, a medical professional must certify that the patient has a life-limiting condition where death is expected within 6 months or less. Patients must sign a statement indicating their choice of hospice care instead of routine Medicare-covered treatment to try to cure an illness. Patients must receive care from an approved hospice program, allowed by Medicare or the private health plan. It is important to note that Medicare will pay for other treatments not associated with the terminal illness. For example, if a cut requires stitches or an infection requires antibiotics, the service would still be covered under the routine benefits of the insurance program. But treatments, such as chemotherapy to cure a cancer, are no longer covered once a patient enters a hospice program. Likewise, Medicare and other insurance companies will not cover prescription drugs that seek to cure the illness, although they may cover prescriptions that relieve pain. That being said, Medicare and most insurance plans will go back to paying for regular healthcare treatment services if, as is sometimes the case, an illness goes into remission (a state of recovery or lessening of the severity).

Insurance companies, including Medicare, may not cover services delivered by a hospice provider if that provider is not part of an approved hospice program. Because all hospice care and services must be approved before reimbursement, it is important that patients and families do not introduce new services, expecting them to be covered, without first discussing the services with the insurance program.

Bereavement services are usually provided to surviving family and loved ones and are covered for a year after death and sometimes longer.

Body and Organ Donation

When you get your driver's license, one question you need to answer is whether or not you agree to be an organ donor. States are not expecting you to be in a fatal crash, but things do happen. By agreeing to be an organ donor, in death you become capable of something really heroic.

Whole Body Donation

As an alternative to burial, some people choose to donate their entire body to medical science. Donated bodies have a number of uses, including in anatomy classes for medical students, in helping train surgeons on new procedures, and in various kinds of medical research. According to one website, each donation, on average, is used for six different medical research or training projects. In the end, the body is cremated and may be returned to the family.[39]

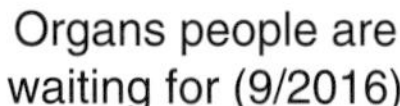

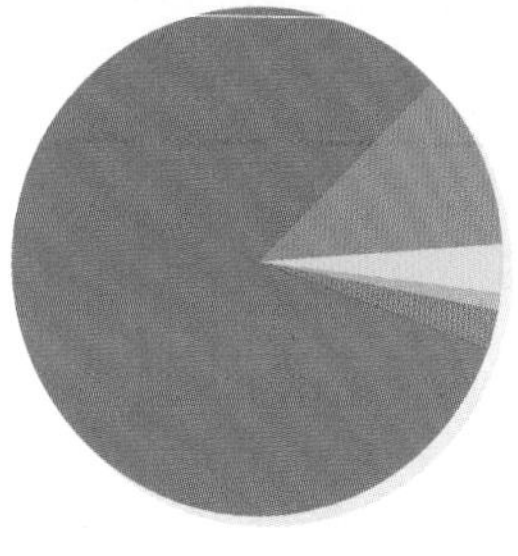

FIGURE 12-4 Distribution of organs for which people are waiting.

U.S. Department of Health and Human Services. (n.d.). Organ donation statistics. Retrieved from https://organdonor.gov/statistics-stories/statistics.html

organ donation The process of surgically removing an organ or tissue from one person (the organ donor) and placing it into another person (the recipient).

You cannot be paid for body donation because federal law prohibits buying bodies.

Organ Donation

You are never too young or too old to be an organ donor. Most major religions approve of organ and tissue donation (there is disagreement in some religions, as noted later in Table 12-3) and consider it an act of charity. There are currently more than 119,000 people waiting for an **organ donation**, and every 10 minutes another name gets added to the list. On average, 22 people who are waiting for a transplant die every day.[40]

The body parts that may be donated include the heart, kidneys, lungs, pancreas, liver, intestines, corneas, skin, tendons, bone, heart valves, hands, and face. Living donors can donate one kidney, one lung, or a portion of their liver, pancreas, or intestine. Blood donation, including bone marrow and stem cells, is also important.[40]

FIGURE 12-4 shows the distribution of organs for which people are waiting.[41]

A small amount of research has been done to determine whether organ donation helps the grieving family come to terms with their loved one's death. One study among parents of children who had died concluded that it was the meaning the parents attributed to the donation that affected their adjustment to their child's death.[42] Another study by the same team found that it was important to the parents to know the outcome for the recipient.[43] In an interview, the director of an organ recovery network reported that the motivation for family members was the idea that "something positive could come out of [their] loss," that "someone else would have a better life," and that, in a way, their "family member would live on."[44]

Donation Process

Registering to donate needed organs is easy. Many states present the option to register when you get a driver's license. Online registration occurs at the state level. From the Health Resources and Services Administration website (part of the federal government), you can link to your state's registry. You can also register through the Donate Life America organization (www.donatelife.net/register/). It is helpful to make your wish to be an organ donor known to your family members or friends.

Even though many people volunteer to be organ donors, only 3 out of 1,000 die in a way that enables the use of their organs. When doctors realize they cannot save a patient's life and the decision is made to donate the organs, the patient is kept on life support to maintain the organs. The Organ Procurement and Transplantation Network maintains the national database of all U.S. patients waiting for an organ transplant. They are the group that matches donated organs to recipients in need.[40]

Determining who gets the organ involves careful consideration by a medical team. The factors that the team considers include the organ(s) to be donated and the match between the donor's and the recipient's blood type and body size.

DONOR STATS

Ninety-five percent of Americans are in favor of being a donor, but only 54% are registered.[45]

The team also considers the severity of the recipient's medical condition and the recipient's availability. The distance between the donor's hospital and the patient's hospital is critical. Different organs can survive (that is, remain viable for transplant) for different lengths of time outside the body. Hearts and lungs can survive for 4 to 6 hours, livers for 12 to 15 hours, kidneys for 36 to 48 hours, and corneas (in the eye) for as long as 14 days. The shorter the organ's viability outside the body, the closer the recipient's hospital needs to be to the donor's hospital.[40]

Funeral Arrangements

A funeral is a ceremony to honor a person who has died. Funeral customs depend on the deceased person's wishes in combination with cultural customs, religion, and the family's desires. The deceased person's body may be buried or cremated. If the body is cremated, it may still be buried, or something else may be done with the ashes. Funerals serve both a religious and a secular (nonreligious) purpose. From a religious viewpoint, they help the soul of the deceased reach the afterlife. From a secular viewpoint, they help family and friends mourn the dead, celebrate the life of the person who has passed, and provide an opportunity for people to offer sympathy to the deceased person's loved ones.

What Does the Average Funeral Cost?

The average funeral in the United States costs between $8,000 and $10,000. The common choice most people make in planning a funeral is to use the services of a funeral home. Customers typically purchase three separate things: the services of the funeral home, the cemetery plot, and the headstone. The usual costs for the services of the funeral home include the basic services fee ($1,500), embalming and preparing the body ($600), the casket ($2,300), the viewing and funeral ceremony ($1,000), and other miscellaneous costs, including the hearse, death certificates, and the obituary ($600). Costs at the cemetery include the plot ($1,000) and the cost to dig the grave ($1,000). Finally, to mark the grave, either a headstone ($2,000) or a grave marker ($1,000), which is a flat granite or bronze plaque that sits on top of the grave site.[47]

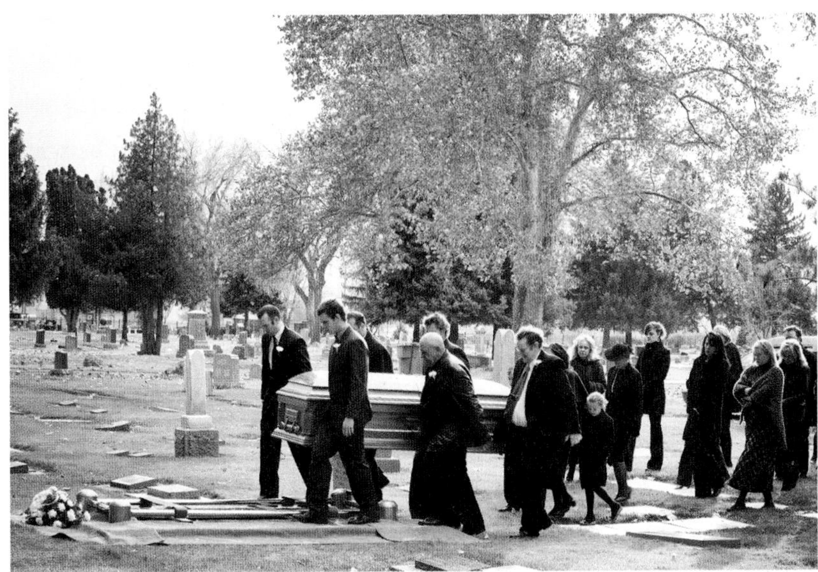

Green Burials

The idea of a green burial is to have as minimal an impact on the environment as possible. Green burials conserve natural resources, preserve the environment by reducing carbon emissions, and protect the health of industry workers. Green burials use only nontoxic and biodegradable materials.

If you work with a green funeral home, they will help you utilize environmentally friendly products, such as a green casket. Varying degrees of green burials are available, depending on your circumstances. For example, you can opt to have the deceased's body refrigerated rather than embalmed. States have different laws depending on whether the person died from an infectious disease, the time between death and burial, and if and how the body is crossing state lines.[48] You may be able to choose a green cemetery, or natural burying ground, or cremation. When burying a body, check the laws in your state, such as whether you must have a casket and what the zoning and permit requirements are.

Cremated Remains

People choose cremation for religious or personal reasons. Once the remains have been cremated, they may be buried in a cemetery, kept, scattered, or enshrined. If the choice is made to scatter the ashes, remember that others may be unhappy that there is no grave to visit and that permission may be needed, depending on the location. If you are having a family member cremated, you need to remove all jewelry before the body is cremated. You must disclose whether the person has any implanted medical devices. One advantage of cremation is that the remains can be divided, so if family members have different ideas about what to do with the ashes, there can be accommodation.

For people whose loved one has been cremated, there are many unique ideas for preserving or scattering the ashes, including the following:

1. *Eternal Reefs.* You can have the ashes mixed into concrete to create a "pearl." The pearls are added to a "reef ball" to help start an ocean habitat. (www.eternalreefs.com)
2. *Angel Flight.* You can have the ashes mixed into fireworks for a one-time display. The family chooses the fireworks' color, brilliance, and display. (www.angels-flight.net)
3. *Holy Smoke.* This organization will take 1 pound of ashes to load into shotgun shells, rifle, or pistol rounds. (www.myholysmoke.com)
4. *Life Gem.* You can have the ashes turned into one or more diamonds. Prices depend on the number, size, and color of the stones. (www.lifegem.com)
5. *Sending ashes up.* You can send ashes into near space to be scattered into the atmosphere (www.mesoloft.com) or into Earth's orbit, to the moon, or into deep space (www.celestis.com).
6. *Memorial tree urns.* Use part of the ashes to nurture a tree. The urns are biodegradable. Depending on where you live, the tree choices include weeping willow, blue spruce, flowering cherry, ponderosa pine, oak, dogwood, coral, *Ginkgo biloba*, Japanese white birch, giant redwood,

COLUMBARIA

A columbarium (plural: *columbaria*) is a building that holds urns with cremated remains.

and 22 other species. The average person's remains will fill seven tree urns. (www.usurnsonline.com/memorials/memorial-tree-urns)

7. *Glass art.* Preserve the memory of your loved one artistically. Have his or her ashes mixed into hand-blown glass artwork. The artist only works with authorized funeral homes. (www.tropicalglassdesign.com)

Make Sure You Know Your Loved One's Wishes

Sometimes we are lucky enough to have the opportunity to say goodbye to our loved one who is dying. Try not to wait until the last minute. Give yourself time to express your love and, if needed, forgiveness.

As discussed earlier in the chapter, make sure you know your loved one's wishes regarding organ donation, cremation or burial, and funeral arrangements. Make sure someone knows and has access to important legal documents, including birth certificate, marriage and divorce certificates (if applicable), Social Security information, any insurance policies, titles to real estate and automobiles owned, financial documents, and keys to a safe-deposit box or home safe.

When a Loved One Dies

When a loved one dies, there are tasks that need to be completed. The following list represents a basic outline of events following the person's death.[48]

1. Immediately

If the person dies at home without a doctor, you need a person to obtain a legal pronouncement of death. If the person is being cared for by a hospice service, the hospice nurse can do this. If a person dies at home, not under hospice care, call 9-1-1. Remember that if the deceased has a living will specifying do not resuscitate, you will need that. Paramedics will arrive and, without the documentation, may try to resuscitate the person. They will take the body to a hospital for a doctor to pronounce the person dead.

There are a number of critical tasks:

- Arrange for the body to go to a mortuary or crematorium.
- Call the person's doctor or the county coroner.
- Call family and close friends. This task is often shared among family members.
- If there are dependent children or pets, finalize a plan for their care.
- If the person was employed, call the employer. You will need information about any benefits or salary due to the person. Ask if there was life insurance through the company.

2. Within a Few Days After Death

Funeral arrangements must be made. Timing and necessary arrangements depend on the religion of the deceased. **TABLE 12-3** reviews the similarities and

THINKING AHEAD

Make sure your parents or guardians put your name on their bank account to prevent it from being frozen when they die.

TABLE 12-3 Funeral Traditions of Different Religions[49]

Religion	Organ Donation	Cremation	Embalming	Timing	Specific Funeral Arrangements	Mourning Period	Notes
Baptist	Acceptable	Acceptable	Acceptable	Within 3 to 5 days	Hymns sung and scripture read	None prescribed	
Buddhist	Acceptable	Acceptable	Acceptable	Services held on days 3, 7, 49, and 100	Simple, solemn, and dignified	Depends on the tie between the deceased and the mourners	Mourners wear white.
Catholic	Some disagreement within the church	Acceptable, but preferably after the funeral mass	Acceptable	There are no funeral masses between Holy Thursday and Easter, nor on Sundays during Advent, Lent, and the Easter Season.	Laypeople may participate as readers, musicians, pallbearers, ushers, and in other usual roles. Music should be appropriate church music.	None prescribed	
Eastern Orthodox	Disagreement within the church	Prohibited	Acceptable	Usually within 2 to 3 days of death but can be up to one week	Open casket. Lit candles are distributed to all present and remain lit throughout the funeral service. Mourners and worshipers stand throughout the service.	40 days	
Episcopalian	Acceptable	Acceptable	Acceptable	Within 2 to 3 days	Closed casket	None prescribed	
Hindu	Acceptable	Traditional for all Hindus except babies, children, and saints	Acceptable	As soon as possible, by next dawn or dusk	A brief wake before cremation	13 days starting with cremation	

Religion	Organ Donation	Cremation	Embalming	Timing	Specific Funeral Arrangements	Mourning Period	Notes
Jewish	Acceptable	Depends on degree of orthodoxy	Not used unless required by law	Preferred within 1 day	No viewing, visitation, or wake. Family members affix a torn black ribbon to clothing.	7 days	Routine autopsies are not acceptable.
Lutheran	Acceptable	Acceptable	Acceptable	Usually within 3 days	May be at church or funeral home.	None prescribed	
Methodist	Acceptable	Acceptable	Acceptable	Within 2 to 3 days	Closed casket	None prescribed	
Muslim	Acceptable	Forbidden	Not used unless required by law	As soon as possible	Prayers are performed by all members of the community. Those praying face Mecca and form at least three lines.	Widows for 4 months and 10 days	Routine autopsies are not acceptable.
Mormon	Acceptable	Allowed but not encouraged	Acceptable	Not on Sunday	Serious but celebratory	None prescribed	
Presbyterian	Acceptable	Generally not supported	Depends	Within a few days	Emphasis placed on scripture reading. May include hymns and a brief sermon.	None prescribed	
Quaker	Acceptable	Acceptable	No specific regulations forbidding, but many Quaker cemeteries do not permit.	Usually within a week of death	No remains are present at funeral. Service follows the format of a customary meeting, beginning with silent meditation followed by speeches by individuals who feel moved to do so.	None prescribed	There is no wake or viewing before the funeral.

Everplans.com. (2016). Funeral traditions of different religions. Retrieved from https://www.everplans.com/articles/funeral-traditions-of-different-religions

differences in the views of major religions regarding aspects of death, funeral arrangements, and mourning.[49]

Prepare an obituary for your local newspaper if that is important to you. Note that many newspapers charge a fee to place an obituary.

Ask a friend or relative to keep an eye on the person's home or apartment, and take care of daily chores, such as answering the phone, collecting mail, and watering plants.

3. Up to 10 Days After Death

Be sure to get death certificates, which usually come from the funeral home. You will need multiple copies for financial institutions, government agencies, and insurers. The deceased person's will may need to go to a city or county office for probate. If necessary, the executor should open a bank account for the estate.

The following organizations or people need to be notified of the death:

- Contact agencies from which the deceased received benefits, such as the Social Security Administration (800-772-1213; www.ssa.gov) and the Department of Veterans Affairs (800-827-1000; www.va.gov). They need to stop paying benefits. Remember to ask about applicable survivor benefits, if any.
- Contact the deceased person's life insurance company or agent to get claim forms.
- Contact the deceased person's bank for details about his or her account(s) and safe-deposit box.
- Contact the deceased person's attorney if needed to transfer assets and if there are probate issues.
- Contact the deceased person's accountant to determine whether there is an estate tax or you need to file a final tax return.
- Contact the police to have them periodically check the deceased person's house, if vacant.
- Contact the deceased person's financial adviser to understand investments and how to access them, if needed.
- Contact utility companies to change or stop services.
- Contact the post office to forward mail.
- If the deceased is receiving a pension, call the issuer to stop the monthly check and determine if there is a beneficiary.

After We Die

It's impossible to know for certain what happens when we die. Because of this uncertainty, people hold a variety of different perspectives about death and the afterlife. Some may follow beliefs of a certain religion, while others may subscribe to their own belief system about what happens to our bodies and souls after death. At one end of the spectrum is the belief that, with death, a person ceases to exist in any form. At the other end, many people believe in some form of an afterlife, where part of an individual's identity continues even after the death of the physical body. Heaven is thought to be one type of afterlife where people can ascend, depending on various standards of their goodness, faith, or other virtues. Heaven is often depicted as a place of peace and joy. Hell is also viewed as one form of the afterlife, but, in contrast, as a place of eternal torment for those who did not meet the standards of Heaven. Some people believe that after your physical body dies, it becomes reincarnated to start a new life in a different body. These beliefs can affect how a person feels about themselves or their loved ones dying, and how they cope with grief. For example, those who

AUTOPSY

An **autopsy** is a medical examination of the body after death. It is usually conducted to determine the cause of death.[50]

When is an autopsy required? Although the requirements vary by state, in general, autopsies are required in the following circumstances:

1. A suspicious death or "foul play" is suspected.
2. The person died of an infectious or contagious disease. (Autopsy is required for public health purposes.)
3. The deceased is an inmate.
4. The death was unexpected, such as that of a healthy child.
5. The death was the result of an injury.
6. The family requests an autopsy.

WebMD. (n.d.). Autopsy. Retrieved from http://www.webmd.com/a-to-z-guides/autopsy-16080#1

autopsy An examination of a body after death to determine the cause of death or the character and extent of changes produced by disease.

do not believe in an afterlife experience more depressive symptoms and anger after a spouse dies. Because there is no factual way to know what happens after death, everyone has a right to their own beliefs about death and the afterlife.

Good Grief?

grief The emotional reaction to a death or loss.

Just as death is complicated, so too is **grief**. Grief is the reaction to a death or loss. It may manifest (meaning show itself) through different outlets, all of which are a normal reaction to the loss of a loved one. After a loss, individuals may have a physical response, such as changes in sleep or appetite. They may have recurring thoughts, such as memories of the deceased person or worries about what will happen without that person. Individuals may experience distressing emotions such as guilt, anger, sadness, or hopelessness, but they may also feel positive emotions such as relief that the loved one is no longer suffering or hopefulness for the future. Individuals may have a spiritual reaction, such as having an increase in faith or questioning of faith. Some may find it therapeutic to talk about the death of a loved one and celebrate that person's life with a memorial or donation. All of these reactions can be part of the grieving process.[51,52]

Everyone experiences the loss of a loved one differently. The nature of a person's relationship with the deceased loved one and the circumstances of death can affect how the person processes the loss. One person might want to talk about his or her grandmother dying, but a sibling may not be ready to accept this reality. Grieving can be a healthy process that involves coming to terms with the loss and adapting to this new situation.[51]

Mental health professionals used to believe that people grieve in stages, where a person first would be in denial, then become angry, try to bargain, become depressed, and finally, accept the death. More recent research has demonstrated that grief does not come in ordered stages. For example, someone may immediately accept the death of a loved one and never become angry or depressed. Professionals also used to think that the grieving process never ended. Of course, the memory of a loved one does not go away, but we now understand that the most intense grief usually occurs in the first 6 months after the loss of a loved one, and most people return to a normal routine within 18 months.[53]

Grief is distinct from depression. However, grief can become depression. If someone feels depressed or suicidal, has been grieving for several months without feeling better, or cannot get back to his or her regular activities because of grief, it is important for that person to seek help.[54] (See Chapter 6 for more information about clinical depression.)

In Summary

This chapter has described how aging affects our bodies and our health, and habits we can embrace to promote healthy aging and, specifically, to reduce the risk of dementia.

You have learned about the importance, both for yourself and for loved ones, of getting things in order to prepare for a death. We have provided some questions to help you initiate these preparations with your parents or elderly family members. You have also learned about the importance and the components of a living will and end-of-life decisions.

As we discussed, palliative care and hospice care can bring immense relief to a person in the late stages of a terminal illness, and to the person's loved ones. We have described for you other end-of-life choices, including organ and whole body donation, the process of making funeral arrangements, and options for cremated remains.

Key Terms

activities of daily living
advance directive
Alzheimer's disease
autopsy
bereavement
cremation
dementia
grief
heroic treatments
hospice
life expectancy
living will
organ donation
palliative care
resuscitation
terminally ill
will

Student Discussion Questions and Activities

1. In the Chicago heat wave of 1995 (see Tales of Public Health box), Black people had significantly higher mortality than Whites. Why do you think this was?
2. Name three things you do currently that will help to promote healthy aging.
3. What grieving mechanisms did/would you find most helpful following the death of a loved one?
4. When you die, what do you want to be done with your body? Why is that your choice?
5. Are you signed up to be an organ donor? Why or why not? In your state, is it noted on the driver's license? Why do you think so many people don't sign up?
6. Assuming your parents are alive, have you discussed their end-of-life wishes with them? Is the idea of having this discussion stressful? Do you believe they have thought about this?
7. Can you describe a scenario in which the decision to transition to hospice care is relatively clear for a patient and the family? What about a situation in which the decision is not so clear? What factors might affect the clarity of this decision, and what can a family do to make the decision easier?

Resources

Grief Share (grief support): https://www.griefshare.org/

Alzheimer's Disease Education and Referral (ADEAR) Center: www.nia.nih.gov/alzheimers
Phone: 1-800-438-4380 (toll-free)
Email: adear@nia.nih.gov

ADEAR caregiver support: https://www.nia.nih.gov/alzheimers/publication/caring-person-alzheimers-disease/about-guide

Alzheimer's Association: www.alz.org
Phone: 1-800-272-3900 (toll-free), 1-866-403-3073 (TTY/toll-free)
Email: info@alz.org

Depression among older adults: https://www.nimh.nih.gov/health/publications/older-adults-and-depression/qf-16-7697_153371.pdf

Funeral Consumers Alliance: https://funerals.org/

References

1. Zitter, J. N. (2017, February 18). First, sex ed. Then death ed. *New York Times*. Retrieved from https://www.nytimes.com/2017/02/18/opinion/sunday/first-sex-ed-then-death-ed.html?_r=0
2. National Vital Statistics System, National Center for Health Statistics, Centers for Disease Control and Prevention. (2018). Mortality Data—2016. Retrieved from https://www.cdc.gov/nchs/nvss/deaths.htm
3. National Vital Statistics System, National Center for Health Statistics, Centers for Disease Control and Prevention. (2016). Ten leading causes of death by age group, United States—2014. Retrieved from https://www.cdc.gov/injury/wisqars/pdf/leading_causes_of_death_by_age_group_2014-a.pdf
4. Mayo Clinic staff. (2015). Aging: What to expect. Retrieved from http://www.mayoclinic.org/healthy-lifestyle/healthy-aging/in-depth/aging/art-20046070
5. Russell, M. A., Hill, K. D., Blackberry, I., Day, L. L., & Dharmage, S. C. (2006). Falls risk and functional decline in older fallers discharged directly from emergency departments. *Journals of Gerontology: Series A, Biological Sciences and Medical Sciences, 61*(10), 1090–1095.
6. United Nations, Department of Economic and Social Affairs, Population Division. (2002.) World population ageing: 1950–2050: IV. Demographic profile of the older population. Retrieved from http://www.un.org/esa/population/publications/worldageing19502050/pdf/90chapteriv.pdf
7. Guinnessworldrecords.com. (n.d.). Oldest person ever (female): Jeanne Louise Calment. Retrieved from http://www.guinnessworldrecords.com/world-records/oldest-person-(female)
8. World Health Organization. (2015). Ageing and health. Retrieved from http://www.who.int/mediacentre/factsheets/fs404/en/
9. Inouye, S. K., Studenski, S., Tinetti, M. E., & Kuchel, G. A. (2007). Geriatric syndromes: Clinical, research, and policy implications of a core geriatric concept. *Journal of the American Geriatric Society, 55*(5), 780–791.
10. Health in Aging. (2015). Eldercare at home: Problems of daily living. Retrieved from http://www.healthinaging.org/resources/resource:eldercare-at-home-problems-of-daily-living/
11. Hebert, L. E., Weuve, J., Scherr, P. A., Evans, D. A. (2013) Alzheimer disease in the United States (2010–2050) estimated using the 2010 census. *Neurology. 80*(19), 1778–1783.
12. Carmeli, E. (2014) The invisibles: Unpaid caregivers of the elderly. Frontiers in Public Health. 2: 91
13. Alzheimer's Association. (n.d.). What is dementia? Retrieved from http://www.alz.org/what-is-dementia.asp
14. Alzheimer's Association. (2017). 2017 Alzheimer's disease facts and figures. Retrieved from http://www.alz.org/facts/
15. National Institute on Aging. (2016). Alzheimer's disease fact sheet. Retrieved from https://www.nia.nih.gov/alzheimers/publication/alzheimers-disease-fact-sheet
16. National Center for Chronic Disease Prevention and Health Promotion, Centers for Disease Control and Prevention. (2016). Alzheimer's disease. Retrieved from https://www.cdc.gov/chronicdisease/resources/publications/aag/alzheimers.htm
17. Alzheimer's Association and Centers for Disease Control and Prevention. (2013). The healthy brain initiative: The public health road map for state and national partnerships, 2013–2018. Retrieved from https://www.cdc.gov/aging/pdf/2013-healthy-brain-initiative.pdf
18. Aldrich, N. CDC promotes public health approach to address depression among older adults. Centers for Disease Control and Prevention. Retrieved from https://www.cdc.gov/aging/pdf/cib_mental_health.pdf
19. Klineberg, E. (2015). *Heat wave: A social autopsy of disaster in Chicago*. Chicago, IL: University of Chicago Press.
20. Centers for Disease Control and Prevention. (2013). Ten great public health achievements in the 20th century. Retrieved from https://www.cdc.gov/about/history/tengpha.htm
21. Murphy, S. L., Xu, J., & Kochanek, K. D. (2013). Deaths: Final data for 2010. Table 22. Life expectancy at birth, at age 65, and at age 75, by sex, race, and Hispanic origin: United States, selected years 1900–2010. Centers for Disease Control and Prevention. Retrieved from https://www.cdc.gov/nchs/data/hus/2011/022.pdf
22. Russell, L. M. (2011). *Reducing disparities in life expectancy: What factors matter?* The National Academies of Sciences, Engineering, and Medicine. Retrieved from http://nationalacademies.org/hmd/~/media/Files/Activity%20Files/SelectPops/HealthDisparities/2011-FEB-24/Commissioned%20Paper%20by%20Lesley%20Russell.pdf
23. Innis, M. (2017, February 25). 'Affordable underground furniture': D.I.Y. coffin clubs catch on in New Zealand. *New York Times*. Retrieved from https://www.nytimes.com/2017/02/25/world/australia/new-zealand-diy-coffins.html

24. *Psychology Today*. (2014). Death and dying. Retrieved from https://www.psychologytoday.com/conditions/death-and-dying
25. Lieber, R. (2013, January 11). A shocking death, a financial lesson and help for others. *New York Times*. Retrieved from http://www.nytimes.com/2013/01/12/your-money/estate-planning/shell-tell-you-its-time-to-think-ahead.html
26. Ashford, K. (2009, December 18). Twelve tough questions to ask your parents. *CBS News*. Retrieved from http://www.cbsnews.com/news/12-tough-questions-to-ask-your-parents/
27. Simmons Hannibal, B. (n.d.). Online estate planning: Do-it-yourself estate planning software. AllLaw.com. Retrieved from http://www.alllaw.com/articles/wills_and_trusts/online-estate-planning-software.htm
28. Mayo Clinic staff. (2014). Living wills and advance directives for medical decisions. Retrieved from http://www.mayoclinic.org/healthy-lifestyle/consumer-health/in-depth/living-wills/art-20046303
29. National Kidney Foundation. (2016). Dialysis. Retrieved from https://www.kidney.org/atoz/content/dialysisinfo
30. Randolph, M. (n.d.). What is a living will? AllLaw.com. Retrieved from http://www.alllaw.com/articles/wills_and_trusts/article7.asp
31. Randolph, M. (n.d.). The witness requirement to execute a will. AllLaw.com. Retrieved from http://www.alllaw.com/articles/nolo/wills-trusts/witness-requirement-execute.html
32. Funeral Consumers Alliance. (n.d.). Home page. Retrieved from https://funerals.org/
33. Abernethy, A. P., Wheeler, J. L., & Bull, J. (2011). Development of a health information technology-based data system in community-based hospice and palliative care. *American Journal of Preventive Medicine, 40*(5 Suppl 2), S217–S224.
34. Teno, J. M., Gozalo, P. L., Bynum, J. P., Leland, N. E., Miller, S. C., Morden, N. E., . . . Mor, V. (2013). Change in end-of-life care for Medicare beneficiaries: Site of death, place of care, and health care transitions in 2000, 2005, and 2009. *JAMA, 309*(5), 470–477.
35. Meghani, S. H. (2004). A concept analysis of palliative care in the United States. *Journal of Advanced Nursing, 46*(2), 152–161.
36. WebMD. (n.d.). Hospice care—topic overview. Retrieved from http://www.webmd.com/balance/tc/hospice-care-topic-overview#1
37. Gray, N. A., Boucher, N. A., Kuchibhatla, M., & Johnson, K. S. (2017). Hospice access for undocumented immigrants. *JAMA Internal Medicine, 177*(4), 579–580.
38. Kelley, A. S., & Morrison, R. S. (2015). Palliative care for the seriously ill. *New England Journal of Medicine, 373*(8), 747–755.
39. Medical research projects. (n.d.). Science Care. Retrieved from http://www.sciencecare.com/medical-research-projects/
40. U.S. Department of Health and Human Services. (n.d.). U.S. government information on organ donation and transplantation. Retrieved from https://organdonor.gov/index.html
41. U.S. Department of Health and Human Services. (n.d.). Organ donation statistics. Retrieved from https://organdonor.gov/statistics-stories/statistics.html
42. Bellali, T., & Papadatou, D. (2006). Parental grief following the brain death of a child: Does consent or refusal to organ donation affect their grief? *Death Studies, 30*(10), 883–917.
43. Bellali, T., Papazoglou, I., & Papadatou, D. (2007). Empirically based recommendations to support parents facing the dilemma of paediatric cadaver organ donation. *Intensive and Critical Care Nursing, 23*(4), 216–225.
44. Final gifts: Organ donation could help families grieve. (2012). *Daily Messenger.* Retrieved from http://www.mpnnow.com/x1224698724/Final-Gifts-Organ-Donation-Could-Help-Families-Grieve
45. organdonor.gov. (2016). Organ Donor Statistics. Retrieved from https://www.organdonor.gov/statistics-stories/statistics.html
46. Parting.com. (2017, January 23). How much does the average funeral cost? Retrieved from https://www.parting.com/blog/how-much-does-the-average-funeral-cost/
47. Funeral Information Society. (2011). State-by-state embalming requirements. Retrieved from http://www.funeralinformationsociety.org/images/laws/Embalming%20by%20State.pdf
48. *Consumer Reports*. (2012, October). What to do when someone dies. Retrieved from http://www.consumerreports.org/cro/magazine/2012/10/what-to-do-when-a-loved-one-dies/index.htm
49. Everplans.com. (2016). Funeral traditions of different religions. Retrieved from https://www.everplans.com/articles/funeral-traditions-of-different-religions
50. WebMD. (n.d.). Autopsy. Retrieved from http://www.webmd.com/a-to-z-guides/autopsy-16080#1
51. KidsHealth by Nemours. (2013). Death and grief. Retrieved from http://kidshealth.org/en/teens/someone-died.html
52. Nordal, K. C. (2011). Grief: Coping with the loss of your loved one. American Psychological Association. Retrieved from http://www.apa.org/helpcenter/grief.aspx
53. Konigsberg, R. D. (2011). New ways to think about grief. *TIME*. Retrieved from http://content.time.com/time/magazine/article/0,9171,2042372,00.html
54. KidsHealth by Nemours. (2013). Getting help for intense grief. Retrieved from http://kidshealth.org/en/teens/intense-grief.html

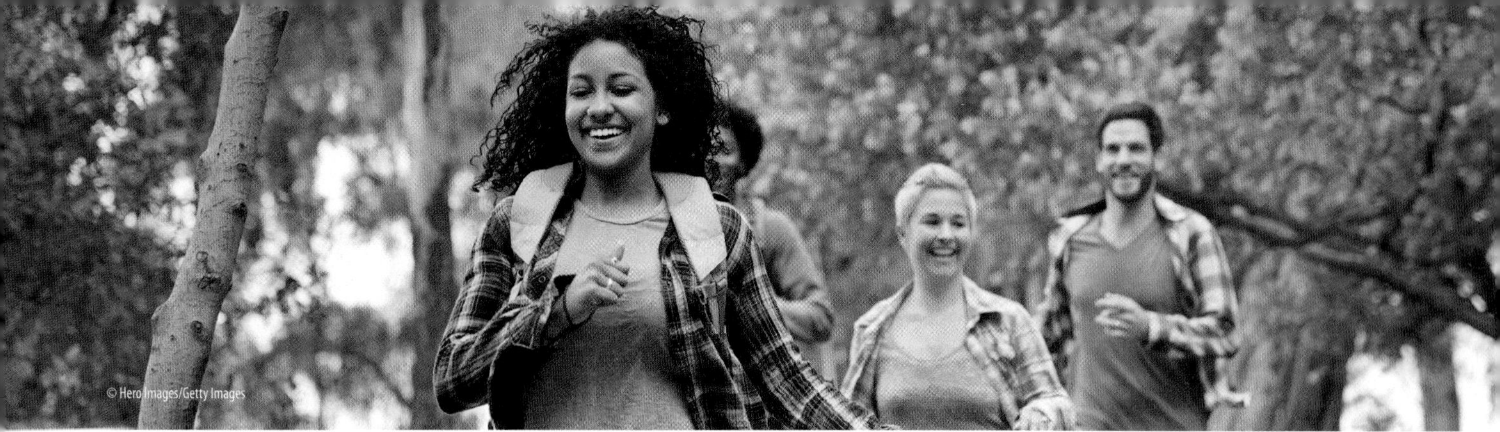

CHAPTER 13

A Growing Challenge: Chronic Diseases

CHAPTER OBJECTIVES

- Explain what chronic and noncommunicable diseases are.
- Discuss different types of chronic conditions.
- Recognize the burden of chronic diseases in the United States and around the world.
- Explore specific chronic disease conditions, including cancer, diabetes, asthma, and cardiovascular diseases, and discuss prevention and treatment strategies for individuals and populations.

Despite the fact that infectious disease outbreaks and epidemics occur all over the world, fewer people are dying from conditions such as tuberculosis, malaria, polio, and AIDS than ever before. That's the good news. The bad news? Chronic conditions—diseases such as heart disease, stroke, cancer, certain respiratory diseases, and diabetes—now cause more deaths globally than infectious diseases.[1]

Chronic diseases are those that persist for a long time, even with treatment. Unlike infectious diseases, they are not contagious, and, for the most part, cannot be prevented by vaccines or quickly cured by drugs or other therapies. Today, the large majority of Americans over 65 years of age has at least one chronic health condition (such as heart disease, cancer, diabetes, obesity, or Alzheimer's disease).[2] Nearly half of all Americans *of any age* have a chronic condition, a prevalence that will worsen as Americans continue to consume unhealthy food and drink, abuse drugs and alcohol, avoid exercise, and lead increasingly stressful lives.[2]

chronic diseases Diseases that last for 3 months or longer.

The reasons chronic, noncommunicable diseases have surpassed infectious diseases as the leading killer around the world are complex. One reason is that food and beverage companies are targeting poorer countries around the world with their marketing, and increasingly targeting poor and vulnerable communities in the United States.[3] Another reason is that tobacco companies show no signs of reducing the aggressive marketing of their products across the world, placing new generations of young people at risk for cancer, heart disease, and other smoking-related illnesses.[4] The increase in the prevalence of conditions such as obesity, diabetes, and heart disease is an ironic byproduct of an increasingly prosperous and Westernized world: more access for more people to processed food, cigarettes, alcohol, and other products that come with an industrialized lifestyle. Consumption of these products is associated with numerous chronic diseases.[5]

In the United States, chronic diseases have long been the leading cause of death because infectious diseases are less prevalent here than they are around the world. Many of the lifestyles that contribute to chronic conditions—dependence on cars; the pervasiveness of fast food and sweetened beverages; and diets high in fat, sugar, and sodium—have been the norm in this country for decades, even though they are now being introduced around the world at increasing rates.

Today, the three leading causes of death in the United States are all chronic conditions: heart disease (around 630,000 deaths per year in the United States), cancer (600,000 deaths), and chronic lower respiratory diseases (155,000 deaths).[6] Living a healthy lifestyle—eating well, exercising, avoiding cigarettes, getting adequate sleep, and so on—can help reduce your risk of acquiring these conditions. Along with individual action, public policies are needed, such as restricting the influence of processed food and tobacco marketing in vulnerable communities. Ultimately, however, none of us can completely prevent the possibility of chronic disease. For example, cancer can strike anyone, healthy or not, at any time.

Cancer: A Collection of Related Diseases

cancer A malignant growth or tumor resulting from the division of abnormal cells.

Cancer is the name given to a category of related diseases, with over 100 specific diseases falling under this umbrella. Cancer occurs when the body's normal mechanism of cell behavior stops working. Normally, cells reproduce at controlled rates and eventually die and are replaced with new cells. Cancer cells grow and divide in an uncontrolled manner.

Cancer cells can invade healthy tissues and spread around the body via the blood and lymph systems. This can compromise the body's healthy functions and, if untreated, eventually lead to death. Usually, these new, abnormal cells form a mass of tissue, called a **tumor**. However, not all cancers present as tumors. **Leukemia**, for example, is a category of cancers that usually begins in the bone marrow and leads to unnaturally high numbers of abnormally undeveloped white blood cells that spread through the body without forming tumors.

tumor A benign or malignant overgrowth of tissues.

leukemia A category of cancers that usually begins in the bone marrow and leads to unnaturally high numbers of abnormally undeveloped white blood cells that spread through the body without forming tumors.

It is also important to know that not all tumors are cancerous; tumors that are cancerous are often referred to as "malignant," while noncancerous tumors are called "benign." Medical tests can determine if a tumor is malignant or benign. These tests may include magnetic resonance imaging (MRI), computerized axial tomography (CAT) scanning, a biopsy, or blood screening.

Cancer Incidence and Mortality

In 2017, there were around 1.8 million new cases of cancer diagnosed in the United States. During the same year, around 600,000 people died from this set of diseases. Cancer mortality does not affect all genders and races equally; mortality is higher for men than women (annual cancer deaths are around 208 per 100,000 for men and 145 per 100,000 women). Among races and ethnicities,

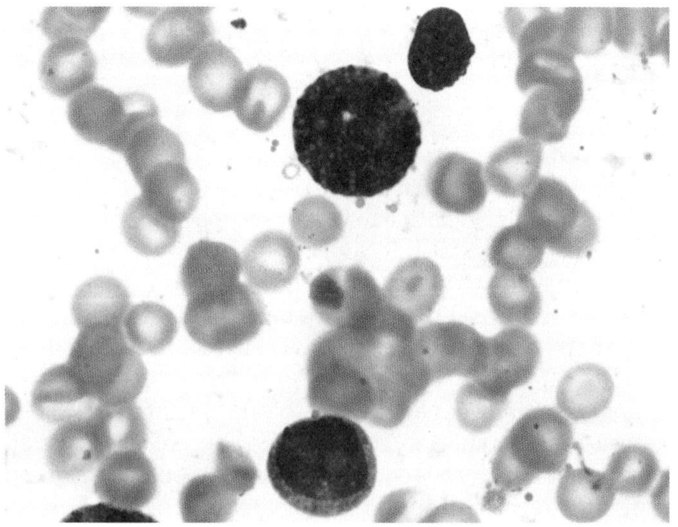

Cancer cells.

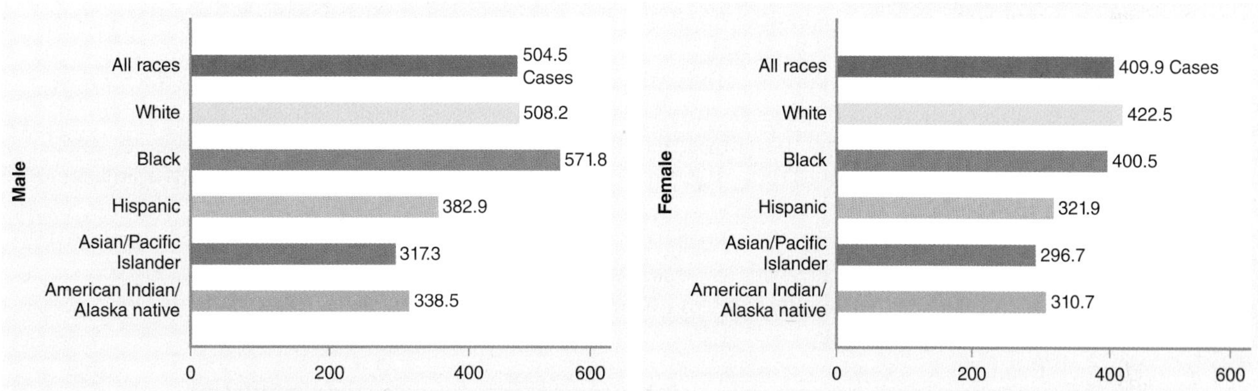

FIGURE 13-1 Cancer rates differ by racial and ethnic groups. For Black men, the chances of getting cancer are higher than they are for White men, for example. Among women, the rate for all cancers is higher for White women than it is for Black women.

Reproduced from Cancer.gov (2014). https://www.cancer.gov/PublishedContent/Images/about-cancer/understanding/disparities/number-new-cases-gender-enlarge.__v30062078.jpg

mortality is highest in African American men at 262 per 100,000, and lowest in Asian and Pacific Islander women at 91 per 100,000.[7] **FIGURE 13-1** shows new cancer incidence among different races and ethnicities and by sex.

The reasons for these differences are complex, and epidemiology researchers continue to investigate the causes. One important factor to these disparate mortality rates is the unequal access to healthcare coverage among Americans. For example, a White person is more likely to have access to insurance coverage than a typical African American. Medically underserved populations are more likely to be diagnosed with late-stage diseases, because they have less access to family practice physicians and diagnostic cancer screenings earlier on.[8]

Another cause is socioeconomic status (SES), whereby poorer populations (African American, Latino, recent immigrants, etc.) tend to have higher rates of cancer. The connection appears to be the fact that communities living in poverty are more likely to be exposed to environmental toxins such as pollution, poor working conditions, access to tobacco, and access to cheaper, highly processed foods; all of these are direct or indirect risk factors for cancer.[9]

TALES OF PUBLIC HEALTH

Betty Gets Cancer

In a powerful episode of the hit television series, *Mad Men*, audiences watched a physician discover cancer tumors on the lung of one of the show's central characters, Betty Draper Francis. But instead of telling 38-year-old Betty, a mother of four children, the doctor contacted her husband to allow him to decide how and how much to tell his wife.

That fictional episode took place in 1970, and cancer diagnosis and treatment has come a long way since. During the 1960s and into the 1970s, there was a stigma around breast cancer. It was not something anyone talked about—even among family members. Later, celebrities such as Shirley Temple and Betty Ford (**FIGURE 13-2**) would make public announcements about their cancers to show others that it's OK to talk about it with the people around you.

Today, there are online and local support groups in communities everywhere, giving patients more access to information and empathetic listeners without geographic restriction. The American Cancer Society and other organizations have partnered with well-known institutions, such as Avon and the National Football League, to raise awareness about breast cancer and encourage annual screenings. Football teams have worn pink uniforms and played with pink game balls to get people to think and talk about breast cancer and how to prevent it. Walks, runs, and other fundraisers have been organized by companies such as Avon, and even KFC, which sold its fried chicken in pink buckets for a time to raise money for Susan G. Komen, a breast cancer advocacy organization. While these kinds of "pink marketing" programs may seem to do more for corporate branding than reducing cancer mortality, they are part of an important trend toward greater awareness and less secrecy about a disease that was once deemed unspeakable.

Decades ago, a patient might have communicated with only a few medical professionals, generally doctors and nurses. Today, a cancer patient will often work closely with several nurses, a medical oncologist, a radiation oncologist, a surgeon, a mental health therapist, physical therapists, and others. New technologies, therapies, and protocols mean that a patient being treated today has a much greater chance of survival than one with a similar diagnosis 50 years ago.

Unfortunately, however, modern cancer treatments are still unavailable to many people in the United States. In 2018, there are still more than 20 million Americans with no health insurance at all, meaning that, despite the progress made, there are still people with cancer who receive less treatment than what the *Mad Men* character Betty Draper Francis would have seen five decades ago.

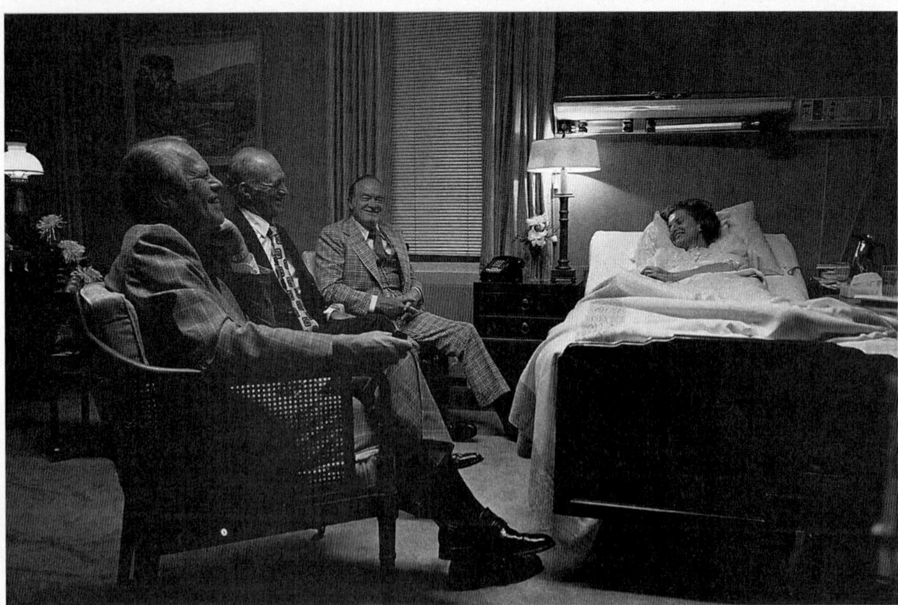

FIGURE 13-2 A first lady shares her cancer with the world: Up until the early 1970s, cancer was highly stigmatized; people were ashamed to admit they had it and were unlikely to discuss it with family and friends. That began to change in the mid-1970s, when U.S. First Lady Betty Ford (pictured here after breast cancer treatment with [*left to right*] President Ford, an unidentified man, and Bob Hope), along with others, openly shared her breast cancer diagnosis through print and electronic media.

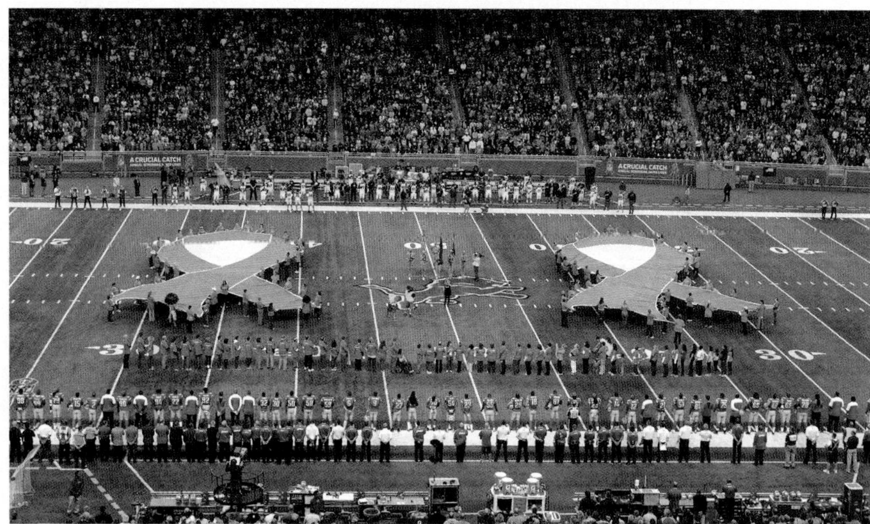

Awareness of cancer and cancer screening options have increased dramatically over the past few decades. Today, even the NFL incorporates breast cancer advocacy into parts of its season by encouraging teams to, among other activities, incorporate pink into their uniforms.

Common Forms of Cancer

Cancer can occur anywhere in the body. As seen in **TABLE 13-1**, the most frequently diagnosed cancers in the United States each year are lung, breast, and prostate cancers. Among men, prostate cancer is the most common form of cancer, while in women breast cancer is most common. Table 13-1 also demonstrates that the most common cancers are not necessarily the most deadly. While breast cancer is the most common type of cancer diagnosed, more people die from lung, colorectal, and pancreatic cancers than from breast cancer.

Survival Rates by Type

The 5-year survival rates are generally used as a measure of how deadly a particular cancer is. These rates indicate the percentage of people with the same type (or type and stage) of cancer who will still be alive 5 years after they were diagnosed. This rule, which originated in the 1930s, determined that once a person survives 5 years after diagnosis, it is unlikely that the cancer will recur. How likely this is depends on the type of cancer, but today, the 5-year survival rate is often used to assume that a patient has "survived" cancer. However despite the fact that it is unusual for cancers to recur after 5 years of remission (the decrease or disappearance of signs of cancer), they can recur at any time.

Currently, the most deadly cancer is considered to be pancreatic cancer; only 7% of those diagnosed will survive 5 years. Other deadly types include liver and lung cancers, both of which have a survival rate of around 17%.[10]

Classification and Stages of Cancer

The usual classification of cancers is by the location in the body where the cancer occurs (as in Table 13-1) or by "histological type," which is the type of tissue in which the cancer originates. Below are the five histological classifications, and the type of tissues in which each cancer originates:

- *Carcinomas*: Originating in the skin or tissues lining the internal organs
- *Sarcomas*: Originating in bone, cartilage, fat, muscle, or other connective tissues

TABLE 13-1 One-Year Cancer Incidence (New Cases) and Death Rates (by Mortality), United States[7]

Cancer Type (Body Site)	Estimated New Cases	Estimated Deaths
Lung	222,500	155,900
Colon and rectal	135,400	50,250
Pancreatic	53,700	43,100
Breast	255,000	42,000
Liver and bile	40,700	28,900
Prostate	161,400	26,700
Leukemia	62,100	24,500
Non-Hodgkin lymphoma	72,240	20,140
Bladder	79,000	16,900
Kidney	64,000	14,400
Endometrial	61,380	10,920
Melanoma	87,110	9,730
Thyroid	56,870	2,010

- *Leukemias*: Originating in the blood or bone marrow
- *Lymphomas*: Originating in the immune system
- *Central nervous system*: Originating in the brain or the spinal cord

carcinomas A type of cancer that develops in the epithelial tissues.

sarcomas A malignant tumor that arises from connective and supporting tissues.

Carcinomas, or tumors that form on the internal or external linings of the body, are the most common classification of cancer, accounting for more than 80% of all cases. Carcinomas tend to affect organs or glands that secrete, such as the breasts, which produce milk, or the lungs, which secrete mucus. **Sarcomas** can originate in bones, tendons, and muscles. Young adults are more likely to be affected by sarcomas, the most common of which occurs in the bone. Leukemias, which are not tumors, are also sometimes referred to as "liquid cancers." Leukemia usually consists of the overproduction of immature white blood cells, which do not function adequately, leading to bruising and infections. Lymphomas originate in the lymphatic glands, which fight infection and clean toxins from your body, and can develop within different organs, such as the breast or the stomach. There are two types of lymphomas, Hodgkin's and non-Hodgkin's lymphoma. The presence of a specific type of cells, called Reed–Sternberg cells, in the lymph indicates Hodgkin's lymphoma, which then leads to different forms of treatment.

Stages of Cancer

Staging is the way oncologists (medical doctors specializing in cancer) describe how extensive a cancer is. A cancer is said to have "metastasized" when the

TABLE 13-2 Stages of Cancer

Stage	Description
0	Relatively small and limited to surface cells
1	Limited or no spread to outside cells; beginning to grow within the original site
2	Limited or no spread, but cancer continues to grow, potentially into a large tumor
3	Cancer is growing significantly and beginning to be seen in the lymph system and other cells in the body
4	Cancer has spread into systems and/or organs in parts of the body that are far from the original site

cancer cells spread beyond the original organ. This is also called metastatic cancer. One of the first places a cancer will spread is into the nearby lymph nodes. Because the lymphatic system is a body-wide network of tissues and organs, it may spread the cancer to other parts of the body. **TABLE 13-2** lists the numerical system used to classify the extent that a cancer has grown and spread throughout the body.

Causes of Cancer

Worldwide, more than one out of every five cancer deaths (about 22%) is caused by tobacco. Another 10% of cancer deaths is due to other preventable causes, including poor diet, lack of exercise, and alcohol abuse.[11] See the Try It! Reducing Your Chances of Getting Cancer box for more on lifestyle causes and what you can do to reduce your risk. There are also environmental associations with cancer, such as being exposed to toxins like radiation, herbicides, pesticides, chemicals in the workplace (e.g., asbestos), and pollutants. While research has demonstrated clear links between hazards such as these and cancers, new studies continue to explore these factors and are helping us to better understand the extent to which getting cancer is simply "bad luck" compared to having specific causes.[12]

Cancer Treatment

Cancer treatment depends on issues such as the type of cancer and its stage. It also depends on the patient. A course of treatment can be determined by a person's age and health, but also an individual's preferences and priorities. Some people are opposed to certain types of treatment, and, increasingly, these preferences are being taken into consideration when determining how to treat cancer. Generally speaking, the goal of treatment is to kill cancer cells and reduce their spread. The following are the three most common cancer treatments. They can be executed alone, or in concert with the others:

- *Surgery*: The tumor is removed from the site of the cancer.
- *Chemotherapy*: Chemicals are injected into the body with the intention of killing cancer cells.
- *Radiation*: High-energy radiation, such as X-rays, gamma rays, and charged particles, are directed at cancer cells.

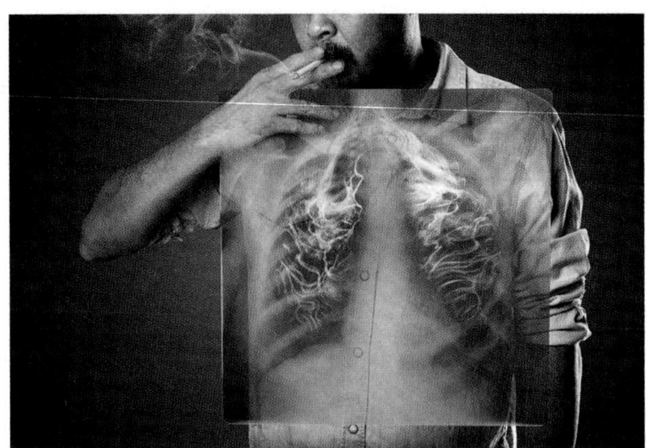

melanoma A malignant tumor formed in the pigment-producing cells (melanocytes).

TRY IT!

Reducing Your Chances of Getting Cancer

While nothing can be done to guarantee that you won't ever get cancer, there is much evidence to show that certain behaviors can reduce your chances. The following is a list of the most widely accepted behaviors for reducing cancer risk:

- *Avoiding tobacco.* Worldwide, more than one out of every five cancer deaths (about 22%) is caused by tobacco,[11] and avoiding tobacco may be the number one most effective behavior for preventing cancer. Tobacco use—especially smoking cigarettes—has been linked to cancer in a variety of sites in the body, including the lungs, mouth, throat, larynx, pancreas, bladder, cervix, and kidneys. In addition to smoking, chewing tobacco and exposure to secondhand smoke are also associated with cancer.
- *Healthy eating.* The National Cancer Institute, the American Cancer Society, and many other cancer-related research and advocacy organizations recommend eating a diet high in vegetables and low in meat. There is evidence of an association between vegetable consumption and reduced cancer risk,[13,14] as well as research connecting red meat and processed foods with increased cancer risk.[15] While overall, experts tend to recommend eating more vegetables and fish and less sugar, processed food, and meat, there is still much research to be done in this area, especially with regard to organic foods, specific types of vegetables, and different types of spices.
- *Exercise.* There is considerable evidence indicating that exercising regularly will reduce your risk of getting cancer—especially breast and colon cancers.[16] In general, rigorous exercise seems to be more protective than moderate exercise. Nevertheless, more research needs to be done to give us better insights on the ideal type, frequency, and intensity of exercise and which forms of cancer can be impacted the most.
- *Vaccination.* Some noncancerous conditions may potentially lead to cancer. These conditions, in turn, can be prevented through vaccinations. This is why vaccination is considered to be an effective means of reducing one's chances of acquiring the disease. Two of these conditions are hepatitis B and the human papillomavirus (HPV). Hepatitis B can increase your risk of developing liver cancer, and HPV, a sexually transmitted virus, has been shown to cause cancers of the cervix, the head, and the neck. While the hepatitis B vaccine is recommended for adults with high risk (such as people with sexually transmitted infections and intravenous drug users), the HPV vaccine is now recommended for adolescent girls and boys or anyone under age 26 who did not receive it earlier.
- *Being careful in the sun.* Skin cancer is the most common form of cancer, especially among the White population, which is 20 times more likely to get it than African Americans. It is not as deadly as other cancers, though, and early detection is important. **Melanoma**, a cancer that begins in the melanocyte cells, counts for only 1% of all skin cancers, but it is the most fatal. To avoid skin cancers of any kind, try to avoid direct sun between 10 a.m. and 4 p.m. Try not to burn. Covering up with a hat or clothing is the best option, but applying sunscreen with a sun protection factor (SPF) of 15 or higher can also help. Finally, avoid tanning beds, as they have also been shown to cause cancer.

Unfortunately, plenty of nonsmokers have acquired lung cancer, and many vegetarians, dedicated exercisers, and otherwise healthy people have been struck with a cancer of some kind. Cancer can strike anyone at any time. However, these activities have been demonstrated to reduce your risk, and for now, that's better than nothing and certainly worth a try.

Reducing Cancer Risk: In Individuals and in Societies

According to data from the American Cancer Society, in the United States fewer people are dying of cancer than ever before. Cancer mortality declined by 23% between 1991 and 2014.[10] This reduction is due to developing new ways to treat the disease, better screening techniques, new understanding about how to prevent the disease from occurring in the first place, and a gradual decrease in smoking among Americans during that period.

While no activities and behaviors are guarantees for preventing cancer, several actions have been empirically demonstrated to reduce your risk of getting cancer. Just as we can each make personal lifestyle decisions to reduce our odds of someday receiving a cancer diagnosis, there are policies to reduce the prevalence of cancer in societies. Placing limits on the sale of tobacco and establishing smoke-free workplace laws are two examples of this. Other examples include policies regulating toxins and pollutants in factories, farms, and other worksites. Because tobacco and processed food marketing, as well as toxic environments, are more likely to affect lower income communities and people of color in the United States,[17] the fight against cancer must address deeper structural inequalities to reduce cancer in total as well as the disproportionate effect is has on the least advantaged among us.

Cardiovascular Diseases

Seemingly out of nowhere, a man starts to have labored breathing; his expression turns to panic as he clutches his chest and then falls to the ground. You've likely seen this portrayal of a **heart attack** on television. In reality, not all heart attacks look alike. There may be important early warning signs, but the person having the heart attack may not understand what is happening (**FIGURE 13-3**). The precursors of a cardiovascular event start long before a heart attack or stroke occurs, and they affect both women and men. In addition, there are many other forms of **cardiovascular disease** (CVD) that fall under the public's radar.

heart attack The sudden cessation of blood supply to the heart, often due to a blocked artery.

cardiovascular disease A range of conditions affecting the heart and blood vessels.

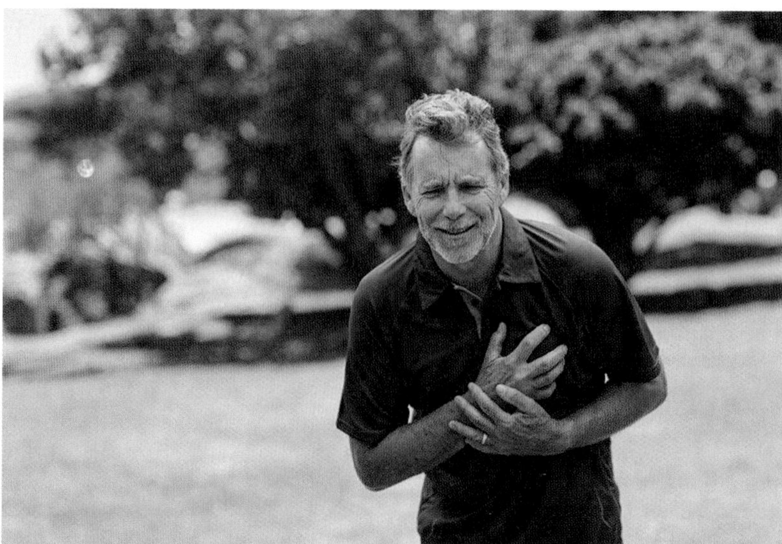

FIGURE 13-3 Chest pain is the most well-known symptom of a heart attack; however, heart attack symptoms can include other things like nausea; pain or discomfort in the arm, jaw, neck, or back; and shortness of breath.

TRY IT!

Steps for Preventing Cardiovascular Disease

- Eat a heart-healthy diet.
- Engage in physical activity (**FIGURE 13-4**).
- Quit tobacco (or even better—don't start!)
- Minimize alcohol intake.
- Manage stress.

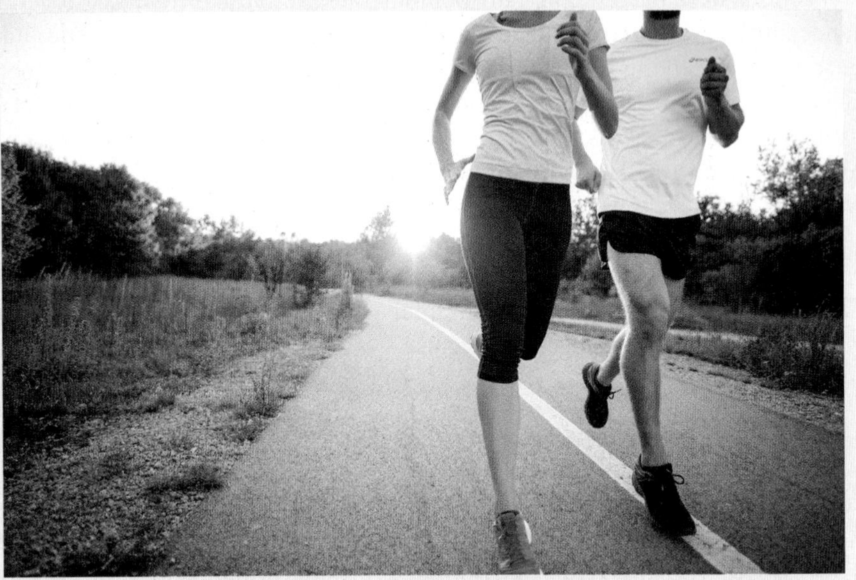

FIGURE 13-4 Regular exercise can help prevent heart disease.

cerebrovascular disease
A disease in which damage to the blood vessels that supply the brain occurs. Interrupted blood flow to the brain can lead to stroke.

CVDs are a group of disorders affecting the heart and blood vessels. These include coronary artery disease, **cerebrovascular disease**, peripheral arterial disease, rheumatic heart disease, congenital heart disease, and deep vein thrombosis. CVDs are the number one cause of death worldwide, with over 17 million people dying prematurely each year. In the United States, about 610,000 people die of heart disease annually (**FIGURE 13-5**).[18,19] The South has the highest rate of heart disease–related deaths.

Many factors contribute to CVDs, including behaviors, environment, and genetics. Health behaviors that affect your risk of developing CVD include diet, level of physical activity, and use of tobacco and alcohol. (See Chapters 2, 3,

TYPES OF CARDIOVASCULAR DISEASES (CVDS)[18]

- *Coronary heart disease*: Disease of the blood vessels supplying the heart muscle
- *Cerebrovascular disease*: Disease of the blood vessels supplying the brain
- *Peripheral arterial disease*: Disease of blood vessels supplying the arms and legs
- *Rheumatic heart disease*: Damage to the heart muscle and heart valves from rheumatic fever, caused by streptococcal bacteria
- *Congenital heart disease*: Malformations of heart structure existing at birth
- *Deep vein thrombosis and pulmonary embolism*: Blood clots in the leg veins, which can dislodge and move to the heart and lungs

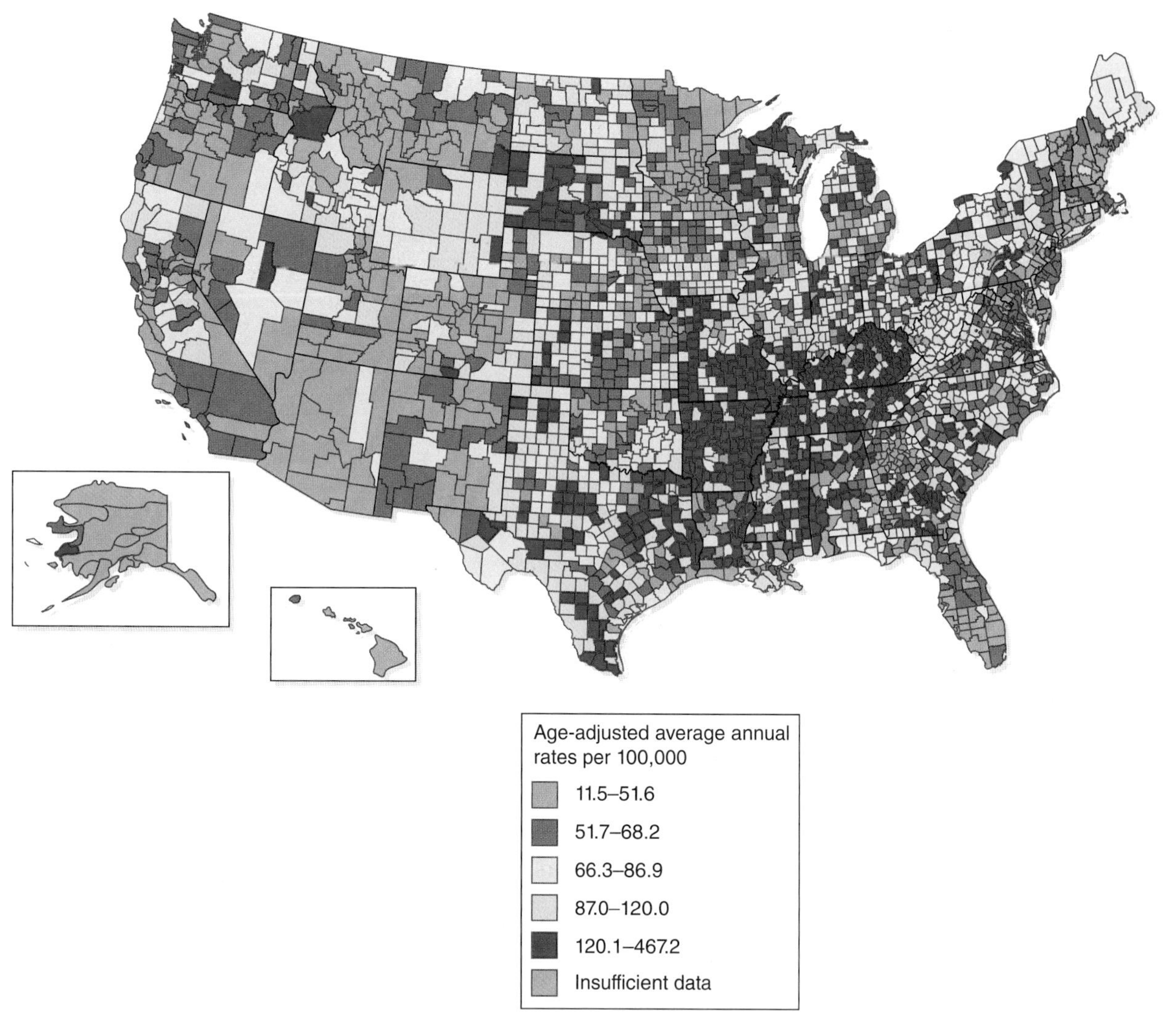

FIGURE 13-5 Heart disease death rates, 2011–2013, adults, ages 35+, by county.

Centers for Disease Control and Prevention (CDC). (2017). Heart disease facts. Retrieved from https://www.cdc.gov/heartdisease/facts.htm

WHAT IS HIGH BLOOD PRESSURE?

High blood pressure, known as **hypertension**, is one of the main causes of cardiovascular diseases (**FIGURE 13-7**). The amount of blood pumping to the heart and size of the arteries determines one's blood pressure. Risk factors for hypertension are the usual suspects: hereditary factors such as family history of hypertension, older age, being male, and being African American; and behavioral risk factors such as lack of physical activity, an unhealthy diet high in sodium, excessive alcohol intake, and being overweight.

hypertension A condition in which blood flows through the blood vessels with greater than normal force, causing blood pressure to be abnormally high.

Unfortunately, hypertension has no symptoms, which means someone could live for years without knowing they have it (Figure 13-7). About one in every three U.S. adults has high blood pressure. Luckily, it can be easily detected by using a blood pressure machine. Usually, when you visit a health clinic, your blood pressure is taken, and many pharmacies have a blood pressure machine available for you to check your own blood pressure. Hypertension is managed with prescription medication and behavior changes, such as a healthy diet and active lifestyle.[20–22]

Blood pressure category	Systolic mm Hg (upper #)		Diastolic mm Hg (lower #)
Normal	Less than 120	and	Less than 80
Prehypertension	120–139	or	80–89
High blood pressure (hypertension) stage 1	140–159	or	90–99
High blood pressure (hypertension) stage 2	160 or higher	or	100 or higher
Hypertensive crisis (emergency care needed)	Higher than 180	or	Higher than 110

FIGURE 13-6 This chart is intended to help you interpret blood pressure readings and understand what is considered a normal blood pressure.

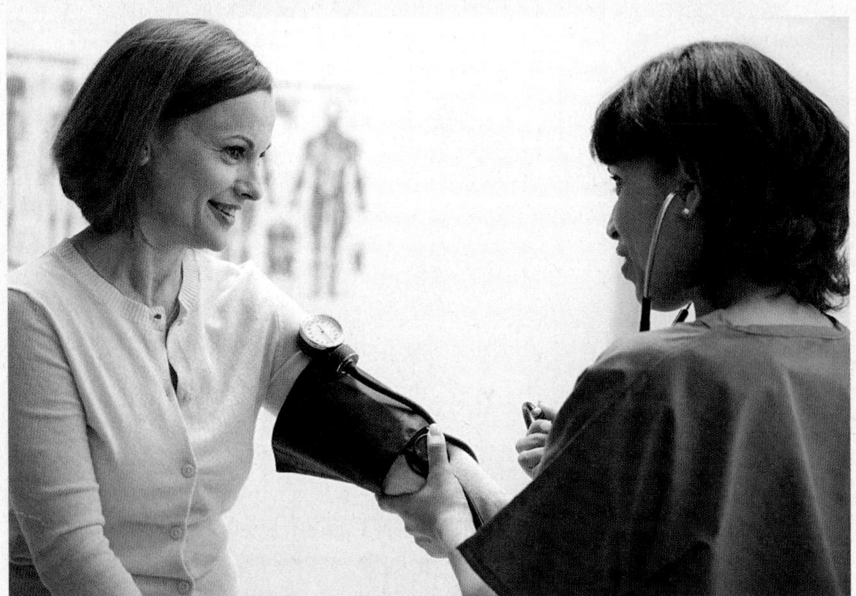

FIGURE 13-7 High blood pressure is often called a "silent killer" because there are often no symptoms; that's why it is important to get your blood pressure checked often.

and 7 for more information.) These behaviors can also lead to hypertension (high blood pressure), diabetes, high cholesterol, and obesity (see the Diabetes section later in this chapter). All of these conditions increase the risk for CVDs.

Behavior is not the only determinant. Some factors outside of your control, such as age, sex, and genetics, can influence your risk. In addition, CVDs are influenced by social, economic, and cultural factors. These include poverty, stress, and racism. For example, as discussed previously, in poor neighborhoods residents may not feel safe enough to exercise outdoors, or the neighborhood may have an abundance of fast-food eateries and liquor stores. Racism can affect heart health in multiple ways. Persistent exposure to racism and internalizing negative stereotypes can cause stress and trigger physical reactions that can harm the heart. In addition, limited opportunities for economic advancement and living in poor conditions can negatively affect cardiovascular health.

Addressing these social determinants is of fundamental importance to preventing CVDs and other health issues.

We will discuss two of the most common types of CVDs: coronary artery disease and cerebrovascular disease.

Coronary Heart Disease

Coronary heart disease is the most common type of CVD. Coronary heart disease occurs when plaque builds up on the walls of the coronary arteries. Heart attacks, also known as myocardial infarctions, result from coronary heart disease. During a heart attack, oxygen-rich blood cannot flow to the heart, usually because fatty deposits have built up on the walls of blood vessels (**FIGURE 13-8**).[23] People can sometimes feel a heart attack coming right before it happens. Symptoms include chest pain and shortness of breath. See (**FIGURE 13-9**) to understand how symptoms differ in men and women.

coronary heart disease A condition in which plaque builds up in coronary arteries, causing them to harden and narrow.

In the United States, about 735,000 people have a heart attack each year (**FIGURE 13-10**). For most people, it is their first heart attack, but about a quarter have had prior heart attacks. Heart attacks are most common among those over 75 years of age and occur more often in men.[19] However, Black men and women have higher rates of heart attacks at almost all ages, compared to White men and women.

Although heart attacks can be fatal, many people do survive. Getting medical treatment quickly is key to not only surviving but having a better quality of life. This means that if you suspect someone is having a heart attack, call 9-1-1 immediately. Most people wait over *2 hours* before seeking medical help for a heart attack. Delaying treatment can result in permanent heart damage or death. Keep in mind that the symptoms of a second heart attack might be different than those experienced in the first attack.[24]

Emergency treatment can help reduce the damage done to the heart muscle. In some cases, coronary artery bypass grafting might be used to treat a heart attack. During this procedure, a surgeon removes a healthy artery and uses it to bypass the section of the coronary artery that is blocked. After a heart attack, a combination of medications and lifestyle changes will aid in returning to an active, full life. Cardiac rehabilitation is often recommended; it involves a combination of education to help identify ways to reduce future heart problems and exercise training to build strength.[25]

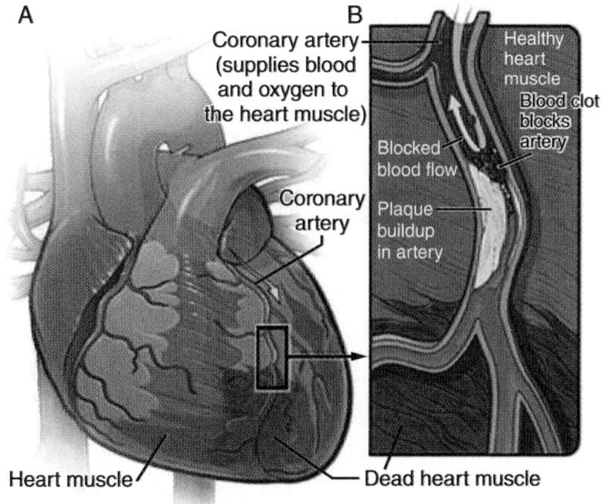

FIGURE 13-8 Heart with muscle damage and a blocked artery.

NIH Medline Plus. (2009). Heart Disease: Symptoms, Diagnosis, Treatment. Retrieved from https://medlineplus.gov/magazine/issues/winter09/articles/winter09pg25-27.html

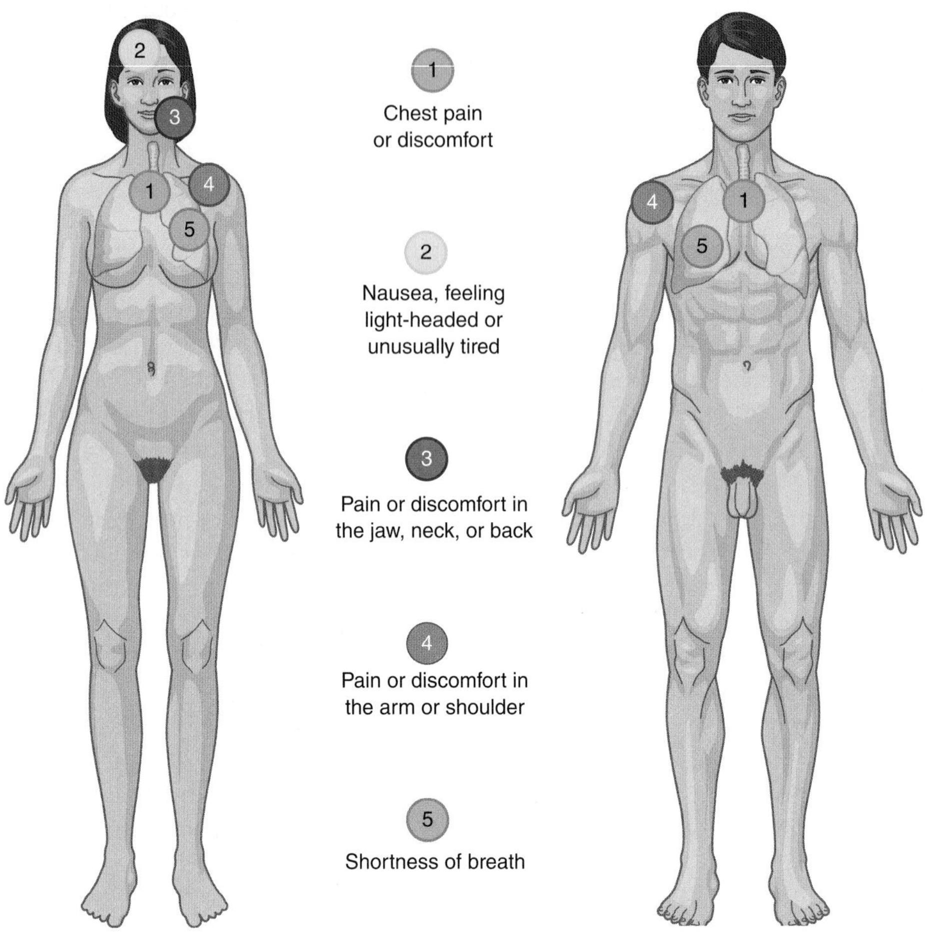

FIGURE 13-9 Major signs and symptoms of a heart attack in women and men.

Centers for Disease Control and Prevention (CDC). (2015). Heart attack signs and symptoms. Retrieved from https://www.cdc.gov/heartdisease/signs_symptoms.htm

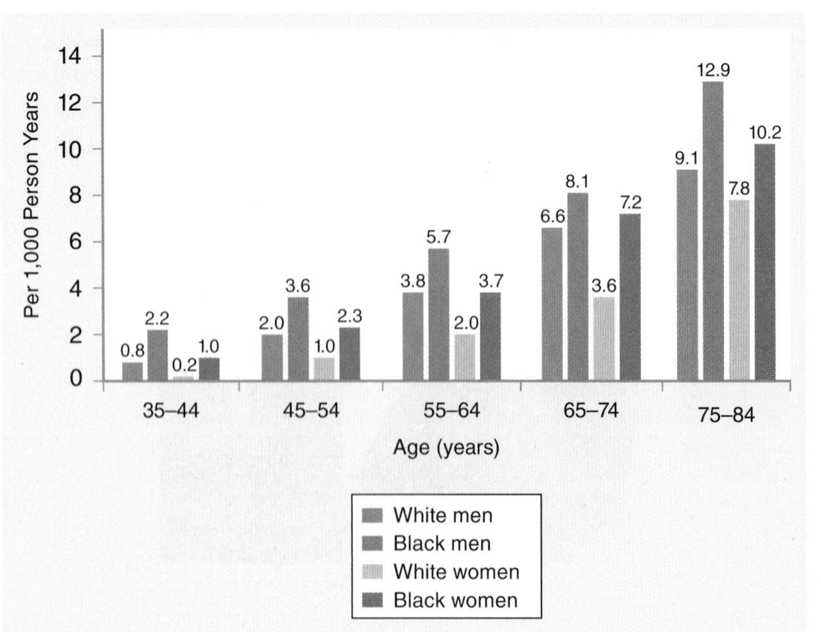

FIGURE 13-10 Incidence of myocardial infarction by age, sex, and race.

Reprinted with permission Circulation. 2015;131:e29-e322 ©2015 American Heart Association, Inc.

What causes a heart attack? There are three categories of risk factors:[26]

- *Major*: risk factors that cannot be changed:
  - Increased age
  - Male sex
  - Heredity
- *Modifiable*: risk factors you can control:
  - Smoking tobacco
  - High cholesterol
  - Hypertension (high blood pressure)
  - Physical inactivity
  - Obesity
  - Diabetes
- *Contributing*: risk factors associated with CVD whose significance is not yet clear:
  - Stress
  - Alcohol intake
  - Nutrition

Don't be fooled by the names of the categories, though. Many of the modifiable risk factors are "major" in that they are a significant contributor to heart disease. The more risk factors someone has, the greater their chance of developing coronary heart disease and having a heart attack. It is essential to manage the modifiable and contributing risk factors to prevent a heart attack. That means quitting smoking; treating high cholesterol, high blood pressure, and diabetes; being physically active; managing stress; minimizing alcohol intake; and eating a heart-healthy diet. A small (81 mg), daily dose of aspirin (**FIGURE 13-11**) in

IS RED WINE "GOOD" FOR YOUR HEART?[27]

It seems ironic that excessive alcohol is one of the main contributors to heart disease, and yet, you may have heard people say that red wine helps to prevent coronary artery disease. So, what's the real story? Evidence suggests that drinking red wine in moderation (1 to 2 drinks daily) protects against coronary artery disease, but it is not clear why. The leading theories are that either the antioxidants or a substance called resveratrol are linked to wine's heart-healthy benefits. It is not clear though, why red wine, and whether other alcoholic substances are equally as beneficial. What is clear is that doctors are *not* recommending that you start drinking wine just to protect your heart. Given the negative effects of moderate to heavy drinking (such as liver damage, cognitive damage, and damage to the nervous system), if you do not drink alcohol you do not need to start. There are plenty of other ways to help out your heart.

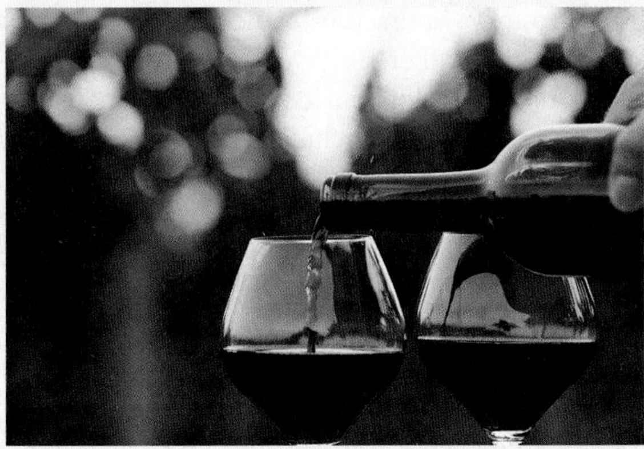

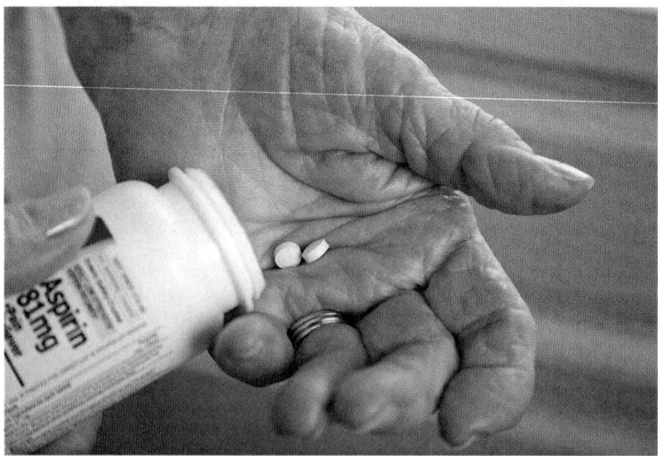

FIGURE 13-11 Aspirin may help lower your risk for heart attack or stroke.

older adults can sometimes help prevent heart attack or stroke, too. Discuss with a doctor what steps to prevent a heart attack are right for you.[28]

BY THE NUMBERS

Heart Attacks in the United States

Every 43 seconds, someone in the United States has a heart attack.[29]

Cerebrovascular Disease

stroke The sudden onset of persistent neurologic deficits resulting from blocked blood flow to the brain.

Cerebrovascular disease comprises a group of disorders in which part of the brain is affected by bleeding or inadequate blood supply. A **stroke** is the most common type of cerebrovascular disease. A stroke occurs when not enough blood reaches the brain (FIGURE 13-12). When there is blockage of blood flow to the brain, brain cells start to die within minutes of not receiving oxygen. Strokes can cause disability, brain damage, paralysis, cognitive problems, and death. There are two types of strokes:[30]

- *Ischemic*: Blood clots, particles, or plaque block the blood vessels to the brain.
- *Hemorrhagic*: A blood vessel in the brain bursts and the resulting buildup of blood damages brain tissue.

The signs of a stroke usually come on suddenly and include numbness, confusion, vision problems, trouble walking, and headache.[30]

Treatment for a stroke usually starts in the ambulance, which is why it is better to call 9-1-1 than to drive yourself or someone else to a hospital if you suspect a stroke. Medication or other surgical procedures may be needed to stop the bleeding or break up blood clots.[32] After providing emergency medical treatment, rehabilitation for strokes may include speech therapy, physical therapy, or

SPOTTING SIGNS OF STROKE[31]

If you think someone may be having a stroke, use the acronym "FAST" to check:

F—Face. Ask the person to smile. Does one side of the face droop?
A—Arms. Ask the person to raise both arms. Does one arm drift downward?
S—Speech. Ask the person to repeat a simple phrase. Is the speech slurred or strange?
T—Time. If you see any of these signs, call 9-1-1 right away.

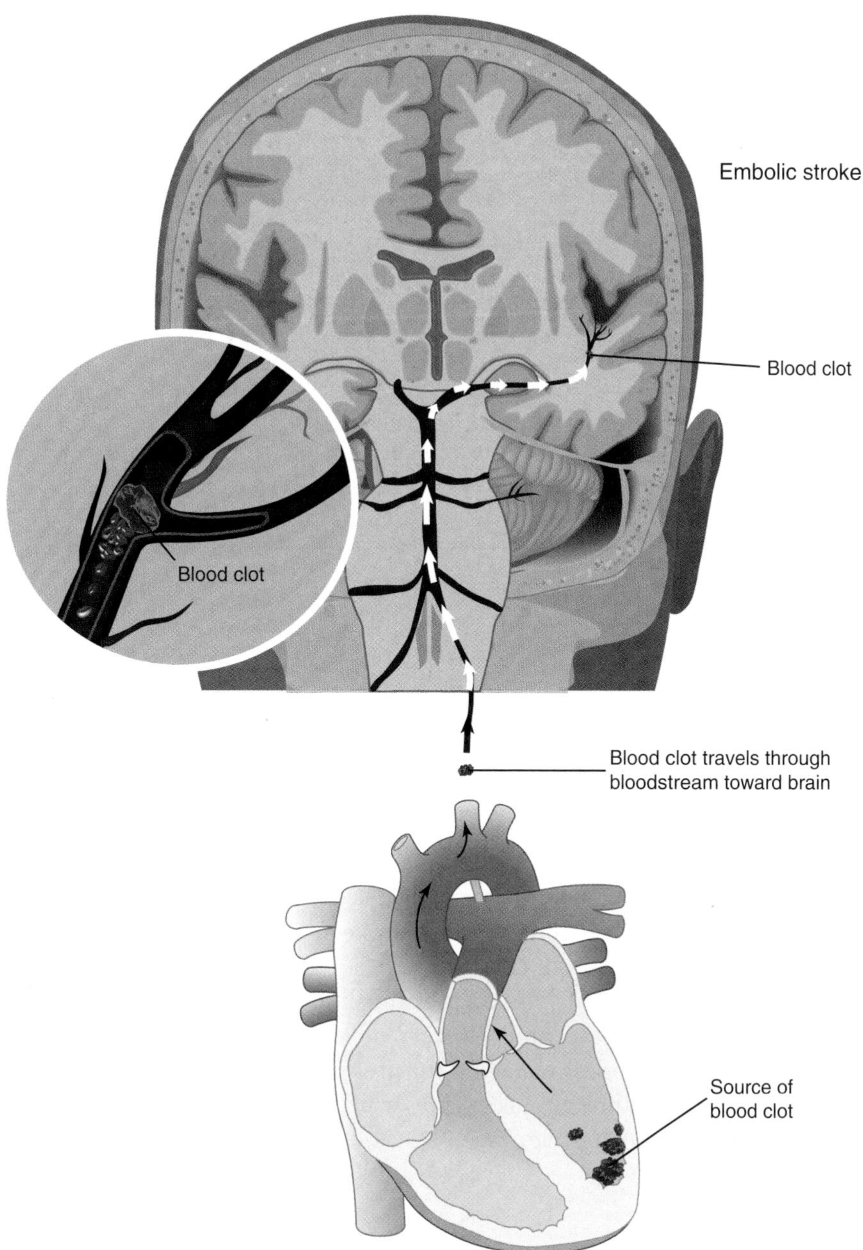

FIGURE 13-12 A stroke happens when a blood clot blocks blood flow to the brain. This causes brain tissue to become damaged or die.

Centers for Disease Control and Prevention (CDC). (2016). About stroke. Retrieved from https://www.cdc.gov/stroke/about.htm

GOING UPSTREAM

Why Are People of Color at Higher Risk for Cardiovascular Diseases?[36]

Several theories exist as to why people of color, particularly Black men and women, are at higher risk of developing cardiovascular diseases and dying from them. One theory is that this population has higher rates of obesity and diabetes, which can lead to CVD. Another theory is that a gene common among African Americans may make this group more sensitive to salt. However, it is clear that a large part of this disparity exists due to barriers to diagnosis and treatment. Social determinants of health, including inequalities in income, education, and access to care, discussed throughout this book, disproportionately affect people of color and contribute to these barriers to cardiovascular care.

Talk to your health care team about the
ABCS
Aspirin when appropriate
Blood pressure control
Cholesterol management
Smoking cessation

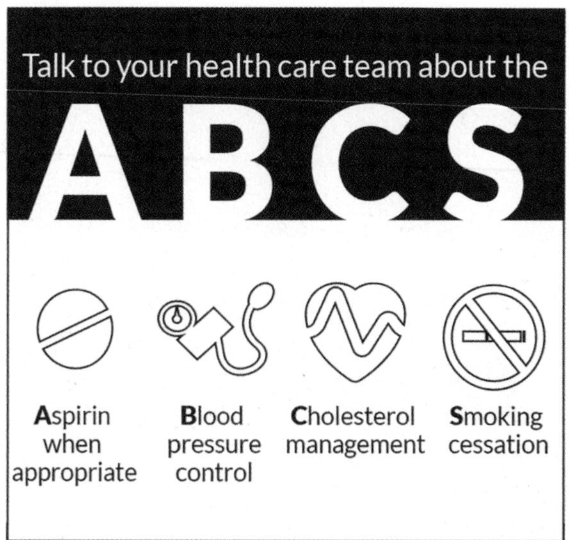

FIGURE 13-13 Lower your risk of stroke and heart attack by following the "ABCS."

Million Hearts. (n.d.). Prevention. Retrieved from https://millionhearts.hhs.gov/learn-prevent/prevention.html

occupational therapy. Speech therapy helps stroke victims to recover their speech. Physical therapy can help people relearn movement and coordination. Occupational therapy can improve daily activities such as eating, dressing, and writing.[33]

In the United States, almost 800,000 people have a stroke each year. Most of these are ischemic strokes among people who have not had a stroke before. Strokes kill more than 130,000 people annually, making it the fifth leading cause of death in the United States. Risk of stroke is nearly twice as high for Blacks than Whites. Blacks are also more likely to die from a stroke compared to Whites. People of Hispanic ethnicity are also at increased risk of stroke compared to Whites.[34,35]

Causes of strokes are high blood pressure, high cholesterol, heart disorders, diabetes, sickle cell disease, and a history of strokes. Much like other CVDs, stroke prevention includes managing (or preventing) hypertension, high cholesterol, and diabetes through taking prescribed medication and engaging in a healthy diet and active lifestyle (**FIGURE 13-13**).

insulin A hormone that is produced and secreted by the pancreas whose role is to regulate the body to either use glucose for energy or to store it for future energy use. It keeps blood sugar levels from getting too high (hyperglycemia) or too low (hypoglycemia).

type 1 diabetes Previously called juvenile diabetes, a condition in which the body's immune system attacks beta cells in the pancreas, causing them to lose the ability to produce insulin.

type 2 diabetes Previously called adult-onset diabetes, a condition that occurs when the cells become resistant to insulin. Blood sugar levels rise, and the pancreas responds by producing more and more insulin. When the pancreas can no longer keep up with the demand and becomes exhausted, it loses control over blood sugar regulation, resulting in the diabetic condition.

Diabetes

Diabetes is a disease that occurs when the levels of glucose in your blood, also called blood sugar, are too high. This affects how your body turns food into energy. Your body turns most of the food you eat into glucose (sugar) and releases it into your bloodstream. Your pancreas releases a hormone called **insulin** that helps regulate the amount of glucose in your blood. Insulin absorbs glucose from your bloodstream and helps move it into cells where it is needed for energy. It also regulates glucose production by your liver and tells your body to switch off production of glucose when the blood levels are too high. Normally, your body produces the right amount of insulin to keep your blood glucose at the right level, by removing extra glucose from the blood and controlling the amount your liver produces.[37]

When you have diabetes, your body cannot regulate the amount of glucose in the blood. There are two main types of diabetes: **type 1 diabetes** and **type 2 diabetes** (**TABLE 13-3**). Gestational diabetes is an additional type that occurs only during pregnancy.

Over time, having too much glucose in your blood can cause other health problems. Some of the potential complications include heart disease, nerve damage, eye problems, and kidney disease. Preventing diabetes or managing it if you have it can help avoid these complications.

TABLE 13-3 Comparison of Type 1 and Type 2 Diabetes[45]

	Type 1 Diabetes	Type 2 Diabetes
Percentage of people with diabetes	5%	90 to 95%
Population	Most common in children, teens, and young adults	Occurs mostly in older adults, although increasingly children, teens, and young adults are being diagnosed
Prevention	An immune reaction that health professionals do not know how to prevent	Lifestyle changes may prevent or delay (losing weight if you are overweight and being physically active three times per week or more)
Onset	Often starts quickly with severe symptoms	Disease develops gradually over many years
Other	Must use insulin to survive	Prediabetes can develop into type 2 diabetes (but not type 1)

TABLE 13-4 Celebrities With Diabetes

Person	Profession	Type of Diabetes
Mariah Carey	American singer, songwriter, record producer, and actress	Gestational diabetes
Randy Jackson	American bassist, singer, record producer, entrepreneur, and television personality	Type 2 diabetes
Nick Jonas	American singer, songwriter, producer, and actor	Type 1 diabetes
Tom Hanks	American actor and filmmaker	Type 2 diabetes
Selma Hayek	Mexican and American film actress, producer, and former model	Gestational diabetes
Bret Michaels	American singer-songwriter and musician	Type 1 diabetes
Sherri Shepherd	American actress, comedian, author, and television personality	Type 2 diabetes
Sonia Sotomayor	First Latina Supreme Court Justice	Type 1 diabetes

Approximately 9.4% of the population has diabetes, and that number is growing. In 2015, there were 30.3 million Americans with diabetes, up from 29.1 million in 2014 (**FIGURE 13-14**). Nearly one in four people with diabetes do not know they have the disease. An estimated 84.1 million people have **prediabetes**, which can lead to diabetes if not treated.[38]

prediabetes A condition of higher-than-normal blood glucose levels; not high enough to establish a diagnosis of diabetes.

Being a celebrity does not protect you from diabetes, nor does having diabetes prevent people from being highly successful. **TABLE 13-4** presents a list of famous people who have diabetes.

Type 1 Diabetes

Type 1 diabetes is a disease in which your pancreas produces little or no insulin. Usually, people who have a diagnosis of type 1 diabetes get it in childhood or adolescence. The exact cause of type 1 diabetes is unknown. Type 1 diabetes is rare, with a prevalence of 2.6 to 3.4/1,000 people.[39] From what doctors know right now, there is no way to prevent type 1 diabetes.

The symptoms of type 1 diabetes include intense thirstiness, dry mouth, nausea and vomiting, stomach pain, frequent urination, unexplained weight

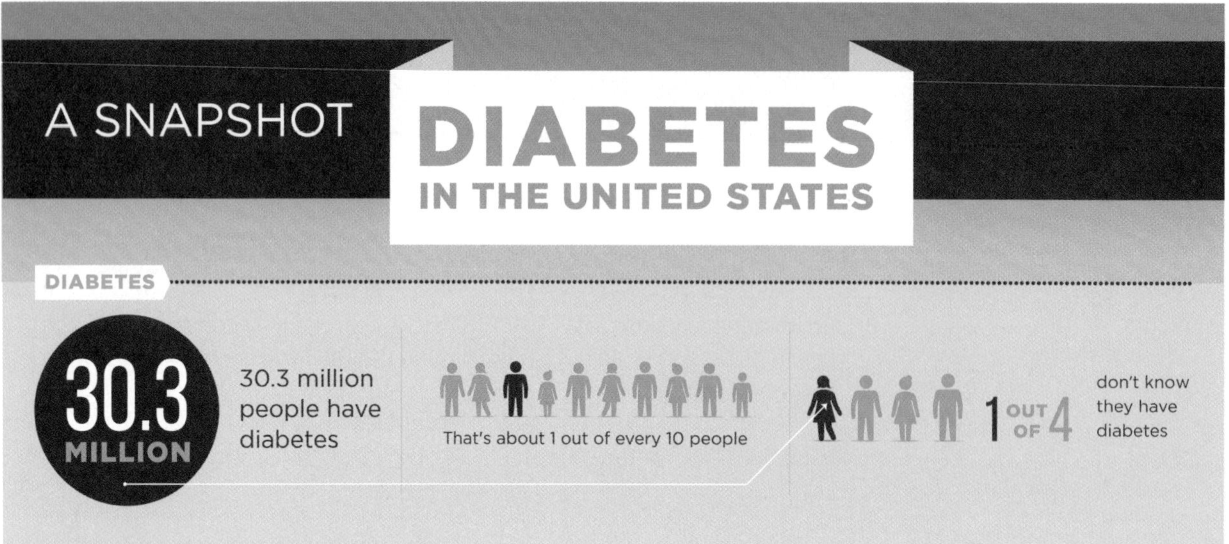

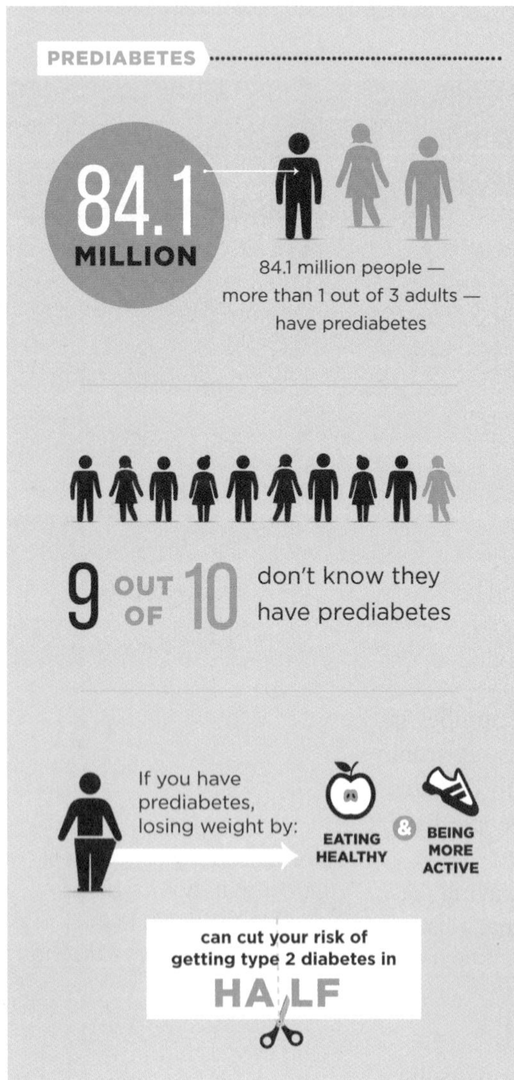

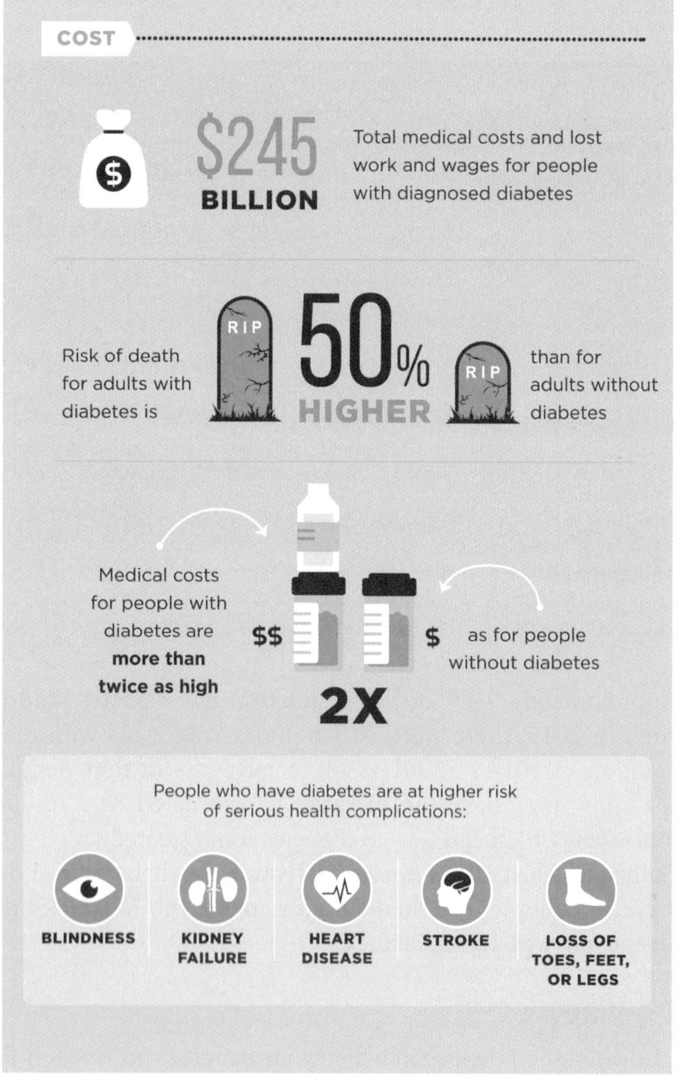

FIGURE 13-14 A snapshot of diabetes in the United States.

TYPES OF DIABETES

TYPE 1

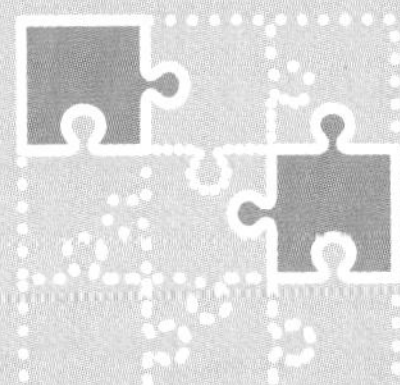

BODY DOESN'T MAKE ENOUGH INSULIN

- Can develop at any age
- No known way to prevent it

Nearly 18,000 youth diagnosed each year in 2011 and 2012

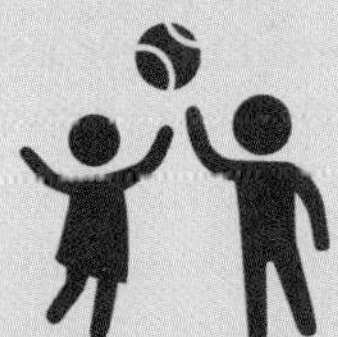

In adults, type 1 diabetes accounts for approximately 5% **of all diagnosed cases of diabetes**

TYPE 2

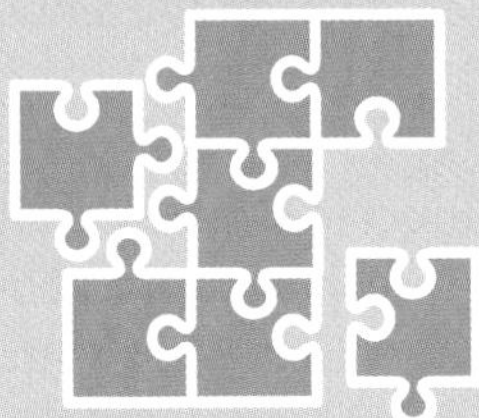

BODY CAN'T USE INSULIN PROPERLY

- Can develop at any age
- Most cases can be prevented

In adults, type 2 diabetes accounts for approximately 95% **of all diagnosed cases of diabetes**

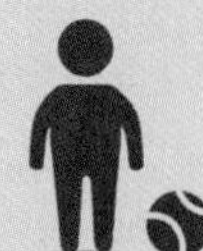

More than 5,000 youth diagnosed each year in 2011 and 2012

1.5 MILLION **People 18 years and older diagnosed in 2015**

RISK FACTORS FOR TYPE 2 DIABETES:

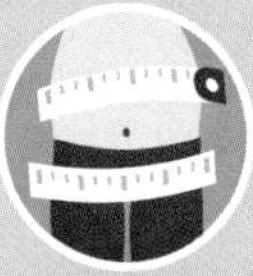

BEING OVERWEIGHT

HAVING A FAMILY HISTORY

BEING PHYSICALLY INACTIVE

BEING 45 AND OLDER

WHAT CAN YOU DO?

You can **prevent** or **delay** type 2 diabetes

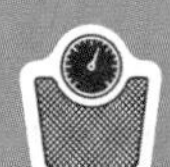

LOSE WEIGHT IF NEEDED

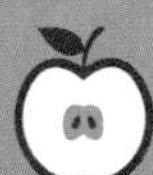

EAT HEALTHY

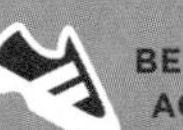

BE MORE ACTIVE

LEARN MORE AT www.cdc.gov/diabetes/prevention OR SPEAK TO YOUR DOCTOR

You can **manage** diabetes

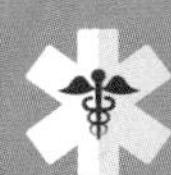

WORK WITH A HEALTH PROFESSIONAL

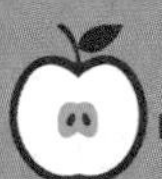

EAT HEALTHY

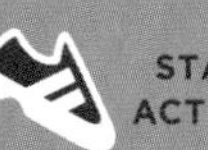

STAY ACTIVE

LEARN MORE AT www.cdc.gov/diabetes/ndep OR SPEAK TO YOUR DOCTOR

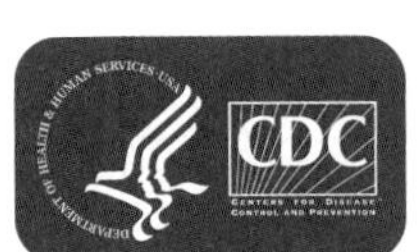

REFERENCES

Centers for Disease Control and Prevention. National Diabetes Statistics Report: Estimates of Diabetes and Its Burden in the United States, 2017. Atlanta, GA: U.S. Department of Health and Human Services; 2017.

American Diabetes Association. Economic Costs of Diabetes in the U.S. in 2012. Diabetes Care. 2013;36(4):1033-1046.

Centers for Disease Control and Prevention, National Center for Health Statistics. Underlying Cause of Death 1999-2015 on CDC WONDER Online Database, released December, 2016. Data are from the Multiple Cause of Death Files, 1999-2015, as compiled from data provided by the 57 vital statistics jurisdictions through the Vital Statistics Cooperative Program. Accessed at http://wonder.cdc.gov/ucd-icd10.html on April 4, 2017.

Mayer-Davis EJ, Lawrence JM, Dabelea D, Divers J, Isom S, Dolan L, et al. Incidence Trends of Type 1 and Type 2 Diabetes among Youths, 2002-2012. N Engl J Med. 2017;376:1419-29.

CDC's Division of Diabetes Translation works toward a world free of the devastation of diabetes.

CS279453B

FIGURE 13-14 A snapshot of diabetes in the United States.

Centers for Disease Control and Prevention (CDC). (2017). A snapshot of diabetes in the United States. Retrieved from https://www.cdc.gov/diabetes/pdfs/library/socialmedia/diabetes-infographic.pdf

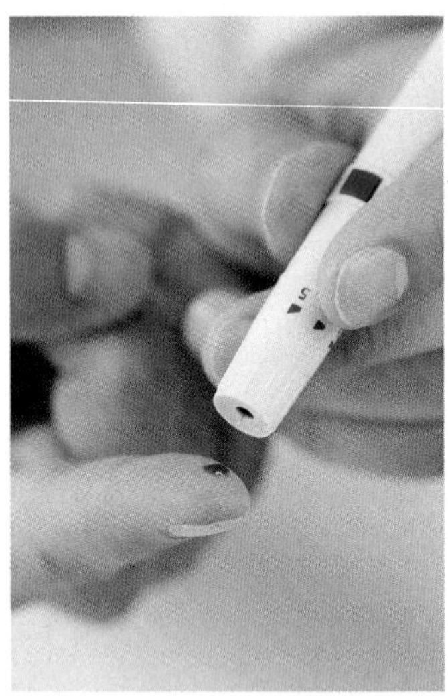

FIGURE 13-15 People with diabetes use a lancing device to draw a drop of blood. This blood sample can then be tested to measure blood sugar.

loss, tiredness, blurred vision, labored breathing, and frequent skin, urinary, or vaginal infections.[40]

Doctors do not yet know what causes type 1 diabetes. We understand that genes play a role, but there must be something that causes the immune system to react. When this happens the pancreas stops making insulin. If you have type 1 diabetes, your healthcare provider will help you figure out how often to test your blood sugar (**FIGURE 13-15**). When and how often you test it depends on your current health, age, and how active you are, the time of day, and other considerations. Your healthcare provider may suggest any of the following times: before every meal and a bedtime snack; 1 to 2 hours after eating; before, during, and after physical activity; when you are sick or under stress; and if you think your blood sugar might be too high, too low, or falling.[41–43]

People with type 1 diabetes must use insulin to manage their blood glucose levels. There are different types of insulin available, which differ in the amount of time they start to work and how long they last (**TABLE 13-5**).

If you have type 1 diabetes, you will feel better day-to-day and prevent long-term health problems if you take your insulin as directed by your healthcare provider (**FIGURE 13-16**), eat a healthy diet, and are physically active. Because being physically active lowers your blood sugar, you must pay attention to adjust your eating or insulin dose to compensate for increased physical activity.

It is important if you have type 1 diabetes to keep it under control. If you don't, you can develop eye problems, kidney damage, poor blood circulation, and nerve damage.

Type 2 Diabetes

Type 2 diabetes, the most common form, occurs when your body does not properly use insulin. When you have type 2 diabetes, at first your pancreas makes extra insulin because your body isn't using it properly. But over time, your body cannot produce enough insulin to keep your blood glucose at normal levels.

Although there are key ways to help prevent getting type 2 diabetes, some risk factors cannot be changed. These include a family history of diabetes, being over the age of 45, and your race/ethnicity. If you are African American, Alaska Native, American Indian, Asian American, Hispanic/Latino, Native Hawaiian

TABLE 13-5 Types of Insulin[44]

Type	Time to Start Working	Time to Peak Effectiveness	Length of Time Continues to Work
Rapid-acting	15 minutes	1 hour	2 to 4 hours
Regular or short-acting	30 minutes	2 to 3 hours	3 to 6 hours
Intermediate-acting	2 to 4 hours	4 to 12 hours	12 to 18 hours
Long-acting	Several hours	6 to 10 hours*	About 24 hours

*Depends on both individual response and which insulin is used.
Note: These times are a general guide, as people have different physiological responses to their insulin.

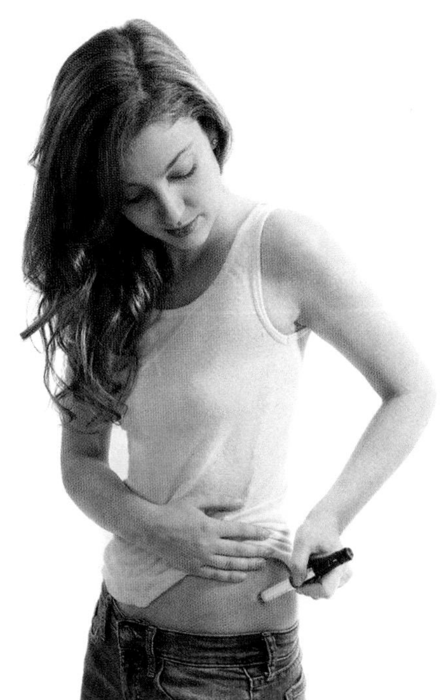

FIGURE 13-16 An autoinjector can be used to deliver insulin when needed.
© LEA PATERSON/Science Photo Library/Getty Images

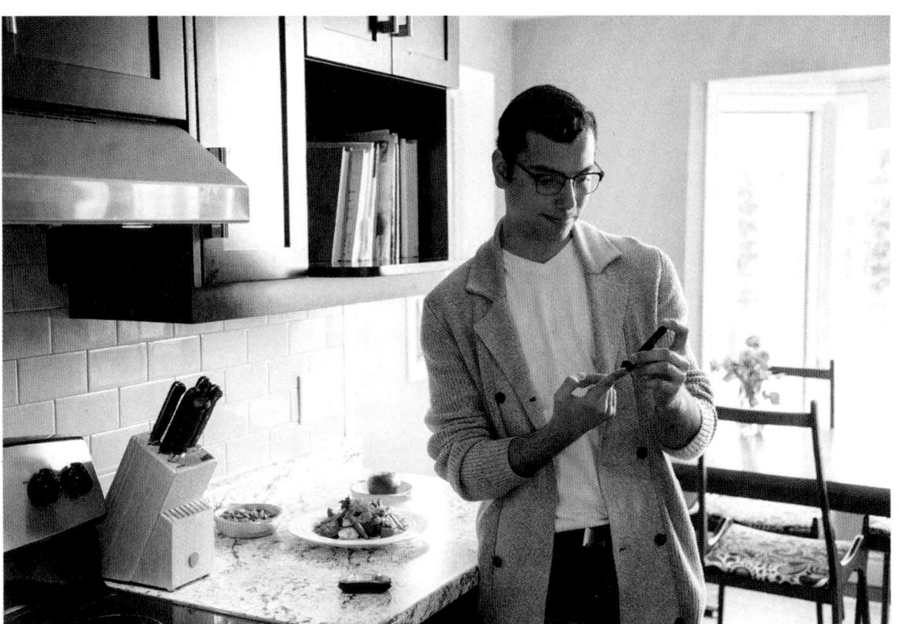

© Fertnig/E+/Getty Images

or Pacific Islander, you are more likely to develop diabetes. But there are risk factors that can be modified, including being overweight or obese, and not being physically active. **TABLE 13-6** helps determine if your weight for your height and ethnicity put you at increased risk. If your weight is equal to or above the weight listed here, you have a greater chance of developing type 2 diabetes.

There are also medical diagnoses that put you at higher risk, including high blood pressure, having low HDL levels (good cholesterol) or high triglyceride

TABLE 13-6 Body Mass Index Chart by Ethnicity to Determine if You Are at Increased Risk for Type 2 Diabetes[46]

Not Asian American or Pacific Islander		Asian American		Pacific Islander	
At-Risk BMI ≥ 25		At-Risk BMI ≥ 23		At-Risk BMI ≥ 26	
Height	**Weight**	**Height**	**Weight**	**Height**	**Weight**
4'10"	119	4'10"	110	4'10"	124
4'11"	124	4'11"	114	4'11"	128
5'0"	128	5'0"	118	5'0"	133
5'1"	132	5'1"	122	5'1"	137
5'2"	136	5'2"	126	5'2"	142
5'3"	141	5'3"	130	5'3"	146
5'4"	145	5'4"	134	5'4"	151
5'5"	150	5'5"	138	5'5"	156
5'6"	155	5'6"	142	5'6"	161
5'7"	159	5'7"	146	5'7"	166
5'8"	164	5'8"	151	5'8"	171
5'9"	169	5'9"	155	5'9"	176
5'10"	174	5'10"	160	5'10"	181
5'11"	179	5'11"	165	5'11"	186
6'0"	184	6'0"	169	6'0"	191
6'1"	189	6'1"	174	6'1"	197
6'2"	194	6'2"	179	6'2"	202
6'3"	200	6'3"	184	6'3"	208
6'4"	205	6'4"	189	6'4"	213

levels, or having a history of heart disease, stroke, depression, or polycystic ovary disease. Managing these health problems may reduce your chances of developing type 2 diabetes.

Symptoms

About 40% of children and adolescents with type 2 diabetes have no symptoms. These individuals receive their diagnosis at the time of a routine physical exam.

Noticeable symptoms of diabetes are excessive thirst and frequent urination. Because there is excess sugar in the bloodstream, the body pulls liquid from tissues. As a result, the person feels thirsty and drinks and urinates more. Fatigue is another symptom because insulin helps move sugar into cells for energy. If the person's blood sugar is high, fluid may also be pulled from the lenses, causing blurred vision. Type 2 diabetes also affects the body's ability to heal and resist infections. Even if you are eating, you may experience weight loss. Without the ability to utilize the sugar, your body burns fat and muscle for energy. See your doctor if you have these symptoms.

Type 2 diabetes used to be called adult-onset diabetes, but over time, more children and teens, in addition to adults, are developing it. This increase in diabetes prevalence is the result of many factors, including better detection, aging of the population, and the increasing numbers of minorities who are at greater risk for diabetes. There are also increases in factors that raise the risk of diabetes, such as obesity and a sedentary lifestyle. Public health advocates point to such factors as increasing dependence on cars, increasing proliferation of fast food and sweet beverages, and reduced physical activity in schools as contributing factors to this concerning trend.[47]

BY THE NUMBERS

Diabetes in the United States

- 30.3 million people in the United States have diabetes (9.4% of the population).
- 7.2 million people with diabetes are undiagnosed (12.8% of people with diabetes).

Prediabetes

As the name suggests, prediabetes is when your blood sugar levels are elevated, but not yet into the range that indicates diabetes. According to the Centers for Disease Control and Prevention (CDC), as of 2017, approximately 84 million American adults have prediabetes, and 90% of them do not realize it.[48] People with prediabetes are at increased risk of developing type 2 diabetes as well as heart disease and stroke. The symptoms and risk factors are the same as for diabetes.

TRY IT!

Find Out if You Are at Risk For Prediabetes

If you want to find out your risk for prediabetes, go to https://doihaveprediabetes.org/prediabetes-risk-test.html.

Note that if you are at increased risk, exercising and changing your diet can lower your risk!

Not surprisingly, the prevention recommendations for type 2 diabetes also apply to prediabetes. If you need to lose weight, losing what the CDC considers a small amount of weight: 5% to 7% of your body weight and increasing the amount of exercise you get to 150 minutes per week of a brisk walk or similar exercise will lower your risk. The goal, of course, is to make these behavior changes permanent. The CDC created a lifestyle change program that is available in all states. Some locations offer the classes in Spanish. To find an in-person class, go to https://nccd.cdc.gov/DDT_DPRP/Programs.aspx.

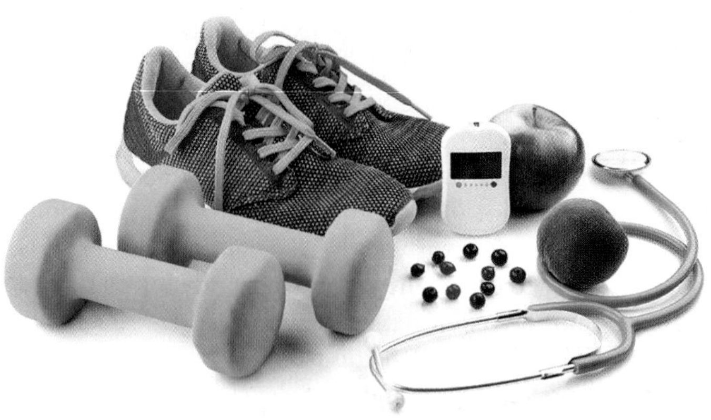

© Africa Studio/Shutterstock.

TABLE 13-7 Blood Glucose Levels[49]

Result	HbA1c Test	Fasting Blood Sugar Test	Glucose Tolerance Test	Random Blood Sugar Test
Normal	Below 5.7%	99 mg/dL or below	140 mg/dL or below	2 hours after eating 140 mg/dL or below
Prediabetes	5.7% to 6.4%	100 to 125 mg/dL	140 to 199 mg/dL	–
Diabetes	6.5% and above	126 mg/dL or above	200 mg/dL or above	200 mg/dL or above

Highlights of these lifestyle change classes include:

- Working with a trained coach to make realistic, lasting lifestyle changes
- Learning how to eat a healthy diet and be more physically active
- Understanding how to manage stress and continue to be motivated
- How to identify others with similar goals to create support

If you have received a diagnosis of prediabetes, take it seriously, as prediabetes is a serious illness. The best thing about it, however, is that it is reversible. Making life changes, even if they are hard, may change the path you are on. Staying active, eating a healthy diet, maintaining a healthy weight, and keeping your blood pressure under control will all help to reduce the likelihood that you will get diabetes.

Getting Tested for Diabetes[49]

To know if you have prediabetes or diabetes, your healthcare provider will have you do one or more of the following tests.

- *HbA1c* measures your average blood sugar over the past 2 or 3 months.
- *Fasting blood sugar* measures your blood sugar after you have not eaten all night.
- *Glucose tolerance test* measures your blood sugar before and after you drink a liquid that contains glucose. You will need to fast before this test. Blood is drawn before you drink the liquid and then again at 1 hour, 2 hours, and possibly 3 hours afterward.
- *Random blood sugar* measures your blood sugar at the time you are tested. You can eat before this test.

TABLE 13-7 lists values indicating normal, prediabetes, and diabetes, by the type of test.

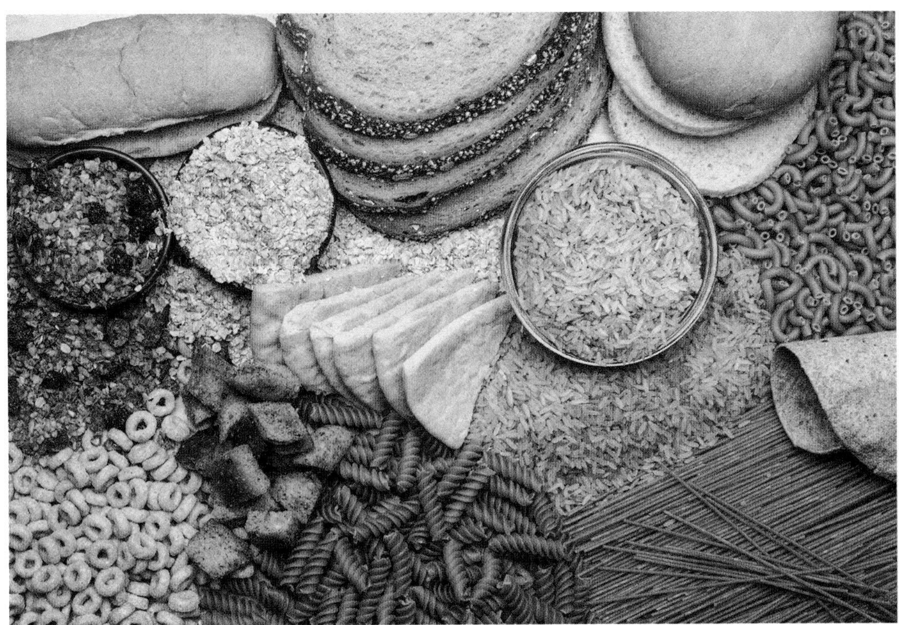

Whole grains.

If your healthcare provider thinks you may have type 1 diabetes, they may do additional tests.

Managing Diabetes

Approximately 29 million people have diabetes. Because we now know more about how to treat and manage diabetes, people with diabetes not only are living longer, but have a better quality of life than in the past.

Eat Right. Eating right goes a long way to helping control diabetes. Eat small portions and eat slowly. This gives your body an opportunity to register the feeling of being full. Eat less saturated fat and less sugar. Think of dividing your dinner plate into quarters. One-quarter has lean protein, one-quarter has a whole grain or small potato, and half your plate has nonstarchy vegetables. If you choose canned or frozen fruit, pick fruit that has juice, not syrup. Fresh fruit is also a good choice.

Eat more 100% whole grains (e.g., oatmeal and cereals made with whole grains), dark green vegetables (e.g., spinach and broccoli), orange vegetables (e.g., carrots, sweet potatoes, winter squash), and beans (e.g., black, garbanzo, kidney, pinto). If you have access to a registered dietitian, they can help you make a meal plan. See the box on dining with diabetes for a guide to how to make healthy choices when you eat out. The guidelines also work well when you are eating at home.

Remember that healthy eating is always a good choice, even if you do not have diabetes.

Be Physically Active. Being physically active has many benefits. Not only does it help control your blood glucose, but it also helps your blood pressure, raises your good cholesterol, and lowers your bad cholesterol. It also helps maintain or lower your weight.

If you are not already physically active, you may want to start with a little exercise and work your way up. Experts recommend moderate exercise 5 or

HOW TO DINE OUT WITH DIABETES[50]

Learning how to decode restaurant menus will help you maintain your healthy diet.

- *Avoid fried foods.* You should avoid anything described as crispy, crunchy, battered, tempura, or breaded. Fried foods have extra carbohydrates, cholesterol, trans fats, and saturated fats.
- *Avoid high-fat foods.* You should avoid anything described as creamy, buttery, smothered, loaded, au gratin, or cheesy. Fats are often used to carry flavor, so many restaurants like to add fat. Creamy salad dressings are also high in fat.
- *Avoid high-sugar foods.* While it is obvious that desserts have lots of sugar, foods described as glazed or sticky may also have added sugar.
- *Avoid high-sodium foods.* Salt is a flavor enhancer. Words that may indicate that a food is high in salt include pickled, smoked, brined, and soy or teriyaki sauces.

There are healthy choices available on most menus.

Look for foods cooked healthily, including foods described as baked, broiled, grilled, poached, steamed, boiled, or roasted. Even using these techniques, foods can have added fats. Watch the descriptions! For example, chicken or fish poached in broth would be a good choice. If you are in doubt, ask the server.

Choose vegetable and lean protein–based foods. Read the descriptions of how the foods are cooked. It is easy to take a lean protein and make it less healthy. Steamed vegetables are a healthy choice. When ordering salads, avoid unhealthy toppings such as cheese and creamy dressings. Ask for the dressing on the side so that you can add it yourself.

Feel empowered to ask for healthy changes to the preparation or serving. Don't beat yourself up if you make an unwise food choice. Just move on and resolve to do better next time.

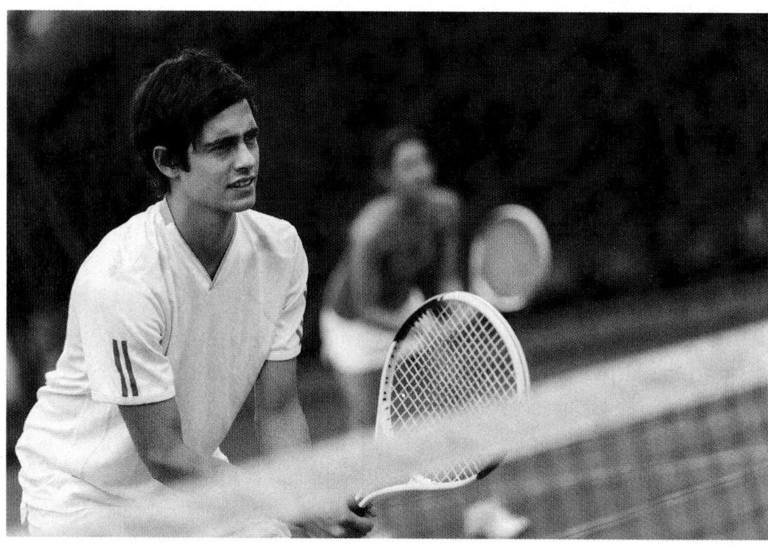

more days per week for at least 30 minutes. It is better to spread your activity out during the week rather than exercising for a long time once per week. Examples of moderate-intensity exercise are walking briskly, ballroom dancing, swimming, playing tennis (doubles), water aerobics, or bicycling slower than 10 mph.

If you have diabetes, the CDC recommends some pre cautions. Check your blood sugar before you are physically active. If your blood sugar is below 100, have a snack before you exercise. If it is above 300 or fasting above 250, do not exercise.

Physical activity can lower your blood glucose level too much; a condition called hypoglycemia. Signs of hypoglycemia include feeling shaky, weak, confused, irritable, anxious, hungry, tired, sweaty, or headachy. Severe hypoglycemia can cause you to lose consciousness.

Remember to drink plenty of water while you are exercising. Wear cotton socks and correctly fitting athletic shoes. After you exercise, be sure to check your feet for sores, blisters, or cuts. This is important because diabetes can cause nerve-related damage, so sometimes people with diabetes are unaware of injuring their feet.

BY THE NUMBERS

A1C Blood Test Results

In general, for every 1% reduction in results of A1C blood tests (e.g., from 8.0% to 7.0%), the risk of developing eye, kidney, and nerve disease is reduced by 40%.[51]

Gestational Diabetes[52]

Gestational diabetes can cause health problems for both the mother and infant. Between weeks 24 and 28 of your pregnancy, your doctor will give you a glucose challenge test. If your blood glucose level is high during the challenge test, the doctor will follow up with the oral glucose tolerance test.

You may have gestational diabetes and have no symptoms or only mild ones, such as being thirstier than normal or needing to urinate more frequently than normal. The hormonal changes that occur during pregnancy may make it more likely to get gestational diabetes. Your genes also play a role in getting gestational diabetes. If you are overweight, losing the extra weight before you become pregnant will lower your chances of getting gestational diabetes. Being physically active before and during pregnancy may also reduce your risk.

If you get a diagnosis of gestational diabetes, your healthcare provider will recommend a healthy meal plan and physical activity. They may also recommend daily blood glucose testing and, if needed, insulin injections.

After you deliver the baby, gestational diabetes usually goes away. But it is more likely that you will have gestational diabetes in future pregnancies. It may also be true that you have type 1 or type 2 diabetes that is discovered during your pregnancy. If you have gestational diabetes, you are more likely to develop type 2 diabetes later.

Children born to mothers with gestational diabetes are more likely to become obese, and those children are more likely to develop type 2 diabetes. Helping your child to have a healthy diet, maintain a healthy weight, and be physically active will lower your child's risk of developing type 2 diabetes.

Diabetes in the United States

Diabetes is a significant public health problem and is the seventh leading cause of death in the United States.[53] A diagnosis of diabetes increases the risk of a heart attack by 1.8 times, increases the risk of dying compared to those without

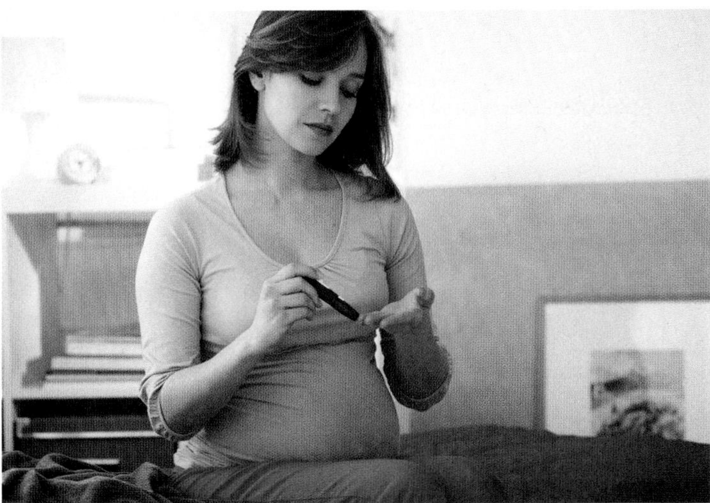

diabetes, and is the leading cause of kidney failure, lower limb amputations, and adult-onset blindness.

While genes do play a role in your risk of developing type 2 diabetes, lifestyle choices are fundamental. The lifestyle choices that affect the likelihood of your developing type 2 diabetes include choosing or not to exercise, food choices, and being overweight or obese. **FIGURE 13-17** shows the age-adjusted prevalence of obesity and diabetes in 1994, and **FIGURE 13-18** shows the age-adjusted prevalence of obesity and diabetes in 2015.[54] It is not a coincidence that as obesity has risen in the United States over time, so has the prevalence of diabetes.

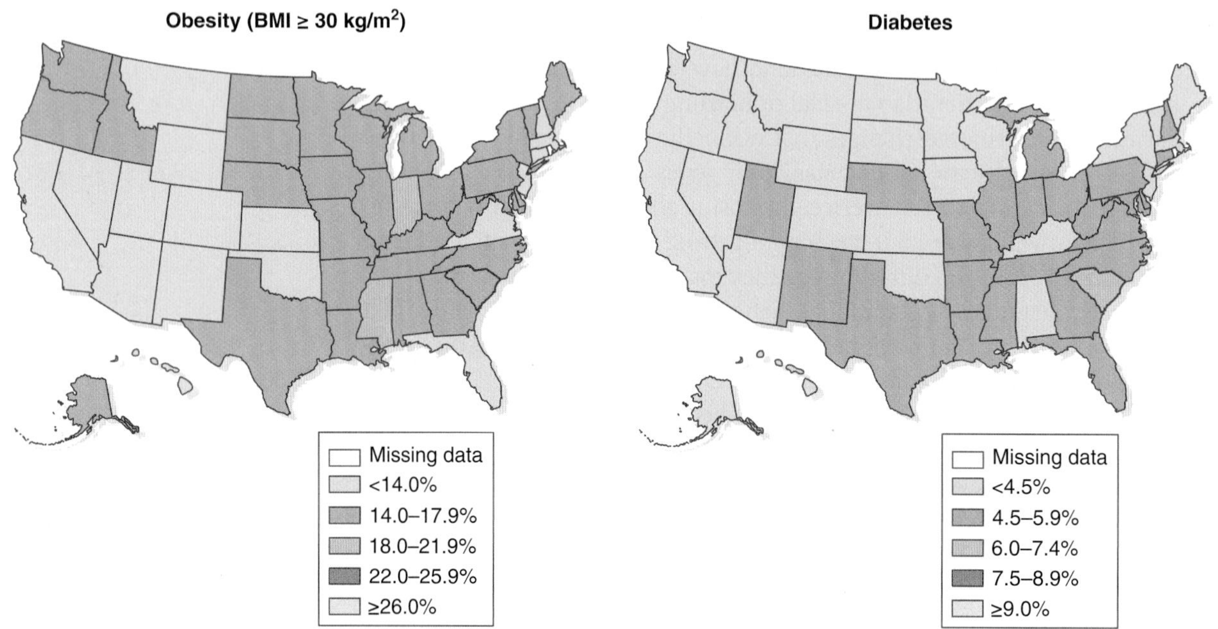

FIGURE 13-17 Age-adjusted prevalence of obesity and diagnosed diabetes among U.S. adults, 1994.

Centers for Disease Control and Prevention (CDC). (2018). Diabetes home: Data and statistics. Retrieved from https://www.cdc.gov/diabetes/pdfs/library/socialmedia/diabetes-infographic.pdf

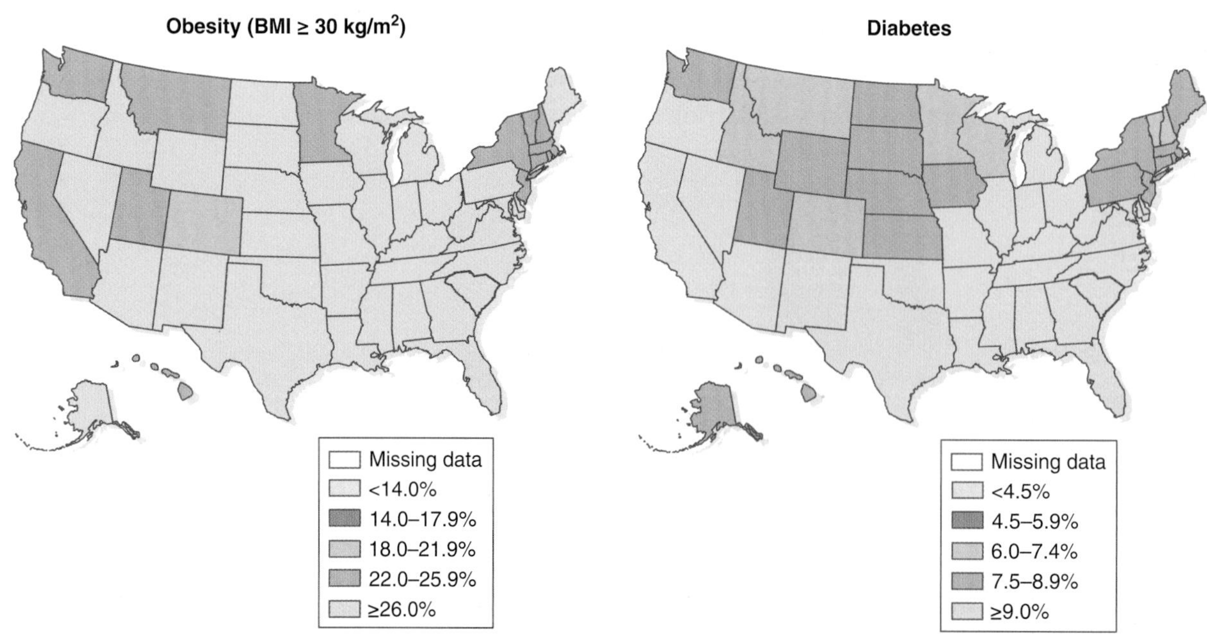

FIGURE 13-18 Age-adjusted percentage of U.S. adults who were obese or who had diagnosed diabetes, 2015.

Centers for Disease Control and Prevention (CDC). (2018). Diabetes home: Data and statistics. Retrieved from https://www.cdc.gov/diabetes/pdfs/library/socialmedia/diabetes-infographic.pdf

TABLE 13-8 World Health Organization Estimates of the Prevalence and Number of Adults with Diabetes[63]

Region	Prevalence (%)		Number (in millions)	
	1980	2014	1980	2014
African region	3.1%	7.1%	4	25
Region of the Americas	5.0%	8.3%	18	62
Eastern Mediterranean region	5.9%	13.7%	6	43
European region	5.3%	7.3%	33	64
Southeast Asia region	4.1%	8.6%	17	96
Western Pacific region	4.4%	8.4%	29	131
Total	4.7%	8.5%	108	422

Social Determinants of Health and Diabetes

Social determinants of health affect conditions in which people are born, grow, live, work, and age.[55] Type 2 diabetes is a disease strongly influenced by social determinants.[56] While healthcare providers and researchers know that lifestyle changes improve the health of individuals with diabetes, at the population level, we have not seen improvements. We know more about how social determinants affect prevention of type 2 diabetes than we do about how these determinants impact disease progression.[57] One study confirmed that financial distress, community disadvantage, and educational attainment significantly affected blood glucose levels.[58] Other studies found that race,[59] social isolation,[60] and low health literacy[61] were also associated with elevated blood glucose levels. If the medical community wants to seriously address the growing epidemic of diabetes, it needs to understand the influence of social determinants of health on the population and focus on addressing those as well as the disease itself.

In the past, diabetes was a disease that predominantly affected wealthy nations. Now the prevalence of diabetes is increasing around the world. Since 1980, the prevalence of diabetes has nearly doubled from 4.7% of the adult population to 8.5%. The World Health Organization estimates that in 2014 there were approximately 422 million adults with diabetes compared to 108 million in 1980 (**TABLE 13-8**). In the past decade, the rise in prevalence has been faster in low- and middle-income countries.[62]

Chronic Respiratory Diseases

Chronic respiratory diseases are chronic diseases of the airways and other parts of the lung. Among the most common ones are **asthma**, **chronic obstructive pulmonary disease** (COPD), respiratory allergies, occupational lung diseases, and pulmonary hypertension. This section will focus on asthma and COPD.

asthma An obstructive airway disease marked by episodic airway narrowing, causing difficulty in breathing.

chronic obstructive pulmonary disease A progressive respiratory disease marked by chronic obstruction of the airflow from the lungs.

Asthma

The World Health Organization estimates that approximately 235 million people suffer from asthma. While asthma occurs all around the globe, 80% of deaths due to asthma occur in low- and lower middle–income countries.[64] For most people with asthma, the disease starts during childhood. In the United States, more than 22 million people have asthma, and more than a quarter of them are children.

Asthma is a chronic lung disease that inflames and narrows your airways, making them swollen and sensitive. Also, the cells in your airways may make more mucus than normal, which makes breathing even harder.

If you have asthma, the symptoms range from a minor nuisance to severe enough to be life threatening. If the symptoms are mild, they may go away on their own or with minimal treatment. Other times, people have asthma attacks, in which the symptoms become more intense. The symptoms of asthma include wheezing (a high-pitched whistling sound made while breathing, often associated with difficulty breathing[65]), chest tightness, shortness of breath, and coughing.

As noted by the National Heart Lung and Blood Institute at the National Institutes of Health, in thinking about asthma, it helps to understand how your airways work. Your airways carry air into and out of your lungs. When a person has asthma, their airways are inflamed, meaning they are swollen and sensitive. In reaction to this sensitivity, the muscles around them tighten, which makes them narrower. As a result, the person's body gets less air into their lungs. If the swelling gets worse, the airways become even narrower, making it harder to get enough air.[66] **FIGURE 13-19** provides a pictorial explanation of asthma.

Everyone who has a diagnosis of asthma should have an asthma action plan (sometimes called an asthma management plan). This is a written plan that you make with your healthcare provider that shows what medications you take for asthma and when to take them. The plan includes what to do if you have an asthma attack and how to control asthma in the long term. Asthma action plans also give details about when to call your healthcare provider and when to go to the emergency room. **FIGURE 13-20** is an example of an asthma action plan. You can also find it online at www.nhlbi.nih.gov/files/docs/public/lung/asthma_actplan.pdf.

For many people, their asthma gets worse under certain circumstances. These situations include exercise-induced asthma, allergy-induced asthma, viral-induced asthma, and work-related (occupational) asthma.

Exercise-Induced Asthma

Exercise-induced asthma is triggered by vigorous or prolonged exercise. Most people with asthma experience symptoms with vigorous exercise, but others experience asthma symptoms only when they exercise. Symptoms may be

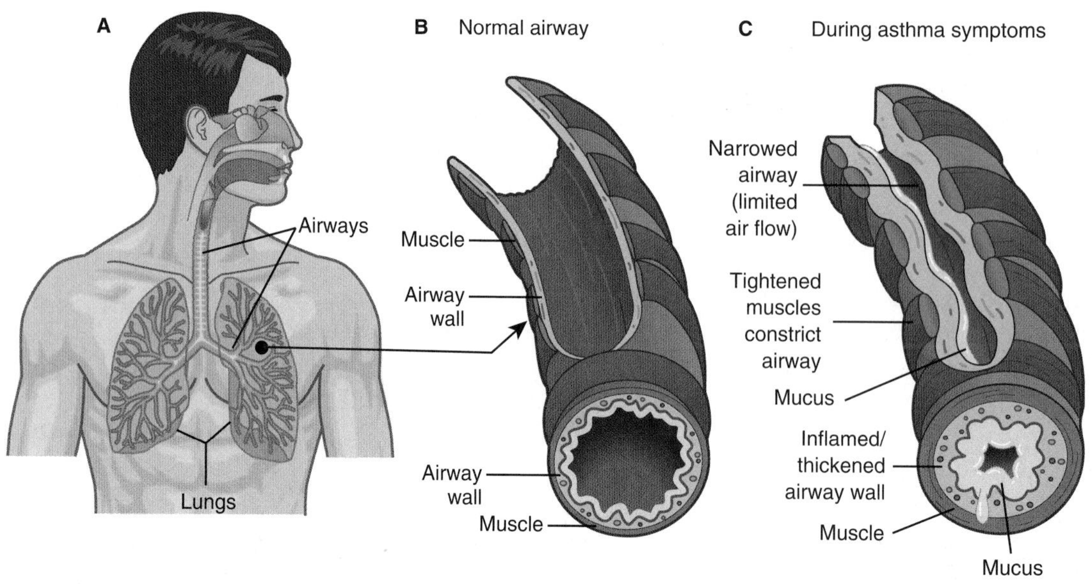

FIGURE 13-19 **A.** Location of the lungs and airways in the body. **B.** Cross section of a normal airway. **C.** Cross section of an airway during asthma symptoms.

National Heart, Lung, and Blood Institute. (2014). Asthma. Retrieved from https://www.nhlbi.nih.gov/health-topics/asthma

Asthma Action Plan

For: ______ Doctor: ______ Date: ______

Doctor's Phone Number ______ Hospital/Emergency Department Phone Number ______

GREEN ZONE

Doing Well

- No cough, wheeze, chest tightness, or shortness of breath during the day or night
- Can do usual activities

And, if a peak flow meter is used,

Peak flow: more than ______
(80 percent or more of my best peak flow)

My best peak flow is: ______

Take these long-term control medicines each day (include an anti-inflammatory).

Medicine	How much to take	When to take it
❒ ______	❒ 2 or ❒ 4 puffs ______	5 minutes before exercise

Before exercise

YELLOW ZONE

Asthma Is Getting Worse

- Cough, wheeze, chest tightness, or shortness of breath, or
- Waking at night due to asthma, or
- Can do some, but not all, usual activities

-Or-

Peak flow: ______ to ______
(50 to 79 percent of my best peak flow)

First: **Add: quick-relief medicine—and keep taking your GREEN ZONE medicine.**

______ (short-acting $beta_2$-agonist) ❒ 2 or ❒ 4 puffs, every 20 minutes for up to 1 hour
❒ Nebulizer, once

Second: **If your symptoms (and peak flow, if used) return to GREEN ZONE after 1 hour of above treatment:**
❒ Continue monitoring to be sure you stay in the green zone.

-Or-

If your symptoms (and peak flow, if used) do not return to GREEN ZONE after 1 hour of above treatment:
❒ Take: ______ (short-acting $beta_2$-agonist) ❒ 2 or ❒ 4 puffs or ❒ Nebulizer
❒ Add: ______ (oral steroid) mg per day For ______ (3–10) days
❒ Call the doctor ❒ before/ ❒ within ______ hours after taking the oral steroid.

RED ZONE

Medical Alert!

- Very short of breath, or
- Quick-relief medicines have not helped, or
- Cannot do usual activities, or
- Symptoms are same or get worse after 24 hours in Yellow Zone

-Or-

Peak flow: less than ______
(50 percent of my best peak flow)

Take this medicine:

❒ ______ (short-acting $beta_2$-agonist) ❒ 4 or ❒ 6 puffs or ❒ Nebulizer
❒ ______ (oral steroid) mg

Then call your doctor NOW. Go to the hospital or call an ambulance if:
- You are still in the red zone after 15 minutes AND
- You have not reached your doctor.

DANGER SIGNS
- **Trouble walking and talking due to shortness of breath**
- **Lips or fingernails are blue**

- **Take ❒ 4 or ❒ 6 puffs of your quick-relief medicine AND**
- **Go to the hospital or call for an ambulance** ______ (phone) **NOW!**

See the reverse side for things you can do to avoid your asthma triggers.

FIGURE 13-20 Asthma action plan.

How To Control Things That Make Your Asthma Worse

This guide suggests things you can do to avoid your asthma triggers. Put a check next to the triggers that you know make your asthma worse and ask your doctor to help you find out if you have other triggers as well. Then decide with your doctor what steps you will take.

Allergens

❐ **Animal Dander**

Some people are allergic to the flakes of skin or dried saliva from animals with fur or feathers.

The best thing to do:

- Keep furred or feathered pets out of your home.

If you can't keep the pet outdoors, then:

- Keep the pet out of your bedroom and other sleeping areas at all times, and keep the door closed.
- Remove carpets and furniture covered with cloth from your home. If that is not possible, keep the pet away from fabric-covered furniture and carpets.

❐ **Dust Mites**

Many people with asthma are allergic to dust mites. Dust mites are tiny bugs that are found in every home—in mattresses, pillows, carpets, upholstered furniture, bedcovers, clothes, stuffed toys, and fabric or other fabric-covered items.

Things that can help:

- Encase your mattress in a special dust-proof cover.
- Encase your pillow in a special dust-proof cover or wash the pillow each week in hot water. Water must be hotter than 130° F to kill the mites. Cold or warm water used with detergent and bleach can also be effective.
- Wash the sheets and blankets on your bed each week in hot water.
- Reduce indoor humidity to below 60 percent (ideally between 30—50 percent). Dehumidifiers or central air conditioners can do this.
- Try not to sleep or lie on cloth-covered cushions.
- Remove carpets from your bedroom and those laid on concrete, if you can.
- Keep stuffed toys out of the bed or wash the toys weekly in hot water or cooler water with detergent and bleach.

❐ **Cockroaches**

Many people with asthma are allergic to the dried droppings and remains of cockroaches.

The best thing to do:

- Keep food and garbage in closed containers. Never leave food out.
- Use poison baits, powders, gels, or paste (for example, boric acid). You can also use traps.
- If a spray is used to kill roaches, stay out of the room until the odor goes away.

❐ **Indoor Mold**

- Fix leaky faucets, pipes, or other sources of water that have mold around them.
- Clean moldy surfaces with a cleaner that has bleach in it.

❐ **Pollen and Outdoor Mold**

What to do during your allergy season (when pollen or mold spore counts are high):

- Try to keep your windows closed.
- Stay indoors with windows closed from late morning to afternoon, if you can. Pollen and some mold spore counts are highest at that time.
- Ask your doctor whether you need to take or increase anti-inflammatory medicine before your allergy season starts.

Irritants

❐ **Tobacco Smoke**

- If you smoke, ask your doctor for ways to help you quit. Ask family members to quit smoking, too.
- Do not allow smoking in your home or car.

❐ **Smoke, Strong Odors, and Sprays**

- If possible, do not use a wood-burning stove, kerosene heater, or fireplace.
- Try to stay away from strong odors and sprays, such as perfume, talcum powder, hair spray, and paints.

Other things that bring on asthma symptoms in some people include:

❐ **Vacuum Cleaning**

- Try to get someone else to vacuum for you once or twice a week, if you can. Stay out of rooms while they are being vacuumed and for a short while afterward.
- If you vacuum, use a dust mask (from a hardware store), a double-layered or microfilter vacuum cleaner bag, or a vacuum cleaner with a HEPA filter.

❐ **Other Things That Can Make Asthma Worse**

- Sulfites in foods and beverages: Do not drink beer or wine or eat dried fruit, processed potatoes, or shrimp if they cause asthma symptoms.
- Cold air: Cover your nose and mouth with a scarf on cold or windy days.
- Other medicines: Tell your doctor about all the medicines you take. Include cold medicines, aspirin, vitamins and other supplements, and nonselective beta-blockers (including those in eye drops).

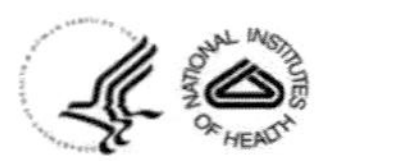

U.S. Department of Health and Human Services
National Institutes of Health

National Heart Lung and Blood Institute

For More Information, go to: www.nhlbi.nih.gov

NIH Publication No. 07-5251
April 2007

FIGURE 13-20 (CONTINUED) Asthma action plan.

National Heart, Lung, and Blood Institute. (2007). Asthma action plan. Retrieved from https://www.nhlbi.nih.gov/files/docs/public/lung/asthma_actplan.pdf

BY THE NUMBERS[67]

Asthma

- Number of adults (18 years or older) with asthma: 18.4 million (2015)
- Number of children (under 18 years) with asthma: 6.2 million (2015)
- Number of emergency room visits with asthma as the primary diagnosis: 1.6 million (2013)
- Percentage of visits to office-based physician with asthma on the medical record: 6.5% (2013)
- Number of deaths due to asthma: 3,651 or 1.1/100,000 people (2014)

worse if the air is cold and dry. During an exercise-induced asthma attack, the airways in the lungs become narrower. The medical term for this is bronchoconstriction. It is this narrowing that causes symptoms.[68]

The symptoms of exercise-induced asthma may begin during or after exercise. The symptoms may continue for 30 minutes or longer if you do not treat them. In addition to the usual asthma symptoms, such as coughing, wheezing, shortness of breath, and chest tightness, there are symptoms related to exercise, such as fatigue during exercise, worse than usual athletic ability, and feeling out of shape, even when you know you are in good physical condition. A sign of exercise-induced asthma in young children is that they may avoid exercising.[69]

If you have exercise-induced asthma, you should see a healthcare provider. If you find that your asthma symptoms, such as shortness of breath or wheezing, are quickly getting worse or using your prescription inhaler (**FIGURE 13-21**) does not improve your symptoms, get emergency medical treatment.[69]

Preventing asthma may be a more useful approach than treating it. To help prevent exercise-induced asthma, warming up prior to exercising and cooling down after exercise can help. It is also important to take your asthma medication. You should also limit outdoor exercise when it is very cold and when air pollution levels are high. If you have a cold, you should consider waiting to exercise until you feel better.

Exercise Choices for People With Asthma. There are exercises that you can do that will not make your asthma worse. We will discuss which exercises are easier or

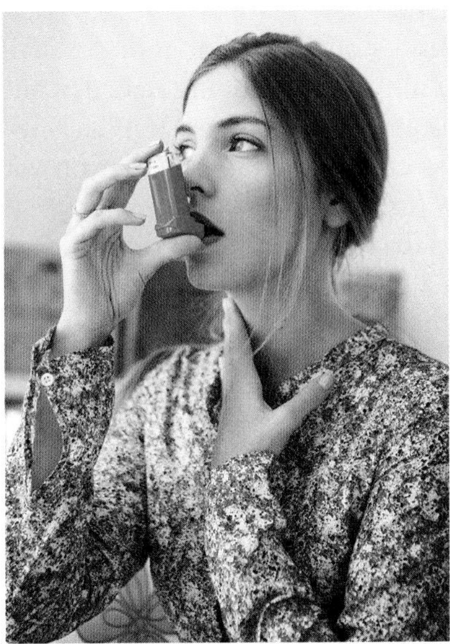

FIGURE 13-21 An inhaler delivers medication to people with asthma during an attack.

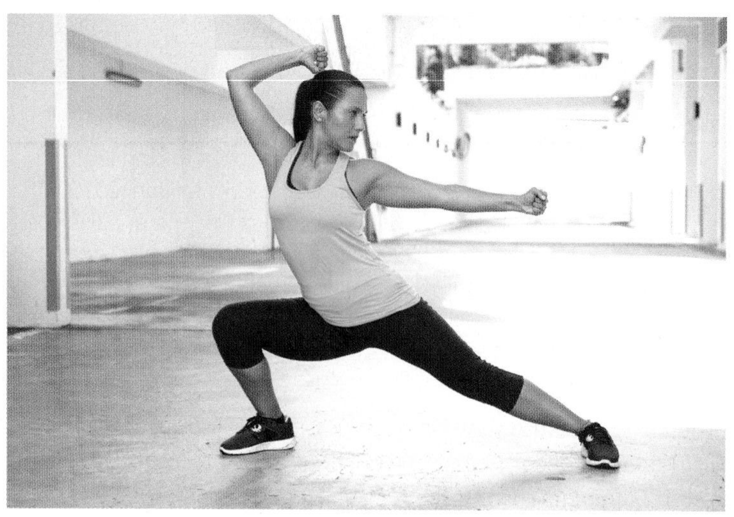

Tai chi.

harder if you have asthma. Because people are more likely to participate in an exercise they enjoy, we are not recommending that you abandon your favorite exercise even if it may make your asthma worse. Follow your healthcare provider's advice to assure that your asthma is under control. If you do not already have a favorite exercise, choosing one of the recommended activities may be a wise choice.

Exercises that help you control your breathing, such as yoga and tai chi, are often good choices. There is some evidence that yoga probably leads to a lessening of symptoms in people with asthma as well as small improvements in quality of life.[70] Activities where your heart rate and breathing rate are continuously raised for a sustained period of time are more likely to trigger asthma than exercises where you start and stop. Activities like baseball or softball where you run the bases and then wait or golf where you take your turn and then walk (or ride) to the next hole are sports that are less likely to induce an asthma attack.

Racquet sports that allow you to be on the court playing but have regular rests between games as well as access to water are good choices. Not surprisingly, doubles tennis is a better choice than singles if you have asthma. Remember that dehydration can worsen exercise-induced asthma, so drink water regularly throughout your exercise.

Running long distances, such as a marathon or a half-marathon, causes you to breathe deeply. The huffing and puffing may dry out your airways, causing irritation. Shorter track and field events are less likely to cause you problems. In a similar manner, cross-country skiing is harder on your lungs than downhill skiing, in general. Easy (green circle) and intermediate (blue square) slopes will be easier on your lungs than difficult (black diamond) slopes.

Swimming is also a good choice because the air you are breathing is very humid. But be aware that if you can smell the chlorine, the water can have too much of the chemical, which can cause an asthma attack.

Sports like soccer and basketball in which players are running up and down the field or court are challenging for people with asthma.

If you have asthma, make sure you take time to warm up sufficiently before you start playing. This will make it easier to breathe during the whole game. Use an inhaler 15 to 30 minutes before you start exercising. It is a good choice for your lungs to avoid exercising when you are sick.

Even if you have exercise-induced asthma, you should exercise. Many accomplished athletes have asthma (**TABLE 13-9**). Even if you have not heard of all of these people, they played a variety of sports, and are all extremely talented.

TABLE 13-9 Accomplished Athletes With Asthma

Name	Sport	Honors
David Beckham	Soccer	Six Premier League (English professional league for men's soccer) titles, two Major League Soccer (U.S. and Canadian) Cup wins, and one win of the Union of European Football Associations Champions League
Jerome Bettis	Football	Halfback for the Los Angeles Rams/St. Louis Rams and Pittsburgh Steelers, including winning Super Bowl XL. Voted into the Pro Football Hall of Fame
Jackie Joyner-Kersee	Track and field	Three gold, one silver, and two bronze medals in heptathlon and long jump at four different Olympic Games
Greg Louganis	Diving	Five Olympic medals, five World Championship titles, and 47 national titles
Paula Jane Radcliffe	Long distance runner	Three London marathons, three New York marathons, and one Chicago marathon; represented Great Britain at four Olympics
Dennis Rodman	Basketball	Five NBA championships, twice an NBA all-star, seven NBA rebounding championships
Peter Vanderkaay	Swimming	Two gold and two bronze medals in four Olympic games, four gold and one silver medal in five World Championship games
Amy Van Dyken	Swimming	Six gold medals in two Olympic games
Kristi Yamaguchi	Figure skating	Gold medals at one Olympic game and two World Championship games

BY THE NUMBERS

Allergies and Asthma

About 90% of children with asthma also have allergies, but among adults with asthma, about 50% also have allergies.[71]

Allergic Asthma or Allergy-Induced Asthma

The same things that cause you to have allergy symptoms, such as pollen, dust mites, and pet dander, may also cause asthma symptoms. Allergies and asthma often occur together. Some people who have skin or food allergies may experience asthma symptoms.

You get an allergic response when your immune system mistakenly identifies a substance like tree or grass pollen as a trespasser. Your body wants to protect you from this trespasser, so antibodies bind to the trespasser, causing an allergic reaction. Common allergy symptoms include nasal congestion, runny nose, itchy eyes, or a skin rash. For some people, their lungs and airways react, leading to asthma symptoms.

If your symptoms are severe, you may need medication to treat your allergies or asthma. One of the major risk factors for allergic asthma is a family history of allergies. If you have allergies, you are at higher risk of getting asthma.

It is useful to know what your allergy and asthma triggers are and learn to avoid or minimize your exposure. Your healthcare provider will help you find the best treatment to manage your symptoms.

Common causes for allergic asthma include tree, grass, and weed pollen, mold spores, animal dander and saliva, dust mite feces, and cockroach feces. Other substances you may encounter do not cause an allergic reaction but can still trigger an asthma attack. These include tobacco smoke or smoke

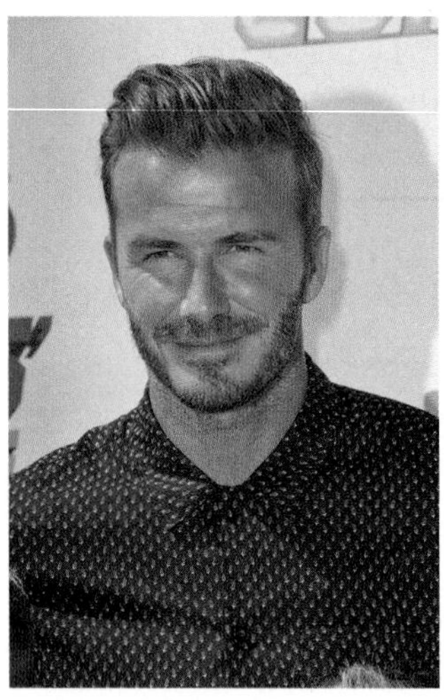

David Beckham.

© Featureflash Photo Agency/Shutterstock.

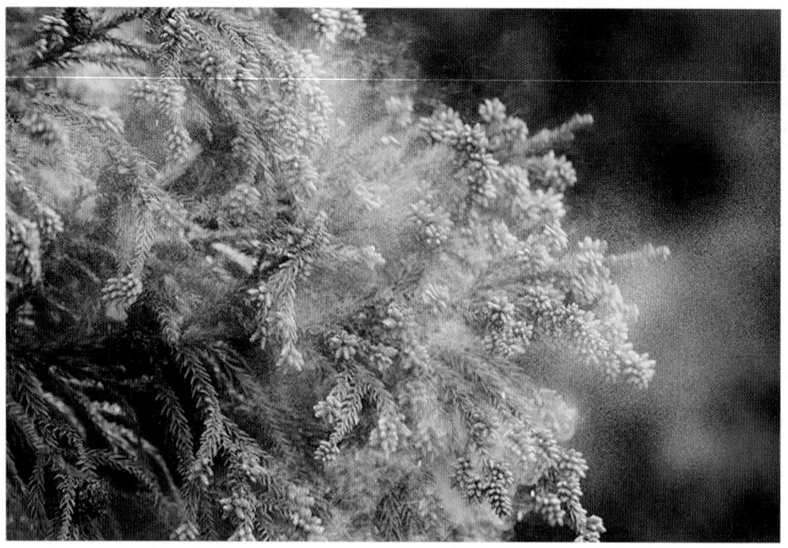

Tree pollen.

© KPG_Payless/Shutterstock.

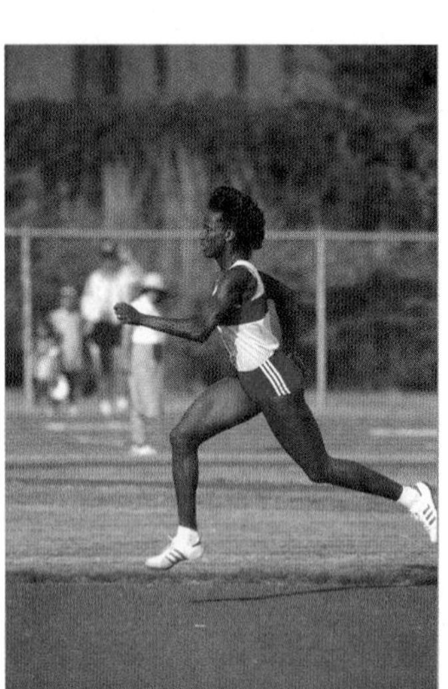

Jackie Joyner-Kersee.

© Focus On Sport/Contributor/Getty Images

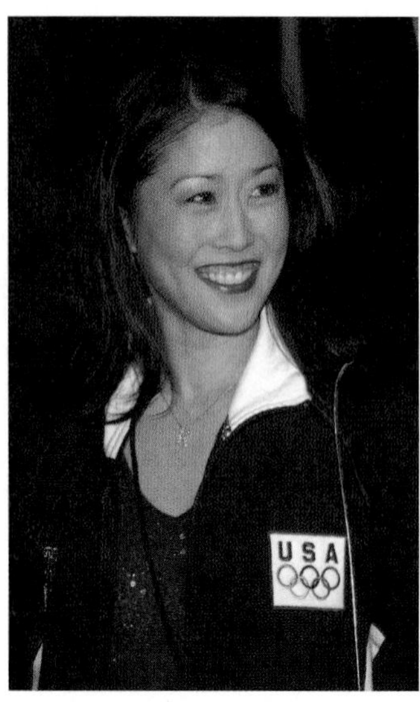

Kristi Yamaguchi.

© Featureflash Photo Agency/Shutterstock.

DOGS AND ALLERGIES[71]

Dog's skin dander causes people to have allergic reactions. Dogs with nonshedding coats are a better choice than dogs that have an undercoat because they shed less dander. The American Kennel Club lists breeds with nonshedding coats, including the Afghan hound, Bedlington terrier, bichon frise, Chinese crested, coton de Tulear, Irish water spaniel, Kerry blue terrier, Maltese, poodle, Portuguese water dog, schnauzer, soft-coated Wheaten terrier, and Xoloitzcuintle (Mexican hairless dog).

There are also hybrids (sometimes called designer dogs), or mixed breeds, where one parent has a nonshedding coat. The two most common dogs in this category are labradoodles (Labrador retriever/poodle) and goldendoodles (golden retriever/poodle). Note that there is no guarantee these pups will have poodle-like (nonshedding) coats.

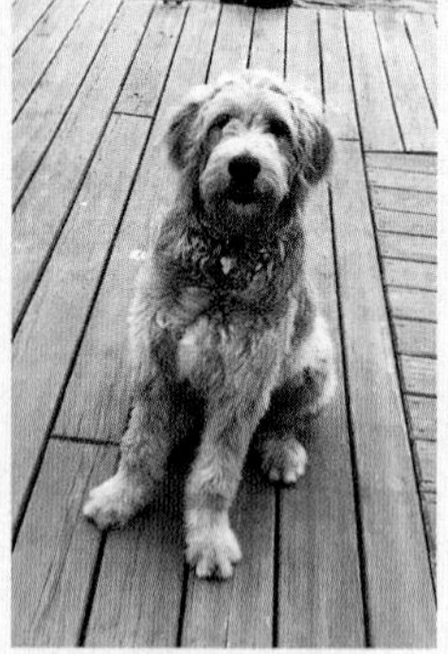

Courtesy of Caitlin Callison.

from fireplaces, candles, incense, or fireworks; air pollution; chemical odors or fumes; perfumes, air fresheners, or other scented products; and dusty rooms.

It may seem obvious, but to control your allergic asthma, you need to avoid breathing in allergens. Weather reports or weather apps often tell you when pollen counts are high. When they are high, stay inside with the windows closed. The filters in air conditioners help reduce exposure to pollen. To avoid dust mites, use allergen-proof covers for your pillows, mattress, and box spring. If you have allergic asthma, you should wash your sheets and other bedding at least once a week in hot water. If you have a choice, do not have wall-to-wall carpeting. Get rid of areas where dust gathers, like piles of clothing. Controlling your indoor humidity will help slow the growth of mold, cockroaches, and dust mites. Air conditioners and dehumidifiers help keep the humidity levels down.

Many times, pets are the cause for allergic responses. If your pets are causing serious problems, you may choose to find them another home or keep them outdoors. If you have pet allergies, at the very least, you should ban them from your bedroom.

If you cannot control your allergy symptoms and they are causing allergic asthma, you may need medication to improve your symptoms. Seek medical attention from a healthcare provider. She or he may start with nasal allergy medications that don't make you sleepy. If these don't work, your healthcare provider may prescribe nasal steroid spray and stronger allergy medications. If none of these help, your healthcare provider may consider allergy shots to help your body become desensitized to allergens.[71]

Viral-Induced Asthma

There are two types of viral-induced asthma: people with no history of asthma, but who develop asthma symptoms with a viral illness; and those who already have asthma and the viral illness makes their symptoms worse. People who have asthma often find that a common cold can make their asthma symptoms worse.[72] Approximately 80% of wheezing episodes and worsening of asthma symptoms occur with viral respiratory infections.[73]

However, people who do not otherwise have asthma can have asthma symptoms when they have a cold. Viruses that cause colds or the flu can also cause asthma symptoms. Treatment is the same as treatment for other types of asthma. Because there are no effective treatments for common viruses, the best approach is to try and prevent them. Limiting contact with people who have upper respiratory infections and frequently washing your hands with soap and water will help limit the spread of viruses (see Chapter 8 for further information).

Work-Related Asthma

Work-related asthma is asthma caused by or made worse by exposure to substances in the workplace. In some cases, the cause may be an allergic reaction, such as an allergy to the powder used in latex gloves. In other cases, workers are employed in industries where they are exposed to substances that irritate their lungs. Substances that may trigger work-related asthma include the following[74]:

- Adhesives
- Shellac
- Lacquer
- Plastics
- Epoxy resins
- Carpeting
- Foam
- Rubber
- Insulation
- Dyes
- Proteins in animal hair
- Grains
- Green coffee beans
- Cotton
- Flax and hemp dust
- Platinum
- Chromium
- Nickel sulfate

Work-related asthma is often identified by symptoms being worse on work days and improving when the person is at home for weekends and vacations.[74]

Chronic Obstructive Pulmonary Disease

In the United States, the two conditions considered to be COPD are emphysema and chronic bronchitis. When you have COPD, it is hard to breathe, and it gets worse over time.

When you breathe in air, it goes down your windpipe and into your lungs where the bronchial tubes branch into thousands of smaller tubes that end in tiny round air sacs (**FIGURE 13-22**). When you are healthy your airways and air sacs are elastic. You breathe in and your air sacs expand and fill with air. When you exhale the air sacs deflate, and the air moves out of your lungs.

Your air sacs are very thin, much like a soap bubble. Oxygen goes through the walls of your air sac and into the blood.

When you have COPD, your airways and air sacs become less elastic. The airways become thick and inflamed, and the walls between many of the air sacs are destroyed, creating larger, but fewer air sacs. This means that the flow of air both into and out of your lungs decreases.[76] When you have COPD, your body has a hard time getting enough oxygen when you breathe in and a hard time getting rid of the carbon dioxide in your body when you breathe out. As the disease progresses, it becomes harder and harder to stay active because you will feel shortness of breath.

The primary cause of COPD is cigarette smoking. Seventy-five percent of people with COPD either smoke or used to smoke. Even if you do not smoke, exposure to other lung irritants may raise your risk for COPD. Other lung irritants include secondhand smoke, air pollution, and chemical fumes or dust from work or the environment. If you have a family history of COPD and smoke, you are more likely to develop the disease.[77]

According to the CDC, the percentage of people with COPD increases with age and varies with race/ethnicity, education, and smoking status (**TABLE 13-10** and **FIGURE 13-23**).

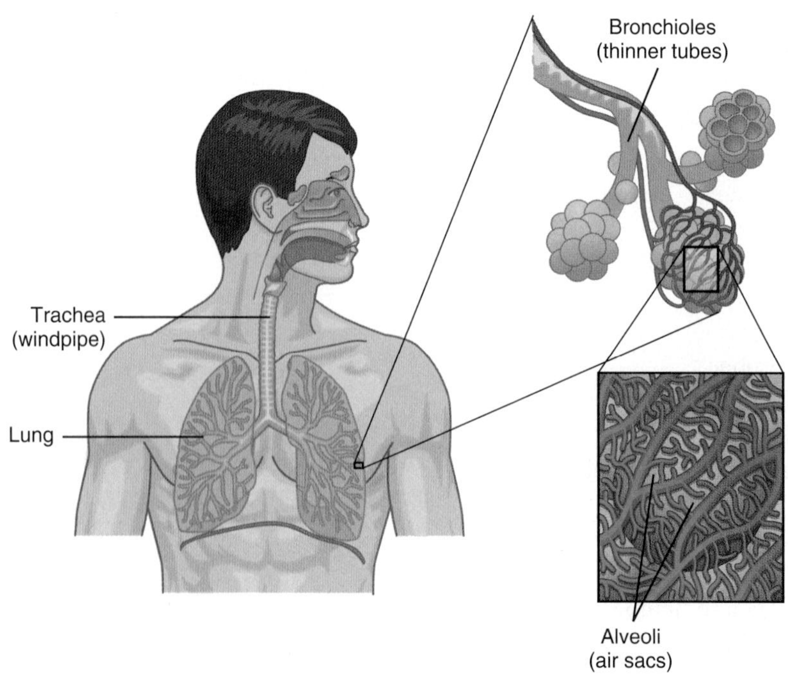

FIGURE 13-22 Lungs.

HEALTHY LUNGS

A healthy adult lung has an estimated 300 million air sacs![75]

TABLE 13-10 Characteristics of People With Physician-Diagnosed COPD from the Behavioral Risk Factor Surveillance System, United States, 2013[78]

Characteristic	Percentage	Estimated Number With COPD
Total	6.0	15,667,000
Age Group (years)		
18–34	2.6	1,931,000
35–44	3.6	1,447,000
45–54	6.7	2,976,000
55–64	9.7	3,823,000
65–74	11.8	3,061,000
≥75	12.3	2,429,000
Race/Ethnicity		
White, non-Hispanic	6.3	11,237,000
Black, non-Hispanic	6.5	1,844,000
American Indian/Alaska Native, non-Hispanic	10.2	267,000
Asian, non-Hispanic	2.0	181,000
Native Hawaiian/Pacific Islander, non-Hispanic	6.2	30,000
Other race, non-Hispanic	4.8	44,000
Multiracial, non-Hispanic	10.7	321,000
Hispanic	4.1	1,414,000
Education Level		
Less than high school diploma or GED	9.8	3,898,000
High school diploma or GED	6.8	5,145,000
At least some college	4.6	6,556,000
*Smoking status**		
Current smoker	14.3	5,754,000
Former smoker	7.0	5,653,000
Never smoker	2.8	3,752,000

* Current smokers smoked ≥100 cigarettes in their life and currently smoke cigarettes some days or every day. Former smokers smoked ≥100 cigarettes in their life but are not current smokers. Never smokers did not smoke ≥100 cigarettes in their life.

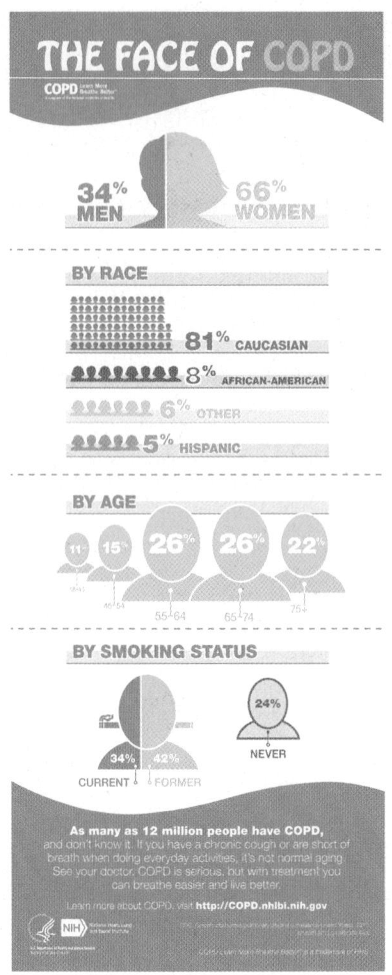

FIGURE 13-23 The face of COPD.

National Heart, Lung, and Blood Institute. (2011). The face of COPD. Retrieved from https://www.nhlbi.nih.gov/health/educational/copd/press-room/media/5782-COPD_Face-Infographic_v11.pdf

Signs of COPD

COPD progresses slowly. At first, you may have mild or even no symptoms. As the disease progresses, the symptoms worsen. The symptoms include an ongoing cough or one that produces a lot of mucus, shortness of breath, especially when physically active, wheezing, and chest tightness. The more damage your lungs have, the more severe your symptoms are likely to be. If you smoke, the damage will occur faster than if you stopped smoking.[79]

Sometimes with COPD you have signs that are so severe, you need to go to a hospital emergency room. If you have any of the following signs, seek emergency care, including lips or fingernails turning blue, having a hard time catching your breath or talking, not being mentally alert, or your heart is beating faster than expected for your level of exertion. Seek medical attention if you have already been treated for COPD, but the treatment for your symptoms is not working.[79]

Treatment

Currently, there is no cure for COPD. The goal of treatment is to help the person feel better, stay active, and slow the progression of the disease, as well as prevent and treat complications and improve overall health. If you or a loved one has COPD, a healthcare professional will help create a treatment plan.

The CDC, the National Institutes of Health, the American Lung Association, and the COPD Foundation all recommend that if you smoke, the most important part of treatment is to stop smoking. In addition, you should avoid other lung irritants such as secondhand smoke, dust, and fumes.

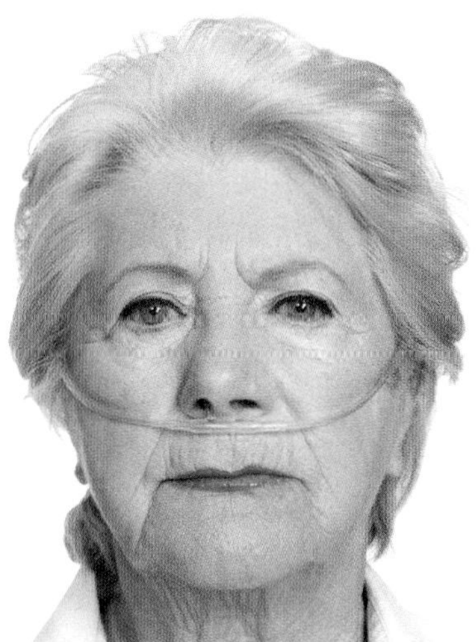

Woman with nasal oxygen.
© STEEX/E+/Getty Images

Your healthcare provider may prescribe medicine to relax the muscles around your airways, which will help you breathe more easily. Because getting the flu is more serious if you have COPD, it is important to get a yearly flu shot. If you have severe COPD, your healthcare provider may recommend oxygen therapy. You may need oxygen some or all of the time.[80]

Managing Your Life With COPD

If you or a loved one are diagnosed with COPD, getting ongoing medical care is important. While it may require adjustment, there are ways to manage COPD symptoms. Do activities slowly. Keep items frequently used close at hand. Learn to ask for help if needed. Keep clothes and shoes comfortable and easy to put on and take off.[81]

In Summary

Chronic diseases, such as cancer, cardiovascular diseases, asthma, and COPD, are common and caused by a combination of behavioral, social, and genetic factors. While the United States and the world have made great strides in reducing death from chronic diseases in the 20th century, there are still millions of people around the world who die each year. While there are policies and behaviors that we know can reduce mortality and improve quality of life, there is still much more we need to understand about chronic diseases.

Key Words

asthma
cancer
carcinomas
cardiovascular disease
cerebrovascular disease
chronic diseases
chronic obstructive pulmonary disease
coronary heart disease
heart attack
hypertension
insulin
leukemia
melanoma
prediabetes
sarcomas
stroke
tumor
type 1 diabetes
type 2 diabetes

Resources

American Diabetes Association: www.diabetes.org
American Heart Association: www.heart.org
American Lung Association: www.lung.org
Cancer Support Community: www.cancersupportcommunity.org/resources
My Life Line: www.mylifeline.org/resources
COPD Foundation: www.copdfoundation.org
National Cancer Institute: www.cancer.gov

Student Discussion Questions and Activities

1. Placing limits on the sale of tobacco and establishing smoke-free workplace laws are two examples of laws and policies intended to reduce cancer rates in the United States. What are some other policies you can think of that may help more people avoid cancer?
2. What would you do or say if a parent or grandparent told you they had cancer? How would you talk to them? Would you feel comfortable making recommendations or offering to help? If so, what might be some ways you might offer to help?
3. Why do you think that CVDs are so highly prevalent in the United States if there are ways to change behavior and lifestyle to effectively reduce one's risk?
4. Think about what you normally eat. Does it include foods high in sugar, fat, and salt? How hard do you think it would be to change to a healthier diet?
5. Consider changes people need to make to lower their risk of type 2 diabetes. Do you need to make those changes? Design a program for yourself or friends to lower the risk of type 2 diabetes.
6. Imagine you have asthma. How do you control the symptoms?
7. Imagine what a day would be like if you had COPD and had to take an oxygen tank with you everywhere you went. How would that effect what you do every day?

References

1. World Health Organization (WHO). Global status report on noncommunicable diseases 2010. Retrieved from http://www.who.int/nmh/publications/ncd_report2010/en/
2. Ward, B.W., Schiller, J. S. & Goodman, R. A. (2014). Multiple chronic conditions among US adults: A 2012 update. *Preventing Chronic Disease*, 2014;11:E62.
3. Popkin, B. M. (2004). The nutrition transition: An overview of world patterns of change. *Nutritional Reviews*, *62*(7 Pt 2), S140–S143.
4. Hafez, N., & Ling, P. M. (2005). How Philip Morris built Marlboro into a global brand for young adults: Implications for international tobacco control. *Tobacco Control*, *14*(4), 262–271.
5. Stuckler, D., McKee, M., Ebrahim, S., & Basu, S. (2012). Manufacturing epidemics: The role of global producers in increased consumption of unhealthy commodities including processed foods, alcohol, and tobacco. *PLoS Medicine*, *9*(6), e1001235.
6. Centers for Disease Control and Prevention (CDC). (2016). Health, United States, 2016: With chartbook on long-term trends in health. Retrieved from https://www.cdc.gov/nchs/data/hus/hus16.pdf
7. American Cancer Society. (2017). Cancer facts and figures. Retrieved from https://www.cancer.org/research/cancer-facts-statistics/all-cancer-facts-figures/cancer-facts-figures-2017.html
8. Chen, J., Vargas-Bustamante, A., Mortensen, K., & Ortega, A. N. (2016). Racial and ethnic disparities in health care access and utilization under the Affordable Care Act. *Medical Care*, *54*(2), 140–146.
9. Breen, N., Scott, S., Percy-Laurry, A., Lewis, D., & Glasgow, R. (2014). Health disparities calculator: A methodologically rigorous tool for analyzing inequalities in population health. *American Journal of Public Health*, *104*(9), 1589–1591.
10. Siegel, R. L., Miller, K. D., & Jemal, A. (2016). Cancer statistics, 2016. *CA: A Cancer Journal for Clinicians*, *66*(1), 7–30.
11. World Health Organization (WHO). (n.d.). Cancer. Retrieved from http://www.who.int/mediacentre/factsheets/fs297/en/
12. Wu, S., Powers, S., Zhu, W., & Hannun, Y. A. (2016). Substantial contribution of extrinsic risk factors to cancer development. *Nature*, *529*(7584), 43–47.
13. Turati, F., Rossi, M., Pelucchi, C., Levi, F., & La Vecchia, C. (2015). Fruit and vegetables and cancer risk: A review of southern European studies. *British Journal of Nutrition*, *113*(Suppl 2), S102–S110.
14. Bradbury, K. E., Appleby, P. N., & Key, T. J. (2014). Fruit, vegetable, and fiber intake in relation to cancer risk: Findings from the European prospective investigation into cancer and nutrition (EPIC). *The American Journal of Clinical Nutrition*, *100*(Suppl 1), 394S–398S.

15. Bouvard, V., Loomis, D., Guyton, K. Z., Grosse, Y., El Ghissassi, F., Benbrahim-Tallaa, L., Guha, N., Mattock, H., Straif, K. (2015). Carcinogenicity of consumption of red and processed meat. *The Lancet Oncology*, *16*(16):1599–1600.
16. Courneya, K. S., & Friedenreich, C. M. (Eds.) (2010). Physical activity and cancer: An introduction. In K. S. Courneya & C. M. Friedenreich (Eds.), *Physical activity and cancer* (pp. 1–10). Berlin, Heidelberg: Springer.
17. Hiatt, R. A., & Breen, N. (2008). The social determinants of cancer: A challenge for transdisciplinary science. *American Journal of Preventive Medicine*, *35*(2 Suppl), S141–S150.
18. World Health Organization (WHO). (n.d.). Cardiovascular diseases (CVDs). Retrieved from http://www.who.int/mediacentre/factsheets/fs317/en/
19. Centers for Disease Control and Prevention (CDC). (2017). Heart disease facts. Retrieved from https://www.cdc.gov/heartdisease/facts.htm
20. Centers for Disease Control and Prevention (CDC). (2017). Conditions that increase risk for stroke. Retrieved from https://www.cdc.gov/stroke/conditions.htm
21. Mayo Clinic. (2016). High blood pressure (hypertension). Retrieved from http://www.mayoclinic.org/diseases-conditions/high-blood-pressure/basics/definition/con-20019580
22. Working Group (2013). Heart disease and stroke statistics—2013 update: A report from the American Heart Association. Retrieved from http://circ.ahajournals.org/content/127/1/e6
23. National Heart, Lung, and Blood Institute. (2015). What is a heart attack? Retrieved from https://www.nhlbi.nih.gov/health/health-topics/topics/heartattack
24. National Heart, Lung, and Blood Institute. (2015). Life after a heart attack. Retrieved from https://www.nhlbi.nih.gov/health/health-topics/topics/heartattack/lifeafter
25. National Heart, Lung, and Blood Institute. (2015). How is a heart attack treated? Retrieved from https://www.nhlbi.nih.gov/health/health-topics/topics/heartattack/treatment
26. American Heart Association. (2016). Understand your risks to prevent a heart attack. Retrieved from http://www.heart.org/HEARTORG/Conditions/HeartAttack/UnderstandYourRiskstoPreventaHeartAttack/Understand-Your-Risks-to-Prevent-a-Heart-Attack_UCM_002040_Article.jsp#.WZxqG8aQzRZ
27. Mayo Clinic. (2016). Red wine and resveratrol: Good for your heart? Retrieved from http://www.mayoclinic.org/diseases-conditions/heart-disease/in-depth/red-wine/ART-20048281
28. National Heart, Lung, and Blood Institute. (2015). How can a heart attack be prevented? Retrieved from https://www.nhlbi.nih.gov/health/health-topics/topics/heartattack/prevention
29. Centers for Disease Control and Prevention (CDC). (2017). Heart attack. Retrieved from https://www.cdc.gov/heartdisease/heart_attack.htm
30. Centers for Disease Control and Prevention (CDC). (2016). About stroke. Retrieved from https://www.cdc.gov/stroke/about.htm
31. Centers for Disease Control and Prevention (CDC). (2017). Stroke signs and symptoms. Retrieved from https://www.cdc.gov/stroke/signs_symptoms.htm
32. Centers for Disease Control and Prevention (CDC). (2017). Stroke treatment. Retrieved from https://www.cdc.gov/stroke/treatments.htm
33. Centers for Disease Control and Prevention (CDC). (2017). Recovering from stroke. Retrieved from https://www.cdc.gov/stroke/recovery.htm
34. Centers for Disease Control and Prevention (CDC). (2017). Stroke facts. Retrieved from https://www.cdc.gov/stroke/facts.htm
35. Centers for Disease Control and Prevention (CDC). (2017). Stroke. Retrieved from https://www.cdc.gov/stroke/index.htm
36. American Heart Association. (2016). High blood pressure and African Americans. Retrieved from https://www.heart.org/HEARTORG/Conditions/HighBloodPressure/UnderstandSymptomsRisks/High Blood Pressure and-African-Americans_UCM_301832_Article.jsp
37. National Institute of Diabetes and Digestive and Kidney Diseases. (2016). What is diabetes? Retrieved from https://www.niddk.nih.gov/health-information/diabetes/overview/what-is-diabetes
38. Centers for Disease Control and Prevention (CDC). (2017). New CDC report: More than 100 million Americans have diabetes or prediabetes. Retrieved from https://www.cdc.gov/media/releases/2017/p0718-diabetes-report.html
39. Menke, A., Orchard, T. J., Imperatore, G., Bullard, K. M., Mayer-Davis, E., & Cowie, C. C. (2013). The prevalence of type 1 diabetes in the United States. *Epidemiology*, *24*(5), 773–774.
40. WebMD. (n.d.). Type 1 diabetes guide. Retrieved from http://www.webmd.com/diabetes/type-1-diabetes-guide/default.htm
41. American Diabetes Association. (2016). Standards of medical care in diabetes—2016 abridged for primary care providers. *Clinical Diabetes*, *34*(1), 3–21.
42. Joslin Diabetes Center. (n.d.). Monitoring your blood glucose. Retrieved from http://www.joslin.org/info/monitoring_your_blood_glucose.html
43. Mayo Clinic. (n.d.). Diabetes and exercise: When to monitor your blood sugar. Retrieved from http://www.mayoclinic.org/diseases-conditions/diabetes/in-depth/diabetes-and-exercise/art-20045697
44. WebMD. (n.d.). Type 1 diabetes. Retrieved from http://www.webmd.com/diabetes/type-1-diabetes
45. Centers for Disease Control and Prevention (CDC). (2017). The surprising truth about prediabetes. Retrieved from https://www.cdc.gov/features/diabetesprevention/index.html
46. National Institute of Diabetes and Digestive and Kidney Diseases. (n.d.). Risk factors for type 2 diabetes. Retrieved from https://www.niddk.nih.gov/health-information/diabetes/overview/risk-factors-type-2-diabetes
47. Centers for Disease Control and Prevention (CDC). (2012). Increasing prevalence of diagnosed diabetes—United States and Puerto Rico, 1995–2010. *Morbidity and Mortality Weekly Report, 61*(45), 918–921.
48. CDC (2017). Prediabetes. Retrieved from: https://www.cdc.gov/diabetes/basics/prediabetes.html
49. Centers for Disease Control and Prevention (CDC). (2017). Getting tested. Retrieved from https://www.cdc.gov/diabetes/basics/getting-tested.html
50. Rodriguez, D. (2016). Dining out with diabetes: Menu words to watch for. Retrieved from https://www.everydayhealth.com/hs/diabetes-guide-managing-blood-sugar/diabetes-dining-menu-words/
51. Centers for Disease Control and Prevention (CDC). (2016). Stay healthy. Retrieved from https://www.cdc.gov/diabetes/managing/health.html
52. National Institute of Diabetes and Digestive and Kidney Diseases. (n.d.). Gestational diabetes. Retrieved from https://www.niddk.nih.gov/health-information/diabetes/overview/what-is-diabetes/gestational

53. Centers for Disease Control and Prevention (CDC). (2014). National diabetes statistics report: Estimates of diabetes and its burden in the United States, 2014. Retrieved from http://www.cdc.gov/diabetes/data/statistics/2014StatisticsReport.html.
54. CDC's Division of Diabetes Translation. (2017). Maps of trends in diagnosed diabetes and obesity. Retrieved from https://www.cdc.gov/diabetes/statistics/slides/maps_diabetesobesity_trends.pdf
55. World Health Organization (WHO). (n.d.). What are social determinants of health? Retrieved from http://www.who.int/social_determinants/sdh_definition/en/
56. Centers for Disease Control and Prevention (CDC). (2011). *National diabetes fact sheet: National estimates and general information on diabetes and prediabetes in the United States.* Atlanta, GA: Centers for Disease Control and Prevention.
57. Walker, R. J., Smalls, B. L., Campbell, J. A., Strom Williams, J. L., & Egede, L. E. (2014). Impact of social determinants of health on outcomes for type 2 diabetes: A systematic review. *Endocrine, 47*(1), 29–48.
58. Kogan, S. M., Brody, G. H., & Chen, Y. F. (2009). Depressive symptomatology mediates the effect of socioeconomic disadvantage on HbA(1c) among rural African Americans with type 2 diabetes. *Journal of Psychosomatic Research, 67*(4), 289–296.
59. Okosun, I. S., & Dever, G. E. (2002). Abdominal obesity and ethnic differences in diabetes awareness, treatment, and glycemic control. *Obesity, A Research Journal, 10*(12), 1241–1250.
60. Kacerovsky-Bielesz, G., Lienhardt, S., Hagenhofer, M., Kacerovsky, M., Forster, E., Roth, R., Roden, M. (2009). Sex-related psychological effects on metabolic control in type 2 diabetes mellitus. *Diabetologia, 52*(5), 781–788.
61. Osborn, C. Y., Bains, S. S., & Egede, L. E. (2010). Health literacy, diabetes self-care, and glycemic control in adults with type 2 diabetes. *Diabetes Technology and Therapeutics, 12*(11), 913–919.
62. World Health Organization (WHO). (2016). Global report on diabetes. Retrieved from http://apps.who.int/iris/bitstream/10665/204871/1/9789241565257_eng.pdf
63. NCD Risk Factor Collaboration (NCD-RisC). (2016). Worldwide trends in diabetes since 1980: A pooled analysis of 751 population-based studies with 4.4 million participants. *The Lancet, 387*(10027), 1513–1530.
64. World Health Organization (WHO). (2017). Asthma. Retrieved from http://www.who.int/mediacentre/factsheets/fs307/en/
65. Mayo Clinic. (2017). Wheezing. Retrieved from http://www.mayoclinic.org/symptoms/wheezing/basics/definition/SYM-20050764
66. National Heart, Lung and Blood Institute. (2014). What is asthma? Retrieved from https://www.nhlbi.nih.gov/health/health-topics/topics/asthma/
67. Centers for Disease Control and Prevention (CDC). (2017). Asthma. Retrieved from https://www.cdc.gov/nchs/fastats/asthma.htm
68. Mayo Clinic. (2014). Exercise-induced asthma: Definition. Retrieved from http://www.mayoclinic.org/diseases-conditions/exercise-induced-asthma/basics/definition/CON-20033156
69. Mayo Clinic. (2014). Exercise-induced asthma: Symptoms. Retrieved from http://www.mayoclinic.org/diseases-conditions/exercise-induced-asthma/basics/symptoms/con-20033156.
70. Yang, Z. Y., Zhong, H. B., Mao, C., Yuan, J. Q., Huang, Y. F., Wu, X. Y., Gao, Y. M., Tang, J. L.. (2016). Yoga for asthma. *Cochrane Database of Systematic Reviews, 4*, CD010346
71. WebMD. (n.d.). Allergic asthma. Retrieved from http://www.webmd.com/asthma/guide/allergic-asthma#1
72. Castillo, J. R., Peters, S. P., & Busse, W. W. (2017). Asthma exacerbations: Pathogenesis, prevention, and treatment. *Journal of Allergy and Clinical Immunology: In Practice, 5*(4), 918–927.
73. Ohrmalm, L., Malinovschi, A., Wong, M., Levinson, P., Janson, C., Broliden, K., Alving, K. (2016). Presence of rhinovirus in the respiratory tract of adolescents and young adults with asthma without symptoms of infection. *Respiratory Medicine, 115*, 1–6.
74. WebMD. (2016). Occupational asthma. Retrieved from http://www.webmd.com/asthma/guide/occupational-asthma-work-related-asthma#2
75. COPD Foundation. (n.d.). Understand your lungs. Retrieved from https://www.copdfoundation.org/What-is-COPD/Living-with-COPD/Understand-Your-Lungs.aspx.
76. American Lung Association. (2016). What is COPD? Retrieved from http://www.lung.org/lung-health-and-diseases/lung-disease-lookup/copd/learn-about-copd/what-is-copd.html
77. National Institute of Diabetes and Digestive and Kidney Diseases. (2017). Risk factors. Retrieved from https://www.nhlbi.nih.gov/health/health-topics/topics/copd/atrisk
78. Wheaton, A. G., Cunningham, T. J., Ford, E. S., Croft, J. B., & Centers for Disease Control and Prevention (CDC). (2015). Employment and activity limitations among adults with chronic obstructive pulmonary disease—United States, 2013. *Morbidity and Mortality Weekly Report, 64*(11), 289–295.
79. National Heart, Lung and Blood Institute. (2017). Signs and symptoms. Retrieved from https://www.nhlbi.nih.gov/health/health-topics/topics/copd/signs
80. National Heart, Lung and Blood Institute. (2017). Treatment. Retrieved from https://www.nhlbi.nih.gov/health/health-topics/topics/copd/treatment
81. National Heart, Lung and Blood Institute. (2017). COPD: Living with. Retrieved from https://www.nhlbi.nih.gov/health/health-topics/topics/copd/livingwith

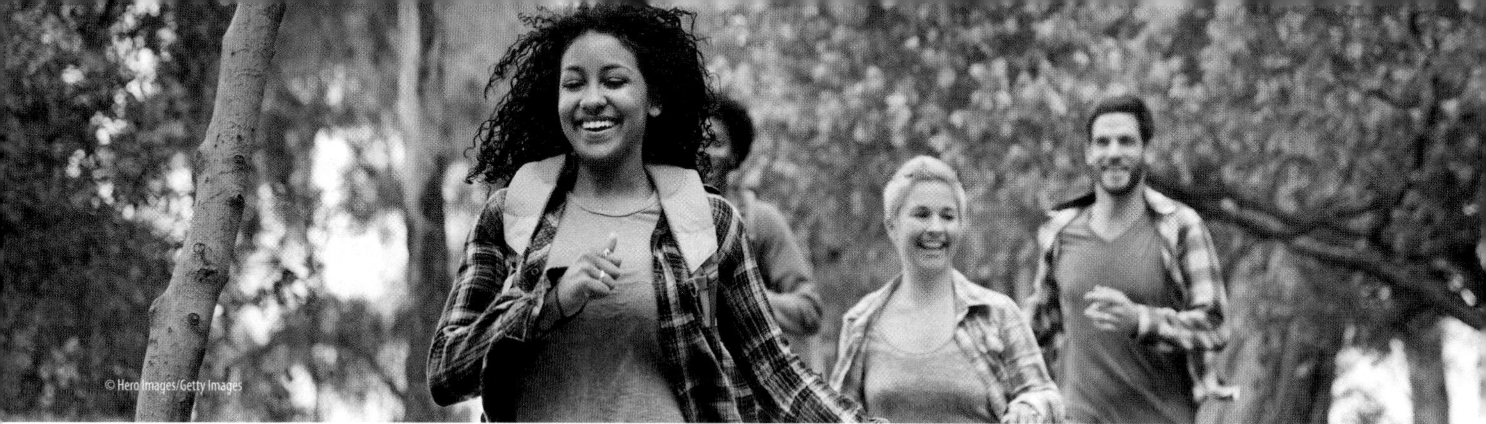

CHAPTER 14

Getting Covered: Healthcare Policy and Health Insurance

CHAPTER OBJECTIVES

- Discuss the history of the United States healthcare system.
- Illustrate why a historical context is important to understanding the healthcare payment and reimbursement structure in the United States and how it differs from the systems in Europe and Canada.
- Describe the current American healthcare system, including systems of payment and providers.
- Describe different models of healthcare insurance in the United States.
- Describe different types of coverage plans among health insurance companies.
- Review options for gaining access to health coverage, especially for college students.

Do you recall President Barack Obama signing the Patient Protection and Affordable Care Act (ACA or "Obamacare") back in 2010? It was a historic moment — the only comprehensive national healthcare plan ever passed in the United States. Although there was strong opposition from republicans in Congress at the time, the bill garnered enough votes in both the Senate and the House of Representatives to advance to the president for approval.

This plan was a sign of hope for those who needed health care, and for the thousands of advocates who worked for decades to achieve a national health system. Finally, our country would have a single system where people would get health care when they needed it, regardless of their ability to pay. Finally, patients and their families would be able to make decisions about health and not be under the control of private insurance companies. Finally, we would live in a society where the need to put food on the table or stay warm would not compete with monthly insurance premiums, doctor visit copays, and annual **deductibles**, and where bureaucracy and paperwork would no longer cause people to throw their hands up in confusion.

deductibles The amount the insurance holder must pay out of pocket before an insurance company will cover costs. For example, if the deductible is $500 and the total bill is $1,000, the insurance holder must pay $500 and the insurance company will cover the remainder.

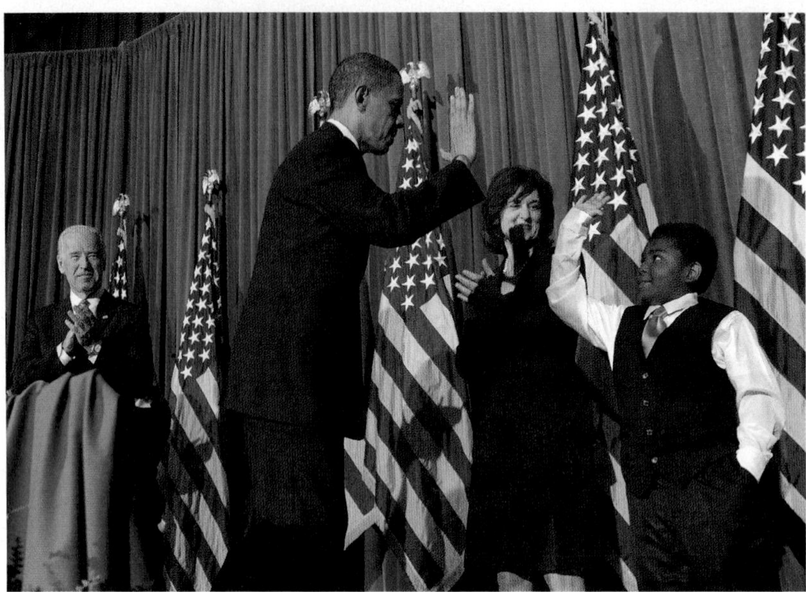

U.S. President Barack Obama gives a high five to 11-year-old Marcelas Owens after signing the Patient Protection and Affordable Care Act into law in 2010.

You may be wondering if you are living in the same world as the optimistic vision just described. Despite the passage of the ACA in 2010, most people still receive coverage from private insurance companies and many of those with private insurance still face significant costs and inconveniences with paperwork and bureaucratic requirements. Despite financial penalties imposed by the ACA on individuals who do not acquire coverage, many people—especially young people—found themselves without any form of health insurance at all.

So what's going on? You might be wondering, "Why am I still not covered if we passed a national insurance program?" Or, "Why do I have to pay so much money for this so-called "national healthcare plan?"

The U.S. Health System in Historical Context

Why is our national health system less comprehensive than that of Canada, Europe, Australia, or Japan? In part, it is due to the traditional values that differ between the United States and other nations. These values have enormous influence over the policy differences between the United States, Canada, and Europe. The emphasis in the United States on rugged individualism throughout its history, and the principles of "life, liberty, and the pursuit of happiness," may play a role. This philosophy may help explain why the United States has long operated without a national health system to serve all of its citizens.[1,2]

All European Union member states have a universal healthcare system for their populations. Some systems, such as in the United Kingdom and Canada, are publicly funded, "single-payer systems." In this type of system, the government, rather than private insurance companies, coordinates all healthcare payments for its citizens.[3] In other countries, such as Germany and Netherlands, insurance coverage is provided to every citizen through private insurance companies. In some countries, nearly everything is paid for, while in others, citizens must cover some portion of healthcare costs themselves. While we may think that European nations all have similar health systems, there are some major differences between them (**TABLE 14-1**).

TABLE 14-1 Health Care Around the World

Country	Funding System
United Kingdom	Universal system funded through a nationwide tax. Approximately 10% of residents purchase additional insurance to get access to doctors more quickly or to receive noncovered treatments through private facilities.
Denmark	Universal system is funded through local taxes. Approximately 40% of residents purchase additional insurance to visit private physicians and receive other services, such as physical therapy.
France	Social health insurance paid by individuals through individual contributions, usually deducted from employees' salaries. Supplemental insurance is offered by private insurance companies for addition benefits.
Germany	Social health insurance paid by employer and employee, with autonomous, competitive third-party payers (insurers).
Switzerland	Compulsory health insurance. All residents required to purchase basic private plans at affordable prices. The government defines the benefit package for the basic plan, so they are very similar, although administered by private companies.
Australia	Universal insurance is provided for basic services. Residents purchase additional health insurance paid by individuals. Regionally, not nationally administered.
Singapore	Medical savings accounts and catastrophic health insurance subsidized by the government and funded through a general tax.
The Netherlands	Compulsory health insurance. All residents are required to purchase private plans through a national exchange (similar to insurance plan under the U.S. ACA)
United States	Health insurance is predominantly paid for by employers through incentivized tax subsidies.

The Commonweath Fund. (2016). International profiles of health care systems, 2015. Retrieved from http://www.commonwealthfund.org/publications/fund-reports/2016/jan/international-profiles-2015

Different countries also experience different population health outcomes with their health systems. As a percentage of total government spending, the United States spends more on healthcare than any other nation (**FIGURE 14-1**); however, our health outcomes are not as good as many other nations. Across most outcomes, the United States ranks below the nations that have had universal health systems in place for several years (**TABLE 14-2**).

Despite the adoption of universal health care in Europe and Canada, the United States never managed to adopt such a policy in the 20th century. The American system still relies mostly on private health insurance—purchased through employers—to cover its citizens.

Historically, businesses used health insurance as a benefit to attract the best workers without paying higher wages. These businesses were able to purchase large group policies to cover all their workers at rates that were much lower per person than if the employees had to purchase the plans for themselves. In addition, business did not have to pay taxes on the insurance premiums.

However, it eventually became very expensive for employers as healthcare costs grew faster than the rate of inflation. Despite the tax advantages enjoyed by businesses, the system still left many Americans (such as self-employed or

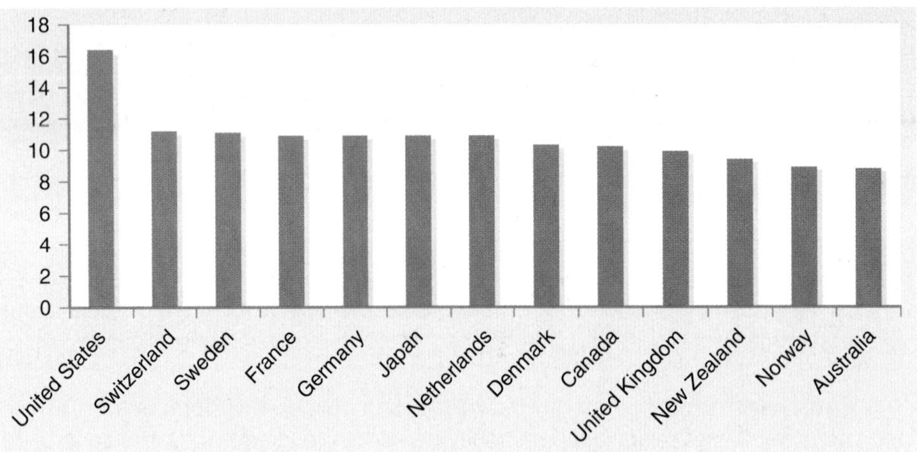

FIGURE 14-1 Percent of gross domestic product spent on health care for selected countries, 2013.

Data from Organization for Economic Cooperation and Development, 2015.

TABLE 14-2 Selected Health Outcomes by Country

	Life expectancy at birth, 2013	Infant mortality per 1,000 live births, 2013	Percentage of population age 65+ with two or more chronic conditions, 2014	Obesity rate (BMI >30), 2013	Percentage of population (age 15+) who are daily smokers, 2013
Australia	82.2	3.6	54	28.3	12.8
Canada	81.5	4.8	56	25.8	14.9
Denmark	80.4	3.5	-	14.2	17.0
France	82.3	3.6	43	14.5	24.1
Germany	80.9	3.3	49	23.6	20.9
Japan	83.4	2.1	-	3.7	19.3
Netherlands	81.4	3.8	46	11.8	18.5
New Zealand	81.4	5.2	37	30.6	15.5
Norway	81.8	2.4	43	10.0	15.0
Sweden	82.0	2.7	42	11.7	10.7
Switzerland	82.9	3.9	44	10.3	20.4
United Kingdom	81.1	3.8	33	24.9	20.0
United States	78.8	6.1	68	35.3	13.7

Data from Organization for Economic Cooperation and Development, 2015.

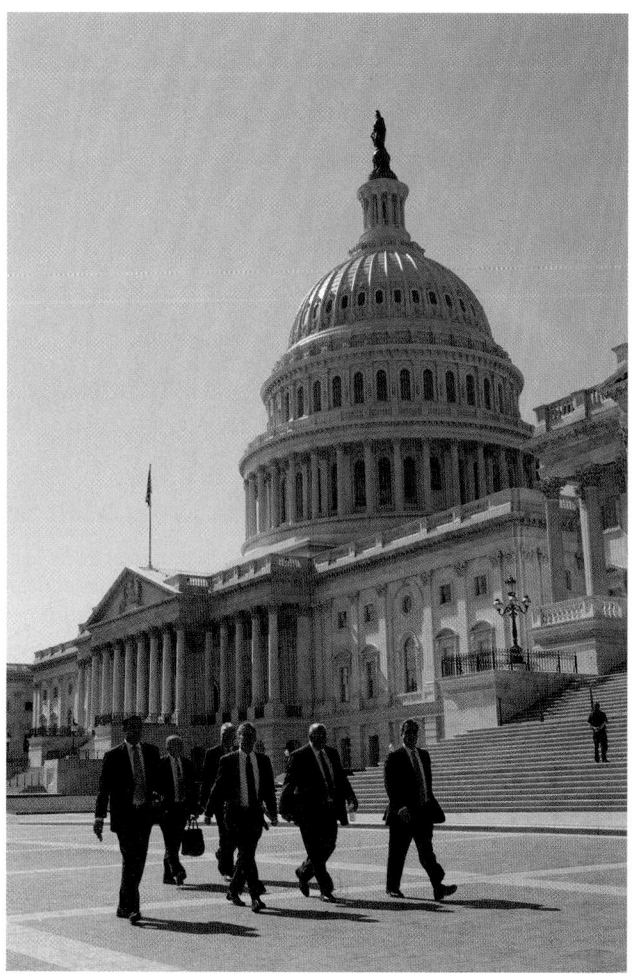

Lobbyists.

part-time workers) without any health insurance at all. This issue became a rallying cry for political and social leaders throughout the 20th century to find a solution for the growing number of Americans without insurance.

During many attempts to pass a U.S. national healthcare system, there has been a great deal of opposition over the years, including the American Medical Association, the Health Insurance Association of America, the pharmaceutical industry, and other business organizations. Historically, business has exerted financial and political influence in the United States and has enjoyed high levels of respect among the American public. Confidence in government, on the other hand, has always been lower among Americans compared to Europeans, which also may help explain why it was so difficult for the United States to pass a single health insurance plan until 2010.[4]

When it was finally passed, the ACA created a nationally coordinated healthcare system that would seek to ensure that all Americans have some form of basic health insurance. And from September 2013 to March 2015 the rate of uninsured people in the United States dropped by 7.5 percentage points. In the first 2 years since the ACA was implemented, 15 million people acquired coverage.[5] Over subsequent years, republicans tried to repeal the act, coming close under the administration of President Donald Trump, who tried and failed to do so in 2017.

There are three ways the ACA attempted to achieve universal coverage for all Americans. First, it expanded the existing **Medicaid** system (originally intended for low-income and disabled individuals). Second, it provided federal subsidies

Medicaid U.S. public health insurance program serving people with low incomes and minimal assets. Medicaid was passed in 1965 as part of the federal Social Security Act. It is jointly funded by state and federal governments, but it is managed by the states.

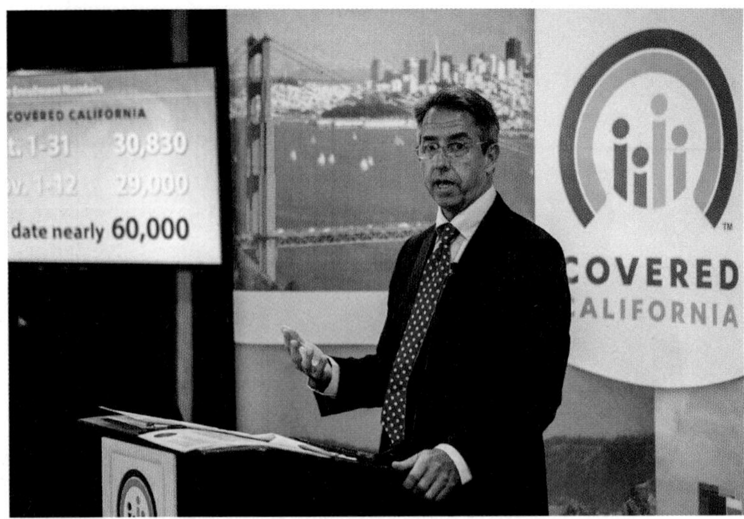

Some states manage their own ACA marketplaces, or "exchanges." The California Exchange is called Covered California. Here, Executive Director Peter Lee reports results at the end of 2013.

to help previously uninsured people and families get health insurance through an expanded healthcare marketplace. Third, it established a financial tax penalty for people who remain uninsured. This provision was repealed in 2018.

While the American healthcare system previously relied on private insurance companies to coordinate health care through a regulated private market, the ACA created government-sponsored marketplaces, also called "exchanges." In some states, the exchanges are run by the state itself, while other states simply use the federal exchange as their marketplace. Later, we will discuss the insurance options that are available to you. The next section provides some basic information about the U.S. healthcare system and how it is organized.

Healthcare Providers and Medical Professionals

Only a few decades ago, most people could name only two categories of medical professionals: doctors and nurses. Today, many types of medical professionals provide care, including the traditional doctors of medicine (MD), doctors of osteopathic medicine (DO), physician assistants (PA), and nurse practitioners (NP). There are also numerous other categories of healthcare providers, including other doctoral-level professions such as psychologists, naturopathic physicians, and chiropractors. There are also nurse-midwives, paramedics, surgeon assistants, clinical social workers, speech pathologists, and radiologists.

The U.S. National Institutes of Health (NIH) defines conventional medicine as that which is practiced by holders of MD and DO degrees and by allied health professionals, such as physical therapists, psychologists, and registered nurses. Although the boundaries between complementary and alternative medicine (CAM) are blurring in the minds of consumers,[6] this chapter discusses only conventional medical practitioners. See Chapter 4 for a discussion of many of the types of practitioners currently defined outside the category of conventional medicine.

Physicians

Generally speaking, the terms *physician* and *doctor* mean the same thing. In the United States, a medical physician is someone who has received an MD or DO degree from an accredited medical school and has passed a licensing examination

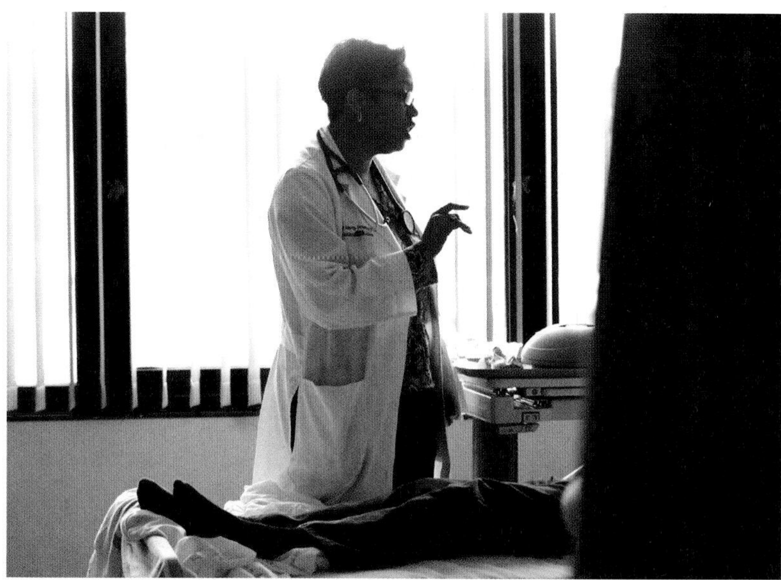

Karen Morris-Prester was the first grandmother to graduate from Yale Medical School. Today, the percentage of males and females graduating from medical school is about equal.

from the National Board of Medical Examiners or the National Board of Osteopathic Medical Examiners. MDs and DOs also must complete intern programs where they continue their training under the supervision of other physicians and residency programs, and work in a facility (usually a hospital) for 2 to 6 years.[7]

The basis of osteopathic medicine is the principle that the well-being of an individual depends on the skeleton, muscles, ligaments, and connective tissues functioning smoothly together.[8] As a contrast, the basis of training for an MD is on counteracting or neutralizing the effects of a disease.[9]

Another important distinction is the difference between a primary care physician (sometimes called a generalist) and a specialist. A primary care physician performs routine checkups and often provides counseling and education to patients, as well as continuing medical care for a variety of conditions. Primary care physicians can practice family medicine, pediatrics, or internal medicine. Gynecologists, who focus their care on women's reproductive health, are often considered primary care physicians. **Internal medicine** doctors, or "internists," focus on preventing, identifying, and treating conditions related to internal systems, such as those of the heart, lungs, or neurologic systems. Pediatricians take care of children, preventing, identifying, and treating many conditions of childhood. In the past, many primary care physicians were called general practitioners.

internal medicine Medical practice concerned with preventing, identifying, and treating conditions related to internal systems, such as those of the heart, lungs, or neurologic systems. Internists are considered "primary care" physicians, although not generalists.

Specialized physicians, or specialists, focus on specific diseases (e.g., cancer is the disease for which oncology is the specialty) or organ systems (the lung is the organ and pulmonology is the specialty). Specialists are required to obtain additional certification in their area of specialization and undergo additional years of training in their specialty.

Nurses

In 2016, there were more than 3 million active nurses in the United States, comprising the largest category of healthcare professionals.[10] While most nurses work in acute-care settings such as hospitals, many nurses work in a wide variety of settings, including physician's offices, schools, prisons, public health environments providing health education, and insurance offices, where they have become a critical component of the administrative functions of our healthcare system.

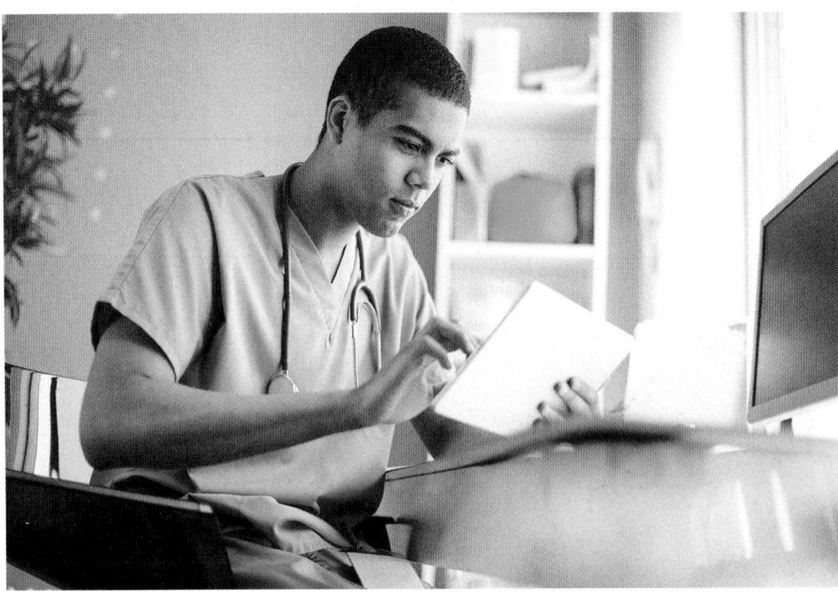

Registered nurses (RNs) require a 2-year associates degree. More advanced levels of nursing include a 4-year bachelor of science in nursing (BSN), and the advanced-practice nurse practitioner, which requires a masters-level degree in nursing. Depending on the state, nurse practitioners are sometimes designated by insurance companies as primary care physicians and can have some level of authority to prescribe medications.

Hospitals and Healthcare Facilities

inpatient care Health care that requires an overnight stay in a hospital or other facility.

More and more, a distinction is made between health care delivered in an "inpatient" setting versus an "outpatient" setting.[11] **Inpatient care** refers to health care that requires an overnight stay in a hospital or other facility. Today, numerous surgeries and procedures that used to require an inpatient stay, now do not. This transformation is both a result of advances in medical technology and due to pressure from managed healthcare insurance organizations that have exerted financial pressure on hospitals to become as efficient as possible.[12] For instance, many hospitals now have "day surgery" departments, where you might go for an operation that can be performed in just a few hours and does not require an overnight hospital stay.

Prescription Drugs

A prescription drug is a pharmaceutical medication or therapy that requires a prescription issued by a licensed medical professional to be dispensed by a licensed pharmacist. "Over-the-counter" drugs do not need a prescription, and include pain medications such as aspirin and allergy medications or ointments such as hydrocortisone. They can be found on the shelves of a pharmacy or even behind the pharmacy counter.

During the 1980s and 1990s, prescription drug spending in the United States grew more rapidly than any other major component of the medical system (**FIGURE 14-2**).[13] Prescription drug usage increased from 4.7% of total U.S. healthcare expenditures in 1980, to 5.6% in 1990, and it currently comprises more than 10% of total U.S. healthcare spending.[14] Per capita, the United States spends the most money on prescription drugs in the world, followed by

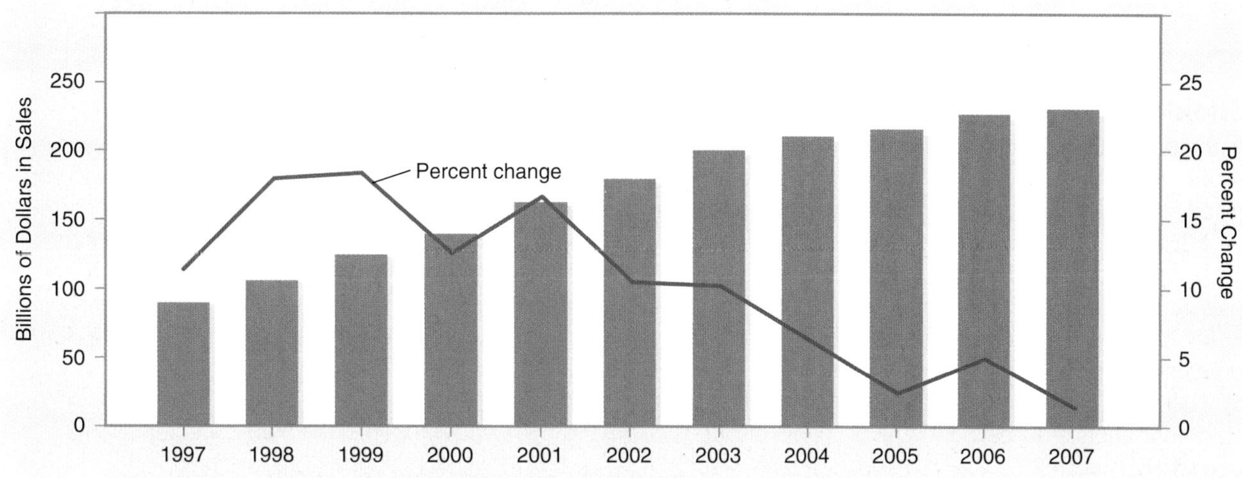

FIGURE 14-2 Size and growth of the U.S. pharmaceutical market, 1997–2007.

Data from Aitken, M., Berndt, E. R., & Cutler, D. M. (2009). Prescription drug spending trends in the United States: Looking beyond the turning point. *Health Affairs, 28*(1), w151–160.

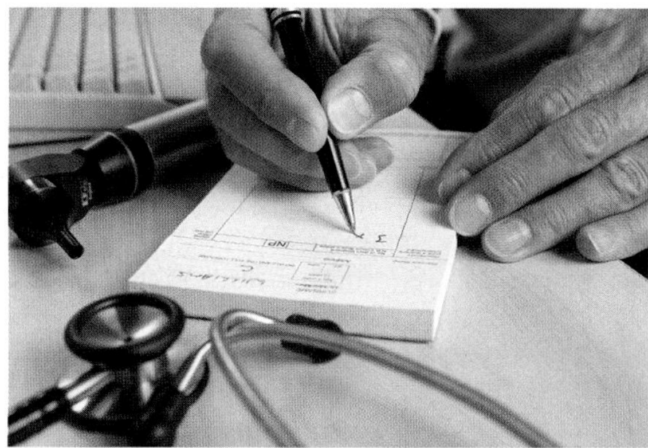

Canada, and then New Zealand.[15] Growth in prescription drug usage has led to increased concerns about the ability of the U.S. healthcare system to sustain the growth in medical and insurance costs.[16]

In the United States, the Food and Drug Administration (FDA) is the agency under the Department of Health and Human Services that makes determinations about which drugs require prescriptions for use. In addition, each state has specific policies for which type of medical professional can prescribe particular drugs based on the class of the medication. Thus, physicians, nurses, naturopathic physicians, and physician assistants have different levels of restrictions based on the laws established in each state.

The process of writing a prescription and sending it to a pharmacy to be filled is changing quickly. In 2016, New York became the first state to require that all prescriptions be created electronically. Computer tablets directly connected to pharmacies are now replacing handwritten prescription pads. This new advancement is expected to reduce the prescription drug abuse that can arise from the sale of such drugs on the black market, which, particularly in the case of opioids such as morphine and oxycodone, is becoming a growing national concern.[17]

Time to Get Covered: Where to Start

It is important to emphasize that the ACA did not create new types of health insurance plans. Instead, it created a new *process* to make it easier for people to

UP FOR DEBATE

Should the United States Allow Direct-to-Consumer Advertising?

In the United States, there are several categories of pharmaceutical drugs that require a prescription, and are unavailable for you to purchase off the shelf from the store. And yet, drug companies can still market those products directly to you by advertising on TV, in magazines, and through social media. What do you think about that?

Nearly every other country in the world bans prescription drug companies from marketing directly to consumers. The United States and New Zealand are the only two countries that allow **direct-to-consumer advertising** (DTC) of prescription drugs. In other nations, if a drug requires a prescription, it cannot be advertised to the public. The reasoning is that because regulations restrict people from buying drugs directly from a store or pharmacy without a prescription, drug companies should not be permitted to "sell" directly to consumers.

Pharmaceutical companies argue that DTC advertising increases knowledge, encourages patient–physician communication, reduces the stigma of certain disorders by placing them widely open in the public, and represents freedom of speech.[18]

Physicians have indicated that direct-to-consumer advertising has both positive and negative effects on patients and on public health.[19] In recent years, the physician community has begun to organize in greater opposition to the practice.

In 2015, the American Medical Association (AMA) voted to ban DTC advertising, citing concerns about the negative impact of commercially driven promotions, and the role marketing costs play in rising drug prices. The AMA also argued that DTC marketing increased demand for new and more expensive drugs, even when these drugs may not be appropriate.[20] Meanwhile, a spokesperson for the pharmaceutical manufacturers trade association (PhRMA) said that DTC advertisers design their advertising to "provide scientifically accurate information to help patients better understand their health care and treatment options."[9]

In many cases, drug companies market their products, not to get patients to seek the medication, but to get them to request their particular brand when generic (non–brand name) versions of the drug are available. The generic drugs are less expensive than the brand name ones being advertised.

Along with issues of treatment, DTC advertising has cost implications, both for individuals and the nation's health system. One drug, Neulasta, for example, can cost $5,000 per injection in the United States, generating $4.6 billion in sales in 1 year for its manufacturer, Amgen.[21] This level of profit makes the total DTC advertising spending in 2015 of approximately $5 billion for the entire industry[21] seem cost-effective!

What do you think? Should prescription drug ads be banned from the eyes of consumers, or do consumers have the right to receive the most professionally produced and effective communications possible from the manufacturers? After all, the call to action is not to "buy," but to "ask your doctor."

direct-to-consumer advertising When drug companies market directly to customers by advertising their products on television, in magazines, and even through social media and the Internet, despite the product being available only by a doctor's prescription.

get access to the existing health insurance system, and to improve the quality of the current system.

As a consumer of health insurance, it helps to understand the existing system of health insurance in the United States. What is available now, and what will likely be available in the near future, will probably be similar to the insurance offerings that employers currently use to cover their workers through group insurance.

Private Insurance and the Evolution to Managed Care

indemnity Protection against loss, as in health insurance. The basic system of indemnity plans is that premiums are collected by the insurance company, usually on a monthly basis. Those funds are added to the "risk pool," from which payments are drawn.

When Americans were being insured in large numbers by their employers during the 20th century, they were mostly being covered by **indemnity** insurance plans. The basic system of indemnity insurance works like this: Premiums are collected by the insurance company, usually on a monthly basis. Those funds go into the "risk pool," from which payments are drawn. Traditionally, the American insurance system has been based on such indemnity plans, which are designed to "indemnify" or "protect" the policyholder from expensive, or catastrophic, procedures (**FIGURE 14-3**).

Another fundamental principle of health insurance is "cost-sharing," which is how insurance companies determine how much the plan member

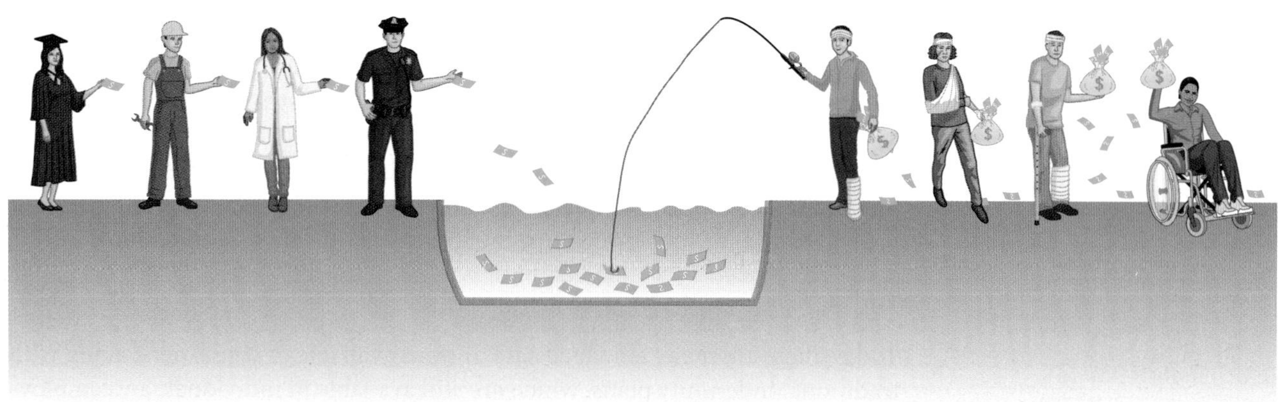

FIGURE 14-3 Insurance risk and how it works.

John's plan deductible: $1,500 **Co-insurance:** 20% **Out-of-Pocket Limit:** $5,000

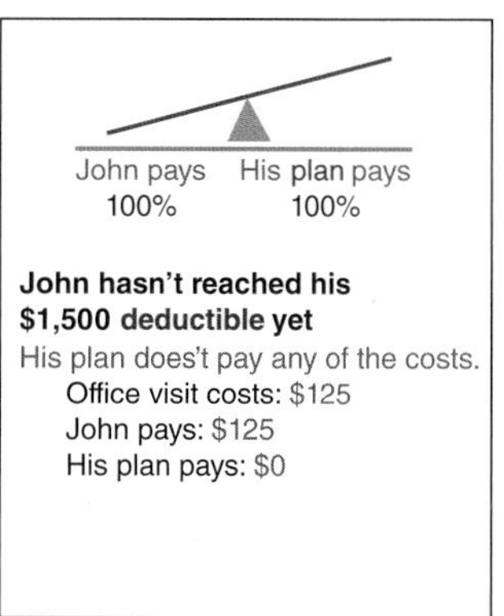

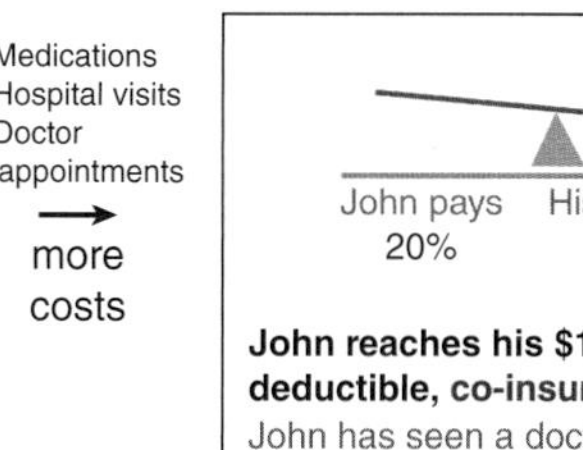

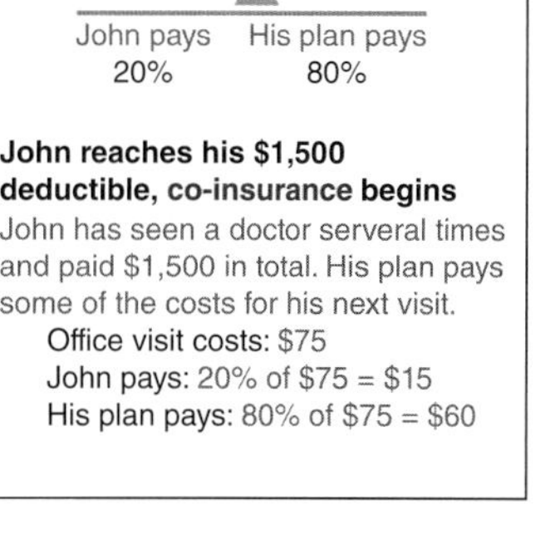

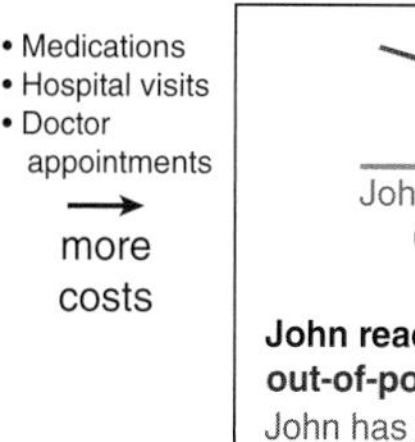

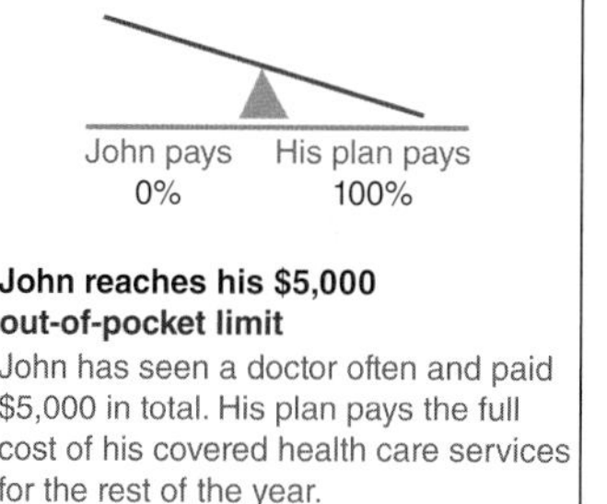

January 1st
Beginning of coverage period

December 31st
End of coverage period

FIGURE 14-4 Cost-sharing example.

pays through premiums compared to how much is spent on deductibles, co-insurance, or copayments (FIGURE 14-4). In cost sharing, patients still have to pay something but not the entire bill.

The late 1980s and early 1990s saw big increases in healthcare costs because of new technologies, new drugs, and the rise in medical malpractice lawsuits, among other factors.[22] During this time, **managed care** insurance entered the scene. Managed care organizations reduced the cost of group insurance premiums by creating contracted **networks** of doctors and hospitals who agreed to offer a discount for services and by reducing unnecessary care and hospitalization. By 1993, most Americans receiving health insurance through their employers were in managed care plans.[9]

managed care A system in which networks of doctors and hospitals agree to offer a discount for services and in which unnecessary care and hospitalization are minimized, thus reducing the cost of group insurance premiums.

network A group of healthcare providers and facilities, which usually includes doctors, hospitals, pharmacists, labs, or other facilities.

prior authorization Approval of payment that health insurers give before healthcare providers proceed with pharmaceutical treatments, medical interventions, and certain healthcare services. Also known as prior approval or precertification.

Prior-Authorization and Networks: The Fundamental Concepts of Managed Care

Two major insurance practices were introduced through managed health care that were not previously in existence under the indemnity models of the 20th century: provider networks and **prior authorization**.

A network is a group of healthcare providers and facilities that usually includes doctors, hospitals, pharmacists, labs, or other facilities. Managed care insurance companies establish discounted rates with these "preferred" facilities. In exchange for the discounts, the providers and facilities get increased revenue from the insurance plan, which channels patients to the network through its policies of only reimbursing for "in-network" facilities. In general, the stricter the policies are for keeping patients in-network, such as a standard health maintenance organization (HMO) plan (see "Types of Managed Care Plans," later), the lower the monthly premiums are. In contrast, the more flexible the network policies are, or how much patients can go "out of network," the more expensive the monthly premiums will be.

Types of Managed Care Plans

health maintenance organizations (HMOs) A type of health insurance in which members typically must have their health needs managed by a primary care physician, and health services are paid for within a limited network of hospitals and clinics and medical professionals. The HMO was the first managed care model and remains at the center of the choices available to employers and to individuals who purchase their plan through the marketplace.

preferred provider organizations (PPOs) A type of health insurance in which members may see physician specialists directly without a referral from a primary care physician, as long as the specialist is within the preferred network of providers. Physicians, medical care providers, and hospitals outside of the network incur an additional fee.

point-of-service (POS) plans Similar to a health maintenance organization, a plan in which members designate an in-network primary care physician to be their care coordinator. However, as with a preferred provider organization, limited coverage is available for care that is received outside the provider network.

Today, there are many managed care options available to consumers, along with traditional indemnity plans, which are still available to individuals and employers through the ACA. **Health maintenance organizations**, **preferred provider organizations**, and **point-of-service plans** are among the most common options available through the marketplace (**TABLE 14-3**), although they are not the only ones.

Health Maintenance Organizations (HMOs)

HMOs remain the most common choice available to employers and individuals who purchase their plan through the marketplace. HMOs usually pay for health services at a limited network of hospitals and clinics and medical professionals. When you stay in the network, your payments at the time of service are often only copayments, which typically range from \$10 to \$50. Despite the limited choice of doctors, many people find this option better than having more choice but having to pay more in up-front costs, such as \$500 deductibles. HMOs usually require patients to select a primary care physician as a care coordinator (or "gatekeeper"). Patients must get approval from this provider to access specialized care, such as surgeries and complex diagnostic services. In addition to provider networks, HMOs also usually feature a "drug formulary," which is a list of prescription drugs that are approved for coverage, often accompanied by a list of drugs not approved. Drugs are listed on the formulary because they may be more effective, or because the HMO received a discount from the pharmaceutical company or a pharmaceutical contracting agency.

Preferred Provider Organization (PPO)

PPOs are more flexible than HMOs, but for that reason, the monthly premium can be more expensive than an HMO. PPOs usually give patients more choice of healthcare providers and hospitals, but the choice is still limited by a "preferred" network. Typically, patients get some reimbursement if they go outside the network, but not the full benefit that they would get if they stayed within the network. One of the biggest advantages of PPOs is that most plans allow members to see physician specialists directly without a referral from a primary care physician, if the specialist is within the preferred network. For example, if you have a painful earache, you can make an appointment directly with an ear, nose, and throat specialist without approval from your primary care provider. However, you only get the full benefit if you select a specialist within the provider network.

Point-of-Service (POS) and Exclusive Provider Organization (EPO) Plans

A POS plan is similar to a HMO plan, where plan members designate an in-network primary care physician to be their care coordinator. However, as with

TABLE 14-3 Differences Among Major Types of Health Plans

	PPO Preferred Provider Organization	**EPO Exclusive Provider Organization**	**POS Point-of-Service Plan**	**HMO Health Maintenance Organization**
Differences in Managed Care Structures	Use of both in-network and out-of-network providers is permitted	Use of only in-network providers is permitted	Use of both in-network and out-of-network providers permitted	Use of only in-network providers is permitted
	Contracted providers only	Contracted providers only	Contracted providers only	Providers on staff and/or contracted providers
	No gatekeeping	Typically no gatekeeping	Unrestricted use of specialty services	Use of gatekeeping Focus on prevention and primary care
	Unrestricted use of specialty services	Unrestricted use of specialty services		Specialty services are obtained upon referral
	Providers are paid according to discounted fee schedules	Fee for service	Combination of capitation and fee for service	Providers are paid mostly under capitation Some fee for service
	No risk sharing	No risk sharing	Some risk sharing	Risk sharing for capitation
Primary Care Physician (PCP) Required?	No	Sometimes	Yes	Yes
Referral required to see a specialist?	No	No	Sometimes	Yes
In-network benefits?	Yes	Yes	Yes	Yes
Out-of-network benefits	Yes	No	Yes	No
Flexibility	Highest	High	Medium	Low
Cost	$$$$	$$$	$$	$

Shi, L., & Singh, D. A. (2015). Essentials of the U.S. health care system. Burlington, MA: Jones & Bartlett Publishers.

a PPO, limited coverage is available for care received outside the provider network.

You would likely pay deductibles or coinsurance costs that are higher than they would be if you had used an in-plan provider coordinated by your primary care physician.[23] **Exclusive provider organization** plans lie somewhere between PPO and POS plans. Usually most similar to a POS plan, EPO plans generally offer the freedom to select a specialist, but with no reimbursement at all if you stray from the provider network.

exclusive provider organization (EPO) A plan that does not require a primary care physician or referral within the established provider network. Emergency and urgent care are the only time out-of-network visits are covered.

Government Health Insurance

Veterans Administration

The Veterans Administration (often referred to as the "VA") system is for retired military veterans. Run through the U.S. Department of Veterans Affairs, the VA system is one of the largest healthcare systems in the world. It provides hospital care, mental health services, and long-term care to approximately 8.76 million individuals each year,[24] and has a budget of around $65 billion.[25]

The VA is unlike other public health insurance financing systems in the United States because it runs its own facilities, including hospitals, clinics, nursing homes, and counseling centers. It is also unlike other systems in its dedication to exclusively serving veterans and their families. Historically, the VA has been known for its high quality of care, but in recent years it has been criticized for long wait times for patients to receive services and poor management of mental health issues of veterans.

Medicare

Medicare A federal government program that covers a portion of the cost of health care and is primarily for Americans who are aged 65 years and older.

President Lyndon Johnson established **Medicare** as part of the Social Security Act of 1965. Medicare covers a portion of the cost of health care for Americans who are aged 65 years and older, which make up the largest portion of Medicare beneficiaries. In addition to older adults, the Medicare program finances medical care for people with a disability that qualifies them for social security benefits, and for individuals who suffer from end-stage renal disease, which is a permanent failure of the kidneys. It is different from Medicaid, discussed previously (**FIGURE 14-5**). In 2016, nearly one in five Americans (approximately 56 million) received their health care through the Medicare system.[26]

Medicare has a four-part structure, comprising separate insurance programs:

- *Medicare Part A*: funds hospital and related services, such as rehabilitation and skilled nursing facilities. The reimbursement process is complicated, and copayments are based on number of days in the hospital.
- *Medicare Part B*: mostly consists of physician care, but also includes other service items, such as ambulance and outpatient services. The monthly rate that an individual pays for Part B Medicare is variable and is based on the person's income.

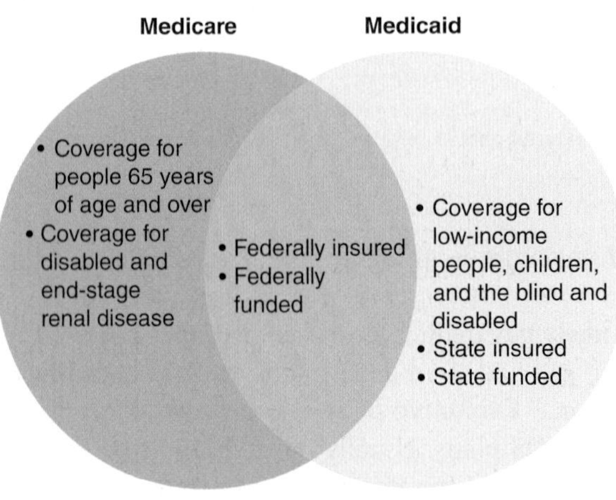

FIGURE 14-5 Medicare-Medicaid difference.

Health Markets. (n.d.). The right plan at the best price. Retrieved from https://www.healthmarkets.com/

- *Medicare Part C*: This option is for Medicare-eligible individuals who wish to receive their benefits through a private company rather than the federal government. The Medicare Part C program (also called Medicare+Choice) enabled managed care companies to enter the Medicare market. By choosing to join a Medicare+Choice plan, individuals become members of the participating HMO or PPO plan. In addition, they receive supplementary coverage not available through standard Medicare; however, they must comply with the managed care policies, such as using network providers and obtaining prior authorization for certain services.
- *Medicare Part D*: the prescription drug component of Medicare. Enrollees pay a monthly premium based on income, and they receive their medications through privately managed prescription drug benefit plans.

Medicaid

Medicaid is the nation's public health insurance program serving people with low incomes. It is funded by both state and federal governments, but managed by the states. For this reason, specific eligibility criteria and policies are different from state to state.

In addition to providing insurance to people who otherwise could not afford insurance, the program also covers individuals with other serious needs, such as those who require institutionalization in psychiatric facilities.

Medicaid is a "means-tested" program, which is the policy of providing a service only to people who fall below a threshold of income or assets. Means-testing is contrasted with insurance systems such as those in Canada, where every citizen gets equal healthcare benefits.

Acquiring Health Insurance: How to Navigate the System

After the passage of the ACA, young adults became able to stay on their parents' plan until age 26. But similar to the way all car drivers must obtain automobile insurance, the ACA required that all Americans acquire health insurance or face penalties. The mandate component was always one of the more controversial elements of the ACA law (**FIGURE 14-6** and **TABLE 14-4**).

The Health Insurance Marketplace system was launched through the ACA to facilitate insurance enrollment for Americans. Each state has a different marketplace, either run by the state or by the federal government, and for most people, the state marketplace is only available during the open enrollment period. The specific dates for the open enrollment period can change from year to year, but the open enrollment is usually from around November 15 of one year to February 15 of the following year (i.e., November 15, 2017, to February 15, 2018).

Options for College Students and Young Adults

There are several options for college students and adults younger than 26 years of age. For many students, the easiest and more affordable option may be to stay on your parent's health plan, which you may do until you reach the age of 26. If you are working, insurance coverage options may be offered through your employer. Your monthly premium can vary dramatically, based on the level cost-sharing the employer decides to take on, so you need to ask about all the options your employer has available to you. Some employers offer an

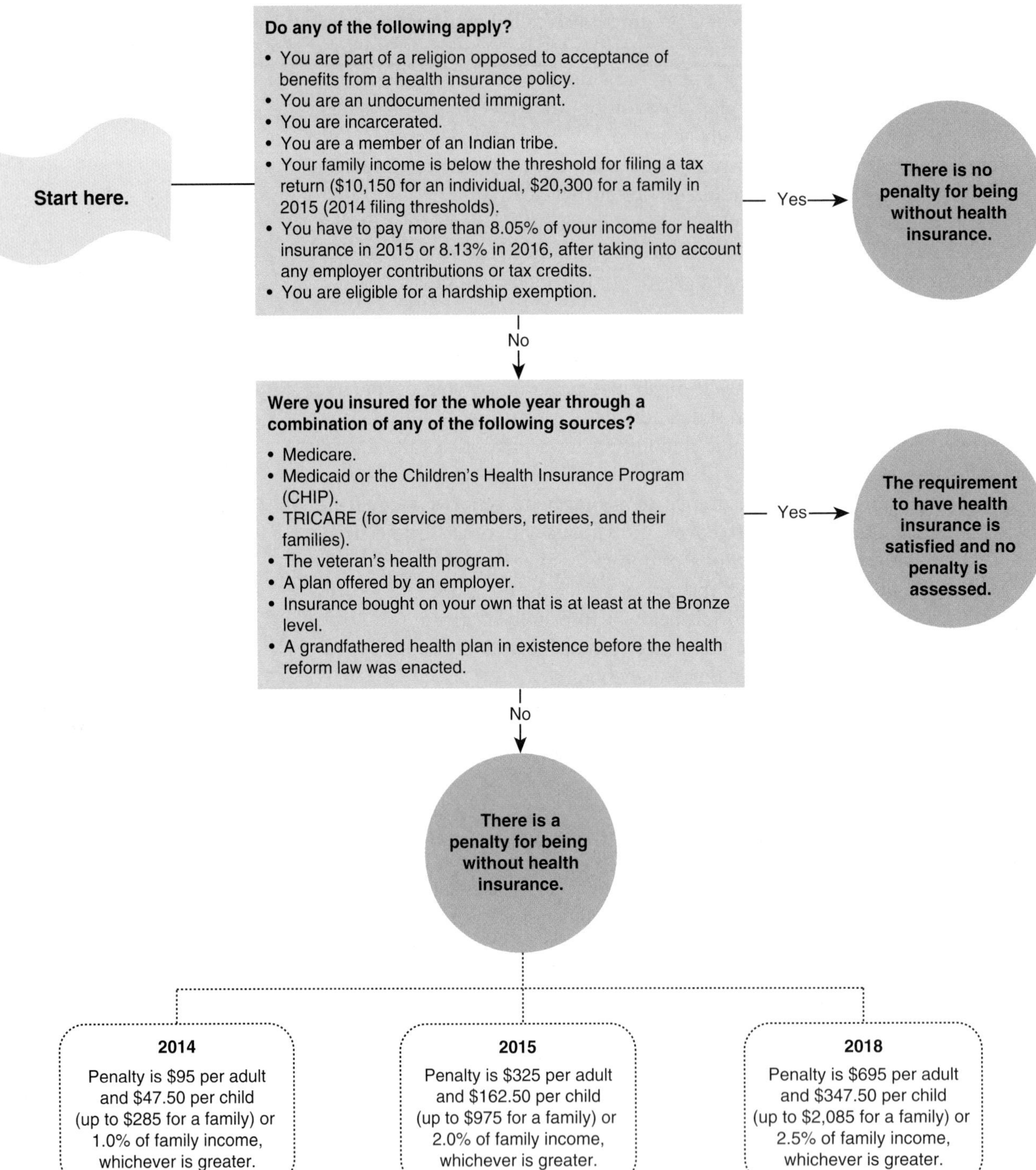

Income is defined as total income in excess of the prior year's filing threshold ($10,150 for an individual and $20,300 for a family in 2014). The penalty is pro-rated by the number of months without coverage, though there is no penalty for a single gap in coverage of less than 3 months in a year. The penalty cannot be greater than the national average premium for Bronze coverage in an Exchange ($2,484 in 2015 for single coverage and $12,420 for a family of three or more children). After 2016, penalty amounts are increased annually by the cost of living.

Key Facts:

- In 2015 employees paid $1,072 on average towards the cost of individual coverage in an employer plan and $4,955 for a family of four.
- A Kaiser Family Foundation subsidy calculator illustrating premiums and tax credits for people in different circumstances is available at http://healthreform.kff.org/subsidycalculator.aspx.

FIGURE 14-6 Requirement to purchase insurance.

The Henry J. Kaiser Family Foundation. (2017). The requirement to buy coverage under the Affordable Care Act. Retrieved from http://kff.org/infographic/the-requirement-to-buy-coverage-under-the-affordable-care-act/

TABLE 14-4 Health Insurance Options for Individuals Younger than Age 26

Option	Why It Might Work	Why It Might Not Work
Your parents' plan	If your are 26 or younger and parents are willing to add you to their plan.	Your parents may not have insurance of their own; they may find it too costly to add you.
Through your job	If your employer offers an affordable health benefit plan, and cost-sharing is affordable to you.	Even if you have a job, your employer may not offer health insurance, or the insurance plan offered through work may be very expensive.
Student health plan	Some campuses provide comprehensive and affordable insurance offerings for students.	Many colleges do not offer student health insurance; but even among those that do, it may still be difficult to find one affordable enough for you.
Purchase a private insurance plan	This may be the only, or least expensive, option available for you.	Even the least expensive ACA options (a Bronze plan, for example) may be expensive. If this is the case you should look into cost-assistance or "hardship" options available through the marketplace.
Medicaid and other government plans	If you have a very low income and are not listed as a dependent, or you are a former foster youth. Note that Medicaid rules differ from state to state, and some offer good options for young and low-income residents.	You may not be eligible, depending on how the state determines eligibility (bank account, real assets, etc.).

array of different insurance options, including medical savings accounts, which are accounts that can be amassed tax free and used for medical expenses only. Medical savings accounts can often be a good choice for people in their 20s who usually have lower healthcare costs while they are still young. Thus, your account can grow significantly if you don't need to spend it.

Individuals with lower incomes (defined differently by each state) can acquire insurance through the Medicaid program. If you qualify, this is probably the most affordable option out there. Medicaid enrollment can happen any time during the year.

State Marketplaces

The state-based marketplaces provide options for shopping and applying for coverage. The marketplaces allow you to compare plans side-by-side and find the best option for you. If you live in one of the states that has its own marketplace, that is where you will go to acquire your health insurance. If your state does not offer a marketplace, you will need to find your options through www.healthcare.gov, which is the federal marketplace.

Precious Metals: What's the Right Choice?

Plans in the Health Insurance Marketplace are presented in four "metal" categories: Bronze, Silver, Gold, and Platinum. These types are not an indication of quality; rather, they are a measure of how you and your plan share the costs of health care. The higher the category of metal, the more money you pay up front in premiums and the less you pay if you need care.

"Catastrophic" plans are available to people under 30 years of age or who have obtained a hardship exemption. These are the cheapest type of plan you can get that counts as minimum essential coverage, but it is important to be aware that you will be trading an inexpensive premium for very high out-of-pocket costs. In other words, despite the relatively cheap premiums, you may still face high out-of-pocket costs if you qualify for these plans.

Some state marketplaces offer their own unique, inexpensive health insurance options, such as the "Essential" plan offered in New York State. This plan is for people with lower incomes, but not low enough to qualify for Medicaid.

Unfortunately, you may find that even the most inexpensive plans available to you are extremely expensive, which can be frightening when you face the prospect of a financial penalty for not having insurance.

Certified Application Counselors Navigators

You can get in-person help applying for coverage and financial assistance from Certified Application Counselors (CACs), also called Marketplace Navigators. These are individuals trained to give you unbiased information about your coverage options. They can help you prepare your applications, establish eligibility, and get you enrolled in the plan that is best for you. They are required to complete comprehensive training and criminal background checks and can be trusted to treat your information confidentially and provide you with honest information.[27] Many colleges and universities fund navigators to provide information for their students, so if you need counseling for healthcare enrollment, you should look into what is available on your campus. College health centers are a good place to start and often have navigators available to help students find the best options available to them.

Platinum	Gold	Silver	Bronze	Catastrophic
90%	80%	70%	60%	Less than 60%
A platinum health plan is a standardized type of health insurance that pays, on average, 90 percent of your health care expenses. This type of plan will have the highest monthly premium, but your co-pays and deductible will be very low.	A gold health insurance plan generally pays 80 percent of your health care expenses. This type of plan will have the high monthly premium. Premiums for this plan will be less than a platinum plan, but the deductible will also be a bit higher.	This type of plan typically pays 70% of your health care expenses. With a medium premium cost, you can expect to pay about 30% of your health care costs.	This plan pays 60% of your health care expenses on average. It is the most affordable premium for those who are not under 30 or do not qualify for a hardship exemption. This plan, although it has the lowest monthly premium, will have the highest deductibles.	Catastrophic coverage plans pay less than 60% of the total average cost of care on average. Deductibles will always be the highest, and the premiums will be the lowest available. Only for people younger than 30 years old or have a hardship exemption.

FIVE STEPS TO BECOME A BETTER ADVOCATE FOR YOUR HEALTH CARE

In addition to becoming knowledgeable about health care and insurance, it is also important to become a "health advocate" for yourself and others who may depend on you. Here are some important tips to get the most out of your healthcare experience — and perhaps help some of your family and friends as well:

Understand Your Insurance Plan and Coverage

This chapter has provided you with some basic information about how Insurance works, but it is very important to learn about your own plan. Understanding your coverage, copayments, provider networks, and referral options can help you to navigate the system with more authority. This will mean less chance of ending up in a situation that makes you feel uncomfortable or out of control.

Learn About Your Condition or Illness

Many people visit the doctor without investigating their symptoms and treatment options on their own. Doing some basic research can allow you to better understand the information your doctor gives you. Because the Internet is so full of information from many different (and often untrustworthy) sources, be sure to check the source of everything you read. Ideally it comes from a government, academic, or medical institution website (look for .gov, .edu, and .org domains).

Keep Track of Your Records and History

Today's medical system is becoming more streamlined and coordinated but that does not mean the patient is always kept in the loop. Ensure you are on top of your records by keeping names, numbers, and emails for your doctors, clinics, and other providers. Getting access to your records, especially when your file has been transferred between providers and institutions, can be difficult, but it is important. Your files have important information about your tests, diagnoses, and treatment plans and you should be aware of all of it. While doctors are not always required to proactively share this information with you, they must do so if asked. So ask.

Check Your Medical Bills for Errors

Medical errors have always been a part of the healthcare system and probably always will be. While medical bills are not always easy to understand, clinic and hospital office staff members are trained to answer any questions you have about them, so if you have a concern, raise your voice. In the end, you will most likely have to pay a portion of the bill, so keep that in mind. This is your money!

Don't Be Afraid to Speak Up, Ask Questions, or Insist on a Second Opinion

There are many reasons you should be prepared to ask for a second opinion. One is the possibility of an error. If a doctor tells you a specific illness or condition is present, you have every reason to ask another provider for another diagnosis. Additionally, keep in mind that not all doctors hold the same values, or share your values. If you feel uncomfortable with anything, speak up, or move to another doctor. It may make the difference between being mistreated and treated fairly. Be ready to ask questions. Have questions prepared before you even walk into a doctor's office; ask more questions based on what you are told; ask questions about different treatment options; and if you desire, ask about getting another perspective from someone else. Taking these actions does not have to be antagonistic; good health care requires teamwork and coordination, and at the center of it all is you. This is also an area where you may be able to help a friend or family member who may not understand the system very well, or for whom English is a second language.

What's Ahead: Improving Quality, Satisfaction, and Affordability

The United States spends more money as a percentage of our economy on medical care, and yet, on many measures of population health, it continues to experience worse outcomes than most European countries on many indicators. In fact, the United States has a lower life expectancy than most Western European nations, and it has one of the highest infant mortality rates among all industrialized nations.

A process called "delivery system reform" seeks to ensure that the system leads to the highest quality outcome for patients at the least possible cost. It seeks to accomplish this in three ways:

1. Changing how we pay for care to focus on quality
2. Improving the coordination of healthcare between patients, employers, insurance, and medical providers
3. Improving the use of health data

Although many insurance companies pay for each test or treatment separately, health policy experts agree that doctors and other practitioners should work as a team. Things are starting to change as medical groups, hospitals, and insurance companies are increasingly looking for ways to coordinate their efforts. It is likely that, as a consumer, you will see more medical care integration in the years ahead.

Although the ACA has allowed many people to gain access to the healthcare system that did not have access before,[28] the United States has a long way to go before healthcare costs are no longer such a crippling concern for many. We can also hope that some day the United States will compare favorably with other developed nations in essential health outcomes, such as child and maternal mortality. While the American health system is evolving in different ways, there are still opportunities to change policies. Good examples of this are to increase subsidies to people to make insurance more affordable and to provide more treatment options.

For students interested in influencing the future of your nation, healthcare policy is an important area. You can volunteer (becoming trained as a Certified Application Counselor, for example) or become an advocate (such as working to influence the policy changes that lie ahead for the ACA). This is an exciting time to get involved, and there is no shortage of work to be done to create a system in which all Americans can take pride.

In Summary

The health insurance system currently in place in the United States is the result of a long series of historical events and the evolution of the value systems of Americans. The United States was founded on principles that included freedom and suspicion of government, and these principles have played a role in preventing a comprehensive national system. While a national program was passed in 2010, there are still many changes that need to take place for the system to cover all Americans.

The American system of delivering care is complex, and it involves several types of medical professionals. Some were discussed in this chapter, while others are covered in Chapter 4. The decisions you make about which types of doctors to see have a lot to do with your personal values and the types of practitioners with whom you feel most comfortable.

Finding the best option for health insurance coverage is a complex process; it can be difficult, especially when you need to do it for yourself or your family. Thankfully, the number and variety of options is greater today than ever before. It takes research to find the best option for yourself, and things are constantly changing, so be sure to thoroughly investigate all of the options available to you.

Key Terms

deductibles
direct-to-consumer advertising
exclusive provider organization (EPO)
health maintenance organizations (HMOs)
indemnity
inpatient care
internal medicine
managed care
Medicaid
Medicare
network
point-of-service (POS) plans
prior authorization
preferred provider organizations (PPOs)

Student Discussion Questions and Activities

1. Do you think that all Americans should have access to medical care at any time, free of charge? Why or why not? Why do you think your opinion may be different from others?
2. What are the best elements of the American health system? What are the worst elements?
3. Do you have health insurance? How is your insurance paid? Is it through your parents, your employer, your school? Would you rather not discuss this?
4. Whether you are covered by insurance or not, imagine for now that you have no insurance coverage. Would you feel the urgent need to acquire it? What would your first steps be to acquire it? What kind of plan do you think you would select?
5. What do you think are the most important changes that need to occur in health insurance and the medical system today? Why? What is something you or someone your age can do to make that happen?

References

1. Lipset, S. M. (1997). *American exceptionalism: A double edged sword*. New York: W.W. Norton & Company.
2. Steinmo, S., & Watts J. (1995). It's the institutions, stupid! Why comprehensive national health insurance always fails in America. *Health Politics Policy Law*, *20*(2), 329–372.
3. McDermott, J. (1994). Evaluating health system reform: The case for a single-payer approach." *JAMA, 27*(10), 782–784.
4. Micklethwait, J., & Wooldridge, A. (2004). *The right nation: Conservative power in America*. New York: Penguin.
5. Long, S. K. (2015). Taking stock: Gains in health insurance coverage under the ACA as of March 2015. Urban Institute. Retrieved from http://hrms.urban.org/briefs/Gains-in-Health-Insurance-Coverage-under-the-ACA-as-of-March-2015.html.
6. National Center for Complementary and Integrative Health. (2017). Complementary, alternative, or integrative health: What's in a name? National Institutes of Health. Retrieved from https://nccih.nih.gov/health/integrative-health.
7. Shi, L., & Singh, D. A. (2015). *Essentials of the U.S. health care system*. Burlington, MA: Jones & Bartlett Learning.
8. General Osteopathic Council. (2016). About Osteopathy. Retrieved from http://www.osteopathy.org.uk/visiting-an-osteopath/about-osteopathy/
9. Iglehart, J. K. (1994). Physicians and the growth of managed care. *N Engl J Med, 331*(17), 1167–1171.
10. The Henry J. Kaiser Family Foundation. (2016). Total number of professionally active nurses. Retrieved from https://www.kff.org/other/state-indicator/total-registered-nurses/?currentTimeframe=0&sortModel=%7B%22colId%22:%22Location%22,%22sort%22:%22asc%22%7D
11. Rosenthal, E. (2016, February 27). Ask your doctor if this ad is right for you. *New York Times*. Retrieved from. https://www.nytimes.com/2016/02/28/sunday-review/ask-your-doctor-if-this-ad-is-right-for-you.html
12. Bernstein, A. B. (2004). Health care in America: Trends in utilization. U.S. Department of Health and Human Services, Centers for Disease Control and Prevention, National Center for Health Statistics. Retrieved from https://www.cdc.gov/nchs/data/misc/healthcare.pdf
13. Aitken, M., Berndt, E. R., & Cutler, D. M. (2009). Prescription drug spending trends in the United States: Looking beyond the turning point. *Health Affairs, 28*(1), w151–160.
14. Morgan, S., & Kennedy, J. (2010). Prescription drug accessibility and affordability in the United States and abroad. *Issue Brief (Commonwealth Fund), 89*, 1–12.
15. Mossialos, E., Wenzl, M., Osborn, R., & Sarnak, D. (2016). 2015 International profiles of health care systems. The Commonwealth Fund. Retrieved from http://www.commonwealthfund.org/publications/fund-reports/2017/may/international-profiles

16. Morgan, S., & Kennedy, J. (2010). Prescription drug accessibility and affordability in the United States and abroad. Commonwealth Fund pub. 1408. Retrieved from http://www.commonwealthfund.org/~/media/Files/Publications/Issue%20Brief/2010/Jun/1408_Morgan_Prescription_drug_accessibility_US_intl_ib.pdf
17. Volkow, N. D. (2014). Prescription opioid and heroin abuse. National Institute on Drug Abuse. The Science of Drug Abuse and Addiction. Bethesda, MD: National Institutes of Health.
18. Abramson, J. (2004). *Overdo$ed America.* New York: HarperCollins.
19. U.S. Food and Drug Administration. (2015, Oct 23). The impact of direct-to consumer advertising. U.S. Food and Drug Administration Information for Consumers. Retrieved from https://www.fda.gov/Drugs/ResourcesForYou/Consumers/ucm143562.htm
20. American Medical Association. (2015 Nov. 17). AMA calls for ban on direct to consumer advertising of prescription drugs and medical devices. AMA News Room. Retrieved from https://www.ama-assn.org/content/ama-calls-ban-direct-consumer-advertising-prescription-drugs-and-medical-devices
21. Picchi, A. (2016, Mar 11). Drug ads: $5.2 billion annually – and rising. *CBS News.* Retrieved from https://www.cbsnews.com/news/drug-ads-5-2-billion-annually-and-rising/
22. Centers for Medicare and Medicaid Services. (2004). National Health Expenditure (NHE) amounts by type of expenditure and source of funds: Calendar years 1965–2013. Centers for Medicare and Medicaid Services 1965–2019. Retrieved from https://www.cms.gov/Research-Statistics-Data-and-Systems/Statistics-Trends-and-Reports/NationalHealthExpendData/NationalHealthAccountsProjected.html
23. HealthCoverageGuide.org. (n.d.). Point-of-Service Plan (POS).
24. Veterans Health Administration. (2016). Veterans Health and Administration. Retrieved from https://www.va.gov/
25. U.S. Department of Veterans Affairs. (2016). Annual budget submission: Office of Budget. Retrieved from https://www.va.gov/budget/products.asp
26. The Henry J. Kaiser Family Foundation. Kaiser Family Foundation. (2015). Total number of Medicare beneficiaries. Retrieved from https://www.kff.org/medicare/state-indicator/total-medicare-beneficiaries
27. Gogan, J. L., Davidson, E. J., & Proudfoot, J. (2016). The HealthCare.gov Project. *Journal of Information Technology Teaching Cases 6*(2), 99-110.
28. Iglehart, J. K. (2013). Implementing the ACA: Onward through the thorns. *Health Affairs (Millwood), 32*(9), 1518.

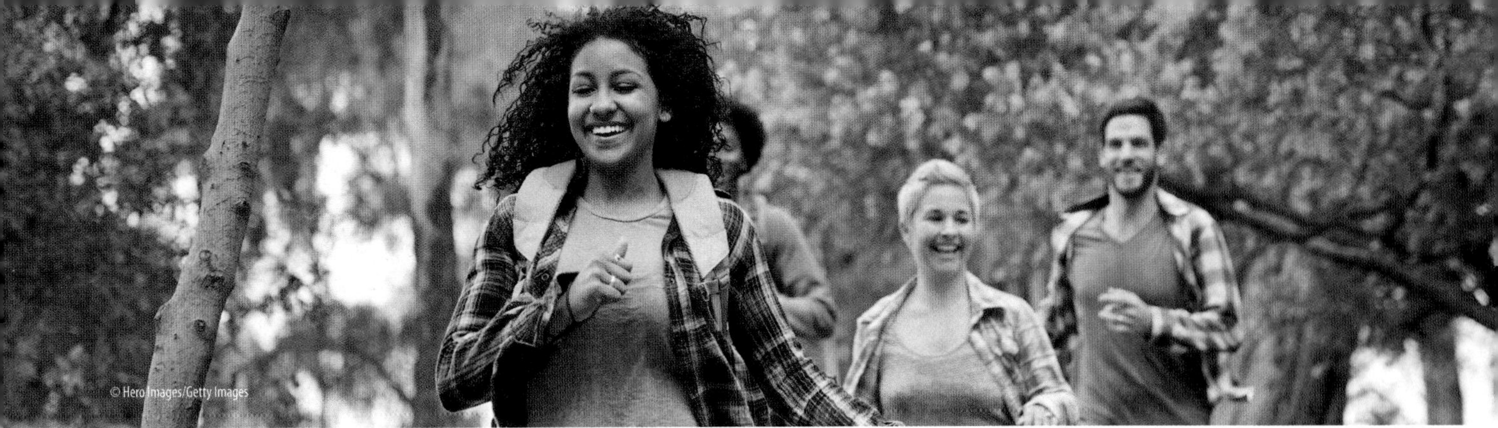
© Hero Images/Getty Images

CHAPTER 15

Global Health: We Are the World

CHAPTER OBJECTIVES

- Understand the importance of having a global perspective when thinking about health issues.
- Discuss social justice in health from an international perspective.
- Identify significant public health issues around the world and their underlying causes.
- Explore how international organizations are addressing the most critical health issues facing populations around the world.
- Identify opportunities for individuals interested in solving some of the world's more pressing global health problems.

What Is Global Health?

Global health is an area of study, research, and practice that places a priority on improving health and achieving health equity for all people worldwide.[1] The term *global health* can describe a concept, such as the health of individuals around the globe, or an objective, such as a healthier, more equitable world.[1] Global health is also an important area of research. Many international universities, institutes, and organizations study the patterns of health conditions affecting people living all around the world. Global health research encompasses **epidemiology**, medical and social sciences, geospatial sciences, economics, and political science, all working to improve health for everyone living on earth. Health in the United States also relates to global health, especially as we consider the ways that health conditions and diseases flow into and out of this and other countries, such as through migration.

global health Health-based research and practice that prioritizes improving global health equity.

epidemiology The branch of public health that studies the cause and distribution of disease among local and global populations, with a focus on preventing and controlling the spread of communicable diseases.

The health of people worldwide is often discussed by comparing "industrialized" or "Westernized" countries with "Third World," "underdeveloped," or "developing" countries. These sorts of labels can be controversial because they make generalizations about different countries and even entire parts of the planet.[2] Also,

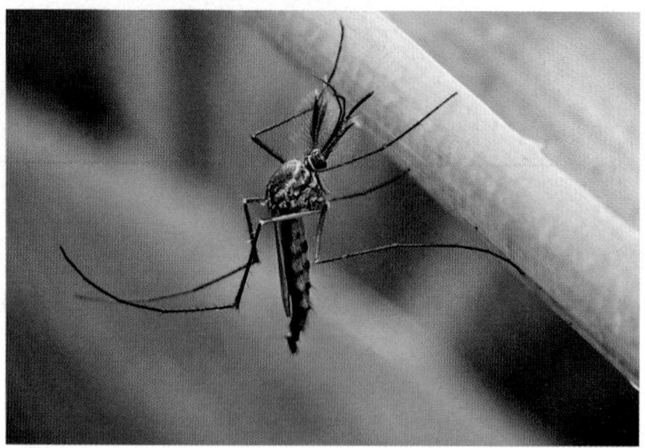

Mosquitos, mostly just an annoying pest in the United States, kill more than 500,000 people each year around the world.

terms like "Third World" or "underdeveloped" can be offensive to people who do not wish for their countries to become "Westernized," especially if that leads to greater consumerism, environmental devastation, and economic inequality.[3]

Nevertheless, it is helpful to be able to distinguish between countries that are more economically advantaged from those less advantaged, because it is through these differences that we can more clearly understand the health inequalities that exist in the world today.[4] This chapter uses the terms "Western," "industrialized," or "developed" to connote wealthier countries and regions and terms like "resource-poor," "developing," and "less developed" to describe the less economically advantaged nations and regions, despite the shortcomings of these labels.

Why Global Health?

Why is it important that we consider health beyond our own political borders? One reason is out of a moral concern for others suffering needlessly in a world that we all share. Because the most disadvantaged people live outside industrialized nations (such as the United States, Canada, Japan, Australia, and countries in Europe), the public health imperative of social justice is an important component of global health. Today, the parts of the world that suffer the most from illnesses such as human immunodeficiency virus/acquired immunodeficiency syndrome (HIV/AIDS), tuberculosis, and malaria are those that lie outside these industrialized countries.[5]

While the average life expectancy for someone born in the United States in 2015 was 79.3 years, in several African countries the life expectancy was less than 55 years in that same year[6] (**TABLE 15-1**).

Many preventable diseases long ago eradicated from the United States still affect people around the world at alarming rates. Tuberculosis, for example, was one of the most deadly diseases in the United States during the early 1900s, killing more than 110,000 Americans per year.[7] Those numbers declined to less than 500 (in a country with 4 times the population) during the early 2000s, as public health departments became established, improving housing conditions and water sanitation. But across the world, more than 1.5 million people are still dying on an annual basis from the same disease.[8]

HIV and AIDS is another area where there are major disparities between the United States and the rest of the world. In 2014, approximately 7,000 people died from AIDS-related diseases in the United States,[9] while across the world, 1.2 million of the more than 40 million people affected by HIV/AIDS died from

TABLE 15-1 Highest and Lowest Life Expectancies by Country and by Gender

Male		Female	
Country	**Years**	**Country**	**Years**
Highest		*Highest*	
Switzerland	81.3	Japan	86.8
Iceland	81.2	Spain	85.5
Australia	80.9	Republic of Korea	85.5
Sweden	80.7	France	85.4
Israel	80.6	Switzerland	85.3
Lowest		*Lowest*	
Sierra Leone	49.3	Sierra Leone	50.8
Angola	50.9	Angola	54.0
Central African Republic	50.9	Central African Republic	54.0
Lesotho	51.7	Chad	54.5
Chad	51.7	Côte d'Ivoire	54.4

World Health Organization. Global Health Observatory Indicator Views. 2015.

AIDS-related illnesses.[10] The reasons for vast global inequities such as these are numerous and complex. They occur in part because of wealth and income differences that exist between countries. They also occur because of differences in access to care. In resource-poor countries, fewer people have access to medical professionals and to treatment facilities.

Addressing unfair conditions is why so many people become dedicated to working in global health. As Martin Luther King once said, "Injustice anywhere is a threat to justice everywhere."[11] This perspective believes it is unacceptable that the poorest people on earth bear the greatest burden of the world's disease. The **social justice imperative** seeks to channel resources to the people that need them the most, recognizing that those dying prematurely from preventable disease in the largest numbers are also the poorest people in the world. Another tragic, but common issue in global health is the large numbers of people who are not receiving even the most simple solutions to preventable conditions. For example, more than one million people around the world suffer from common eye issues that can be corrected by a $1.50 pair of glasses. This can lead to problems in school, inability to perform basic job functions, and greater vulnerability to accidents.

social justice imperative The effort to channel resources to the populations that need them the most—the populations suffering the highest rates of death from preventable disease—populations that are among the poorest in the world.

Another reason to be concerned about global health and international patterns of health and disease is the fact that these patterns can affect each of us in many different ways. Today, people are more connected to each other throughout the world than ever before. For most of the span of human civilization, nearly everyone stayed close to their towns, cities, or countries for their entire lives. Today, more people migrate from country to country than ever before. More than 215 million people (over 3.2% of the world's population) now migrate in any given year.[12] The reasons people leave their countries today include weather-related events such as droughts, as well as conflicts, such as wars and ethnic violence. Many people migrate for economic reasons, such as the opportunity to find a new job. Despite political efforts to oppose or limit immigration into specific countries, global migration is a fact of life in the 21st century, and it has serious implications on the health of everyone living in every country around the world.

Compared to previous centuries, when nations could exist in relative isolation, today, no country or region is immune from the effects of a more interconnected world. Diseases now have a greater ability to spread from country to country than ever before—by foot, by bus, and by plane. For this reason alone, governments and individuals must take global health issues more seriously than ever before. Countries such as the United States, and even major cities, are now spending more effort preparing for the prevention and for the arrival of diseases such as Zika, severe acute respiratory syndrome (SARS), and deadly flu varieties (H1N1), all of which were diseases that once remained mostly confined to a single country or a single region. (See Tales of Public Health: Ebola? Here?). Working to address health issues and health disparities across the world is one component to ensuring the long-term health of your own community, because we are more interconnected in more ways than we ever were before.

A third perspective from which to think about the importance of global health is the economic, or structural, perspective. This point of view emphasizes the effect that improved global health can have on the international economy, including the U.S. economy. Unhealthy people who do not reach their full potential represent a threat to the world economy. More people suffering from preventable disease means fewer people working productively, fewer people solving social problems, and fewer people gaining an education and moving ahead in the world. Also, as economic and political instability are related to the rise in terrorism across the world,[13] improving opportunities for health across the world helps political stability and can be a method for addressing the underlying causes of global terrorism.[14,15]

Understanding and Measuring Global Health

global burden of disease (GBD) Developed in 1990 as a collaboration between hundreds of global health institutions, including the World Health Organization and the World Bank. This project seeks to measure, and then find solutions to, the causes and costs of all diseases around the world.

How do we know what the most pressing illnesses, diseases, and opportunities for improving health are in the world? One way is to examine the **global burden of disease (GBD)**, a process developed in 1990 as a collaboration between hundreds of worldwide institutions and individual experts, including the World Health Organization (WHO) and the World Bank. The global burden of disease project seeks to measure and find solutions to the causes and costs of the world's worst diseases. One unit of measurement used by this effort is "disability-adjusted life years" (DALYs),[16] a measure now commonly used by global health researchers. This unit measures the overall disease burden of a condition on society, in terms of number of years lost due to poor health, disability, or death. It is calculated using a formula that includes prevalence and incidence. Some conditions, such as Alzheimer's disease, cause many DALYs in a country. Countries with high rates of preventable disease and premature death have a higher number of DALYs than healthier countries.

The most recent Global Burden of Disease (GBD) report, from 2013, showed that global life expectancy increased from 65.3 years in 1990 to 71.5 years in 2013. This increase was largely due to organizations working globally to reduce cardiovascular disease, cancer, and diarrhea-related child deaths.

Globally, the number of DALYs caused by communicable, maternal, neonatal, and nutritional disorders has declined from 1.19 billion in 1990 to 769.3 million in 2013, while DALYs for **noncommunicable diseases** have increased from 1.08 billion to 1.43 billion during the same time period.[17]

noncommunicable diseases A chronic health condition that is nontransmissible. The four major categories of noncommunicable diseases are cardiovascular diseases, cancers, chronic respiratory conditions, and diabetes.

Women in the World: A Global Health Challenge and Opportunity

Women and girls suffer the effects of discrimination throughout the world in ways that might be unbelievable to many people living in the United States or Europe. Sex-based health inequalities are particularly severe in the poorest countries around the world. In those countries, the majority of women lack basic health care and face life-threatening health issues. In some cases, these problems are related to poverty and a lack of medical infrastructure: not enough doctors, lack of feminine hygiene resources, and more.

Lack of government policies, poor infrastructure, and cultural stigma lead to numerous health problems for women around the world. Around the world, mothers are dying while giving birth at rates that far exceed those in Western nations. Medical issues such as cervical cancer are also preventable challenges faced by women all over the globe.[18] Many sexually transmitted diseases, such as HIV/AIDS, disproportionally affect women.

In other cases, the problems can be connected to culture: Intimate partner violence is common throughout the world, as approximately 35% of all women have experienced either violence or rape from an intimate partner.[19] Lack of control in sexual relationships can lead to decreased contraceptive use and increased risk of sexually transmitted diseases. In many nations, especially Egypt, Sudan, Djibouti, and Eritrea, female genitals are ceremoniously cut and mutilated. In others, such as Niger, Mali, and Bangladesh, child marriage of girls as young as 12 years of age is common. (This issue is discussed in more detail in Chapter 10.) These are just a few examples of how cultural norms around the world can lead to high rates of morbidity and mortality from numerous issues.

TABLE 15-2 includes more specific instances of the particularly difficult burden placed on women in the realm of global health.

Refugees and Migrant Health: 60 Million People in Need

According to the United Nations High Commissioner for Refugees, 60 million people in the world were forcibly displaced from their homes due to armed conflict in 2016 alone.[22] That's greater than the entire population of Spain! The world is now experiencing the highest rate of displacement since World War II.

As of 2018, the largest source of forced migration came from the brutal civil war in Syria, from which more than 10 million refugees have escaped since 2011. The other largest sources of conflict-generated migration were Afghanistan, Somalia, and Sudan.

The WHO estimates that as many as 1 billion people have experienced some form of involuntary migration; the majority of these involve people forced to leave their home, but not their country. Most of these individuals have major health needs. Health concerns facing refugees include accidental

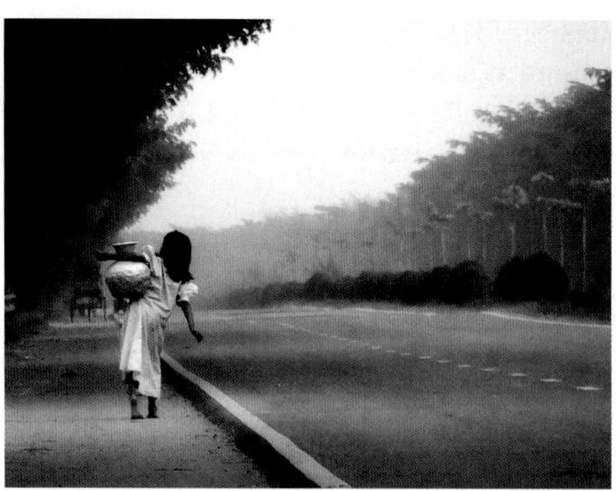

Bangladesh has higher than average rates of child labor, preteen marriage, and childhood malnutrition.

TABLE 15-2 Critical Issues in Women's Health

Issue	Evidence
Violence toward women	▪ 1 in 3 women are treated violently[20]
Maternal morbidity	▪ Around 300,000 women die needlessly each year while giving birth due to lack of infrastructure[20]
Reproductive justice	▪ Reproductive restrictions ▪ Genital mutilation
HIV/AIDS	▪ Young women die of HIV/AIDS at the highest rate of all
Sexual discrimination and abuse	▪ 15 million girls 17 years or younger married each year[21] (half of all marriages in some countries) ▪ Forced prostitution ▪ Sexual slavery ▪ Forced marriage
Breast cancer	▪ 1.7 million new cases diagnosed each year ▪ Low- and middle-income countries have twice the burden of disease than wealthier nations.
Political inequalities	▪ Voting discrimination ▪ Property ownership discrimination ▪ Lack of legal rights upon marriage

injuries, heat- and cold-related trauma, gastrointestinal illnesses, and complications related to pregnancy and childbirth.[23] Other issues that are more difficult to track include depression and other mental health problems (see the Going Upstream: Refugee and Migrant Health box). Violence is always a concern with migration, as migrants are continually facing threats such as assault, robbery, and rape.

The WHO works closely with other organizations around the world to address this area of global public health. Guided by the 2008 Resolution on the Health of Migrants, the WHO works closely with governments and international

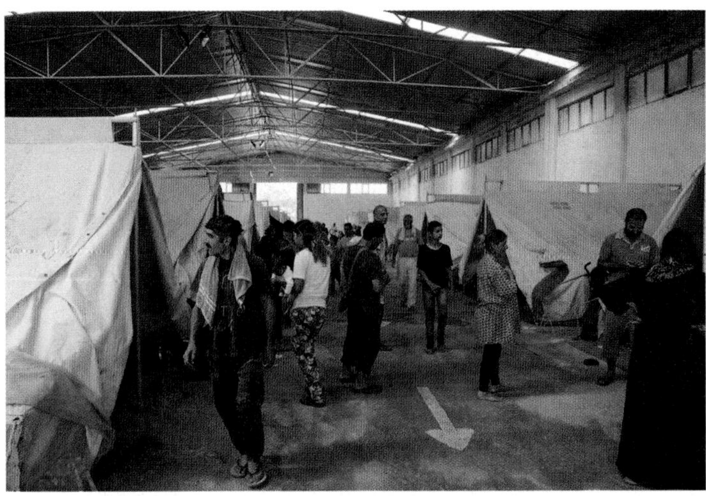

The camp in Vasilika, Greece, in 2016. The camp houses refugees fleeing from Afghanistan, as well as from other countries.

© NurPhoto / Contributor/Getty Images.

organizations, such as the International Rescue Committee, to help address the health issues faced by these vulnerable, resilient, and admirable human beings.

Leading Causes of Death Worldwide and Among the Poor

According to the WHO, the leading causes of death in the world in 2015 were coronary heart disease, stroke, lower respiratory infections, and chronic obstructive lung disease. However, when you look at death by wealth levels (**TABLE 15-3**), a new picture emerges. People with lower income in resource-poor countries not only suffer more, but they also die from different causes. Unfortunately, many of these underlying factors are interrelated—poverty is associated with poor sanitation, which often leads to diarrhea-related illness, also more likely to occur in impoverished countries.

Childhood Underweight and Malnutrition

Poor childhood nutrition, or **malnutrition**, is a leading cause of disease and death, especially among children, in many countries around the world. The countries with the highest prevalence of childhood death from malnutrition include India, Bangladesh, Vietnam, Myanmar, and Ethiopia.[24] These conditions are referred to as wasting (exceedingly low weight based on the child's height), stunting (short height based on a child's age), and underweight (low weight based on a child's age). Children suffer from these conditions as a result of poor or restricted nutrition for pregnant mothers, vitamin deficiency, and general starvation, all of which are related to broader issues of extreme weather, drought, poor sanitation, and poverty.

malnutrition A condition in which a person's diet lacks the necessary nutrients to sustain fundamental physiological and cognitive functions. It increases the risk of morbidity and mortality.

HIV/AIDS

HIV, which causes AIDS, remains one of the leading health concerns in many parts of the world.[25] Worldwide, nearly 37 million people were living with HIV/AIDS in 2014, of which 2.6 million were children under 15 years of age. Despite reductions in the spread of the disease, HIV/AIDS killed 1.2 million people in 2014.[26]

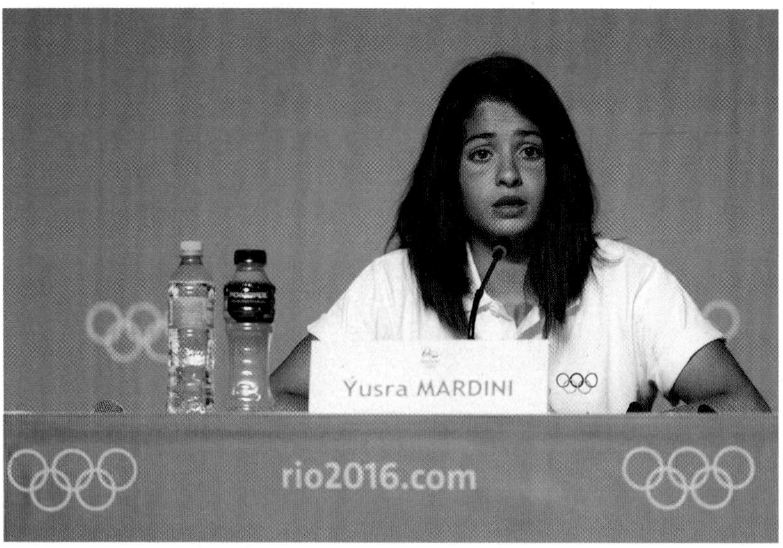

Yusra Mardini, a refugee from Syria and 18-year-old swimmer, was a member of the 2016 Refugee Olympic Team.

TABLE 15-3 Causes of Death by Different Sub-Regions (Based on Income)

Western Sub-Saharan Africa (Low-Income)		Southern Latin America (Middle-Income)		Western Europe (High-Income)		Global	
Disease	**% of Total Deaths**	**Disease**	**% of Total Deaths**	**Disease**	**% of Total Deaths**	**Disease**	**% of Total Deaths**
Malaria	16.9	Ischemic heart disease	13.5	Ischemic heart disease	17.8	Ischemic heart disease	14.4
Lower respiratory	9.9	Stroke	9.4	Stroke	9.8	Stroke	11.5
HIV/AIDS	9.3	COPD	7.3	Alzheimer's disease and other dementias	8.4	COPD	5.2
Diarrheal diseases	5.9	Lower respiratory infections	7.0	Tracheal, bronchial, and lung	5.8	Lower respiratory infections	4.9
Road injuries	4.0	Alzheimer's disease and other dementias	5.8	COPD	4.7	Tracheal, bronchial, and lung	2.9
Stroke	3.9	Tracheal, bronchial, and lung	3.3	Lower respiratory infections	3.9	HIV/AIDS	2.8
Preterm birth complications	3.5	Diabetes	2.8	Colon and rectum cancers	3.7	Alzheimer's disease and other dementias	2.8

Hemoglobinopathies and hemolytic anemias	3.4	Chronic kidney disease	2.7	Other cardiovascular and circulatory diseases	2.3	Road injuries	2.6
Neonatal encephalopathy	3.2	Colon and rectum cancers	2.7	Diabetes	2.3	Diarrheal diseases	2.5

University of Washington, Institute for Health Metrics and Evaluation. (2016). GBD compare: Viz hub. Retrieved from https://vizhub.healthdata.org/gbd-compare/

Most of the people in the world affected by HIV live in poor countries. Sub-Saharan Africa is the most affected region in the world, where 25.8 million people were living with HIV in 2014. In fact, almost 70% of new HIV infections occur in sub-Saharan Africa. In that part of the world, where most of the children affected by the disease live, HIV/AIDS is still the third leading cause of death. Children affected by AIDS include not only those who contract the disease but also those who become orphaned because one or both of their parents die prematurely.

Women are particularly vulnerable to HIV/AIDS. In sub-Saharan Africa, 66% of new infections among those aged 15 to 24 years occur in women.[27] Unfortunately, the countries most affected by HIV also suffer from other health conditions, such as **communicable diseases**, poor sanitation, hunger, and poverty.

Nevertheless, there are definite signs of progress in the fight to end HIV/AIDS around the world. Cooperative efforts by world leaders, governments, and **nongovernmental organizations (NGOs)**, such as UNAIDS, have successfully addressed some of the root causes of the virus, especially unsafe sex practices. Education campaigns in churches, workplaces, and community centers have resulted in the reduction of multiple sexual partnerships, for example. In some areas, these campaigns have reduced extra-marital relationships by as much as 30 percent, leading to significant slowdowns in HIV transmission.[28]

Antiretroviral therapy (ART), the combination of several medicines used to slow the rate that HIV grows in the body, has been effective in preventing the onset of AIDS.[29] By 2015, nearly 16 million people living with HIV around the world were using ART, up from less than 14 million the year before.[30] It has been estimated that increased access to ART has resulted in a 42% decline in HIV/AIDS-related deaths between 2004 and 2014.[31] One of the barriers to more widespread dissemination of ART therapies is cost. The price paid by insurance companies and other purchasers can often run to more than $3,000 for a month's supply of a single medication.[32]

communicable diseases An infectious disease transmitted indirectly or directly from person to person. Zoonotic diseases are infectious diseases transmitted from animal to human.

nongovernmental organizations (NGOs) A not-for-profit organization that is independent from states and international governmental organizations. They are usually funded by donations, but some avoid formal funding altogether and are run primarily by volunteers.

Tuberculosis

Tuberculosis (TB) is an infectious bacterial disease that mostly affects the lungs. It is highly contagious, and is transmitted from person to person via small water droplets from the throat and lungs of people with the active disease. For most people exposed to tuberculosis droplets, their immune system fights off the disease and prevents infection. However, for those with less robust immune systems, TB can take a toll on health and even lead to death. TB symptoms include severe coughing (often including blood), fever, and chest pain. TB is treatable with a course of antibiotics that can last 6 months to 2 years,[33] and is largely preventable. Nevertheless, it remains a serious health problem facing countries throughout the less developed world. People with compromised immune systems, such as those living with HIV or suffering from malnutrition, are particularly susceptible, which is why the TB/HIV combination is a public health issue for millions of people around the world. Globally, 12% of the 9.6 million individuals who became infected with TB in 2014 were also HIV-positive.[34]

Because of how contagious it is, a single person affected by TB will often infect as many as 15 other people during a period of a few months, or as long as a year. Without treatment, around two-thirds of people who get TB will die.[35] Nearly one-third of the entire world's population is at risk of acquiring TB at any time, and each year, more than 9.5 million people develop active TB. More than 4,000 people die from TB every day. Fewer than 20% of these people receive the drugs they need to combat the disease.[36] In other words, TB is one of the world's most preventable public health problems. This is why many institutions, such as the United Nations (UN), the World Bank, and the WHO, have declared it a global health priority.

The largest number of cases of TB in the world are in India, Indonesia, and China. In 2014, 58% of the nearly 10 million new cases were in Southeast Asia and Western Pacific regions.[37] In the United States, most people who contract TB come from one of seven countries (Mexico, Philippines, Vietnam, India, China, Haiti, and Guatemala).[38]

Because TB mostly occurs in less developed countries, treatment can be inadequate due to lack of medical professionals and high quality medical centers. Also problematic are the new strains of the bacteria that become highly resistant to drugs used to treat the disease. Drug-resistant TB is a serious component of the global TB problem, and one that is high on the global health agenda today.[39]

Malaria and Mosquito-borne Diseases

Malaria (also discussed in Chapter 8) is another example of a highly preventable disease that, due to poverty and lack of infrastructure, still kills around a half-million people around the world every year. As with the Zika virus (first discovered in 1947), malaria (discovered in 1880) is transmitted by the bite of an infected female mosquito (**FIGURE 15-1**). Children and pregnant women are particularly vulnerable, and represent around 70% of all malaria deaths worldwide.[40] Although malaria was once common all over the world, even in the southern United States, it is now mostly found in developing countries, especially those close to the Equator. Fortunately, new testing methods, the marketing and distribution of insecticide-treated mosquito nets, and new drugs have resulted in a reduction of global malaria cases between 2000 and 2015.

However, these positive trends did not happen randomly. They came from significant global investments—from individual countries and from international NGOs such as the Global Fund and the Bill and Melinda Gates Foundation. If funding is reduced, malaria may increase once again. As with TB, drug resistance to malaria is a problem, as new mutations of the parasite continue to appear, resisting the treatments of the previous strains, and leading to new mutations that can spread widely across the world.

Malaria is not the only disease transmitted by mosquito bites, although it is the most common, with around 60% of all mosquito-borne disease deaths coming from malaria.[41] Another emerging global health epidemic is the mosquito-transmitted virus called Zika. In February 2016, the WHO declared Zika a global public health emergency, as the disease has now been found in nearly every country in the world. Although mosquitos transmit most cases of Zika, transmission of the virus also occurs through sexual contact.[42]

Mosquito-transmitted diseases, such as malaria and Zika, are examples of how our increasingly connected globe, growing urbanization, and accelerating climate change have led to the spread of previously restricted vectors from small geographic pockets to locations all around the world.[43]

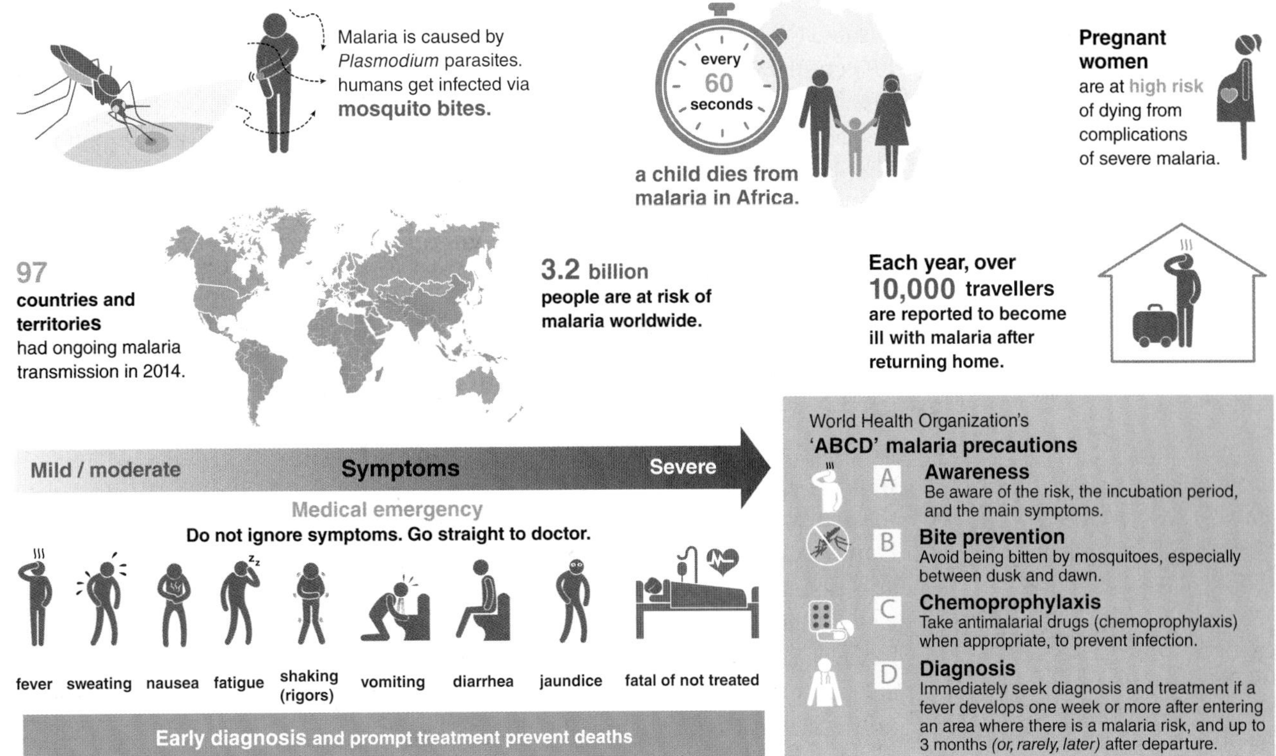

FIGURE 15-1 Malaria, a disease resulting from a parasite that is transmitted by mosquito bites, is a common disease in populations close to the Equator, even though it is relatively unseen in the United States.

Reproduced from World Malaria Day. Courtesy of Centers for Disease Control and Prevention.

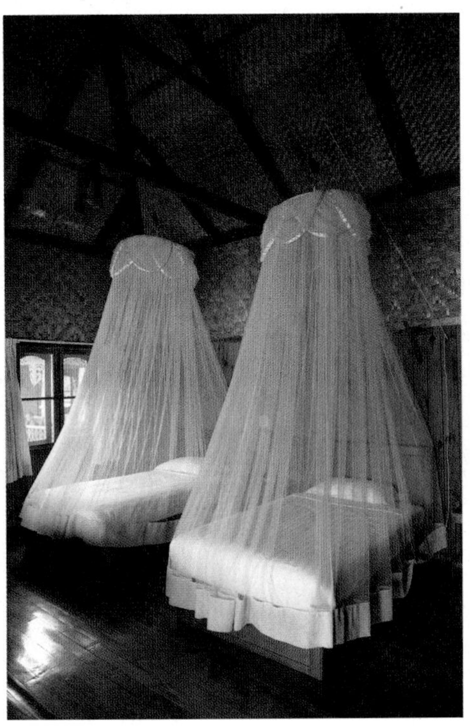

Many hotels throughout Africa and Asia are equipped with quality mosquito nets like these to help prevent malaria; however, millions of families throughout the region remain unprotected in their homes.

Other Communicable Diseases

While HIV/AIDS has been affecting humans for decades, and TB and malaria for centuries, new infectious diseases appear on the scene each year. Often, these diseases can be a threat to the health of the entire world. In 2002, the world witnessed the outbreak of SARS, a disease that researchers believe emerged from people in South China eating civets, a wild mammal native to tropical Asia and Africa.[44] While the disease eventually killed nearly 800 people in 37 countries, it was eradicated through a coordinated effort by researchers, medical professionals, and international aid organizations.

Another disease that recently reappeared is the Ebola virus. Ebola is a fast-acting disease that causes an acute, serious illness which is often fatal. The recent epidemic emerged in the West African country of Guinea in December of 2013. In August 2014, the WHO declared the outbreak to be a public health emergency of international concern.[45] By 2016, more than 11,000 deaths were attributable to **Ebola virus disease**, which is one of five viruses within the genus Ebolavirus referred to as Ebola (see the Tales of Public Health: Ebola? Here? box). In December 2015, after intense treatment, epidemiologic research, and isolation of infected people, Guinea, the last country still seeing patients, was declared Ebola-free. By March 2016, the outbreak was declared to be no longer a global health emergency. Before that, there were cases in many different parts of the world, including the United States.[46] Nevertheless, it is likely only a matter of time before it reappears.

Ebola virus disease A deadly viral disease transmitted from animals to humans that spreads rapidly among humans. It causes flulike symptoms, followed by internal and external bleeding. It has a 21-day incubation period and is contagious only when a person is expressing symptoms.

vaccinations A medical treatment that stimulates the immune system to respond to a specific disease. This creates a response that protects the immune system from future exposure to the specific disease. They are administered through injections, nasally, or orally.

A global health infrastructure consisting of research institutions, well-funded medical organizations, and robust national medical programs in each country are necessary to control new and emerging diseases. Hygiene, hand washing, and clean water play critical roles in protecting people from infectious diseases. **Vaccinations** continue to be an important tool in preventing and eradicating diseases affecting the most vulnerable populations. Vaccinations have seen great success in eliminating or severely reducing diseases such as polio and smallpox.[47]

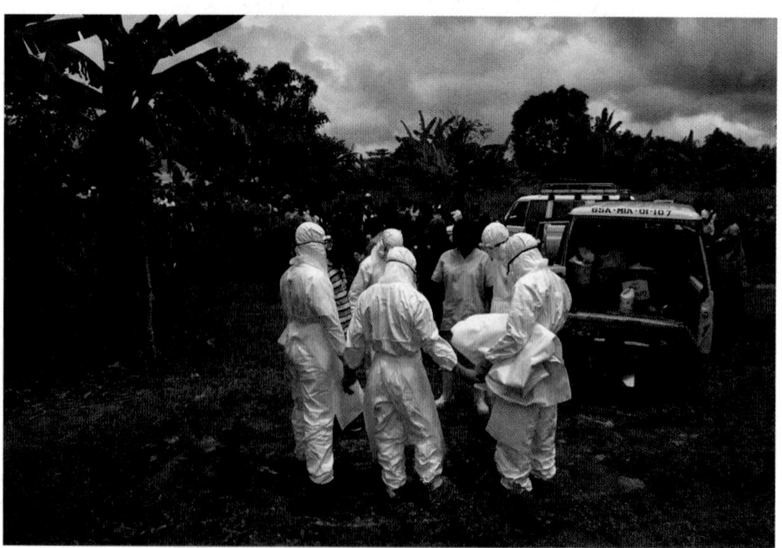

An International Red Cross burial team prays before collecting the body of an Ebola victim from his home near Monrovia, Liberia, in October of 2014.

TALES OF PUBLIC HEALTH

Ebola? Here?

It was 1976, and the United States was celebrating its bicentennial—200 years old!

Meanwhile, in West Africa, a new virus, called Ebola, emerged from deep in the jungle. People were dying by the dozens in two small villages located on the Ebola river: Nzara, South Sudan, and Yambuku, Zaire. It starts with flulike symptoms, followed by decreased appetite, muscular pain, and joint pain. Finally, vomiting, diarrhea, and abdominal pain lead to shortness of breath and chest pain, followed by death.

In all, 280 local people would lose their lives to the disease before global health researchers, medical professionals, and international relief agencies contained it a few months later. Epidemiologists traced the virus to the handling and eating of "bushmeat," primarily bats and monkeys. Burial ceremonies that involved direct contact with infected bodies also transmitted the spread of the virus, leading to deaths beyond those who ate the poorly handled meat. Caregivers also died, as contaminated bedding, hospital supplies, equipment, and surfaces were sources of infection. Because unsafe sex spreads the virus, the sexual practices of the affected communities also became significant factors in its spread.

On March 23, 2014, the Ministry of Health of Guinea informed the WHO of 49 confirmed Ebola cases in the country. It was not particularly shocking news because Ebola outbreaks had been occurring regularly over the years, sometimes killing dozens, sometimes as many as 300 people (**TABLE 15-4**). But before long, cases were being reported in neighboring countries of Liberia and Sierra Leone.

A public health alarm soon sounded. In August 2014, the WHO declared the Ebola outbreak in West Africa an international public health emergency, after thousands of people had died—in Guinea, Liberia, and Sierra Leone. People traveling across borders were spreading it to Senegal and Mali. Through air travel, it ended up in Nigeria.

Then it hit the United States.

On September 30, 2014, Liberian Eric Duncan was diagnosed at Presbyterian Hospital in Dallas, Texas. One month later, Dr. Craig Spencer, a volunteer with Doctors Without Borders), who had been treating Ebola patients in Guinea, was diagnosed, quickly treated, and cured. The news media made his evening front page news: He went out on the town, rode multiple New York City subway lines, grabbed some coffee and some dinner, and went bowling in Brooklyn. People in the city were on edge, and for a while, it seemed to be the biggest topic of the day.

Dallas and NYC medical staff monitored, responded, and ultimately, ensured that it did not spread beyond these two patients. Eventually it was controlled in West Africa as well, along with the countries around the world to which it had spread during this outbreak.

Nevertheless, public health researchers were left with the following questions: How did it happen? After dozens of relatively minor outbreaks (200 infections, 100 deaths), why did this particular outbreak reach foreign lands and ultimately kill 11,000 Africans? Were mistakes made in the medical treatment stage and at the international agency level? What if more money had been available? How much of a role did sexual culture and transmission play? These are some of the questions currently faced by the world today as it gets ready for the next big outbreak of tomorrow.

TABLE 15-4 Biggest Ebola Outbreaks, 1976–2014[46]

Emergence	Country	Number of Cases	Number of Deaths
1976	Zaire	318	280
1995	Zaire	315	254
2000	Uganda	425	224
2007	Congo	264	187
2014	Multiple	28,657	11,325

Data from: Centers for Disease Control and Prevention. (2018). Ebola (Ebola Virus Disease). Retrieved from: https://www.cdc.gov/vhf/ebola/history/chronology.html

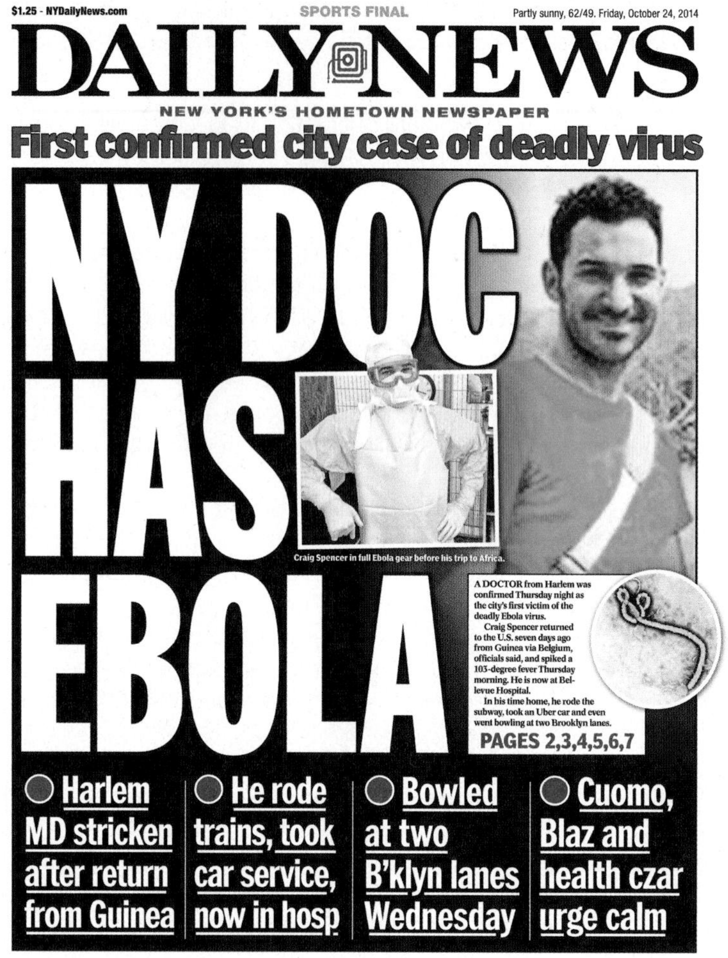

$1.25 - NYDailyNews.com SPORTS FINAL Partly sunny, 62/49. Friday, October 24, 2014

DAILY NEWS

NEW YORK'S HOMETOWN NEWSPAPER

First confirmed city case of deadly virus

NY DOC HAS EBOLA

Craig Spencer in full Ebola gear before his trip to Africa.

A DOCTOR from Harlem was confirmed Thursday night as the city's first victim of the deadly Ebola virus.

Craig Spencer returned to the U.S. seven days ago from Guinea via Belgium, officials said, and spiked a 103-degree fever Thursday morning. He is now at Bellevue Hospital.

In his time home, he rode the subway, took an Uber car and even went bowling at two Brooklyn lanes.

PAGES 2,3,4,5,6,7

- Harlem MD stricken after return from Guinea
- He rode trains, took car service, now in hosp
- Bowled at two B'klyn lanes Wednesday
- Cuomo, Blaz and health czar urge calm

Ebola comes to New York.

Chronic Noncommunicable Diseases: No Longer a "First World" Problem

Although the disease burden around the world has mostly been experienced through communicable diseases (those spread from person to person), that is rapidly changing. With economic and social development, technological advancements, and aging populations, more people are now affected by chronic, noncommunicable diseases than by infectious diseases.

Heart Disease, Cancer, and Other Noncommunicable Diseases

Heart disease, now the world's number one killer, includes among its causes tobacco use, poor diet, and lack of exercise—all problems facing today's world. Today, the only part of the world where communicable disease remains the primary burden of disease is sub-Saharan Africa.[48]

The leading chronic diseases facing the world's population are cardiovascular diseases, cancers, chronic respiratory diseases, and diabetes. These four illnesses are all closely associated with tobacco and alcohol use, salt intake, obesity, high blood pressure, and excessive sugar consumption.[49] As countries such as India and China grow wealthier, more companies seek to gain customers in those countries for their

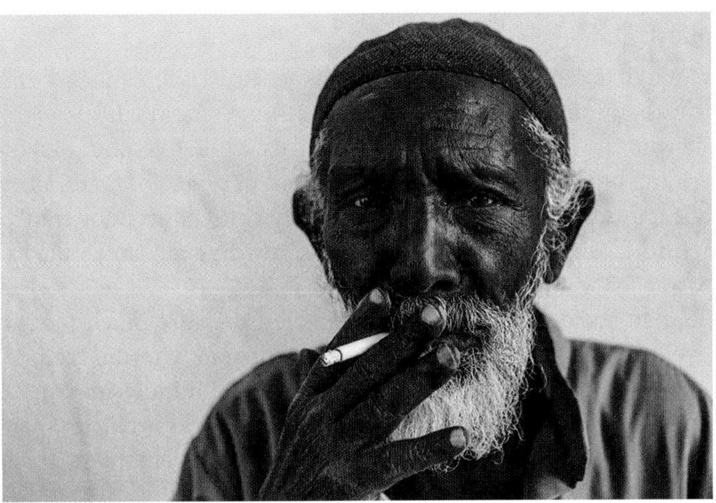

Noncommunicable diseases are becoming more significant causes of morbidity (sickness) and mortality (death) around the world, with tobacco a leading cause, as it may be for this smoker from Egypt.

© hadynyah/E+/Getty Images.

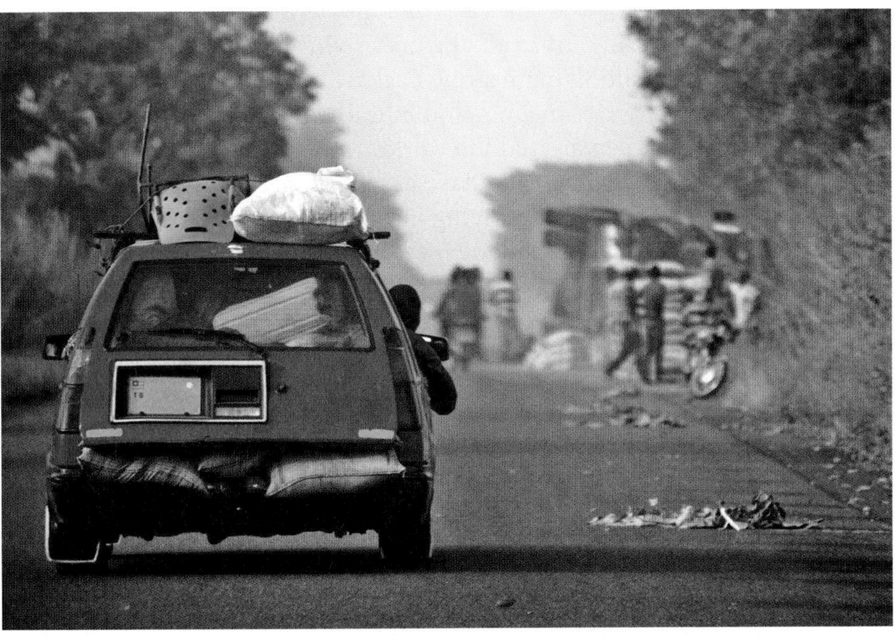

Road accidents are a much more serious health issue in Africa and in Asia than they are in the United States.

© peeterv/E+/Getty Images.

fast food, alcohol, and tobacco products. As a result, chronic, noncommunicable diseases are affecting these populations at larger rates than before.

The WHO now identifies tobacco, alcohol, and unhealthy food as leading causes of disease.[50] These factors are among the primary contributors to the world's premature deaths, preventable illnesses, and national and international inequalities in health.[51] Modernization and industrialization cause injuries and illnesses for people around the world that are debilitating but not always mortal. In other words, they hurt people but do not necessarily kill them. Around the world, more and more people are suffering from iron-deficiency anemia, hearing loss, back pain, sexual diseases, and diabetes. Each of these conditions now affects more than 400 million people globally, causing unnecessary pain and suffering, and lost potential.[52]

Road Accidents

Highway injury is a major global health issue. Road accidents are the leading cause of death among young people (15 to 29) internationally. Roughly half of the people who die in road accidents are in cars while the other half are pedestrians or riding bicycles or motorcycles. The direct causes of road injury include unsafe roads, unsafe driving, and lack of safety belts.[53] But poor transportation infrastructure, lack of regulation, and urban crowding all contribute to the high rates of road accidents.[54]

While road accidents occur in all countries, they are much more common in the developing world. Of the 1.25 million people who die from road traffic accidents, 90% of those deaths occur in low- and middle-income countries, even though those countries have only half of the world's vehicles. For all these reasons, road safety is an important UN sustainable development goal. The UN seeks to achieve a 50% reduction in road traffic fatalities by 2020.

The Social Causes of Disease

Medical and epidemiologic research, vaccine programs, new treatments, and innovative distribution approaches are all important to reduce the amount of global death and suffering. After all, the underlying cause of a case of malaria is more than a mosquito flying nearby. Lack of water infrastructure leading to stagnant and dirty water in a hot and humid country all contribute to the high rates of malaria seen around the world. Another issue is access to medication and treatment. People who have access to medication and treatment have a much better chance of surviving malaria when they contract it. Many factors can improve access to medicines. These include a country's medical system, the number and quality of healthcare professionals available to administer the medications, and availability of the drugs. A country's medical education system, and whether it produces the required number of medical professionals to adequately serve the population, is an underlying factor to these issues as well.

The fundamental infrastructure of the country has an influence on whether people can receive preventive medication or treatment. Are there good roads and enough transportation to bring medications from a big city to a remote, mosquito-infested area? Is it safe to travel, or is it one of the many war-torn lands that the world is witnessing today? Can people afford to travel or see doctors, or are they too drained by poverty to see beyond daily subsistence? These are some of the critical issues that underlie whether people receive treatment. All these problems are complex and interconnected.

We discuss many of the underlying causes of global health challenges here. Following this discussion is a listing of some of the critical institutions and global partnerships that are working to address these underlying factors that influence the health of the world's most vulnerable people.

Poverty and Income Inequality

Poverty may be considered the number one underlying cause of preventable morbidity (illness) and mortality (death) around the world.[55] The *wealth* of a community, family, or person directly relates to the *health* of that community, family, or individual. This is just as true in the United States as it is across the world. There are impoverished and unhealthy people and communities in every major city in the US, just as there are in every major city across the world.[56]

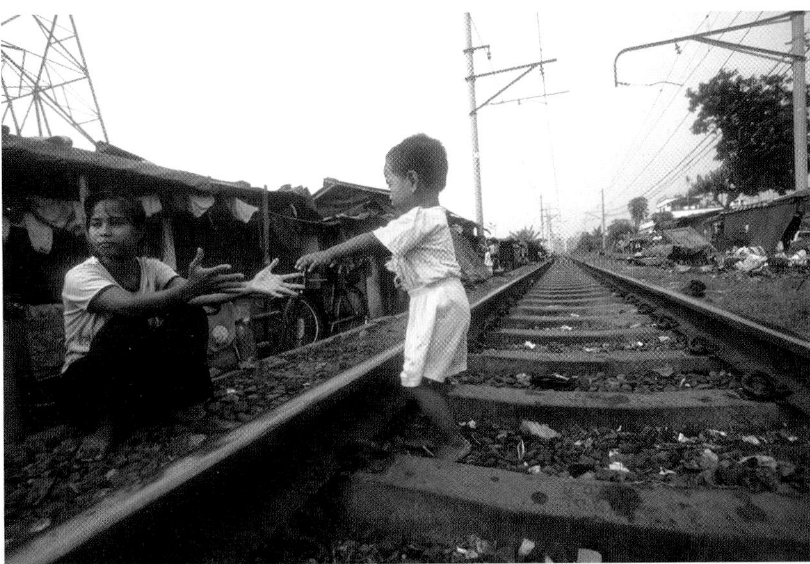

Living conditions, such as these in Jakarta, Indonesia, are an important determinant of health for millions of people all over the world.

© Paula Bronstein/Contributor/Hulton Archive/Getty Images.

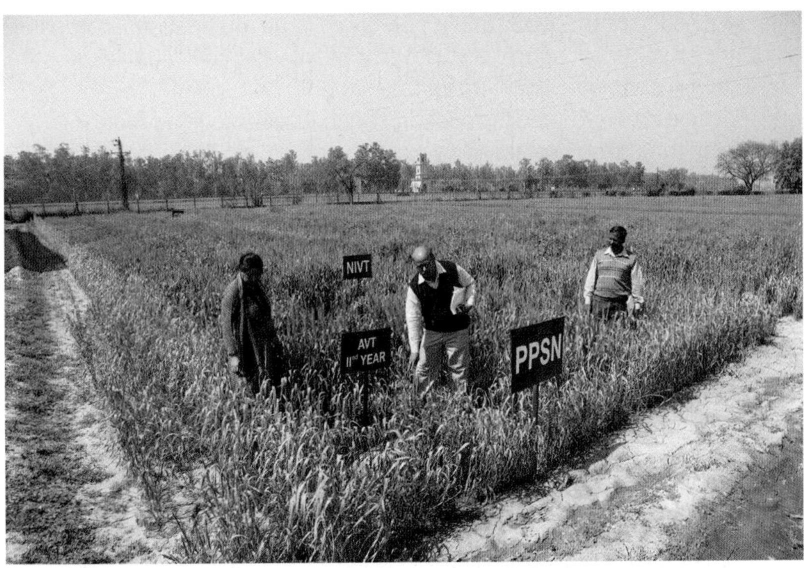

Scientists work to increase food yields by breeding new varieties of wheat at a breeding research station in Karnal, India.

© Pallava Bagla / Contributor/Getty Images.

However, the levels of extreme poverty seen around the world are much less commonly experienced by Americans. Approximately 1.2 billion people in the world (more than three times the population of the United States) live on less than one dollar of family income per day. These human beings—most of whom are children—also tend to live in polluted environments without decent shelter, clean water, or flush toilets.[57]

War and Conflict

Unfortunately, we live in a world filled with armed conflict. Wars have a significant impact on global health, particularly the health of the world's children. Throughout the world, one in six children live where there is some form of war.[61] The United Nations International Children's Education Fund (UNICEF)

UP FOR DEBATE

GMOs as a Solution to World Hunger?

Hunger is a global health priority that is closely related to poverty. It is also a problem that can be improved through science and technology. Some scientists believe that biotechnology and **transgenic** (i.e., genetically modified) crops represent the greatest opportunities to solve the world hunger problem.[58] For example, a transgenic sweet potato has been created to resist a virus in Africa that was previously able to destroy an entire harvest. In Southeast Asia, rice has been modified to include more iron and vitamins that may alleviate chronic malnutrition. Numerous plant modifications have been developed to survive weather extremes. Bioengineers have even modified bananas to contain a vaccine protecting against hepatitis C, a disease that kills around 750,000 people per year, mostly in Africa and Asia.[59]

Many people all over the world, including scientists, are concerned about genetic modification of food, often called **genetically modified organisms (GMOs)**. One example is "golden rice," a transgenic grain fortified with vitamin A. More than 100 Nobel laureate scientists support its production and distribution as a means to reduce malnutrition around the globe. However, the international environmental justice organization Greenpeace opposes it. Greenpeace argues that the release of GMOs into the natural world is a form of "genetic pollution." Greenpeace has contended that genetically engineered organisms can spread through nature and disrupt natural ecosystems, leading to unforeseen challenges for future generations, the way products such as plastics and Styrofoam are seen as environmental contaminants today.

Scientists concerned about global health counter that golden rice, for example, can reduce vitamin A deficiency among the poorest people living in Africa and Southeast Asia. Vitamin A deficiencies can cause childhood blindness and reduce immune function, which can lead to many other diseases.[60]

Greenpeace is concerned that corporate domination of the food supply, notably by large multinational companies such as Monsanto, is not a sustainable solution to solve global hunger and poverty. People and communities, not the elite (politicians, bureaucrats, and scientists), they say, should be in charge of the human food supply.[59]

What do you think? Should greater restrictions be placed on the production of genetically modified food worldwide? Does the immediate benefit outweigh the unknown risks? Do you understand what happens when corporations, NGOs, and governmental organizations own the intellectual property rights of our food supply and set the price of production?

Should genetically modified food be more actively encouraged? If you have a compromise position, can you articulate how both sides of the debate can be satisfied to a greater degree than they are now?

transgenic See genetically modified organisms (GMOs).

genetically modified organisms (GMOs) A living organism that has undergone genetic modification to serve the needs of humans. Also referred to as *transgenic*.

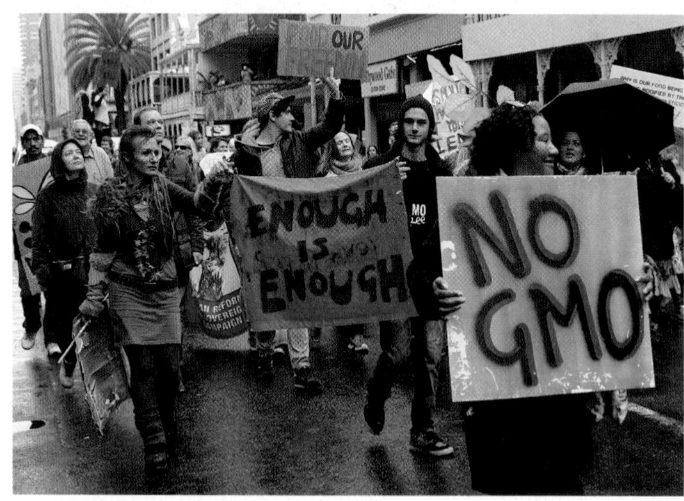

Anti-GMO protesters in South Africa.

estimates there are 230 million children living in countries and areas where there is armed conflict.[62] Right now, there are civil wars in Syria, Afghanistan, Iraq, Libya, and South Sudan. There is sectarian conflict in Lebanon. Sectarian violence occurs throughout Nigeria and in the Democratic Republic of the Congo. For decades, there has been a territorial dispute between Israel and Palestine, which leads to death and destruction on both sides.

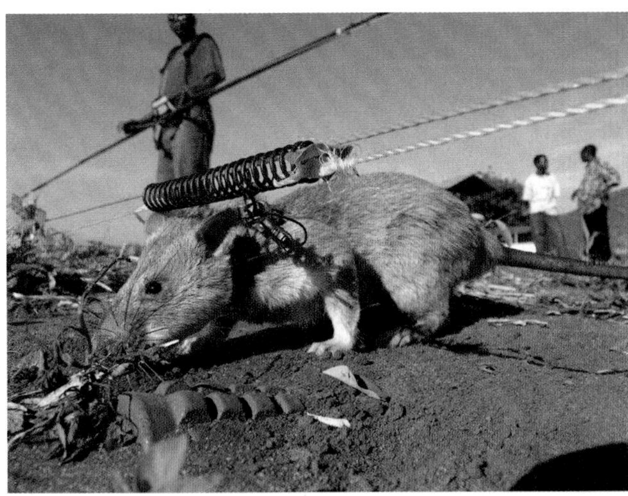

In some countries, rats are used to sniff out dangerous landmines at risk of exploding at any time. Here a rat works at the Anti-Personnel Landmines Removal Product Development (APOPO) organization's training field in Tanzania.

Training rats to detect land mines. (2012, March). *The Solutions Journal, 3*(2), 7–8. Retrieved from https://www.thesolutionsjournal.com/article/training-rats-to-detect-land-mines/

Along with the risk of premature death and disability from violence, war also leads to severe malnutrition, malaria, and other diseases. War often damages or destroys what little health infrastructure that may exist in a country before the violence. This includes clinics, hospitals, and other healthcare centers, as well as water treatment and electrical systems.[63] These breakdowns can affect vaccination programs, as well as maternal and child health programs.

There are also serious psychological effects of being exposed to violence. People, especially children, who are even indirectly exposed to war and conflict can have mental and emotional injuries for the rest of their lives. These include post-traumatic stress disorder and other psychological and physical stresses. They also include behavioral problems, such as acting violently toward others, which often extends into the next generation of children and then the generation beyond that.[64]

Another of the residual effects of war is remaining landmines. Estimates of the number of landmines still in the ground range between 80 to 110 million. These landmines result in between 15,000 and 25,000 new casualties each year. Even decades after the end of wars, anyone who strays into a minefield is at risk. Most minefields are unmarked, making them even more dangerous. Half the people who step onto a landmine will die, and children die at a higher rate because their vital organs are closer to the blast. Cambodia, Iraq, Angola, Iran, and Laos each may have more than 10 million landmines in place today.[62]

GOING UPSTREAM

Refugee and Migrant Health

Zozan Qerani has a 4-inch scar on her wrist. Thankfully, the original cut was treated by a medical team trained to treat people in her situation. But what caused the scar? Was there anything that could be done to prevent such an accident from happening again?

Unfortunately, the question is not an easy one. The scar was the result of a suicide attempt. What led to the attempt was a sustained compound of depression, anxiety, and posttraumatic stress disorder. What caused these depressive symptoms? Zozan was one of the hundreds of thousands of refugees fleeing into Europe from years of war and conflict in Iraq. The trauma began for her and her husband, Atoo, both Yazidi Kurds, after they witnessed war crimes in Kurdistan, where her town was destroyed by Islamic State terrorist militias in 2014.

Zozan and Atoo's story was first told in the *Columbia Journalism Review*,[65] where reporter Marc Herman described them both as seeming to appear to be "the picture of health." But the reality was much different, as the couple struggled with 2 years of displacement. Conditions such as trauma-induced psychosis and other issues set in during their traumatic journey into Greece, where humanitarian relief efforts were in place, but little hope could be seen for a productive future.

It was estimated that half of the 1.2 million new refugees that entered Europe in 2015 needed help for depression, anxiety, or posttraumatic stress disorder.[66] When conditions such as these go untreated, they can lead to numerous downstream problems, including poverty, despair, and, ultimately, suicide.

So where can we intervene upstream, to address the root cause and prevent these mental health challenges from getting worse? While governments and organizations are working at all levels to prevent wars from happening in the first place and reduce their devastating effects, there are no easy answers. What do you think? From an international health perspective, what actions can be taken? Is it easier to ignore refugees entering Europe and the United States? How are effects of conflict-induced migration felt in the United States, and what U.S.-based policies can be enacted to reduce these effects? Since the United States led the invasion of two of the countries producing the greatest number of migrants (Iraq and Afghanistan), what responsibility should the United States have to protect and treat refugees from these countries? Do you think there is an adequate discussion of these downstream issues when a nation considers going to war?

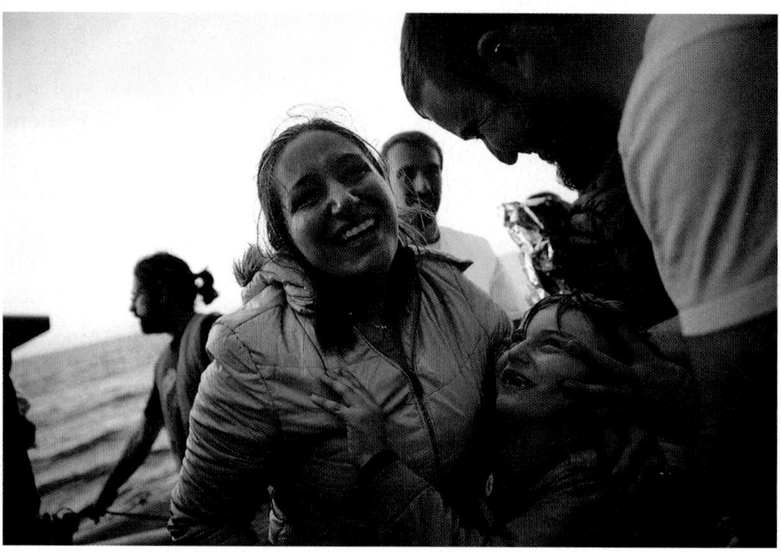

Syrian refugees escaping a brutal civil war are facing psychological issues along with physical health stresses.

Political Infrastructure

Political systems have had an enormous effect on the health of people around the world. Governments, when run poorly or only with the interest of certain members of its population in mind, can inflict serious harm and illness on their populations. Cambodia, China, the Soviet Union, and Nazi Germany are extreme examples within the last 100 years, but many governments today are sacrificing the health of their people for political gain. Other countries have functioning political institutions but an unwillingness to make changes to prioritize health care or public health systems. Even the United States is an example of this, leaving its population less healthy than it could be, despite research showing how money can be better spent on the public's health.

Weather and Climate Change

Public health problems, whether it is the Zika virus or childhood obesity, are always harder on people who are already suffering—poverty, neglect,

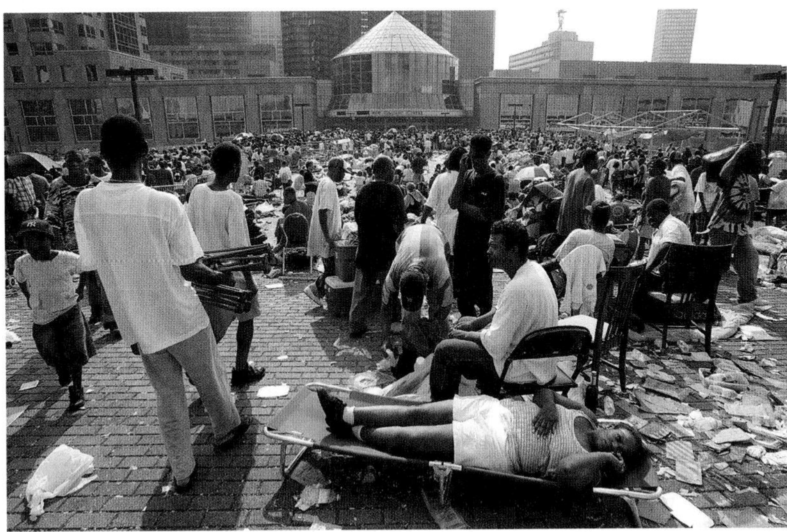

Although Hurricane Katrina occurred in the United States, it had many of the same devastating effects of a natural disaster in other parts of the world—it disproportionally affected lower-income residents and exposed an inequitable public infrastructure.

illness, etc. Weather and global warming are both issues where the poor suffer most. Tornados, tropical hurricanes, flooding, and drought happen every year. In addition to devastation of buildings, crops, and energy systems, most lead to health problems. These can be stress-related psychological issues or diseases like malaria. Poor people around the world often lose everything they own in these catastrophes. They continue to live in poverty and perpetuate the cycle. Hurricane Katrina, which occurred in Mississippi and Louisiana in 2005, is one example of this phenomenon. Another is the 2010 earthquake in Haiti, one of the worst natural disasters in recent history. That event killed 160,000 people and devastated the lives of nearly everyone in the country.[67]

Global warming and climate change are already making weather-related events more plentiful. These are typhoons, hurricanes, droughts, and floods. They are all expected to get worse over time, and, again, disproportionally affect the poorest and most vulnerable. See Chapter 11 for a more complete discussion about climate change.

Corporate Practices

Each year the tobacco, alcohol, and food and beverage industries spend billions of dollars marketing their products to people all over the world.[68] Companies are now investing more money on marketing than ever before, and there is no sign that this will change soon. Coca-Cola has announced plans to spend $8.2 billion in Mexico alone between 2015 and 2020, while PepsiCo said it would invest around $5 billion. In Africa, Coca-Cola pledged to increase its total investment by $17 billion over the same period. In fact, Coca-Cola is now the largest employer on the continent of Africa.[69]

All of these investments increase the number of people consuming these products and the amount they consume.[70,71] This development in global public health deserves the attention of anyone with an interest in the health of the world's people. Paradoxically, while more than one billion people around the world suffer from hunger, there are two billion people who are overweight.[72] Both of these unfortunate statistics indicate that our food systems, while efficient in delivering profits to multinational corporations, are not efficient in maximizing public health.

Who is in charge of international food systems? One answer is "big food," the name given to multinational food and beverage companies like PepsiCo, Coca-Cola, Tyson, Nestle, Kraft, Unilever, Danone, and ConAgra. The 10 largest food companies in the world control about 15% of all food sales, and that percentage is rising each day.[73] Meanwhile, millions of people living in poverty are either faced with a lack of food, or with low-cost, highly processed foods low in nutrition but high in sugar, salt, and saturated fats.

Global Health: The Good News

Despite the challenges, the health of the world is actually getting better. The childhood mortality rate has improved each year, all around the world, although it remains a problem in low-income countries. The TB death rate dropped 47% between 1990 and 2015.[74] Water sanitation gradually improved through modernization and infrastructure improvements, although diarrhea and sanitation still kill more than a million children each year.[75] Conditions like AIDS and malaria, while not being eliminated, are being contained more effectively through health education and social marketing campaigns. Vaccination programs have also saved the lives of millions around the world. The medical infrastructure in many countries gets better each year. Thanks to governments, nongovernmental organizations, and tireless volunteers, more and more people around the world are beginning to live healthier and more productive lives.

Who Is Making A Difference?

Numerous institutions and individuals are dedicated specifically to improving the world's health. They come in different sizes and structures.

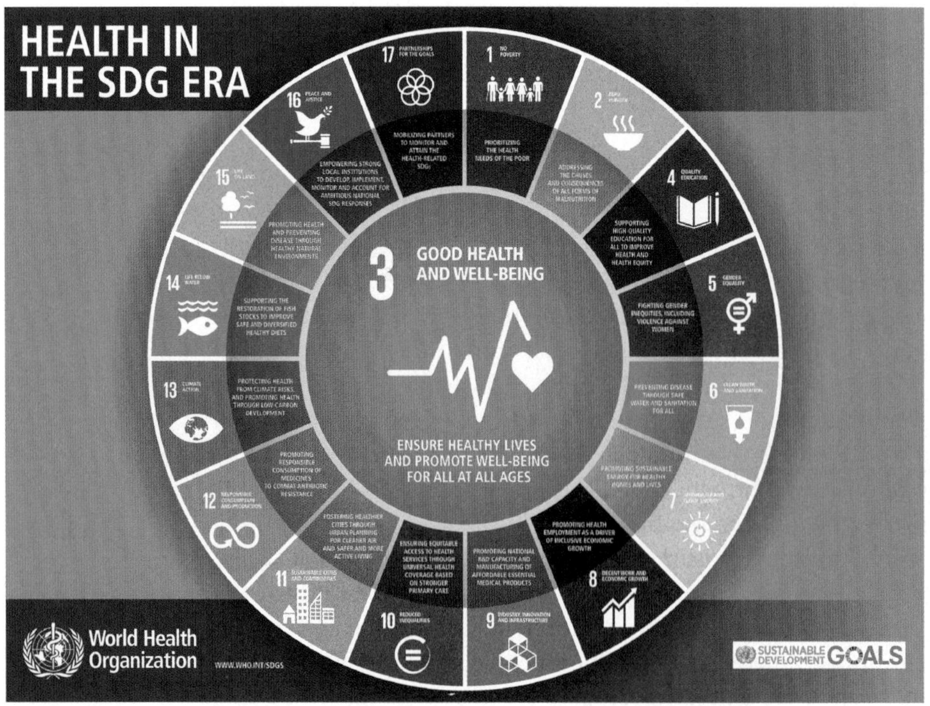

FIGURE 15-2 Sustainable development goals.

Health in SDG Era. Reprinted with permission from World Health Organisation.

International Agencies

A few large international aid organizations are focused specifically on global health. These institutions have a significant impact on the health of people around the world, particularly in resource-poor countries. The UN oversees the largest of these, which include the World Bank and the WHO. The World Bank is an international entity consisting of five agencies providing financial and technical assistance to developing countries around the world to reduce global poverty. In the 1980s and 1990s, the World Bank's Global Fund was a leader in making major investments in controlling HIV/AIDS and TB. Among many of its current programs is an international effort to address mental health, especially depression and anxiety across the world. Research shows that every dollar invested in scaling up treatment for depression and anxiety leads to a return of four dollars in better health and ability to work,[76] and the World Bank is learning to make wiser and more impactful investments in global health.

The WHO is a specialized agency of the UN that is concerned with international public health. Established in 1948 and based in Geneva, Switzerland, the WHO has played a leading role in the eradication of smallpox and is intimately involved in responding to global outbreaks. A great deal of its work includes providing accurate information on the latest global health issues. Its current priorities include HIV/AIDS, Ebola, malaria, TB, sexual and reproductive health, and global health nutrition. With a budget of $4 billion per year, it hires staff throughout the world for leadership positions that require various levels of technical expertise and skills.

The UN oversees both the World Bank and the WHO, and it has established a global agenda, which includes its Sustainable Development Goals. These goals address poverty, hunger, disease, gender inequality, and access to water and sanitation. The goals are then carried forward by organizations, large and small, all over the world. All of the Sustainable Development Goals directly relate to health or contribute to health indirectly. Health is the focus of Sustainable Development Goal 3: Ensure healthy lives and promote well-being for all at all ages.

social entrepreneurship Use of business techniques and private sector approaches to solve social and environmental problems.

Social Entrepreneurial Organizations

Social entrepreneurship uses business techniques and private sector approaches to solve social and environmental problems, and there are thousands

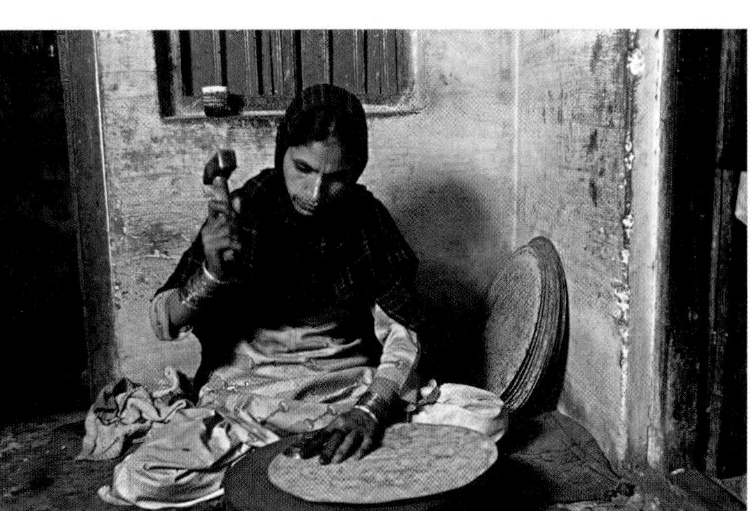

Grameen Bank is helping to reduce poverty and improve the health of women in India and other countries, including the United States.

microfinance A practice in which banking organizations provide small loans to low-income people. The goal is for the loan recipients to start businesses that generate income and break the cycle of poverty.

of social entrepreneurship organizations working to improve health, mostly at the local level, all around the globe. One example of this is the Grameen Bank, a Nobel Peace Prize–winning **microfinance** organization and community development bank founded in Bangladesh. It makes very small loans to very poor people, mostly women. When Grameen Bank was awarded the Peace Prize in 2006, more than 7 million borrowers had been granted such loans. The average amount borrowed was 100 dollars and the repayment percentage was very high. Muhammad Yunus, Grameen's founder, earned a doctoral degree at Vanderbilt University, and was inspired during the Bangladesh famine of 1974 to make small loans to people to avoid predatory lending. Grameen's loans are reducing widespread rural poverty in Bangladesh and serving as a model for related organizations all around the world. There is likely a similar organization working near where you live, that makes small loans or provides grants to organizations dedicated to health and social justice.

The American Assistance for Cambodia is another social entrepreneur, which provides business opportunities for women previously exploited as sex workers. Small investments of as little as $400 can result in a formerly abused child becoming a mother, wife, and business owner.[77]

PATH (previously the Program for Appropriate Technology in Health, but now simply called PATH), is an organization that seeks to take advantage of innovation and entrepreneurism to improve global health. Based in Seattle, PATH is particularly concerned with the health of women and children. It focuses primarily on vaccines, drugs, diagnostic technologies, and other devices and works in partnership with organizations all over the world to deliver therapies to people with the greatest need. The Institute for OneWorld Health is a nonprofit pharmaceutical company and medical research organization based in San Francisco and associated with PATH. Recognizing that the high cost of pharmaceutical drugs is a major barrier to improvements in global health, the institute develops medicines intended for poor patients in the developing world.

Foundations

A foundation is a nonprofit organization that donates funds and support to other public or private organizations. One of the largest of these is the Bill and Melinda Gates Foundation, which dedicates most of its resources toward global health. Their global development division works to help the world's poorest people lift themselves out of hunger and poverty. Recognizing that global health can only be successfully improved through partnership and collaboration, the foundation also builds strategic relationships and promotes health-supporting policies. The Gates foundation is especially focused on gender equality. Melinda Gates once said, "In the developing world, its about time women are on the agenda. For instance, 80% of small subsistence farmers in sub-Saharan Africa are women, and yet all of the programs in the past were predominantly focused on men.[78]

Nongovernmental and Nonprofit Organizations

A nongovernmental organization (NGO) is a not-for-profit organization that is independent from states and international governmental organizations. NGOs are usually funded by donations, but some avoid formal funding altogether and are run primarily by volunteers. Médecins Sans Frontières, or Doctors Without Borders, is an international humanitarian-aid NGO and Nobel Peace Prize laureate, which works to improve the health of people in war-torn regions and developing countries facing endemic diseases.

Research and Academic Institutions

Several institutions were formed as partnerships and dedicated to improving international public health. For example, the Centre for Global Health Research is an independent, not-for-profit organization in Toronto co-sponsored by a hospital and major university, and founded on the principle that effective health initiatives must be supported by reliable, evidence-based research. The centre was created to conduct large-scale epidemiologic studies in developing countries and has offices in Toronto, Bangalore, and New Delhi. Funding is provided by grants from the Canadian and United States Institutes of Health Research, and foundations including the Bill and Melinda Gates Foundation, St. Michael's Hospital, and the University of Toronto.

The U.S. National Institutes of Health (NIH) is has also invested in making inroads in global health. The Fogarty International Center seeks to advance the NIH mission by supporting global health research throughout the world. More than 5,000 scientists have received training from the center. Research projects have been conducted at more than 100 universities in the United States.

Global health research institutes and centers exist at academic institutions throughout the nation. Pursuing a degree in public health is one way to participate in global health research or practice. Along with staff positions in these institutions, research assistant positions are often available for people who do not have a masters or doctoral degree.

Large international organizations, social entrepreneurs, research institutions, and foundations can be exciting places to work. These institutions are always seeking curious, bright people to travel to far away places and improve the health of the people around the globe, and, today, job opportunities at these organizations are easy to find on the Internet and social media.

Individuals

Many individuals dedicate themselves to and succeed in improving the state of global health. Paul Farmer is a physician best known for his humanitarian work, such as providing health care to rural and under-resourced areas in developing countries, starting in Haiti, and proceeding to several African nations, including Rwanda and Kenya. Co-founder of the international social justice and health organization Partners in Health, he serves as a role model for individuals working to create global health impact.

Nice Nailantei Leng'ete is someone who has changed the face of global health for the better. Growing up among the Maasai tribe in Kenya, Nice was told that as a young girl at around 10 years of age, she would have to endure female genital cutting and early marriage. The cutter might use an unsterile razor or a knife, without anything to deaden the pain of removing the labia and clitoris. The wound would then be sewn up so sex would not be enjoyable, and very likely be painful, for the rest of her life.

But unlike the other girls, Nice ran away from home and hid in a tree. Although she was beaten, she was able to talk her way out of the ritual. As the days went on, she relentlessly argued with every authority who came before her: her parents, her grandparents, and eventually Maasai elders, who rarely heard the appeals of women, let alone girls. After months of perseverance in the face of hostility and disdain from her entire society, she was successful. In the wake of her unlikely achievement, and eventually with the endorsement of her community, she became a sexual health educator, teaching youth about HIV, early pregnancy, and marriage, and the importance of staying in school. As an adolescent, she personally prevented 150 girls from forcible genital mutilation.

Seven years later, her work resulted in more than 15,000 girls being saved from the procedure.

Nice subsequently joined an international agency, and is now a world-renowned leader in helping villages transition to holding coming-of-age rituals without including injury to girls.

Another individual who has positively impacted the lives of millions is Malala Yousafzai, a Pakistani activist for female education. As a 15-year-old returning home from school in Pakistan's Swat Valley one day, she was shot by members of the Taliban political group and was severely wounded. Although she was targeted for her advocacy of girls' education, the attack propelled her to international fame and led to a global outcry to address the issue of gender inequality. She was awarded the Nobel Peace Prize in 2014 and has launched her own foundation, called the Malala Fund. The goal of the fund is to ensure that all girls all over the world are able to complete at least 12 years of safe, quality education so they can achieve their potential and be positive change-makers in their families and communities.

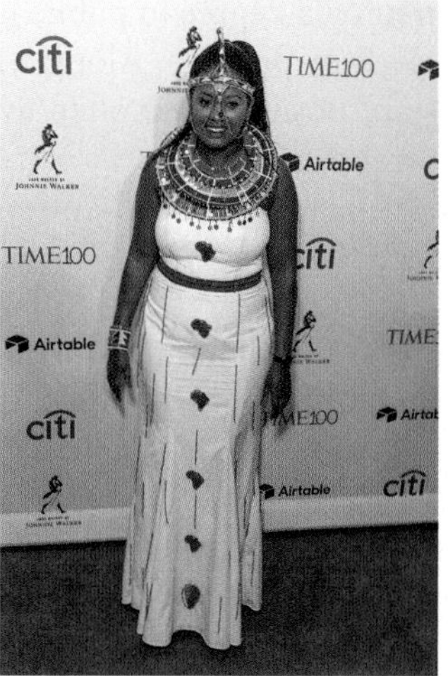

Nice Nailantei is now a global ambassador for helping villages transition away from female genital cutting in their ceremonies that celebrate the passage from girlhood to womanhood.

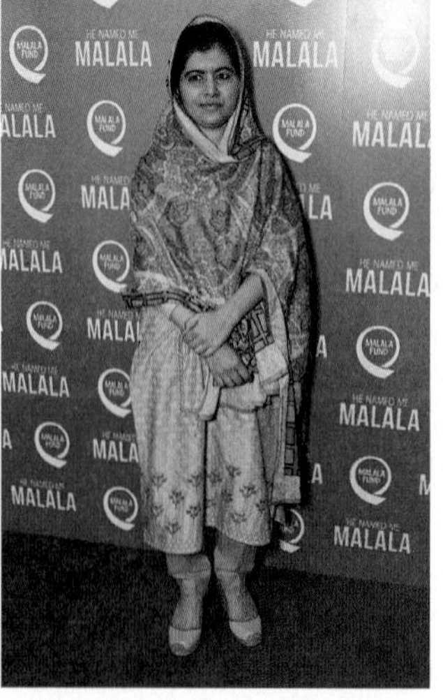

Malala Yousafzai attends a 2015 London screening of a film about her life called *He Named Me Malala*.

It's Your World: Make a Difference!

All over the globe, organizations are working to design and implement programs intended to improve the health of the people who need it the most. More than ever before, poverty assistance programs and innovative health policies are in place that specifically prioritize the needs of poor people. This includes global advocacy, regional initiatives, and direct support to ministries of health in developing countries.[79] Public interest in the health and well-being of people all around the world, especially poor and marginalized individuals, has grown. Complex diseases recently held to be untreatable, are now being solved with greater success.

Global health research is also growing rapidly. More and more research programs are emerging and focusing on scientific discovery, development of new clinical resources (preventive, diagnostic, and therapeutic), and evaluation of the different interventions being used to improve public health. More resources, increasingly coordinated efforts, and new young people joining the commitment every day to a more just and socially equitable global society, give us reasons to be optimistic. Opportunities abound. The world is yours. Embrace it.

In Summary

Global health is a complex and challenging area of research, practice, and engagement. The influences on the health of the people in other parts of the world are numerous and complex, and they range from new microbes being discovered in laboratories to enduring factors such as poverty, war, culture, sanitation, and extreme weather conditions. These factors work together to create complex challenges faced by individuals, communities, and nations that seek to improve global health.

Today, our world is more interconnected than ever before. The field of global health is as relevant to people living in the United States as it has ever been in world history. For these and other reasons discussed in this chapter, global health is an area of work that many Americans choose to pursue for their professional careers. There are countless opportunities to become involved in improving global health. Doing so is social justice work and can be both challenging and fulfilling.

Key Terms

communicable diseases
Ebola virus disease
epidemiology
genetically modified organisms (GMOs)
global burden of disease (GBD)
global health
malnutrition
microfinance
noncommunicable diseases
nongovernmental organizations (NGOs)
social entrepreneurship
social justice imperative
transgenic
vaccinations

Student Discussion Questions and Activities

1. How are you "globally connected"? Do you have relatives living in other countries? Do you communicate with people across the world? Do these people experience health issues that are different from the ones you experience? How and what are they?

2. This chapter discussed three perspectives on why studying global health is important: (1) the moral perspective ("It's the right thing to do"), (2) the interconnectivity and personal perspective ("Diseases spread across the world can affect me"), and (3) the economic perspective ("Improving global health improves the world economy and world security"). While you may agree with all of these perspectives, does one resonate with you more than others? Why?
3. This chapter discussed several critical areas of global health, including communicable and noncommunicable diseases, poverty, and global warming. What do you see as the important issues facing people around the world? What do you see as the most important global health issues in the future?
4. If you were to pursue one global health challenge, what would it be? Why? If you were to start today, what would you do?
5. Find a YouTube video about a social entrepreneur/entrepreneurial organization in global health. What is the issue or problem the organization seeks to solve? Why is it important to global health? What is the solution offered?

References

1. Koplan, J. P., Bond, T. C., Merson, M. H., Reddy, K. S., Rodriguez, M. H., Sewankambo, N. K., and Wasserheit, J. N. Koplan, J. P., et al. (2009). Towards a common definition of global health. *The Lancet, 373*(9679), 1993–1995.
2. Solarz, M. W. (2014). *The language of global development: A misleading geography*. Vol. 39. London, UK: Routledge.
3. Ura, K. (2015). The Experience of Gross National Happiness as Development Framework. *ADB South Asia Working Paper Series,* 42(2015), 6.
4. Sullivan, A., & Sheffrin, S. M. (2003). *Economics: Principles in action*. Upper Saddle River, NJ: Pearson Prentice Hall.
5. Murray, C. J., Ortblad, K. F., Guinovart, C., Lim, S. S., Wolock, T. M., Roberts, D. A., Dansereau, E. A., Graetz, N., Barber, R. M., Brown, J. C. and Wang, H. (2014). Global, regional, and national incidence and mortality for HIV, tuberculosis, and malaria during 1990–2013: A systematic analysis for the Global Burden of Disease Study 2013. *The Lancet, 384*(9947), 1005–1070.
6. World Health Organization. (2015). *International statistical classification of disease and related health problems.* 10th revision. Geneva: World Health Organization.
7. Stragnell, G., ed. (1922). *International record of medicine and general practice clinics*. Vol. 116. New York: MD Publications.
8. Glaziou, P., et al. (2016). TB deaths rank alongside HIV deaths as top infectious killer. *The International Journal of Tuberculosis and Lung Disease*, 20(2), 143–144.
9. Centers for Disease Control and Prevention. (2015). HIV Surveillance Report 2015 (p. 26), Retrieved from https://www.cdc.gov/hiv/pdf/library/reports/surveillance/cdc-hiv-surveillance-report-2015-vol-27.pdf
10. World Health Organization. (2015). Global Health Observatory (GHO) data. Retrieved from http://www.who.int/gho/hiv/en/
11. Chafey, L. (2012). Injustice anywhere is a threat to justice everywhere—internal vs. international armed conflicts: should the distinction be eliminated. *University of Baltimore Journal of International Law,* 1, 184.
12. The World Bank. (2011). *Migration and Remittances Factbook 2011*. http://www.who.int/en/news-room/fact-sheets/detail/hepatitis-c
13. Tucker, J. B. (2003). Strategies for countering terrorism: Lessons from the Israeli experience. *Journal of Homeland Security* 3 (2003).
14. Canetti, D., Hall, B. J., Greene, T., Kane, J. C. and Hobfoll, S. E. (2014). Improving mental health is key to reduce violence in Israel and Gaza. *The Lancet, 384*(9942), 493–494.
15. Kerridge, B. T., Khan, M. R., Rehm, J. and Sapkota, A. (2014). Terrorism, civil war and related violence and substance use disorder morbidity and mortality: A global analysis. *Journal of Epidemiology and Global Health, 4*(1), 61–72.
16. Lopez, A. D., & Murray, C. J. L. (1998). The global burden of disease 1990–2020.
17. Murray, C. J. L., et al. (2015). Global, regional, and national disability-adjusted life years (DALYs) for 306 diseases and injuries and healthy life expectancy (HALE) for 188 countries, 1990–2013: quantifying the epidemiological transition. *The Lancet, 386*(10009), 2145–2191.
18. Nour, N, M. (2008). An introduction to global women's health. *Reviews in Obstetrics and Gynecology, 1*(1), 33.
19. García-Moreno, C. (2013). *Global and regional estimates of violence against women: prevalence and health effects of intimate partner violence and non-partner sexual violence.* Geneva: World Health Organization.
20. World Health Organization. (2015). Ten top issues for women's health. Retrieved from http://www.who.int/life-course/news/2015-intl-womens-day/en/
21. Girls Not Brides. (2002). About child marriage. Retrieved from http://www.girlsnotbrides.org/about-child-marriage/
22. Hatton, T. J. (2016). 60 Million refugees refugees, asylum seekers, and policy in OECD countries. *The American Economic Review, 106*(5), 441–445.
23. World Health Organization. (2016). Migrant and refugee health: Key issues. Retrieved from http://www.euro.who.int/en/health-topics/health-determinants/migration-and-health/migrant-health-in-the-european-region/migration-and-health-key-issues.
24. De Onis, M., Monteiro, C., Akré, J. and Clugston, G. (1993). The worldwide magnitude of protein-energy malnutrition: An

overview from the WHO Global Database on Child Growth. *Bulletin of the World Health Organization, 71*(6), 703–712.

25. Ortblad, K. F., Lozano, R., & Murray, C. J. L. (2013). The burden of HIV: Insights from the Global Burden of Disease Study 2010. *AIDS, 27*(13), 2003–2017.
26. World Health Organization. (2018). Fact Sheet on HIV/AIDS. Retrieved from: http://www.who.int/mediacentre/factsheets/fs360/en/.
27. UN Women. (2016). Facts and Figures: HIV and AIDS. Retrievedfrom.http://www.unwomen.org/en/what-we-do/hiv-and-aids/facts-and-figures#sthash.fRBCchUC.dpuf
28. Halperin, D. T., Mugurungi, O., Hallett, T. B., Muchini, B., Campbell, B., Magure, T., Benedikt, C., and Gregson, S. (2011). A surprising prevention success: Why did the HIV epidemic decline in Zimbabwe? *PLoS Medicine, 8*(2), e1000414.
29. WebMD: "How do you treat HIV?" Retrieved from http://www.webmd.com/hiv-aids/tc/hiv-highly-active-antiretroviral-therapy-haart-topic-overview
30. World Health Organization. (2018). Fact Sheet on HIV/AIDS. Retrieved from http://www.who.int/mediacentre/factsheets/fs360/en/
31. World Health Organization. (2018). Fact Sheet on HIV/AIDS. Retrieved from http://www.who.int/mediacentre/factsheets/fs360/en/
32. AIDSinfo, Access. (2013). Guidelines for the use of antiretroviral agents in HIV-1-infected adults and adolescents. K8-12. Retrieved from https://aidsinfo.nih.gov/contentfiles/AdultandAdolescentGL003371.pdf
33. World Health Organization. (2017). Tuberculosis (TB). Retrieved from: http://www.who.int/topics/tuberculosis/en/
34. World Health Organization. (2015). Global Health Tuberculosis Report 2015. Retrieved from http://www.who.int/tb/publications/global_report/gtbr2015_executive_summary.pdf?ua=1
35. World Health Organization. (2018). What is TB? How is it treated?. Retrieved from http://www.who.int/features/qa/08/en/
36. The White House. (2015). FACT SHEET: Obama Administration Releases National Action Plan for Combating Multidrug-Resistant Tuberculosis. Retrieved from https://obamawhitehouse.archives.gov/the-press-office/2015/12/22/fact-sheet-obama-administration-releases-national-action-plan-combating
37. Glaziou, P., Floyd, K., Weil, D., and Raviglione, M. (2016). TB deaths rank alongside HIV deaths as top infectious killer. *The International Journal of Tuberculosis and Lung Disease, 20*(2), 143–144.
38. Centers for Disease Control and Prevention. (2016). Latent tuberculosis infection: A guide for primary health care providers. Retrieved from http://www.cdc.gov/tb/publications/ltbi/appendixb.htm.
39. World Health Organization. (2014). Companion handbook to the WHO guidelines for the programmatic management of drug-resistant tuberculosis.
40. The Global Fund. (2018). Malaria. Retrieved from https://www.theglobalfund.org/en/malaria/
41. Handwerk, B. (2016, May 31). Malaria, Zika and Dengue could meet their match in mosquito-borne bacteria. *Smithsonian.* Retrieved from https://www.smithsonianmag.com/science-nature/malaria-zika-and-dengue-could-meet-their-match-mosquito-borne-bacteria-180959271/
42. McCarthy, M.. (2016). Zika virus was transmitted by sexual contact in Texas, health officials report. *BMJ, 352*, i720.
43. Chan, J. F., Choi, G. K., Yip, C. C., Cheng, V. C., and Yuen, K. Y. (2016). Zika fever and congenital Zika syndrome: an unexpected emerging arboviral disease. *Journal of Infection, 72*(5), 507–524.
44. Sutton, T. C., & Subbarao, K. (2015). Development of animal models against emerging coronaviruses: From SARS to MERS coronavirus. *Virology, 479*, 247–258.
45. World Health Organization. (2018). WHO Director-General addresses the Executive Board. Retrieved from http://www.who.int/dg/speeches/2018/142-executive-board/en/
46. Centers for Disease Control and Prevention. (2018). Ebola (Ebola Virus Disease). Retrieved from: https://www.cdc.gov/vhf/ebola/history/chronology.html
47. World Health Organization. (2018). Questions and Answers on Vaccine Safety. Retrieved from: http://www.who.int/features/qa/84/en/
48. Skolnik, R. (2015). *Global health 101*. Burlington, MA: Jones & Bartlett Learning.
49. Kontis, V., et al. (2015). Regional contributions of six preventable risk factors to achieving the 25 × 25 noncommunicable disease mortality reduction target: A modelling study. *The Lancet, Global Health, 3*(12), e746–e757.
50. World Health Organization. (2011). *Global status report on noncommunicable diseases, 2010. Description of the global burden of NCDs, their risk factors and determinants*. Geneva, Switzerland: WHO.
51. Yach, D., Hawkes, C., Gould, C. L., & Hofman, K. J. (2004). The global burden of chronic diseases: overcoming impediments to prevention and control. *JAMA, 291*(21), 2616–2622.
52. Smith, J. (2015, July 16). Lives grow longer, and health care's challenges change. *New York Times*. Retrieved from: https://www.nytimes.com/2015/07/17/upshot/lives-grow-longer-and-health-cares-challenges-change.html
53. Stoker, P., Garfinkel-Castro, A., Khayesi, M., Odero, W., Mwangi, M. N., Peden, M., and Ewing, R. 2015). Pedestrian safety and the built environment: A review of the risk factors. *Journal of Planning Literature, 30*(4), 377–392.
54. Stoker, P., Adkins, A. and Ewing, R., 2017. Pedestrian safety and public health. In *Walking: Connecting Sustainable Transport with Health* (pp. 211–229). Emerald Publishing Limited.
55. Cohen, L. (2016). Building a thriving nation: 21st-century vision and practice to advance health and equity. *Health Education & Behavior, 43*(2), 125–132.
56. Jamison, D. T., Summers, L. H., Alleyne, G., Arrow, K. J., Berkley, S., Binagwaho, A., Bustreo, F., Evans, D., Feachem, R. G., Frenk, J., and Ghosh, G. (2013). Global health 2035: A world converging within a generation. *The Lancet, 382*(9908), 1898–1955.
57. Olinto, P., Beegle, K., Sobrado, C., and Uematsu, H. (2013). The state of the poor: Where are the poor, where is extreme poverty harder to end, and what is the current profile of the world's poor? *Economic Premise, 125*, 2.
58. Achenbach, J. (2016, Jun 30). 107 Nobel laureates sign letter blasting Greenpeace over GMOs. *Washington Post*. Retrieved from https://www.washingtonpost.com/news/speaking-of-science/wp/2016/06/29/more-than-100-nobel-laureates-take-on-greenpeace-over-gmo-stance/
59. World Health Organization. (2017). Hepatitis C. Retrieved from http://www.who.int/en/news-room/fact-sheets/detail/hepatitis-c
60. Alberts, B., Beachy, R., Baulcombe, D., Blobel, G., Datta, S., Fedoroff, N., Kennedy, D., Khush, G. S., Peacock, J., Rees, M., and Sharp, P. (2013). Standing up for GMOs. *Science, 341*(6152), 1320–1320.
61. Rieder, M., & Choonara, I. (2012). Armed conflict and child health. *Archives of Disease in Childhood. 97*(1), 59–62.

62. UNICEF. (2015). A Post-2015 World Fit For Children. Retrieved from http://www.unicef.org/post2015/files/P2015_issue_brief_set.pdf
63. Ghobarah, H. A., Huth, P., & Russett, B. (2004). The post-war public health effects of civil conflict. *Social Science & Medicine, 59*(4), 869–884.
64. Leavitt, L. A., & Fox Nathan, A. (2014). *The psychological effects of war and violence on children.* London, UK: Psychology Press.
65. Herman, M. (2016). Why reporting on refugee crises requires empathy for mental health issues. *Columbia Journalism Review.* Retrieved from http://www.cjr.org/first_person/refugee_crisis_mental_health_journalism.php
66. Imm-Bazlen, U. (2016). *Trauma und traumafolgestörungen. Begleitung von flüchtlingen mit traumatischen erfahrungen.* Berlin/Heidelberg: Springer; 35–76.
67. Oliver-Smith, A. (2010). Haiti and the historical construction of disasters. *NACLA Report on the Americas, 43*(4), 32–36.
68. Moodie, R., Stuckler, D., Monteiro, C., Sheron, N., Neal, B., Thamarangsi, T., Lincoln, P., and Casswell, S. (2013). Profits and pandemics: Prevention of harmful effects of tobacco, alcohol, and ultra-processed food and drink industries. *Lancet, 381*(9867), 670–679.
69. Cohen, D. (2013). *A big fat crisis: The hidden forces behind the obesity epidemic and how we can end it.* New York: Nation Books.
70. Grier, S. A., & Kumanyika, S. (2010). Targeted marketing and public health. *Annual Review of Public Health, 31*, 349–369.
71. Stuckler, D., McKee, M., Ebrahim, S., & Basu, S. (2012). Manufacturing epidemics: The role of global producers in increased consumption of unhealthy commodities including processed foods, alcohol, and tobacco. *PLoS Medicine, 9*(6), e1001235.
72. Stein, A. D., Thompson, A. M., & Waters, A. (2005). Childhood growth and chronic disease: evidence from countries undergoing the nutrition transition. *Maternal Child Nutrition, 1*, 177–184.
73. Stuckler, D., & Nestle, M. (2012). Big food, food systems, and global health. *PLoS Medicine, 9*(6), e1001242.
74. World Health Organization. (2016). WHO International Factsheet. Retrieved from http://www.who.int/mediacentre/factsheets/fs104/en/
75. Das, J. K., Salam, R. A. and Bhutta, Z. A. (2014). Global burden of childhood diarrhea and interventions. *Current Opinion in Infectious Diseases, 27*(5), pp. 451–458.
76. World Health Organization. (2016). Press release: Investing in treatment for depression and anxiety leads to fourfold return. Retrieved from http://www.who.int/mediacentre/news/releases/2016/depression-anxiety-treatment/en/
77. Kristof, N. D., & WuDunn, S. (2010). *Half the sky: Turning oppression into opportunity for women worldwide.* New York: Vintage Books.
78. Solomon, D. (2010, Oct. 22). The Donor. *New York Times.* Retrieved from https://www.nytimes.com/2010/10/24/magazine/24fob-q4-t.html
79. World Health Organization. (n.d.). Health and Development. Retrieved from http://www.who.int/hdp/poverty/en/

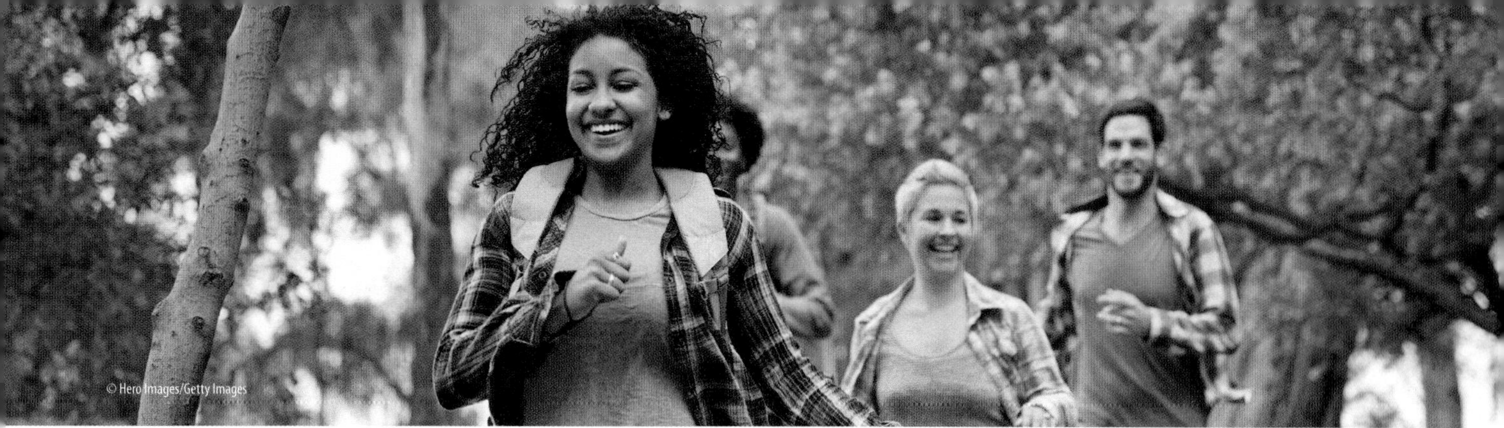
© Hero Images/Getty Images

CHAPTER 16

From Information to Action

CHAPTER OBJECTIVES

- Apply the social-ecological model to public health issues.
- Describe cultural competence and respect.
- Understand the organizations that shape health and have a sense of the system of organizations.
- Identify methods for advocacy and using a community organization in addressing a public health issue.
- Build a plan to change a behavior to improve your health.
- Apply methods to build happiness.

▶ Revisiting the Social-Ecological Model

Throughout this textbook, you have read about factors that affect your health and the health of your family, your community, and our society as a whole. As we have learned, where we live, the friends we have, our cultural background, and many other factors affect our health.

Public health institutions take an ecological approach to understanding and improving individual, family, and community health. Embracing the **social-ecological model** helps us to understand the necessity of individual-level, family-level, community-level, and policy-level interventions (**FIGURE 16-1**). Individual, interpersonal, institutional, community, population health, and public policy factors all play a part in influencing health. These levels interconnect to provide a multifaceted view of health. What happens on your campus—as defined by the physical settings, the political atmosphere, the social climate, and other considerations—will affect your individual behavior and consequently your health and well-being.

social-ecological model A theory-based framework for understanding the multifaceted and interactive effects of personal and environmental factors that determine behaviors, and for identifying behavioral and organizational leverage points and intermediaries for health promotion within organizations.

Let's pick a common health problem to consider how the social-ecological model applies in real life. In the United States, 9.4% of people of all ages (30.3 million) have diabetes.[1]

At an *individual* level, factors that influence diabetes include genetics, weight, diet, exercise, and consistency in taking medication (if diagnosed with diabetes).

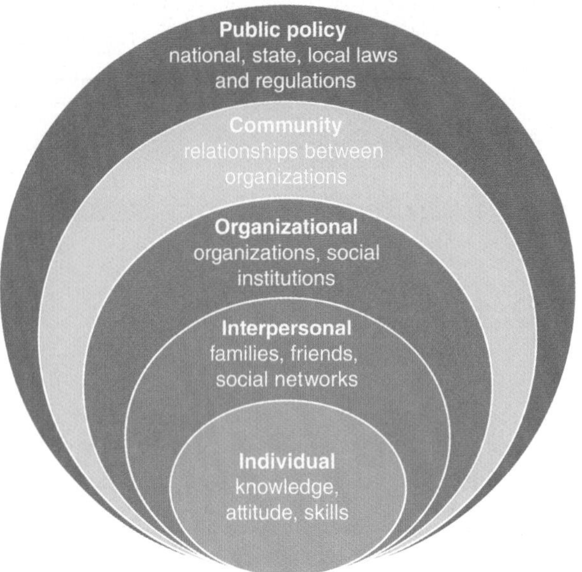

FIGURE 16-1 The social-ecological model.

On an *interpersonal* level, cultural factors affect both food choices and beliefs about medication. The role of food within family relationships, traditions, cultural norms, and values regarding food influences the choices we make. How our family and friends feel about medications can also influence our beliefs and willingness to use them to control diabetes.

At the *institutional* level, food choices at your school limit or expand your options. Do the vending machines offer healthy choices? Does your school have programs to promote healthy food choices? What are the options at your school for physical activities that you enjoy? Is there a student health clinic to provide access to quality health care, medication, and education about diabetes?

At the *community* level, what are the availability and options for making healthy food choices? If the only options are fast food, it is certainly harder to make healthy choices. Are there safe places available for you to exercise?

At the *society* level, policies affect our access to health care and the choices we have about what foods are available. On September 13, 2012, the New York City Board of Health voted unanimously to approve a ban on sweetened drinks larger than 16 ounces at any establishment that received a health grade from the health department.[2] (In this instance, health "grades" rate compliance in food handling, food temperature, personal hygiene, and vermin control.[3]) The ban was to take effect 6 months after the board of health passed the law. Twice, courts ruled against the ban, and it then went to the state supreme court. Less than 2 years later, after being approved by the board of health, New York State's Supreme Court made a final ruling that overturned the ban.[4] The ruling was a blow to public health advocates and a major victory for the American soft drink industry.

Cultural Competence and Respect

Culture comprises the characteristics and knowledge of a particular group of people, including their language, religion, cuisine, social habits, thoughts, actions, customs, music and arts, beliefs, and values.[5,6] As these factors pertain to health, culture influences the beliefs and belief systems surrounding health, healing, wellness, illness, and disease.

In 1998, a team of social service professionals issued a monograph supporting the idea that understanding the inherent strengths of all cultures makes delivery of health care more effective.[7] Although the focus of this text is not the delivery of health care, the idea of cultural competence or cultural relevance provides a critical lens through which to view the world. **Cultural competence** can be defined as "a set of values, behaviors, attitudes, and practices within a system, organization, program or individuals" that allows the parties involved to work effectively across cultures.[8] It refers to the ability to honor and respect the beliefs, language, interpersonal styles, and behaviors of individuals and families. To be culturally competent requires a long-term commitment. At the individual level, this effort requires examining one's own attitudes and values, and the acquisition of the values, knowledge, skills, and attributes that will allow an individual to work appropriately in cross-cultural situations.[8] The monograph's authors chose the word *competence* because it implies the ability to function effectively.[7] Many public health professionals believe that cultural competence and relevance are critical to having a healthier population.

cultural competence A set of values, behaviors, attitudes, and practices within an organization or program or among individuals that allows them to work effectively cross-culturally.

To be culturally competent, you must first value diversity. "You" can be an individual, a group, or part of an organization. You must have the capacity for cultural self-assessment. You must be conscious of the dynamics when people or groups of people from different cultures interact. The last two factors necessary for cultural competence apply to organizations and include (1) having institutionalized cultural knowledge and (2) adapting to reflect an understanding of cultural diversity.

Why is cultural respect important? Cultural respect and competence are critical to reducing health disparities. The United States is the most diverse country in the world. The people who live here are of many backgrounds, cultures, languages, races, ethnicities, and beliefs. The ability to communicate effectively across barriers of language and culture directly affects how we see others and how others see us.

Knowledge of the broad differences between various cultures is not, by itself, enough. Two people of the same ethnicity can have very different experiences, based on their individual socioeconomic status, education level, cultural traditions, religious or spiritual beliefs, and personal histories, all of which affect who they are as individuals. Cultural competence requires sensitivity to

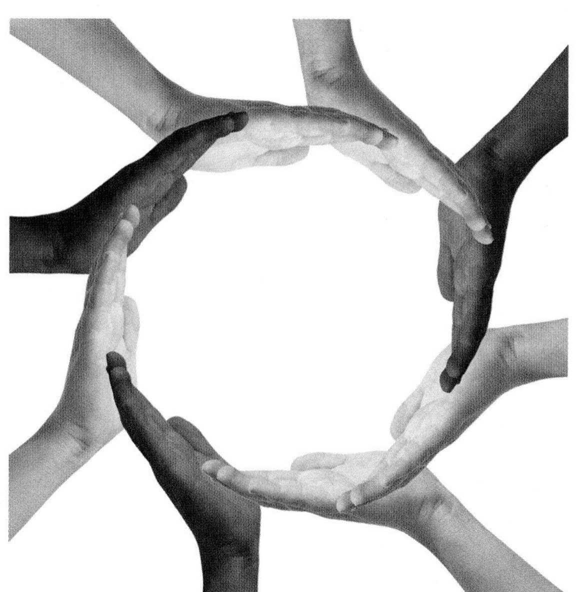

© Arcady/Shutterstock.

intercultural differences, but culture is only part of a large and interconnected array of factors that influence our health.

Organizations That Shape Health

At every level of society, there are organizations that shape and protect your health. Their mandate, funding, and organization determine what they do and what their focus is. These organizations may be governmental, quasi-governmental, or nongovernmental. You are probably already familiar with many of the agencies and organizations discussed in the following section. This section will help you understand how they fit together and give you a sense of the system as a whole. **FIGURE 16-2** provides an illustration of how all of the components of the health system interact.

Governmental Organizations

governmental organizations A type of social organization that exists at all levels of government, from the international level all the way down to the local level, or your county or township, to serve the needs of its citizens.

World Health Organization (WHO) Established in 1948, an international organization that works with local offices in more than 150 countries and governments to achieve global health.

Governmental organizations can exist at all levels of government, from the international level all the way down to the local level, or your county or township.

International Organizations

The most important international health agency is the **World Health Organization (WHO)**.[9] The goal of WHO is to build a better, healthier future for people all over the world. The WHO has played a major part in the control and eradication of many infectious diseases, including smallpox, Chagas disease, lymphatic filariasis, onchocerciasis, and leprosy.[10]

The WHO was founded under the auspices of the United Nations. Any country that ratifies the WHO constitution and receives a majority vote from members may join. In 2016 there were 194 member countries.[9] Delegates from the member nations meet and approve the program and budget, as well as major policy decisions. Nations pay dues to support the WHO (partially) financially. The amount each country pays is calculated based on the country's wealth and population. Additional funding comes from voluntary contributions.

The WHO has six leadership priorities[9]:

1. *Advancing universal health coverage.* This priority involves enabling countries to sustain or expand access to all needed health services and financial protection, and promoting universal health coverage.[9]

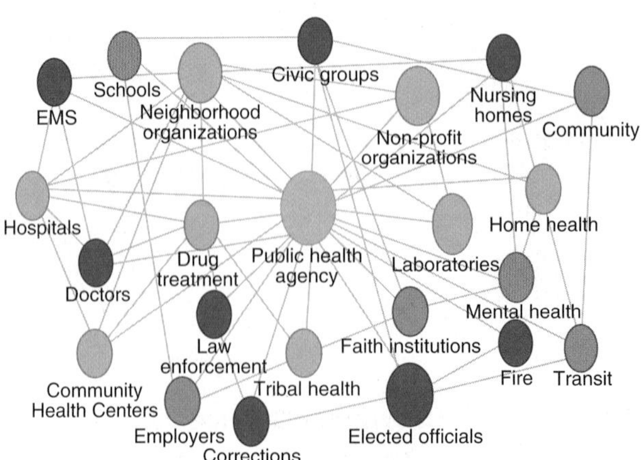

FIGURE 16-2 Web of public health components.

Centers for Disease Control and Prevention (CDC). (2017). National Public Health Performance Standards. Retrieved from http://www.cdc.gov/nphpsp/essentialservices.html

The idea of universal health coverage combines access to the services needed with financial protection to promote health and prevent diseases, and ensure that poor health does not lead to poverty. The WHO will respond by providing practical advice to countries on how to promote universal health coverage.

2. *Achieving health-related development goals.* This priority focuses on addressing unfinished and future challenges relating to maternal and child health; combating human immunodeficiency virus (HIV), malaria, and tuberculosis; and completing the eradication of polio and a number of neglected tropical diseases.[9] In 2000, the United Nations made a public commitment to combat poverty, hunger, disease, illiteracy, environmental degradation, and discrimination against women. The intention was to achieve these Millennium Development Goals by 2015. The WHO is working to sustain the gains made toward these goals. These goals are now transitioning into 17 Sustainable Development Goals, to be completed by 2030.
3. *Addressing the challenge of noncommunicable diseases and mental health, violence, and injuries and disabilities.*[9] Noncommunicable diseases, or chronic diseases, have devastating health consequences for individuals, families, and communities, and they threaten to overwhelm health systems. The four main types of noncommunicable diseases are cardiovascular diseases (including heart attacks and stroke), cancers, chronic respiratory diseases (such as asthma), and diabetes. The WHO will coordinate a broad response at global, regional, and local levels.
4. *Ensuring that all countries can detect and respond to acute public health threats under the International Health Regulations.*[9] The WHO will support countries to prevent and respond to acute public health risks and to report certain disease outbreaks and public health events.
5. *Increasing access to quality, safe, efficacious, and affordable medical products (medicines, vaccines, diagnostics, and other health technologies).*[9] Because equity in public health depends on access to essential, high-quality, and affordable medical technologies, The WHO will continue to improve access to safe, quality, affordable, and effective medicines. They will also support innovation for affordable health technology, local production, and national regulatory authorities.
6. *Addressing the social, economic, and environmental determinants of health as a means to promote health outcomes and reduce health inequalities within and between countries.*[9] The unit within the WHO responsible for coordinating the efforts on social determinants of health supports countries' actions to address health inequities. The group supports, guides, and strengthens the abilities of countries to develop, engage, study, and evaluate initiatives to promote health equity through addressing the **social determinants of health**.

social determinants of health The circumstances in which people are born, grow, live, work, and age. They are shaped by the distribution of money, power, and resources at global, national, and local levels.

National Organizations

The Department of Health and Human Services. The Department of Health and Human Services (DHHS) is part of the executive branch of the federal government and is the overarching department responsible for the health of the citizens of the United States, including the U.S. territories. Other parts of the

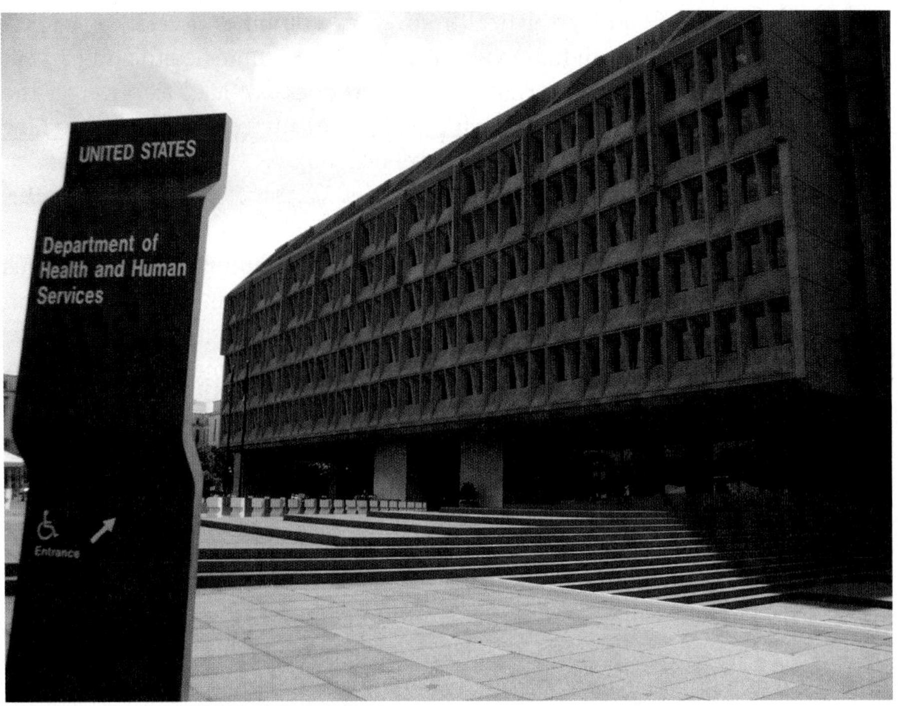

The U.S. Department of Health and Human Services building, Washington, D.C.

Wikimedia Commons. (2011.) Retrieved from https://commons.wikimedia.org/wiki/File:Department_of_Health_%26_Human_Services_-_Stierch.jpg

Administration for Children and Families The operating division within the Department of Health and Human Services that targets children, youth, families, and communities. This department administers a broad range of programs that include income assistance, child support enforcement, adoption assistance, foster care, and child care, as well as services for people with developmental disabilities, refugees, migrants, victims of child abuse, and American Indians.

Administration for Community Living The operating division within the Department of Health and Human Services that focuses on people with disabilities and older adults. The agency works to ensure that individuals with disabilities and the elderly can live where they choose, with the people they want, and that they can fully participate in their communities. Programs also support family caregivers, address issues of elder abuse, address the needs of American Indians, provide community services, and offer individualized support for individuals with disabilities.

Agency for Healthcare Research and Quality The operating division within the Department of Health and Human Services that supports research to improve the quality of health care, minimize its costs, ensure patient safety, respond to medical errors, and increase access to essential services.

government are also responsible for parts of the health agenda. The Department of Agriculture oversees food production and safety. The Environmental Protection Agency is responsible for ensuring that our environment is safe, and the Department of Labor oversees the Occupational Health and Safety Administration, which protects people in the workplace.

The DHHS is the largest department in the government, with a budget of over $1.112 billion in 2018 and more than 80,000 full-time employees.[11] There are 11 operating divisions within the department:

- The **Administration for Children and Families** has programs that target children, youth, families, and communities. This department administers a broad range of programs that include income assistance, child support enforcement, adoption assistance, foster care, and child care, as well as services for people with developmental disabilities, refugees, migrants, victims of child abuse, and American Indians.[12]
- The **Administration for Community Living** has two primary foci: people with disabilities and older adults. The agency works to ensure that individuals with disabilities and the elderly can live where they choose, with the people they want, and that they can fully participate in their communities. Programs also support family caregivers, address issues of elder abuse, address the needs of American Indians, provide community services, and offer individualized support for individuals with disabilities.[12]
- The **Agency for Healthcare Research and Quality** supports research to improve the quality of health care, minimize its costs, ensure patient safety, respond to medical errors, and increase access to essential services.[12]
- The **Agency for Toxic Substances and Disease Registry** is responsible for prevention of exposure to toxic substances and the resulting health problems and reduced quality of life due to exposure to harmful substances from waste sites, unplanned releases, and other causes of environmental pollution.[12]

- The **Centers for Disease Control and Prevention (CDC)** is the leading public health institute in the United States. Its primary goal is to protect public health and safety through the control and prevention of disease, injury, and disability. The CDC focuses on infectious disease, foodborne pathogens, environmental health, occupational safety and health, health promotion, injury prevention, and public education to improve the health of U.S. citizens.[12]
- The **Centers for Medicare and Medicaid Services** administers several programs, including the Medicare program, and works with state governments to administer Medicaid, the State Children's Health Insurance Program, and health insurance portability standards.[12] (Portability means that when individuals change or lose their job, if they have a preexisting medical condition, they can still get health insurance.)
- Medicare provides health insurance for U.S. workers aged 65 years and older who have paid into the system. Medicare also provides health insurance to younger people with disabilities, end-stage renal disease, and amyotrophic lateral sclerosis.

  Medicaid is an insurance program for persons of all ages whose income and resources are insufficient to pay for health care.

  The State Children's Health Insurance Program provides matching funds to states for health insurance to families with children. The program covers uninsured children in families with modest incomes that are too high to qualify for Medicaid.[12]
- The **Food and Drug Administration** ensures that food is safe, pure, and wholesome; human and animal drugs, biological products, and medical devices are safe and effective; and electronic products that emit radiation are safe.[12]
- The **Health Resources and Services Administration** is the agency responsible for improving access to healthcare services for uninsured, isolated, or medically vulnerable individuals, including people living with HIV/acquired immunodeficiency syndrome (AIDS), and pregnant women, mothers, and children. This department supports the training of health professionals and works to improve rural health care. It also oversees organ, bone marrow, and cord blood donation. It supports programs that prepare against bioterrorism, compensates individuals harmed by vaccination, and works to protect against healthcare malpractice and healthcare waste, fraud, and abuse.[12]
- The **Indian Health Service** provides American Indians and Alaska Natives with comprehensive health services by developing and managing programs to meet their health needs.[12]
- The **National Institutes of Health** (NIH) is the premier health research organization in the United States. This agency supports biomedical and behavioral research within the United States and abroad, trains researchers, and promotes collecting and sharing of medical knowledge. The NIH both conducts its own scientific research and provides significant biomedical research funding to other research facilities.[12]

  The NIH is composed of 27 institutes and centers, each with a specific research agenda, often organized by particular diseases or body systems, such as the National Cancer Institute, National Institute of Allergy and Infectious Diseases, or by population such as the National Institute on Minority Health and Health Disparities. A full description of the scope of each institute is available at the NIH's website (www.nih.gov/institutes-nih/list-nih-institutes-centers-offices).[13]

Agency for Toxic Substances and Disease Registry The operating division within the Department of Health and Human Services that is responsible for prevention of exposure to toxic substances and the resulting health problems and reduced quality of life due to exposure to harmful substances from waste sites, unplanned releases, and other causes of environmental pollution.

Centers for Disease Control and Prevention (CDC). The operating division within the Department of Health and Human Services that protects public health and safety through the control and prevention of disease, injury, and disability.

Centers for Medicare and Medicaid Services. The operating division within the Department of Health and Human Services that administers several programs, including the Medicare program, and works with state governments to administer Medicaid, the State Children's Health Insurance Program, and health insurance portability standards.

Food and Drug Administration The operating division within the Department of Health and Human Services that ensures that food is safe, pure, and wholesome; human and animal drugs, biological products, and medical devices are safe and effective; and electronic products that emit radiation are safe.

Health Resources and Services Administration The operating division within the Department of Health and Human Services that is responsible for improving access to healthcare services for uninsured, isolated, or medically vulnerable individuals, including people living with HIV/AIDS, and pregnant women, mothers, and children.

Indian Health Service The operating division within the Department of Health and Human Services that provides American Indians and Alaska Natives with comprehensive health services by developing and managing programs to meet their health needs.

National Institutes of Health The operating division within the Department of Health and Human Services that supports biomedical and behavioral research within the United States and abroad, trains researchers, and promotes collecting and sharing of medical knowledge.

Substance Abuse and Mental Health Services Administration The operating division within the Department of Health and Human Services that improves the quality and availability of prevention, treatment, and rehabilitative services.

National Science Foundation An independent federal agency whose mission is "to promote the progress of science; to advance the national health, prosperity, and welfare; [and] to secure the national defense."

- The **Substance Abuse and Mental Health Services Administration** improves the quality and availability of prevention, treatment, and rehabilitative services. The agency aims to reduce illness, death, disability, and the cost to society resulting from substance abuse and mental health disorders. It also supports programs and services to families and communities.[12]

The National Science Foundation. The **National Science Foundation** is an independent federal agency whose mission is "to promote the progress of science; to advance the national health, prosperity, and welfare; [and] to secure the national defense." The National Science Foundation funds research and education in most fields of science and engineering. Its goals are discovery, learning, research infrastructure, and stewardship.[14]

State Health Agencies

Each U.S. state and territory has a health department. Visit the following site, provided by the CDC, for a link to each state's health department: www.cdc.gov/mmwr/international/relres.html.

In 1988, the National Academy of Medicine (at the time called the Institute of Medicine) issued a report titled, *The Future of Public Health,* to ensure that public health programs are efficient and effective. State health departments, whose purpose is to promote, protect, and maintain the health and welfare of their citizens, embraced the core functions of public health. There are three core functions: assessment, policy development, and assurance. Within each function are essential public health services that help health departments fulfill their purpose.[15]

The 10 essential public health services are listed here and categorized under the appropriate core function[15]:

I. Assessment
   1. Track health status to identify and solve community health problems (e.g., vital statistics and health status of citizens).
   2. Study and investigate health problems and health hazards in the community (e.g., epidemiologic surveillance and laboratory support).

II. Policy development
   3. Inform, educate, and vest the people with the power to address health issues (e.g., health promotion campaigns and social marketing).
   4. Organize community partnerships and action to identify and solve health problems (e.g., facilitating community and project advisory groups to promote health).
   5. Advance policies and plans that support individual and community health efforts (e.g., leadership development and health system planning).

III. Assurance
   6. Enforce laws and regulations that protect health and ensure safety (e.g., enforcement of health codes for restaurants).

THE NATIONAL SCIENCE FOUNDATION GETS RESULTS!

In the past few decades, researchers funded by the National Science Foundation have won some 217 Nobel Prizes.[14]

7. Connect people to needed personal health services and ensure the provision of health care when otherwise unavailable (e.g., increase access to care).
8. Guarantee a competent public and personal healthcare workforce (e.g., education and training for all public healthcare providers).
9. Assess the effectiveness, accessibility, and quality of personal and population-based health services (e.g., continuous evaluation of programs).
10. Investigate innovative solutions to health problems (e.g., links with academic institutions and capacity building).

State public health agencies often have divisions that are responsible for the following areas:

- Administration
- Communicable disease prevention and control
- Vital statistics
- Public health nursing
- Health education or promotion
- Maternal and child health
- Mental health
- Occupational and industrial health
- Laboratory services
- Health services
- Veterinary public health

Depending on the size of the state, the budget, and state politics, sometimes the areas are combined.

Local Health Departments

Your local health department is part of the city or county where you live. For most people, especially those living outside the major cities, county health departments provide the public health services to their population. County health departments inspect restaurants and public buildings for cleanliness, collect information on births and deaths in the population, dispense immunizations, and are responsible for reporting certain infectious diseases.

Quasi-Governmental Organizations

Quasi-governmental health agencies receive funding from both public and private sources. They perform functions expected of government agencies without government supervision. Because federal bureaucracies have a tendency to grow over time, one reason to create a **quasi-governmental organization** is that it avoids creating another bureaucracy. It encourages agencies to develop new sources of revenues and exempts the organization from the laws that govern central management, especially personnel and compensation laws. Another reason is to allow management flexibility, even at the cost of less accountability to representative institutions.[16]

Although there are quasi-governmental organizations in areas other than health, the main health-related organization is the **American Red Cross**. The American Red Cross is a humanitarian organization that provides emergency assistance and disaster relief; blood and blood product donation and distribution; services for military members and their families; educational programs on preparedness, health, and safety; and international relief and development. It responds to more than 65,000 disasters every year or about one every 8 minutes.

quasi-governmental organization An agency that receives funding from both public and private sources. They perform functions expected of government agencies without government supervision.

American Red Cross A humanitarian organization that provides emergency assistance and disaster relief; blood and blood product donation and distribution; services for military members and their families; educational programs on preparedness, health, and safety; and international relief and development.

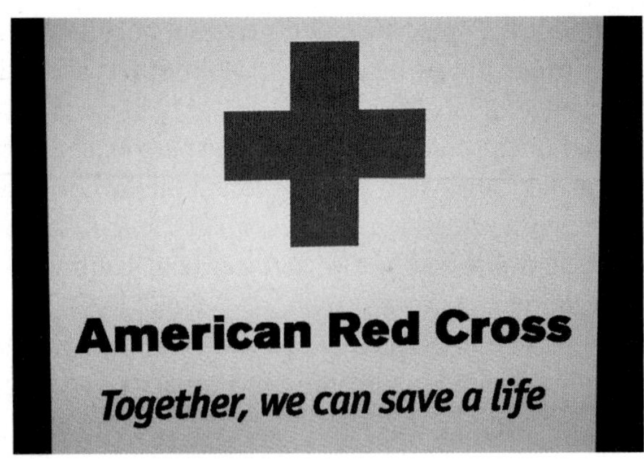

© 360b/Shutterstock.

It is also the nation's largest blood collection organization. The American Red Cross supplies approximately 40% of the country's blood and blood products.[17]

Nongovernmental Organizations

nongovernmental organizations (NGOs) A not-for-profit organization that is independent from states and international governmental organizations. They are usually funded by donations, but some avoid formal funding altogether and are run primarily by volunteers.

Nongovernmental organizations (NGOs) are funded mainly by private donations. In the field of public health, these entities often deliver public health services. There are 1.5 million NGOs in the United States, of which more than 102,000 focus on health issues. NGOs date from the time of the French Revolution[18] and have had a critical role in public health. Some are well known, like the American Cancer Society, the American Lung Association, and the American Diabetes Association.

The focus of many nonprofit agencies is health, including about 60% of community hospitals, all community health centers, and an estimated 17% of home healthcare agencies. Nonprofit health plans serve at least 40% of all private health insurance enrollees.[19]

TALES OF PUBLIC HEALTH

A Nongovernmental Organization Wins the 1999 Nobel Peace Prize[20]

Médecins Sans Frontières (Doctors Without Borders) is a private, international NGO. The association provides assistance to populations in distress, to victims of natural or man-made disasters, and to victims of armed conflict, irrespective of race, religion, creed, or political convictions. It treats patients with dignity and with respect for their cultural and religious beliefs. Doctors Without Borders gives priority to those in the gravest and most immediate danger. Its work spans the globe, including Africa, Asia, the Middle East, the Caribbean, and Central America. In 2015, over 30,000 mostly local

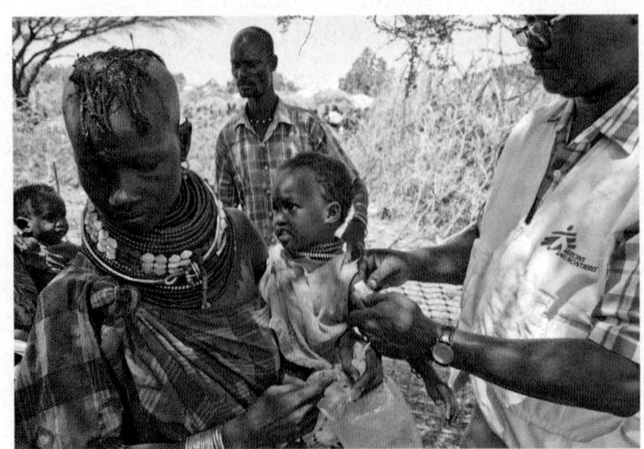

Nigeria 2010 © John Heeneman/MSF.

doctors, nurses, and other medical professionals, logistical experts, water and sanitation engineers, and administrators provided medical aid in over 70 countries.

In 1999, Doctors Without Borders received the Nobel Peace Prize for its "pioneering humanitarian work on several continents." In his acceptance speech on behalf of Doctors Without Borders, Dr. James Orbinski, then president of the organization, discussed the victims of the Rwandan genocide. During this period, hundreds of people came to the hospital every day. The hospital was so crowded that patients lay in the streets. In his speech, the doctor described the gutters as running red with blood. He spoke of one of his patients in particular:

> She was one among many—living an inhuman and simply indescribable suffering. We could do little more for her at that moment than stop the bleeding with a few necessary sutures. We were completely overwhelmed, and she knew that there were so many others.... She said to me in the clearest voice I have ever heard, "Allez, allez... ummera, ummera-sha"—"Go, go... my friend; find and let live your courage."

Dr. Orbinski affirmed the right to humanitarian assistance and of the road the organization has taken: to remain outspoken, passionate, and deeply committed to its core principles of volunteerism, impartiality, and its belief that every person deserves both medical assistance and the recognition of his or her humanity.

Professional Health Organizations

Professional health organizations' members are health professionals who have completed degrees and/or training programs and have met the qualifications required by their discipline. The missions of these organizations are often to improve health and strengthen the discipline. The American Public Health Association, which represents all fields that come under the public health umbrella, has more than 25,000 members, including public health researchers, educators, and advocates. The American Medical Association (AMA) represents doctors of medicine, doctors of osteopathic medicine, and medical students in the United States. In 2013, the AMA had approximately 228,000 members.[21] The National Medical Association is the largest and oldest national organization representing African American physicians and their patients in the United States, with more than 30,000 African American physicians as members.[22] The American Academy of Pediatrics is the professional association of pediatricians. It has 64,000 members in primary care and subspecialty areas.[23] The American Academy of Family Physicians was instrumental in establishing family medicine as a recognized medical specialty and has approximately 125,000 members.[24] There are hundreds of other professional organizations in the United States.

Improving Social Determinants of Health

Our health status is intricately related to our society, including dimensions such as the healthcare system, academic and occupational settings, economic productivity, social welfare expenditures, public safety, and criminal justice systems. Good health enhances society. When many members of the population are in poor health, that fact affects the functioning of communities and institutions within the society. It is imperative for public health to address problems in the most comprehensive manner possible. We must identify and champion strategies that will improve health and behavioral health status. These strategies should occur at all the levels of the social-ecological model—individual, community, and society.

Comparing the performance of the U.S. healthcare system with those of other countries can help highlight areas of competence and weakness, and assist in determining areas that hinder or help improvement. Briefly, we will compare data from 13 high-income countries: Australia, Canada, Denmark, France, Germany, Japan, the Netherlands, New Zealand, Norway, Sweden, Switzerland, the United Kingdom, and the United States. Because of the length of time it takes for data to be collected, analyzed, and made publicly available, almost all data are for years before the major insurance provisions of the Affordable Care Act (ACA) in the United States; most are for 2013.[25]

What the United States spends on health care greatly exceeds the expenses of other high-income countries. It isn't just that the United States has the most expensive health care, but it is also the least effective.[26] Even before the ACA, the United States was spending more on health care than most other countries. If the ratio between public health spending and health care spending was the same in 2014 as it was in 2009, the United States spent about $300 per person on public health and more than $9,500 per person on medical care in 2014.[27] Much of the spending of U.S. healthcare dollars is on expensive technologies like magnetic resonance imaging machines.[28] In comparison, only a small portion of the economy goes to social services, such as housing assistance, employment programs, and disability benefits.[29]

Of all the countries in the comparison and despite its larger investment in health, the United States has the lowest life expectancy, the highest infant mortality rate, the highest percentage of people older than 65 years with two or more chronic conditions, and the highest rate of obesity. Comparison data can be seen in Table 14-2. The only health measure in which the United States does better than most of the other high-income countries is the percentage of population 15 years and older who are daily smokers. (The U.S. has the third lowest percentage of smokers.)

Because we spend so much money on health care, we have less to spend on social services. These services contribute to society's health and well-being and help eliminate health disparities. In particular, countries where there was a higher ratio of social services spending compared to healthcare spending had lower infant mortality rates and longer life expectancy.[30,31] Another way is to look at how we spend our health dollars. In the United States, we spend a trillion dollars annually on health care. Approximately 95% of that goes to direct medical care and about 5% to prevention efforts.[32] Forty percent of deaths are due to behaviors that prevention efforts might have the ability to change. But only 10% to 15% of deaths could be avoided with more or better-quality medical care. The obvious answer to this set of facts is that we need to reprioritize how our society spends its healthcare dollars and focus more on disease and injury prevention.

Determinants of Health

Many things influence the health of an individual, including genetics, the environment, behavioral choices, medical care, and the social context in which we live. The genes you inherited from your parents directly relate to only about 2% of deaths. Other diseases such as diabetes, cancer, and cardiovascular diseases also have a genetic component.[33,34] There were, on average 178,700 deaths annually from 2000 to 2014 due to environmental causes.[35] The causes of death include traffic fatalities, falls, fires, extremes of temperature, assault, and poisoning. Some of these deaths were due to structural hazards, but all contribute to the overall burden of mortality. Adding illness or disability due to environmental causes would increase the number significantly.

There was a time when improvements in medical care had an enormous impact on health—for example, the discovery of antibiotics. But currently, in the United States, the use of medical care has a surprisingly limited impact on reducing deaths. Some medical professionals realize that there is a need to put more emphasis on preventive medicine, because until the behavioral issues are addressed, drugs and medical interventions are doing little to change the causes of death.

Behavioral choices people make have the largest influence on health. Every day we choose what we eat, whether we exercise, if we overuse legal and illegal drugs, how attentive we are to safety, and how well we cope with stress, all of which are important determinants of health.[32] However, these choices and most diseases are complex and are embedded in a larger social context.[36] Education, employment, poverty (or having sufficient income), housing, crime rates where you live, and the neighborhood and its cohesion all have a powerful impact on health. Having a connection to other people is an important health predictor. Individuals who are socially isolated are two to five times more likely to die than those who have a community of individuals around them.[37] This finding is even more true among patients who have severe chronic diseases.[38]

So Why Aren't We Redirecting Healthcare Dollars to Prevention?

Previously, there was a lack of consensus about how to address behavioral choices, social conditions, and the physical environment. In 2000, the National Academy of Medicine published a book examining social, behavioral, and clinical interventions backed by scientific evidence about effectiveness.[39]

We know that some prevention efforts have resulted in huge public health gains. Childhood vaccines are extremely effective at preventing a broad range of childhood diseases, some of which have devastating consequences. Policies aimed at reducing exposure to tobacco smoke, including raising taxes, increased enforcement of not selling to minors, and smoking restrictions in many public places, have significantly reduced the number of people who smoke. Broadly advertised benefits of physical activity combined with increased walking and biking paths have encouraged more people to exercise.

A Social-Ecological Approach to Health and Health Interventions

As previously discussed, the social-ecological model explains the interaction between the individual, the community, and the physical, social, and political environments.[40–42] The dynamic interaction among the levels of the model helps explain the differences in health among various populations. It is important to remember that the model is dynamic, recognizing that personal choices and family, institutional, community, and societal priorities change over the course of an individual's life.

As noted in the National Academy of Medicine book *Promoting Health*, things that happen at a societal level are critical determinants of health.[39] Many people share risk factors (stress, insufficient income, poor social support, poor diet, environmental exposures, etc.). Thus, strategies that help prevent diseases at the community or society level will be more cost-effective than those made at the individual level. Many populations share risks within their society or community, making health-promotion efforts at those levels more efficient. Another reason for a higher-level approach is that many individual-level behavioral interventions have not been terribly successful. Asking people to change behaviors is asking a lot. The success of an intervention requires people to do things that they have not been doing and to stop doing things that they have been doing. There are many individual, interpersonal, family, and cultural behaviors that are part of people's everyday lives. For a program focused on disease prevention and health promotion to be successful, it must fit within the circumstances in which people live.

For disease prevention and health promotion programs to be successful, they should broadly address the social and behavioral determinants of disease, injury, and disability. Approaches should address multiple levels within the social-ecological model simultaneously. They should also employ a variety of avenues, such as education and social support. Programs must be mindful of target groups and tailor approaches to their needs. Working in tandem with sectors of society (law, justice, education, the media) that are not traditionally part of public health has been successful in the past and likely will be so in the future.

Advocacy and Community Organizations

Achieving optimum health of a population requires an artful combination of preventing disease and disability while caring for those with diseases. Because there is a finite amount of resources, achieving the correct balance is difficult. Policy and political priorities often overtake equity and efficiency.

Community-Based Organizations

community-based organizations Organizations, often led by community members themselves, that provide numerous programs and services for the betterment of the community.

Community-based organizations, which are often led by community members themselves, are important because they provide numerous programs and services to the community. Often the recipients are marginalized and disadvantaged; that is, society has put them in a position of powerlessness.[43] Because these organizations often grow out of the community, they are integral to the community and understand and are connected to the community.[44] Community-based organizations often function as advocates for the population with which they work. The organizations work with policy and decision makers to promote programs and services for their community.

The essential organizational features of community-based organizations are fluid. Community organizations are geographically based and represent the residents.[45] They should be volunteer-driven, spring from the community, and be flexible. Other essential characteristics of community-based organizations include that they are organized to some degree, private (nongovernmental), nonprofit, and self-governing.[46]

Community-based organizations must be financially and socially supported to improve the health systems in which they work. The goal is for these community-based organizations to turn research into advocacy and action to participate in research.

Community-based participatory research is one approach to addressing the complex health, social, and environmental problems on which community-based organizations focus. This method is a collaborative approach to research that involves all partners in the research process (trained researchers, community members, advocates, etc.). Each partner brings its own perspective, strengths, and expertise to the research question.[47] The focus of this research is often on influencing policy and practice.

Advocacy

advocacy Strategic use of the news and other media outlets to advance a public health policy agenda.

The history of public health **advocacy** demonstrates that there will likely always be some people who oppose new ideas. We know that seat belt use saves lives. When laws mandating seat belts were enacted, there was opposition from people who felt seat belt laws infringed on their individual liberty and from people who claimed proponents overestimated the benefits of seat belts. The tobacco industry strongly opposed controls and supported scientists who discredited findings of tobacco's harmfulness.[48]

Public health advocacy strategically uses the news and other media outlets to advance a public health policy agenda. The goal is to craft a story, so the message builds public support and influences politicians to change or enact laws and fund interventions that improve the public's health.[49] Using the media for advocacy has been applied to promoting HIV testing,[50] obesity prevention,[51] and physical activity,[52] and in discussing the link between food insecurity and health disparities.[53]

Media advocacy is not always successful, however. Researchers analyzed data from the CDC's National Behavioral Risk Factor Surveillance System from 1993 to 2007 combined with content analysis to estimate how well HIV/AIDS newspaper coverage predicted later HIV testing behavior. They found that as press coverage increased, fewer people got tested for HIV—the exact opposite of what public health advocates hoped to achieve.[50]

To successfully advocate for a public health policy, you must plan strategically. The following are 10 essential questions a public health advocate should be able to answer[49]:

1. *What are your public health objectives with this issue?* You must understand the importance of what you want to change or safeguard.
2. *Can there be a "win-win" outcome for both the public health advocate and the decision maker (the politician or government official)?*[49] Politicians want the public to view them as leaders. As an advocate, you should work with government officials to help them understand that helping you helps them as well. Keep criticism of the official private.
3. *How do you influence key decision makers?* All up and down the political (or organizational) structure, people are answerable to others: to the electorate or others in the system. As an advocate, you need to understand that access and influence go beyond the immediate person you are trying to reach.
4. *What are the strengths and weaknesses of your and your opposition's position (assuming there is an opposition)?*[49] You must think carefully about your position and all the aspects of it. You must also understand your opposition's position. Be self-critical. If you must present in public, rehearse the worst questions you may face and practice making your most compelling arguments.

   During an interview, think carefully before you answer a question. Have three main points you want to make and stick to those. Do not get into an argument with the interviewer.
5. *What decision(s) do you want to change or influence?*[49] Your activities, such as media campaigns and public speaking, should always serve the public health objective(s) you are trying to meet.
6. *How will you frame what is at issue here?*[49] Framing is a way to present a problem or issue. Framing includes explaining and describing the problem so that you get the most support from your audience. Knowing who the people in your audience are is crucial. The way you describe the problem, or frame it, should attend to the attitudes and beliefs of your audience. It is a core skill to help people figure out why they should support your position.

   An example of framing in a recent public health debate can be found in the controversy over whether parents should have their children immunized for measles, mumps, and rubella. Realize that immunizations rarely cause serious complications and are mainly limited to local reactions. A doctor in England first put forth the idea that this vaccination caused autism. This doctor was later found to have used false data and has been widely discredited.[54] But people who have a child with autism are looking for an explanation. (Autism is a developmental disorder in which the child has trouble communicating and understanding what people think and feel. Thus, individuals with autism often do not respond to others' touch, facial expressions, or body language.) Because of the way the doctor framed his idea regarding the measles, mumps, and rubella vaccination, a segment of the population believes that this vaccination caused their child's autism. The people who believe in the doctor's claims overemphasize the risk of the vaccine and underemphasize the risk of measles, mumps, and rubella. So that you understand this idea isn't correct, measles vaccine is very safe; it causes acute encephalitis about once in a million doses. In contrast, about 1 in 1,000 people who do not receive the vaccination will get measles. Severe complications from measles include pneumonia and encephalitis (swelling of the brain).[55]

7. *What symbols or word pictures can be brought into this frame?*[49] Because people's attention span for news stories is short, the goal is to leave a lasting impression with the public. Many public health issues seem too technical and boring to those not involved with the matter. To engage the public, associate the change you would like to happen with ideas that people already like and value. For example, if there is a vacant lot that you would like the city to donate to your group, promote turning it into a public park with ideas about using it as a place where activities for community children can be held and friends can gather.
8. *What sound bites can be used to convey agenda items 6 and 7?* Because the news cycle is short, powerful sound bites are critical. As the Berkeley Media Study Group says, "They make us stop and reflect on an issue, and they stay in our heads long after the news cycle has moved on to the next big thing."[56]

   As an example, Nicholas Kristof, an op-ed journalist from the *New York Times,* wrote the following: "To protect the public, we regulate toys and mutual funds, ladders, and swimming pools. Shouldn't we regulate guns as seriously as we regulate toys?"[57] This sound bite is effective because it compares a controversial issue to a familiar issue, making it common sense.
9. *Can the issue be personalized?*[49] Giving a human face to the story helps the public identify with it.
10. *How can large numbers of people be quickly organized to express their concerns?*[49] Politicians are concerned about what their constituents think and feel about an issue. Using the Internet allows for mass dissemination. Providing the public with an email template describing the problem, providing relevant information, and suggesting the desired action is a quick way to mobilize thousands of people.

Advocacy, public health policy, your community, and where you live all matter. The environment in which you live, including the housing conditions, the air quality, and the water quality, affects your health. Public health policies that focus on reducing the gaps in the social determinants of health represent necessary changes to ensure everyone is as healthy as possible. In addition to policy, change can occur at a personal level. With effort, you can make positive changes that will improve your health.

Change for Health

When it comes to health recommendations, we have all heard similar messages:

- Aim to exercise at least 30 minutes a day.
- Walk at least 10,000 steps a day.
- Eat a varied and nutritious diet, including plenty of fresh fruits and vegetables daily.
- Maintain your body mass index at between 18.5 and 24.9.
- Get enough sleep.
- Get the screenings your healthcare professional recommends: blood pressure; cholesterol; blood sugar; for women, mammograms and Pap smears, as recommended.
- Don't smoke.
- Limit alcohol to one drink per day.
- Reduce stress, improve relationships, and develop new interests.

Behavior change is hard, and some people find it harder than others. Even individuals with a strong intention to change a behavior are only successful about 50% of the time.[58] Positive, informative strategies that people can use to set specific health goals are more effective in helping people change behavior than fear, guilt, or regret.[59]

A behavioral researcher at Stanford University, Dr. B. J. Fogg, developed an approach to behavior change. His theory says that for behavior to change, three elements must come together at the same time[60]:

Behavior = Motivation × Ability × Trigger, abbreviated B = MAT

All three elements are necessary for most behaviors to change. Things that occur above the action line (**FIGURE 16-3**) happen, while things that occur below the action line do not. If we suggest that you do something hard, like performing a big trick on the flying trapeze (Search "Triple Twisting Double Layout - Flying Trapeze" on YouTube), and you are afraid of heights, you will feel minimal motivation to do it; thus, it likely won't happen, even with a trigger. Similarly, if we suggest you walk around the block, even with little motivation it is easy enough to do, and it is therefore likely to happen.

The goal is to create positive health habits. Dr. Fogg suggests that there are two important parts to help make this happen. One part is to start small. Don't start out deciding to do 100 push-ups. If you don't already do them regularly, a goal of 100 is likely too physically challenging. Start with a small number and

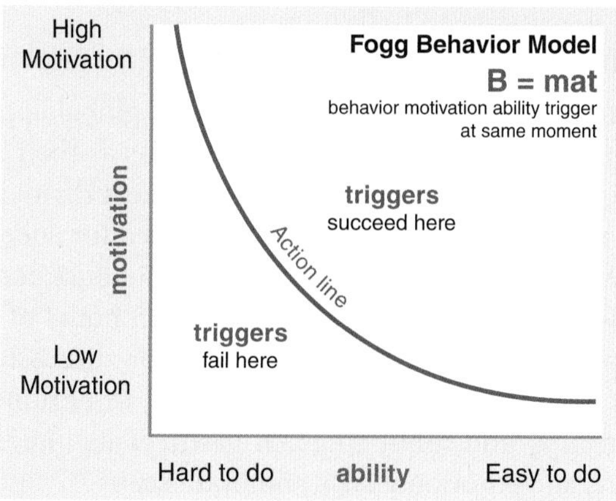

FIGURE 16-3 Fogg Behavior Model.

BJ Fogg. (2007). [Graphic Illustration of the Fogg Behavior Model]. BJ Fogg's Behavior Model. Retrieved from http://behaviormodel.org/

congratulate yourself when you succeed. Tiny steps are easier than huge ones. The other part of the idea is to develop triggers for your behavior. As Dr. Fogg describes in his TED Talk (www.foggmethod.com), developing triggers for your behavior makes the behavior change easier. The trigger does not have to be logically linked to the behavior, but it does need to be something that you regularly do. Dr. Fogg started out doing two push-ups every time after he peed. As he did more, the push-ups got easier, so that now he is doing eight every time he pees, resulting in many push-ups over the course of a day.[61]

How Technology May Help Change Behavior

People can use technology to help change a health behavior, either to take away a bad one or to create a new one. One device markets itself as smart technology to break bad behavior.[62] This device uses a variety of stimuli (vibration, beep, tap, or zap) to train your brain to create a negative association of the stimuli with the behavior you want to change, including smoking, nail biting, overeating or unhealthy eating, and overspending. Another device is worn like a pager.[63] You choose a word, phrase, or image that will remind you what behavior you want to change. Every time this device vibrates, you are supposed to think about your personal message. You program the frequency with which you want the device to vibrate, or you can set it to vibrate at random intervals. A similar device was designed for students with attention problems and has no display to distract the wearer.[64] This device uses a vibration to remind the wearer to get back to the task at hand. Yet another device uses a gyroscope (a gyroscope is a device that uses the earth's gravity to help determine orientation) to measure the user's posture and track the person's activity.[65] [The authors have not personally tried any of these devices. Please do not take this description as an endorsement of any of them.] These gadgets are not without their critics. Physicians are less comfortable with do-it-yourself options and encourage professional oversight.

Many people use a fitness tracker to motivate them to exercise. Some work independently, and others use smart technology in combination with a smartphone to encourage users during workouts and record their fitness routine. A 2016 study compared four randomly chosen fitness trackers.[66] What the tracker measures varies depending on the device, but likely includes distance, step counting, calories, fitness analytics, and goal tracking. Although there are many options available, given the growth of the industry, the future will likely bring even more, with an estimate for 2017 of 90 million fitness trackers shipped.[67] Some research shows that fitness trackers significantly increased activity over the use of a pedometer.[68]

We May Be More Capable of Changing Than You Think

A small but carefully done study examined a more global approach to behavior change. The research team chose college students as their subjects because they have relatively flexible schedules. The researchers divided the group into an intervention arm and a comparison arm, balanced for age, gender, and college grade point average. The intervention covered 5 hours per day, Monday to Friday, over a 6-week period. Each day included 2.5 hours of exercise, 1 hour of mindfulness practice, and a 1.5-hour lecture or discussion. The lecture/discussion topics included sleep, nutrition, exercise, mindfulness, compassion, gratitude, relationships, and well-being. All participants underwent a series of physical, cognitive, and emotional tests and brain scans.[69]

The intervention group was advised to eat a healthy diet, by limiting alcohol and carbohydrates not derived from produce, and to eat primarily whole foods. They were also supposed to sleep 8 to 10 hours per night. Their exercise routine was Pilates twice per week, yoga once per week, and body weight circuit training once per week. The students were offered an anatomy and movement workshop once per week. Twice during the intervention, each student met privately with an instructor. The intervention group was also supposed to complete high-intensity interval training twice per week and to engage in random acts of kindness each day. At the end of the 6-week period, the participants received no additional instruction or support. The approach for the comparison group was to live as usual.[69]

At the end of the intervention period, all of the preliminary tests were redone. The test results for the comparison group showed no changes over the 6-week period. The intervention group showed substantial improvement in physiology (stronger, fitter, and more flexible), cognition (improved on thinking, focus, and working memory), and affect (feeling happier, calmer, and higher self-esteem).[69]

The magnitude of the changes within the intervention group was more than 2.5 times that seen for mindfulness training alone. The researchers concluded that the results indicate that well-designed, multifaceted intervention can help make large improvements in health. Additionally, the authors suggest that one change may amplify the effects of another. Six weeks after the end of the study, the intervention group was not exercising or meditating as much as during intervention. They still scored higher than baseline on measures of fitness, mood, thinking skills, and well-being.[69]

Happiness

In the first chapter, we talked about the importance of happiness to your health. Happiness is a condition that you can work to create. It may surprise you to learn that happiness does not come from external factors. While you may be briefly happy with that perfect grade you got on a term paper or your new relationship, you will soon go back to your baseline level of happiness. Research has shown that being focused on external factors actually increases stress and depression.[70]

It is true that some people have naturally positive personalities, but even if you don't, you can build happiness skills.[71] Appreciating what you have is a simple way to boost optimism and reduce stress. You may have heard people describe a person's approach to life as the glass being "half empty or half full." This is a common measure of optimism (half full) or pessimism (half empty). Decide to view the glass as half full. While changing one's perspective is easier said than done, it is possible. Remind yourself of positive things and remember to be grateful for what you have. Be mindful and notice beautiful things around you. Regardless of what you are doing, try to make the feeling of happiness and enjoyment last. Dr. Fred Bryant, a professor at Loyola University, describes this process as "savoring."[72]

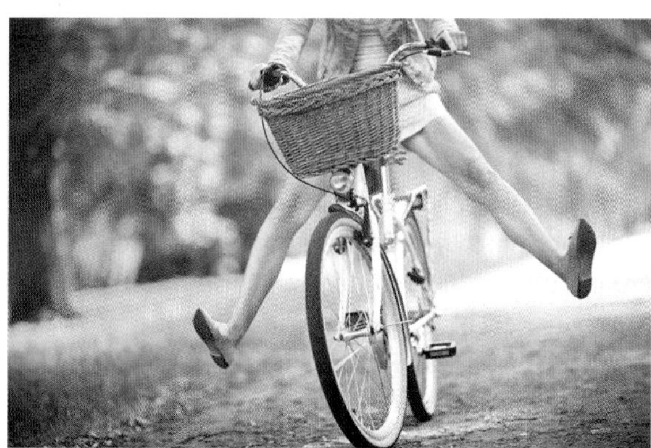

As part of appreciating what you have, Dr. Bryant has distilled his idea into 10 steps[72]:

1. Share your good feelings with others.
2. Take a mental photograph.
3. Congratulate yourself.
4. Get in touch with your senses (smell, taste, etc.).
5. When something good happens, express it joyfully.
6. Compare the current outcome to something worse.
7. Enjoy the moment.
8. Count your blessings and be thankful.
9. Avoid negative thinking.
10. Relish the present because time passes quickly.

Be Thankful

Gratitude is a positive response to the appreciation of others and what they do for us. Research shows that gratitude improves emotional and physical health, as well as bolsters relationships and communities. By appreciating others, we get kindness in return.[73] Research demonstrates that the practice of gratitude increases happiness and decreases depression. Dr. Robert Emmons, a professor of psychology at the University of California–Davis, recommends that writing a gratitude journal over a 3-week period will increase happiness for at least 6 months. The practice not only increases happiness by about 25% but also improves quality of sleep.[73]

Strive

Working to create a meaningful life makes people happy.[74] Being optimistic attracts other people, so that not only do you feel better, but you also reduce your stress and increase self-esteem. You will have an easier time attaining your goals so that you will feel successful, and you will be more successful. A person's level of hope correlates with how well he or she manages tasks. This approach to life also makes people healthier. A 2007 study that followed more than 6,000 people for 20 years found that a sense of hopefulness and enthusiasm reduced the risk of coronary heart disease. The protective effect was real, even when considering smoking and exercise.[75]

Believing that your goals are obtainable promotes a sense of meaning and purpose in life—a key ingredient of happiness.[74,75]

Empathize

Empathy is the ability to put yourself in someone else's shoes. It is the capacity to care genuinely about others, to imagine and understand how others think and feel, including when it is different from how we would naturally feel. The ability to empathize makes us less judgmental, less frustrated, less angry, and more patient. If you listen to others' points of view, they are likely to reciprocate. Friends don't always have to agree with one another, but it is important to acknowledge your friend's point of view.

The ability to listen to others helps strengthen the bonds of friendship. According to Dr. Emma Seppala, the Associate Director of the Center for Compassion and Altruism Research and Education at Stanford University's School of Medicine, people are hardwired for empathy. Practicing this type of understanding will help nurture your relationships with others.[76]

Like happiness in general, compassion and empathy are skills we can learn.[77] In addition, there is self-compassion—that is, extending compassion to one's self in instances of perceived inadequacy, failure, or general suffering.[78] People who have more self-compassion lead healthier, more rewarding, and more productive lives than those who are self-critical.

Give

Psychologists have a term they call "helper's high." When individuals donate money, the part of the brain that controls reward reinforcement is activated. This area of the brain is involved in social bonding and releases "feel good" neurotransmitters. These neurotransmitters can be addictive (in a good way!) so that doing something beneficial for others makes the person feel good.[79] This is a somewhat complicated explanation of why when you give someone something or do something for someone, you reap benefits as well; in other words, kindness counts. A research team asked two groups of participants over a 6-week period to perform five acts of kindness each week either for themselves or for others. Those assigned to the group doing acts of kindness for themselves had a reduction in well-being, while those who did acts of kindness for others had a 42% increase in happiness.[80] Altruistic emotions and behaviors are associated with greater well-being, health, and longevity. When we give, we are more satisfied with our lives, and our physical health improves.[81] Giving connects us to other people, helps create stronger communities, and contributes to a happier and healthier society.

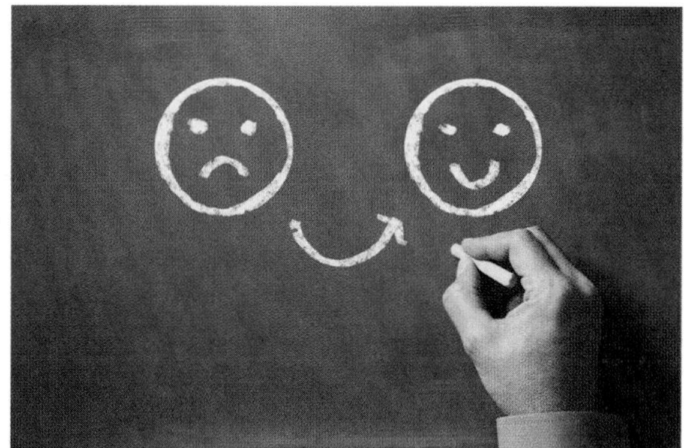

In Summary

The social-ecological model provides a broad framework for health. It describes the interaction between the individual, the community, and the physical, social, and political environments, and it explains how each of these factors has an impact on health. Additionally, you have read how these factors apply to many health issues.

Embracing diversity and cultural competence, both as an individual and within an organization, helps to reduce health disparities.

At every level of society, there are organizations that shape and protect your health, from international, to national, to state and local governments. In addition, quasi-governmental, nongovernmental, and professional organizations directly or indirectly affect your health.

A comparison of health measures in the United States to measures in other high-income countries helps to highlight areas of strength and weakness in our healthcare system. Our resources and efforts would be most beneficial if redirected toward prevention.

Community-based organizations can effectively improve the health of the people they serve. Public health advocacy strategically uses the available resources and knowledge to advance public health policy initiatives.

Changing one's behavior is hard but possible. You can employ tangible strategies to improve your happiness.[82]

Key Terms

Administration for Children and Families
Administration for Community Living
advocacy
Agency for Healthcare Research and Quality
Agency for Toxic Substances and Disease Registry
American Red Cross
Centers for Disease Control and Prevention (CDC)
Centers for Medicare and Medicaid Services
community-based organizations
cultural competence
Food and Drug Administration
governmental organizations
Health Resources and Services Administration
Indian Health Service
National Institutes of Health
National Science Foundation
nongovernmental organizations (NGOs)
quasi-governmental organization
social determinants of health
social-ecological model
Substance Abuse and Mental Health Services Administration
World Health Organization (WHO)

Student Discussion Questions and Activities

1. Pick a disease or health problem and apply the social-ecological model. Describe how each level within the model might impact the disease.
2. Choose a culture with which you are not familiar. Research the culture's language, religion, cuisine, social habits, customs, music, arts, beliefs, and values. Report on your findings. Is there a way to meet someone from this culture (perhaps another student)? If so, interview the person and describe what you have learned.
3. Select one of the institutes within the National Institutes of Health. Go to the institute's website and write a brief description of their mission and what they do.
4. Select a common U.S. health condition other than infant mortality, obesity, or percentage of smokers. See how the rates of the conditions compare with rates in other high-income countries. (Limit yourself to data available on the Internet.)
5. Choose a public health problem for which you would like to advocate. Imagine you are going to be interviewed about this topic. What are your three main points?
6. Write a gratitude journal every day for 3 weeks. You can include more than just big things. Being grateful for small things is effective, too.

References

1. Centers for Disease Control and Prevention. (2017). 2015 national diabetes statistics report. Retrieved from https://www.cdc.gov/media/releases/2017/p0718-diabetes-report.html
2. Sadeghi-Nejad, N. (2012, September 13). NYC's soda ban is a good idea, but a tax would be better. *Forbes*. Retrieved from https://www.forbes.com/sites/natesadeghi/2012/09/13/nycs-soda-ban-is-a-good-idea-but-a-tax-would-be-better/#c7d38642b3a4
3. NYC Health. (n.d.). Restaurant grades. Retrieved from http://www1.nyc.gov/site/doh/services/restaurant-grades.page
4. Grynbaum, M. M. (2014, June 24). New York's ban on big sodas is rejected by final court. *New York Times*.
5. Zimmerman, K. A. (2015, February 19). What is culture? Definition of culture. Live Science [website]. Retrieved from http://www.livescience.com/21478-what-is-culture-definition-of-culture.html
6. National Institutes of Health. (2017, February 15). Cultural respect. Retrieved from https://www.nih.gov/institutes-nih/nih-office-director/office-communications-public-liaison/clear-communication/cultural-respect
7. Cross, T. L., Bazron, B. J., Dennis, K. W., & Isaacs, M. R. (1989). *Towards a culturally competent system of care: A monograph on effective services for minority children who are severely emotionally disturbed.* Washington, DC: Georgetown University Child Development Center.

8. Denboba, D., U.S. Department of Health and Human Services, Health Services and Resources Administration. (1993). *MCHB/DSCSHCN guidance for competitive applications, maternal and child health improvement projects for children with special health care.* Retrieved from https://culturalcompetenceac.wordpress.com/definitions/
9. World Health Organization. (2016). Global guardian of public health. Retrieved from http://www.who.int/about/what-we-do/global-guardian-of-public-health.pdf
10. Remme, J. H. F., Feenstra, P., Lever, P. R., Medici, A. C., Morel, C. M., Noma, M., . . . Vassall, A. (2006). Tropical diseases targeted for elimination: Chagas disease, lymphatic filariasis, onchocerciasis, and leprosy. In D. T. Jamison, J. G. Breman, A. R. Measham, G. Alleyne, M. Claeson, D. B. Evans . . . P. Musgrove (Eds.), *Disease control priorities in developing countries* (2nd ed., pp. 433–450). New York, NY: Oxford University Press.
11. U.S. Department of Health and Human Services. (2018). HHS FY 2018 budget in brief. Retrieved from http://www.hhs.gov/about/budget/fy2018/budget-in-brief/index.html
12. U.S. Department of Health and Human Services. (2015). HHS agencies and offices. Retrieved from http://www.hhs.gov/about/agencies/hhs-agencies-and-offices/index.html
13. National Institutes of Health. (2017). List of NIH institutes, centers, and offices. Retrieved from https://www.nih.gov/institutes-nih/list-nih-institutes-centers-offices
14. National Science Foundation. (2017). The National Science Foundation: Where discovery begins—homepage. Retrieved from https://www.nsf.gov/
15. Institute of Medicine, Committee for the Study of the Future of Public Health, Division of Health Care Services. (1988). *The future of public health* (p. 225). Washington, DC: National Academy Press.
16. Kosar, K. R. (2011, June 22). The quasi government: Hybrid organizations with both government and private sector legal characteristics. Congressional Research Service. Retrieved from https://fas.org/sgp/crs/misc/RL30533.pdf
17. American Red Cross. (2016). Help those affected by disasters. Retrieved from http://www.redcross.org/what-we-do/blood-donation
18. Davies, T. (2014). *NGOs: A new history of transnational civil society* (p. 23). New York, NY: Oxford University Press.
19. Alliance for Advancing Nonprofit Health Care. (2016). The value of nonprofit health care. Retrieved from http://www.nonprofithealthcare.org/reports/5_value.pdf
20. NobelPrize.org. (1999). Médecins Sans Frontières—Nobel lecture. Retrieved from http://www.nobelprize.org/nobel_prizes/peace/laureates/1999/msf-lecture.html
21. Smith, E. (2015, February 27). Medical association: What's behind its membership surge. Associations Now. Retrieved from http://associationsnow.com/2015/02/medical-association-heres-whats-behind-our-member-surge/
22. National Medical Association. (2017). National Medical Association—homepage. Retrieved from http://www.nmanet.org/
23. American Academy of Pediatrics. (2017). About the AAP. Retrieved from https://www.aap.org/en-us/about-the-aap/Pages/About-the-AAP.aspx
24. American Academy of Family Physicians. (2017). American Academy of Family Physicians—homepage. Retrieved from http://www.aafp.org/home.html
25. Commonwealth Fund. (2015). U.S. health care from a global perspective: Spending, use of services, prices, and health in 13 countries. Retrieved from http://www.commonwealthfund.org/publications/issue-briefs/2015/oct/us-health-care-from-a-global-perspective
26. Bernstein, L. (2014, June 14). Once again, U.S. has most expensive, least effective health care system in survey. *The Washington Post.* Retrieved from https://www.washingtonpost.com/news/to-your-health/wp/2014/06/16/once-again-u-s-has-most-expensive-least-effective-health-care-system-in-survey/?noredirect=on&utm_term=.a69d71373044.
27. Centers for Medicaid and Medicare Services. (2015). National health expenditures 2015 highlights. Retrieved from https://www.cms.gov/research-statistics-data-and-systems/statistics-trends-and-reports/nationalhealthexpenddata/downloads/highlights.pdf
28. Bradley, E. H., & Taylor, L. A. (2013). *The American health care paradox: Why spending more is getting us less.* New York, NY: Public Affairs.
29. Squires, D., & Anderson, C. (2015). U.S. health care from a global perspective: Spending, use of services, prices, and health in 13 countries. *Issue Brief (Commonwealth Fund), 15,* 1–15.
30. Avendano, M., & Kawachi, I. (2014). Why do Americans have shorter life expectancy and worse health than do people in other high-income countries? *Annual Review of Public Health, 35,* 307–325.
31. Bradley, E. H., Elkins, B. R., Herrin, J., & Elbel, B. (2011). Health and social services expenditures: Associations with health outcomes. *BMJ Quality and Safety, 20*(10), 826–831.
32. McGinnis, J. M., Williams-Russo, P., & Knickman, J. R. (2002). The case for more active policy attention to health promotion. *Health Affairs, 21*(2), 78–93.
33. Strohman, R. C. (1993). Ancient genomes, wise bodies, unhealthy people: Limits of a genetic paradigm in biology and medicine. *Perspectives in Biology and Medicine, 37*(1), 112–145.
34. Baird, P. A. (1994). *The role of genetics in population health.* In R. G. Evans, M. L. Barer, & T. R. Marmor (Eds.), *Why are some people healthy and others not?* (pp. 133–159). New York, NY: Aldine de Gruyter.
35. Centers for Disease Control and Prevention. (2017). CDC Wonder. Retrieved from http://wonder.cdc.gov/
36. Baird, P. A. (2000). Genetic technologies and achieving health for populations. *International Journal of Health Services, 30*(2), 407–424.
37. Berkman, L. F., & Glass, T. (2000). Social integration, social networks, social support, and health. In L. F. Berkman & I. Kawachi (Eds.), *Social epidemiology* (pp. 137–173). New York, NY: Oxford University Press.
38. Rutledge, T., Reis, S. E., Olson, M., Owens, J., Kelsey, S. F., Pepine, C. J., . . . National Heart, Lung, and Blood Institute. (2004). Social networks are associated with lower mortality rates among women with suspected coronary disease: The National Heart, Lung, and Blood Institute-sponsored women's ischemia syndrome evaluation study. *Psychosomatic Medicine, 66*(6), 882–888.
39. Division of Health Promotion and Disease Prevention, Institute of Medicine. (2000). *Promoting health: Strategies from social and behavioral research* (Vol. 2016). Washington, DC: National Academies Press.
40. Israel, B. A., Schulz, A. J., Parker, E. A., Becker, A. B., Allen, A. J., & Guzman, J. R. (2003). Critical issues in developing and following community based participatory research principles. In M. Minkler & N. Wallerstein (Eds.), *Community-based participatory research for health* (pp. 53–76). San Francisco, CA: Jossey-Bass.
41. Sallis, J. F., Owen, N., & Fisher, E. B. (2008). Ecological models of health behavior. In M. Minkler, B. K. Rimer, & K. Viswanath

(Eds.), *Health behavior and health education* (4th ed., pp. 465–485). San Francisco, CA: John Wiley & Sons.
42. Wallerstein, N., & Duran, B. (2003). The conceptual, historical and practice roots of community-based participatory research and related participatory traditions. In M. Minkler & N. Wallerstein (Eds.), *Community-based participatory research for health* (pp. 27–52). San Francisco, CA: Jossey-Bass.
43. Carey, G. E., & Braunack-Mayer, A. J. (2009). Exploring the effects of government funding on community-based organizations: "Top-down" or "bottom-up" approaches to health promotion? *Global Health Promotion, 16*(3), 45–52.
44. Chillag, K., Bartholow, K., Cordeiro, J., Swanson, S., Patterson, J., Stebbins, S., . . . Sy, F. (2002). Factors affecting the delivery of HIV/AIDS prevention programs by community-based organizations. *AIDS Education and Prevention, 14*(3 Suppl A), 27–37.
45. Chavis, D. M., & Florin, P. (1990). Nurturing grassroots initiatives for health and housing. *Bulletin of the New York Academy of Medicine, 66*(5), 558–572.
46. Wilson, M. G., Lavis, J. N., & Guta, A. (2012). Community-based organizations in the health sector: A scoping review. *Health Research Policy and Systems, 10*(1), 36.
47. Cacari-Stone, L., Wallerstein, N., Garcia, A. P., & Minkler, M. (2014). The promise of community-based participatory research for health equity: A conceptual model for bridging evidence with policy. *American Journal of Public Health, 104*(9), 1615–1623.
48. Yerushalmy, J. (1973). Letter: Smoking in pregnancy. *Developmental Medicine and Child Neurology, 15*(5), 691–693.
49. Chapman, S. (2004). Advocacy for public health: A primer. *Journal of Epidemiology and Community Health, 58*(5), 361–365.
50. Stevens, R., & Hornik, R. C. (2014). AIDS in black and white: The influence of newspaper coverage of HIV/AIDS on HIV/AIDS testing among African Americans and White Americans, 1993–2007. *Journal of Health Communication, 19*(8), 893–906.
51. Millstein, R. A., & Sallis, J. F. (2011). Youth advocacy for obesity prevention: The next wave of social change for health. *Translational Behavioral Medicine, 1*(3), 497–505.
52. Richards, R., Murdoch, L., Reeder, A. I., & Amun, Q. T. (2011). Political activity for physical activity: Health advocacy for active transport. *International Journal of Behavioral Nutrition and Physical Activity, 8*, 52.
53. Rock, M. J., McIntyre, L., Persaud, S. A., & Thomas, K. L. (2011). A media advocacy intervention linking health disparities and food insecurity. *Health Education Research, 26*(6), 948–960.
54. Wakefield, A., Murch, S., Anthony, A., Linnell, J., Casson, D. M., Malik, M., . . . Walker-Smith, J. A. (1998). RETRACTED: Ileal-lymphoid-nodular hyperplasia, non-specific colitis, and pervasive developmental disorder in children. *Lancet, 351*(9103), 637–641.
55. Atkinson, W., Wolfe, C., & Hamborsky, J. (Eds). *Epidemiology and prevention of vaccine-preventable diseases* (12th ed.). Washington, DC: Public Health Foundation.
56. Gehlert, H. (2015, December 22). Top 10 public health media bites of 2015. Berkeley Media Studies Group. Retrieved from http://www.bmsg.org/blog/top-10-public-health-media-bites-2015
57. Kristof, N. (2015, August 26). Lessons from the Virginia shooting. *New York Times*. Retrieved from https://www.nytimes.com/2015/08/27/opinion/lessons-from-the-murders-of-tv-journalists-in-the-virginia-shooting.html
58. Orbell, S., & Sheeran, P. (1998). "Inclined abstainers": A problem for predicting health-related behaviour. *British Journal of Social Psychology*, 37(Pt 2), 151–165.
59. Sheeran, P., Maki, A., Montanaro, E., Avishai-Yitshak, A., Bryan, A., Klein, W. M., . . . Rothman, A. J. (2016). The impact of changing attitudes, norms, and self-efficacy on health-related intentions and behavior: A meta-analysis. *Health Psychology, 35*(11), 1178–1188.
60. Fogg, B. J. (2016). What causes behavioral change? B. J. Fogg's Behavior Model [website]. Retrieved from http://behaviormodel.org/
61. Fogg, B. J. (2013). Three steps to changing behavior. Fogg Method [website]. Retrieved from http://www.foggmethod.com/
62. Pavlok.com. (n.d.). Pavlok—break bad habits with classical Pavlovian conditioning. Retrieved from http://pavlok.com.ourssite.com/
63. MotivAider. (2017). The MotivAider in healthcare. Retrieved from http://habitchange.com/healthcare/index.php
64. RE-vibe. (2017). RE-vibe: Anti-distraction Wristwear. Retrieved from http://fokuslabs.com/
65. Lumo Bodytech. (2016). Lumo lift posture coach. Retrieved from http://www.lumobodytech.com/lumo-lift/
66. Kaewkannate, K., & Kim, S. (2016). A comparison of wearable fitness devices. *BMC Public Health, 16*(1), 433.
67. ABI Research. (2012). Wearable sports and fitness devices will hit 90 million shipments in 2017. Retrieved from https://www.abiresearch.com/press/wearable-sports-and-fitness-devices-will-hit-90-mi/
68. Cadmus-Bertram, L. A., Marcus, B. H., Patterson, R. E., Parker, B. A., & Morey, B. L. (2015). Randomized trial of a Fitbit-based physical activity intervention for women. *American Journal of Preventive Medicine, 49*(3), 414–418.
69. Mrazek, M. D., Mooneyham, B W., Mrazek, K. L., & Schooler, J. W. (2016). Pushing the limits: Cognitive, affective, and neural plasticity revealed by an intensive multifaceted intervention. *Frontiers in Human Neuroscience, 10*, 117.
70. Auerbach, R. P., Webb, C. A., Schreck, M., McWhinnie, C. M., Ringo Ho, M.-H., Zhu, X., & Yao, S. (2011). Examining the pathway through which intrinsic and extrinsic aspirations generate stress and subsequent depressive symptoms. *Journal of Social and Clinical Psychology, 30*(8), 856–886.
71. Gander, F., Proyer, R. T., & Ruch, W. (2016). Positive psychology interventions addressing pleasure, engagement, meaning, positive relationships, and accomplishment increase well-being and ameliorate depressive symptoms: A randomized, placebo-controlled online study. *Frontiers in Psychology, 7*, 686.
72. Kennelly, S. (2012, July 23). 10 steps to savoring the good things in life. Greater Good [website]. Retrieved from http://greatergood.berkeley.edu/article/item/10_steps_to_savoring_the_good_things_in_life
73. Emmons, R. A. (2008). *Thanks! How the art of gratitude can make you happier.* New York, NY: Mariner Books.
74. Steger, M. F., Kashdan, T. B., & Oishi, S. (2008). Being good by doing good: Daily eudaimonic activity and well-being. *Journal of Research in Personality, 42*(1), 22–42.
75. Kubzansky, L. D., & Thurston, R. C. (2007). Emotional vitality and incident coronary heart disease: Benefits of healthy psychological functioning. *Archives of General Psychiatry, 64*(12), 1393–1401.
76. BeWell Stanford. (n.d.). Compassion's curative powers. Retrieved from http://web.stanford.edu/group/bewell/cgi-bin/bewell-wp/compassions-curative-power/
77. Davidson, R. J., & Begley, S. (2012). *The emotional life of your brain: How its unique patterns affect the way you think, feel and*

live—and how you can change them. New York, NY: Hudson St. Press.

78. Neff, K. D., & Germer, C. K. (2013). A pilot study and randomized controlled trial of the mindful self-compassion program. *Journal of Clinical Psychology, 69*(1), 28–44.
79. Moll, J., Krueger, F., Zahn, R., Pardini, M., de Oliveira-Souza, R., & Grafman, J. (2003). Human fronto–mesolimbic networks guide decisions about charitable donation. *Proceedings of the National Academies of Sciences, 103*(42), 15623–15628.
80. Nelson, S. K., Layous, K., Cole, S. W., & Lyubomirsky, S. (2016). Do unto others or treat yourself? The effects of prosocial and self-focused behavior on psychological flourishing. *Emotion, 16*(6), 850–861.
81. Post, S. G. (2005). Altruism, happiness, and health: It's good to be good. *International Journal of Behavioral Medicine, 12*(2), 66–77.
82. Therapist Aid. (2016). Building happiness (exercises). Retrieved from http://www.therapistaid.com/therapy-worksheet/building-happiness-exercises

Glossary

abortion A procedure that a woman undergoes to end a pregnancy; there are two types of abortion: the "abortion pill" and clinical procedures, which include aspiration, and dilation and evacuation (D&E).

abstinence In the context of sex, refers to the practice of abstaining (or not having) vaginal, anal, or oral sex.

abuse The cruel and violent treatment of a person (or animal).

active living An expanded definition of physical activity that includes normal daily activities, such as using stairs, walking to work, gardening, or performing housework.

activities of daily living Routine activities that people usually do every day without needing assistance, such as eating and bathing.

acupuncture An ancient Chinese medicinal practice where practitioners use thin needles to stimulate certain points on the body.

Administration for Children and Families The operating division within the Department of Health and Human Services that targets children, youth, families, and communities. This department administers a broad range of programs that include income assistance, child support enforcement, adoption assistance, foster care, and child care, as well as services for people with developmental disabilities, refugees, migrants, victims of child abuse, and American Indians.

Administration for Community Living The operating division within the Department of Health and Human Services that focuses on people with disabilities and older adults. The agency works to ensure that individuals with disabilities and the elderly can live where they choose, with the people they want, and that they can fully participate in their communities. Programs also support family caregivers, address issues of elder abuse, address the needs of American Indians, provide community services, and offer individualized support for individuals with disabilities.

advance directive A legal document that outlines a patient's end-of-life care preferences.

advocacy Strategic use of the news and other media outlets to advance a public health policy agenda.

aerobic exercise Exercise that helps improve how the body uses oxygen. The word *aerobic* literally means "relating to or requiring oxygen" and aerobic activity is commonly defined as continuous activity that elevates the heart rate to around 75% of its maximum rate.

Agency for Healthcare Research and Quality The operating division within the Department of Health and Human Services that supports research to improve the quality of health care, minimize its costs, ensure patient safety, respond to medical errors, and increase access to essential services.

Agency for Toxic Substances and Disease Registry The operating division within the Department of Health and Human Services that is responsible for prevention of exposure to toxic substances and the resulting health problems and reduced quality of life due to exposure to harmful substances from waste sites, unplanned releases, and other causes of environmental pollution.

air pollution A condition in which toxic chemicals or compounds are in the air, at levels that pose a health risk.

alcohol A substance that results from the fermentation of yeasts, sugars, and starches that is an ingredient in beer, wine, and other liquors.

Alzheimer's disease A progressive type of dementia in which people suffer damage to brain cells that causes loss of memory and other important mental functions.

American Red Cross A humanitarian organization that provides emergency assistance and disaster relief; blood and blood product donation and distribution; services for military members and their families; educational programs on preparedness, health, and safety; and international relief and development.

anaerobic exercise Short-duration and high-intensity exercise that activates fast-twitch muscle fibers and strengthens muscles through activities such as sprinting, body building, and jumping.

anorexia nervosa An eating disorder characterized by restriction of energy intake to the point of resulting in significantly low body weight; fear of gaining weight; and inability to recognize that perceptions of their body are out of touch with reality and that they are putting themselves in danger due to their low body weight.

antibiotics Substances, such as penicillin, that are capable of destroying or weakening certain microorganisms, especially bacteria or fungi, that cause infections or infectious diseases.

arousal The onset of sexual desire; it consists of four stages: excitement, plateau, orgasm and ejaculation, and resolution.

asthma An obstructive airway disease marked by episodic airway narrowing, causing difficulty in breathing.

athlete exposures A unit of susceptibility to injury equal to one athlete participating in one game or practice in which the athlete is exposed to the possibility of athletic injury. For college-aged individuals, this measure does not include injuries among those participating in recreational team or individual sports activities.

attention deficit hyperactivity disorder (ADHD) A disorder in which the inability to pay attention and/or hyperactive and impulsive behavior is persistent and affects daily functioning.

autism spectrum disorder (ASD) A spectrum of disorders that includes a continued deficiency in social interaction and restricted patterns of behavior that occur early in life.

autopsy An examination of a body after death to determine the cause of death or the character and extent of changes produced by disease.

bacteria Microscopic living organisms, usually one-celled, that can be found everywhere. Bacteria can be dangerous, such as when they cause infection, or beneficial, as in the process of fermentation (such as in wine) or decomposition.

bereavement The process of dealing with death through grieving, challenging, accepting, and/or letting go of someone who has died.

binge eating disorder An eating disorder characterized by binging (eating large quantities of food, in a discrete period of time, without having control over one's eating during that episode).

bioplastics A type of biodegradable plastic derived from biological substances rather than from petroleum.

bipolar disorder A disorder that causes extreme changes in mood and includes mania or hypomania, and sometimes depression as well; formerly known as manic-depression.

body composition The amount of body fat in proportion to overall weight. Body composition is improved through losing fat, increasing lean muscle, or a combination of both.

body dysmorphic disorder A disorder in which a person becomes preoccupied with perceived flaws in physical appearance that other people may not notice or consider to be an issue, which escalates to a point that the individual performs repetitive behaviors or mental acts that cause distress or impairment in functioning.

borderline personality disorder A personality disorder characterized by a pervasive pattern of instability of interpersonal relationships, self-image, and affect, with marked impulsivity.

built environment The physical environments where communities live and interact, including parks, sidewalks, green space, and housing.

bulimia nervosa An eating disorder characterized by binging and purging (inappropriate compensatory behavior designed to prevent weight gain from the excessive eating).

bullying The abuse and mistreatment of someone vulnerable by someone else who is stronger or more powerful.

cancer A malignant growth or tumor resulting from the abnormal division of cells.

capital punishment The lawful infliction of death as a punishment; the death penalty.

carbon dioxide A colorless, odorless gas produced by burning carbon and organic compounds and by respiration. It is naturally present in air (about 0.03%) and is absorbed by plants in photosynthesis. It traps heat in the atmosphere and, as such, contributes to the warming of the earth.

carcinogens A substance capable of causing cancer in living tissue.

carcinomas A type of cancer that develops in the epithelial tissues.

cardiac muscle A type of involuntary muscle tissue found only in the heart. This muscle constricts to remove blood from the heart and relaxes to fill the heart with blood.

cardiorespiratory endurance The ability of the heart, blood vessels, and lungs to deliver oxygen and essential nutrients to the working muscles and remove waste products during vigorous physical activity.

cardiovascular disease A range of conditions affecting the heart and blood vessels.

Centers for Disease Control and Prevention (CDC) The operating division within the Department of Health and Human Services that protects public health and safety through the control and prevention of disease, injury, and disability.

Centers for Medicare and Medicaid Services The operating division within the Department of Health and Human Services that administers several programs, including the Medicare program, and works with state governments to administer Medicaid, the state Children's Health Insurance Program, and health insurance portability standards.

cerebrovascular disease A disease in which damage to the blood vessels that supply the brain occurs. Interrupted blood flow to the brain can lead to stroke.

child neglect A form of child abuse that occurs when a person who is responsible for the child fails to care for the minor's emotional or physical needs.

Child Protective Services A state governmental agency that responds to reports of child abuse or neglect. Different states use different names, such as Department of Children and Family Services or Department of Social Services.

chiropractic A process that involves physically adjusting the body, primarily the spine, to improve functioning, correct alignment problems, and alleviate pain.

chronic diseases Diseases that last for 3 months or longer.

chronic obstructive pulmonary disease A progressive respiratory disease marked by chronic obstruction of the airflow from the lungs.

chronic traumatic encephalopathy A progressive degenerative disease of the brain found in athletes (and others) with a history of repetitive brain trauma, including symptomatic concussions and hits to the head.

cocaine A white powdery or crystalline stimulant derived from the leaves of the coca plant. Also known as coke, blow, snow, or crack.

communicable diseases An infectious disease transmitted indirectly or directly from person to person. Zoonotic diseases, by contrast, are infectious diseases transmitted from animal to human.

community-based organizations Organizations, often led by community members themselves, that provide programs and services for the betterment of the community.

complementary and alternative medicine (CAM) An approach used in conjunction with conventional medicine or an approach that employs nonmainstream practices instead of traditional medicine.

complementary health approach A group of diverse medical and health care interventions, practices, products, or disciplines that are not generally considered part of conventional medicine.

complex carbohydrates Sometimes referred to as "good" carbohydrates because they provide useful nutrients to the body, as compared to simple ("bad") carbohydrates, which are more easily converted to fat.

condom Barrier device used during sexual intercourse to help prevent pregnancy or STDs.

congenital anomalies A structural or functional anomaly (e.g., metabolic disorders) that occurs during intrauterine life and can be identified prenatally, at birth, or later in life. Also known as a birth defect, congenital disorder, or congenital malformation.

contact transmission A transmission mechanism in which the infectious agent is transferred via direct transmission, indirect transmission, or droplet transmission.

contraception Medications, devices, and behaviors that can reduce the risk of becoming pregnant by either preventing sperm from getting to an egg or preventing the ovaries from releasing an egg; also known as birth control.

conventional farming Farming techniques that make use of synthetic chemical fertilizers, pesticides, and herbicides and may include genetically modified organisms.

coronary heart disease A condition in which plaque builds up in coronary arteries, causing them to harden and narrow.

cremation To reduce a body to ashes by fire, especially as a funeral rite.

cultural competence A set of values, behaviors, attitudes, and practices within an organization or program or among individuals that allows them to work effectively cross-culturally.

cutoff value The level at which the result of a diagnostic test is determined to be positive or negative.

cyberbullying A form of bullying that takes place over digital devices like cell phones, computers, and tablets. It can occur through SMS, text, and apps, or online in social media, forums, or gaming where people can view, participate in, or share content. It includes sending, posting, or sharing negative, harmful, false, or mean content about someone else. It can include sharing personal or private information about someone else that is intended to cause embarrassment or humiliation.

date rape Forcible sexual intercourse by a male acquaintance of a woman, during a date or other voluntary social engagement. The fact that the parties knew each other or that the woman willingly accompanied the man are not legal defenses to a charge of rape. In instances of date rape, the woman did not intend to submit to the sexual advances and resisted verbally and/or physically.

dead zone A low-oxygen area within the world's oceans or lakes. Because most organisms need oxygen to live, in these areas organisms cannot survive.

deductibles The amount the insurance holder must pay out of pocket before an insurance company will cover costs. For example, if the deductible is $500 and the total bill is $1,000, the insurance holder must pay $500 and the insurance company will cover the remainder.

defense mechanisms Subconscious thoughts that we use to avoid feeling anxious or guilty when we are confronted with situations in which we feel threatened.

dementia A chronic or persistent disorder of the mental processes caused by brain disease or injury and marked by memory disorders, personality changes, and impaired reasoning.

depression Mood disorder characterized by symptoms that include feelings of sadness, worthlessness, or hopelessness; diminished pleasure in activities; and thoughts of death or suicide.

determinants of health See *Social determinants of health.*

direct transmission A transmission mechanism in which the infectious agent is transferred directly into the body via touching, biting, kissing, or sexual intercourse or by droplets entering the eye, nose, or mouth.

direct-to-consumer advertising When drug companies market directly to customers by advertising their products on television, in magazines, and even through social media and the Internet, despite the product being available only by a doctor's prescription.

discrimination Unfair treatment of a person based on the person's race, ethnicity, gender, religious beliefs, sexual orientation, or other personal characteristics.

dissociative drugs A class of drugs that can distort one's perception of reality. The sensations experienced when taking these types of drugs are referred to as "tripping."

drug overdose Taking too much of a substance, whether it is a prescription drug, over-the-counter medication, or a supplement. It may be legal or illegal. It can be intentional or unintentional. If you have taken enough of the substance to have a harmful effect, you have overdosed. The severity of the overdose is dependent upon the individual (physical and medical history), the drug, and the amount of the drug consumed. It can cause serious medical complications, the most severe being death.

Ebola virus disease A deadly viral disease transmitted from animals to humans that spreads rapidly among humans. It causes flulike symptoms, followed by internal and external bleeding. It has a 21-day incubation period and is contagious only when a person is expressing symptoms.

electronic cigarettes Battery-powered devices that deliver nicotine via a vaporizer. Also known as e-cigarettes, e-cigs, or electronic nicotine delivery systems.

emotional abuse Any act, including confinement, isolation, verbal assault, humiliation, intimidation, or any other treatment that may diminish the sense of identity, dignity, and self-worth of the victim.

endemic A disease or condition regularly found among particular people or in a certain area.

endorphins Hormones that improve neurologic function and produce feelings of well-being and happiness.

environmental tobacco smoke exposure Exposure to tobacco smoke from being exposed to someone else's cigarette, cigar, or pipe smoke. It can also be described as the material in indoor air that originates from tobacco smoke.

epidemic A widespread occurrence of an infectious disease in a community at a particular time.

epidemiologists Individuals who study the causes and distributions of disease among local and global populations. They not only focus on preventing and controlling the spread of communicable diseases, but also on understanding how to prevent chronic diseases.

epidemiology The branch of public health that studies the cause and distribution of disease among local and global populations, with a focus on preventing and controlling the spread of disease.

epigenetics The process by which our genes respond to environmental cues, and while the genetic code does not change, the epigenetic biological responses, or "switches," can change as a result of nutritional scarcity or abundance in the womb.

etiology The study of the cause or causes of a disease.

exclusive provider organization (EPO) A plan that does not require a primary care physician or referral within the established provider network. Emergency and urgent care are the only time out-of-network visits are covered.

exercise A form of physical activity that is usually planned, structured, and repetitive.

fast-twitch Muscle fibers that are effective for quick movements like jumping and sprinting. They contract quickly, but fatigue is felt sooner than when using slow-twitch muscles.

fatty acids Saturated or unsaturated carboxylic acids with an even number of carbon atoms.

fitness The ability to perform required activities to complete a task or a job.

flexibility The range of motion of a person's joints, the ability of the joints to move freely, and the mobility of the muscles, which allows for more movement throughout the person's body.

focus groups Small number of people brought together with a moderator to discuss a specific topic. They aim at generating discussion instead of on individual responses to formal questions, and produce preferences and beliefs that may be expected from a larger population. The group may be deliberately selected.

Food and Drug Administration The operating division within the Department of Health and Human Services that ensures that food is safe, pure, and wholesome; human and animal drugs, biological products, and medical devices are safe and effective; and electronic products that emit radiation are safe.

food deserts An area high in fast-food outlets but low in grocery stores.

food fortification A method used for nearly a century in industrialized countries to restore micronutrients lost by food processing. In the United States, examples of supplementation include adding vitamin D to milk, folic acid to bread, and iodine to salt.

fossil fuels Natural fuels formed in the geological past from remains of ancient plants and animals and used as fuel.

fungi Simple, aerobic organisms (such as mildews, molds, mushrooms, smuts, toadstools, and yeast) that can grow in low moisture and low pH environments and that have their genetic material bound in a membrane.

gender identity The attitudes, feelings, and behaviors a society associates with someone's biological sex; some people identify as transgender, which means that their identity does not conform to typical associations of their biological sex.

generalized anxiety disorder A disorder that includes excessive anxiety and worry for at least 6 months that causes significant distress and impedes social or occupational functioning.

genetically modified organisms (GMOs) A living organism that has undergone genetic modification to serve the needs of humans. Also referred to as *transgenic*.

global burden of disease (GBD) Developed in 1990 as a collaboration between hundreds of global health institutions, including the World Health Organization and the World Bank. This project seeks to measure, and then find solutions to, the causes and costs of all diseases around the world.

global health Health-based research and practice that prioritizes improving global health equity.

glycemic index A system that ranks food from 1 to 100 to indicate the food's effect on blood sugar (glucose) levels.

glycogen A converted form of glucose that is stored in muscles and the liver.

governmental organizations A type of social organization that exists at all levels of government, from the international level all the way down to the local level, or your county or township, to serve the needs of its citizens.

Great Pacific Garbage Patch A concentration of marine debris in the North Pacific Ocean. It has exceptionally high concentrations of plastics, chemical sludge, and other debris. Most of the debris is suspended beneath the surface of the ocean.

greenhouse gases A group of gases, including carbon dioxide, methane, nitrous oxide, ozone, and fluorocarbons, that allow sunlight to pass through the atmosphere and reach the earth's surface. These gases trap the sun's heat like a blanket, warning the earth. They need to be present in specific amounts; however, when too much is present, the earth warms more than is needed.

grief The emotional reaction to a death or loss.

gyre A large system of rotating ocean currents. They rotate clockwise in the Northern Hemisphere and counterclockwise in the Southern Hemisphere.

hallucinogens A class of drugs that causes hallucinations—profound distortions in a person's perceptions of reality; can be found in some plants and mushrooms (or their extracts) or can be man-made.

harm reduction A movement based in social justice and respect for those with substance use disorder that employs approaches to reduce harm and consequences associated with drug use rather than promote abstinence; includes tactics such as needle exchange and safe injection sites.

hate crimes A violent crime motivated because of the victim's perceived membership in a specific group.

hazing Any action or situation, with or without the consent of the participants, which recklessly, intentionally, or unintentionally endangers the mental, physical, or academic health or safety of a student.

health maintenance organizations (HMOs) A type of health insurance in which members typically must have their health needs managed by a primary care physician, and health services are paid for within a limited network of hospitals and clinics and medical professionals. The HMO was the first managed care model and remains at the center of the choices available to employers and to individuals who purchase their plan through the marketplace.

Health Resources and Services Administration The operating division within the Department of Health and Human Services that is responsible for improving access to healthcare services for uninsured, isolated, or medically vulnerable individuals, including people living with HIV/AIDS and pregnant women, mothers, and children.

health-related fitness Fitness measures intended to ensure overall health.

heart attack The sudden cessation of blood supply to the heart, often due to a blocked artery.

heart disease A broad category of conditions relating to disease of the cardiovascular system, including vessels and heart structures. Coronary artery disease is the most common type, and it is the leading cause of death for both men and women in the United States—and across the world.

herd immunity A form of immunity that occurs when the vaccination of a significant portion of a population (or herd) provides a measure of protection for individuals who have not developed immunity.

heroic treatments Health care or therapy that is likely to be ineffective or, worse, that may cause increased pain or further damage to a patient's health. Heroic procedures are usually undertaken as a last resort, recognizing that lesser treatment will result in death.

heroin An opioid drug that is synthesized from morphine, a powder or tar-like substance extracted from the seed pod of the Asian opium poppy plant.

high-fructose corn syrup a popular sweetener used in sodas and other beverages. Inexpensive production of corn led to its development.

hospice A program or facility designed to provide palliative care and emotional support to the terminally ill patient in a home or homelike setting so that quality of life is maintained and family members may be active participants in care.

host A person or other living organism that can be infected by an infectious agent under natural conditions.

hypertension A condition in which blood flows through the blood vessels with greater than normal force, causing blood pressure to be abnormally high.

hypnotherapy A process by which trained clinicians guide clients into a relaxed state. While in this state, sometimes called a "trance," the person's sense of awareness is heightened, and this allows the person to focus attention on specific thoughts.

immunity Resistance developed in response to stimulus by an antigen (infecting agent or vaccine) and usually characterized by the presence of antibodies produced by the host.

incidence The number of new cases of a disease over a specified period of time.

indemnity Protection against loss, as in health insurance. The basic system of indemnity plans is that premiums are collected by the insurance company, usually on a monthly basis. Those funds are added to the "risk pool," from which payments are drawn.

Indian Health Service The operating division within the Department of Health and Human Services that provides American Indians and Alaska Natives with comprehensive health services by developing and managing programs to meet their health needs.

inpatient care Health care that requires an overnight stay in a hospital or other facility.

insulin A hormone that is produced and secreted by the pancreas whose role is to regulate the body to either use glucose for energy or to store it for future energy use. It keeps blood sugar levels from getting too high (hyperglycemia) or too low (hypoglycemia).

integrative health An approach to health that seeks to bring together conventional and complementary treatments in a coordinated way.

internal medicine Medical practice concerned with preventing, identifying, and treating conditions related to internal systems, such as those of the heart, lungs, or neurologic systems. Internists are considered "primary care" physicians, although not "generalists."

intimate partner violence A pattern of assaultive and coercive behaviors that includes the threat or infliction of physical, sexual, or psychological abuse that is used by a current or former intimate partner for the purpose of intimidation and control over the victim.

ketosis A metabolic process involving raised ketone body levels; it may occur in people with diabetes or those who follow a low-carb diet.

leukemia A category of cancers that usually begins in the bone marrow and leads to unnaturally high numbers of abnormally undeveloped white blood cells that spread through the body without forming tumors.

life expectancy The number of years that an average person will live.

living will A written statement, such as an advance directive, detailing a person's desires regarding medical treatment should the person lose his or her ability to express informed consent.

macronutrients Carbohydrates, proteins, and fats that serve as the primary components of a healthy diet.

malnutrition A condition in which a person's diet lacks the necessary nutrients to sustain fundamental physiological and cognitive functions. It increases the risk of morbidity and mortality.

managed care A system in which networks of doctors and hospitals agree to offer a discount for services and in which unnecessary care and hospitalization are minimized, thus reducing the cost of group insurance premiums.

marijuana A psychoactive drug used recreationally and in some medical contexts. It is the most commonly used illegal drug in the United States. It consists of dried leaves, flowers, stems, and seeds of the plant, *Cannabis sativa*.

massage Various types of movements utilized by trained therapists, usually with their hands, to apply pressure, rub, or manipulate muscle and other soft tissues.

Medicaid U.S. public health insurance program serving people with low incomes and minimal assets. Medicaid was passed in 1965 as part of the federal Social Security Act. It is jointly funded by state and federal governments, but it is managed by the states.

Medicare A federal government program that covers a portion of the cost of health care and is primarily for Americans who are aged 65 years and older.

meditation A group of techniques used to focus one's attention and promote relaxation and mental calmness.

melanoma A malignant tumor formed in the pigment-producing cells (melanocytes).

mental health A component of well-being in which the individual realizes his or her abilities, copes with the normal stresses of life, works productively and fruitfully, and makes a contribution to the community; also defined as having emotional, psychological, and social well-being.

mental illness The collective group of mental disorders or health conditions that are characterized by alterations in thinking, mood, or behavior (or some combination thereof) associated with distress and/or impaired functioning.

metabolism The process that occurs inside the body at the cellular and the physiological levels to generate energy and maintain life. Metabolism consists of two fundamental stages—catabolism and anabolism.

methamphetamine An extremely addictive stimulant chemically similar to amphetamine. Also known as meth, crystal, chalk, and ice.

methane A colorless, odorless flammable gas that is the main constituent of natural gas. It traps heat in the atmosphere and, as such, contributes to the warming of the earth.

microbiome The environment created by the trillions of microscopic organisms living in our gut, which have an enormous influence on our health. They have been found to produce vitamins from our food, fight disease, and control our weight.

microfinance A practice in which banking organizations provide small loans to low-income people. The goal is for the loan recipients to start businesses that generate income and break the cycle of poverty.

micronutrients Nutrients, mostly vitamins and minerals, that are essential for optimal health, although only in miniscule amounts. Micronutrients are important for the normal functioning of the body and enable many of the important chemical reactions that promote good health.

mind–body An approach that utilizes techniques, such as yoga and meditation, that seek to enhance health and well-being by living in the present moment.

muscle protein myofibrils A threadlike fiber that composes skeletal and cardiac muscle fibers.

muscular endurance The ability of a muscle to exert force against resistance over repeated and long periods. Compared to muscular strength, which draws on strength and power for short activities requiring quick bursts, muscular endurance is the body's ability to perform activities of long duration but low intensity, such as doing repetitions of push-ups or sit-ups.

muscular strength The ability of a muscle to exert force against resistance, which comes from the cells providing energy to the muscle fibers for different forms of contractions (concentric, eccentric, and isometric) that initiate power and strength.

National Institutes of Health (NIH) The operating division within the Department of Health and Human Services that supports biomedical and behavioral research within the United States and abroad, trains researchers, and promotes collecting and sharing of medical knowledge.

National Science Foundation An independent federal agency whose mission is "to promote the progress of science; to advance the national health, prosperity, and welfare; [and] to secure the national defense."

neglect Not meeting the basic needs of a person who requires care: physical, medical, educational, and emotional.

network A group of healthcare providers and facilities, which usually includes doctors, hospitals, pharmacists, labs, or other facilities.

noncommunicable diseases A chronic health condition that is nontransmissible. The four major categories of noncommunicable diseases are cardiovascular diseases, cancers, chronic respiratory conditions, and diabetes.

noncontact transmission A transmission mechanism in which the infectious agent is transferred indirectly into the body; includes airborne, vehicle-borne, and vector-borne methods.

nongovernmental organizations (NGOs) A not-for-profit organization that is independent from states and international governmental organizations. They are usually funded by donations, but some avoid formal funding altogether and are run primarily by volunteers.

nuclear energy Energy released during nuclear fission, especially when used to generate electricity.

nutritional environments The environment where people purchase and eat food.

obsessive-compulsive disorder (OCD) A disorder in which an individual has either obsessions, compulsions, or both; obsessions are recurrent and persistent thoughts, urges, or images that are intrusive and unwanted and cause anxiety and distress. In an attempt to reduce distress, an individual may perform compulsions, which consist of repetitive behaviors that are clearly excessive.

organ donation The process of surgically removing an organ or tissue from one person (the organ donor) and placing it into another person (the recipient).

organic farming A type of farming that takes a holistic approach that is both sustainable and harmonious with the environment. It includes, but is not limited to, not using pesticides, fertilizers, genetically modified organisms, antibiotics, or growth hormones.

overuse injury Muscle or joint injury caused by repetitive trauma.

ozone A gas composed of three atoms of oxygen. It is harmful to breathe. The layer in the atmosphere composed of this gas prevents most harmful short-wave ultraviolet B sun rays from reaching the ground.

palliative care Specialized medical care for people with serious illness. This type of care is focused on providing relief from the symptoms and stress of a serious illness.

pandemic An epidemic occurring over a very wide area (several countries or continents) and usually affecting a large proportion of the population.

panic disorder A disorder that causes a person to experience panic attacks, that is, an abrupt surge of intense fear or intense discomfort that reaches a peak within minutes.

paranoid personality disorder A personality disorder characterized by excessive distrust and suspicion.

parasite An organism that lives in or on another organism (its host) and benefits by deriving nutrients at the host's expense.

particulates Tiny particles in the air, including dust, dirt, soot, and smoke. Once a person inhales these particles, they can cause serious health effects.

pathology The study of diseases and the changes that they cause; the way a disease works.

pesticides Substances used for destroying insects or other organisms harmful to cultivated plants or animals.

physical abuse The intentional use of force against a child that has a high likelihood of harm for the child's health, survival, development, or dignity. This includes hitting, beating, kicking, shaking, biting, strangling, scalding, burning, poisoning, and suffocating. Much physical violence against children in the home is inflicted with the object of punishment. This type of abuse often does not occur in isolation, but as part of a constellation of behaviors including authoritarian control, anxiety-provoking behavior, and a lack of parental warmth.

physical activity The broad category of bodily movement that results in energy expenditure.

plantar fasciitis An inflammation of the tissue that runs across the bottom of the foot and connects the heel bone to the toes (plantar fascia).

point-of-service (POS) plans Similar to a health maintenance organization, a plan in which members designate an in-network primary care physician to be their care coordinator. However, as with a preferred provider organization, limited coverage is available for care that is received outside the provider network.

poison A substance that can cause illness or death of a living organism when introduced or absorbed.

population health The health outcomes of a group of individuals, including the distribution of such outcomes within the group. This field of study includes health outcomes, patterns of health determinants, and policies and the interventions that link them. It is an approach that aims to improve the health of an entire human population.

posttraumatic stress disorder (PTSD) The development of specific symptoms after being exposed to one or more traumatic events.

prediabetes A condition of higher-than-normal blood glucose levels; not high enough to establish a diagnosis of diabetes.

predigestive process The process by which the stomach churns, grinds, and applies hydrochloric acid and enzymes to ingested food to prepare it for digestion.

preferred provider organizations (PPOs) A type of health insurance in which members may see physician specialists directly without a referral from a primary care physician, as long as the specialist is within the preferred network of providers. Physicians, medical care providers, and hospitals outside of the network incur an additional fee.

prevalence The total number of cases of a health condition, exposure, or other variable related to health, known to have existed over a period of time.

prions Misfolded proteins that are considered "infectious" because they cause normal proteins to misfold.

prior authorization Approval of payment that health insurers give before healthcare providers proceed with pharmaceutical treatments, medical interventions, and certain healthcare services. Also known as prior approval or precertification.

prognosis The prediction of the future course of a disease and how likely a person is to recover.

qigong A moving meditation that originated in China as a martial art that is designed to be a meditative, healing motion.

quasi-governmental organization An agency that receives funding from both public and private sources. They perform functions expected of government agencies without government supervision.

race A sociocultural concept, not a biological one, that has emerged as a way to categorize and rank groups.

racism Prejudice, discrimination, or antagonism directed against someone of a different race based on the belief that one's own race is superior.

radon A colorless, gaseous radioactive element produced by the decay of radium.

randomized controlled trials A study design that randomly assigns participants to either an intervention group or a control group. The control may be a standard practice, a placebo ("sugar pill"), or no intervention at all. As the study is conducted, the only expected difference between the control and experimental groups is the outcome variable being studied.

refined sugar A form of sugar made from sugar cane or sugar beets. Once the sugar is extracted, it is processed into white sugar. Also known as sucrose.

regional-level eating patterns The diet typical to a given region. Studies of regional-level eating patterns indicate that some cultures can have better overall health outcomes than other cultures due, in large part, to their diets.

Reiki A subtle form of energy work where hands are placed gently on or above certain parts of the body used to help relieve stress and increase relaxation.

religion Beliefs, practices, and rituals related to the transcendent, where the transcendent is a High Power, designed to bring one closer to the High Power and clarify our responsibility to others in our society.

repetitive motion injuries Temporary or permanent injuries to muscles, nerves, ligaments, and tendons caused by doing the same motion over and over again; also called repetitive stress injuries.

reproductive justice A movement dedicated to the human right to have children, not have children, and parent the children people already have in safe and healthy environments and to bodily autonomy from any form of reproductive oppression.

resuscitation The action or process of reviving someone from unconsciousness or apparent death.

safe haven laws Laws that allow any person statutorily defined by law, usually a parent, to abandon an unharmed newborn baby at a designated location. These laws were enacted in response to an increased number of infant abandonments and infanticides.

sarcomas A malignant tumor that arises from connective and supporting tissues.

saturated fats Dietary fats that are solid at room temperature and often referred to simply as "fat."

schizophrenia A disorder that affects how people think and behave and may include delusions, hallucinations, disorganized speech, grossly disorganized or catatonic behavior, and negative symptoms.

screening tests A simple test usually performed to identify those in a population who have or are likely to develop a specified disease.

self-injury The act of deliberately harming one's body; also called self-harm.

sexual abuse Unwanted sexual activity, with perpetrators using force, making threats, or taking advantage of victims not able to give consent.

sexual orientation Refers to the gender or genders to which a person is sexually attracted; includes heterosexual, homosexual, and bisexual.

sexually transmitted diseases (STDs) Diseases that are transmitted through sexual contact; includes HIV/AIDS, human papilloma virus (HPV), chlamydia, gonorrhea, syphilis, genital herpes, hepatitis, and trichomoniasis.

sick building syndrome A situation in which the occupants of a building experience acute health- or comfort-related effects that seem to be linked directly to the time spent in the building. The complainants may be localized in a particular room or zone or may be widespread throughout the building.

simple carbohydrates Sometimes referred to as "bad" carbohydrates because they are more easily converted to fat, as compared to complex ("good") carbohydrates, which provide useful nutrients to the body.

skeletal muscle The muscle associated with muscle strength and endurance. These muscles contract when they receive signals from motor neurons, which direct the muscles to activate through contraction.

skill-related fitness A set of attributes that allows someone to respond to the physical demands of a particular skill or activity, such as construction or textile work. These attributes can be measured with specific tests, such as those measuring agility, speed, reaction time, and balance.

slow-twitch Muscle fibers that contract more slowly, are smaller, and have more oxidative (aerobic) capacity, and less glycolytic (anaerobic) capacity than fast-twitch fibers. They are needed for endurance activities like long-distance running, cycling, and cross-country skiing. They can work for a longer time than fast-twitch muscles without getting tired.

social determinants of health The circumstances in which people are born, grow, live, work, and age. They are shaped by the distribution of money, power, and resources at global, national, and local levels.

social entrepreneurship Use of business techniques and private sector approaches to solve social and environmental problems.

social justice imperative The effort to channel resources to the populations that need them the most—populations suffering the highest rates of death from preventable disease—populations that are among the poorest in the world.

social-ecological model A theory-based framework for understanding the multifaceted and interactive effects of personal and environmental factors that determine behaviors, and for identifying behavioral and organizational leverage points and intermediaries for health promotion within organizations.

social-ecological model of violence A framework for understanding the multifaceted and interactive effects between individual, relationship, community, and societal factors to recognize the reasons that put people at risk for violence or protect them from experiencing or perpetrating violence.

solar power Power obtained by harnessing the energy of the sun's rays.

spirituality A concept similar to religion or a moral and individual experience of believing in something higher than oneself that may not be through an organized set of practices or beliefs.

stalking Repeated visual or physical proximity, nonconsensual communication, and/or verbal, written, or implied threats directed at a person to arouse fear. It is unusual in that the individual behaviors may be legal, such as sending flowers, writing love notes, or waiting outside a person's place of work.

stigma A mark of disgrace; can manifest as either public stigma or self-stigma.

stroke The sudden onset of persistent neurologic deficits resulting from blocked blood flow to the brain.

subclinical infection An infection that is nearly or completely asymptomatic (no signs or symptoms).

Substance Abuse and Mental Health Services Administration The operating division within the Department of Health and Human Services that improves the quality and availability of prevention, treatment, and rehabilitative services.

substance use disorder A term used by the *Diagnostic and Statistical Manual of Mental Disorders* to characterize and diagnose problems with substance use. This term is used rather than terms such as *abuse* or *dependence*.

sudden infant death syndrome (SIDS) The sudden unexplained death of an infant younger than 1 year old. The cause remains unexplained after a complete investigation.

sugar-sweetened beverage-free zones An initiative to eliminate the sale of sugar-sweetened beverages from school campuses.

suicide The act of killing oneself; the desire to commit suicide is often expressed first by suicidal ideation (thinking about killing oneself) and then attempts (trying to kill oneself).

sweatshops According to the U.S. Department of Labor definition, a factory that violates two or more labor laws.

systematic review A focused literature review that identifies, appraises, selects, and synthesizes all of the high-quality research relevant to a particular question.

tai chi A moving meditation that originated in China that is focused and grounded in martial art movement.

tennis elbow Soreness or pain on the outer part of the elbow that occurs when a person damages the tendons that connect the muscles in the forearm to the elbow.

terminally ill A patient with a disease that cannot be cured and will likely cause death within approximately 6 months of diagnosis.

Title IX A comprehensive federal law that prohibits discrimination on the basis of sex in any federally funded education program or activity.

tobacco A product that contains the addictive substance nicotine used for cigarettes, cigars, pipes, and smokeless tobacco; consists of dried leaves from the tobacco plant.

transgenic See genetically modified organisms (GMOs).

traumatic brain injury Damage to the brain caused by an external physical force that may produce a diminished or altered state of consciousness and causes diminution of cognitive abilities or physical functioning. A person who has experienced this type of injury may have trouble with cognitive, emotional, and behavior functioning and may have permanent physical or psychosocial impairments.

tumor A benign or malignant overgrowth of tissues.

type 1 diabetes Previously called juvenile diabetes, a condition in which the body's immune system attacks beta cells in the pancreas, causing them to lose the ability to produce insulin.

type 2 diabetes Previously called adult-onset diabetes, a condition that occurs when the cells become resistant to insulin. Blood sugar levels rise and the pancreas responds by producing more and more insulin. When the pancreas can no longer keep up with the demand and becomes exhausted, it loses control over blood sugar regulation, resulting in the diabetic condition.

unsaturated fats Fats that remain liquid at room temperature, referred to as "oils."

vaccinations A medical treatment that stimulates the immune system to respond to a specific disease. This creates a response that protects the immune system from future exposure to the specific disease. They are administered through injections, nasally, or orally.

virus An organism that relies on a host organism to replicate and survive.

will A legal declaration of a person's wishes regarding the disposal of his or her property, or estate, after death.

wind power Power obtained by harnessing the energy of the wind.

Women, Infants, and Children (WIC) A federal nutrition assistance program for pregnant women and their newborn babies. The program provides vouchers for mothers, which can be spent only on nutritious foods.

World Health Organization (WHO) Established in 1948, an international organization that works with local offices in more than 150 countries and governments to achieve global health.

yoga An ancient practice, originating approximately 2,500 years ago, in what is now India. It combines physical, mental, and spiritual elements, and comes in numerous forms, through different schools, practices, and environments.

© Hero Images/Getty Images

Index

Note: Page numbers followed by *f* and *t* indicate figures, and tables respectively.

B

C

D

E

F

G

H

N

O

P

Q

R

S

T

U

V

W

Z